**Inderbir Singh's Textbook of**

# ANATOMY

**for AYUSH Students**

*(Ayurveda, Yoga & Naturopathy, Unani, Siddha and Homeopathic Students)*

# *Inderbir Singh's Textbook of*

# ANATOMY

## *for AYUSH Students*

*(Ayurveda, Yoga & Naturopathy, Unani, Siddha and Homeopathic Students)*

Upper Extremity ◆ Lower Extremity ◆ Thorax ◆ Abdomen and Pelvis ◆ Head and Neck ◆ Central Nervous System

*Edited by*

***Meera K Bhojani*** MD PhD (Ayur)
Assistant Professor
Department of Basic Principles
All India Institute of Ayurveda
Sarita Vihar, New Delhi, India

***Pranab Kumar Chakraborty*** MD (Homeopathy)
Vice Principal and Head of the Department of Anatomy
Sri Ganganagar Homeopathic Medical College, Hospital and Research Institute
Sri Ganganagar, Rajasthan, India

*Foreword*

***Prof Abhimanyu Kumar***

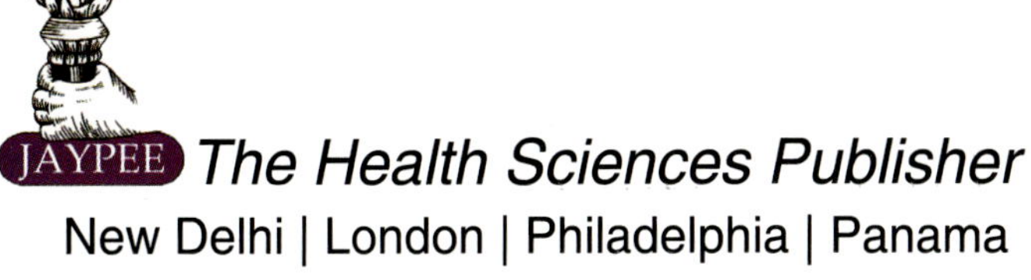


*The Health Sciences Publisher*
New Delhi | London | Philadelphia | Panama

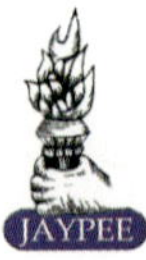

**Jaypee Brothers Medical Publishers (P) Ltd**

**Headquarters**

Jaypee Brothers Medical Publishers (P) Ltd
4838/24, Ansari Road, Daryaganj
New Delhi 110 002, India
Phone: +91-11-43574357
Fax: +91-11-43574314
Email: jaypee@jaypeebrothers.com

**Overseas Offices**

J.P. Medical Ltd
83, Victoria Street, London
SW1H 0HW (UK)
Phone: +44 20 3170 8910
Fax: +44 (0)20 3008 6180
Email: info@jpmedpub.com

Jaypee-Highlights Medical Publishers Inc
City of Knowledge, Bld. 235, 2nd Floor, Clayton
Panama City, Panama
Phone: +1 507-301-0496
Fax: +1 507-301-0499
Email: cservice@jphmedical.com

Jaypee Medical Inc
325 Chestnut Street
Suite 412, Philadelphia, PA 19106, USA
Phone: +1 267-519-9789
Email: support@jpmedus.com

Jaypee Brothers Medical Publishers (P) Ltd
17/1-B Babar Road, Block-B, Shaymali
Mohammadpur, Dhaka-1207
Bangladesh
Mobile: +08801912003485
Email: jaypeedhaka@gmail.com

Jaypee Brothers Medical Publishers (P) Ltd
Bhotahity, Kathmandu, Nepal
Phone +977-9741283608
Email: kathmandu@jaypeebrothers.com

Website: www.jaypeebrothers.com
Website: www.jaypeedigital.com



**Inquiries for bulk sales may be solicited at:** jaypee@jaypeebrothers.com

***Inderbir Singh's Textbook of Anatomy for AYUSH Students***

*First Edition:* **2017**

ISBN 978-93-86150-22-6

Printed at: Paras Offset Pvt. Ltd., New Delhi

# Foreword

About twenty years before medical students found a new book of Human Anatomy "Textbook of Anatomy by Inderbir Singh" with a difference. Today any one may see its presence in almost every library of medical and AYUSH colleges of the country. With its long journey, it improved a lot in many ways, like its presentation, subject matter, illustrations, clinical correlation section etc.

Prof Inderbir Singh is a legend in the field of Human Anatomy with extraordinary caliber as teacher and author. The way he starts chapter and concludes is remarkable. I can't resist myself to quote his words from the preface to the first edition of his textbook "Textbooks of Anatomy have the unenviable reputation of being dull and boring. This book makes an attempt to change this image. The emphasis throughout the book is on a picture memory rather than verbal one; and on understanding of facts rather than their cramming. The author tries to take his young readers by the hand; and lead him or her, through a journey of discovery that is as interesting as it is informative."

Now the authors Dr Meera K Bhojani and Dr Pranab Kumar Chakraborty have poured their expertise and experience in this new creation *Inderbir Singh's Textbook of Anatomy for AYUSH Students*. It has all the features, which students studying in AYUSH institution require. It also covers essential components of syllabus recommended by CCIM.

I am very much confident that this book is going to become one of the favorite books for AYUSH students.

**Prof Abhimanyu Kumar**
Director
All India Institute of Ayurveda
New Delhi

# Preface

Anatomy forms the plinth of all medical subjects. There is an awakening of the importance of anatomy with the realization that sound knowledge of anatomy is the backbone of safe medical practice. Learning anatomy in a short span of time is a Herculean task. Therefore, though it is not conceptually difficult; its sheer bulk makes anatomy overwhelming. In this context, a shift towards teaching / learning basic anatomy along with clinical correlation is a progressive step. This book is a condensed version of Prof. Inderbir Singh's three volumes of Textbook of Anatomy, which will help the young minds grasp anatomy better in the stipulated time. The book now is in a new presentable and up dated form with clinical correlation on the anatomical structures at the end of each topic.

However, the principles that guided the preparation of its previous editions remain valid even today. The overall effort can be a big success as it presents Anatomy in a relatively small volume while retaining all essential facts. The text has been illustrated by good quality color diagrams, tables, flow charts, graphs etc. which are easily reproducible and written in very simple language, so that the students of AYUSH, nursing and other allied health sciences can easily understand, retain and reproduce the same in their theory, practical and viva voce examinations and could have a sufficient knowledge of Anatomy for intelligent study of clinical subjects of the medical curriculum.

It is my pleasure and privilege to edit and revise this book. This task was undertaken bowing down to the request of Jaypee Brothers Medical Publishers, New Delhi, India. I acknowledge Shri Jitendar P Vij (Group Chairman), Ms Chetna Malhotra Vohra (Associate Director-Content Strategy), Dr Arjun Sharma (Marketing Manager) of Jaypee Brothers Medical Publishers, New Delhi, India for entrusting me this responsible job.

I convey my sincere tribute to acclaimed anatomist and educator, Prof Inderbir Singh whose enormous and tireless efforts in the field of Anatomy has favored and blessed the students and teachers as well of AYUSH and other health sciences all through.

**Meera K Bhojani**

# Preface

Professor Inderbir Singh, a legendary Anatomist, an authority, has created a "Textbook of Anatomy" which is providing enormous knowledge to the medical fraternity since many decades. The simplest language and comprehensiveness has made this book most popular amongst Medical students. The general format of the book is completely fresh and new look with the addition of clinical correlations on most of the anatomical structures at the end of each topic. Most of the text on important topics has been tabulated in an easy-to-grasp and readily comprehensible format, which would make it pretty interesting for the undergraduate students to understand the concepts of anatomy.

It is my proud privilege to make this standard textbook in a single volume to fulfil the needs of today's generation of students, especially for AYUSH, nursing and allied students. This book contains numerous high quality, hand-drawn simple illustrations, which would be self-explanatory for undergraduate students and can be easily drawn at the time of examination.

Last but not the least, I extend my heartfelt thanks to Shri Jitendar P Vij (Group Chairman) and Mr. Ankit Vij (Group President), Ms Chetna Malhotra Vohra (Associate Director-Content Strategy) for providing me the opportunity to edit the Textbook of Anatomy for their persistent support in publication of this book.

Dr Arjun Sharma (Marketing Manager) deserves a special thanks for her tireless efforts.

I convey my tribute to a legendary Anatomist, Professor Inderbir Singh for being a pillar in the education of generations of doctors throughout the world.

**Pranab Kumar Chakraborty**

# Contents

## PART 1: UPPER EXTREMITY

## PART 3: THORAX

## PART 4: ABDOMEN AND PELVIS

## PART 5: HEAD AND NECK

# PART 1

## Upper Extremity

# 1 CHAPTER

# Some Essential Terms

## THE SUBJECT OF ANATOMY

Anatomy is the science that deals with the structure of the human body. Different aspects of the subject are as follows:

1. ***Gross anatomy*** or ***morphological anatomy*** is the study of structure that can be seen by naked eye.
2. ***Microscopic anatomy*** or ***histology*** is the study of structure that can be observed only under a microscope.
3. ***Cytology*** is the study of details of the structure of cells.
4. ***Histochemistry*** is the study of chemical processes going on in cells and tissues.
5. ***Ultrastructure*** is the study of tissues using an electron microscope. It provides very high magnification.
6. ***Embryology*** is the study of the development of tissues and organs before birth.
7. ***Applied anatomy*** or ***clinical anatomy*** is the study of aspects of anatomy that are useful in diagnosis and treatment of disease.

## MAIN SUBDIVISIONS OF THE HUMAN BODY

For convenience of description the human body is divided into a number of major parts.

1. The uppermost part of the body is the ***head***. The ***face*** is part of the head.
2. Below the head, there is the ***neck***.
3. Below the neck, there is the region that we call the chest. In anatomical terminology the chest is referred to as the ***thorax***. The thorax is in the form of a bony cage within which the heart and lungs lie.
4. Below the thorax, there is the region we commonly refer to as 'stomach' or 'belly'.
   a. Its proper name is ***abdomen***. The abdomen contains several organs of vital importance to the body.
   b. Traced downwards, the abdomen extends to the hips. A part of the abdomen present in the region of the hips is called the ***pelvis***.
5. The thorax, the abdomen, the neck, and the head together form the ***trunk***.
6. Attached to the trunk, there are the upper and lower ***limbs***, or the upper and lower ***extremities***.

## SOME COMMONLY USED DESCRIPTIVE TERMS

1. The study of anatomy is like the learning of a new language. The learning of anatomical terms is the basic foundation on which all subsequent studies in various subjects of the medical curriculum depend.
2. Of all the terms to be learnt the most fundamental are those used for precise descriptions of the mutual relationships of various structures within the body.
3. In describing such relationships, we usually use terms like 'in front', 'behind', 'above', 'below', etc. However, in a study of anatomy, such terms are found to be inadequate; and the student's first task is to become familiar with the specialised terms used.

## Anatomical Position

1. In describing relationships within the body, we presume that the person is standing upright, looking directly forward, with the arms held by the sides of the body, and with the palms facing forwards.
2. This posture is referred to as the ***anatomical position***. We will now consider some descriptive terms one by one.
   a. When structure **A** lies nearer the front of the body as compared to structure **B**, **A** is said to be ***anterior*** to **B** (1.1).
   The opposite of anterior is ***posterior***. In the above example, it follows that **B** is posterior to **A**.
   b. When structure **C** lies nearer the upper end of the body as compared to structure **D**, **C** is said to be ***superior*** to **D** (1.1). The opposite of superior is ***inferior***. In the above example **D** is inferior to **C**.
   c. The body can be divided into two equal halves, right and left, by a plane passing vertically through it. The plane separating the two halves is called the ***median plane*** (1.2).
      i. When a structure lies ***in*** the median plane it is said to be ***median*** in position (e.g., **G** in 1.2).
      ii. When structure **E** lies nearer the median plane than structure **F**, **E** is said to be ***medial*** to **F**.
      iii. The opposite of medial is ***lateral***. In the above example **F** is lateral to **E**.
   d. In the anatomical position the palm faces forwards and the thumb lies along the outer side of the hand. Starting from the side of the thumb (or first digit) the fingers are named:
      i. Index finger (second digit)
      ii. Middle finger (third digit)
      iii. Ring finger (fourth digit)
      iv. Little finger (fifth digit).
   e. Various combinations of the descriptive terms mentioned above are frequently used.
      i. For example, each eye is anterior to the corresponding ear; and is also medial to it. Therefore, the eye can be said to be ***anteromedial*** to the ear.
      ii. The tip of the nose is inferior and medial to each eye: we can say the nose is ***inferomedial*** to the eye.
   f. We must now consider terms that are sometimes used as equivalent to some of the terms introduced above.
      i. The anterior aspect of the body corresponds to the ventral aspect of the body of four-footed animals. Hence, the term ***ventral*** is often used as equivalent to anterior. (However, we shall see later that the two terms are not always equivalent e.g., in the thigh).
      ii. In the hand, the palm is on the anterior or ventral aspect. This aspect of the hand is often called the ***palmar*** aspect.
      iii. The opposite of ventral is ***dorsal***. The back of the hand is the dorsal aspect, or simply the ***dorsum***, of the hand.
      iv. In the case of the foot, the surface towards the sole is ventral: it is called the ***plantar aspect***. The upper side of the foot is the ***dorsum*** of the foot.
      v. While referring to structures in the trunk the term ***cranial*** (= towards the head) is sometimes used instead of superior; and ***caudal*** (= towards the tail) in place of inferior.

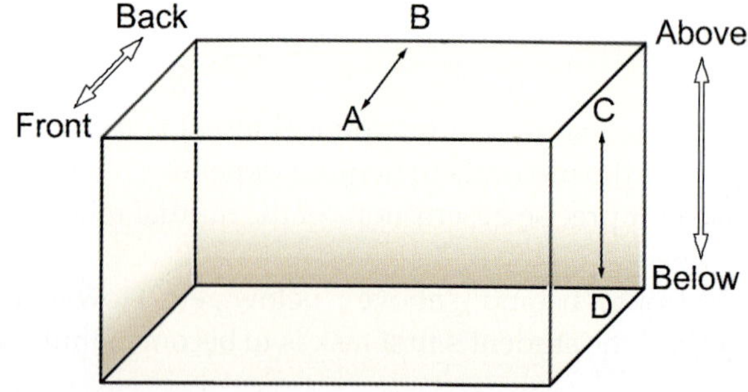


**1.1:** Scheme to explain the terms anterior, posterior, superior, and inferior

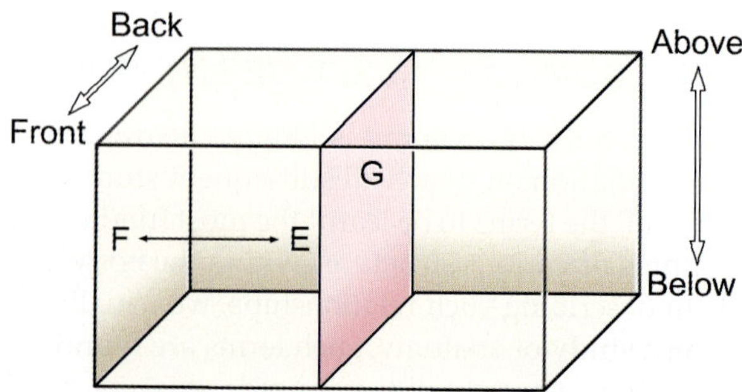


**1.2:** Scheme to explain the terms medial, lateral and median

vi. In the limbs, the term superior is sometimes replaced by ***proximal*** (= nearer) and inferior by ***distal*** (= more distant). Using this convention the phalanges of the hands are designated proximal, middle and distal.

vii. In the case of the forearm (or hand), the medial side is often referred to as the ***ulnar*** side, and the lateral side as the ***radial*** side.

viii. Similarly, in the leg (or foot) we can speak of the ***tibial*** (= medial) or ***fibular*** (= lateral) sides.

In addition to the terms described above there are some terms that are used to define planes passing through the body.

1. We have already seen that a plane passing vertically through the midline of the body, so as to divide the body into right and left halves, is called the ***median plane***. It is also called the ***mid-sagittal plane***.
2. Vertical planes to the right or left of the median plane, and parallel to the latter, are called ***paramedian*** or ***sagittal planes*** (1.3).
3. A vertical plane placed at right angles to the median plane (dividing the body into anterior and posterior parts) is called a ***coronal plane*** or a ***frontal plane*** (1.4).
4. Planes passing horizontally across the body (i.e., at right angles to both the sagittal and coronal planes) and dividing it into upper and lower parts, are called ***transverse*** or ***horizontal planes*** (1.5).
5. There are innumerable oblique planes intermediate between those described above.
6. Sections through any part of the body in any of the planes mentioned above are given corresponding names. Thus, we speak of:
   a. Median sections
   b. Sagittal sections

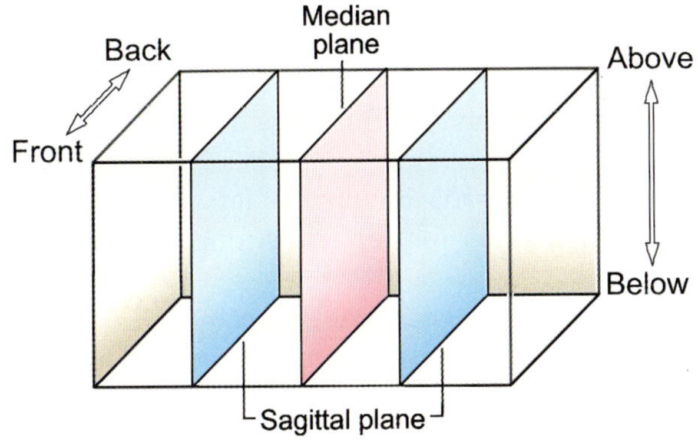


**1.3:** Scheme showing median and paramedian planes

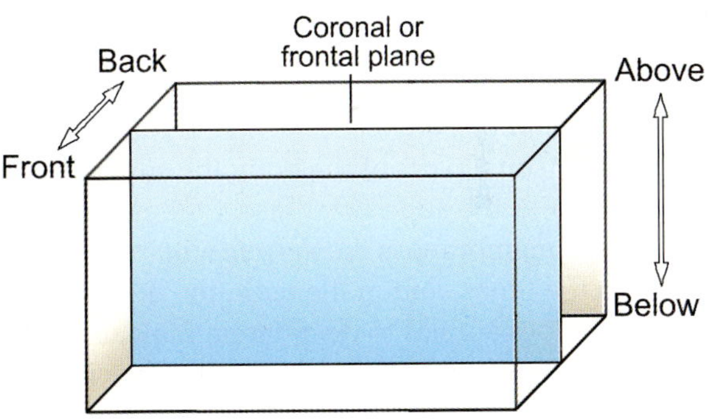


**1.4:** Scheme showing a frontal or coronal plane

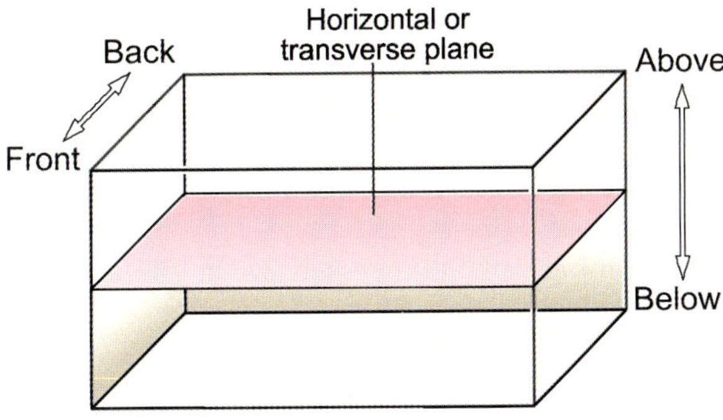


**1.5:** Scheme showing a horizontal or transverse plane

c. Coronal or frontal sections
d. Transverse sections
e. Oblique sections.

## STRUCTURES CONSTITUTING THE HUMAN BODY

When we dissect up any part of the body we encounter various elements.

1. The basic framework of the body is provided by a large number of ***bones*** that collectively form the ***skeleton***. As bones are hard they not only maintain their own shape, but also provide shape to the part of the body within which they lie.
2. In some situations (e.g., the nose or the ear) part of the skeleton is made up, not of bone but of, a firm but flexible tissue called ***cartilage***.
3. Bones meet each other at ***joints***, many of which allow movements to be performed. At joints, bones are united to each other by fibrous bands called ***ligaments***.
4. Overlying (and usually attached to) bones we see ***muscles***.
   a. Muscles are what the layman refers to as flesh. In the limbs, muscles form the main bulk.
   b. Muscle tissue has the property of being able to shorten in length. In other words muscles can contract, and by contraction they provide power for movements.
   c. A typical muscle has two ends, one (traditionally) called the ***origin***, and the other called the ***insertion***.
   d. Both ends are attached, typically, to bones.
5. The attachment of a muscle to bone may be a direct one, but quite often the muscle fibres end in cord like structures called ***tendons*** which convey the pull of the muscle to bone. Tendons are very strong structures.
6. Sometimes a muscle may end in a flat fibrous membrane. Such a membrane is called an ***aponeurosis***.
7. When we dissect a limb we find that the muscles within it are separated from skin, and from each other, by a tissue in which fibres are prominent. Such tissue is referred to as ***fascia***.
   a. Immediately beneath the skin the fibres of the fascia are arranged loosely and this loose tissue is called ***superficial fascia***.
   b. Over some parts of the body the superficial fascia may contain considerable amounts of fat.
   c. Deep to the superficial fascia the muscles are covered by a much better formed and stronger membrane. This membrane is the ***deep fascia***.
   d. In the limbs, and in the neck, the deep fascia encloses deeper structures like a tight sleeve.
8. Membranes similar to deep fascia may also intervene between adjacent muscles forming ***intermuscular septa***. Such septa often give attachment to muscle fibres.
9. Running through the intervals between muscles (usually in relation to fascial septa) there are ***blood vessels***, ***lymphatic vessels***, and ***nerves***.
   a. Blood vessels are tubular structures through which blood circulates.
   b. The vessels that carry blood from the heart to various tissues are called ***arteries***.
   c. Those vessels that return this blood to the heart are called ***veins***.
   d. Within tissues, arteries and veins are connected by plexuses of microscopic vessels called ***capillaries***.
10. ***Lymphatic vessels*** are delicate, thin walled tubes. They are difficult to see. They often run alongside veins.
11. Along the course of these lymphatic vessels small bean-shaped structures are present in certain situations. These are ***lymph nodes***.
12. Lymphatic vessels and lymph nodes are part of a system that plays a prominent role in protecting the body in various ways that you will study later.
13. Running through tissues, often in the company of blood vessels, we have solid cord like structures called ***nerves***.
    a. Each nerve is a bundle of a large number of ***nerve fibres***.
    b. Each nerve fibre is a process arising from a ***nerve cell*** (or ***neuron***).
    c. Most nerve cells are located in the brain and in the spinal cord.
    d. Nerves transmit impulses from the brain and spinal cord to various tissues. They also carry information from tissues to the brain.

   e. Impulses passing through nerves are responsible for contraction of muscle, and for secretions by glands. Sensations like touch, pain, sight and hearing are all dependent on nerve impulses travelling through nerve fibres.
14. Bones, muscles, blood vessels, nerves etc., which we have spoken of in the previous paragraphs are to be seen in all parts of the body. In addition to these many parts of the body have specialized ***organs***, also commonly called ***viscera***.
15. Some of the viscera are solid (e.g., the liver, or the kidney), while others are tubular (e.g., the intestines) or sac like (e.g., the stomach).
16. The viscera are grouped together in accordance with function to form various organ systems.
    a. Some examples of organ systems are the ***respiratory system*** responsible for providing the body with oxygen.
    b. The ***alimentary or digestive system*** responsible for the digestion and absorption of food.
    c. The ***urinary system*** responsible for removal of waste products from the body through urine; and the ***genital system*** which contains organs concerned with reproduction.
17. From the discussions in the previous paragraphs, it will be clear that in the study of the anatomy of any part of the body we have to consider the following:
    a. The skeletal basis of the part including bones and joints.
    b. The muscles and fasciae.
    c. The blood vessels and nerves.
    d. The lymph nodes and their areas of drainage.
    e. Viscera present in the region.

## HOW MUSCLES ARE NAMED

1. The human body contains a very large number of muscles, and each has a name. The student spends a great deal of time learning these names.
2. A muscle may be named on the basis of its action, its shape and size, and the region in which it lies.
3. The name of a given muscle usually consists of two or more words based on these characteristics.
4. How muscles are named will be clear from the following examples.

### Some Names Based on Region

1. The region on the front of the chest is called the ***pectoral region***. There are two muscles in this region. The larger of the two is called the ***pectoralis major***. The smaller one is called the ***pectoralis minor***.
2. The region of the buttock is called the ***gluteal region***. It contains three large muscles that are given the names ***gluteus maximus*** (largest), ***gluteus medius*** (intermediate in size) and ***gluteus minimus*** (smallest).
3. In each of the above examples note that the first word in the name refers to the region concerned, and the second to relative size.

### Some Names Based on Shape

1. Muscles that are straight are given the name ***rectus*** (compare with 'erect'). One such muscle present in the wall of the abdomen is called the ***rectus abdominis***. Another in the thigh is called the ***rectus femoris***. (Femoris = thigh—that is why the bone of the thigh is the femur).
2. Over the shoulder there is a strong triangular muscle called the ***deltoid*** (after the Greek letter *delta*, which is shaped like a triangle).
3. A quadrilateral muscle present in the lumbar region is called the ***quadratus lumborum***.
4. Most muscles have a fusiform shape. The central thicker part is muscular and is called the ***belly***. The ends are usually tendinous.
5. Some muscles have two (or more) bellies each with a distinct origin (or head). A muscle having two heads is given the name ***biceps***.

6. There is one such muscle in the arm and another in the thigh. The one in the arm is the ***biceps brachii*** (brachium = arm) and that in the thigh is the ***biceps femoris***.
7. On the back of the arm, there is a muscle that arises by three heads. It is called the ***triceps***.
8. On the front of the thigh, there is a muscle that has four heads. It is called the ***quadriceps femoris***. (Distinguish carefully between quadriceps and quadratus).

### Some Names Based on Action

1. Muscles that produce flexion may be named ***flexors***; and those that cause extension may be called ***extensors***.
2. Similarly, a muscle may be an ***abductor***, an ***adductor***, a ***supinator*** or a ***pronator***.
3. In each case, the word indicating action is followed by another word indicating the part on which the action is produced. For example, on the back of the forearm there is a muscle that is an extensor of the digits: it is called the ***extensor digitorum***.
4. Sometimes, we can have more than one muscle that qualifies for such a name. In that case we add a third word indicative of position.
   a. On the front of forearm there are two muscles that produce flexion at the wrist (or carpus).
   b. One of them, which lies towards the medial (or ulnar) side is called the ***flexor carpi ulnaris*** (= ulnar flexor of the carpus).
   c. The second muscle lies towards the lateral (or radial) side and is called the ***flexor carpi radialis***.
5. Sometimes, it is necessary to add a fourth word to the name. On the back of the forearm there are two radial extensors of the wrist: we call the longer one the ***extensor carpi radialis longus*** and the shorter one is named the ***extensor carpi radialis brevis***.
6. On the medial side of the thigh, there are three muscles that adduct it. Because of variations in size they are called the ***adductor longus***, the ***adductor brevis***, and the ***adductor magnus*** (magnus = largest).
7. Appreciation of these principles, used in naming muscles, can go a long way in easing the burden of remembering the names of muscles and their actions.

## SOME FEATURES OF JOINTS

1. Joints are formed where two (or more) bones meet.
2. Some joints are merely bonds of union between different bones and do not allow movement. Joints of the skull (sutures) belong to this category.
3. Some joints allow slight movement, while some (like the shoulder joint) allow great freedom of movement.
4. In describing movements, we use certain terms that the student must understand clearly.
   a. Movements at any joint can take place in various planes.
      i. Movements taking place in a sagittal plane are referred to as ***flexion*** (= bending), and ***extension*** (= straightening).
      ii. For example, when we bend the upper limb at the elbow joint so that the front of the forearm tends to approach the front of the arm this movement is called flexion (1.6).
      iii. Straightening the limb at elbow is called extension.
      iv. Bending the neck forwards is flexion of the neck, and straightening it, is extension. Similarly, when we bow, the vertebral column is being flexed, and when the body is made upright the spine is being extended.
   b. Movements in the coronal plane are referred to as ***abduction*** (= taking away) or ***adduction*** (= bringing near).
      i. When a limb is moved laterally so that it moves away from the trunk it is said to undergo abduction (1.7).
      ii. For example, such a movement takes place at the shoulder joint when the upper limb is raised sidewards.
      iii. A similar movement takes place at the hip joint. Adduction and abduction can also take place at the wrist and at some other joints.

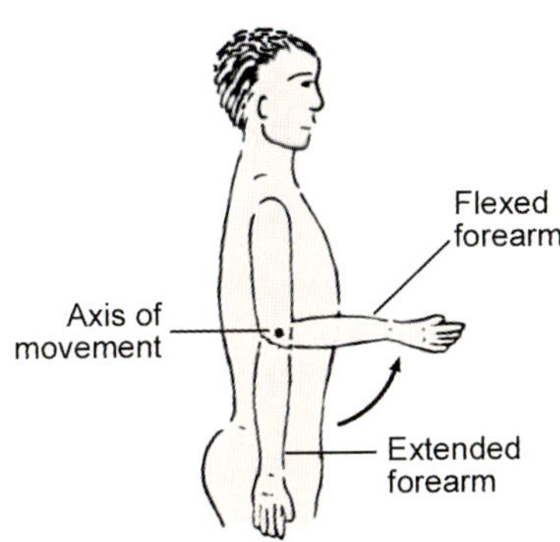


**1.6:** Diagram to explain the movement of flexion of the forearm

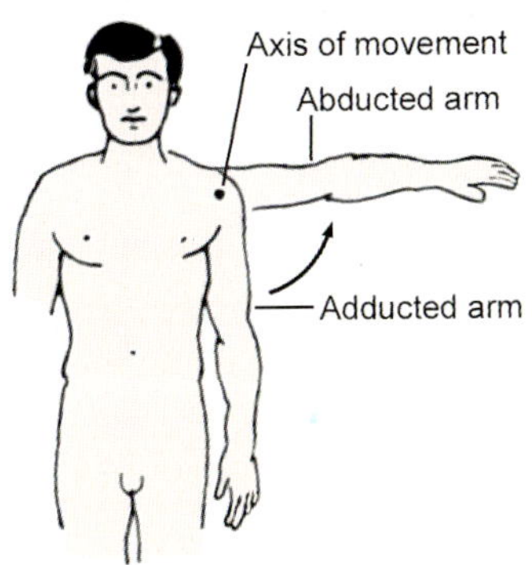


**1.7:** Diagram to explain the movement of abduction of the arm

c. Some joints allow ***rotatory movements***.
   i. When the forearm is rotated so that the palm comes to face forwards, the movement is called ***supination***.
   ii. The opposite movement is called ***pronation***.
   iii. Side-to-side movements of the neck are also rotatory movements.
   iv. The movement of the arm performed by a cricketer in bowling is a rotatory movement at the shoulder.
   v. Note that during this movement the hand moves in a circle. This movement is, therefore, called ***circumduction***.

d. When the foot is turned so that the sole looks somewhat inwards, the movement is called ***inversion***. The opposite movement is called ***eversion***.

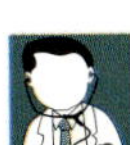

## CLINICAL CORRELATION

### INTRODUCTION

1. A medical student in India spends the first 12 months in the study of what are called the basic sciences of anatomy, physiology and biochemistry.
2. This study is an essential preparation for the understanding and treatment of disease.
3. The purpose of this section is to give students a preliminary glimpse of some facets of clinical practice that make the study of anatomy meaningful and relevant.
4. A patient may come to a doctor with various kinds of problems that may pertain to any part of the body. Some of these are as follows.

### INJURY (TRAUMA)

1. Any part of the body may be affected by injury.
2. The mechanical force inflicting injury may be direct or indirect.
3. It may be produced by a sharp object, or may be a blunt injury.
4. The effects of injury will depend on the tissues injured, and on the severity of injury.

#### Fractures

1. Injury to a bone can break it—breaking of a bone is *fracture*.
   a. The line along which a bone fractures may be ***transverse***, ***oblique***, or ***spiral***.
   b. A fracture in which a bone breaks into several small pieces is called a ***comminuted fracture***.
   c. Sometimes a bone, made up mainly of cancellous bone, (e.g., body of a vertebra) may be compressed (***compression fracture***).
   d. In young children, with soft bones, fractures are often incomplete (i.e., the two parts of a fractured bone may remain together). These are referred to as ***green-stick fractures***.

2. The two fragments of a fractured long bone may sometimes retain their normal relative position, but quite commonly there is ***displacement***. Displacement is produced by the actions of muscles on the two fragments.
3. In treating a fracture, the surgeon tries to bring the fragments back to their normal relative position. This is called ***reduction*** of the fracture.
4. Thereafter, measures are taken to prevent the fragments from being displaced again (***immobilisation***).
   a. Immobilisation can be done by applying a suitable ***plaster cast*** round the limb, or by operation in which the two fragments are united using metal appliances of various types (***internal fixation*** and ***external fixation***).
   b Immobilisation aids the process of healing, and relieves pain.

*Fracture Healing*

1. Immediately after a fracture, there is bleeding from vessels within the bone. This collection of blood (***haematoma***) surrounds the site of the fracture.
2. The bone contains cells that help in repair.
   a. These cells proliferate and invade the haematoma. Cells growing out of the two bone ends meet to form a single mass of cells. New bone is formed within the mass.
   b. This bone forms a covering for the two bone ends and unites them. This covering is called the ***callus***.
3. Immature bone of the callus is gradually replaced by mature bone. In this way the bone becomes one again, but the region of the fracture is thick and may be irregular.
4. As the newly formed bone becomes strong, excess bone around the fracture site is gradually removed. This is called ***remodelling***.
5. Following remodelling in the bones of children, no trace of the fracture site may remain. However, in adults, the fracture site usually shows a recognisable irregularity.

**Injuries to Joints and Ligaments**

1. Severe injury can result in separation of the two bones taking part in a joint. This is called ***dislocation***.
   a. Dislocation is more likely to occur in joints that allow free movement e.g., the shoulder joint.
   b. Dislocation usually involves damage to the capsule and to some ligaments.
2. In some cases, the two articular surfaces are displaced from their normal position but retain some contact with each other. This condition is called ***subluxation***.
3. When dislocation at a joint is combined with fracture of one of the bones within the joint the condition is called ***fracture-dislocation***.
4. A force that strongly stretches a ligament can cause its rupture. This usually leads to displacement of the joint surfaces.
5. However, injury to a ligament short of rupture can be a cause of serious pain at a joint, specially during movements that tend to stretch the ligament. Such a condition is referred to as ***sprain***, or ***strain***.
6. Ligaments can also be damaged by prolonged mild stress and some authorities use the term ***strain*** only for such injury.

**Injuries to Blood Vessels**

1. Injury to an artery is dangerous because loss of blood can, if unchecked, lead to death.
   a. Bleeding from an artery can be stopped by applying pressure over a suitable point.
   b. Knowledge of points where major arteries can be palpated and pressure applied on them is therefore of importance.
2. Injuries to large veins can also be serious.
   a. In some veins the pressure can be lower than atmospheric pressure and air can be sucked into them.
   b. This air travels into the heart and lungs and can block small vessels and capillaries there (***air embolism***).
3. Injured vessels have to be ***ligated*** (tied up). In the case of large vessels repair of the vessel may be possible.
4. Ligation of an artery carries the risk of necrosis (death) of the part supplied if its blood supply through alternative channels (***collateral circulation***) is not adequate.

5. For this reason, a knowledge of anastomoses established by various arteries becomes of importance.
6. Anastomoses are most abundant in regions where the main artery is subjected to compression because of movements e.g., around joints.

**Injuries to Nerves**

1. Injuries to nerves, if complete, can lead to ***paralysis*** (loss of the power of movement) of all muscles supplied, and ***anaesthesia*** (loss of sensations) over the area of sensory supply.
2. When a nerve is injured all structures supplied by branches arising distal to the point of injury are affected. However, injury may be partial and only some of the structures are then affected.
3. The extent of sensory loss is usually less than the area supplied by the nerve, because of overlap in the territories supplied by adjoining cutaneous nerves.

**Injuries to Other Tissues**

1. A ***muscle*** may be injured by any kind of direct violence.
   a. It may also be injured during rigorous exercise (as in athletes).
   b. In persons following sedentary occupations, and in old age, even mild unaccustomed movement can lead to strain within a muscle leading to pain and discomfort.
   c. However, the most serious effects on muscles are seen following injury to the nerves supplying them.
   d. Muscles can also be paralysed as a result of injury to the brain, to the spinal cord, or to nerve roots.
2. ***Tendons*** can be injured as a result of injury.
   a. A sharp injury can cut right through a tendon.
   b. A tendon can be damaged by a fractured bone.
   c. A tendon weakened by degenerative changes may rupture with relatively mild force.
3. The ***skin*** is the tissue most commonly affected by injury.
   a. However, because of great regenerative capacity superficial injuries are easily repaired.
   b. When large areas of skin are lost these areas can be covered with skin taken from other parts of the body. This process is called ***skin grafting***.
   c. Injury to skin may also be caused by extreme heat (burns), or by extreme cold; by chemicals (e.g., strong acids or alkalis); electrical currents; and by various kinds of radiations.
   d. Large areas of skin can be lost as a result of burns. In such cases death can occur because of loss of large amounts of water from the body, or because of infection.
4. Injuries to ***internal organs*** are usually serious and require urgent surgery.
   a. An injured organ may bleed into a body cavity.
   b. Such an ***internal haemorrhage*** can lead to death if it is not recognised and treated in time.
5. Injury to the brain is always very serious and often a cause of death. Damaged nerve cells cannot regenerate and if the patient survives some effects of injury may persist.

**INFLAMMATION AND INFECTIONS**

1. Any tissue or organ in the body can be infected with bacteria or viruses.
   a. Infection may be acute or chronic.
   b. In acute infection the tissue usually shows signs of ***inflammation***.
   c. The part becomes red in colour and warm because of greater blood flow.
   d. Accumulation of fluid causes swelling; and pressure on nerves in the area causes pain.
2. Infection can lead to pus formation. If the pus is in an enclosed space (as on the tip of a finger) it can cause considerable pain.
3. Infection often spreads along fascial planes. Its spread can be limited by fascial septa (as in the palm). In the treatment of infections knowledge of the anatomy of the part is, therefore, important.
4. Many of the terms used to describe infections are made up of the name of the part followed by the suffix 'itis'.
   a. Infection of the tonsil is ***tonsillitis***.
   b. Infection of the vermiform appendix is called ***appendicitis***.

5. Such terms are often used to describe inflammation of the organ that may be caused by agents other than infection.
   a. For example, inflammation of the mucosa of the stomach (***gastritis***) can be caused by any substance that irritates it (e.g. alcohol, or a drug).
   b. A common cold (***rhinitis***) can result from a virus infection, but it can also be caused by ***allergy*** (undue sensitivity of the tissue to some foreign substance).
   c. Inflammation can also be caused by physical agents like heat, cold, mechanical trauma and radiations. Some infections are caused by protozoa.
   d. Infection by ***amoeba histolytica*** can cause ***colitis*** (inflammation of the colon) or ***hepatitis*** (inflammation in the liver).
   e. Another important infection caused by protozoa is ***malaria.***
   f. When there is infection in any part of the body, lymph nodes draining the area may enlarge and become painful. This condition is called ***lymphadenitis***. Lymph vessels may also get inflamed (***lymphangitis***) and may be seen as red streaks over the skin.

## NEOPLASIA

1. In our body, cells in various tissues are constantly multiplying to replace dead cells.
2. The rate of multiplication varies from tissue to tissue and is strictly controlled.
3. Under certain circumstances the mechanisms that control cell proliferation do not work. As a result, there can be uncontrolled multiplication of cells leading to the formation of a ***neoplasm*** or ***tumour***.
4. Some tumours remain confined to their original site. Such tumours are said to be ***benign***, and their surgical removal leads to complete cure.
5. In the case of other tumours, some cells that get detached from the main tumour spread to distant sites (through lymphatic vessels, or sometimes through veins), and start multiplying forming new tumours. Such tumours are said to be ***malignant***.
6. The original tumour is the primary tumour, while the ones formed by spread from it are called ***secondaries***.
7. The spread of malignant tumours greatly adds to the difficulty of treating them, and once secondaries form complete eradication of the tumour may become impossible.
8. A surgeon examining a malignant tumour examines the lymph nodes of the region very carefully, as such examination can provide vital clues about the degree to which the growth has spread.
9. Because of the spread of malignant growths and of infections through lymphatics a knowledge of the lymphatic drainage of various parts of the body is of great importance.
10. Malignant growths fall into two major categories.
    a. A malignant growth arising from epithelial cells is called a ***carcinoma*** (cancer). Carcinoma can arise in the skin, in any tube or cavity lined with epithelium, and from epithelia of glands.
    b. A malignant tumour arising from non-epithelial tissue is usually referred to as ***sarcoma***.
    c. Such tumours can arise from connective tissue (***fibrosarcoma***), from muscle (***myosarcoma***), from bone (***osteosarcoma***) etc.

## OTHER CAUSES OF DISEASE

Apart from trauma, inflammation due to various causes, and neoplasms, some other causes that can lead to disease are as follows:

1. An individual may be born with physical defects that may affect the exterior or interior of the body.
   a. Such defects are called ***congenital malformations***.
   b Many diseases can be traced to genetic causes.
   c. Genetic defects can result in biochemical alterations that can lead to various disorders.
2. Diseases can also be produced as a result of ***malnutrition***, and can be a feature of normal ageing processes.
3. With increasing age there is narrowing of the arteries. Lack of adequate blood supply to the heart or to the brain can lead to serious consequences.
4. Wear and tear in joints is a common cause of joint pains in old persons.
5. Abnormal outgrowths from bone ends can reduce mobility at joints and can also cause pain (***osteoarthritis***).

CHAPTER

# 2 Bones of Upper Extremity

## SKELETON OF THE UPPER LIMB

The bones of the upper limb are shown in 2.1 and 2.2.

The bones join each other at a number of joints.

1. The upper end of the humerus is joined to the scapula at the shoulder joint (2.2).
2. The lower end of the humerus is joined to the upper ends of the radius and ulna to form the elbow joint.
3. The wrist joint is formed where the lower ends of the radius and ulna meet the carpal bones.
4. The upper and lower ends of the radius and ulna are united to one another at the superior and inferior radioulnar joints.
5. There are numerous small joints in the hand:
   a. The intercarpal joints between the carpal bones themselves.
   b. The carpometacarpal between the carpal and metacarpal bones.
   c. The metacarpo-phalangeal between each metacarpal bone and the proximal phalanx.
   d. The interphalangeal joints between the phalanges themselves.

During embryonic development most bones of the body are first seen in the form of cartilage. The replacement of these cartilages by bone is called ***ossification.***

1. In most bones, ossification begins during intrauterine life at an area called the ***primary centre of ossification***.
2. The part of the bone formed by extension of bone formation from the primary centre is called the ***diaphysis***.
3. However, the ends of long bones are still cartilaginous at birth. These are ossified from ***secondary centres*** that (as a rule) appear after birth.
4. Each part ossified from a secondary centre is called an ***epiphysis***.

**2.1: Bones of upper extremity**

| | *Name* | *Location* |
|---|---|---|
| BONES ATTACHED TO TRUNK FORMING PECTORAL GIRDLE | Clavicle | Rod-like bone lying in front of upper part of thorax |
| | Scapula | Triangular plate of bone behind upper part of thorax behind upper part of thorax |
| BONES OF FREE LIMB | Humerus | Arm |
| | Radius | Forearm (laterally) |
| | Ulna | Forearm(medially) |
| | Carpal bones (8) | Wrist (arranged in 2 rows) |
| | Metacarpal bones (5) | Palm |
| | Phalanges | Fingers or digits (3 in each finger and 2 in the thumb) |

5. For many years after birth, the bone of the epiphysis and diaphysis is separated by a plate of cartilage called the ***epiphyseal plate***.
6. This plate is a site of active bone growth. Growth in length of a bone is possible only as long as the plate exists.
7. When a bone has attained its full length the epiphyseal plate disappears and the diaphysis and epiphysis fuse with each other. This is referred to as ***fusion of the epiphysis***.
8. Knowledge of the ages at which various centres of ossification appear, and the ages at which epiphyses fuse to the diaphysis is of practical importance in determining the age of a person.

### *Determination of the Side to which a Limb Bone Belongs*

1. The first step in the study of any bone is to orientate it as it lies in the body.
2. To do this, we have to distinguish the anterior aspect from the posterior; the upper end from the lower; and the medial side from the lateral.
3. Once, we have this information we can find out whether the bone belongs to the right limb or the left one.

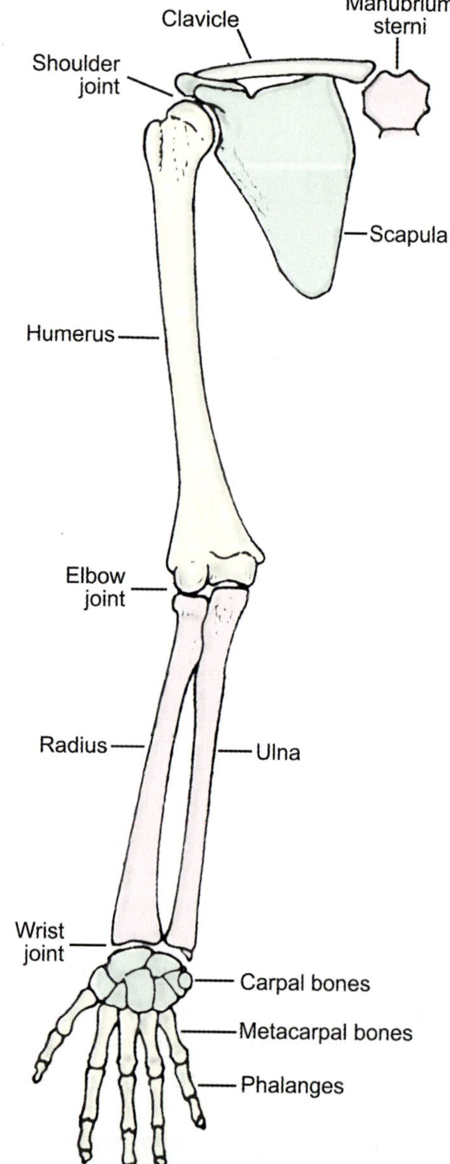


**2.2:** Drawing showing bones and joints of upper extremity

## The Clavicle

### *Determination of Side*

The clavicle is a long bone having a shaft, and two ends (2.3 and 2.4).

1. The medial end is much thicker than the shaft and is easily distinguished from the lateral end that is flattened.
2. The anterior and posterior aspects of the bone can be distinguished by the fact that the shaft (which has a gentle S-shaped curve) is convex forwards in the medial two-thirds, and concave forwards in its lateral one-third.
3. The inferior aspect of the bone is distinguished by the presence of a shallow groove on the shaft, and by the presence of a rough area near its medial end.

For purposes of description it is convenient to divide the clavicle into the lateral one-third that is flattened, and the medial two-thirds that are cylindrical.

1. The ***lateral one-third*** has two surfaces i.e., superior and inferior.
   a. These surfaces are separated by two borders: anterior and posterior.
   b. The anterior border is concave and shows a small thickened area called the ***deltoid tubercle***.
   c. The lower surface (of the lateral one-third) shows a prominent thickening near the posterior border; this is the ***conoid tubercle***.
   d. Lateral to the tubercle, there is a rough ridge that runs obliquely up to the lateral end of the bone, and is called the ***trapezoid line***.
2. The ***medial two-thirds*** of the shaft has four surfaces: anterior, posterior, superior and inferior, that are not clearly marked off from each other.
   a. The large rough area present on the inferior aspect of the bone near the medial end forms part of the inferior surface.

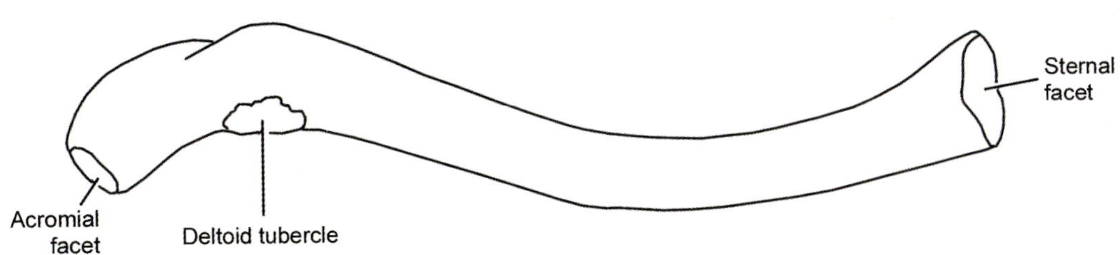


**2.3:** Right clavicle seen from above

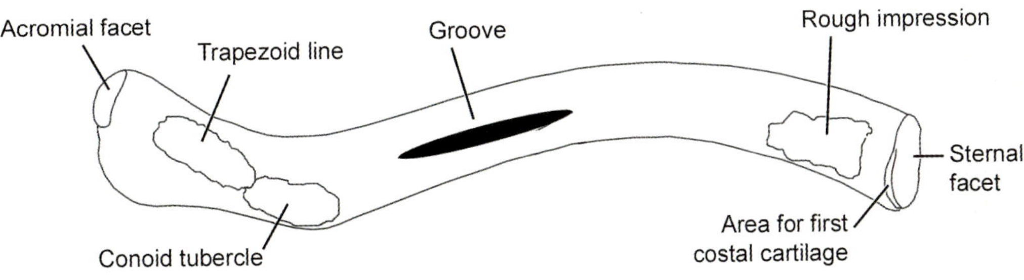


**2.4:** Right clavicle seen from below

   b. The middle-third of the inferior aspect shows a longitudinal groove, the depth of which varies considerably from bone to bone.
3. The ***lateral or acromial end*** of the clavicle bears a smooth facet which articulates with the acromion of the scapula to form the acromioclavicular joint.
4. The ***medial or sternal end*** of the clavicle articulates with the manubrium sterni, and also with the first costal cartilage.
   a. The articular area is smooth and extends on to the inferior surface of the bone for a short distance.
   b. The uppermost part of the sternal surface is rough for ligamentous attachments.
5. The clavicle can be easily felt in the living person as it lies just deep to the skin in its entire extent. The sternal end of the bone forms a prominent bulge that extends above the upper border of the manubrium sterni.

## WANT TO KNOW MORE?

### Attachments on the Clavicle

*The muscles attached to the clavicle are as follows:*

1. The ***pectoralis major*** (clavicular head) arises from the anterior surface of the medial half of the shaft.
2. The ***deltoid*** arises from the anterior border of the lateral one-third of the shaft.
3. The ***sternocleidomastoid*** (clavicular head) arises from the medial part of the upper surface.
4. The ***sternohyoid*** (lateral part) arises from the lower part of the posterior surface just near the sternal end.
5. The ***trapezius*** is inserted into the posterior border of the lateral one-third of the shaft.
6. The ***subclavius*** is inserted into the groove on the inferior surface of the shaft.

   See 2.5 and 2.6.

### Ossification of the Clavicle

1. The clavicle is the first bone in the body to start ossifying.
2. The greater part of the clavicle is formed by ***intramembranous ossification.***
3. The sternal and acromial ends are preformed in cartilage.
4. Two primary centres appear in the shaft during the 6th week of fetal life and soon fuse with each other.
5. The sternal end ossifies from a secondary centre that appears between 15 and 20 years of age, and fuses with the shaft by the age of 25 years.
6. An additional centre may appear in the acromion.

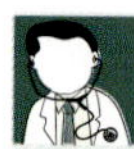

## CLINICAL CORRELATION

### Fractures of the Clavicle

Most fractures of the clavicle are caused by indirect violence.

1. The bone is most commonly fractured at the junction of its middle and outer one-thirds (2.12), this being the weakest point of the bone.
   a. In this fracture, the outer fragment is pulled downwards by the weight of the upper limb. It is pulled medially by the pectoralis major.
   b. The inner segment is pulled upwards by the sternocleidomastoid.
2. Less commonly, the clavicle is fractured near its lateral end.

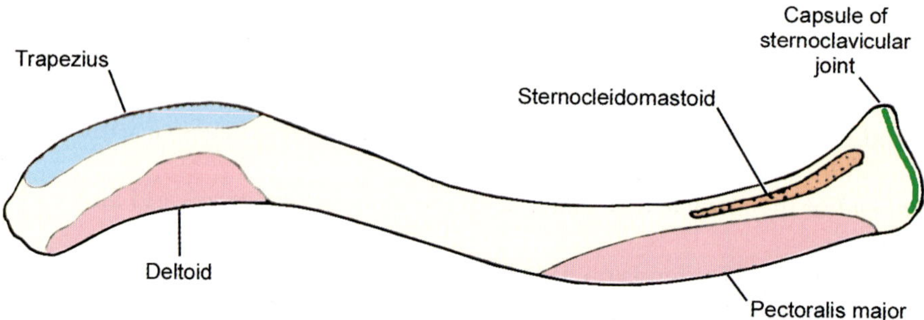


**2.5:** Right clavicle showing attachments, seen from above

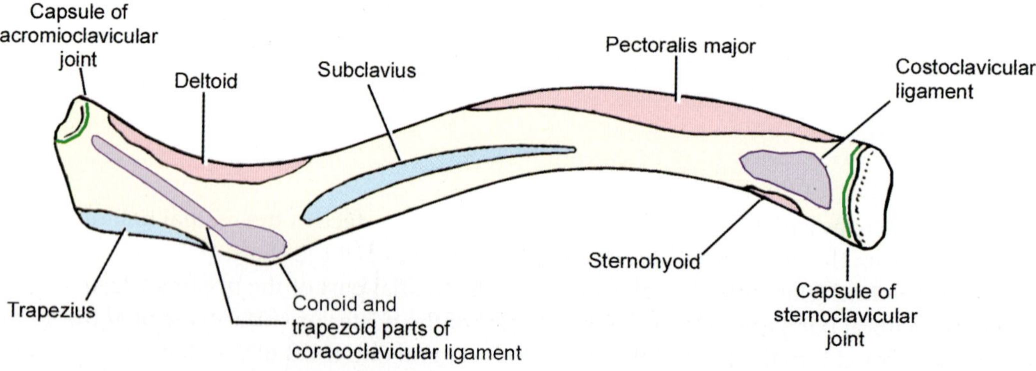


**2.6:** Right clavicle showing attachments, seen from below

## The Scapula

### *Determination of Side*

1. The greater part of the scapula (2.7 to 2.11) consists of a flat triangular plate of bone called the ***body***.
   a. The upper part of the body is broad, representing the base of the triangle.
   b. The inferior end is pointed and represents the apex.
2. The body has anterior (or costal) and posterior (or dorsal) surfaces which can be distinguished by the fact that the anterior surface is smooth, but the upper part of the posterior surface gives off a large projection called the ***spine***.
3. At its lateral angle, the bone is enlarged and bears a large shallow oval depression called the ***glenoid cavity*** which articulates with the head of the humerus.

The side to which a given scapula belongs can be determined from the information given above.

1. In addition to its costal and dorsal surfaces the body has three angles: superior, inferior and lateral; and three borders: medial, lateral and superior.
2. Arising from the body, there are three processes. In addition to the spine already mentioned, there is an acromion process and a coracoid process.
   a. The ***lateral border*** runs from the glenoid cavity to the inferior angle.
   b. The ***medial border*** extends from the superior angle to the inferior angle.
   c. The ***superior border*** passes laterally from the superior angle, but is separated from the glenoid cavity (representing the lateral angle) by the root of the coracoid process. A deep ***suprascapular notch*** is seen at the lateral end of the superior border.
3. The ***costal surface*** lies against the posterolateral part of the chest wall. It is somewhat concave from above downwards.
4. The ***dorsal surface*** gives attachment to the spine.
   a. The part above the spine forms the ***supraspinous fossa,*** along with the upper surface of the spine.
   b. The area below the spine forms the ***infraspinous fossa,*** along with the lower surface of the spine.
   c. The supraspinous and infraspinous fossae communicate with each other through the ***spinoglenoid notch*** that lies on the lateral side of the spine.
5. The part of the body adjoining the lateral border is thickened to form a longitudinal bar of bone. The dorsal aspect of the scapula adjoining the lateral border is rough for muscular attachments.
6. The ***glenoid cavity*** (2.11) is pear shaped and forms the shoulder joint along with the head of the humerus.
   a. Just below the cavity the lateral border shows a rough raised area called the ***infraglenoid tubercle***.
   b. Immediately above the glenoid cavity there is a rough area called the ***supraglenoid tubercle***.
7. The region of the glenoid cavity is often regarded as the head of the scapula. Immediately medial to it there is a constriction which constitutes the ***neck***.
8. The ***spine*** of the scapula is triangular in form.
   a. Its anterior border is attached to the dorsal surface of the body.
   b. Its posterior border is free: it is greatly thickened and forms the ***crest of the spine***.
   c. The medial end of the spine lies near the medial border of the scapula: this part is referred to as the ***root of the spine***.
   d. The lateral border of the spine is free and forms the medial boundary of the ***spino-glenoid notch***.
9. The ***acromion*** is continuous with the lateral end of the spine. It forms a projection that is directed forwards and partly overhangs the glenoid cavity.
   a. It has a lateral border and a medial border that meet anteriorly at the tip of the acromion.
   b. The lateral border meets the crest of the spine at a sharp angle termed the ***acromial angle***.
   c. The medial border of the acromion shows the presence of a small oval facet for articulation with the lateral end of the clavicle.
   d. The acromion has upper and lower surfaces.

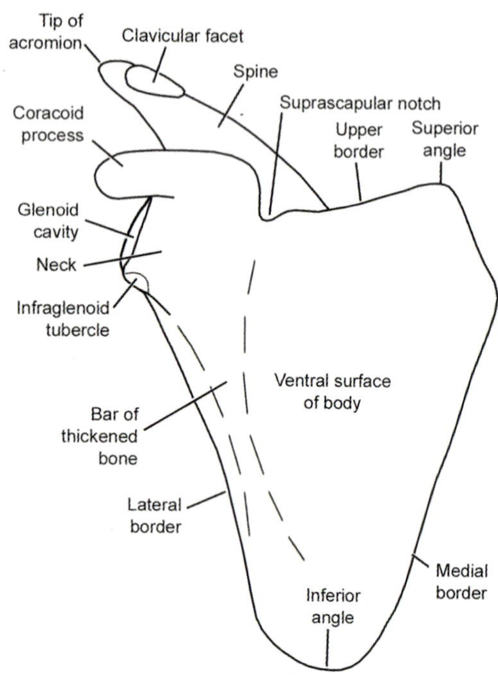


2.7: Right scapula, seen from the front

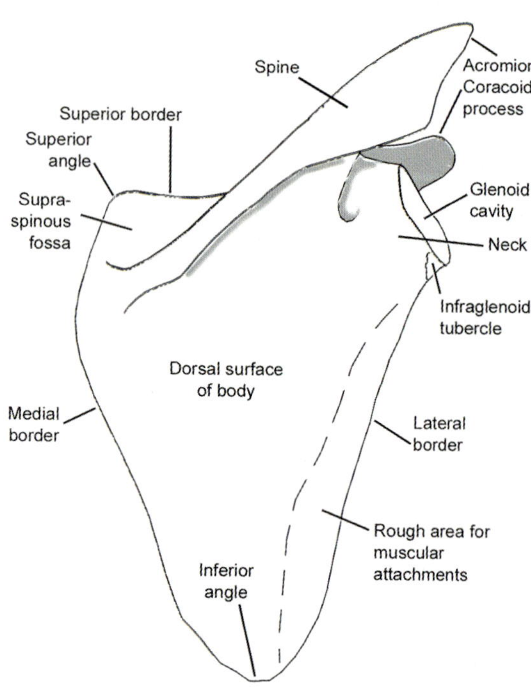


2.8: Right scapula, seen from behind

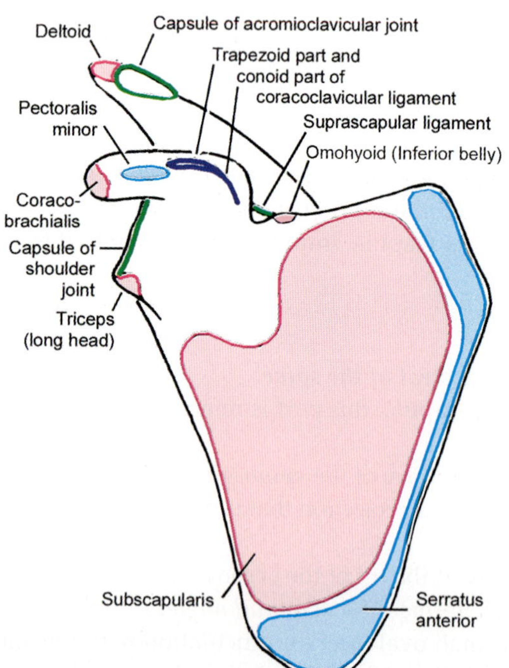


2.9: Right scapula, showing attachments seen from the front

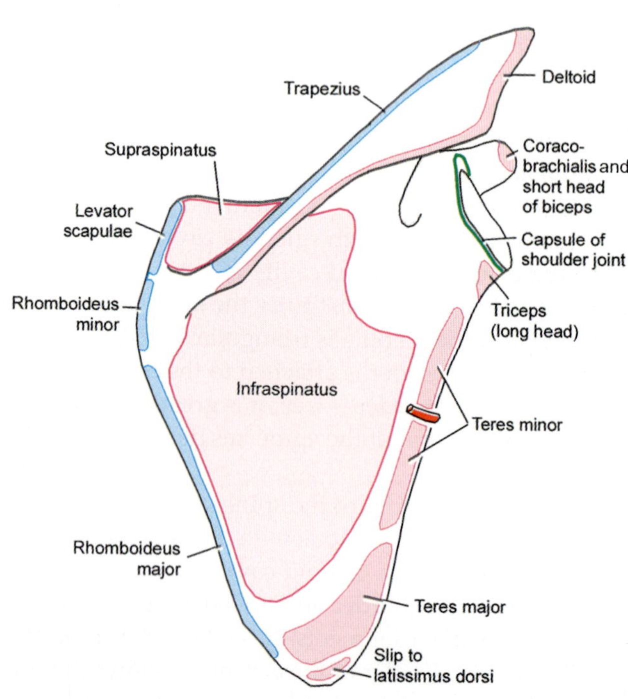


2.10: Right scapula, showing attachments seen from behind

10. The ***coracoid process*** is shaped like a bent finger.
    a. The root of the process is attached to the body of the scapula just above the glenoid cavity.
    b. The lower part of the root is marked by the supraglenoid tubercle.
    c. The tip of the coracoid process is directed straight forwards.
    d. At the point where the coracoid process bends forwards, its dorsal surface is marked by a ridge.

## WANT TO KNOW MORE?

### Attachments on the Scapula

*The muscles attached to the scapula are as follows ( 2.9 to 2.11):*

1. The ***deltoid*** takes origin from the lower border of the crest of the spine; and from the lateral margin, tip and upper surface of the acromion.
2. The ***trapezius*** is inserted into the upper border of the crest of the spine, and into the medial border of the acromion.
3. The short head of the ***biceps brachii*** arises from the (lateral part of the) tip of the coracoid process; and the long head from the supraglenoid tubercle.
4. The ***coracobrachialis*** arises from (the medial part of) the tip of the coracoid process.
5. The long head of the ***triceps*** arises from the infraglenoid tubercle.
6. The ***pectoralis minor*** is inserted into the superior aspect of the coracoid process.
7. The inferior belly of the ***omohyoid*** arises from the upper border near the suprascapular notch.
8. The ***subscapularis*** arises from the whole of the costal surface, but for a small part near the neck.
9. The ***serratus anterior*** is inserted on the costal surface along the medial border.
    a. The first digitation of the muscle is inserted from the superior angle to the root of the spine.
    b. The next two or three digitations are inserted into a narrow line along the medial border.
    c. The lower 4 or 5 digitations are inserted into a large triangular area over the inferior angle.
10. The ***supraspinatus*** arises from the medial two-thirds of the supraspinous fossa, including the upper surface of the spine.
11. The ***infraspinatus*** arises from the greater part of the infraspinous fossa, but for a part near the lateral border and a part near the neck.
12. The ***teres minor*** arises from the upper two-thirds of the rough strip on the dorsal surface, near the lateral border. There is a gap in the area of origin for passage of the circumflex scapular vessels.
13. The ***teres major*** arises from the lower one-third of the rough strip along the dorsal aspect of the lateral border. The area is wide and extends over the inferior angle.
14. The ***levator scapulae*** is inserted into a narrow strip along the dorsal aspect of the medial border, extending from the superior angle to the level of the root of the spine.
15. The ***rhomboideus minor*** is inserted into the dorsal aspect of the medial border, opposite the root of the spine.
16. The ***rhomboideus major*** is inserted into the dorsal aspect of the medial border, from the root of the spine to the inferior angle.
17. The ***latissimus dorsi*** receives a small slip from the dorsal surface of the inferior angle.

*Some ligaments attached to the scapula are as follows:*

1. The ***capsule of the shoulder joint*** and the ***glenoidal labrum*** are attached to the margins of the glenoid cavity. In its upper part the attachment of the capsule extends above the supraglenoid tubercle so that the origin of the long head of the biceps is within the capsule.
2. The ***suprascapular ligament*** bridges across the supra-scapular notch and converts it into a foramen which transmits the suprascapular nerve. The suprascapular vessels lie above the ligament.

**Ossification of the Scapula**

The scapula usually has eight centres of ossification.

1. A centre appears in the body during the 8th week of fetal life.
2. The spine is ossified by extension from this centre.
3. The greater part of the coracoid process is ossified from a centre that appears in the first year.
4. The remaining centres appear about the age of puberty.

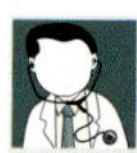

## CLINICAL CORRELATION

1. ***Fractures of the scapula*** are uncommon. They can occur in automobile accidents. Usual sites of fracture are:
   a. Body of the scapula.
   b. Fracture through the neck.
   c. Fracture of the acromion process.
   d. Fracture of the coracoid process (2.12).
2. ***Sprengles shoulder*** is a condition in which the scapula is placed higher than normal.
3. ***Winging of the scapula*** is a condition in which the medial border of the scapula is lifted off the chest wall. It is caused by paralysis of the serratus anterior.

## The Humerus

### *Determination of Side*

1. The humerus is a long bone. It has a cylindrical central part called the ***shaft***, and enlarged ***upper*** and ***lower ends*** (2.13 and 2.14).
2. The upper end is easily distinguished from the lower by the presence of a large rounded head.

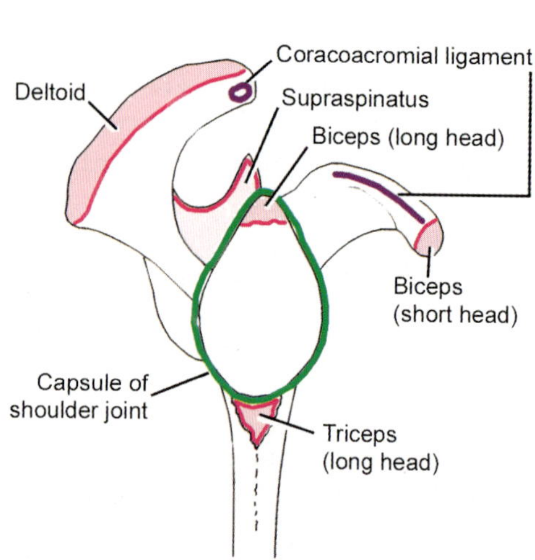


**2.11:** Right scapula, showing attachments seen from the lateral side

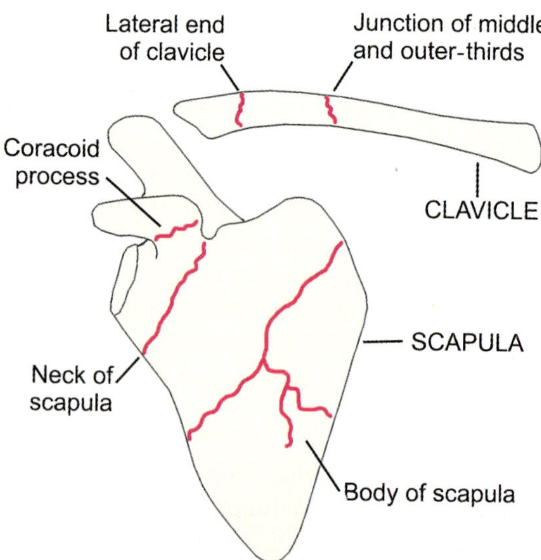


**2.12:** Fractures of clavicle and scapula

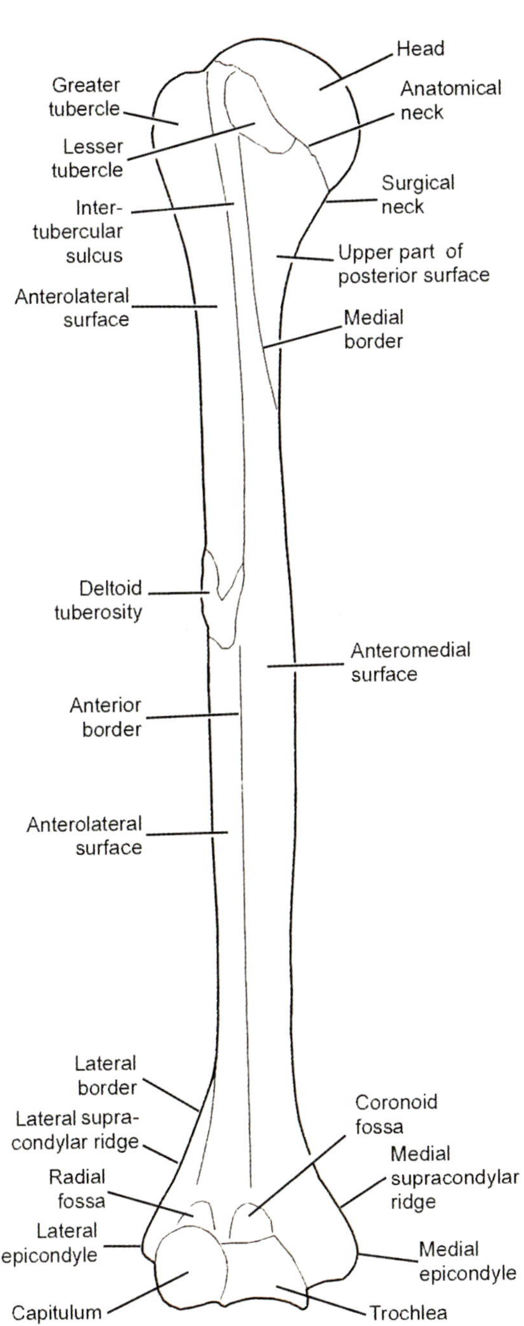


2.13: Right humerus seen from the front

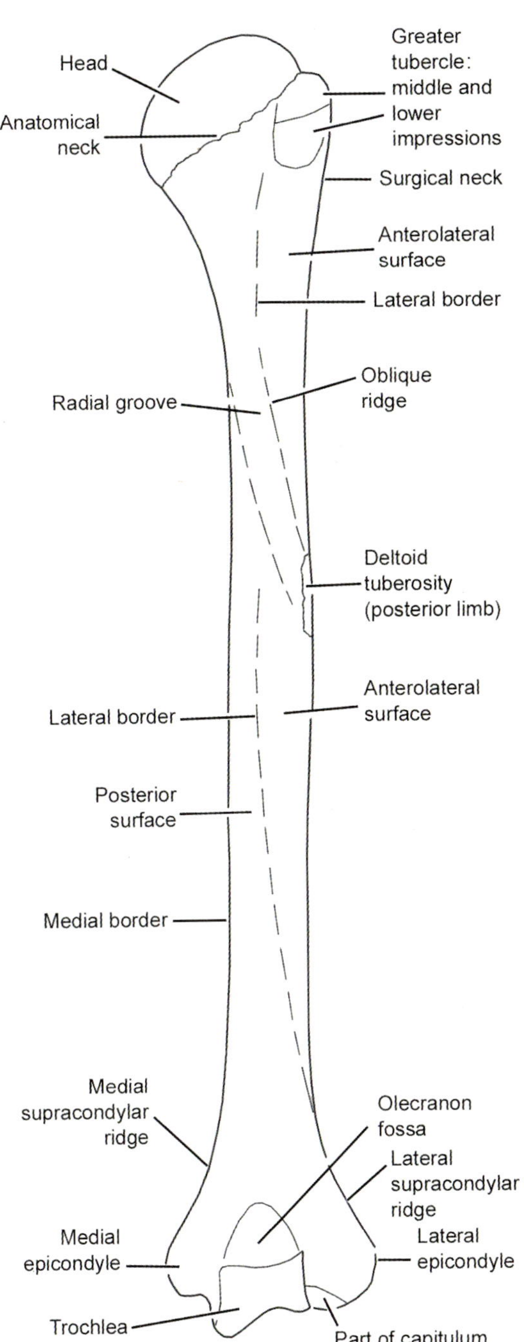


2.14: Right humerus seen from behind

3. The medial and lateral sides can be distinguished by the fact that the head is directed medially.
4. The anterior aspect of the upper end shows a prominent vertical groove called the ***intertubercular sulcus***.

The side to which a given bone belongs can be determined from the information given above.

1. The ***head*** is rounded and has a smooth convex articular surface.
   a. It is directed medially, and also somewhat backwards and upwards.
   b. It forms the shoulder joint along with the glenoid cavity of the scapula.
   c. It may be noted that the articular area of the head is much greater than that of the glenoid cavity.
2. In addition to the head, the upper end of the humerus shows two prominences called ***the greater*** and ***lesser tubercles*** (or tuberosities).
3. These two tubercles are separated by the ***intertubercular sulcus*** (also called the bicipital groove). This is the vertical groove on the anterior aspect of the upper end mentioned above.
   a. The ***lesser tubercle*** lies on the anterior aspect of the bone medial to the sulcus, between it and the head. It has a smooth upper part and a rough lower part.
   b. The ***greater tubercle*** is placed on the lateral aspect of the upper end and parts of it can, therefore, be seen from both the anterior and posterior aspects.
4. The anterior part of the greater tubercle forms the lateral boundary (or lip) of the intertubercular sulcus.
5. The tubercle shows three areas (or impressions) where muscles are attached. The uppermost of these is placed on the superior aspect, the lowest on the posterior aspect, and the middle is in between them.
6. There are two distinct regions of the upper end of the humerus that are referred to as the ***neck***.
   a. The junction of the head with the rest of the upper end is called the ***anatomical neck***.
   b. The junction of the upper end with the shaft is called the ***surgical neck***.
7. The ***shaft*** of the humerus has three borders: anterior, medial and lateral. These are readily identified in the lower part of the bone.
   a. When traced upwards the ***anterior border*** becomes continuous with the anterior margin of the greater tubercle (or ***crest of the greater tubercle***, or ***lateral lip of the intertubercular sulcus***).
   b. The ***medial border*** is indistinct in its upper part, but it can be traced to the lower end of the lesser tubercle, and to its sharp lateral margin (crest of the lesser tubercle, or medial lip of the intertubercular sulcus).
   c. The lower part of the ***lateral border*** can be seen from the front, but its upper part runs upwards on the posterior aspect of the bone.
   d. The three borders divide the shaft into three surfaces:
      i. The ***anterolateral surface*** lies between the anterior and lateral borders.
      ii. The ***anteromedial surface*** between the anterior and medial borders.
      iii. The ***posterior surface*** between the medial and lateral borders.
   e. We may now note certain additional features of the shaft.
      i. The anterolateral surface has a V-shaped rough area called the ***deltoid tuberosity*** that is present near the middle of this surface.
      ii. The anterior limb of the tuberosity lies along the anterior border of the shaft while the posterior limb lies above the lower part of the radial groove (see below).
   f. The medial border also bears a roughened strip near its middle.
      i. When the shaft is observed from behind we see that its upper part is crossed by a broad and shallow ***radial groove*** which runs downwards and laterally across the posterior and anterolateral surfaces.
   g. The radial groove interrupts the lateral border of the shaft.
      i. The part of the lateral border below the groove is indistinct.
      ii. The part of the border above the groove is also not well marked, but can be traced to the posterior part of the greater tuberosity.
      iii. The upper margin of the radial groove is formed by a roughened ridge that runs obliquely across the shaft.
      iv. The lower end of the ridge is continuous with the posterior limb of the deltoid tuberosity.

8. The lower end of the humerus is irregular in shape and is also called the ***condyle***.
   a. The lowest parts of the medial and lateral borders of the humerus form sharp ridges that are called the ***medial*** and ***lateral supracondylar ridges*** respectively.
      i. Their lower ends terminate in two prominences called the ***medial*** and ***lateral epicondyles***.
      ii. The medial epicondyle is the larger of the two.
   b. Between the two epicondyles the lower end presents an irregular shaped articular surface which is divisible into medial and lateral parts.
   c. The lateral part is rounded and is called the ***capitulum***. It articulates with the head of the radius.
   d. The medial part of the articular surface is shaped like a pulley and is called the ***trochlea***.
      i. It is separated from the capitulum by a faint groove.
      ii. The medial margin of the trochlea projects downwards much below the level of the capitulum, and of the epicondyles.
      iii. The trochlea articulates with the upper end (***trochlear notch***) of the ulna.
   e. The anterior aspect of the lower end of the humerus shows two depressions: one just above the capitulum and another above the trochlea.
      i. The depression above the capitulum is called the ***radial fossa.***
      ii. The one above the trochlea is called the ***coronoid fossa*** (2.13).
      iii. Parts of the head of the radius and of the coronoid process of the ulna lie in these depressions when the elbow is fully flexed.
   f. Another depression is seen above the trochlea on the posterior aspect of the lower end (2.14). This depression is called the ***olecranon fossa*** as it lodges the olecranon process of the ulna when the elbow is fully extended.

## WANT TO KNOW MORE?

### Attachments on the Humerus

*The muscles attached to the humerus are as follows (2.15 to 2.17):*

1. The ***supraspinatus*** is inserted into the upper impression on the greater tubercle.
2. The ***infraspinatus*** is inserted into the middle impression on the greater tubercle.
3. The ***teres minor*** is inserted into the lower impression on the greater tubercle.
4. The ***subscapularis*** is inserted into the lesser tubercle.
5. The ***pectoralis major*** is inserted into the lateral lip of the intertubercular sulcus.
6. The ***latissimus dorsi*** is inserted into the floor of the intertubercular sulcus.
7. The ***teres major*** is inserted into the medial lip of the intertubercular sulcus.
   Of the three insertions into the intertubercular sulcus that of the pectoralis major is the most extensive, and that of the latissimus dorsi is the shortest.
8. The ***deltoid*** is inserted into the deltoid tuberosity.
9. The ***coracobrachialis*** is inserted into the rough area on the middle of the medial border.
10. The ***brachialis*** arises from the lower halves of the anteromedial and anterolateral surfaces of the shaft. Part of the area of origin extends onto the posterior aspect.
11. The ***pronator teres*** (humeral head) arises from the anteromedial surface, near the lower end of the medial supracondylar ridge.
12. The ***brachioradialis*** arises from the upper two-thirds of the lateral supracondylar ridge.
13. The ***extensor carpi radialis longus*** arises from the lower one-third of the lateral supracondylar ridge.
14. The ***superficial flexor muscles*** of the forearm arise from the anterior aspect of the medial epicondyle. This origin is called the ***common flexor origin***.
15. The ***common extensor origin*** for the superficial extensor muscles of the forearm is located on the anterior aspect of the lateral condyle.

16. The lateral head of the ***triceps*** arises from the oblique ridge on the upper part of the posterior surface, just above the radial groove.
    a. The medial head of the muscle arises from the posterior surface below the radial groove.
    b. The upper end of the area of origin extends onto the anterior aspect of the shaft.
17. The ***anconeus*** arises from the posterior surface of the lateral epicondyle.

*Some other structures attached to the humerus are as follows*

1. The ***capsular ligament of the shoulder joint*** is attached on the anatomical neck.
    a. On the medial side, the line of attachment dips down by about a centimetre to include a small area of the shaft within the joint cavity.
    b. The line of attachment of the capsule is interrupted at the intertubercular sulcus to provide an aperture through which the tendon of the long head of the biceps leaves the joint cavity.
2. The ***capsular ligament of the elbow joint*** is attached to the lower end of the bone.
    a. Anteriorly the line of attachment reaches the upper limits of the radial fossa and the coronoid fossa.
    b. Posteriorly the line reaches the upper limit of the olecranon fossa.
    c. These fossae therefore lie within the joint cavity.
3. The medial and lateral epicondyles give attachment to the ***ulnar*** and ***radial collateral ligaments*** respectively.

**Important Relations**

1. The intertubercular sulcus lodges the tendon of the long head of the biceps brachii. The ascending branch of the anterior circumflex humeral artery also lies in this sulcus.
2. The surgical neck of the bone is related to the axillary nerve and to the anterior and posterior circumflex humeral vessels.
3. The radial nerve and the profunda brachii vessels lie in the radial groove between the attachments of the lateral and medial heads of the triceps.
4. The ulnar nerve crosses behind the medial epicondyle.

**Ossification of the Humerus**

1. A primary centre appears in the shaft during the 8th fetal week. The greater part of the bone is formed from this centre.
2. Secondary centres at the upper end appear as follows:
    a. For the head appears early in the first year.
    b. For the greater tubercle in the second year.
    c. For the lesser tubercle in the fifth year.
    d. These three parts fuse with each other in the sixth year to form a single epiphysis for the upper end that fuses with the shaft around 18 to 20 years of age.
3. Secondary centres at the lower end are as follows:
    a. In the capitulum during the first year.
    b. In the medial part of the trochlea in the ninth or tenth year.
    c. In the lateral epicondyle around the twelfth year.
    d. These fuse to form a single epiphysis which fuses with the shaft around 15 years of age.
    e. A separate centre appears in the medial epicondyle around the fifth year; and fuses with the shaft about the twentieth year.

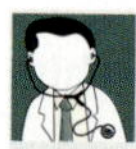

## CLINICAL CORRELATION

**Fractures of the Humerus**

The sites of fracture of the humerus are shown in 2.18.

1. The shaft may be fractured:
   a. Through the surgical neck.
   b. Through the middle of its shaft.
   c. Just above the lower end (supracondylar fracture).
2. Other fractures are:
   a. Through the greater tuberosity.
   b. Through one of its condyles (usually lateral).
   c. Through an epicondyle (usually medial).
3. In children the most common fracture is ***supracondylar***. Fractures through the neck are common in old women. Fracture through the middle of the shaft usually occurs in adults.

***Nerves that can be damaged***

1. The humerus is related to several nerves and these may be damaged because of fracture.
   a. Fracture through the surgical neck of the humerus can damage the axillary nerve.
   b. Fracture through the middle of the shaft can damage the radial nerve (which lies in the radial groove).
   c. In supracondylar fracture the median nerve can be injured, and there is danger of damage to the brachial artery as well.
   d. The ulnar nerve can be damaged in a fracture of the medial epicondyle.

***Non-union***

1. The humerus has a poor blood supply at the junction of its upper and middle-thirds.
2. Fractures at this site may, therefore, heal poorly resulting in delayed union or in non-union.

## The Radius

### *Determination of Side*

1. The radius is a long bone having a shaft and two ends: upper and lower (2.19 to 2.22).
2. The upper end bears a disc shaped head. In contrast the lower end is much enlarged.
3. The lateral and medial sides of the bone can be distinguished by examining the shaft which is convex laterally and has a sharp medial (or interosseous) border.
4. The anterior and posterior aspects of the bone may be identified by looking at the lower end: it is smooth anteriorly, but the posterior aspect is marked by a number of ridges and grooves.

The side to which a given radius belongs can be determined from the information given above.

1. The ***upper end*** of the bone consists of a head, a neck and a tuberosity.
   a. The ***head*** is disc shaped. Its upper surface is slightly concave and articulates with the capitulum of the humerus.
   b. The circumference of the head (representing the edge of the disc) is also smooth and articular.
   c. Medially it articulates with a notch on the ulna: the remaining part is enclosed by the annular ligament (2.21).
   d. This joint between the radius and ulna is the ***superior radioulnar joint***.
2. The region just below the head is constricted to form the ***neck***.
   a. Just below the medial part of the neck there is an elevation called the ***radial tuberosity***.
   b. The tuberosity is rough in its posterior part, and is smooth anteriorly.
3. The shaft of the radius has three borders (anterior, posterior, and interosseous) and three surfaces (anterior, posterior, lateral) (2.22).
   a. The ***interosseous or medial border*** is easily identified as it forms a sharp ridge which extends from just below the tuberosity to the lower end of the shaft. Near the lower end this border forms the posterior margin of a small triangular area.

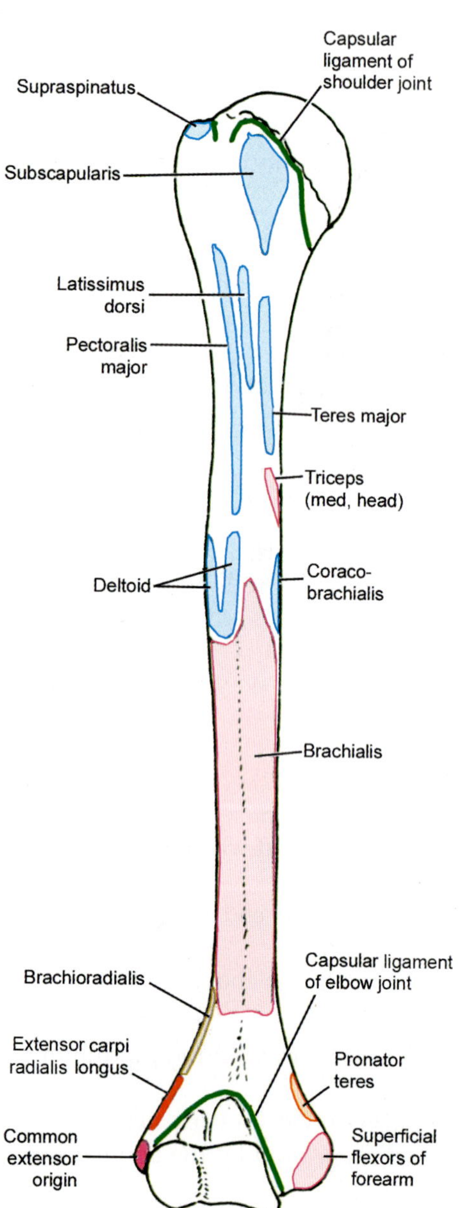


**2.15:** Right humerus, showing attachments seen from the front

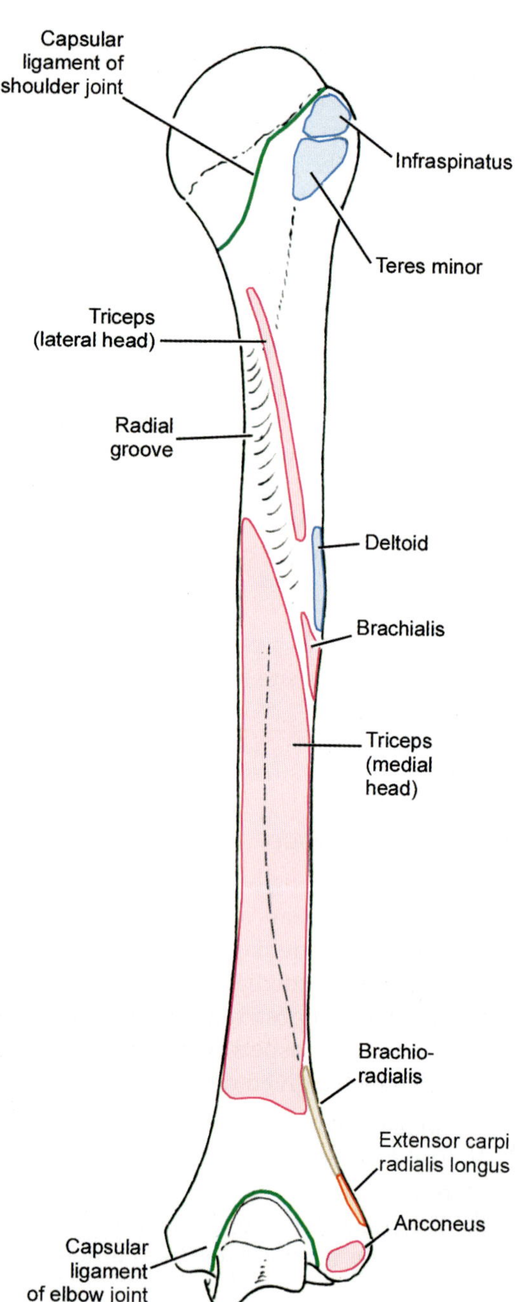


**2.16:** Right humerus, showing attachments seen from behind

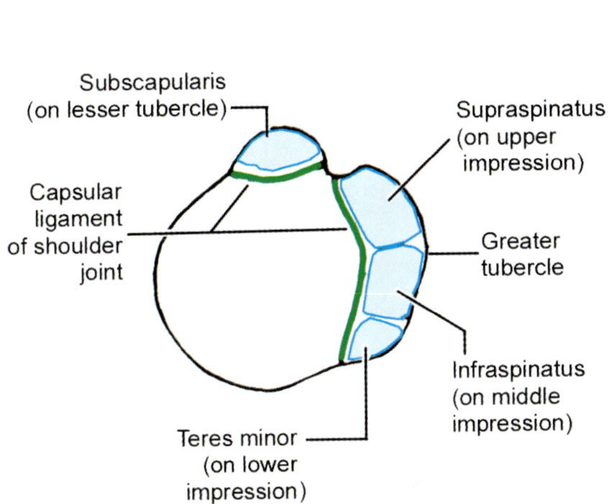


**2.17:** Upper end of right humerus, showing attachments seen from above

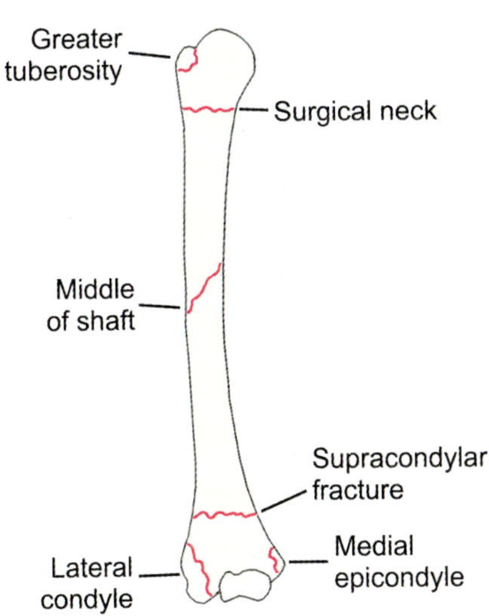


**2.18:** Fractures of humerus

b. The ***anterior border*** begins at the radial tuberosity and runs downwards and laterally across the anterior aspect of the shaft.
   i. This part of the anterior border is called the ***anterior oblique line***.
   ii. It then runs downwards and forms the lateral boundary of the smooth anterior aspect of the lower part of the shaft.
c. The upper part of the ***posterior border*** runs downwards and laterally from the posterior part of the tuberosity. The lower part of the posterior border runs downwards along the middle of the posterior aspect of the shaft to the lower end.
d. The ***anterior surface*** lies between the interosseous and anterior borders; the ***posterior surface*** between the interosseous and posterior borders.
e. The ***lateral surface*** between the anterior and posterior borders.
   i. In the upper part of the bone the lateral surface expands into a wide triangular area as it extends onto the anterior and posterior aspects of the bone.
   ii. The lateral surface shows a rough area near the middle (and most convex) part of the shaft.

4. The lower end of the radius has anterior, lateral and posterior surfaces continuous with the corresponding surfaces of the shaft. In addition it has a medial surface and an inferior surface.
   a. The lateral surface is prolonged downwards as a projection called the ***styloid process***.
   b. The medial aspect of the lower end has an articular area called the ***ulnar notch***.
      i. It articulates with the lower end of the ulna to form the ***inferior radioulnar joint***.
      ii. Just above the notch there is a triangular area bounded posteriorly by the interosseous border.
   c. The posterior aspect of the lower end is marked by a number of vertical grooves separated by ridges.
      i. The most prominent ridge is called the dorsal tubercle that is placed roughly midway between the medial and lateral aspects of the lower end.
      ii. Immediately medial to the tubercle there is a narrow oblique groove, and still more medially there is a wide shallow groove.
      iii. The area lateral to the dorsal tubercle shows two grooves separated by a ridge.
   d. The inferior surface of the lower end is articular. It takes part in forming the wrist joint. It is subdivided into a medial quadrangular area that articulates with the lunate bone, and a lateral triangular area that articulates with the scaphoid bone.

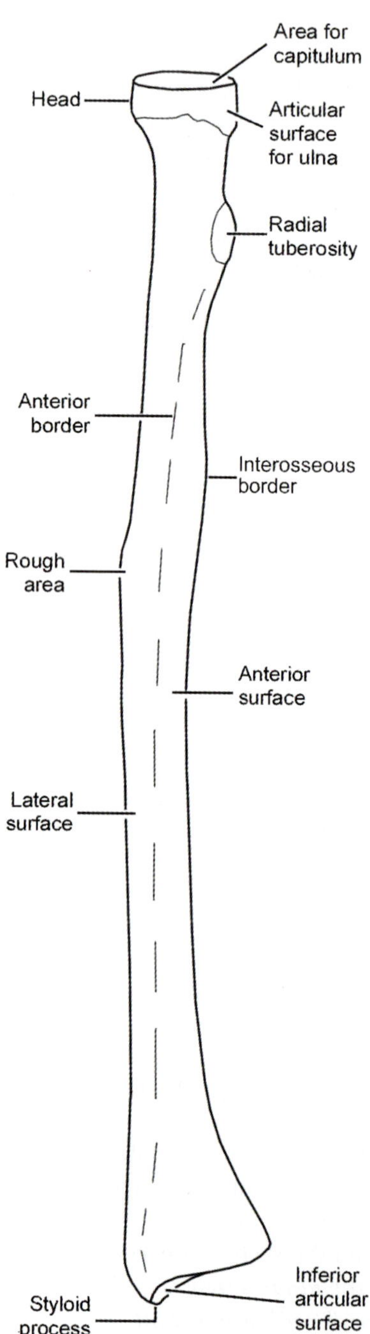


**2.19:** Right radius seen from the front

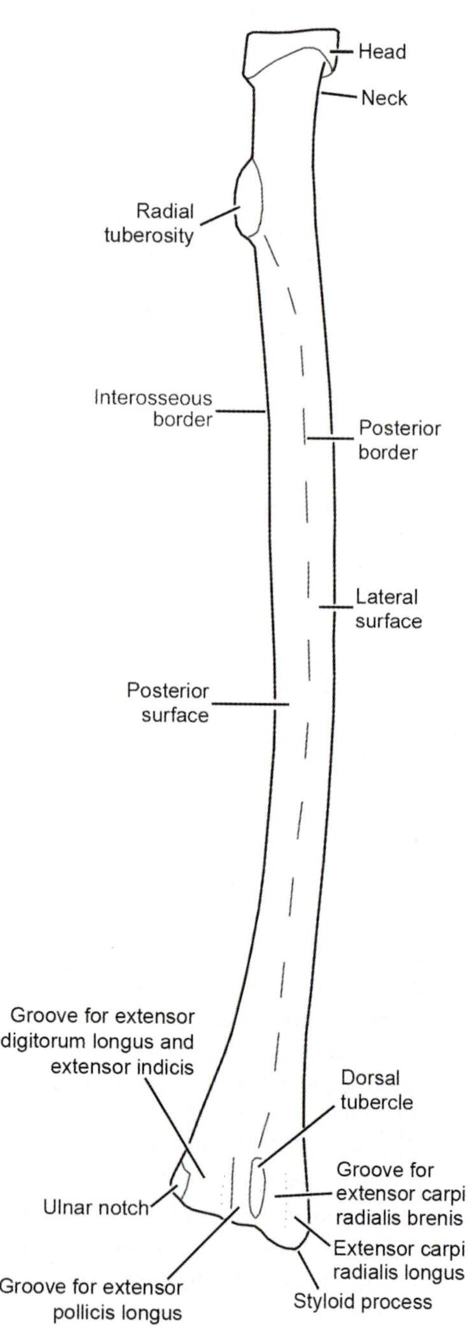


**2.20:** Right radius seen from behind

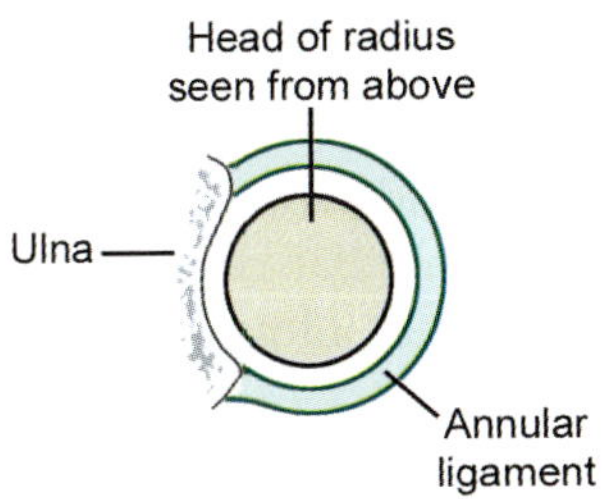


**2.21:** Scheme to show the relationship of the head of the radius to the ulna and to the annular ligament

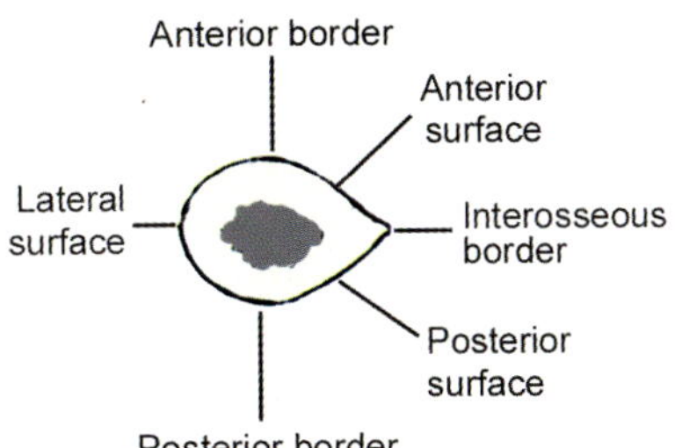


**2.22:** Transverse section across the middle of the shaft of the radius to show its borders and surfaces

## WANT TO KNOW MORE?

### Attachments on the Radius

*The following muscles are inserted into the radius (2.23 to 2.25):*

1. The ***biceps brachii*** is inserted into the rough posterior part of the radial tuberosity.
2. The ***supinator*** is inserted into the upper part of the lateral surface. The area of insertion extends onto the anterior and posterior aspects of the shaft.
3. The ***pronator teres*** is inserted into the rough area on the middle of the lateral surface, at the point of maximum convexity of the shaft.
4. The ***brachioradialis*** is inserted into the lowest part of the lateral surface just above the styloid process.
5. The ***pronator quadratus*** is inserted into the lower part of the anterior surface, and into the triangular area on the medial side of the lower end.

*The following muscles take origin from the radius:*

1. The ***flexor digitorum superficialis*** (radial head) arises from the upper part of the anterior border (oblique line).
2. The ***flexor pollicis longus*** arises from the upper two-thirds of the anterior surface.
3. The ***abductor pollicis longus*** arises from the upper part of the posterior surface.
4. The ***extensor pollicis brevis*** arises from a small area on the posterior surface below the area for the abductor pollicis longus.

The ***tendons*** related to the lower end of the radius are shown in 2.25.

### Ossification of the Radius

1. A primary centre appears in the shaft during the 8th week of fetal life.
2. A secondary centre appears in the lower end in the first year and joins the shaft around 18 years of age.
3. A secondary centre appears in the head of the bone during the 4th or 5th year and fuses with the shaft around the 16th year. Occasionally, the radial tuberosity may ossify from a separate centre.

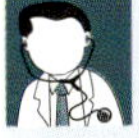

## CLINICAL CORRELATION

### Fractures of the Radius

1. The radius may be fractured through the middle of its shaft (either alone or along with the shaft of the ulna). It may also be fractured either through the upper end (or head) or through the lower end (2.26).
2. Fracture of the lower end of the radius is called *Colles's fracture*.
   a. This fracture is very common in older persons, especially women.

b. Usually, the lower fragment is displaced backwards and laterally resulting in what has been called a ***'dinner-fork'*** deformity.
c. The radial styloid process which normally lies distal to the ulnar styloid process becomes proximal.
d. Complications of this fracture include injury to or compression of the median nerve, rupture of the tendon of the extensor pollicis longus and subluxation of the inferior radioulnar joint.

3. Occasionally, fracture of the lower end of the radius is associated with forward displacement (as against backward displacement in Colles's fracture). This is called ***Smith's fracture*** or ***Barton's fracture***.

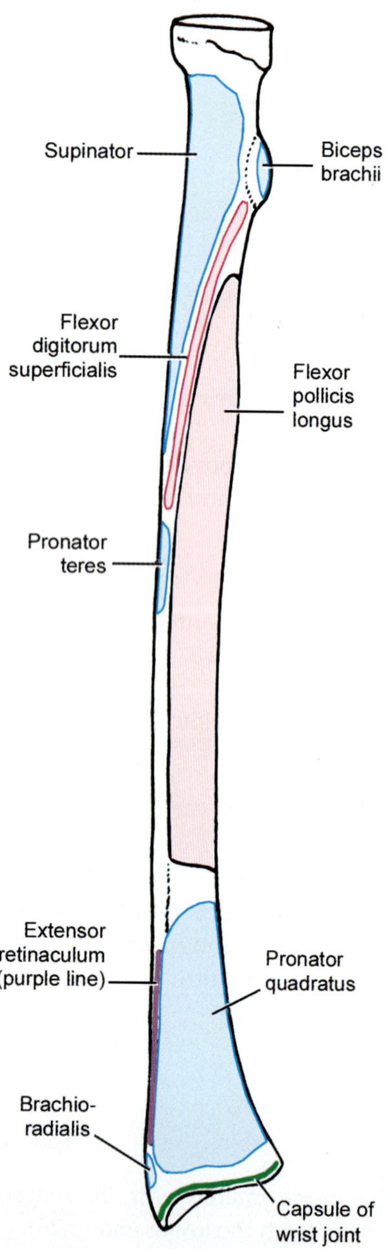


**2.23:** Right radius, showing attachments seen from the front

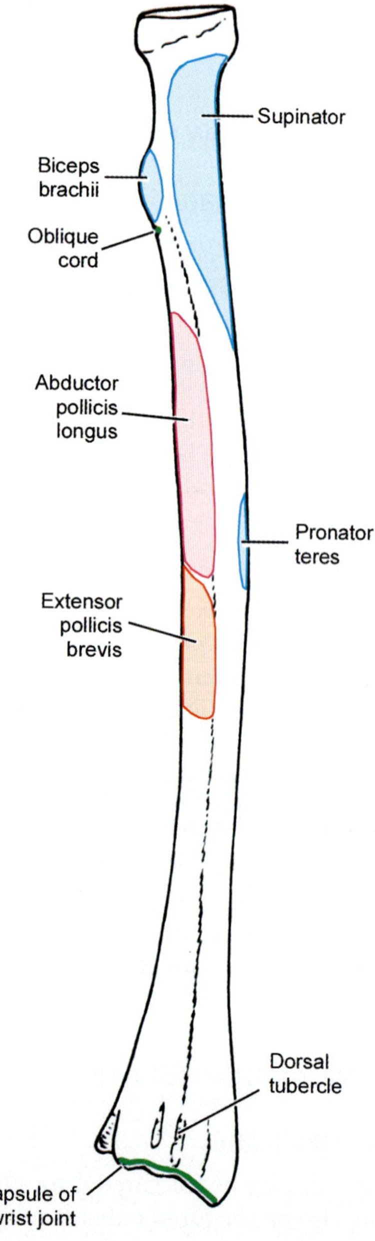


**2.24:** Right radius, showing attachments seen from behind

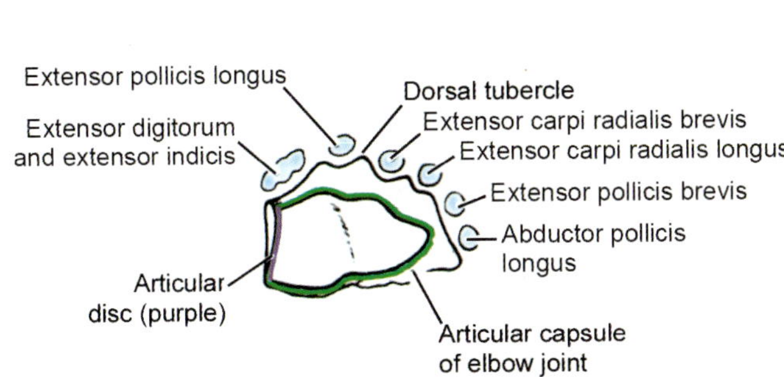


**2.25:** Lower end of right radius seen from below. The related tendons are shown

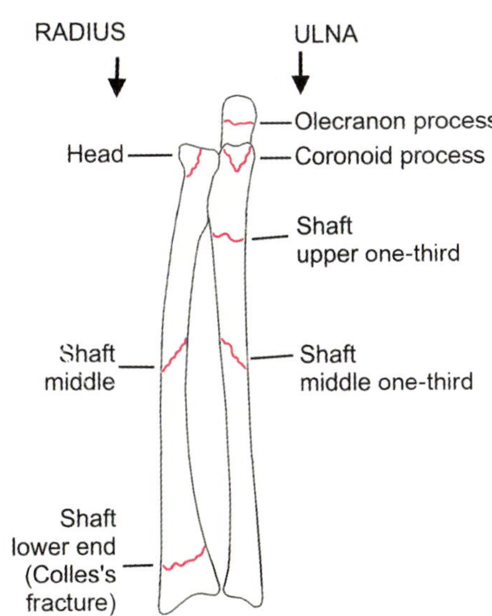


**2.26:** Fractures of radius and ulna

## The Ulna

1. The ulna has a ***shaft***, an ***upper end*** and a ***lower end*** (2.27 and 2.28). The upper end is large and irregular, while the lower end is small.
2. The upper end has a large ***trochlear notch*** on its anterior aspect.
3. The medial and lateral sides of the bone can be distinguished by examining the shaft: its lateral margin is sharp and thin, while its medial side is rounded.

The side to which an ulna belongs can be determined from these facts.

### *The Upper End*

1. The ***upper end*** of the ulna consists of two prominent projections called the ***olecranon process*** and the ***coronoid process***.
   a. When seen from behind the olecranon process appears to be a direct upward continuation of the shaft and forms the uppermost part of the ulna.
   b. The coronoid process projects forwards from the anterior aspect of the ulna just below the olecranon.
2. The trochlear notch covers the anterior aspect of the olecranon process and the superior aspect of the coronoid process.
   a. It takes part in forming the elbow joint and articulates with the trochlea of the humerus.
   b. The upper and lower parts of the notch may be partially separated from each other by a non-articular area.
   c. The trochlear notch is also divisible into medial and lateral areas corresponding to the medial and lateral flanges of the trochlea.
3. In addition to its anterior surface which forms the upper part of the trochlear notch, the olecranon process has superior, posterior, medial and lateral surfaces (2.27). When viewed from the lateral side the uppermost part of the olecranon is seen projecting forwards beyond the rest of the process.
4. The coronoid process has an upper surface that forms the lower part of the trochlear notch. In addition, it has anterior, medial and lateral surfaces.
   a. The anterior surface is triangular. Its lower part shows a rough projection called the ***tuberosity*** of the ulna. The medial margin of the anterior surface is sharp and shows a small tubercle at its upper end.

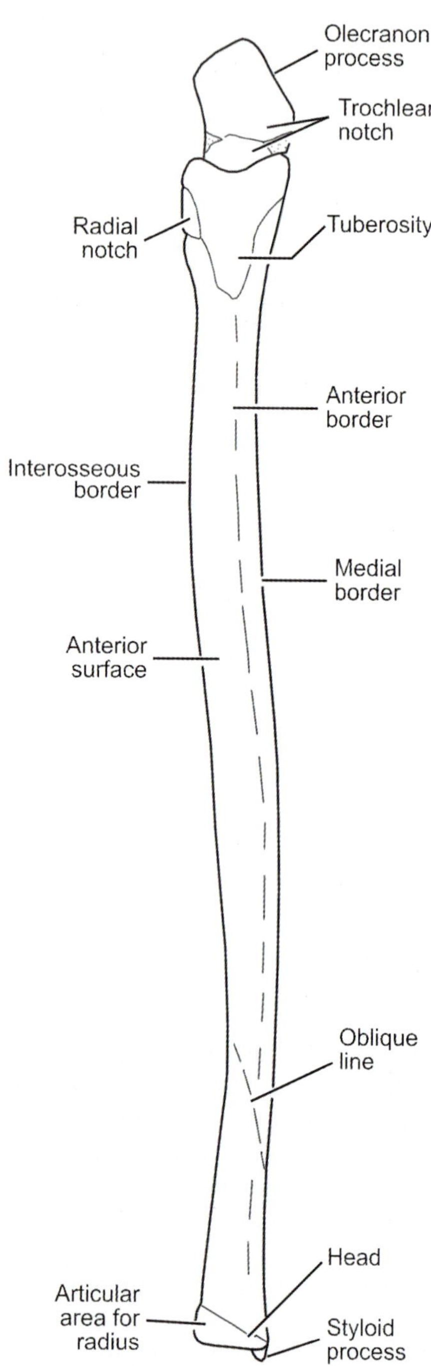


**2.27:** Right ulna seen from the front

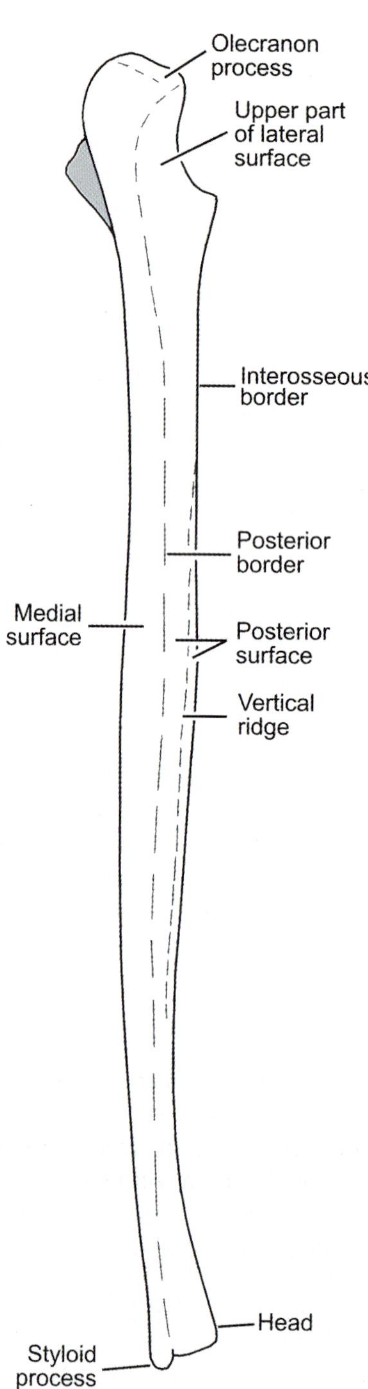


**2.28:** Right ulna seen from behind

b. The upper part of the lateral surface of the coronoid process shows a concave articular facet called the radial notch. The radial notch articulates with the head of the radius forming the superior radio-ulnar joint.
c. The bone shows a depression just below the radial notch. The posterior border of this depression is formed by a ridge called the ***supinator crest***.

### The Lower End

The lower end of the ulna consists of a disc-like ***head*** and a ***styloid process***.

1. The head has a circular inferior surface. This surface is separated from the cavity of the wrist joint by an articular disc.
2. The head has another convex articular surface on its lateral side. This surface articulates with the ulnar notch of the radius to form the inferior radioulnar joint.
3. The styloid process is a small downward projection that lies on the posteromedial aspect of the head.
   a. Between the styloid process and the head the posterior aspect is marked by a vertical groove.
   b. It is of importance to note that in the intact body the tip of the styloid process of the ulna lies at a higher level than the styloid process of the radius.

### The Shaft

The shaft of the ulna has a sharp lateral or interosseous border, and less prominent anterior and posterior borders. It has anterior, posterior and medial surfaces.

1. The upper part of the ***interosseous border*** is continuous with the supinator crest mentioned above.
   a. Its central part forms a prominent ridge on the lateral aspect of the shaft.
   b. The lower part of this border is indistinct and ends on the lateral side of the head.
2. The ***anterior border*** begins at the tuberosity of the ulna (2.27) and runs downwards. Near its lower end it curves backwards to end in front of the styloid process.
3. The ***posterior border*** begins at the apex of the triangular area on the posterior aspect of the olecranon process (2.28) and ends at the styloid process.
4. The ***anterior surface*** of the ulna lies between the interosseous and anterior borders. Its lower part shows an oblique ridge that runs downwards and medially from the interosseous border.
5. The ***medial surface*** lies between the anterior and posterior borders.
6. The ***posterior surface*** is bounded by the interosseous and posterior borders.
   a. It is marked by two lines that divide it into three areas.
   b. The upper of these lines runs obliquely downwards and medially across the upper part of the surface. It starts at the posterior end of the radial notch and terminates by joining the posterior border.
   c. The part of the posterior surface above the line is triangular.
   d. The part below the oblique line is subdivided into medial and lateral parts by a vertical ridge.

### WANT TO KNOW MORE?

**Attachments on the Ulna**

*Some muscles inserted into the ulna are as follows (2.29 to 2.32):*

1. The ***brachialis*** is inserted into the anterior surface of the coronoid process including the tuberosity.
2. The ***triceps*** is inserted into the posterior part of the superior surface of the olecranon process (2.32).

*The muscles taking origin from the ulna are as follows:*

1. The ***flexor digitorum profundus*** arises from the upper three-fourths of the anterior and medial surfaces.
   a. The muscle also takes origin from the posterior border through an aponeurosis common to it, the flexor carpi ulnaris and the extensor carpi ulnaris.
2. The ***supinator*** arises from the supinator crest and from the triangular area in front of it.

3. The ***flexor pollicis longus*** (occasional ulnar head) arises from the lateral border of the coronoid process.
4. The ***flexor digitorum superficialis*** (ulnar head) arises from the tubercle at the upper end of the medial margin of the coronoid process.
5. The ***pronator teres*** (ulnar head) arises from the medial margin of the coronoid process.
6. The ***pronator quadratus*** arises from the oblique ridge on the lower part of the anterior surface of the shaft.
7. The ***flexor carpi ulnaris*** (ulnar head) arises from the medial side of the olecranon process (2.31), and from the upper two-thirds of the posterior border through an aponeurosis common to it, the extensor carpi ulnaris and the flexor digitorum profundus.
8. The ***extensor carpi ulnaris*** (ulnar head) arises from the posterior border by an aponeurosis common to it, the flexor carpi ulnaris and the flexor digitorum profundus.
9. The posterior surface of the ulna is divided into medial and lateral parts by a vertical ridge. The lateral part lies between the vertical ridge and the interosseous border. This part of the posterior surface may be divided into four parts.
   a. The uppermost part gives origin to the ***abductor pollicis longus***.
   b. The next part gives origin to the ***extensor pollicis longus***.
   c. The third part gives origin to the ***extensor indicis***.
   d. The lowest part is devoid of attachments.

**Ossification of the Ulna**

1. A primary centre appears in the shaft in the 8th fetal week and forms the greater part of the ulna.
2. A centre for the lower end appears around the 5th or 6th year and joins the shaft by the 18th year.
3. The greater part of the olecranon is ossified by extension from the primary centre. The proximal part of the process is ossified from two centres that appear about the 10th year and join the shaft around the 15th year.

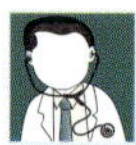

**CLINICAL CORRELATION**

**Fractures of the Ulna**

1. Fracture through the middle of the shaft of the ulna may occur alone or in combination with a similar fracture of the radius (2.26).
2. Fracture through the upper one-third of the shaft is often accompanied with forward dislocation of the head of the radius. This is called ***Monteggia fracture dislocation***.
3. Fracture of the olecranon can occur because of direct injury through a fall. The fracture usually involves the trochlear articular surface.
4. Fracture of the coronoid process is rare, and is usually associated with posterior dislocation of the elbow joint.

## THE SKELETON OF THE HAND

The skeleton of the hand consists of the bones of the wrist, the palm, and of the digits.

1. The skeleton of the wrist consists of eight; small, roughly cuboidal carpal bones.
2. The skeleton of the palm is made up of five metacarpal bones. These are miniature 'long' bones.
3. The skeleton of the fingers is made up of the phalanges. There are three phalanges (proximal, middle and distal) in each digit except the thumb that has only two phalanges (proximal and distal).

### The Carpal Bones

The carpal bones are arranged in two rows, proximal and distal (2.33 and 2.34).

1. The proximal row is made up (from lateral to medial side) of the scaphoid, lunate, triquetral and pisiform bones.
2. The distal row is made up (from lateral to medial side) of the trapezium, trapezoid, capitate and hamate bones.
3. The carpal bones of the proximal row (except the pisiform) take part in forming the wrist joint.

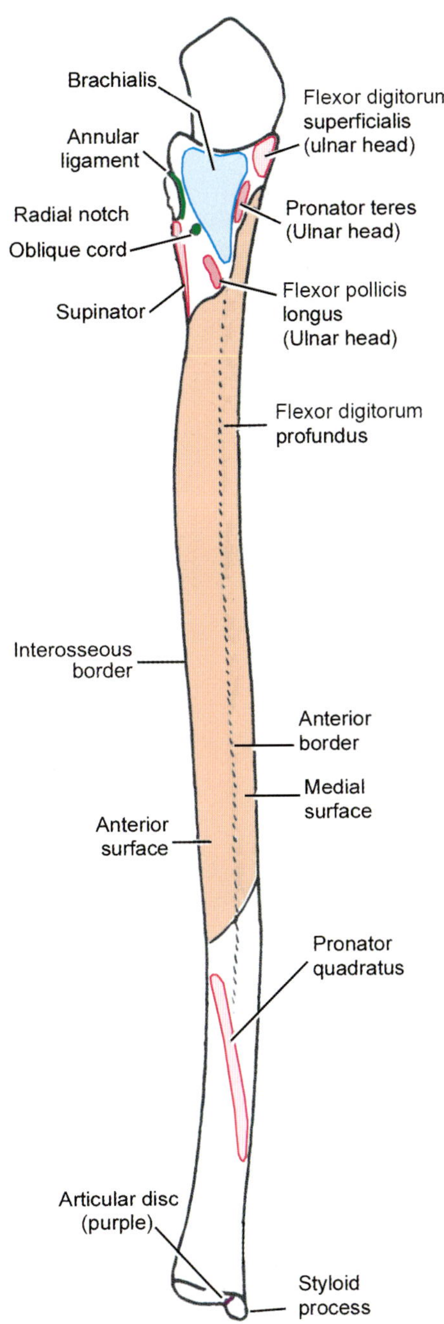


**2.29:** Right ulna, showing attachments, seen from the front

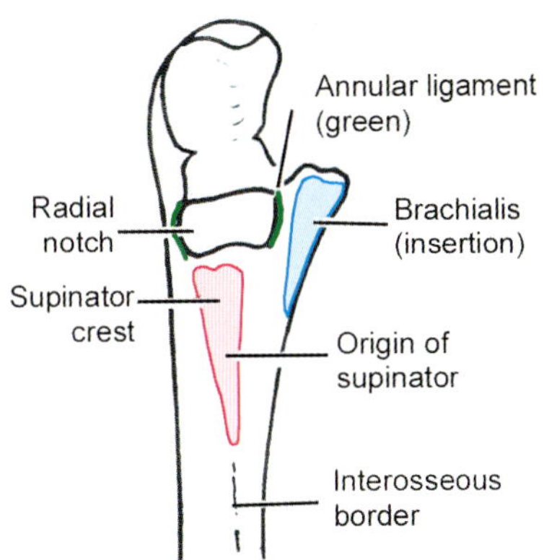


**2.30:** Upper end of right ulna showing attachments seen from the lateral side

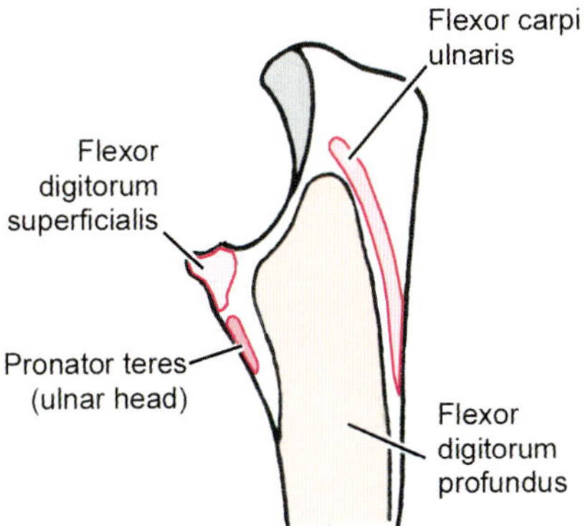


**2.31:** Upper end of right ulna, showing attachments seen from the medial side

4. The distal row of carpal bones articulate with the metacarpal bones. Each carpal bone articulates with neighbouring carpal bones to form intercarpal joints.

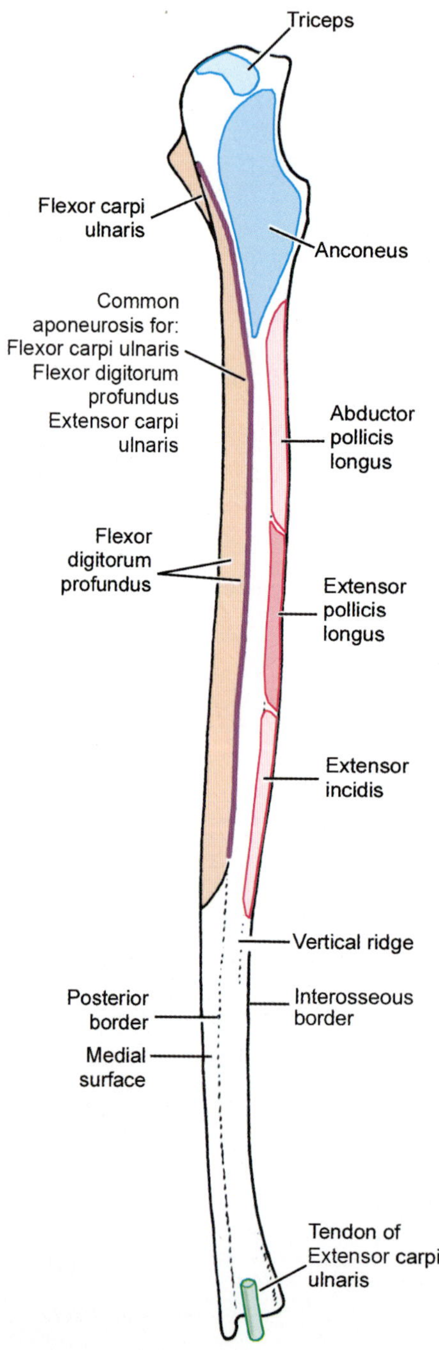


**2.32:** Right ulna, showing attachments seen from behind

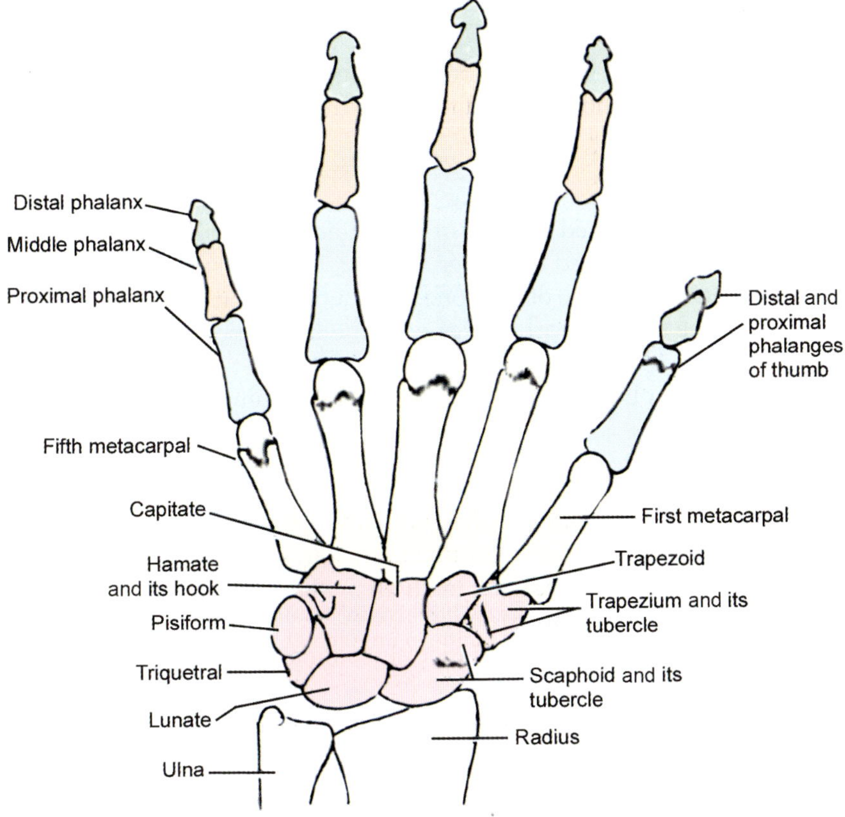


**2.33:** Skeleton of the hand, seen from the palmar aspect

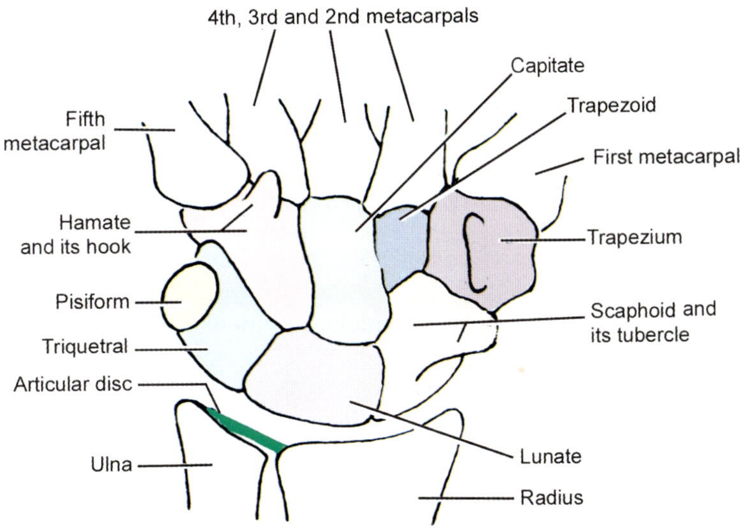


**2.34:** Right carpus, seen from the front

## WANT TO KNOW MORE?

We will now take up the consideration of individual bones of the hand. Many of the features to be described can be identified in the articulated hand (2.33 and 2.34), and these are the ones that need to be known for understanding the attachments of various structures.

### *The Scaphoid Bone*

1. The scaphoid bone can be distinguished because of its distinctive ***boat-like shape***.
2. The proximal part of the bone is covered by a large, convex, articular surface for the radius.
3. Distally and laterally the palmar surface of the bone bears a projection called the ***tubercle***.
   a. The medial surface of the scaphoid articulates with the lunate bone (proximally) and with the capitate (distally).
   b. The distal surface of the scaphoid articulates with the trapezium (laterally) and with the trapezoid bone (medially).

### *The Lunate Bone*

The lunate bone can be distinguished because it is shaped like a ***lunar crescent.***

1. Proximally, the bone has a convex articular facet that takes part in forming the wrist joint.
2. The bone articulates laterally with the scaphoid; medially with the triquetral.
3. Distally, it articulates distally with the capitate.
4. Between the areas for the capitate and for the triquetral the lunate may articulate with the hamate bone.

### *The Triquetral Bone*

1. The triquetral bone can be distinguished from other carpal bones by the fact that it is a small roughly ***cuboidal bone***.
2. It has palmar, dorsal, proximal, distal, medial and lateral surfaces.
3. Note the following in 2.33 and 2.34:
   a. The distal part of its palmar surface articulates with the pisiform bone.
   b. The medial surface is directed as much proximally as medially. It bears a slightly convex surface that takes part in forming the wrist joint: it comes into contact with the articular disc of the inferior radioulnar joint.
   c. Its lateral surface is also directed distally. It articulates with the hamate bone.
   d. The proximal surface is also directed laterally. It articulates with the lunate bone.

### *The Pisiform Bone*

1. This bone is easily distinguished as it is ***shaped like a pea*** (2.33 and 2.34).
2. Its dorsal aspect bears a single facet for articulation with the triquetral bone. It is difficult to determine the side of this bone.

### *The Trapezium*

1. This bone can be distinguished because it bears a thick prominent ***ridge*** on its palmar aspect (2.33 and 2.34).
2. This ridge is called the ***tubercle***.
3. Note the following in 2.33 and 2.34:
   a. The trapezium articulates proximally and medially with the scaphoid.
   b. Distally and laterally it articulates with the first metacarpal bone.
   c. Medially it articulates with the trapezoid bone.
   d. Distally and medially it articulates with the base of the second metacarpal bone.

### *The Trapezoid Bone*

1. This bone can be distinguished from other carpal bones because of its small size and its irregular shape.
2. Its shape resembles that of a ***shoe*** (2.33 and 2.34).
   a. The trapezoid articulates distally with the base of the second metacarpal bone.
   b. Laterally, it articulates with the trapezium.
   c. Medially, it articulates with the capitate bone.
   d. Proximally, it articulates with the scaphoid bone.

### *The Capitate Bone*

1. The capitate bone is easily recognised as it is the largest carpal bone, and bears a rounded ***head*** at one end (2.33 and 2.34).
2. The capitate lies right in the middle of the carpus.
   a. Proximally, it articulates with the lunate bone, the rounded head fitting into a socket formed by the lunate and scaphoid bones.
   b. Distally, the capitate bone articulates mainly with the third metacarpal bone, but it also articulates with the second and fourth metacarpal bones.
   c. Its lateral aspect articulates with the scaphoid (proximally) and with the trapezoid (distally).
   d. Medially, it articulates with the hamate bone.

### *The Hamate Bone*

1. The hamate is easy to recognise as it has a prominent ***hook-like process*** attached to the distal and medial part of its palmar aspect (2.33 and 2.34).
2. When viewed from the palmar aspect the hamate is triangular in shape, the apex of the triangle being directed proximally.
   a. Proximally, the apex of the bone may articulate with the lunate bone.
   b. Distally, the hamate articulates with the fourth and fifth metacarpal bones.
   c. Medially, and proximally the hamate articulates with the triquetral bone.
   d. Laterally, the hamate bone articulates with the capitate bone.

### *The Carpal Tunnel*

1. The carpal bones are so arranged that the dorsal, medial and lateral surfaces of the carpus form one convex surface.
2. On the other hand, the palmar surface is deeply concave with overhanging medial and lateral projections.
3. This concavity is converted into the carpal tunnel by a band of fascia called the ***flexor retinaculum*** (2.35).
4. The flexor retinaculum is attached, medially to the pisiform bone and to the hook of the hamate; and laterally to the tubercle of the scaphoid and to the tubercle of the trapezium.

## The Metacarpal Bones

1. The hand has five metacarpal bones (2.36). They are numbered from lateral to medial side so that the bone related to the thumb is the first metacarpal, and that related to the little finger is the fifth.
2. Each metacarpal is a miniature long bone having a shaft, a distal end and a proximal end.
3. The distal end forms a rounded head. It bears a large convex articular surface for articulation with the proximal phalanx of the corresponding digit.
4. The shaft is triangular in cross section and has medial, lateral and dorsal surfaces.
5. The bases (or proximal ends) of the metacarpal bones are irregular in shape. They articulate with the distal row of carpal bones.
6. The bases of the second and third, third and fourth, and fourth and fifth metacarpal bones also articulate with each other.

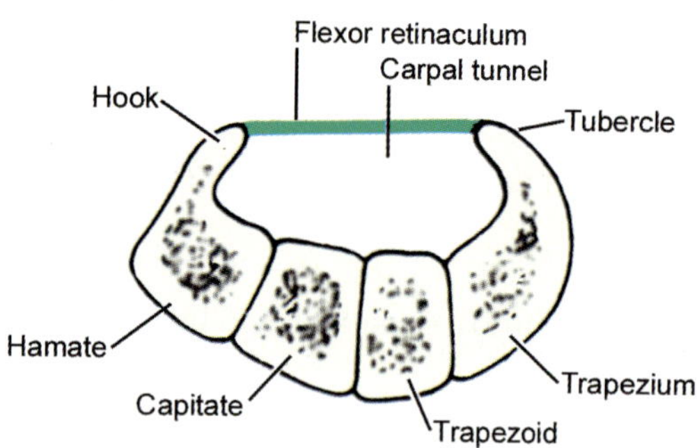


**2.35:** Schematic section across the distal row of carpal bones

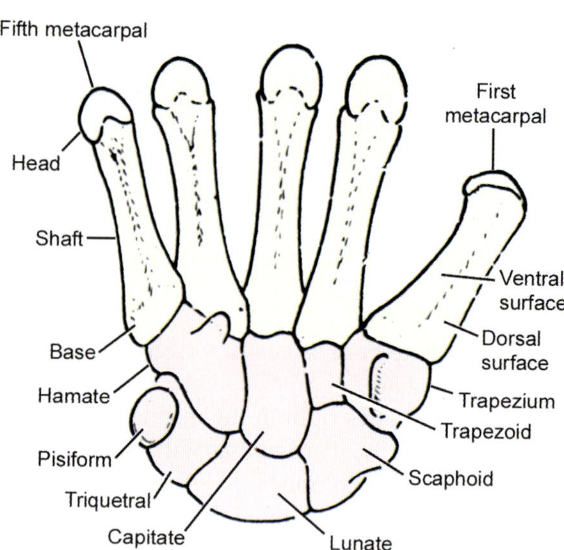


**2.36:** Carpal and metacarpal bones seen from the front

7. The base of each of the metacarpal bones has certain characteristics that enable us to distinguish them from each other as shown in 2.37.

## The Phalanges of the Hand

1. Each digit of the hand, except the thumb, has three phalanges: proximal, middle and distal (2.33 and 2.38).
2. The thumb has only two phalanges: proximal and distal.
3. Each phalanx has a distal end or head, a proximal end or base, and an intervening shaft or body.

 **WANT TO KNOW MORE?**

**Ossification of the Bones of the Hand**

1. Each carpal bone is ossified from one centre that (as a rule) appears before birth as follows:

| | | |
|---|---|---|
| Capitate | : | 2nd month |
| Hamate | : | 3rd month |
| Triquetral | : | 3rd year |
| Lunate | : | 4th year |
| Scaphoid | : | 4th to 5th year |
| Trapezium | : | 4th to 5th year |
| Trapezoid | : | 4th to 5th year |
| Pisiform | : | About 10th year |

2. Metacarpals
   a. Each metacarpal has a primary centre for the shaft that appears in the 9th fetal week.
   b. The first metacarpal has a secondary centre for the base that appears in the 2nd or 3rd year, and unites with the shaft at about 16 years.
   c. The other metacarpal bones have secondary centres (not in the base but) in the heads. These appear at about two years of age and unite with the shaft between 16 and 18 years of age.

3. Phalanges
   a. Each phalanx has a primary centre for the shaft and a secondary centre for its proximal end.
   b. The primary centre appears first in the distal phalanges (about the 8th week); next in the proximal phalanges (about the 10th week); and last in the middle phalanges (about the 12th fetal week).
   c. The secondary centres appear first in the proximal phalanges (2nd year) and later in the middle and distal phalanges (3rd or 4th year). They unite with the shafts between 16 to 18 years of age.

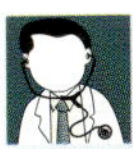

## CLINICAL CORRELATION

**Fractures of Bones of the Hand**

1. The scaphoid bone is the most commonly fractured carpal bone. Clinical examination shows tenderness over the anatomical snuff box. Fractures of other carpal bones are rare.
2. The first metacarpal bone is usually fractured near its base. The fracture often involves the carpometacarpal joint.
3. Other metacarpal bones, and phalanges are fractured by direct injury.
   a. A metacarpal bone may be fractured through the base, the shaft or the neck (i.e., just proximal to the head).
   b. Phalanges may be fractured through the shaft or through either end.

**Development and Congenital Anomalies of Limbs**

1. Up to the end of the first month of intrauterine life the human embryo shows no signs of limbs.
2. At the beginning of the second month paddle-shaped outgrowths called ***limb buds*** arise from the sidewall of the embryo.
   a. The ***forelimb buds*** appear a little earlier than the ***hindlimb buds***.
   b. As each forelimb bud grows, it becomes subdivided by constrictions into arm, forearm and hand.
   c. The hand itself soon shows outlines of the digits, which then separate from each other.
   d Similar changes take place in the lower limb bud.
3. The forelimb bud grows out from the part of the body wall that is innervated by segments C4 to T2 of the spinal cord. That is why the upper limb is innervated by these segments. The corresponding segments for the hind limb are T12 to S3.
4. The limb buds are at first directed forwards and laterally from the body of the embryo.
   a. Each bud has a preaxial (or cranial) border and postaxial (or caudal) border.
   b. The radius is the preaxial bone of the forearm.
   c. In later development the forelimb is adducted to the side of the body. The original ventral surface forms the anterior surface of the arm, forearm and palm.
5. In the case of the lower limb, the tibia is the preaxial bone of the leg.
   a. Adduction of this limb is accompanied by medial rotation so that the great toe and tibia come to lie on the medial side.
   b. The original ventral surface of the limb is represented by the inguinal region, the medial side of the lower part of the thigh, the popliteal surface of the knee, the back of the leg, and the sole of the foot.

*Anomalies of limbs*

The anomalies of the upper and lower limbs are similar and will therefore be considered together.

1. One or more limbs of the body may be partially, or completely, absent (***phocomelia, amelia***).
   a. This condition may be produced by harmful drugs, and is seen characteristically in the children of mothers who have received the drug ***thalidomide*** during pregnancy.
   b. Absence of limb bones, in whole or in part, may also occur independently and may be the cause of deformities of the limb.
   c. One or more muscles of the limb (e.g., pectoralis major) may be absent.

2. Part of a limb may be deformed (e.g., ***club foot, club hand***).
3. There may be abnormal fusion between different bones of a limb.
   a. Adjoining digits may be fused (***syndactyly***).
   b. The phalanges of a digit may be fused to one another (***synphalangia***).
   c. The radius and ulna may be fused to each other, or to the humerus.
4. A digit may be abnormally large (***macrodactyly***) or abnormally short (***brachydactyly***). Supernumerary digits may be present (***polydactyly***).
5. The limbs may remain short in ***achondroplasia***.
6. Sometimes bone ends are not properly formed leading to ***congenital dislocation*** at joints.
7. There may be abnormality of position. A condition in which the scapula placed higher than normal is called ***Sprengel's shoulder***.

| FACETS SEEN ON BASES OF METACARPAL BONES (RIGHT) | | |
|---|---|---|
| | LATERAL SIDE | MEDIAL SIDE |
| ORIENTATION | DIST<br>VENT + DORS<br>PROX | DIST<br>DORS + VENT<br>PROX |
| FIRST METACARPAL | Facet for trapezium | Facet for trapezium |
| SECOND METACARPAL | For trapezoid<br>For trapezium | For third metacarpal<br>For capitate |
| THIRD METACARPAL | For second metacarpal | For fourth metacarpal<br>Styloid process |
| FOURTH METACARPAL | For third metacarpal | For fifth metacarpal |

*Contd...*

*Contd...*

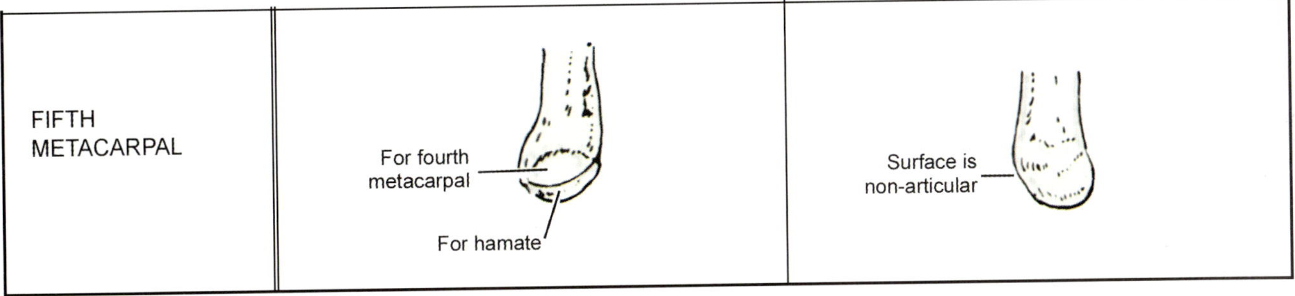


**2.37:** Facets seen on bases of metacarpal bones (right)

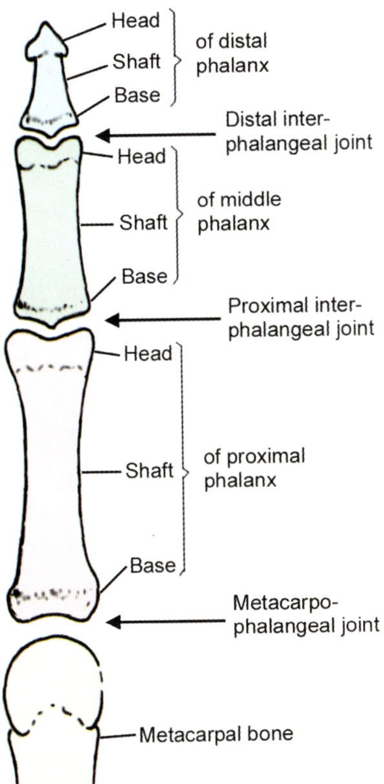


**2.38:** The phalanges of a typical digit of the hand

# 3 CHAPTER

# Pectoral Region, Axilla and Breast

## THE PECTORAL REGION

The pectoral region lies on the front of the thorax. In the mature female the breasts lie over this region.

### Spinal Segments and Dermatomes

1. Areas of skin supplied by individual spinal nerves are called ***dermatomes***.
2. As a rule, the arrangement of dermatomes is simple over the trunk, as successive horizontal strips of skin are supplied by each spinal nerve of the region (i.e., thoracic and lumbar nerves) (3.1).
3. However, the arrangement is unusual over the pectoral region.
   a. The skin of the upper part of the pectoral region is supplied by spinal segments C3 and C4 (upto the level of the sternal angle).
   b. The area just below the level of the sternal angle is supplied by segment T2.
   c. The explanation for this is to be found in the development of the upper limb.
      i. The limb has developed from the region of the trunk supplied by segments C5 to T1.
      ii. As the limb grows the areas of skin supplied from these segments get 'pulled away' into the limb leaving the area for segment C4 in direct continuity with that for segment T2.
4. Normally, the areas of skin supplied by adjoining spinal segments overlap. However, there is no overlap between the areas supplied by C4 and T2 for the reason explained above.

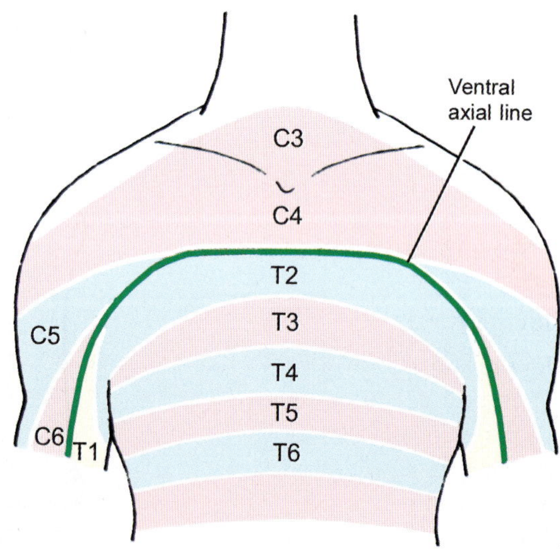

**3.1:** Dermatomes on the front of the thorax

## CUTANEOUS NERVES OF THE PECTORAL REGION

### Supraclavicular Nerves

1. The supraclavicular nerves (C3, 4) arise in the neck from the cervical plexus (as one ramus).
2. The origin lies deep to the sternocleidomastoid muscle. The nerve trunk runs downwards and backwards deep to this muscle and appears at its posterior border.
3. Here the trunk divides into three branches called the medial, intermediate and lateral supraclavicular nerves.
4. These branches descend over the posterior triangle of the neck giving some branches to the skin here.

5. They pierce the deep fascia a little above the clavicle and then run downwards across this bone to reach the pectoral region.
   a. The ***medial supraclavicular nerve*** supplies the skin of the upper and medial part of the thorax. A branch from the nerve supplies the sternoclavicular joint.
   b. The ***intermediate supraclavicular nerve*** supplies the skin over the upper part of the pectoralis major. The area of supply of the medial and intermediate supraclavicular nerves extends up to the level of the second rib.
   c. The ***lateral supraclavicular nerve*** supplies the skin over the shoulder.

### *Cutaneous Branches of Intercostal Nerves*

1. Skin below the level of the sternal angle is supplied by ***anterior cutaneous branches*** of the 2nd to 6th intercostal nerves.
2. More laterally it is supplied by ***lateral cutaneous branches*** of the 3rd to 6th intercostal nerves.

## MUSCLES OF THE PECTORAL REGION

The muscles belonging to the pectoral region proper are:
1. Pectoralis major (3.2 and 3.3)
2. Pectoralis minor (3.4 and 3.5)
3. Subclavius (3.4 and 3.6).

We also see two other muscles parts of which are seen in the region and are described here. These are:
1. Platysma
2. Serratus anterior (3.7 and 3.8).

The pectoralis major is described in 3.2 and shown in 3.3. The pectoralis minor is shown in 3.4 and described in 3.5. The subclavius is shown in 3.4 and described in 3.6.

### WANT TO KNOW MORE?

**Clavipectoral fascia**

1. As its name implies the fascia fills the gap between the clavicle (above) and the medial edge of the pectoralis minor (below). Along with the latter it forms a partition that separates the upper part of the pectoralis major from the contents of the axilla.
2. Near its upper end the fascia splits to enclose the subclavius.
3. At the medial edge of the pectoralis minor it splits to enclose the pectoralis minor.
4. At the lower (lateral) edge of the pectoralis minor the fascia becomes continuous with the axillary fascia (forming the dome-shaped floor of the axilla). It helps to keep the axillary fascia raised up into the hollow of the axilla.
5. When traced medially, the fascia reaches the first and second ribs and the upper two intercostal spaces. Traced laterally, it reaches the coracoid process.
6. Between the coracoid process and the first rib it forms a thickened band called the ***costocoracoid ligament.***
7. The clavipectoral fascia is pierced by:
   a. The thoracoacromial artery and vein, the cephalic vein.
   b. The lateral pectoral nerve.
   c. Some lymphatics of the breast and pectoral region passing to the apical lymph nodes of the axilla also pass through it.

| 3.2: Pectoralis major | |
|---|---|
| Origin | 1. Clavicle: Medial half of anterior surface<br>2. Sternum: Anterior surface<br>3. Upper seven costal cartilages (medial parts)<br>4. Aponeurosis of external oblique muscle |
| Insertion | Lateral lip of intertubercular sulcus. The tendon of insertion is bilaminar. The anterior lamina receives the clavicular fibres and upper sternocostal fibres. The posterior lamina receives the lower fibres |
| Nerve supply | Lateral and medial pectoral nerves (C5, 6, 7, 8, T1) |
| Action | 1. Adductor and medial rotator of arm<br>2. Flexion of the arm (clavicular fibres with anterior fibres of deltoid)<br>3. Extension of flexed arm (against resistance) (with latissimus dorsi)<br>4. When the arm is raised above the head and fixed, the muscle can raise the thorax (as in climbing) (helped by latissimus dorsi)<br>5. Helps in forced inspiration (arm has to be fixed) |
| Notes | 1. Forms anterior fold of axilla<br>2. Mammary gland lies in front of it<br>3. The muscle is in front of the pectoralis minor, the clavipectoral fascia, and upper parts of biceps brachii, the coracobrachialis and serratus anterior |

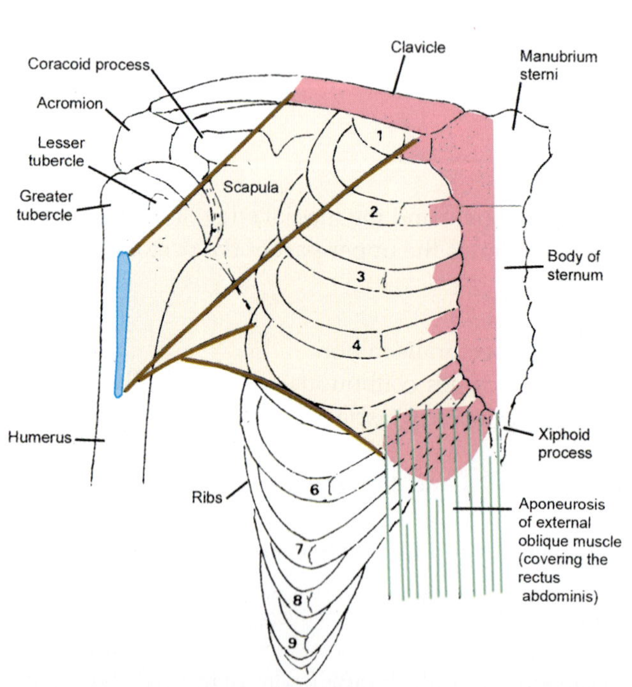


3.3: The pectoralis major

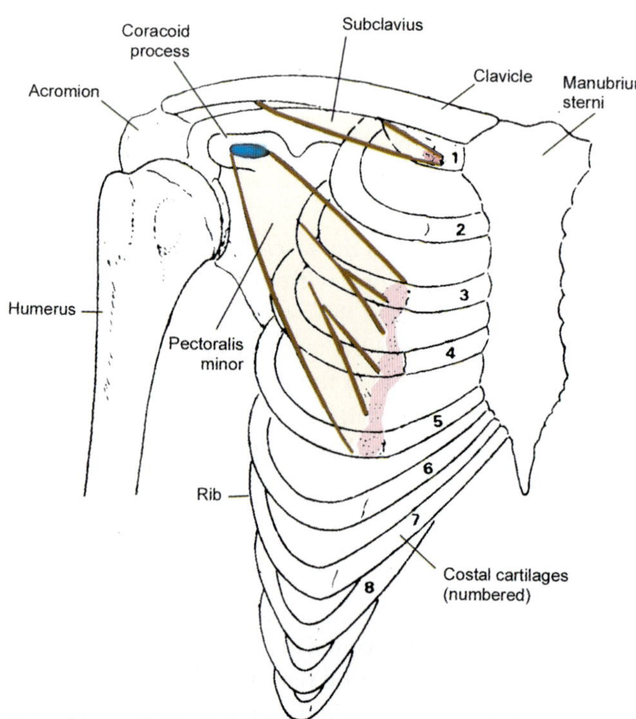


3.4: Attachments of the pectoralis minor and of the subclavius

| 3.5: Pectoralis minor | |
|---|---|
| Origin | 1. 3rd, 4th and 5th ribs (near junction with costal cartilages)<br>2. Fascia covering intercostal spaces |
| Insertion | Coracoid process of scapula. (medial border and upper surface) |
| Nerve supply | Lateral and medial pectoral nerves (C6, 7, 8) |
| Action | 1. Forward movement of scapula (along with serratus anterior)<br>2. Backward rotation of scapula (along with levator scapulae and rhomboids)<br>3. Helps in forced respiration (if the scapula is fixed by the person tightly holding a horizontal bar) |
| Notes | 1. It separates the pectoralis major from the contents of the axilla<br>2. It lies in front of the axilary artery and is used to divide the artery into first, second and third parts<br>3. It is attached to the clavicle by the clavipectoral fascia |

| 3.6: Subclavius | |
|---|---|
| Origin | Clavicle: into groove on middle-third of inferior surface |
| Insertion | Clavicle: into groove on middle-third of inferior surface |
| Nerve supply | Nerve to subclavius (C5, 6) arising from Erb's point (on upper trunk of brachial plexus) |
| Action | 1. Depression of clavicle<br>2. Keeps medial end of clavicle pressed against articular disc of sternoclavicular joint, and smoothens movements |

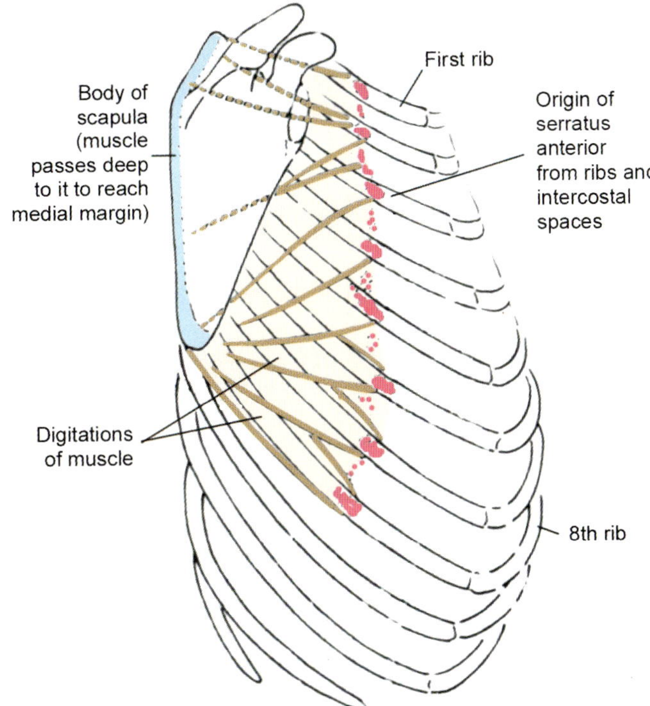


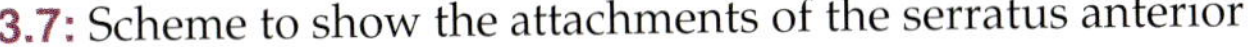
3.7: Scheme to show the attachments of the serratus anterior

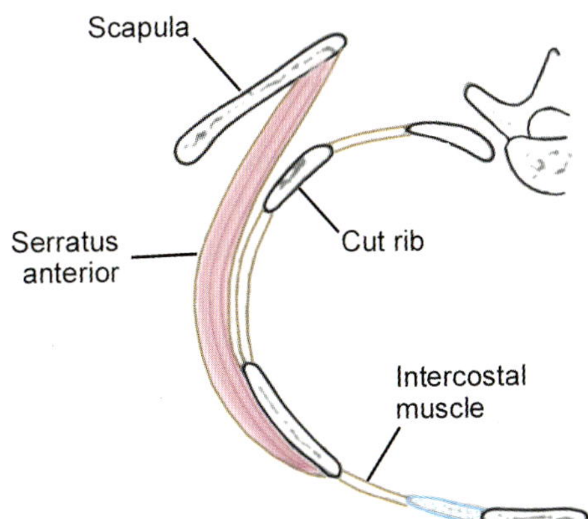


Fig. 3.8: Schematic diagram to show the relationship of the serratus anterior to the thoracic wall and to the scapula

## Platysma

1. This muscle lies in superficial fascia.
2. The platysma arises from the deep fascia over the upper part of the pectoralis major and the anterior part of the deltoid.
3. The fibres form a broad sheet that passes upwards and forwards across the clavicle to enter the neck.
   a. It passes upwards and forwards to reach the lower border of the mandible.
   b. Here it merges with superficial muscle in the lower part of the face.

The ***serratus anterior*** is shown in 3.7 and is described in 3.9.

| | **3.9: Serratus anterior** |
|---|---|
| Origin | Upper eight or nine ribs (outer surfaces) |
| Insertion | Costal surface of scapula (along medial border) |
| Nerve supply | Long thoracic nerve (branch from roots C5, 6, 7 of brachial plexus). |
| Action | 1. Pulls scapula forwards around chest wall (with pectoralis minor). As a result the upper limb moves forwards as in giving a blow.<br>2. Forward rotation of scapula (with trapezius). The glenoid cavity is turned upwards and leads to overhead abduction of the arm. |
| Clinical Notes | The muscle is tested by making the patient place his palms against a wall and pushing against it. If the muscle is paralysed the medial margin of the scapula is lifted off from the ribs. This is called winging of the scapula. Overhead abduction of the arm is not possible. |

## THE AXILLA

The axilla is the region of the armpit. Its boundaries are as follows (3.10):

1. The ***anterior wall*** is formed by the pectoralis major, the pectoralis minor and the clavipectoral fascia. The ***anterior fold*** of the axillla is formed mainly by the pectoralis major.
2. The ***posterior wall*** is formed by muscles lying in front of the scapula.
   a. In the upper part there is the subscapularis.
   b. Lower down there are the teres major and the latissimus dorsi.
   c. Note that the latissimus dorsi winds round the lower margin of the teres major, the two together form the thick ***posterior fold*** of the axilla.
3. The ***medial wall*** is formed by the upper few ribs and intercostal spaces. They are covered by the upper part of the serratus anterior.
4. The ***lateral wall*** is formed by the humerus in the region of the intertubercular sulcus.
5. If we cut a coronal section through the axilla we see that it is conical.
   a. The ***base*** of the cone faces downwards and corresponds to the floor of the axilla.
   b. The ***floor*** is formed by axillary fascia, covered by skin. The axillary fascia has an aperture through which the axillary tail of the breast enters the axilla.
   c. The ***apex*** of the axilla faces upwards and somewhat medially and lies at the level of the outer border of the first rib.
      i. Behind the apex there is the upper border of the scapula, and in front of it there is the clavicle.
      ii. These three structures form the boundaries of an opening through which the axillary vessels and the brachial plexus pass from the neck into the axilla.
      iii. The opening is, therefore, called the ***cervicoaxillary canal***.
6. The ***contents of the axilla*** are the axillary artery and vein, and the axillary lymph nodes. The remaining space is filled with fat. We will consider these contents one by one.

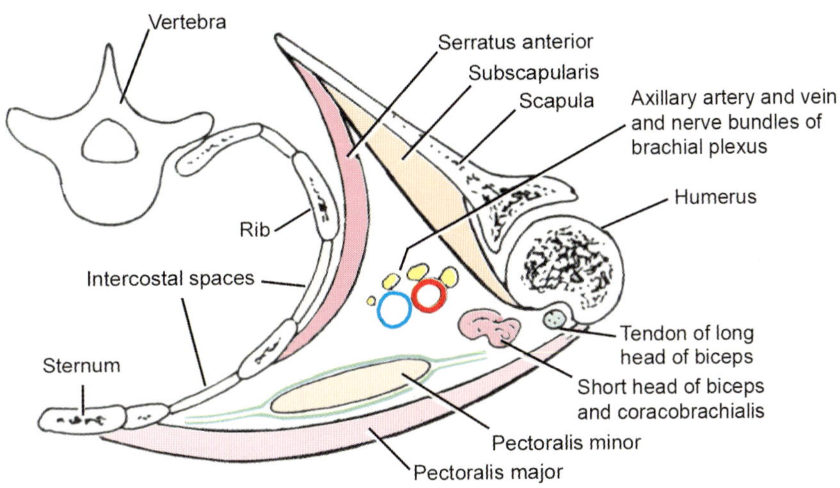


**3.10:** Transverse section through the axilla to show its walls

## THE AXILLARY ARTERY

1. The axillary artery is a continuation of the subclavian artery.
2. It begins at the outer border of the first rib and ends at the lower border of the teres major (by becoming the brachial artery).
3. The artery is crossed by the pectoralis minor. This divides it into first, second and third parts.

The artery has numerous relationships that are given below.

### *Relationship to Muscles*

(See 3.11 and 3.12)

1. The first part of the artery rests (posteriorly) on the muscles of the first intercostal space and the upper part of the serratus anterior.
2. The second part and the upper portion of the third part of the artery lie on the subscapularis muscle. The lower portion of the third part lies on the teres major muscle and the tendon of the latissimus dorsi.
3. The entire artery (except its lowermost part) is overlapped by the pectoralis major.
4. The second part is also covered by the pectoralis minor.
5. The first part is also covered by the clavipectoral fascia (which extends from the pectoralis minor to the clavicle).
6. The coracobrachialis is lateral to the second and third parts of the artery.
7. In addition to muscles the artery is covered superficially by superficial and deep fascia and by skin. Part of the platysma is present in the superficial fascia.

### *Relationship to Veins*

1. The axillary artery is accompanied by the axillary vein: the vein lies anteromedial to the artery (3.15).
2. The first part of the artery is crossed by two tributaries of the axillary vein, namely the cephalic vein and the thoracoacromial vein.

### *Relationship to Brachial Plexus*

1. The first and second parts of the artery are related to the cords of the plexus; and the third part of the artery to their branches (3.13).
2. The first part of the artery is also related to the lateral pectoral nerve that crosses anterior to the artery; and to the medial pectoral nerve that lies behind it. A loop passing in front of the artery joins the two nerves.

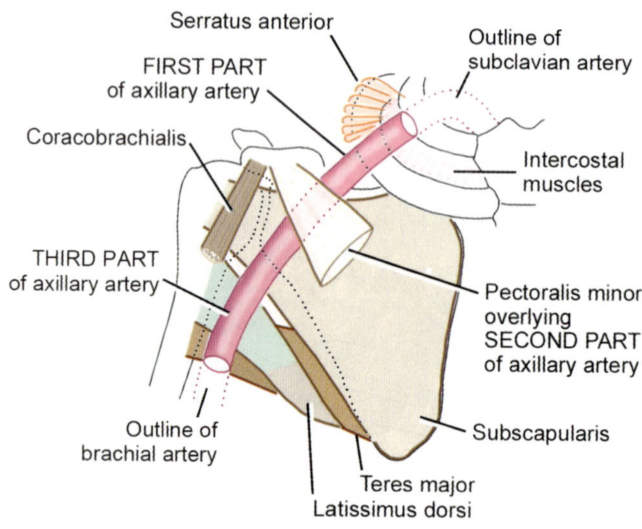


**3.11:** Muscles related to the axillary artery

| | | | |
|---|---|---|---|
| ANTERIOR RELATIONS | Skin<br>Platysma<br>Deep fascia | | |
| | Pectoralis major | | |
| | Clavipectoral fascia | Pectoralis minor | |
| ARTERY | **1st part** | **2nd part** | **3rd part** |
| POSTERIOR RELATIONS | Serratus anterior<br>First intercostal space | Subscapularis | Tendon latissimus dorsi<br>Teres mojor |

**3.12:** Anterior and posterior relations of the axillary artery

3. The third part of the artery is crossed anteriorly by the medial root of the median nerve as the latter passes laterally to join the lateral root.

## Branches of the Axillary Artery

### *Branch of First Part*

1. Superior thoracic artery

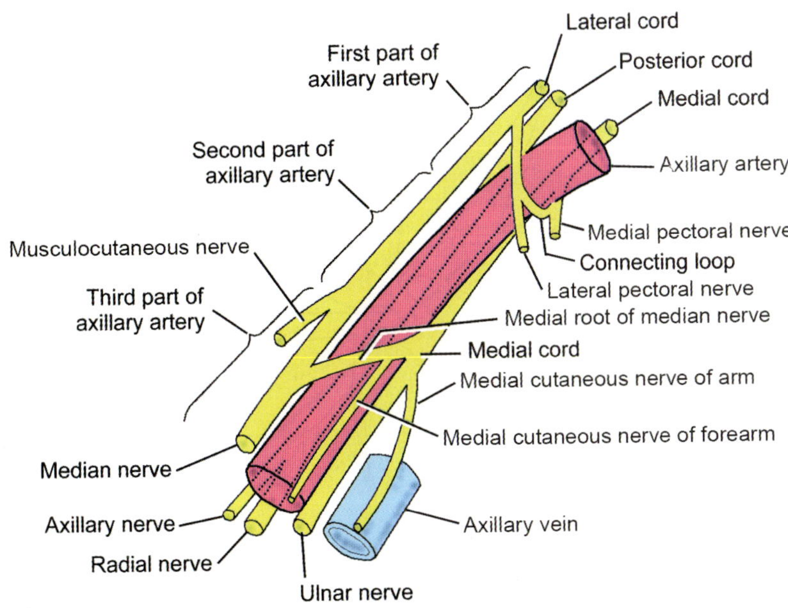


**3.13:** Relations of axillary artery to cords and branches of the brachial plexus

### *Branches of Second Part*

2. Thoracoacromial artery
3. Lateral thoracic artery

### *Branches of Third Part*

4. Subscapular artery
5. Anterior circumflex humeral artery
6. Posterior circumflex humeral artery.

These are described below.

1. The ***superior thoracic artery*** arises from the first part of the axillary artery. It supplies the pectoral muscles and part of the thoracic wall (3.14).
2. The ***thoracoacromial artery*** arises from the second part of the axillary artery deep to the medial margin of the pectoralis minor. It runs upwards and becomes superficial by piercing the clavipectoral fascia. It divides into four branches: pectoral, acromial, clavicular and deltoid.
   a. The ***pectoral branch*** descends between the pectoral muscles, supplying them and the chest wall.
   b. The ***acromial branch*** passes laterally. It first lies deep to the deltoid muscle and then pierces it to reach the acromion where it anastomoses with various other arteries.
   c. The ***clavicular branch*** runs upwards to supply the subclavius and the sternoclavicular joint.
   d. The ***deltoid branch*** runs laterally in the groove between the deltoid and the pectoralis major.
3. The ***lateral thoracic artery*** runs downwards near the lateral margin of the pectoralis minor supplying pectoral muscles, the serratus anterior and the axillary lymph nodes. In the female it gives off prominent branches to the breast.
4. The ***subscapular artery*** runs downwards along the lateral border of the scapula supplying muscles in the region and anastomosing with various other arteries. In its lower part it is accompanied by the nerve to the latissimus dorsi.
   a. The artery gives off a large ***circumflex scapular*** branch.

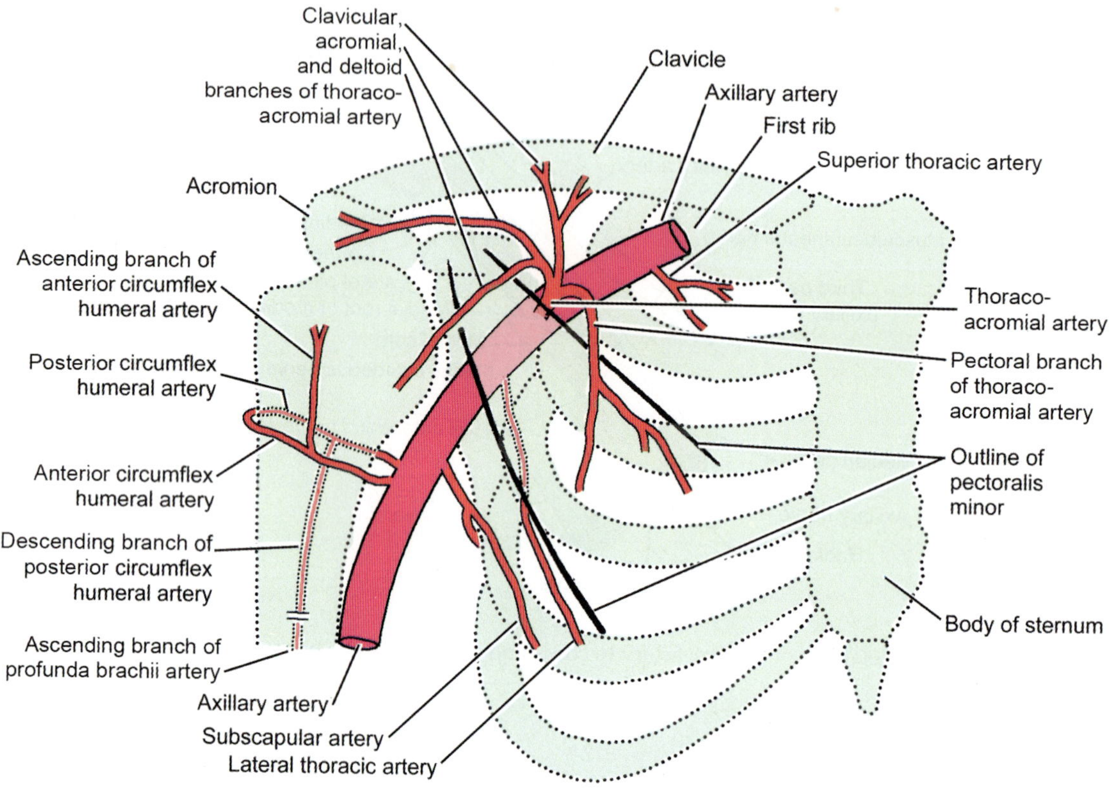


**3.14:** Branches of the axillary artery

b. This branch winds round the lateral border of the scapula passing backwards through the triangular space.
c. It gives branches to muscles on both the ventral and dorsal aspects of the scapula. It takes part in forming the anastomoses round the scapula.

5. The ***anterior circumflex humeral artery*** runs laterally in front of the surgical neck of the humerus.
   a. It anastomoses with the posterior circumflex humeral artery (see below) to form an arterial circle round the neck.
   b. It gives off a branch that ascends in the intertubercular sulcus to the shoulder joint.
6. The ***posterior circumflex humeral artery*** runs backwards (accompanied by the axillary nerve) through the quadrangular space.
   a. It then passes laterally behind the surgical neck of the humerus to anastomose with the anterior circumflex humeral artery.
   b. It gives off a descending branch that anastomoses with a branch of the profunda brachii artery.

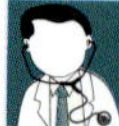

## CLINICAL CORRELATION

1. To stop bleeding, pressure can be applied over the axillary artery near its lower end.
   a. Pressure is applied laterally, at a level just above the lower border of the posterior fold of the axilla.
   b. The artery is compressed against the humerus.
2. The artery can also be compressed against the first rib but this is difficult.
3. The anastomoses around the scapula links the subclavian artery with the third part of the axillary artery and serves to maintain circulation in case of blockage of the axillary artery. The collateral circulation is effective in gradual obstruction, but in sudden ligation it is inadequate.

## THE AXILLARY VEIN

The axillary vein accompanies the axillary artery through the axilla.

1. It is formed at the lower border of the teres major by joining together of the venae comitantes of the brachial artery and the basilic vein.
2. It ends at the outer border of the first rib by becoming continuous with the subclavian vein.
3. The axillary vein receives the cephalic vein and veins accompanying the branches of the axillary artery.
4. The vein lies medial to the axillary artery. The following structures intervene between the artery and vein (3.15):
   a. Medial cord of the brachial plexus.
   b. Medial pectoral nerve.
   c. Ulnar nerve.
   d. Medial cutaneous nerve of the forearm.
5. The medial cutaneous nerve of the arm is medial to the axillary vein (3.15).

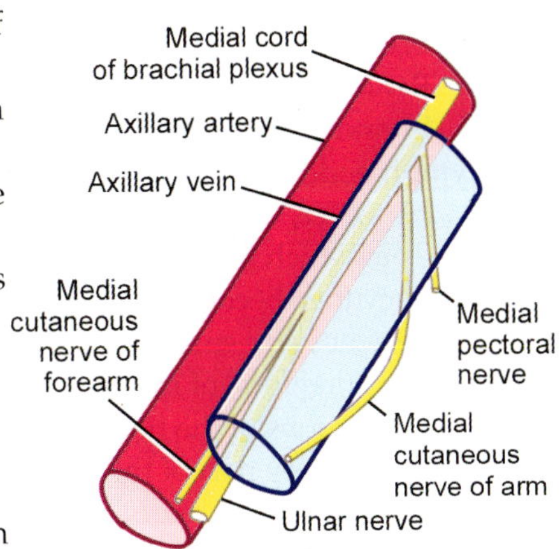


**3.15:** Some relations of the axillary vein

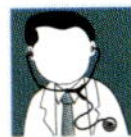

### CLINICAL CORRELATION

1. Fracture of the clavicle may damage a vein that runs across it and connects the upper part of the cephalic vein (deltopectoral vein) with the external jugular vein (lying in the neck). In case of injury to the axillary vein (or surgical removal of a segment) this communication helps to maintain venous drainage of the upper limb.
2. Direct injury to the axillary vein is dangerous. Bleeding is profuse. There is the risk of air being sucked into the vein producing air emboli.

## LYMPH NODES AND LYMPHATIC DRAINAGE

Before taking up the lymph nodes and lymphatic drainage of the upper limb it is desirable to consider certain facts about the lymphatic system in general.

1. When circulating blood reaches the capillaries, part of its fluid content passes through them into the surrounding tissue as tissue fluid.
   a. Most of this tissue fluid re-enters the capillaries at their venous ends.
   b. Some of it is, however, returned to the circulation through ***lymphatic vessels***.
2. These vessels begin as lymphatic capillaries that drain into larger lymph vessels.
   a. Along the course of these lymph vessels there are groups of ***lymph nodes***.
   b. These nodes consist predominantly of lymphoid tissue.
   c. The lymph vessels and lymphatic nodes together constitute the ***lymphatic system***.
3. Lymph vessels are difficult to see and require special techniques for their visualization. Lymph nodes are small bean-like structures that are usually present in groups.
4. The lymphatic system includes other organs consisting predominantly of lymphoid tissue.
   a. Spleen.
   b. Thymus.
   c. Bone marrow.
   d. Tonsils and other aggregations of lymphoid tissue present in relation to the alimentary tract.

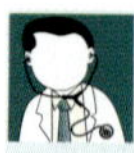

## CLINICAL CORRELATION

1. Apart from the transport of fluid the lymphatic system is concerned with the following:
   a. Production of blood cells.
   b. Removal of unwanted material (including dead cells and bacteria) by phagocytosis.
   c. Immune responses against foreign proteins including bacteria.
2. Lymph nodes are not normally palpable in the living subject.
   a. However, they often become enlarged in disease (particularly by infection, or by malignancy, in the area from which they receive lymph).
   b. They then become palpable; and examination of these nodes provides valuable information regarding the presence and spread of disease.
   c. It is, therefore, of importance for the medical student to know the lymphatic drainage of different organs and regions of the body.
3. Infection in any part of the upper limb can lead to ***lymphadenitis*** or ***lymphangitis***.
4. Infection from the fingers and palm can pass to the dorsum of the hand through lymphatics and can produce oedema, or an abscess there.

## LYMPH NODES OF UPPER LIMB

As the lymph nodes draining the upper limb lie mainly in the axilla it is convenient to give a complete account of the lymph nodes and lymphatic drainage of the upper limb here.

### The Lymph Nodes

1. The chief lymph nodes of the upper limb are located in the axilla: these ***axillary lymph nodes*** are considered below.
2. One or two ***supratrochlear nodes*** lie just above the medial epicondyle of the humerus, along the basilic vein.
3. One or two ***infraclavicular nodes*** lie just below the clavicle, along the cephalic vein, in the groove between the pectoralis major and the clavicle.
4. Some isolated nodes are scattered along the main blood vessels of the limb.

### The Axillary Lymph Nodes

These are divided into the following groups (3.17):

1. The ***lateral group*** of nodes lies along the axillary vein.
2. The ***anterior (or pectoral) group*** of nodes lies along the lateral thoracic vessels i.e., along the lower border of the pectoralis minor.
3. The ***posterior (or subscapular) group*** of nodes lies along the course of the subscapular vessels.
   Note that the lateral, anterior and posterior groups lie on the corresponding walls of the axilla.
4. The ***central group*** of nodes lies in the centre of the axilla embedded in fat.
5. The ***apical group*** is so called because it lies near the apex of the axilla.

The areas of drainage of these groups are shown in 3.16.

## WANT TO KNOW MORE?

**Lymphatic Drainage of The Upper Limb**

Most of the lymphatic vessels of the limbs are superficial (3.18).

1. Plexuses on the palm and the dorsum of the hand give rise to vessels that ascend into the forearm on both its ventral and dorsal aspects.

2. The vessels on the dorsal side of the forearm gradually wind round its medial and lateral borders and join the vessels in front. All these vessels that collect on the front of the forearm can be divided into medial, intermediate and lateral sets.
3. The medial vessels run along the basilic vein; the intermediate set along the median vein of the forearm; and the lateral set along the cephalic vein.
4. After crossing the elbow the vessels of the intermediate and lateral sets also turn medially to join those of the medial set. Ultimately almost all of them end in the lateral group of axillary lymph nodes.
5. Some of the lymphatic vessels running along the basilic vein end in the supratochlear nodes from which new vessels arise to take their place. Some vessels of the lateral set continue upwards along the cephalic vein and end in the infraclavicular nodes.
6. The deep vessels of the limb run along the main arteries (radial, ulnar, interosseous, brachial) and their venae comitantes. Like the superficial vessels these also end in the lateral group of axillary nodes. The lateral group of axillary nodes are, therefore, the main nodes of the upper limb.
7. Lymph from the lateral group drains into the central group of axillary nodes; and from them to the apical group (3.16).
8. The subclavian lymphatic trunk arises from the apical group and conveys the lymph to the thoracic duct (on the left side) or to the right lymphatic duct through which it reaches the bloodstream.

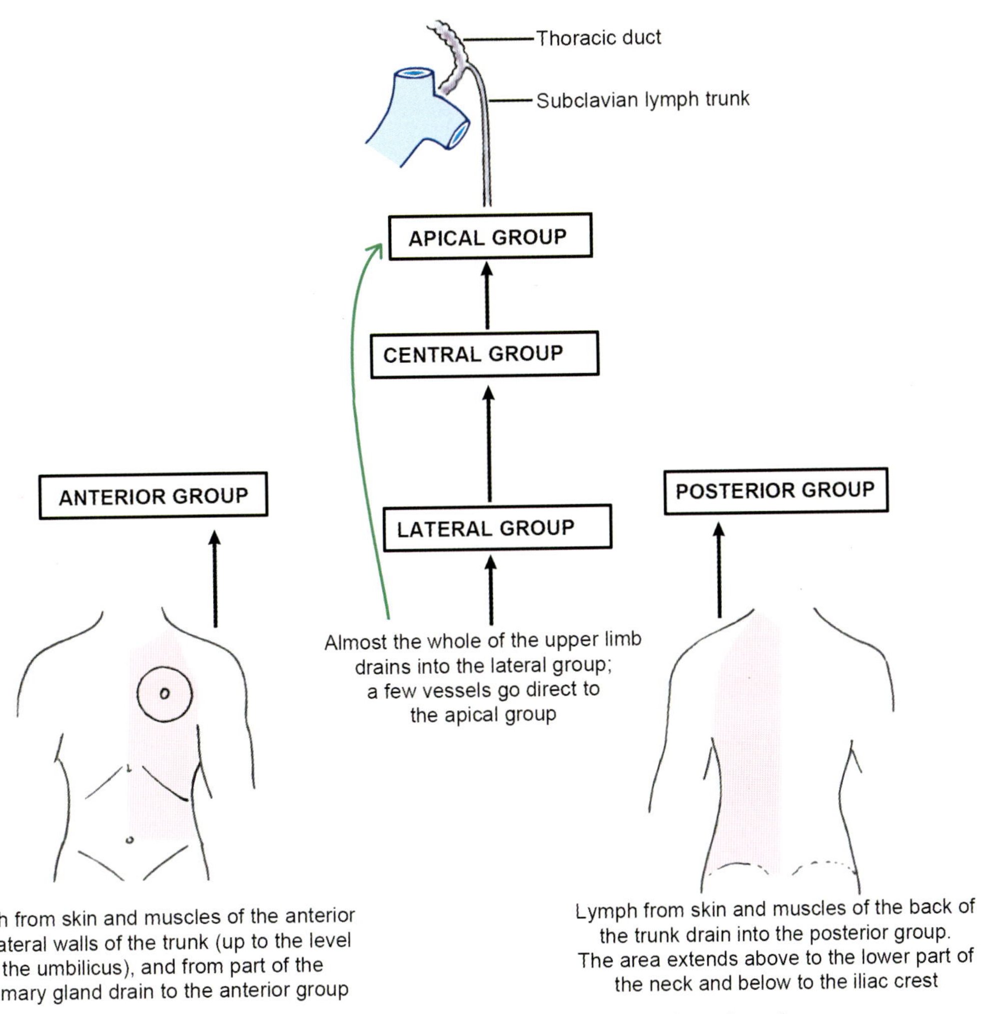


**3.16:** Scheme to show areas drained by the axillary lymph nodes

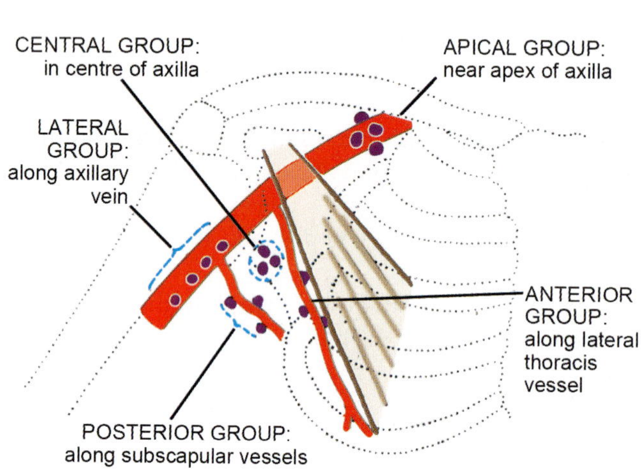


**3.17:** Axillary lymph nodes seen from the front

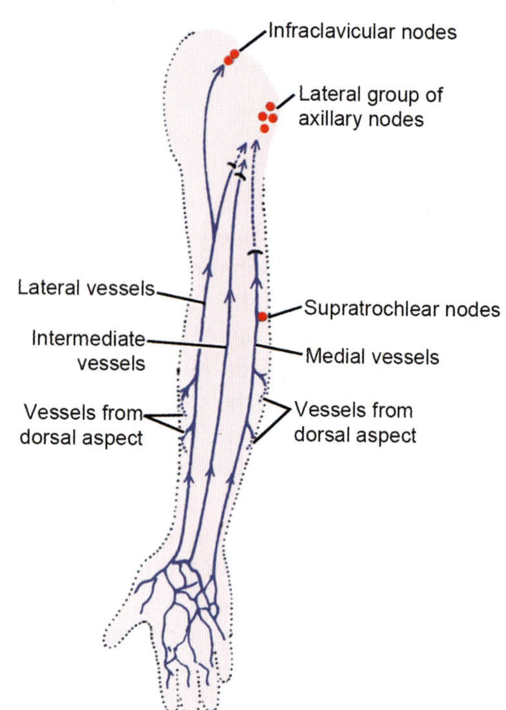


**3.18:** Scheme to show the lymphatic drainage of the upper limb

## THE BRACHIAL PLEXUS AND ITS BRANCHES

### Basic Plan of Brachial Plexus

1. The basic plan of the brachial plexus is shown in 3.19.
2. The plexus consists of roots, trunks (and their divisions) and cords.
3. The main branches arise as continuations of the cords; branches also arise from other parts of the plexus.

#### *Roots of Brachial Plexus*

The ***roots*** of the plexus are the ventral rami of spinal nerves C5, C6, C7, C8 and T1.

#### *Trunks of Brachial Plexus*

1. The roots from C5 and C6 join to form the ***upper trunk*** of the plexus.
2. The root from C7 continues as the ***middle trunk***.
3. The roots from C8 and T1 join to form the ***lower trunk***.

#### *Divisions and Cords of Brachial Plexus*

1. Each trunk divides into an ***anterior*** and a ***posterior division***.
2. The anterior divisions of the upper and middle trunks join to form the ***lateral cord***.

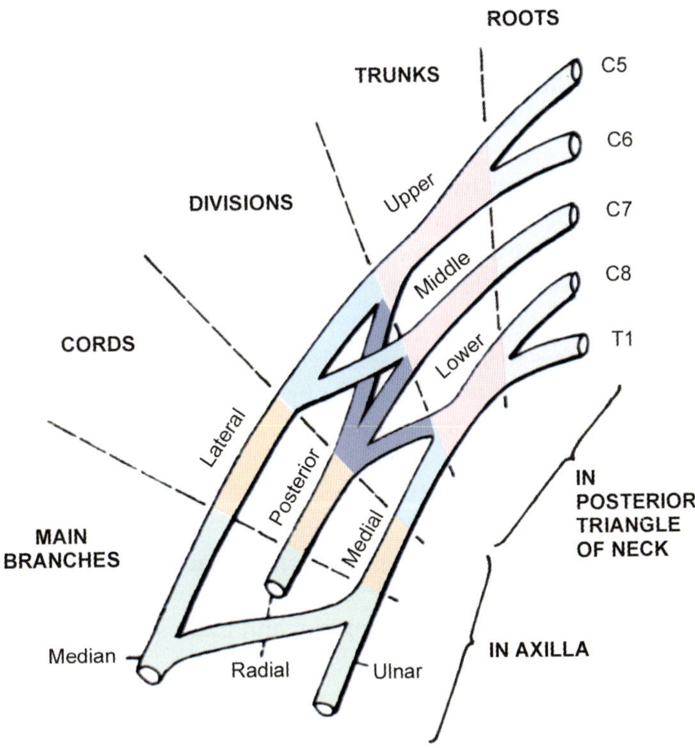


**3.19:** Basic plan of the brachial plexus

3. The anterior division of the lower trunk continues as the ***medial cord***.
4. The posterior divisions of all the three trunks join to form the ***posterior cord***.

### *Branches of Brachial Plexus*

The main branches of the brachial plexus are the ***median***, the ***ulnar*** and the ***radial*** nerves.

1. The median nerve is formed by union of lateral and medial roots arising from the lateral and medial cords, respectively.
2. The ulnar nerve arises from the medial cord.
3. The radial nerve arises from the posterior cord.

### *Some Relationships of Brachial Plexus*

1. The brachial plexus lies partly in the neck and partly in the axilla.
2. The roots and trunks lie in the neck (in the posterior triangle).
3. The cords and their branches lie in the axilla. In the axilla the cords and their main branches are closely related to the axillary artery.
4. To reach the axilla from the neck the plexus passes:
   a. Behind the medial part of the clavicle.
   b. Through the ***cervicoaxillary canal***.

## Branches of Brachial Plexus

1. Branches of the brachial plexus supply the entire upper limb. They also supply some structures in the neck. In this section we will list all the branches, but will describe only those that are seen in the pectoral region or axilla. The other branches will be described where such description is relevant.
2. The branches of the brachial plexus arise from roots, trunks or cords.
3. The branches arising from the roots and trunks arise in the neck and are, therefore, called ***supraclavicular branches*** (not to be confused with the supraclavicular nerves that we have seen in the pectoral region ).
4. The branches from the cords arise in the axilla and are called ***infraclavicular branches***.

### *Branches Arising from Roots*

1. Each root of the plexus gives branches to some muscles lying in the neck (scalene muscles and longus colli).
2. Root C5 gives a contribution to the ***phrenic nerve***. The phrenic nerve descends into the thorax to supply the diaphragm. The diaphragm is the most important muscle of respiration.
3. The ***dorsal scapular nerve*** arises from root C5.
4. The ***long thoracic nerve*** is the nerve to the serratus anterior.
   a. It arises from roots C5, C6 and C7.
   b. The nerve runs downwards first in the neck over the scalene muscles; and then on the medial wall of the axilla over the serratus anterior.
   c. It reaches up to the lower border of the serratus anterior and gives separate twigs to its digitations.

### *Branches Arising from Trunks*

1. The branches arising from the trunks of the brachial plexus are:
   a. Nerve to the subclavius and
   b. Suprascapular nerve.
   Both of these nerves arise from the upper trunk.
2. The ***nerve to the subclavius*** descends in front of the brachial plexus and in front of the third part of the subclavian artery. It passes behind the clavicle to reach the deep surface of the subclavius that it supplies.
3. The ***suprascapular nerve*** runs laterally and backwards over the shoulder.

### *Branches from Cords*

1. The ***lateral pectoral nerve*** is the main nerve supplying the pectoralis major.
   a. It also gives some fibres to the pectoralis minor through a communication with the medial pectoral nerve.
   b. After its origin from the lateral cord the nerve runs medially across the axillary artery.
   c. It then pierces the clavipectoral fascia to enter the pectoralis major.
2. The ***medial pectoral nerve*** is the main nerve of supply for the pectoralis minor. It also sends a few fibres to the pectoralis major.
   a. At its origin from the medial cord the nerve lies behind the axillary artery.
   b. Passing medially and forward it emerges from behind the artery and enters the pectoralis minor.
   c. Some branches pass through this muscle to reach the pectoralis major.
3. The ***upper subscapular nerve*** arises from the posterior cord and supplies the subscapularis (which lies behind the brachial plexus in the posterior wall of the axilla) (3.20).
4. The ***lower subscapular nerve*** arises from the posterior cord. It supplies the teres major and also gives a branch to the subscapularis.
5. The ***thoracodorsal nerve*** is the nerve to the latissimus dorsi. (The latissimus dorsi is a large muscle of the back. The muscle ends in a broad tendon that takes part in forming the posterior fold of the axilla).
   a. The nerve arises from the posterior cord between the upper and lower subscapular nerves.
   b. It passes downwards on the subscapularis to reach the anterior (or deep) surface of the latissimus dorsi (3.20).
6. The ***axillary nerve*** supplies the deltoid and the teres minor (lying in the scapular region).

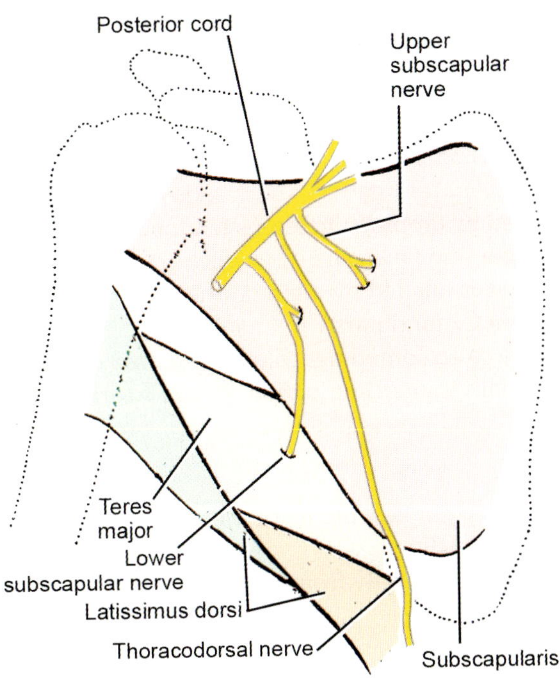


**3.20:** Course of upper and lower subscapular nerves, and of the thoracodorsal nerve

7. The ***musculocutaneous nerve*** is a branch of the lateral cord. It descends into the arm.
8. The ***medial cutaneous nerve of the arm*** is a branch of the medial cord. It runs downwards first on the medial side of the axillary vein and then enters the arm lying on the medial side of the basilic vein.
9. The ***medial cutaneous nerve of the forearm*** is a branch of the medial cord. The nerve runs downwards on the medial side of the axillary artery (between it and the axillary vein) and then enters the arm on the medial side of the brachial artery.
10. The ***ulnar nerve*** is the main continuation of the medial cord. In the axilla the nerve lies medial to the third part of the axillary artery. It then enters the arm, the forearm and the hand.
11. The ***radial nerve*** is the main continuation of the posterior cord. In the axilla it lies posterior to the third part of the axillary artery. It then enters the arm, the forearm and the hand.
12. The ***median nerve*** is a continuation of the lateral cord and lies lateral to the third part of the axillary artery. It also receives a root from the medial cord. It descends into the arm, forearm and hand.

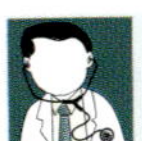

## CLINICAL CORRELATION

### Applied Anatomy of the Brachial Plexus and its Branches

*Causes of disease*

1. The brachial plexus or its branches may be affected by injury or by disease.
2. Injury may be direct e.g., by stabs or gun shots; or indirect through fractured bones, stretching of the neck, etc.
3. Symptoms in the area supplied by the plexus may also be produced by injury or disease of the spinal cord in the segments concerned. In this case it is of importance to determine the exact segments of the cord that are affected. This is done as follows:
   a. By testing the muscles and finding out which ones are paralysed.
   b. By mapping out areas of skin in which sensations are lost or diminished.

4. From this point of view it is necessary to know the nerve supply of both muscles and skin segment wise (or root wise), rather than nerve wise.

*Tendon reflexes*

In examining the nervous system use is often made of ***tendon reflexes*** which can help to localise segmental levels of lesions.

1. The ***biceps tendon reflex*** is elicited by tapping the biceps tendon. This leads to flexion of the elbow. A positive reflex confirms integrity of segment C5 (and partly of C6).
2. Similarly the ***triceps tendon reflex*** is elicited by a tap on the triceps tendon: it causes extension of the elbow and confirms integrity of segment C7 (and partly of C6 and C8).
3. The ***brachioradialis tendon reflex*** (also sometimes called ***supinator jerk***) is elicited by a tap over the insertion of the brachioradialis. This normally causes supination of the forearm, and confirms integrity of segment C6 (and partly C5 and C7).

*Dermatomes*

1. The areas of skin supplied by individual segments of the spinal cord (i.e., by individual spinal nerves) are referred to as ***dermatomes*** (3.21 and 3.22).
2. In the early embryo the limb projects laterally from the body wall and has a cranial or ***preaxial border*** and a caudal or ***postaxial border***.
3 The region adjoining the preaxial border is supplied by the most cranial spinal segments and the region of the postaxial border by the most caudal ones.
4. Parallel strips between the borders are supplied by intervening segments (3.21).

*Effects of Injury*

Injury to a motor nerve results in ***paralysis*** of the muscles supplied by it. This is manifested in two ways.

1. The patient is unable to perform movements dependent on the muscles concerned.
2. Normal posture of a limb, or part of a limb, is disturbed.
   a. It depends upon the balance between the tone of opposing muscles.
   b. For example, the resting forearm is in the semipronated position because of the balance between the tone of the supinators and pronators.
   c. If the supinators are paralysed the unopposed tone of the pronators leads to pronation of the forearm.
   d. Such effects account for the characteristic deformities that are associated with injury to different nerves.

*Erb's Point and Erb's Paralysis*

1. The region where roots C5 and C6 of the brachial plexus meet to form the upper trunk is often referred to as ***Erb's point***. Six nerves meet here (3.25). These are:
   a. Roots C5 and C6
   b. Anterior and posterior divisions of the upper trunk
   c. Suprascapular nerve
   d. Nerve to the subclavius .
2. Injury in this region produces a syndrome that is referred to as ***Erb's paralysis*** (or as ***Erb-Duchenne palsy***).
3. The muscles paralysed are those supplied by nerves C5 and C6, these are:
   a. The deltoid
   b. The biceps brachii
   c. The brachialis
   d. The brachioradialis
   e. The supraspinatus
   f. The infraspinatus
   g. The supinator.

4. The features of paralysis are as follows:
   a. Because of paralysis of the deltoid and of the supraspinatus the arm cannot be abducted: it hangs by the side of the body.
   b. Paralysis of the infraspinatus (a lateral rotator) leads to medial rotation of the arm.
   c. As a result of paralysis of the biceps brachii and of the brachialis (flexors of forearm) the forearm cannot be flexed: it remains extended.
   d. Because of paralysis of the biceps and of the supinator (both supinators) the forearm becomes pronated.
   e. As a result of the combination of medial rotation of the arm and pronation of the forearm the palm faces backwards (***waiter's tip position***) (3.23).
5. Erb's paralysis can occur as a result of any injury that forcibly stretches the region of the upper trunk of the brachial plexus.
6. An example of such injury is a fall on the side of the head.
7. Undue pull upon the neck during birth of a child may cause such a paralysis in the newborn.

*Klumpke's Paralysis*

1. This is caused by injury to roots C8 and T1, or to the lower trunk of the brachial plexus.
2. The flexors of the wrist and all the small muscles of the hand are paralysed.
3. Because of paralysis of the flexors of the wrist, the joint remains extended.
4. Because of paralysis of the interossei the proximal phalanges are extended while the middle and distal phalanges are flexed. This gives rise to a deformity known as a 'claw hand' similar to that seen in ulnar nerve paralysis (See below).
5. Sensory loss, similar to that in ulnar nerve injury (see below) may also be present.

*Cervico-axillary canal and Scalenus Anticus Syndrome*

1. In passing from the neck into the axilla the brachial plexus and the subclavian artery pass through a triangular space called the ***cervico-axillary canal***. The boundaries of this canal are:
   a. Medially by the first rib.
   b. Anteriorly by the clavicle.
   c. Posteriorly by the upper border of the scapula.
2. The structures passing through the canal can be compressed leading to neurological and vascular symptoms.
3. The neurological symptoms are those of compression of the lower trunk and resemble those of Klumpke's paralysis.
4. Because of irritation of the trunk by pressure against the first rib, pain radiating to the medial side of the arm is a conspicuous feature.
   a. To understand the genesis of these symptoms it is necessary to note that the root to the brachial plexus from T1 has to curve over the first rib to join the root from C8 (3.24A and B).
   b. This does not cause problems in the normal person, but when the shoulders begin to sag with age, or in persons who have to lift heavy weights, the pressure of the nerve trunk on the rib may be sufficient to cause symptoms.
   c. Similar symptoms can also be produced by pressure of the scalenus anterior muscle (Scalenus anticus syndrome or scalene syndrome).

*Cervical Rib*

1. Occasionally, a rudimentary rib may be present in relation to the seventh cervical vertebra: this is called a cervical rib. The anterior part of the rib may be represented by a fibrous cord.
2. When a cervical rib is present root T1 has to curve over this rib (or over the fibrous band) (3.26).
3. This results in considerably greater pressure on the nerve root as compared to that from a normal first rib.
4. The same symptoms as described above occur with greater intensity and at an earlier age. However, a cervical rib may exist without producing any symptoms, especially in the young.

*Prefixed and Postfixed Brachial Plexus*

1. We have seen that normally the brachial plexus is formed mainly by roots C5 to T1 and that there are small contributions from C4 and T2 (3.27A to C).
2. Sometimes the contribution from C4 is large; root T1 is small; and the contribution from T2 is absent. This is called a ***prefixed plexus***: because the plexus appears to be 'fixed' one segment higher than normal (3.27).
3. The reverse condition is one in which the plexus appears to be 'fixed' one segment too low: i.e., it is ***postfixed*** (3.27C). In this case the contribution from C4 is missing; root C5 is small; and the contribution from T2 is large.
4. By comparing 3.27C with 3.26, it will be seen that the relationship of a postfixed brachial plexus to a normal first rib is the same as that of a normal plexus to a cervical rib. Hence the symptoms associated with a cervical rib can be present in the absence of such a rib if the brachial plexus is postfixed.

*Injury to Long thoracic nerve*

1. The long thoracic nerve (which supplies the serratus anterior) can be injured in persons who carry heavy weights on the shoulders.
   a. Normally, the serratus anterior (along with the trapezius) helps in overhead abduction of the arm by rotating the scapula forwards.
   b. This movement is not possible when the nerve is injured.
2. The serratus anterior can be tested by asking the patient to stretch his upper limbs forwards, place his palms against a wall and push them against it. When the muscle is paralysed the medial margin of the scapula projects backwards: this is called ***winging of the scapula***.

*Brachial plexus block*

Injection of local anaesthetic into the axillary sheath blocks all branches of the brachial plexus. Operations can then be performed on the upper limb.

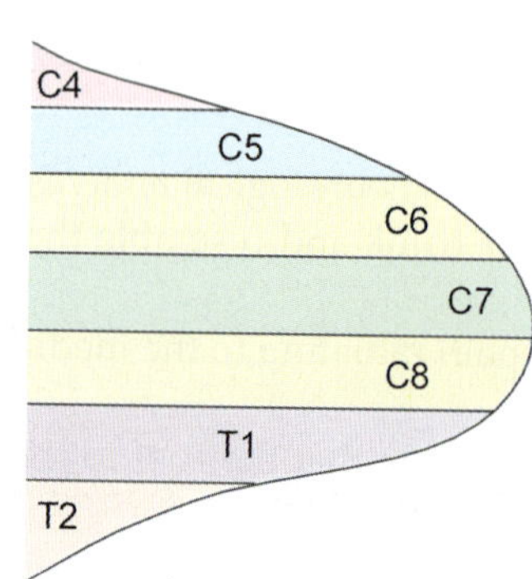


**3.21:** Dermatomes of upper limb in an embryo

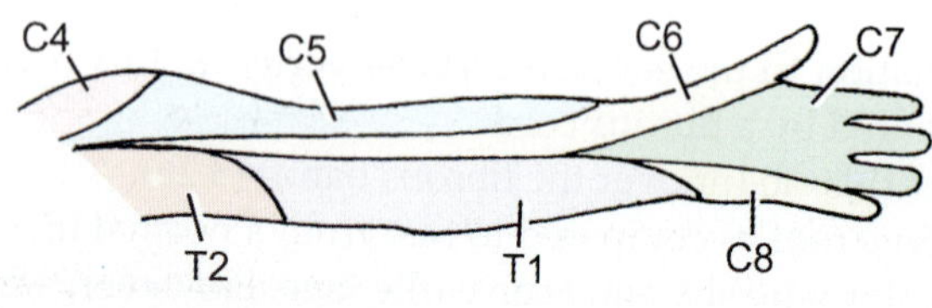


**3.22:** Dermatomes of upper limb in an adult

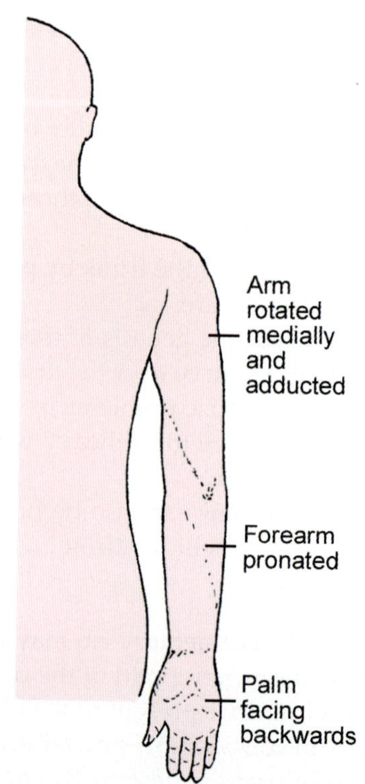


**3.23:** Waiter's tip position of upper limb in Erb's paralysis

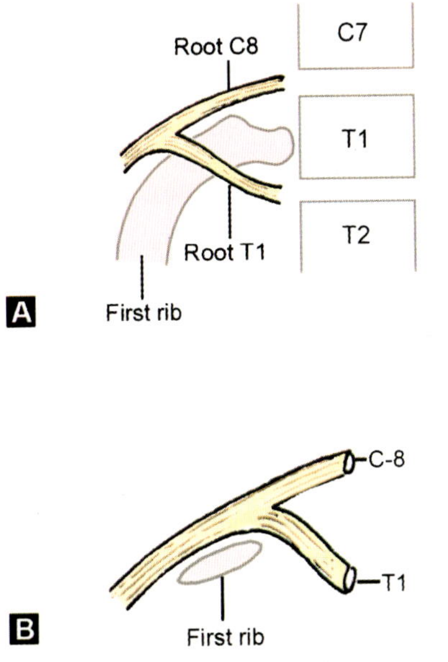


**3.24A and B:** Relation of root T1 of brachial plexus to the first rib

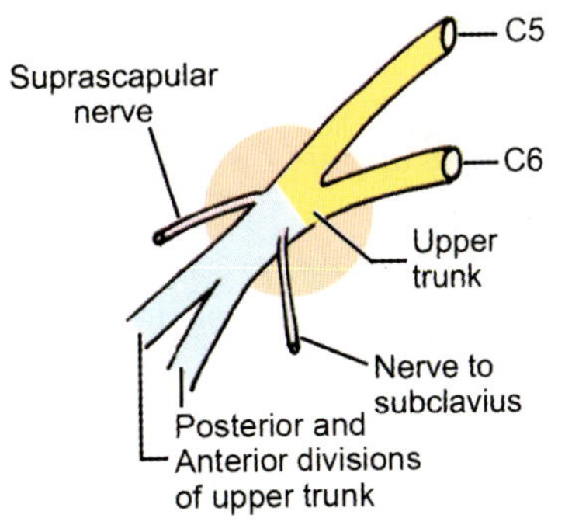


**3.25:** Nerves meeting at Erb's point

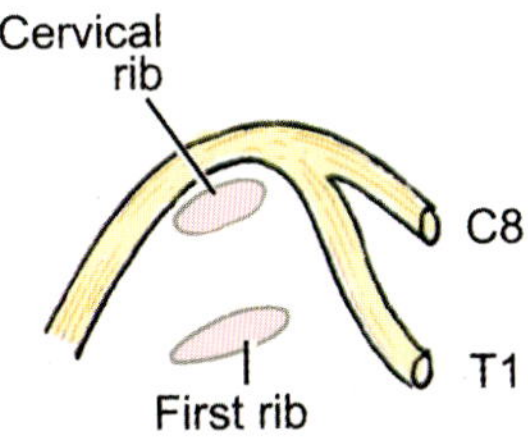


**3.26:** Relation of root T1 of brachial plexus to a cervical rib

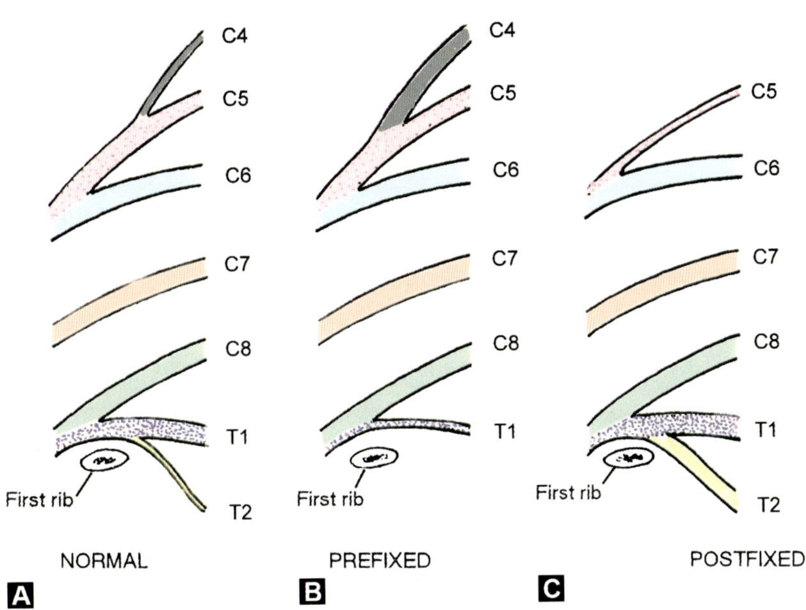


**3.27A to C:** Some variations in the origin of the brachial plexus

# THE MAMMARY GLANDS (BREASTS)

## INTRODUCTION

1. Although the mammary glands (also called the breasts) play no direct role in reproduction, they are included amongst the organs of the reproductive system as they provide essential nourishment to the newborn and infant in the form of milk.
2. They are well developed only in the female after the age of puberty and the description that follows applies only to the mature female (3.28).
3. Each breast (right or left) is a rounded elevation present on the front of the upper part of the thorax, over the pectoral region.
4. Over the centre of the breast the skin shows a dark circular area that is called the ***areola***.
5. In the centre of the areola there is a conical projection called the ***nipple*** (or papilla) (3.28).
6. Deep to the skin, the breast lies in the superficial fascia (i.e., between the skin and the deep fascia).
   a. It consists of a mass of glandular tissue embedded in connective tissue and fat.
   b. The glandular tissue is irregular and the rounded appearance of the breast is due to the presence of abundant subcutaneous fat.
7. The breast extends upwards to the level of the second rib, and downwards to the sixth rib (3.28).
   a. Medially, it extends to the right or left margin of the sternum.
   b. Laterally, its extent is variable, but it may reach the midaxillary line.

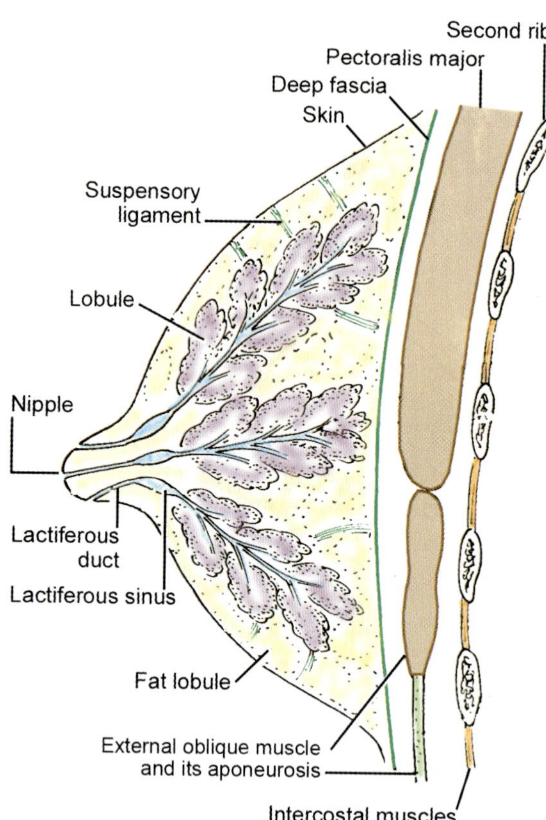


**3.28:** Schematic vertical section through the breast

8. From the upper lateral part of the gland an extension of glandular tissue passes through an aperture in the deep fascia over the axilla to enter the latter (The aperture is the ***foramen of Langer***). This extension is called the ***axillary tail***.
9. The greater part of the breast lies over the pectoralis major.
   a. More laterally it lies on the serratus anterior.
   b. Inferiorly, it overlaps the external oblique muscle of the abdomen, and its aponeurosis.

### WANT TO KNOW MORE?

10. The glandular tissue of the breast consists of acini that are aggregated to form lobules. Several lobules collect to form a lobe. There are about fifteen to twenty such lobes in each breast.
11. The acini of each lobe are drained by small ducts which ultimately end in one ***lactiferous duct*** for each lobe. The ducts open on the surface of the nipple.
12. A little proximal to the opening, each duct shows a dilation called a ***lactiferous sinus***.
13. Deep to the areola there are numerous modified ***sebaceous glands***.
    a. These glands become enlarged during pregnancy and produce surface elevations or tubercles.
    b. The secretions of these glands provide a protective covering for the areola and nipple during lactation.

14. Breast tissue is held in place by bundles of fibrous tissue that connect it to the skin and to the underlying deep fascia.
    a. These bands are referred to as the ***suspensory ligaments*** (or ligaments of Cooper).
    b. In spite of these bands the normal breast has reasonable mobility over the deep fascia and its skin can be pinched up.
15. In the male, and in the female before the age of puberty, the mammary glands are rudimentary.
    a. The areola and a poorly developed nipple can be recognised.
    b. Deep to them there are a few ducts only; there are no acini.
16. In the female, the initial enlargement of the breast at puberty is mainly due to accumulation of fat.
    a. It is later that the duct system proliferates and acini appear.
    b. Considerable further proliferation takes place during pregnancy.
17. There is partial atrophy of glandular elements after the end of lactation. The breast atrophies in old age.

## Blood Vessels, Lymphatics and Nerves of the Breasts

1. The breast is supplied by perforating branches of the internal thoracic artery.
    a. These branches are large in the female, and this explains why the internal thoracic artery was earlier called the internal mammary artery.
    b. This artery lies within the thorax and runs downwards vertically, a short distance from the margin of the sternum.
2. The lateral thoracic branch of the axillary artery also gives several branches to the breast (and is sometimes called the external mammary artery).
3. Branches are also given off to the breasts from the intercostal arteries.
4. Blood from the breast is drained by veins corresponding to the arteries.
5. As the mammary glands are frequent sites of carcinoma, their lymphatic drainage is of considerable importance. It is described below.
6. The sensory innervation of the breast is derived from the anterior and lateral cutaneous branches of the fourth, fifth, and sixth thoracic nerves.
    a. The sensory innervation is richest in the areola and nipple.
    b. The nerves supplying the glandular tissue are sympathetic.

## Lymphatic Drainage of the Breast

1. The lymph vessels of the breast are usually divided into:
    a. Those of the parenchyma, along with those of the skin covering the areola and nipple; and
    b. Those of the skin (excluding those of areola and nipple).
2. This scheme will be followed here. However, it is necessary to state at the outset that the two sets of vessels are not distinct: they communicate and drain predominantly into the same sets of lymph nodes.
3. The lymphatic drainage of the parenchyma, and of the areola and nipple is shown in 3.29.
    a. The parenchyma is permeated by a plexus of lymph vessels.
    b. Many of these vessels communicate with a dense subareolar plexus lying beneath the skin of the areola and nipple. Vessels from the plexus in the parenchyma, and from the subareolar plexus drain as follows.
4. Most of the vessels pass in a lateral direction into the axillary lymph nodes.
    a. These vessels end mainly in the anterior group of axillary lymph nodes: a few drain into the posterior group.
    b. Lymph from the anterior and posterior groups passes to the central group, and from there to the apical group of axillary lymph nodes.
    c. Some vessels from the upper part of the parenchyma pass direct to the apical group: some of these vessels are interrupted by the infraclavicular lymph nodes (3.18).

5. Several vessels drain in a medial direction into the parasternal nodes present within the thorax near the lateral margins of the sternum. These vessels pass along the perforating branches of the intercostal arteries.
6. Some lymph vessels reach the intercostal nodes lying within the thorax near the posterior ends of the intercostal spaces. These vessels travel backwards along the lateral cutaneous branches of the posterior intercostal arteries (3.30).
7. The lymphatic drainage of the skin of the breast (excluding that of the areola and nipple) is shown in 3.31.
   a. The main drainage is into the same nodes that drain in parenchyma viz., the anterior group of axillary nodes laterally; and the parasternal nodes medially.
   b. Some vessels from the upper part of the skin cross the clavicle and reach the lowest nodes of the deep cervical chain: these nodes lie just above the clavicle and are, therefore, called the supraclavicular lymph nodes (3.31).

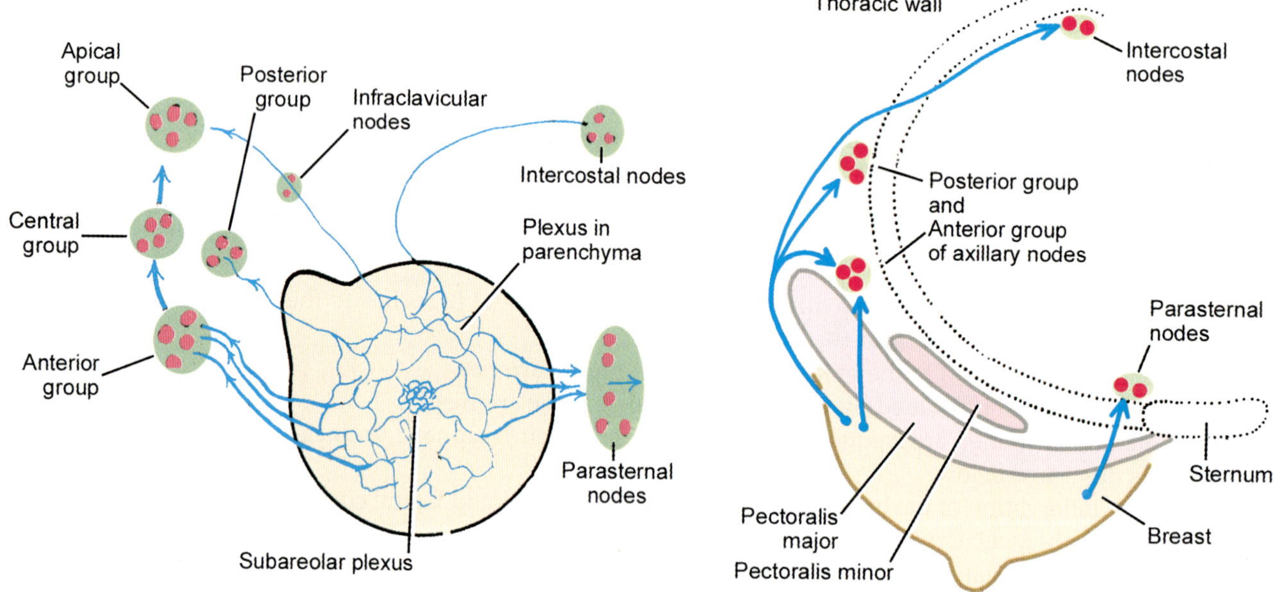


**3.29:** Scheme to show the lymphatic drainage of the parenchyma of the breast, and of the skin of the areola and nipple

**3.30:** Scheme to show some routes followed by lymphatic vessels draining the breast

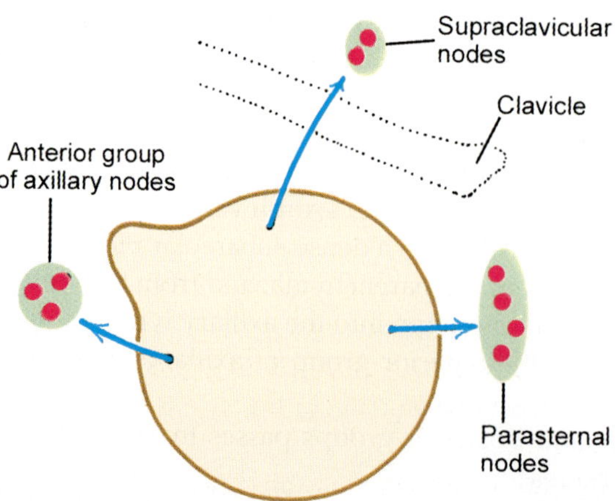


**3.31:** Lymphatic drainage of the skin of the breast (excluding that over the areola and nipple)

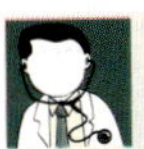

## CLINICAL CORRELATION

### Breast

1. Inflammation of the breast is called ***mastitis***. It may be acute or chronic. Mastitis can lead to abscess formation.
   a. Traditionally, radial incisions have been advised for drainage of an abscess in the breast (to avoid injury to the ducts).
   b. However, such incisions are disfiguring and incisions along the junction of the areola and nipple are now preferred.
2. ***Cysts***, multiple or single, may be formed by obstruction of ducts. A milk-containing cyst is called a ***galactocele***.
3. Masses in the breast may be caused by ***neoplasms*** (***tumours***). The breast is a common site of ***carcinoma***.
4. An operation for removal of the breast is called ***mastectomy***. Removal of the breast alone is called ***simple mastectomy***.
5. In the past an extensive operation involving removal of axillary lymph nodes, the pectoralis major and pectoralis minor used to be performed in an effort to remove all cancer cells. Such an operation is called ***radical mastectomy***.
6. Most surgeons have now given up the traditional radical operation.
   a. In most cases only simple removal of the breast along with removal of axillary lymph nodes is undertaken.
   b. Sometimes, the pectoralis minor is removed.
   c. Surgery is followed by radiotherapy (exposure to X-rays which kill cancer cells).
7. Some factors of importance in the diagnosis of carcinoma are as follows:
   a. Periodic palpation of the breast (which can be done by a woman herself) can lead to early detection of any mass. Early detection of carcinoma is also facilitated by a procedure called ***mammography***.
   b. We have seen that the normal breast is movable over underlying tissues. In carcinoma of the breast the suspensory ligaments may be invaded by cancer cells and may shorten. When this happens the breast becomes fixed and skin may get retracted at the attachments of the ligaments.
   c. Knowledge of the lymphatic drainage of the breast is very important in dealing with carcinoma of the breast. The following additional facts about lymphatic drainage may be noted.
   d. The vessels to the axillary nodes pass laterally over the pectoralis major, and wind around its lateral margin to reach the nodes. Some vessels from the parenchyma may reach the nodes by piercing the pectoralis major.
   e. The lymph nodes of the anterior group are in direct contact with the axillary tail of the breast and cancer may spread to them without having to pass through the lymph vessels.
   f. Lymphatics of the skin over the breast cross the midline and carcinoma of one breast can spread to the other breast through them.
   g. Some vessels from the inferomedial part of the breast probably communicate with lymphatics within the abdominal cavity (subperitoneal plexus). Cancer of the breast has been known to spread to the peritoneum, to the liver and to pelvic organs.
   h. Although the lymphatics of the breast communicate with those lying on the deep fascia (covering the pectoralis major) this is not a normal route for drainage of lymph from the breast. However, if the superficial channels are blocked (by carcinoma) lymph may pass through these communications. Obstruction of superficial lymphatics can lead to oedema of the skin resulting in an appearance like that of an orange peel (***peau d' orange*** appearance).
   i. In addition to spread through lymphatic vessels, cancer of the breast can occasionally spread through veins. Through this route metastases can be formed in vertebrae.

# 4 CHAPTER The Back and Scapular Region

## THE BACK

1. The posterior aspect of the thorax and abdomen is referred to simply as the ***back***.
2. Here, there is a deep layer of muscles belonging to the back proper (studied along with the head and neck).
3. Superficial to them there are several muscles that belong to the upper limb, but are placed on the back. Some of these are inserted into the scapula while others reach the humerus.
4. The muscles of the upper limb present on the back and in the shoulder region produce important movements of the upper limb. To understand their actions properly it is necessary to explain some facts about these movements before we study the muscles.

### Movements of the Arm

1. The basic movements to be seen at any joint are flexion, extension, abduction, adduction, and rotatory movements. In the case of the arm, these movements are somewhat different than at most joints. Note the following.
2. Movements of the arm take place at the shoulder joint that is formed by articulation of the head of the humerus with the glenoid cavity of the scapula.
3. In relation to the wall of the thorax the scapula is placed obliquely so that its costal surface faces forwards ***and medially***, while the dorsal surface faces backwards ***and laterally***. Because of this orientation the glenoid cavity does not face directly laterally, but faces ***forwards and laterally***.
4. As movements of the arm are described with reference to the plane of the scapula (and not in relation to the trunk) the definition of some movements is somewhat different from that for other joints as follows:
   a. In the neutral position the arm hangs vertically by the side of the trunk.
   b. Flexion and extension take place in a plane ***at right angles to the plane of the scapula***.
   c. In ***flexion*** the arm moves forwards (4.1) ***and somewhat medially***.
   d. Reversal of this movement (i.e., bringing it back to the side of the trunk) is ***extension***.
   e. Continuation of extension beyond the vertical position of the arm is called ***hyperextension***.
   f. The movements of abduction and adduction take place ***in the plane of the scapula***.
   g. In this movement the arm moves laterally, and somewhat forwards (4.2).
   h. After reaching the horizontal position (i.e., from 1 to 2 in 4.2) the movement can be continued to raise the arm to a vertical position (3): this is referred to as ***overhead abduction***.
   i. Bringing the arm back to the neutral position (i.e., back to 1) is called ***adduction***.
   j. Further adduction brings the arm in front of the chest (4). Abduction and adduction take place partly at the shoulder joint, and partly by rotation of the scapula.
   k. The rotatory movements of the arm are ***medial rotation*** and ***lateral rotation*** (4.3A and B).
   l. A rotation of the humerus that carries the flexed forearm medially is medial rotation.
   m. The opposite movement in which the forearm is carried laterally is lateral rotation.
   n. Note further that rotation is named with reference to the the ***front*** of the humerus.
   o. It follows that any muscle passing from the trunk (or scapula) to the front of the humerus will be a medial rotator. A muscle passing to the back of the humerus will be a lateral rotator.

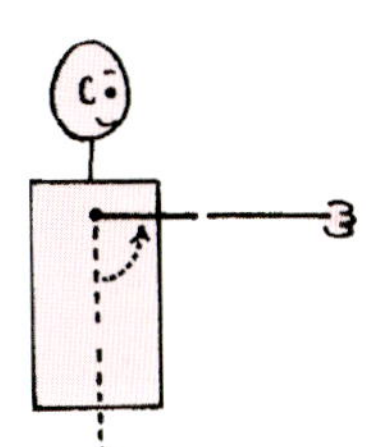

4.1: Scheme to illustrate the movement of flexion of the arm

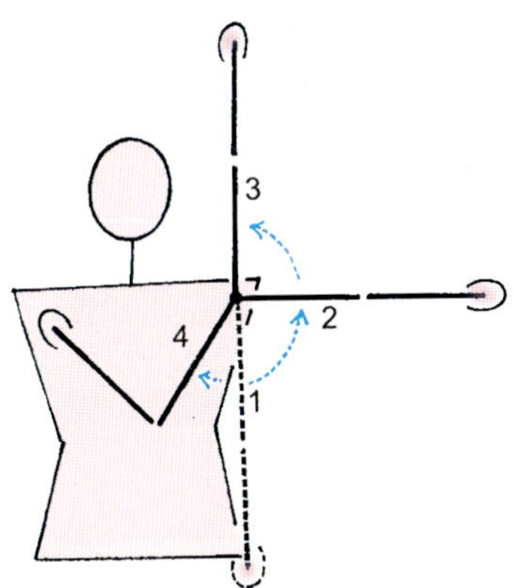


4.2: Scheme to illustrate abduction and adduction of the arm

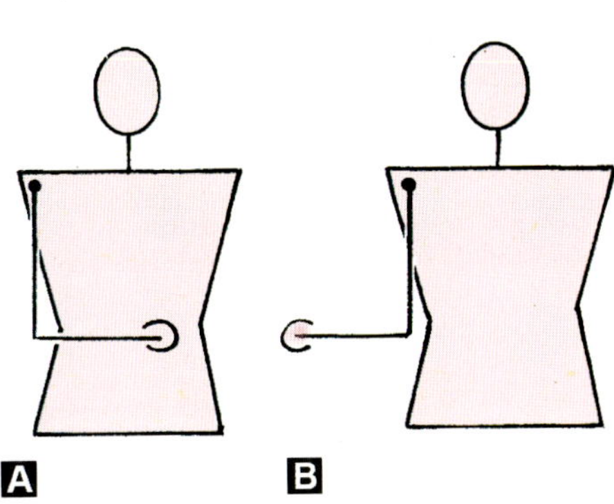


4.3A and B: (A) Medial rotation of the arm (B): Lateral rotation of the arm

## Movements of the Scapula

These are as follows:

1. In ***protraction,*** the entire scapula slides forwards over the chest wall. Reversal of this movement is ***retraction***.
2. In ***elevation,*** the entire scapula moves upwards (as in shrugging the shoulders); and the opposite movement is called ***depression***.
3. In addition to these simple movements the scapula can undergo rotation.
   a. To understand this movement imagine that the scapula is transfixed by an imaginary nail passing through the centre of its body (4.4A and B).
   b. Rotation is named in terms of movement of the inferior angle of the scapula.
4. In ***forward rotation*** (also called ***lateral rotation***) the inferior angle of the scapula passes forwards and somewhat laterally (4.4B).
   a. Simultaneously, the superior angle and the acromion pass backwards and medially.
   b. The glenoid cavity comes to face upwards.
   c. This movement takes place during abduction of the arm, and is essential for raising the arm above the head.
5. Reversal of this movement constitutes ***backward (or medial) rotation***.

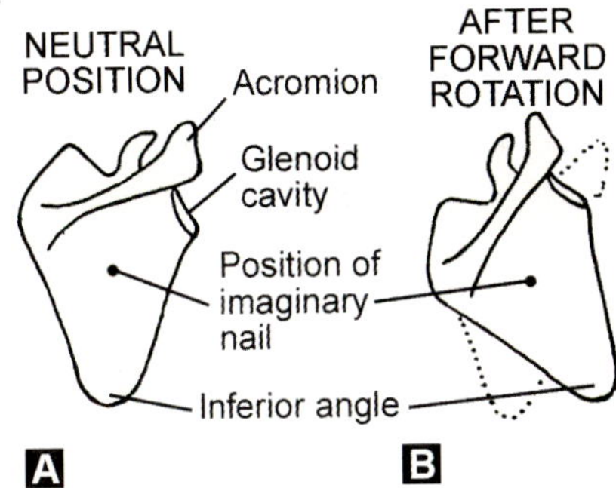


4.4A and B: (A) Neutral position of the scapula (B): Position of the scapula after forward rotation

## MUSCLES OF THE BACK

1. The trapezius is described in 4.5 and illustrated in 4.6.
2. The latissimus dorsi is described in 4.7 and illustrated in 4.8.
3. Three muscles: the levator scapulae, the rhomboideus minor and rhomboideus major are described in 4.9 and the attachments of the levator scapulae are shown in 4.10.

## NERVES OF THE BACK

### Cutaneous Nerves of the Back

1. The skin of the back is supplied mainly by cutaneous branches arising from dorsal rami of spinal nerves (4.11). The lateral parts of the back are innervated by cutaneous branches from ventral rami. Note that dorsal rami make no contribution to the cutaneous supply of the free upper limb.

| 4.5: Trapezius | |
|---|---|
| Origin | 1. Superior nuchal line (medial one-third)<br>2. External occipital protuberance<br>3. Ligamentum nuchae<br>4. Spines of vertebrae C7 to T12<br>5. Intervening supraspinous ligaments |
| Insertion | 1. Clavicle (posterior border of lateral one-third)<br>2. Acromion (medial margin)<br>3. Scapula (crest of spine and tubercle on it) |
| Nerve supply | 1. Accessory nerve, spinal part (motor)<br>2. Branches from nerves C3, 4 (sensory) |
| Action | 1. Forward rotation of scapula (with serratus anterior)<br>2. Elevation of scapula (with levator scapulae)<br>3. Retraction of scapula (with rhomboids)<br>4. Draws head backwards and laterally. When muscles of both sides act the head is drawn directly backwards |

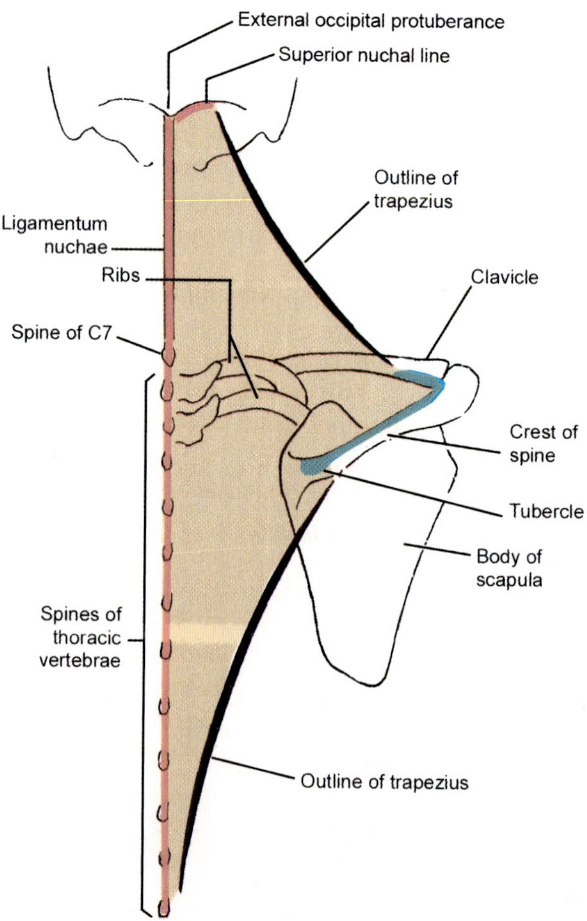


**4.6:** Scheme to show the attachments of the trapezius

| 4.7: Latissimus dorsi | |
|---|---|
| Origin | 1. Spines of vertebrae T7 to T12<br>2. Intervening supraspinous ligaments<br>3. Lumbar fascia<br>4. Slip from iliac crest<br>5. Slips from lowest 3 or 4 ribs<br>6. Slip from inferior angle of scapula |
| Insertion | Muscle ends in a tendon which is inserted into anterior aspect of upper end of humerus, in floor of intertubercular sulcus |
| Nerve supply | Thoracodorsal nerve (C6, 7, 8) |
| Action | 1. Adduction and medial rotation of arm<br>2. Extension of flexed arm, against resistance<br>3.Depression of raised arm against resistance (with pectoralis major)<br>4. Elevation of trunk (when the arms are raised and fixed) (with pectoralis major) |
| Notes | Fibres of the muscle converge towards axilla and end in a tendon that winds round the lower border of the teres major. The two form the posterior fold of the axilla |

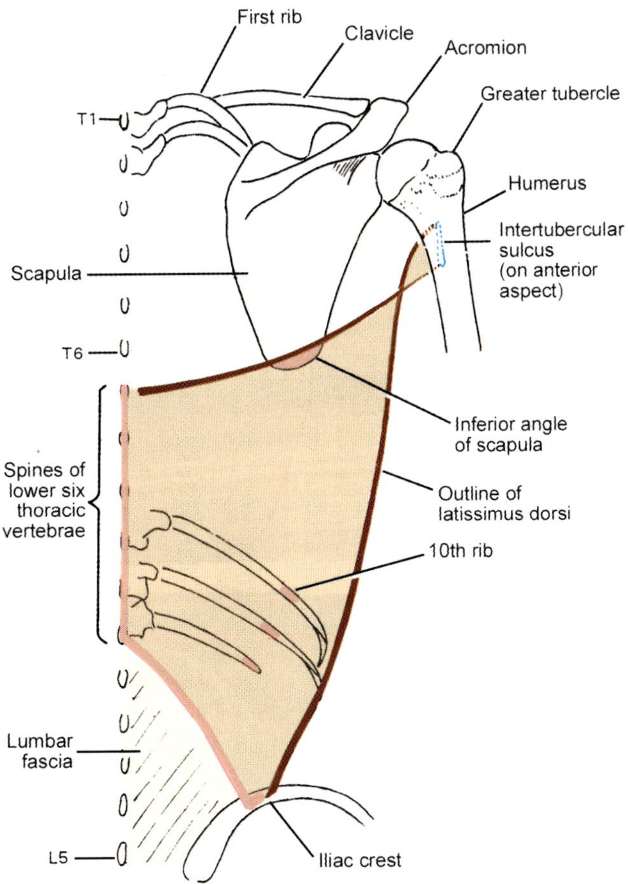


4.8: Scheme to show the attachments of the latissimus dorsi

**4.9: Levator scapulae, rhomboideus minor and rhomboideus major**

| *Muscle* | *Levator Scapulae* | *Rhomboideus Minor* | *Rhomboideus Major* |
|---|---|---|---|
| Origin | Transverse processes of upper four cervical vertebrae | 1. Lowest part of ligamentum nuchae<br>2. Spines of vertebrae C7 and T1 | 1. Spines of vertebrae T2 to T5.<br>2. Intervening supraspinous ligaments |
| Insertion | Medial border of scapula from superior angle to root of spine | Medial border of scapula opposite root of spine | Medial border of scapula, from root of spine up to inferior angle |
| Nerve supply | 1. Branches from spinal nerves C3, C4.<br>2. Dorsal scapular nerve | Dorsal scapular nerve (C4, 5) | Dorsal scapular nerve (C4,5) |
| Action | 1. Elevation of scapula<br>2. Backward rotation of scapula<br>3. Stabilization of scapula during movements of upper limb<br>4. Bends neck to its own side | 1. Retraction of scapula<br>2. Backward rotation of scapula<br>3. Stabilization of scapula during movements of upper limb | 1. Retraction of scapula<br>2. Backward rotation of scapula<br>3. Stabilization of scapula during movements of upper limb |

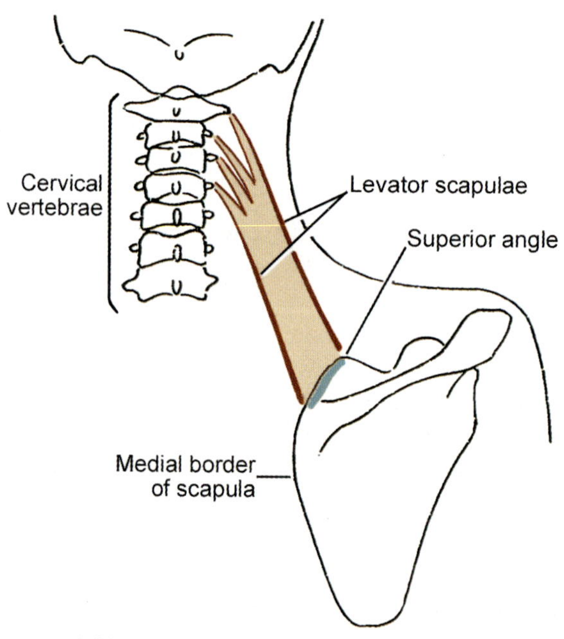


**4.10:** Attachments of the levator scapulae

2. Each dorsal ramus divides into medial and lateral branches. These branches supply deep muscles of the back (erector spinae). [These muscles do not belong to the upper limb. In fact, no muscle of either the upper or lower limb is innervated by dorsal rami].
3. Of the two branches of a dorsal ramus only one gives off cutaneous branches.
   a. In the cervical and upper thoracic region these arise from the medial branches, and become superficial near the middle line of the back.
   b. In the lower thoracic and lumbar region the cutaneous branches arise from the lateral branch, and become superficial along a line corresponding to the lateral edge of the erector spinae.

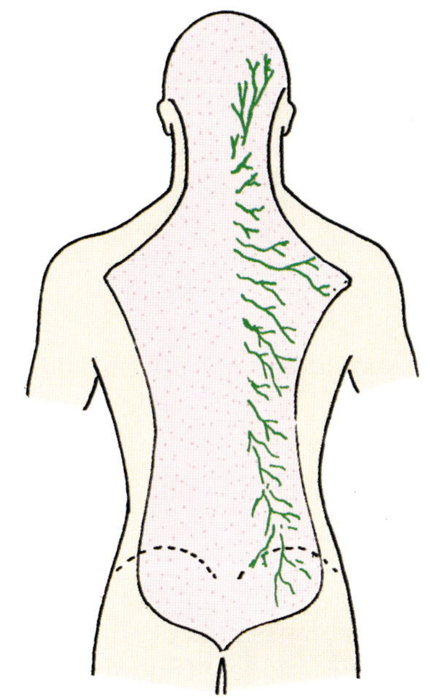

**4.11:** Area of skin of the back supplied by dorsal rami of spinal nerves

## Nerves Supplying Muscles

### *Spinal part of accessory nerve*

1. Running downwards deep to the trapezius, and supplying it, there is the spinal part of the accessory nerve.
2. The accessory nerve is the eleventh cranial nerve. It has a cranial part arising from the medulla oblongata of the brain, and a spinal part arising from the upper part of the spinal cord.
3. The two parts unite for a short part of their course and again separate.
4. This nerve will be studied in detail when we consider the head and neck.
   a. Here we may note that the spinal part of the nerve reaches the trapezius in the lower part of the neck and descends into the back, deep to this muscle.
   b. We have already seen that the trapezius also receives branches from the cervical plexus (C3, C4) but these probably carry only proprioceptive fibres.

## Dorsal Scapular Nerve

1. The dorsal scapular nerve arises from root C5 of the brachial plexus.
2. It passes backwards and downwards through the lower part of the neck (through the scalenus medius) to reach the anterior aspect of the levator scapulae.
3. It then descends into the back to reach the anterior (i.e., deep) aspect of the rhomboideus muscles. Here, it is accompanied by the dorsal scapular artery (or the deep branch of the transverse cervical artery).
4. The dorsal scapular nerve supplies the rhomboideus major and minor and may give a branch to the levator scapulae.

# THE SCAPULAR REGION

In the scapular region we see several muscles that take origin from the scapula and gain insertion into the humerus These are:

1. The deltoid muscle (4.12 and 4.13)
2. The supraspinatus (4.14)

3. The infraspinatus (4.15 and 4.16)
4. The teres minor (4.15 and 4.17)
5. The teres major (4.15, 4.18 and 4.20)
6. The subscapularis (4.19 and 4.20).

**WANT TO KNOW MORE?**

*Relations of the deltoid muscle*

The deltoid muscle covers the region of the shoulder joint from the lateral side, the front and the back. It therefore covers a large number of structures. These are:

1. Upper end of the humerus.
2. Coracoid process.
3. Coracoacromial ligament.
4. Pectoralis minor.
5. Origins of the long and short heads of the biceps brachii and of the coracobrachialis.
6. Insertion of the pectoralis major, teres major, latissimus dorsi, and the long head of the triceps.
7. Insertions of the supraspinatus, infraspinatus and teres minor (by posterior part of deltoid).
8. Origin of the lateral head of the triceps (by posterior part of deltoid).
9. Axillary nerve.
10. Anterior and posterior circumflex humeral arteries.
11. There are a number of bursae deep to the deltoid, the most important of which is the subacromial bursa (also called the subdeltoid bursa).

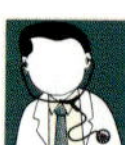

**CLINICAL CORRELATION**

*Paralysis of the deltoid*

1. Paralysis of the deltoid, followed by atrophy, occurs when the axillary nerve is injured.
   a. Because of atrophy, the rounded contour of the shoulder is lost and there may be a slight hollow below the acromion.
   b. There is loss of sensation on the lateral side of the upper part of the arm.
2. To test the deltoid muscle the examiner first abducts the patient's arm to 15 degrees. He then asks the patient to continue abduction against resistance.
3. Injury to the axillary nerve can occur in fracture through the surgical neck of the humerus.

## Mechanism of Abduction of the Arm

1. Abduction of the arm is a complicated movement and the deltoid is one of the most important muscles for it.
2. The supraspinatus also has an important role.
3. This is, therefore, an appropriate place for us to examine the contribution of various muscles to this movement.
4. Abduction of the arm takes place partly at the shoulder joint, and partly by rotation of the scapula as explained below.
   a. The first few degrees of abduction at the shoulder joint are produced by the supraspinatus.
   b. The deltoid produces abduction of the arm at the shoulder joint up to about 90 degrees.
   c. Further abduction is produced by forward rotation of the scapula. The muscles responsible for this action are the serratus anterior and the trapezius acting together.

| 4.12: Deltoid | |
|---|---|
| Origin | 1. Clavicle: upper surface and anterior border of lateral one-third<br>2. Acromion: lateral margin and upper surface<br>3. Spine of scapula: lower lip of crest |
| Insertion | Deltoid tuberosity on lateral aspect of shaft of humerus |
| Nerve supply | Axillary nerve (C5, 6) |
| Action | 1. Abduction of arm at shoulder joint up to 90 degrees (This is by acromial fibres)<br>2. Flexion and medial rotation of humerus (anterior fibres)<br>3. Extension and lateral rotation of humerus (posterior fibres) |
| Notes | See notes on mechanism of abduction of arm and relations of deltoid given below |

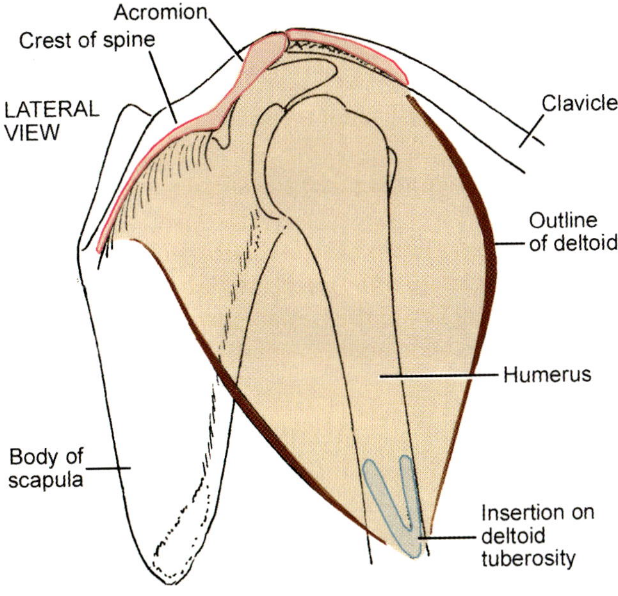


**4.13:** Attachments of the deltoid muscle

| 4.14: Supraspinatus | |
|---|---|
| Origin | Posterior aspect of scapula (medial two-thirds of supraspinous fossa) |
| Insertion | Greater tubercle of humerus (uppermost impression) |
| Nerve supply | Suprascapular nerve (C4, 5, 6) |
| Action | 1. Stabilises shoulder joint (along with other muscles around the joint)<br>2. Abduction of arm (first few degrees) |
| Notes | 1. The muscle passes under the coracoacromial arch<br>2. See clinical note below |

| 4.15: Infraspinatus , teres major and teres minor | | | |
|---|---|---|---|
| *Muscle* | *Infraspinatus* | *Teres Minor* | *Teres Major* |
| Origin | Scapula, posterior aspect (medial two-thirds of infraspinous fossa) | Scapula, posterior aspect (along upper two-thirds of lateral border) | Scapula, posterior aspect (Inferior angle, and lower one-third of lateral border) |
| Insertion | Posterior aspect of upper end of humerus, middle impression on greater tubercle | Posterior aspect of upper end of humerus, lowest impression on greater tubercle | Anterior aspect of upper end of humerus, on medial lip of intertubercular sulcus |
| Nerve supply | Suprascapular nerve (C4, 5, 6) | Axillary nerve | Lower subscapular nerve (C6, 7) |
| Action | 1. Both these muscles are adductors and lateral rotators of the humerus<br>2. They stabilise the shoulder joint and strengthen the posterior part of the capsule<br>3. During abduction of the arm (by deltoid and supraspinatus) their downward pull neutralises the upward pull of the deltoid and prevents the head of the humerus from getting stuck under the coracoacromial arch. (The subscapularis has a similar role) | | 1. Adductor and medial rotator of arm<br>2. Helps in extension of arm<br>3. Aids abduction of the arm just like the infraspinatus<br>4. Strengthens capsule of shoulder joint and stabilises it |

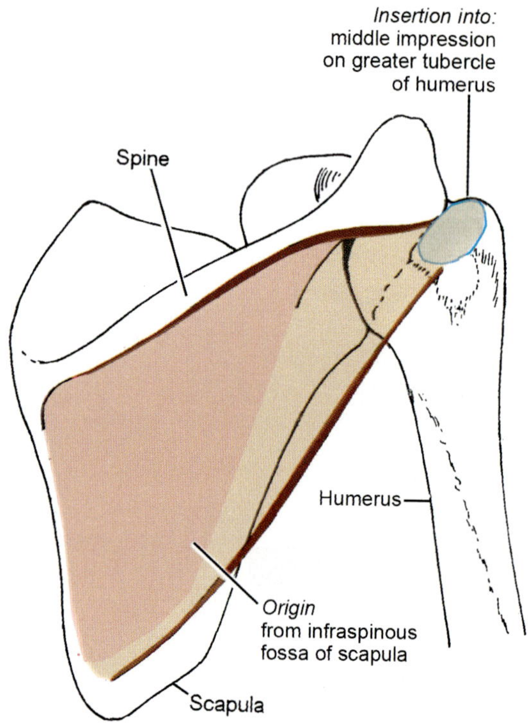


**4.16:** Attachments of the infraspinatus

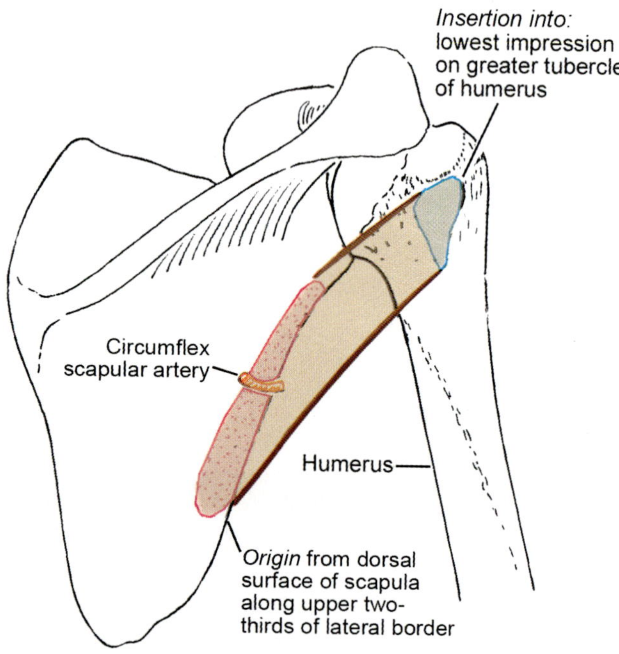


**4.17:** Attachments of the teres minor

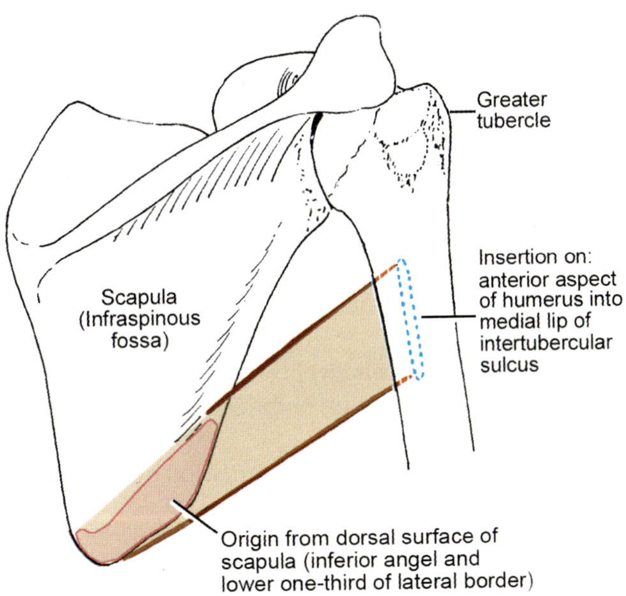


**4.18:** Attachments of the teres major

| **4.19: Subscapularis** | |
|---|---|
| Origin | Scapula, costal surface (medial two-thirds of subscapular fossa) |
| Insertion | Lesser tubercle of humerus |
| Nerve supply | Upper and lower subscapular nerves (C5, 6, 7) |
| Action | 1. Adductor and medial rotator of arm<br>2. Helps in extension of arm<br>3. Its downward pull on the humerus cancels the upward pull of the deltoid and allows smooth abduction of the arm<br>4. Strengthens capsule of shoulder joint and stabilises it<br>These actions are the same as those of the teres major |
| Notes | The subscapularis and teres major form the posterior wall of the axilla. The contents of the axilla lie over them |

## Musculotendinous Cuff of Shoulder

1. As the tendons of the subscapularis, teres minor, supraspinatus and infraspinatus approach their insertions they flatten and their edges unite with each other.
2. In this way a strong cuff (covering) is formed for the shoulder joint. This is an important factor in giving strength to the joint.
3. As these muscles are all rotators of the humerus, this structure is also called the ***rotator cuff***.

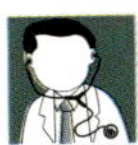

### CLINICAL CORRELATION

1. The cuff does not extend on to the inferior aspect of the shoulder joint, leaving a weak region through which dislocation of the head of the humerus can take place more easily than in any other direction.

2. ***Rupture of the tendinous cuff*** involves injury mainly to the supraspinatus tendon.
   a. It is more likely to occur in old persons because of degeneration with age.
   b. The patient is unable to initiate abduction at the shoulder joint, but can maintain it once the arm is partially abducted.
3. ***Strain of the supraspinatus*** is common in persons who have to work for long periods with the arms in slight abduction (e.g., typists). It can cause distressing and persistent pain.
4. The ***subacromial bursa*** lies deep to the coracoacromial arch and the adjoining part of the deltoid muscle.
   a. The bursa facilitates abduction at the shoulder joint.
   b. During overhead abduction, the greater tuberosity slips below the bursa and comes to lie deep to the acromion.
   c. When the bursa is inflamed (***subacromial bursitis***) pressure over the deltoid, just below the acromion elicits pain, but pain cannot be elicited after abduction of the arm (because the bursa is now under the acromion. This is called ***Dawbarn's sign***.
   d. Subacromial bursitis is usually associated with inflammation of the supraspinatus tendon.

## Quadrangular and Triangular Spaces

In 4.21 note the following:

1. The lower border of the teres minor is separated by a gap from the upper border of the teres major.
2. More anteriorly, the lower border of the subscapularis forms the upper boundary of the gap.
3. The gap mentioned above is divided into medial and lateral parts by the long head of the triceps.
4. The medial part is quadrangular in shape and is called the ***quadrangular space***. The lateral part of the gap is triangular in shape and is called the ***triangular space***.

### *The Quadrangular Space*

It boundaries are formed as follows:

1. Upper border, by the teres minor and the subscapularis.
2. Lower border, by the teres major.

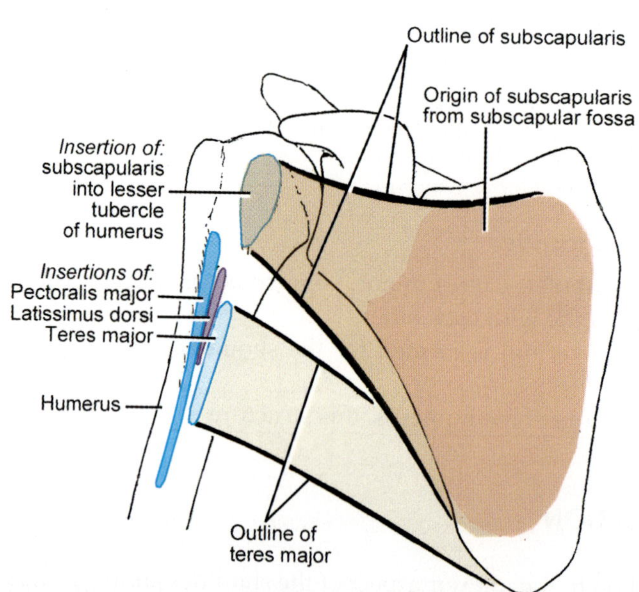


**4.20:** Attachments of the subscapularis. The teres major is also shown. Note the various insertions in the intertubercular sulcus

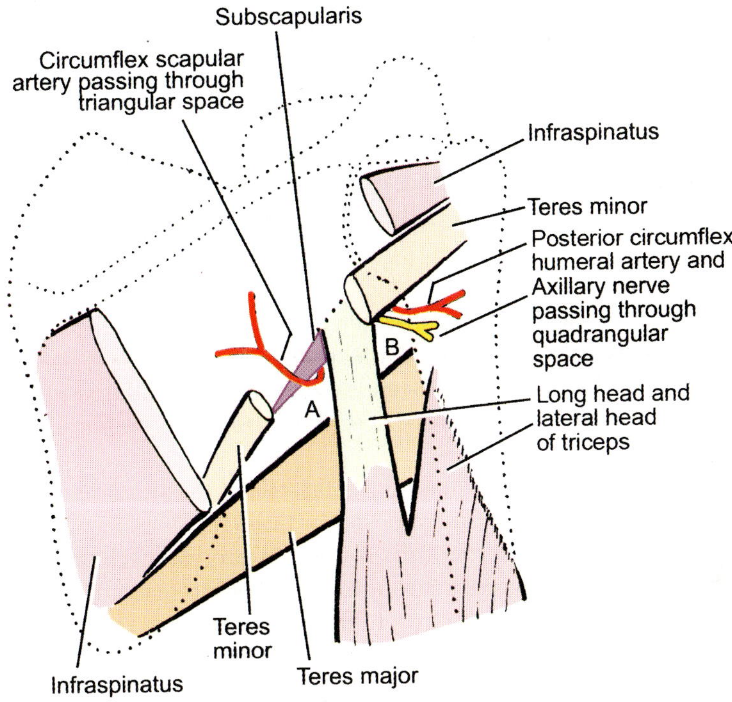


**4.21:** Diagram to show the triangular space (A), and the quadrangular space (B), of the scapular region

3. Medial border by the long head of the triceps.
4. Lateral border by the surgical neck of the humerus.

The structures passing through this space are:

1. The axillary nerve
2. The posterior circumflex humeral artery.

### *The Triangular Space*

1. Its upper and lower boundaries are the same as those of the quadrangular space.
2. Its lateral boundary is formed by the long head of the triceps.
3. The circumflex scapular branch of the subscapular artery passes through this space.

### *Lower Triangular Space*

1. Just below the teres major (in the arm) we see another triangular space between the humerus (laterally) and the long head of the triceps (medially).
2. Note that two very important structures i.e., the radial nerve and the profunda brachii artery pass through this space to reach the back of the arm.

## NERVES OF SCAPULAR REGION

1. The nerves of the scapular region are the upper and lower subscapular nerves, the suprascapular nerve and the axillary nerve.
2. The ***upper subscapular nerve*** arises from the posterior cord and supplies the subscapularis.
3. The ***lower subscapular nerve*** arises from the posterior cord. It supplies the teres major and also gives a branch to the subscapularis.

### The Suprascapular Nerve

1. The suprascapular nerve runs laterally and backwards over the shoulder (4.22). As it does so, it lies deep to the trapezius.
2. Reaching the upper border of the scapula it passes backwards through the suprascapular notch (below the transverse scapular ligament) to enter the supraspinous fossa and supplies the supraspinatus.
3. The nerve then enters the infraspinous fossa where it ends by supplying the infraspinatus. The nerve also gives branches to the shoulder joint ('a' in 4.22) and to the acromioclavicular joint ('b' in 4.22).

### The Axillary Nerve

1. The axillary nerve (4.23) supplies the deltoid and the teres minor. It is also called the circumflex humeral nerve and is a branch of the posterior cord of the brachial plexus.
2. At its origin it lies behind the axillary artery. It descends over the subscapularis, and reaching its lower border it passes backwards through the quadrangular space described above, in company with the posterior circumflex humeral artery.
3. As it passes through the space it is closely related to the capsule of the shoulder joint which lies above it.
4. The nerve ends by dividing into an anterior and a posterior branch.
   a. The ***anterior branch*** passes laterally and forwards round the surgical neck of the humerus and ends by supplying the deltoid. Some ramifications pass through the deltoid to reach the skin.
   b. The ***posterior branch*** supplies the posterior part of the deltoid and also the teres minor.
   c. Its terminal part becomes the ***upper lateral cutaneous nerve of the arm***. This nerve supplies the skin over the lower part of the deltoid muscle. (The skin over the upper part of the deltoid is supplied by the lateral supraclavicular nerves). The axillary nerve also gives a branch to the shoulder joint ('c' in 4.23).

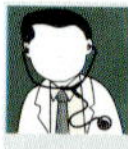

#### CLINICAL CORRELATION

The axillary nerve can be injured in a fracture through the surgical neck of the humerus. The deltoid is paralysed (See below).

## ARTERIES OF SCAPULAR REGION

1. In the back and scapular region we see some arteries that begin in the neck as (direct or indirect) branches of the subclavian artery.
2. Like the axillary artery, the subclavian artery is divided into first, second and third parts (by a muscle called the scalenus anterior).
3. A short artery called the ***thyrocervical trunk*** arises from the junction of the first and second parts of the subclavian artery (4.24A and B). The thyrocervical trunk divides into three branches as follows:
   a. The ***inferior thyroid artery*** is distributed only within the neck. It supplies the thyroid gland.
   b. The ***suprascapular artery*** descends into the scapular region and is described below.
   c. The distribution of the third branch of the thyrocervical trunk is variable, and depending on this, the artery is given alternative names. Both variants described below are almost equally common.
   d. In the first variant the third branch is called the ***transverse cervical artery***. It divides into a ***superficial branch***, (which is confined to the neck), and a ***deep branch*** which descends into the back in company with the dorsal scapular nerve.
   e. In the second variant the third branch of the subclavian artery is called the ***superficial cervical artery***.
      i. This artery supplies the same territory as the superficial branch of the transverse cervical artery.
      ii. When this is the case we find that the dorsal scapular nerve is accompanied by an artery arising directly from the third part of the subclavian artery: this is the ***dorsal scapular artery***.

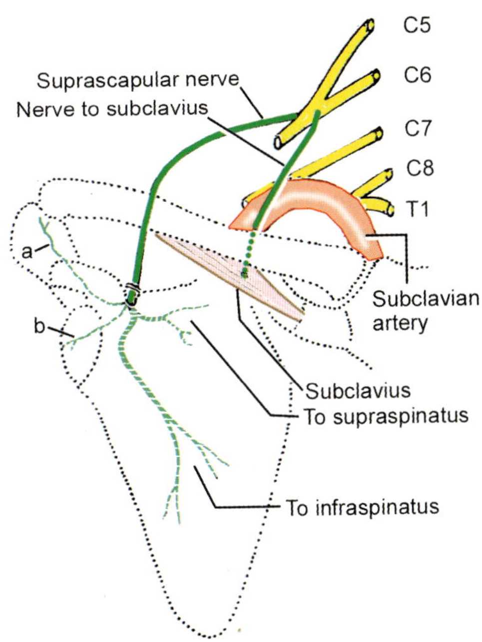


**4.22:** Scheme to show the course of the suprascapular nerve, and the nerve to the subclavius

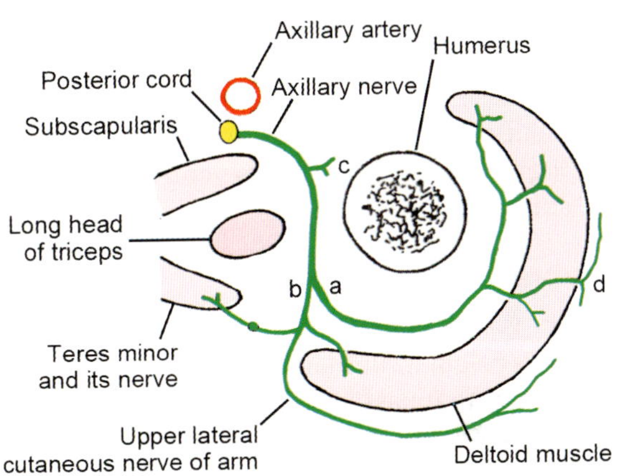


**4.23:** Scheme to show the course and distribution of the axillary nerve. a: anterior branch; b: posterior branch; c: branch to shoulder joint; d: cutaneous twig from anterior branch

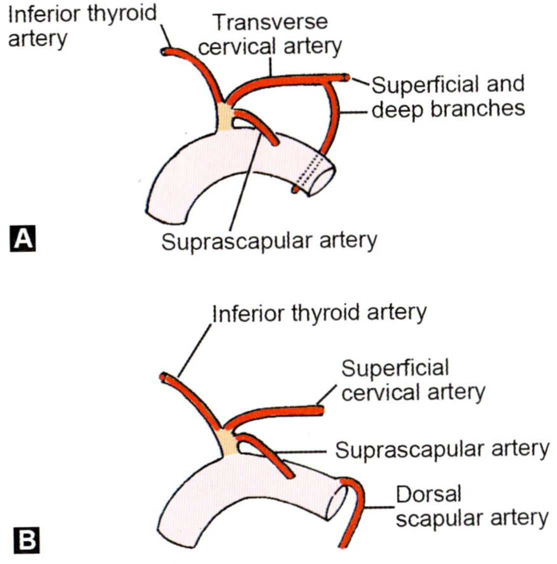


**4.24A and B:** Two patterns of branching of the thyrocervical trunk

### The Transverse Cervical Artery

This artery divides into superficial and deep branches.

1. The ***superficial branch*** of the artery (or, alternatively, the superficial cervical artery) runs laterally across the posterior triangle of the neck to reach the trapezius. It then ascends deep to the trapezius, supplying it and neighbouring structures.
2. The ***deep branch*** of the transverse cervical artery (or the dorsal scapular artery) passes laterally and backwards in the lower part of the posterior triangle of the neck to reach the upper angle of the scapula.
   a. It then runs along the medial border of this bone up to the inferior angle: in this part of its course it lies, at first deep to the levator scapulae, and then deep to the rhomboideus muscles.
   b. It supplies these muscles and the trapezius.
   c. It gives branches that pass ventral or dorsal to the scapula to anastomose with the suprascapular and subscapular arteries.

### The Suprascapular Artery

This artery is seen in both the neck and the upper limb.

1. From its origin it runs laterally behind the clavicle. It then passes backwards to reach the superior border of the scapula: here it passes above the transverse scapular ligament and enters the supraspinous fossa. After giving some branches to the supraspinatus it passes into the infraspinous fossa.
2. The muscles supplied by this artery are:
   a. Supraspinatus
   b. Infraspinatus
   c. Sternocleidomastoid
   d. Subclavius.
   e. A branch enters the subscapular fossa and supplies the subscapularis.
3. The suprascapular artery gives off cutaneous branches to the upper part of the chest (suprasternal branch) and to the acromial region (acromial branch).
4. Articular branches supply the shoulder joint and the acromioclavicular joint.
5. The artery also establishes several anastomoses as described below.

#### *Anastomosis around the Scapula*

1. On the back of the body of the scapula the suprascapular artery anastomoses with the deep branch of the transverse cervical artery and with the circumflex scapular branch of the subscapular artery (4.25).
2. On the ventral surface of the body of the scapula, branches of the suprascapular artery anastomose with the subscapular artery and with the deep branch of the transverse cervical artery.
3. Over the acromion branches of the suprascapular artery anastomose with the thoracoacromial and posterior circumflex humeral arteries.

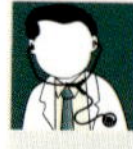

### CLINICAL CORRELATION

1. It may be noted that the anastomoses around the scapula described above connect the first part of the subclavian artery to the third part of the axillary artery.
2. They serve as collateral channels in case of obstruction to the arterial trunk between these levels.
3. The collaterals take time to become effective and are useful in gradual obstruction of the artery.
4. If the axillary artery has to be ligated the collateral circulation may be inadequate.

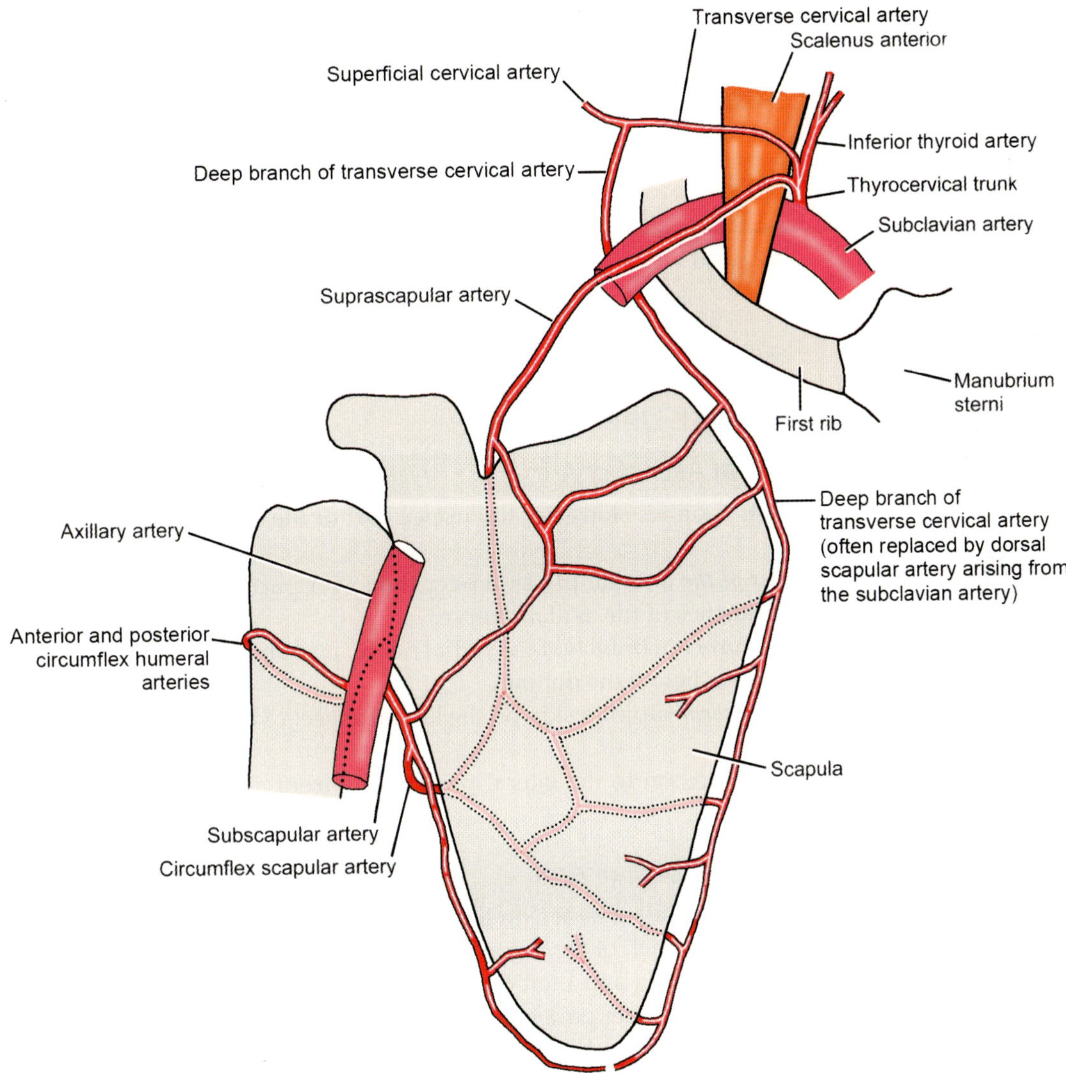


**4.25:** Anastomoses around the scapula

# 5 CHAPTER

# Cutaneous Nerves and Veins of the Free Upper Limb

## CUTANEOUS NERVES OF THE FREE UPPER LIMB

### *Cutaneous Nerves Supplying Lateral Aspect of Arm*

1. The ***lateral supraclavicular nerve***. It supplies skin over the upper part of the deltoid muscle (5.1 and 5.2).
2. The ***upper lateral cutaneous nerves of the arm*** supply skin over the lower part of the deltoid. These are terminal branches of the axillary nerve.
3. The ***lower lateral cutaneous nerve of arm*** is a branch of the radial nerve. It supplies skin over the lateral aspect of the arm below the deltoid.
4. The ***lateral cutaneous nerve of the forearm*** supplies skin on the lateral aspect of the arm near the cubital fossa (See below).

The area of supply of these nerves extends on to the lateral parts of the front and back of the arm also.

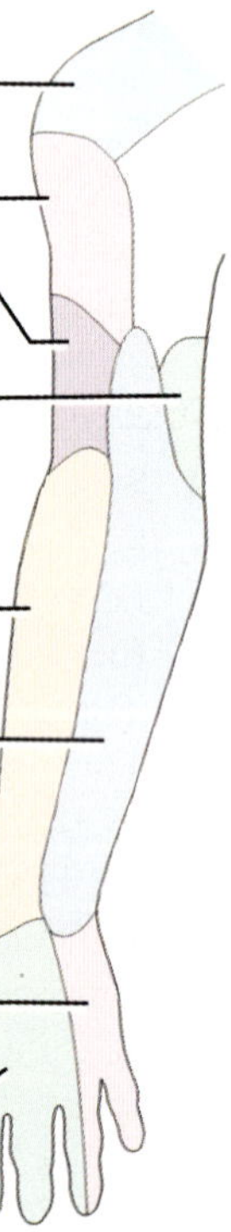

**5.1:** Cutaneous nerve supply of the front of the upper extremity

### *Cutaneous Nerves Supplying Medial Aspect of Arm*

1. The ***intercostobrachial nerve*** supplies a small area of skin adjoining the axilla.
   a. This nerve is the lateral cutaneous branch of the second intercostal nerve.
   b. It supplies skin on the floor of the axilla and then descends into the arm to supply skin on the medial side of the upper part of the arm.
2. The ***medial cutaneous nerve of the arm*** is a branch of the medial cord of the brachial plexus.
   a. It runs downwards first on the medial side of the axillary vein and then on the medial side of the basilic vein.
   b. It supplies skin on the medial side of the lower one-third of the arm.
3. The ***medial cutaneous nerve of the forearm*** supplies the medial aspect of the arm near the cubital fossa (See below).

### *Cutaneous Nerves Supplying the Front of the Arm*

1. The greater part of the skin on the front of the arm is supplied by the nerves supplying the lateral and medial aspects (as noted above).
2. A broad strip on the front of the arm is supplied by branches of the medial cutaneous nerve of the forearm.

### *Cutaneous Nerves Supplying the Back of the Arm*

1. On the posterior aspect of the arm also the main supply is by nerves supplying the medial and lateral aspects (named above).
2. Over the middle of the back of the arm a strip of skin is innervated by the posterior cutaneous nerve of the arm (branch of radial nerve), and lower down by the posterior cutaneous nerve of the forearm (branch of radial nerve).

### Cutaneous Nerves Supplying the Front of the Forearm

1. The ***lateral cutaneous nerve of the forearm*** is a continuation of the musculocutaneous nerve. It supplies skin over the lateral aspect and front of the forearm. Its lowest part supplies the skin of the thenar eminence.
2. The ***medial cutaneous nerve of the forearm*** is a branch of the medial cord of the brachial plexus.
   a. The nerve runs downwards on the medial side of the axillary artery (between it and the axillary vein), and then on the medial side of the brachial artery.
   b. It becomes superficial in the middle of the arm. It gives some branches to the skin on the front of the arm and then divides into anterior and posterior branches that run on the corresponding aspects of the medial part of the forearm.

### Cutaneous Nerves Supplying the Back of the Forearm

1. The medial and lateral parts of the back of the forearm are supplied by the nerves already seen from the front (medial and lateral cutaneous nerves of the forearm).
2. The greater part of the skin of the back of the forearm is supplied by the posterior cutaneous nerve of the forearm. Small areas of skin of the forearm supplied by other nerves are shown in 5.1 and 5.2.

Supraclavicular nerves from cervical plexus
Upper lateral cutaneous nerve of arm
Medial cutaneous nerve of arm
Posterior cutaneous nerve of arm
Lower lateral cutaneous nerve of arm
Posterior cutaneous nerve of forearm
Medial cutaneous nerve of forearm
Lateral cutaneous nerve of forearm
Dorsal digital branch of radial nerve
By ulnar nerve
By branch from median nerve

**5.2:** Cutaneous nerve supply of the back of the upper extremity

### Cutaneous Nerve Supply of the Hand

1. Small parts of the hand near the wrist are supplied by cutaneous nerves of the forearm (5.1 and 5.2). In front, these are the lateral and medial cutaneous nerves of the forearm; and behind there is the posterior cutaneous nerve of the forearm.
2. The greater part of the hand is, however, supplied by cutaneous branches of the ***median***, ***ulnar*** and ***radial*** nerves.
3. The skin on the palmar aspect of the hand is supplied mainly by branches of the ulnar and median nerves (5.3A).
   a. The ulnar nerve supplies the medial one and half digits and the corresponding part of the palm.
   b. The rest of the palmar aspect is supplied by branches of the median nerve.
4. The nerve supply of the skin on the dorsum of the hand is shown in 5.3B.
   a. Note that the dorsal aspects of the terminal phalanges of each digit are supplied by nerves that wind round from the palmar aspect. As a result the nerve supply of these phalanges is the same as on the palmar aspect as follows.

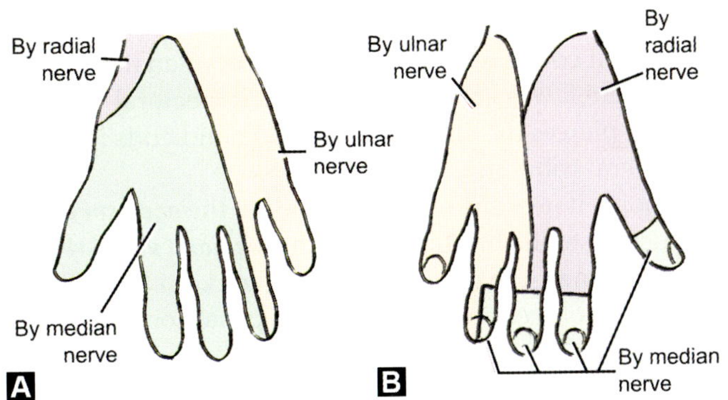


**5.3A and B:** Cutaneous nerve supply of the hand. (A) Palmar aspect; (B) Dorsal aspect

b. Over the medial one and a half fingers the supply is by the ulnar nerve, and over the other digits it is by the median nerve.
c. The rest of the dorsum of the hand is supplied in its lateral half (or so) by the radial nerve, and in its medial half (or so) by the ulnar nerve (See 5.2 carefully).

5. Finally, note that the ulnar nerve supplies the medial part of the hand, on both the palmar and dorsal aspects. The supply to the lateral part of the hand is by the median nerve on the palmar aspect, and mainly by the radial nerve on the dorsal aspect.

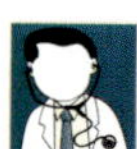

**CLINICAL CORRELATION**

1. Testing the integrity of the nerves supplying the skin is helpful in diagnosis of injury to a peripheral nerve.
2. When the integrity of spinal nerve roots or of the spinal cord itself is to be investigated it is more useful to know the segmental nerve supply of the skin. This has been considered in Chapter 3.

## VEINS OF THE UPPER LIMB

The venous drainage of the limbs is carried out through two separate sets of veins.

a. Most of the blood is returned through ***superficial veins*** that lie in the superficial fascia and have no relationship to the arteries of the limb.
b. The other set, the ***deep veins***, run along the arteries.

### Superficial Veins

The superficial veins of the upper limb are subject to considerable variation. The descriptions below refer to the commonest patterns only.

1. The fingers are drained by two sets of digital veins: dorsal and ventral (5.4).
   a. The ***dorsal digital veins*** from the adjoining sides of the medial four digits end by forming three ***dorsal metacarpal veins*** which in turn join each other to form a ***dorsal venous network*** over the dorsum of the hand.
   b. The network is joined by digital veins from the thumb, the radial side of the index finger and from the ulnar side of the little finger (5.4).
   c. The palmar digital veins drain into a superficial plexus in the palm.
   d. The veins of the hand are further drained by two main superficial veins. These are the cephalic and basilic veins.
2. The ***cephalic vein*** begins from the lateral side of the venous network on the dorsum of the hand (5.5).
   a. It ascends along the radial border of the forearm: in the lower part of the forearm it is on the posterior aspect, but winds round the radial border to reach the anterior surface.
   b. Crossing in front of the lateral part of the elbow it runs upwards in the arm along the lateral side of the biceps brachii.
   c. In the upper part of the arm, it comes to lie in the groove between the anterior margin of the deltoid muscle and the pectoralis major (Here it was earlier called the deltopectoral vein).
   d. A little below the clavicle it pierces the clavipectoral fascia and ends in the axillary vein.
3. The cephalic vein receives several tributaries along its course.
   a. One of these is large and joins it near the elbow: it is called the ***accessory cephalic vein*** (5.5).
   b. The cephalic vein is connected to the basilic vein by the ***median cubital vein*** (See below).
4. The ***basilic vein*** begins from the ulnar side of the venous network on the dorsum of the hand (5.4, 5.5).
   a. It ascends along the ulnar side of the forearm, first on its posterior aspect and then winding round the ulnar border to reach the anterior aspect.
   b. Crossing in front of the medial part of the elbow it runs upwards along the medial side of the biceps brachii muscle.
   c. At about the middle of the arm it pierces the deep fascia and comes to lie medial to the brachial artery. It ascends in this position up to the lower border of the teres major where it becomes the axillary vein.

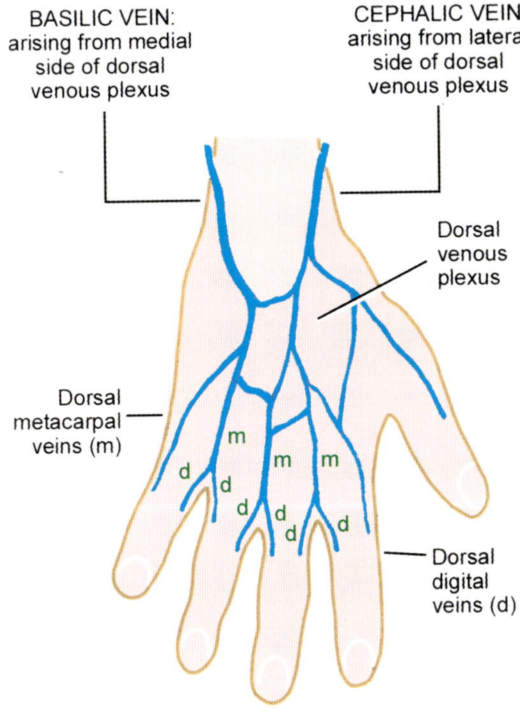


5.4: Veins on the dorsum of the hand

5. The ***median cubital vein*** (5.5) lies in front of the elbow joint.
   a. It passes upwards and medially from the cephalic vein to the basilic vein.
   b. It is often the largest vein in the region and is frequently used for taking blood samples or for giving intravenous injections and blood transfusions.
6. The ***palmar venous plexus*** is drained by the ***median vein of the forearm*** (5.5). This vein ascends on the front of the forearm and ends in the basilic vein or the median cubital vein.

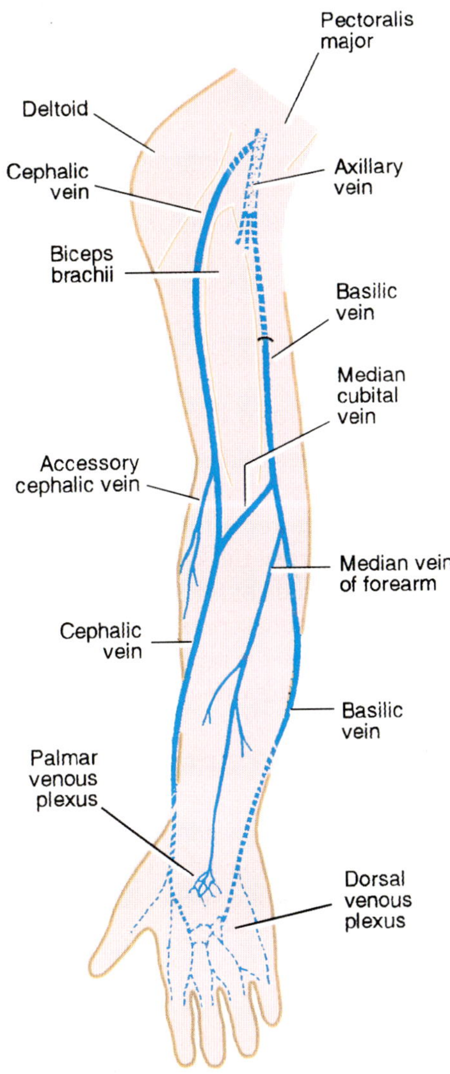


5.5: Superficial veins of the upper limb

## Deep Veins

1. The deep veins accompany the arteries of the limb. They are small in calibre and are often paired and may form plexuses around the arteries they accompany. Such veins are called ***venae comitantes***.
2. They are found in relation to the palmar digital and palmar metacarpal arteries, the dorsal metacarpal arteries, the superficial and deep palmar arches, the radial and ulnar arteries, anterior and posterior interosseous arteries and the brachial artery.
3. The veins accompanying the brachial artery are joined (near the lower border of the teres major) by the basilic vein to form the axillary vein.

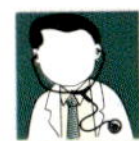

### CLINICAL CORRELATION

1. The anatomy of the superficial veins of the upper limb is important as they are commonly used for withdrawal of blood, intravenous infusions, and more sophisticated procedures like cardiac catheterization. The median cubital vein is frequently used but any other easily located vein may be used.

2. After serious injury (and some other causes) a patient goes into a state of shock. The blood pressure falls and veins may not be visible. In such a case it is useful to remember that the cephalic vein lies just behind the styloid process of the ulna.
3. A vein canulated for infusion may develop ***thrombosis*** (clot formation).
4. Thrombosis accompanied by inflammation is called ***thrombophlebitis***. In this condition the vein concerned is seen as a painful cord-like inflamed area.
5. A vein can be damaged by direct injury or even by unaccustomed movement. For example, working for long periods with an arm raised can result in thrombosis in the axillary vein.

## ANTERIOR COMPARTMENT OF THE ARM

### Compartments of the Arm

1. For purposes of description the arm can be divided into anterior and posterior compartments. These are best visualised in a transverse section (5.6).
2. Deep structures in the arm are enveloped by deep fascia that keeps them in place.
3. In the centre of the section we see the humerus that has been cut across.
   a. Two bands of fascia, the ***medial*** and ***lateral intermuscular septa***, pass from the deep fascia to the humerus.
   b. These septa separate structures lying in the anterior compartment from those in the posterior compartment.
   c. However, the septa extend proximally only to about the middle of the arm, and above this level separation of the compartments is incomplete.

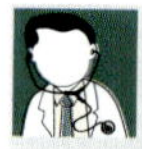

### CLINICAL CORRELATION

1. In a condition called ***compartment syndrome*** increasing oedema in a fascial compartment of a limb can lead to severe ischaemia, which is characterised by much pain.
2. Failure to recognise the condition can lead to destruction of muscle tissue and fibrosis.
3. The condition is treated by giving incisions in fascia enclosing the compartment, to relieve pressure.

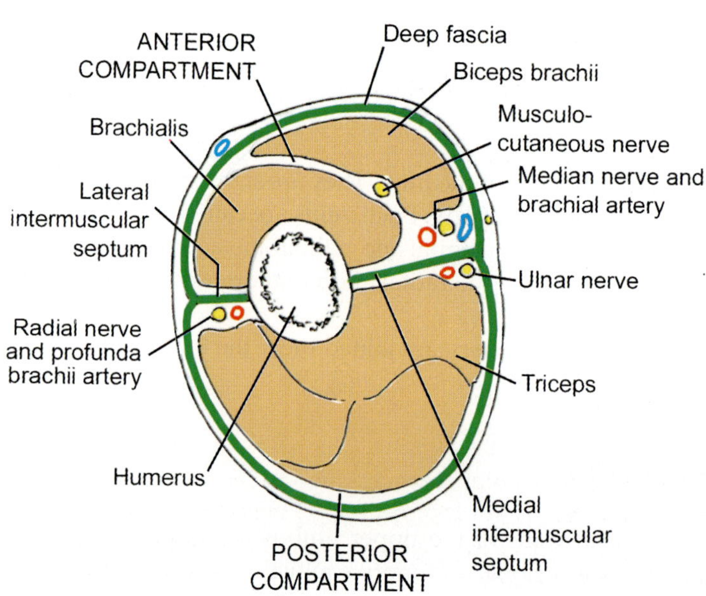


**5.6:** Compartments of the arm

## Muscles of the Anterior Compartment of the Arm

These are listed in 5.7. For illustrations see figures 5.8 and 5.9.

### *Notes on Biceps Brachii*

1. The tendon of the long head arches over the head of the humerus to enter the intertubercular sulcus.
   a. This part of the tendon lies within the cavity of the shoulder joint and is surrounded by a tubular sheath of synovial membrane.
   b. This sheath is prolonged into the intertubercular sulcus.
2. At its lower end the tendon of the biceps brachii dips backwards to be inserted into the posterior part of the tuberosity of the radius. A bursa intervenes between the tendon and the anterior part of the tuberosity and facilitates movement.
3. The muscle crosses three joints viz., shoulder, elbow, and superior radioulnar. It can, therefore, act on all of them.
4. Supination is powerful only when the forearm is semiflexed (because in this position the lowest part of the tendon is in straight line with the rest of the muscle).

**5.7: Muscles of the anterior compartment of the arm**

| *Muscle* | *Biceps Brachii* | *Coracobrachialis* | *Brachialis* |
|---|---|---|---|
| Origin | 1. Long head from supraglenoid tubercle (on scapula)<br>2. Short head from tip of coracoid process (together with coracobrachialis)<br>The two heads fuse to form a large belly which ends in a tendon | Tip of coracoid process (scapula) (in common with short head of biceps brachii) | 1. Front of lower half of humerus (anteromedial and anterolateral surfaces)<br>2. Intermuscular septa |
| Insertion | Tuberosity of radius (posterior part) | Medial border of humerus (near middle of shaft) | Anterior surface of coronoid process of ulna, including tuberosity. |
| Nerve supply | Musculocutaneous nerve (C5,6) | Musculocutaneous nerve (C5, 6, 7) | 1. Musculocutaneous nerve (C5,6).<br>2. Radial nerve (C7) (lateral part) |
| Action | 1. Flexion of arm at shoulder (short head)<br>2. Long head keeps head of humerus in place during movements of the arm<br>3. Flexion of forearm (at elbow)<br>4. Supination of forearm | Flexor of arm | Flexor of forearm at elbow joint |

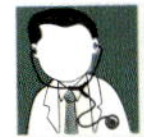

### CLINICAL CORRELATION

1. The tendon (of origin) of the long head of the biceps brachii lies within the capsule of the shoulder joint. In osteoarthritis of this joint abnormal irregular projections develop from the bones concerned and friction against them can lead to inflammation (***tendinitis***). There is pain in the shoulder.
2. Damage to the tendon can end in ***rupture***.

3. The ***biceps tendon reflex*** is elicited by a tap on the biceps tendon.
   a. The examiner places his thumb over the tendon and gives a tap on his thumb.
   b. There is reflex contraction of the biceps.
   c. The reflex is lost in injury to the musculocutaneous nerve, or to spinal segments: C5 and C6. It is exaggerated in upper motor neuron paralysis (hemiplegia).

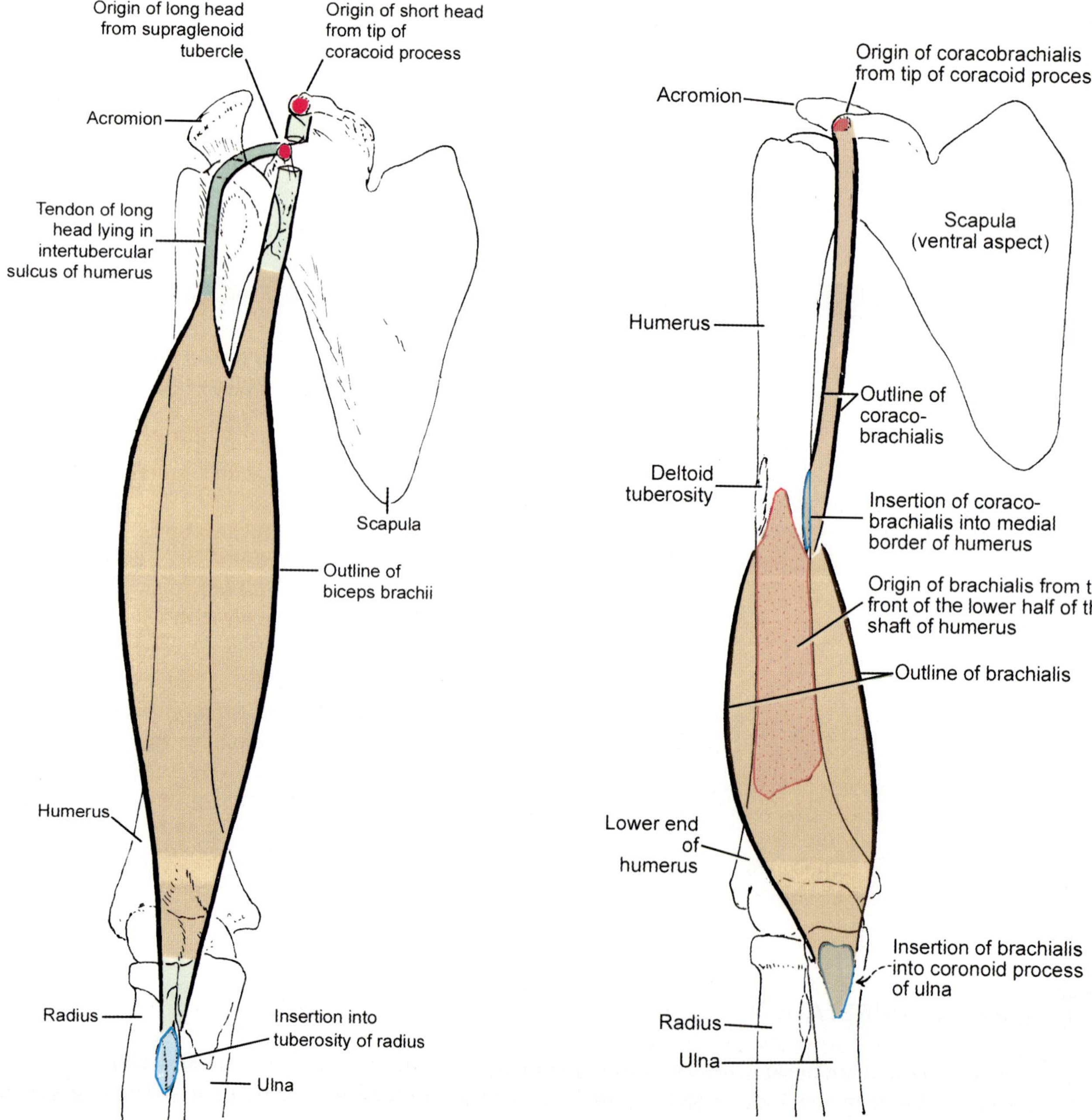


**5.8:** Scheme to show the attachments of the biceps brachii

**5.9:** Scheme to show the attachments of the coracobrachialis and brachialis muscles

## THE BRACHIAL ARTERY

1. This is the main artery of the arm. It begins at the lower border of the teres major as the continuation of the axillary artery.
2. Its upper part lies on the medial aspect of the arm. As it descends it gradually passes forwards, so that its lower end lies in front of the elbow.
3. Here it terminates (at the level of the neck of the radius) by dividing into the radial and ulnar arteries.
4. The relations of the artery are considered below.

### Relationship to Muscles

1. From above downwards the artery lies successively on:
   a. The long head of the triceps.
   b. The medial head of the triceps.
   c. The brachialis.
2. Anterolaterally, it is related to the coracobrachialis and the medial margin of the biceps brachii.
   a. Its lowest part lies medial to the biceps tendon.
   b. The bicipital aponeurosis, passes medially across the artery.
   c. The lowest part of the artery lies in the cubital fossa.

### Relationship to Nerves

1. The uppermost part of the artery is related to the same nerves that surround the third part of the axillary artery.
   a. The radial nerve is posterior to it.
   b. The median nerve is lateral to it.
   c. The ulnar nerve is medial to it (5.10).
2. The radial nerve is related only to the uppermost part of the brachial artery: it separates from the artery by passing posterior to the humerus.
3. The median nerve descends along the lateral side of the upper half of the artery. It then crosses in front of the artery and comes to lie along its medial side.
4. The ulnar nerve lies medial to the upper half of the artery. Lower down it parts company from the artery as it pierces the medial intermuscular septum to enter the posterior compartment of the arm.

### Relationship to Veins

1. The brachial artery is accompanied throughout its length by small veins (venae comitantes).
2. The basilic vein comes to lie medial to the artery a little above the elbow (5.11), but is separated from it by deep fascia.
   a. The vein pierces the deep fascia near the middle of the arm, and thereafter ascends in close company with the artery.
   b. At the upper end of the brachial artery the venae comitantes join the basilic vein to form the axillary vein.
3. Note that there is no 'brachial' vein.

### Branches of the Brachial Artery

The branches given off by the brachial artery are the following (5.12):

1. The ***profunda brachii artery*** lies mainly in the posterior compartment of the arm. It is described here to provide a compact account of the branches of the brachial artery.
   a. This artery arises a little below the upper end of the brachial artery.
   b. Accompanying the radial nerve it passes laterally and downwards behind the humerus, where it lies in the radial groove. It gives off the following branches:
      i. A ***nutrient artery*** is given off to the humerus.
      ii. The ***ascending branch*** anastomoses with the descending branch of the posterior circumflex humeral artery.

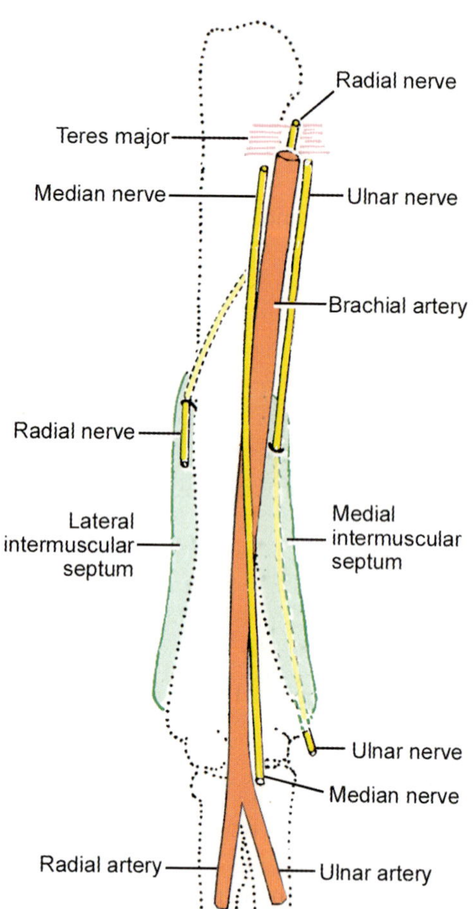


**5.10:** Diagram showing nerves related to the brachial artery

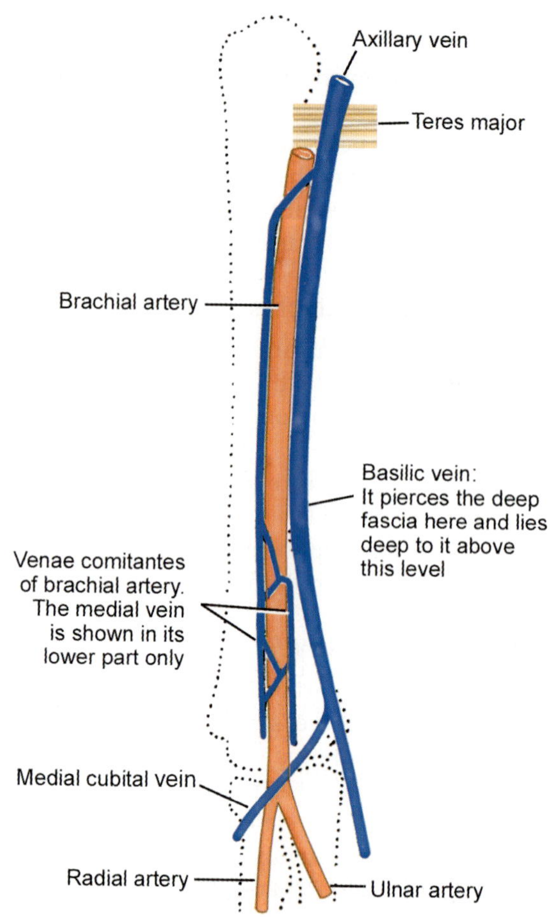


**5.11:** Diagram showing veins related to the brachial artery

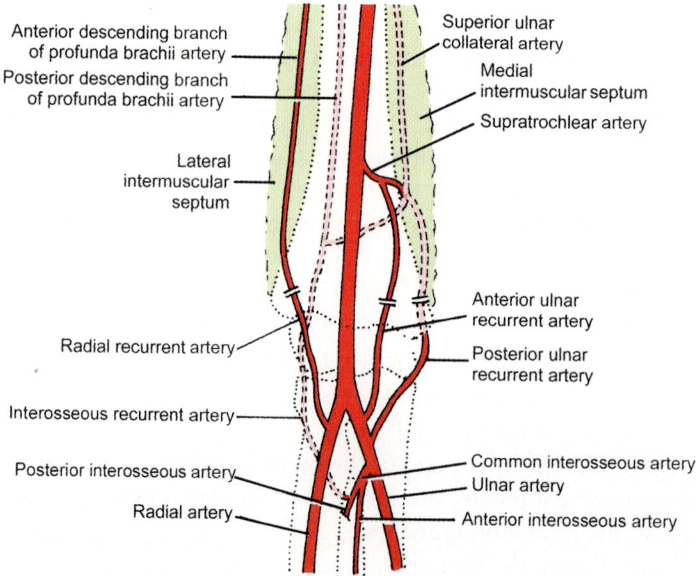


**5.12:** Anastomoses around the elbow

iii. ***The posterior descending*** (or middle collateral) branch descends in the substance of the medial head of the triceps and anastomoses with the recurrent branch of the posterior interosseous artery.
iv. The ***anterior descending*** (or radial collateral) artery pierces the lateral intermuscular septum and enters the anterior compartment of the arm. It runs along the radial nerve in the lower lateral part of the arm and ends by anastomosing with the recurrent branch of the radial artery.

2. The ***superior ulnar collateral artery*** arises near the middle of the arm.
   a. Accompanying the ulnar nerve this artery pierces the medial intermuscular septum to enter the posterior compartment of the arm.
   b. It runs downwards to reach the back of the medial epicondyle.
   c. The artery ends by anastomosing with the posterior recurrent branch of the ulnar artery and with the supratrochlear artery.
3. The ***supratrochlear artery*** (or inferior ulnar collateral artery) arises from the brachial artery a little above the elbow (5.12).
   a. It first passes medially and then backwards (piercing the medial intermuscular septum).
   b. It then runs laterally behind the humerus and anastomoses with the posterior descending branch of the profunda brachii artery and with the interosseous recurrent artery.
   c. Before piercing the medial intermuscular septum it gives off a branch that descends to anastomose with the anterior recurrent branch of the ulnar artery.
4. In addition to the branches described above the brachial artery and its branches give off numerous ***muscular branches***.
5. ***Nutrient arteries*** to the humerus are given off by the brachial artery itself and by the profunda brachii branch.
6. At its lower end the brachial artery terminates by dividing into the ***radial and ulnar arteries***. These descend into the forearm and will be studied there.

In 5.12 note the arteries helping to form the arterial anastomoses around the elbow joint.

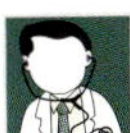

## CLINICAL CORRELATION

1. To compress the ***brachial artery*** apply lateral pressure over the medial side of the arm immediately posterior to the medial margin of the biceps brachii. The artery is pressed against the humerus.
2. Compression of the brachial artery may occur in fracture of the shaft of the humerus (especially in supracondylar fracture) or in dislocation of the elbow joint.
3. Fractures are very often immobilised by applying plaster casts around the affected part. A plaster cast that is too tight can be a cause of ischaemia and results can be serious if the condition is not recognised in time.
4. The anastomoses around the elbow joint (5.12) are of importance in the event of obstruction to the brachial artery near its lower end.
5. The brachial artery is used for measurement of blood pressure.
   a. An inflatable cuff is tied round the arm.
   b. A stethoscope is placed on the brachial artery as it lies in the cubital fossa.
   c. The cuff is inflated until the brachial artery is compressed and blood flow is cut off.
   d. The pressure is slowly decreased till blood begins to flow again.
   e. Characteristic sounds heard through the stethoscope enable estimation of systolic and diastolic pressure.

***Volkmann's Ischaemic Contracture***

1. Spasm of the brachial artery can follow fractures in the region of the elbow. This reduces blood supply to muscles of the forearm, and ultimately leads to their fibrosis.
2. A similar condition can occur if the brachial artery is occluded for any reason.
3. Ischaemia caused by sudden occlusion of the artery results in paralysis of muscles.
   a. Fibrosis shortens muscles and leads to deformities of the wrist and digits.

b. The deformity seen depends on the relative extent to which the flexor and extensor muscles are shortened.
c. Typically, there is greater shortening of flexors. The wrist is flexed, but the fingers are extended. Other types of deformity may exist.

## NERVES OF THE FRONT OF THE ARM

The main nerves to be seen on the front of the arm are the musculocutaneous nerve, the median nerve, the ulnar nerve and the upper part of the radial nerve.

### Musculocutaneous Nerve

1. The ***musculocutaneous nerve*** is a branch of the lateral cord of the brachial plexus. The nerve pierces the coracobrachialis and then runs downwards and laterally through the front of the arm: here the biceps is superficial to it and the brachialis is deep to it (5.13).
2. Reaching the lateral side of the arm it crosses in front of the lateral side of the elbow to enter the forearm. Here the nerve becomes superficial and is called the ***lateral cutaneous nerve of the forearm***. As implied by its name the musculocutaneous nerve is distributed partly to muscles and partly to skin.
   a. The muscles supplied are the coracobrachialis, the biceps brachii (both heads) and the brachialis. (Note that the brachialis also receives a supply from the radial nerve).
   b. As the lateral cutaneous nerve of the forearm it supplies the skin of the lateral half of the front of the forearm, and also along its lateral border. Its lowest part supplies the skin of the thenar eminence.

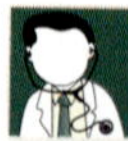

**CLINICAL CORRELATION**

Injury to the musculocutaneous nerve results in paralysis of muscles supplied. The bicipital tendon reflex is lost. There is loss of sensation over the lateral side of the forearm.

### The Median Nerve

1. The ***median nerve*** is formed by union of lateral and medial roots that arise from the corresponding cords of the brachial plexus.
2. Its upper end lies in the axilla, lateral to the axillary artery. It continues into the arm lateral to the brachial artery.
3. Near the middle of the arm it crosses superficial to the artery to reach its medial side, and descends in this position to the cubital fossa.
4. The nerve leaves the cubital fossa by passing between the superficial and deep heads of the pronator teres. Its course and distribution in the forearm and hand will be considered in Chapter 6.
5. The branches given off in the arm are as follows:
   a. A branch to the pronator teres ( a muscle of the forearm) arises in the lower part of the arm.
   b. Articular branches arising near the elbow supply the elbow joint and the superior radioulnar joint.
6. Note that the median nerve does not supply any muscle in the arm.

### The Ulnar Nerve

1. The ***ulnar nerve*** is a branch of the medial cord of the brachial plexus. It extends from the axilla to the hand.
2. At its origin the nerve lies medial to the axillary artery (between it and the axillary vein). It runs down into the front of the arm where it lies medial to the brachial artery.

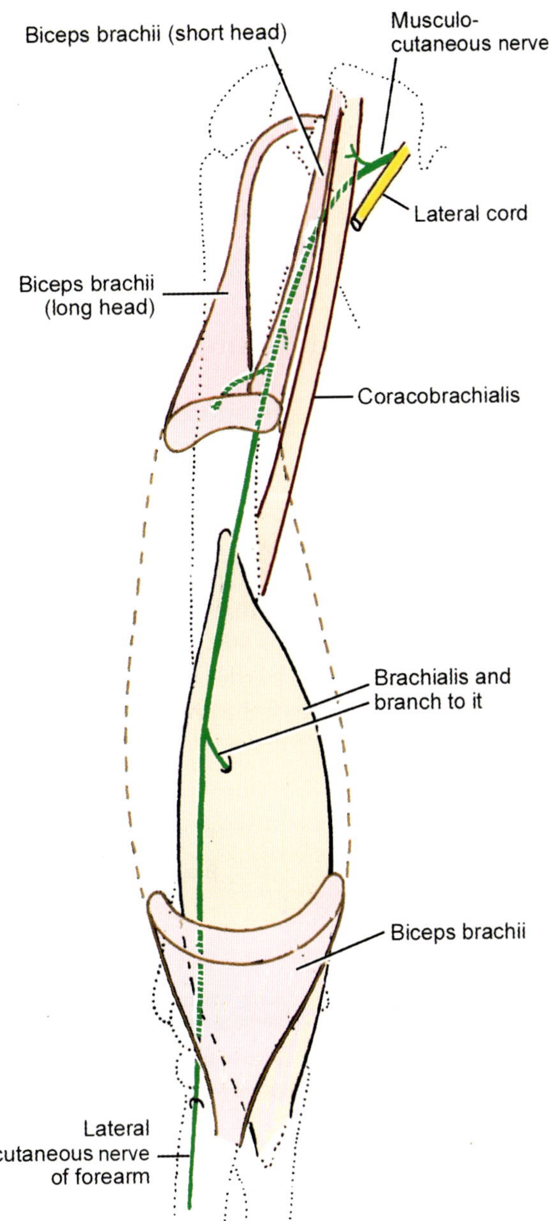


**5.13:** Scheme to show the course and distribution of the musculocutaneous nerve. For areas of skin supplied by the lateral cutaneous nerve of the forearm see 5.1

3. At the middle of the arm the nerve passes into the posterior compartment by piercing the medial intermuscular septum, and descends between this septum and the lower part of the triceps (medial head).
4. Passing medially as it descends it passes behind the medial epicondyle of the humerus.
5. The nerve enters the forearm by passing deep to the tendinous arch joining the humeral and ulnar heads of the flexor carpi ulnaris (a muscle of the forearm).
6. The ulnar nerve does not give off any branches in the arm. Its course and distribution in the forearm and hand will be considered in Chapter 6.

## The Radial Nerve

The ***radial nerve*** is seen for a short distance in the front of the arm. It then enters the back of the arm. Its complete course and branches in the arm will be considered while describing the posterior compartment of the arm.

## CUBITAL FOSSA

1. The region where the front of the arm becomes continuous with the front of the forearm is marked by a triangular depression called the cubital fossa. (Cubit = elbow).
2. In the fossa we will see some structures belonging to the arm (described in this chapter) and some belonging to the forearm (considered in Chapter 6).
3. For descriptive purposes the fossa can be said to have a roof, a floor, and superior, medial and lateral boundaries (5.14 and 5.15).
4. The ***roof*** of the fossa is formed by overlying fascia. The structures that lie within this fascia are:
   a. The cephalic vein
   b. The basilic vein
   c. The median cubital vein
   d. The median vein of the forearm
   e. We also see the medial and lateral cutaneous nerves of the forearm.
5. The ***superior boundary*** of the fossa is formed by an imaginary line connecting the medial and lateral epicondyles of the humerus (5.14).
6. ***Laterally***, the cubital fossa is bounded by the medial border of the ***brachioradialis***.
7. ***Medially***, the fossa is bounded by the lateral margin of the ***pronator teres***.

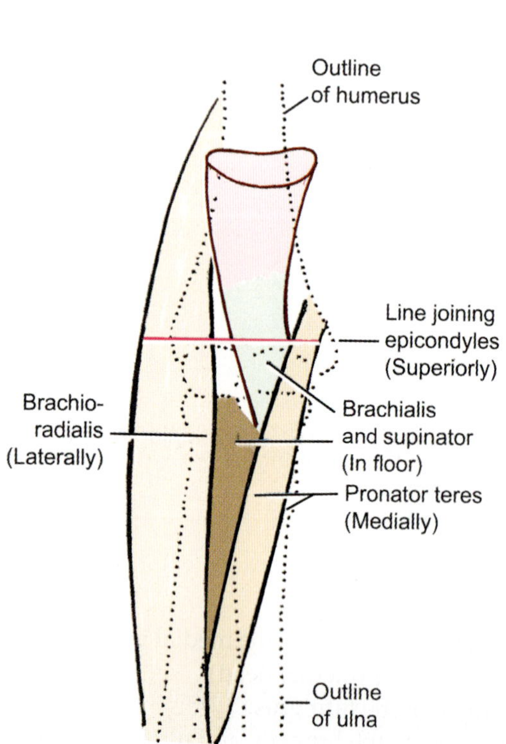


**5.14:** Boundaries of the cubital fossa

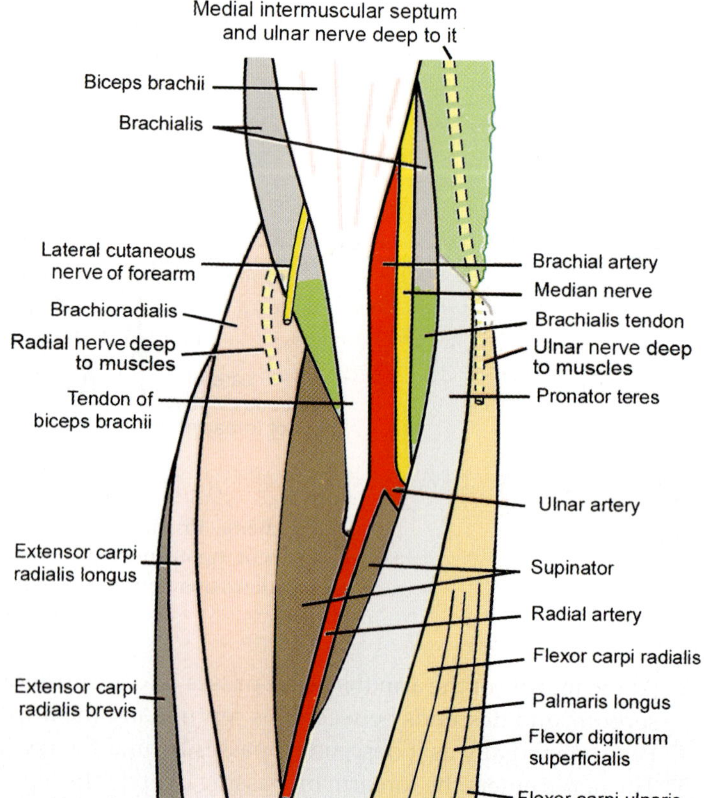


**5.15:** Cubital fossa after removal of superficial structures. The radial nerve and the ulnar nerve lie deep to muscles. Their position is indicated diagrammatically

8. The ***apex*** of the fossa lies inferiorly and is formed by crossing of the brachioradialis across the front of the pronator teres (5.14).
9. The ***floor*** of the fossa is formed by the lower end of the brachialis, above, and by the ***supinator*** muscle, below.
10. The ***contents of the fossa*** are as follows:
    a. The most prominent content of the fossa is the tendon of the biceps brachii (along with the bicipital aponeurosis).
    b. Medial to the tendon there is the lower end of the brachial artery. The brachial artery divides into the radial and ulnar arteries within the fossa. Note that the ulnar artery is the larger of the two. The radial artery runs downwards to reach the apex of the fossa.
    c. The median nerve lies medial to the brachial artery. The median nerve gives off several branches in the cubital fossa. They supply several muscles of the front of the forearm (including the pronator teres).
    d. The pronator teres has two heads. The main part of the muscle is called the superficial head. The deep head is in the form of a small slip. The median nerve descends into the forearm ***through the interval between*** the superficial and deep heads.
    e. As the ulnar artery descends, it passes ***deep to*** the deep head of the pronator teres. The deep head separates the median nerve from the ulnar artery.
    f. In the lateral part of the fossa we see the radial nerve and some of its branches.
11. The radial nerve enters the region by passing forwards in the interval between the brachialis (medially) and the ***brachioradialis*** (laterally).
    a. Here it gives branches to both these muscles, and also to the ***extensor carpi radialis longus***.
    b. The radial nerve then divides into superficial and deep branches.
    c. The superficial branch descends into the front of the forearm.
    d. The deep branch enters the substance of the supinator muscle (and while within the muscle) winds round the radius to reach the back of the forearm. (The deep branch is also called the posterior interosseous nerve).
12. Many structures mentioned above will be described fully in Chapter 6. The radial nerve is considered further below.

## POSTERIOR COMPARTMENT OF THE ARM

1. The cutaneous nerves present in the back of the arm have already been considered.
2. The back of the arm is occupied by one large muscle: the ***triceps***. It is described below (5.16 and 5.17). Other structures seen in the back of the arm are as follows:
3. The ***profunda brachii artery*** has already been described.
4. The ***radial nerve*** is described in this chapter.

| 5.16: Triceps | |
|---|---|
| Origin | 1. Long head from infraglenoid tubercle of scapula<br>2. Lateral head from ridge on posterior aspect of humerus<br>3. Medial head from posterior surface of humerus below the radial groove, and from intermuscular septa. |
| Insertion | Olecranon process of ulna (posterior part of superior surface) |
| Nerve supply | Radial nerve (C6, 7, 8) |
| Action | 1. Extension of forearm at elbow joint<br>2. Long head helps in bringing back the abducted or extended arm to the side of the body |
| Note | The ridge from which the lateral head arises corresponds to the upper part of the lateral border of the bone. The ridge extends from the greater tubercle to the deltoid tuberosity. It lies above the radial groove. |

## Notes about the Triceps

1. The upper part of the triceps is overlapped by the deltoid muscle.
2. The long head descends passing anterior to the teres minor, but posterior to the teres major. Here the long head forms the lateral boundary of the quadrangular space. Note that the axillary nerve passes backwards through this space, accompanied by the posterior circumflex humeral branch of the axillary artery.
3. Just above the origin of the medial head, the posterior aspect of the humerus bears the ***radial groove***. The groove is so called because the radial nerve lies in it. It is accompanied by the profunda brachii artery.

## The Radial Nerve

1. The ***radial nerve*** is the main continuation of the posterior cord of the brachial plexus. At its upper end (i.e., in the axilla) it lies behind the third part of the axillary artery.
2. In the upper part of the arm it lies behind the upper part of the brachial artery. It leaves the front of the arm by passing backwards (between the long and medial heads of the triceps).
3. This nerve enters the back of the arm through the interval between the long head of the triceps and the humerus. This interval is sometimes called the ***lower triangular space***. The nerve passes downwards and laterally lying in the radial groove.
4. Finally, it passes through an aperture in the lateral intermuscular septum to reach the cubital fossa. Here it descends between the brachialis (medially) and the brachioradialis and the extensor carpi radialis longus (laterally). It ends in front of the lateral epicondyle of the humerus by dividing into superficial and deep terminal branches.

Branches of radial nerve given off in the arm are as follows:

### *Muscular Branches*

1. Branches arising from the radial nerve near its upper end (while the nerve is medial to the humerus) supply the long and medial heads of the triceps. The branch to the medial head descends along the medial side of the humerus close to the ulnar nerve (5.18).
2. In the radial groove the nerve gives another branch to the medial head of the triceps, and also supplies the lateral head. One branch descends through the medial head to reach the anconeus muscle.
3. Branches arising from the radial nerve after it has pierced the lateral intermuscular septum (i.e., as it lies in the lateral part of the front of the arm) supply the brachialis (lateral part), the brachioradialis and the extensor carpi radialis longus.

### *Cutaneous Branches*

1. The ***posterior cutaneous nerve of the arm*** is given off by the radial nerve while the latter is in the axilla. Its area of supply is shown in 5.2.
2. The ***lower lateral cutaneous nerve of the arm*** (5.1) arises from the radial nerve while the latter lies in the radial groove.
   a. It becomes superficial by piercing the lateral head of the triceps, and curving round the lateral side of the arm it reaches the front of the elbow.
   b. It supplies the skin of the lower part of the lateral surface of the arm (5.1, 5.2).
3. The ***posterior cutaneous nerve of the forearm*** also arises from the radial nerve while the latter lies in the radial groove. It becomes superficial by piercing the lateral head of the triceps, and descends into the posterolateral part of the forearm reaching up to the wrist. It supplies an extensive area of skin on the back of the arm and on the back of the forearm (5.2).

   Further details of the course of the radial nerve in the forearm and hand will be considered in Chapter 6. Effects of injury to this nerve will also be considered in that chapter.

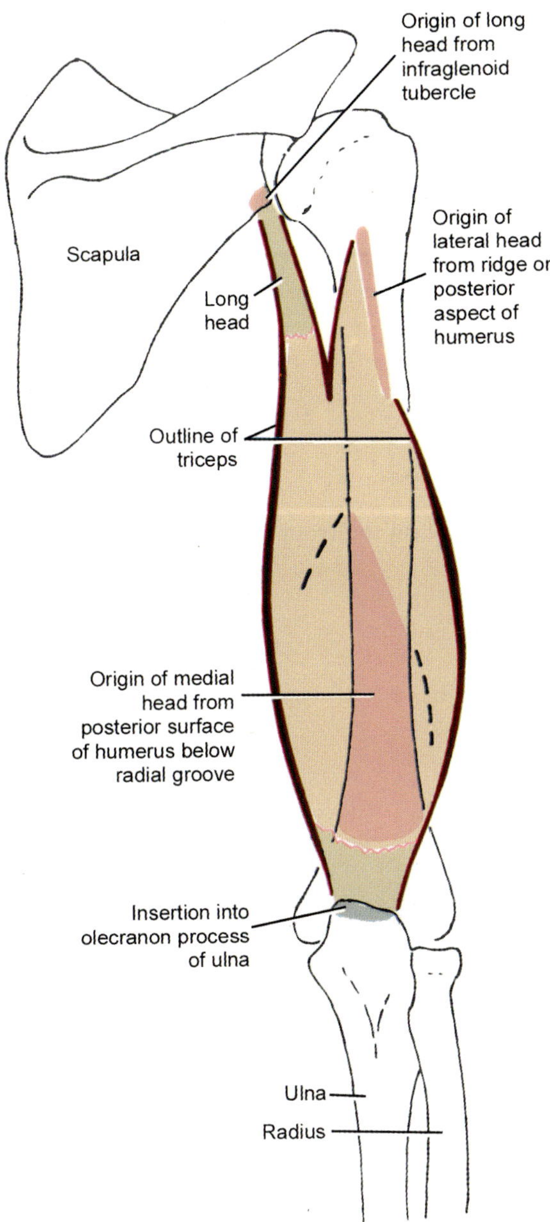


**5.17:** Scheme to show the attachments of the triceps muscle

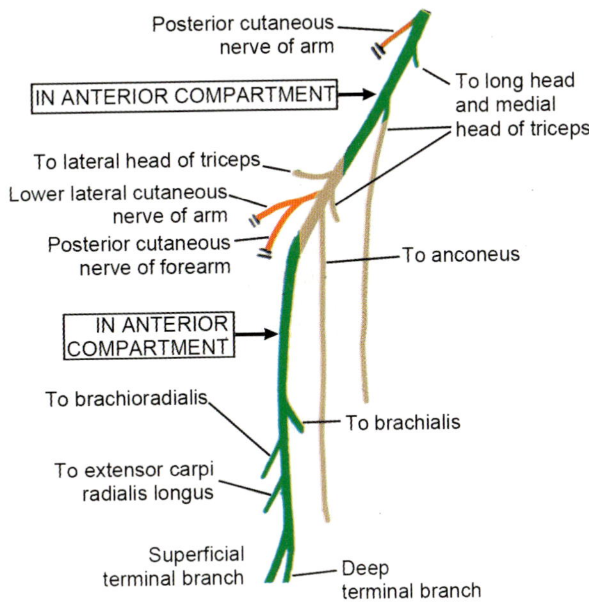


**5.18:** Branches given off by the radial nerve in the arm

6

CHAPTER

# The Forearm and Hand

## FRONT OF FOREARM AND HAND

### Superficial Structures

The superficial structures (cutaneous nerves and superficial veins) present on the front of the forearm have been described in Chapter 5.

## MUSCLES OF THE FRONT OF THE FOREARM

The muscles of the front of the forearm are arranged in three layers as follows:

*Superficial layer*

1. Pronator teres
2. Flexor carpi radialis
3. Flexor carpi ulnaris

*Intermediate layer*

4. Flexor digitorum superficialis (6.3)

*Deep layer*

5. Flexor digitorum profundus
6. Flexor pollicis longus
7. Pronator quadratus.

The main facts about these muscles are given in 6.1. The relationship of the flexor carpi radialis tendon to the flexor retinaculum is illustrated in 6.2. Some important additional facts about the muscles are given below.

### Pronator Teres

1. The insertion is at the site of maximum convexity of the shaft of the radius.
2. The lateral border of the pronator teres forms the medial boundary of the cubital fossa.
3. The median nerve passes between the humeral and ulnar heads.
4. The ulnar artery passes deep to the ulnar head. In other words, the ulnar head separates the ulnar artery from the median nerve.

### Flexor Carpi Radialis

1. The muscle ends in a tendon that passes anterior to the wrist in its lateral part.
2. Here the tendon passes through a tunnel, bounded laterally by a groove in the trapezium, and medially by two slips of the flexor retinaculum that are attached to the margins of the groove.
3. The radial artery lies just lateral to the tendon of this muscle (between it and the brachioradialis).

**6.1: Muscles of the front of the forearm**

| *Muscle* | *Origin* | *Insertion* | *Action* | *Nerve Supply* |
|---|---|---|---|---|
| Pronator teres | 1. Humeral head from (a) lowest part of supracondylar ridge and (b) medial epicondyle<br>2. Ulnar head (deep head) from medial side of coronoid process | Lateral surface of shaft of radius, at about its middle | 1. Pronates the forearm.<br>2. Weak flexor of elbow | Median nerve (C6,7) |
| Flexor carpi radialis | Medial epicondyle of humerus<br>The tendon passes through a tunnel bounded laterally by a groove in the trapezium, and medially by two slips of the flexor retinaculum | Palmar surface of base of second metacarpal bone. A slip reaches the third metacarpal bone | Flexion and abduction of wrist | Median nerve (C6, 7) |
| Flexor carpi ulnaris | 1. Humeral head: medial epicondyle.<br>2. Ulnar head:<br>a. Medial side of olecranon process<br>b. Upper two-thirds of posterior border<br>3. Tendinous arch passing from medial epicondyle to olecranon process. | Pisiform bone<br>Pull is transmitted to the hamate bone through piso-hamate ligament and to the fifth metacarpal through the piso-metacarpal ligament | Flexion and adduction of wrist | Ulnar nerve (C7, 8) |
| Palmaris longus | Medial epicondyle of humerus | 1. Flexor retinaculum<br>2. Palmar aponeurosis | Flexion of hand at wrist<br>Makes palmar aponeurosis tense | Median nerve (C7, 8) |
| Flexor digitorum superficialis | 1. Humero-ulnar head from<br>a. Medial epicondyle of humerus.<br>b Ulnar collateral ligament of elbow joint<br>c. Medial margin of olecranon process<br>2. Radial head from anterior border of radius (oblique line) | Tendon splits into four parts, one for each digit except the thumb. Opposite the terminal phalanx the tendon for each digit splits to form two slips, medial and lateral. Each slip is inserted on the corresponding side of the middle phalanx. | Flexion of middle and proximal phalanges of digits concerned | Median nerve (C7, 8, T1) |
| Flexor digitorum profundus | 1. From following parts of ulna:<br>a. Medial surface of coronoid process<br>b. Upper three-fourths of anterior surface<br>c. Upper three-fourths of medial surface<br>d. Upper three-fourths of posterior border<br>2. Medial half of interosseus membrane | Tendon splits into four parts, one for each digit other than the thumb. The tendon for each digit is inserted into the base of the distal phalanx. | 1. Flexion of distal phalanges<br>2. Helps in flexing the wrist | 1. Medial part by ulnar nerve.<br>2. Lateral part by median nerve (ant. int. branch) (C8, T1) |
| Flexor pollicis longus | 1. Anterior surface of radius (below oblique line (excluding lower one-fourth)<br>2. Lateral part of interosseus membrane<br>3. Occasionally slip from margin of coronoid process | Base of distal phalanx of thumb (ventral aspect) | Flexion of phalanges of thumb | Median nerve (ant. int. branch) (C8, T1) |
| Pronator quadratus | Oblique ridge on lower part of anterior surface of ulna | 1. Anterior surface of shaft of radius in its lower one-fourth<br>2. Medial surface of radius (triangular area above ulnar notch) | 1. Chief pronator of the forearm<br>2. Prevents separation of radius and ulna | Median nerve (ant. int. branch) (C8, T1) |

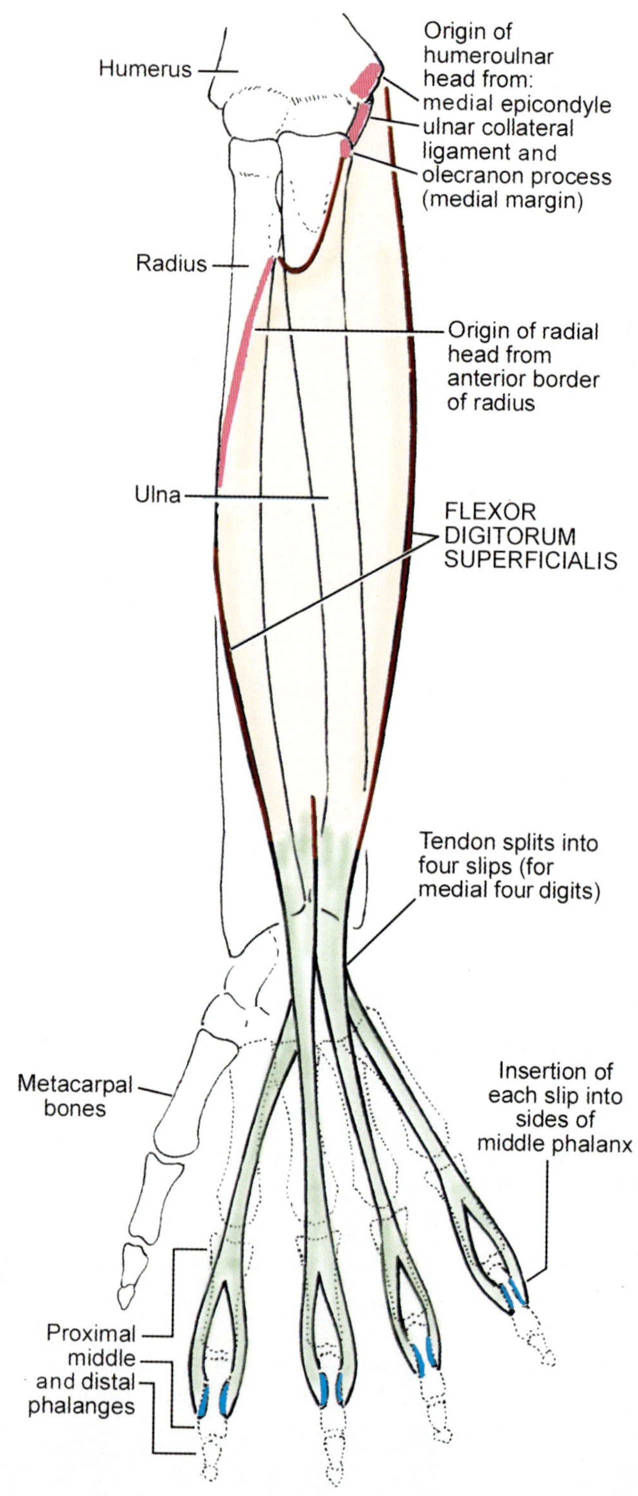


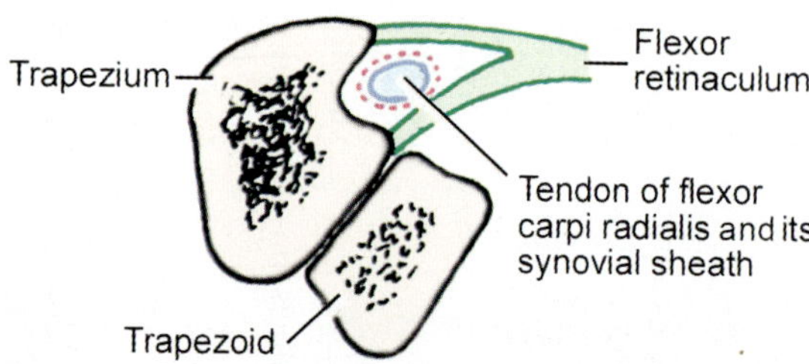


**6.2:** Transverse section across the lateral part of the wrist showing the relationship of the flexor carpi radialis tendon to the flexor retinaculum

**6.3:** Attachments of the flexor digitorum superficialis

## Flexor Carpi Ulnaris

1. The ulnar nerve enters the forearm by passing deep to the tendinous arch connecting the humeral and ulnar heads of origin.
2. At the wrist the ulnar artery and nerve lie lateral to the tendon of this muscle.

## Flexor Digitorum Superficialis and Profundus

### WANT TO KNOW MORE?

**Further Details of Arrangement in the Digits**

1. Over the base of the proximal phalanx the profundus tendon lies deep to that of the superficialis (6.4A to C).
2. Over the middle of the proximal phalanx the superficialis tendon splits into two slips.
3. The profundus tendon passes through the interval between these slips.

**Fibrous Flexor Sheath**

1. During their course over the ventral aspect of the digits, the tendons of the flexor digitorum superficialis and profundus (for that digit) lie in a common canal bounded posteriorly, by the phalanges and anteriorly (and on the sides) by a fibrous membrane.
2. This membrane is called the fibrous flexor sheath (6.9). It holds the tendons in place.

### *Synovial Sheaths*

1. At the wrist the four tendons of the flexor digitorum superficialis lie superficial to the four tendons of the profundus.
2. All the eight tendons pass through the ***carpal tunnel*** which is bounded, in front by the flexor retinaculum; and behind by the carpal bones.
3. Here the tendons are surrounded by a common synovial sheath (also called the ***ulnar bursa***)(6.5A and B).
4. Over the digits the tendons are surrounded by a common digital synovial sheath, which lines the inside of the fibrous flexor sheath.
5. The digital sheath of the little finger is continuous proximally with the ulnar bursa. For description of the radial bursa see below.

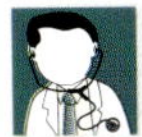

### CLINICAL CORRELATION

1. Normally the ***flexor digitorum superficialis and profundus*** act together to flex the fingers at all interphalangeal joints. These muscles can be tested individually by putting the other out of action. Remember that each muscle acts on all four fingers. If a muscle is prevented from acting on three fingers the fourth also does not move.
   a. To test the superficialis the patient tries to flex the middle phalanx of one finger while the other three fingers are held in extended position to inactivate the profundus.
   b. To test the profundus, hold the middle phalanx in extended position and ask the patient to flex the distal phalanx.
2. Sometimes a rounded swelling is seen on the back of the wrist. It is called ***ganglion***.
   a. The swelling is really a cyst walled by synovial membrane.
   b. The cyst is filled by fluid.
   c. The swelling is often in close relationship to the synovial sheath of a tendon.

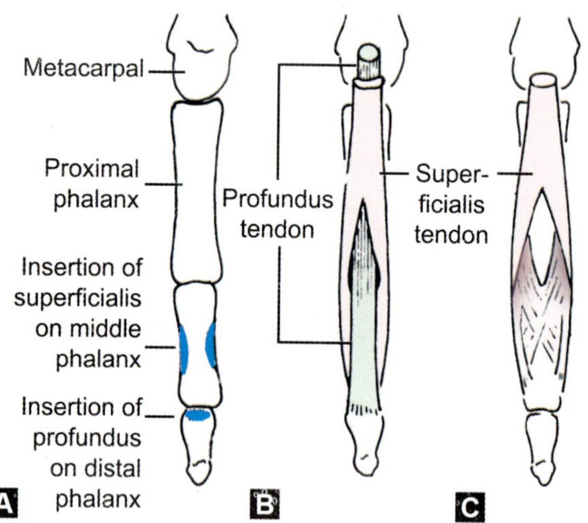


**6.4A to C:** Drawings to show the arrangement of tendons on the palmar aspect of a typical finger.(A) Areas of insertion of flexor digitorum superficialis and profundus; (B) View with both tendons in place; (C) View with profundus tendon removed

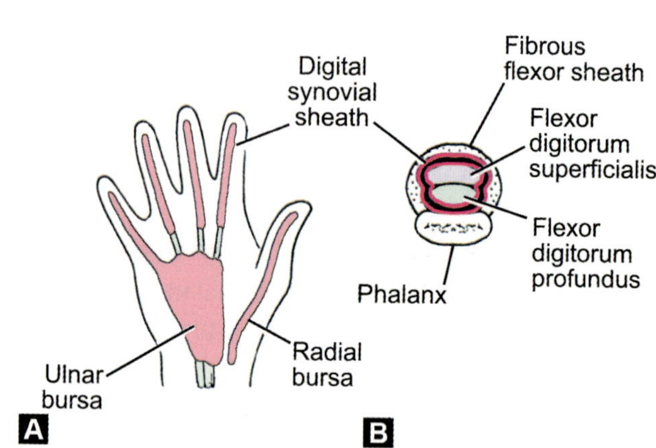


**6.5A and B:** (A) Synovial sheaths of tendons on the front of the wrist and hand;(B) TS across a digit showing the arrangement of flexor tendons. Note the common synovial sheath for the superficialis and profundus

### Flexor Pollicis Longus

1. The muscle ends in a tendon which runs across the front of the wrist (lateral part). Here, it lies in the carpal tunnel. The tendon then passes into the thumb.
2. Here it is surrounded by a synovial sheath, and a fibrous flexor sheath, just like tendons of the digital flexors.
3. The synovial sheath surrounding the tendon is called the ***radial bursa*** (6.5A). It surrounds the tendon as it passes through the carpal tunnel and extends up to the insertion of the tendon.
4. In the carpal tunnel, the radial bursa sometimes communicates with the ulnar bursa.

### Vessels and Nerves of the Forearm

These are considered in chapter 5.

## IMPORTANT FASCIA IN THE WRIST AND HAND

### Flexor Retinaculum

1. This is a strong band of fascia stretching across the ventral aspect of the carpus.
2. The space between the retinaculum and the carpal bones is called the ***carpal tunnel***. It transmits the tendons of the flexor digitorum superficialis and profundus, the tendon of the flexor pollicis longus and the median nerve (6.7A and B).

#### WANT TO KNOW MORE?

3. The retinaculum is attached medially to the pisiform bone, and to the hook of the hamate bone (6.6). Laterally, it splits into a superficial and a deep layer.
   a. The superficial layer is attached to the tubercle of the scaphoid, and to the tubercle of the trapezium.
   b. The deep layer is attached to the trapezium posterior to the groove for the flexor carpi radialis.

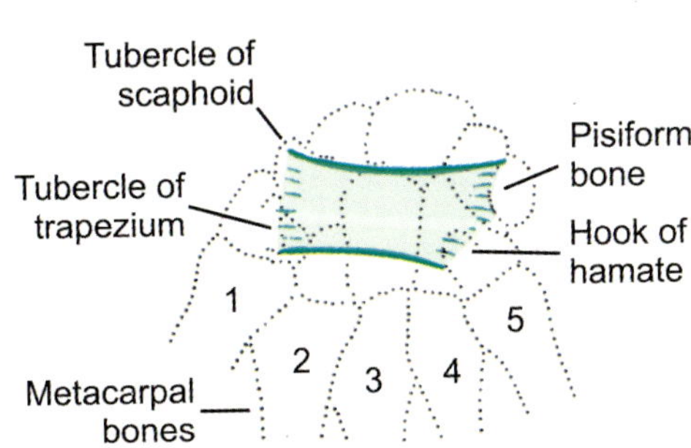


6.6: Attachments of the flexor retinaculum

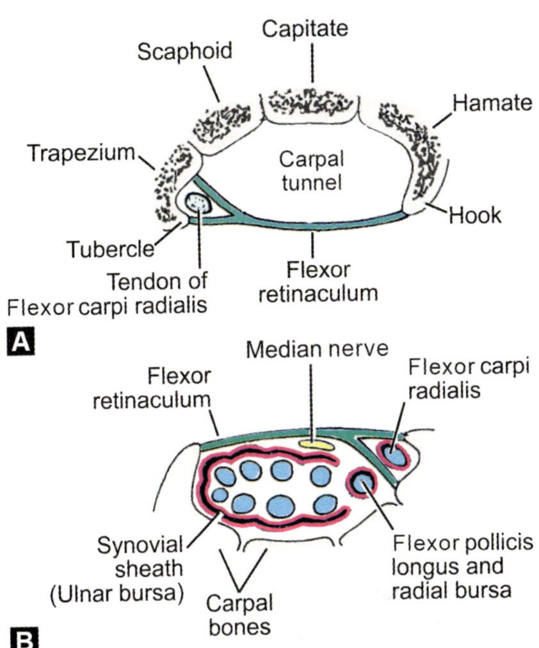


6.7A and B: (A) Boundaries of the carpal tunnel; (B) Structures passing through the carpal tunnel

*Carpal Tunnel Syndrome*

See page 112.

## Palmar Aponeurosis

1. This is a triangular structure consisting of thickened deep fascia that covers the central part of the palm (See later in the text).
2. Several important structures lie under cover of the palmar aponeurosis.
   a. These include the flexor tendons, the lumbrical muscles and the superficial palmar arch.
   b. Digital arteries arising from the arch, and digital branches of the median and ulnar nerves, pass distally under cover of the aponeurosis and enter the digits by passing under the free distal edge of the aponeurosis in the intervals between the digits.

### WANT TO KNOW MORE?

3. The apex of the triangle is directed proximally. It is continuous with the tendon of the palmaris longus.
4. Distally, the aponeurosis is broad. It divides into four processes, one for each finger.
   a. Each process again divides into two slips that diverge to be attached to the two sides of the digit concerned.
   b. In this way an aperture is formed between the two slips, and the tendons of the flexor digitorum superficialis and profundus (for the digit) pass through this aperture.
5. The lateral edge of the aponeurosis is connected to the first metacarpal bone by the ***lateral palmar septum***. The medial edge of the aponeurosis is connected to the fifth metacarpal bone by the ***medial palmar septum***. These septa divide the palm into compartments.

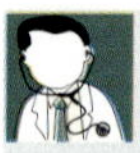

### CLINICAL CORRELATION

1. The fibres of the palmar aponeurosis may undergo progressive shortening. This results in deformities of the hand and restriction of finger movements.
2. The fourth and fifth digits remain in a state of flexion at the metacarpophalangeal and proximal interphalangeal joints. Operative removal of restricting fibres can give relief.
3. The condition is called ***Dupuytren contracture.***

## MUSCLES IN THE PALM

These are:

1. A superficial muscle: the palmaris brevis.
2. A set of four small ***lumbrical muscles***.
3. ***Thenar muscles*** (6.10) that move the thumb are as follows:
   a. Abductor pollicis brevis
   b. Flexor pollicis brevis
   c. Opponens pollicis
   d. Adductor pollicis.
4. ***Hypothenar muscles*** that move the little finger are as follows:
   a. Abductor digiti minimi
   b. Flexor digiti minimi
   c. Opponens digiti minimi.
5. ***Interosseous*** muscles
   a. Palmar interossei
   b. Dorsal interossei of palm.

For comparison of palmar and dorsal interosseous muscles, see 6.11.

### WANT TO KNOW MORE?

**Palmaris Brevis**

1. This is a subcutaneous muscle.
2. Laterally, it is attached to the flexor retinaculum and the palmar aponeurosis.
3. Medially, it is attached to skin along the ulnar border of the hand.
4. It is supplied by the superficial branch of the ulnar nerve.
5. It causes wrinkling of the skin over the medial side of the palm and may thus help in providing a better grip.

The lumbrical muscles are described in 6.8. They are illustrated in 6.9.

| 6.8: Lumbricals | |
|---|---|
| These are four small muscles that take origin from the tendons of the flexor digitorum profundus. | |
| Origin | 1. First lumbrical from radial side of tendon for index finger<br>2. Second lumbrical from radial side of tendon for middle finger<br>3. Third lumbrical from contiguous sides of tendons for middle and ring fingers<br>4. Fourth lumbrical from contiguous sides of tendons for ring and little fingers |

*Contd...*

*Contd...*

| | |
|---|---|
| Insertion | Each muscle ends in a tendon that passes backwards on the radial side of one metacarpo-phalangeal joint and is inserted into the lateral basal angle of the extensor expansion for that digit in the following order:<br>1. Tendon of first lumbrical into second digit<br>2. Tendon of second lumbrical into third digit<br>3. Tendon of third lumbrical into fourth digit<br>4. Tendon of fourth lumbrical into fifth digit |
| Nerve supply | 1. First and second lumbricals from median nerve (C8, T1)<br>2. Third and fourth lumbricals from ulnar nerve deep branch (C8,T1) |
| Action | 1. Flexion of metacarpo-phalangeal joint, and<br>2. Extension of interphalangeal joint of digit concerned |
| Notes | Help in fine movements of fingers, as in writing or threading a needle |

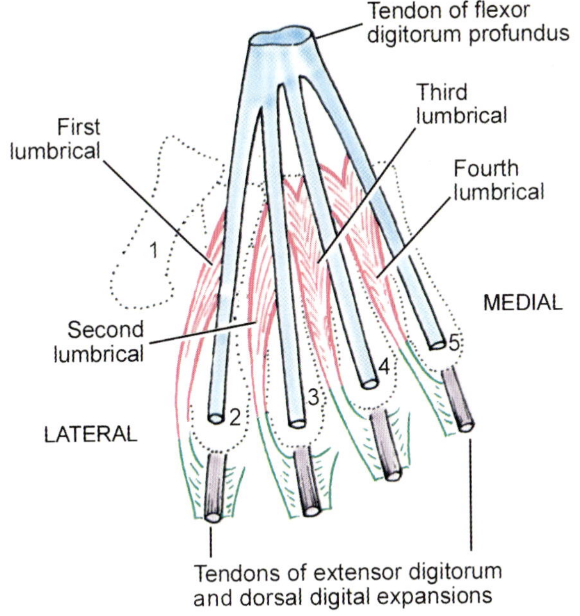


**6.9:** Diagram to show attachments of lumbrical muscles

| **6.10: Thenar muscles** | | | | |
|---|---|---|---|---|
| *Muscle* | *Origin* | *Insertion* | *Action* | *Nerve Supply* |
| Abductor pollicis brevis | 1. Tubercle of scaphoid<br>2. Tubercle of trapezium<br>3. Adjoining part of flexor retinaculum | 1. Lateral side of base of proximal phalanx of thumb<br>2. Some fibres to dorsal digital expansion | Abduction of thumb at metacarpophalangeal and carpometacarpal joints. Abduction is associated with medial rotation | Median nerve (C8, T1) |

*Contd...*

*Contd...*

| *Muscle* | *Origin* | *Insertion* | *Action* | *Nerve Supply* |
|---|---|---|---|---|
| Flexor pollicis brevis | *Superficial head:*<br>1. Tubercle of trapezium (distal part)<br>2. Flexor retinaculum (adjoining part)<br>*Deep head:*<br>Trapezoid and capitate bones | Lateral side of base of proximal phalan of thumb | Flexion of thumb | *Superficial head:* Median nerve. (C8, T1)<br>*Deep head:* Deep branch of ulnar nerve (C8, T1) |
| Opponens pollicis | 1. Tubercle of trapezium<br>2. Flexor retinaculum (adjoining part) | Lateral half of palmar surface of first metacarpal bone | Opposition of thumb (flexion plus medial rotation) | Median nerve. (C8, T1) Sometimes from deep branch of ulnar nerve also |
| Adductor pollicis | *Oblique head:*<br>1. Capitate bone<br>2. Bases of 2nd and 3rd metacarpals<br>*Transverse head:*<br>Palmar aspect of 3rd metacarpal bone (distal two-thirds) | 1. Medial side of base of proximal phalanx of thumb<br>2. Some fibres intodorsal digital expansion | Adducts the thumb from flexed or abducted position The movement is forceful in gripping | Deep branch of ulnar nerve (C8,T1) |
| | | Hypothenar Muscles | | |
| Abductor digiti minimi | 1. Pisiform bone<br>2. Tendon of flexor carpi ulnaris<br>3. Pisohamate ligament | Ulnar side of base of proximal phalanx of little finger | Abducts little finger at metacarpophalangeal joint | Deep branch of ulnar nerve (C8, T1) |
| Flexor digiti minimi | 1. Hook of hamate (proximal part)<br>2. Adjoining part of flexor retinaculum | Ulnar side of base of proximal phalanx of little finger | Flexion of little finger at metacarpophalangeal joint | Deep branch of ulnar nerve (C8, T1) |
| Opponens digiti minimi | 1. Hook of hamate (distal part)<br>2. Adjoining part of flexor retinaculum | Medial surface of 5th metacarpal bone | Flexes the fifth metacarpal bone and rotates it laterally (makes palm hollow) | Deep branch of ulnar nerve (C8, T1) |

**6.11: Palmar and dorsal interosseous muscles compared**

| | *Palmar Interossei* | *Dorsal Interossei* |
|---|---|---|
| FEATURES COMMON TO BOTH | 1. Four palmar interossei<br>2. Numbered from lateral to medial side<br>3. Insertion of each muscle into dorsal digital expansion of one digit<br>4. Movements described with reference to the third digit<br>5. Nerve suppy from deep branch of ulnar nerve (C8, T1)<br>6. They flex the metacarpo-phalangeal joint and extend the interphalangeal joints of the digit concerned | 1. Four dorsal interossei<br>2. Numbered from lateral to medial side<br>3. Insertion of each muscle into dorsal digital expansion of one digit<br>4. Movements described with reference to the third digit<br>5. Nerve suppy from deep branch of ulnar nerve (C8, T1)<br>6. They flex the metacarpo-phalangeal joint and extend the interphalangeal joints of the digit concerned |

*Contd...*

*Contd...*

| | *Palmar Interossei* | *Dorsal Interossei* |
|---|---|---|
| FEATURES DIFFERENT IN THE TWO | 1. Each muscle arises from one metacarpal<br>2. The third digit does not give origin to, or receive the insertion of any palmar interosseus muscle<br>3. These are ADDUCTORS of the digit towards the line of the middle finger (6.12B)<br>4. A palmar interosseus muscle may or may not be inserted into the base of the proximal phalanx<br>5. Palmar interossei take origin from, and are inserted into the first, second, fourth, and fifth digits (not the third) | 1. Each muscle arises from two adjoining metacarpals<br>2. The third digit gives origin to, and receives insertions of two muscles (one on each side, medial and lateral)<br>3. These are ABDUCTORS of digits away from the line of the middle finger (6.12A)<br>4. A dorsal interosseus muscle is always inserted into the base of the proximal phalanx of the digit concerned<br>5. Dorsal interossei take origin from all five metacarpals and are inserted into the second, third and fourth digits (not first and fifth) |

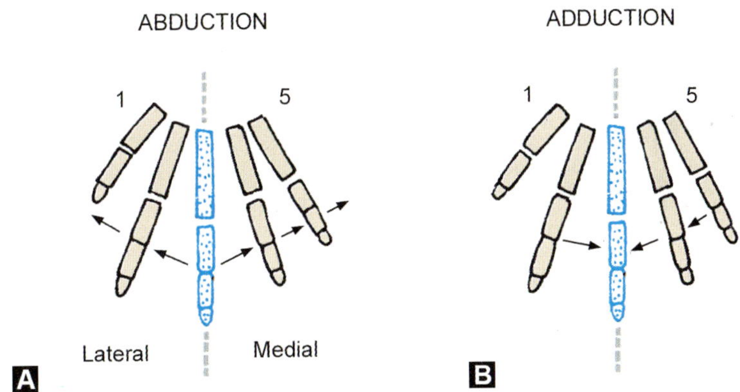


**6.12A and B:** Scheme to illustrate abduction and adduction of the digits of the hand

## NERVES OF THE FOREARM AND HAND

### The Median Nerve

1. The median nerve is formed by union of lateral and medial roots that arise from the corresponding cords of the brachial plexus.
2. Its upper end lies in the axilla, lateral to the axillary artery.
3. It continues into the arm lateral to the brachial artery. Near the middle of the arm it crosses superficial to the artery to reach its medial side, and descends in this position to the cubital fossa.
4. The nerve leaves the cubital fossa by passing between the superficial and deep heads of the pronator teres.
5. It runs down the forearm in the plane between the flexor digitorum superficialis and the flexor digitorum profundus.
6. At the wrist the nerve lies between the tendons of the flexor digitorum superficialis (medially) and the flexor carpi radialis (laterally).
7. The nerve enters the hand by passing deep to the flexor retinaculum.
8. The nerve is distributed as illustrated in 6.13.

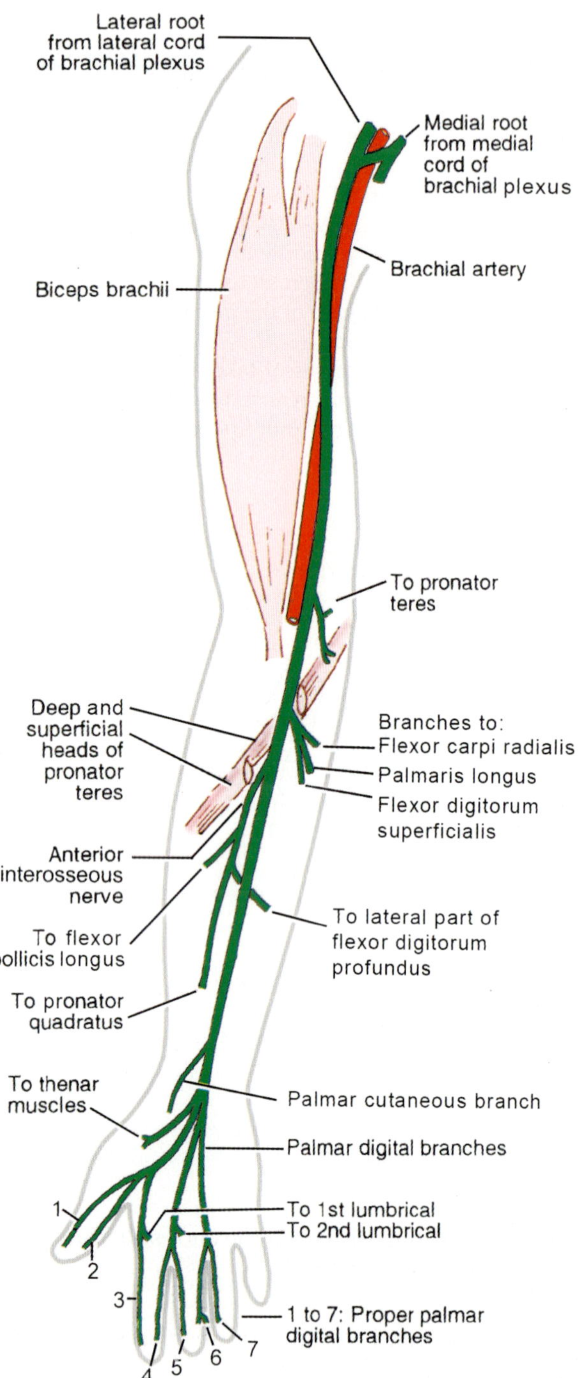


**6.13:** Scheme to show the course and branches of the median nerve

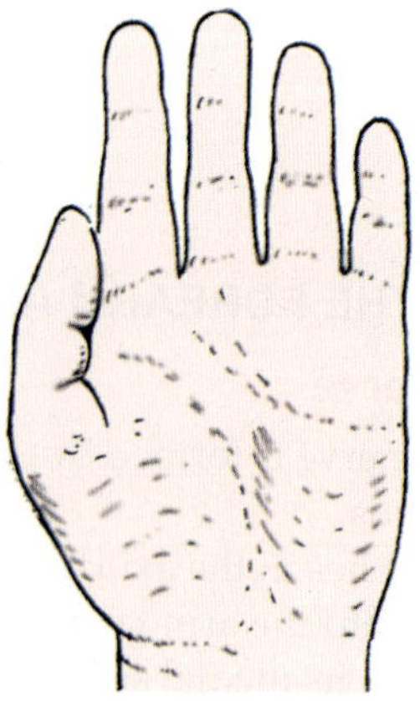

**6.14:** Ape-like hand in median nerve palsy. Note the flattened thenar eminence and the adducted and extended thumb

### Muscular Branches

1. The pronator teres is supplied by a branch that arises in the lower part of the arm.
2. Direct branches arising in the upper part of the forearm supply the flexor carpi radialis, the palmaris longus and the flexor digitorum superficialis.
3. The ***anterior interosseous nerve*** arises from the median nerve as the latter passes between the two heads of the pronator teres.
   a. It runs down the forearm in front of the interosseous membrane.
   b. The muscles supplied through it are the flexor pollicis longus, the lateral part of the flexor digitorum profundus and the pronator quadratus.
4. A muscular branch arising in the palm supplies the thenar muscles namely the flexor pollicis brevis, the abductor pollicis brevis and the opponens pollicis.
5. The first and second lumbrical muscles of the hand are supplied by branches from the digital nerves.

### Cutaneous Branches

1. The ***palmar cutaneous branch*** (superficial palmar branch) arises in the lower part of the forearm, and passes into the hand superficial to the flexor retinaculum. It supplies the skin over the thenar eminence and over the middle of the palm.
2. The median nerve ends by dividing into a variable number of ***palmar digital branches*** that subdivide so that ultimately seven ***proper palmar digital nerves*** are formed: two each (one medial and one lateral) for the thumb, the index and the middle fingers, and one for the lateral half of the ring finger.
   a. Through these branches the median nerve supplies the palmar surface of the lateral three and a half digits.
   b. It also supplies the dorsal surfaces of the terminal parts of the same digits including the nail beds, the skin over the terminal phalanx of the thumb, and over the middle and terminal phalanges of the index and middle fingers and the lateral half of the ring finger.
   c. Apart from skin the digital nerves also supply deeper tissues. The digital nerves lie in front of the palmar digital arteries.

### Articular Branches

1. Articular branches arising directly from the median nerve near the elbow supply the elbow joint and the superior radioulnar joint
2. The distal radioulnar joint and the wrist joint are supplied through the anterior interosseous nerve.
3. The metacarpophalangeal and interphalangeal joints are supplied through the digital branches.

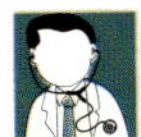

## CLINICAL CORRELATION

**Effects of Injury to the Median Nerve**

The effects of injury to the median nerve vary depending upon the level of injury, the effects being confined to structures supplied by branches distal to the injury. The ***muscles paralysed*** and the effects thereof are as follows (Consult 6.13):

1. ***Flexor carpi radialis***: Flexion and abduction of the wrist are weak. Unopposed action of the flexor carpi ulnaris adducts the hand when flexion is attempted.
2. ***Pronator teres*** and ***pronator quadratus***: Power of pronation is lost. However, the brachioradialis (supplied by the radial nerve) can bring the forearm to the midprone position.
3. ***Flexor digitorum superficialis***: Middle phalanges cannot be flexed: all fingers are affected.
4. Because of the paralysis of the lateral part of the ***flexor digitorum profundus*** the terminal phalanges of the index and middle fingers cannot be flexed.
   a. Those of the ring and little fingers can be flexed because the medial part of the muscle is supplied by the ulnar nerve.
   b. Note that the proximal phalanges can be flexed by the interossei (ulnar nerve).

5. ***Flexor pollicis longus***: The thumb cannot be flexed at the interphalangeal joint.
6. ***Thenar muscles***: The thumb cannot be abducted or opposed at the carpometacarpal joint: it remains in a position of extension (produced by the extensor pollicis longus) and adduction (produced by the adductor pollicis). This is referred to as an *'**ape-like**'* hand (6.14).
7. There is ***sensory loss*** in the area supplied by the median nerve.

*Carpal Tunnel Syndrome*

1. The carpal tunnel is a passage between the carpal bones and the flexor retinaculum (6.7A).
2. Most of it is occupied by the flexor tendons and their synovial sheaths (6.7B).
3. The median nerve passes through the tunnel.
4. Any increase in the volume of contents of the tunnel can compress the median nerve. This may occur because of inflammation in the synovial sheaths (ulnar bursa).
5. Pressure on the nerve gives rise to burning pain in the lateral three and a half digits.
6. Skin over the thenar eminence is spared because it is supplied by the palmar cutaneous branch of the median nerve that arises above the level of the flexor retinaculum and descends superficial to it.
7. The carpal tunnel syndrome can be treated by incising the flexor retinaculum.

## The Ulnar Nerve

1. This nerve is a branch of the medial cord of the brachial plexus. It extends from the axilla to the hand (6.15).
2. At its origin it lies medial to the axillary artery (between it and the axillary vein).
3. It runs down into the front of the arm where it lies medial to the brachial artery.
4. At the middle of the arm the nerve passes into the posterior compartment by piercing the medial intermuscular septum, and descends between this septum and the lower part of the triceps (medial head).
5. Passing medially as it descends, it passes behind the medial epicondyle of the humerus.
6. The nerve enters the forearm by passing deep to the tendinous arch joining the humeral and ulnar heads of the flexor carpi ulnaris.
7. The nerve runs down the medial side of the front of the forearm lying superficial to the flexor digitorum profundus.
8. In the lower two-thirds of the forearm the nerve is accompanied by the ulnar artery which lies lateral to it.
9. In the upper part of the forearm the nerve is deep to the flexor carpi ulnaris and to the flexor digitorum superficialis.
10. The nerve becomes superficial in the lower one-third of the forearm: here it lies between the tendons of the flexor carpi ulnaris (medially) and that of the flexor digitorum superficialis (laterally).
11. The nerve enters the hand by passing between the superficial and deep layers of the flexor retinaculum, lying just lateral to the pisiform bone.
12. The ulnar nerve is distributed to skin, muscle and joints through the following branches (6.15).

### *Cutaneous Branches*

1. The ***palmar cutaneous branch*** arises near the middle of the forearm. It supplies the skin of the medial one-third of the palm.
2. The ***dorsal branch*** arises from the ulnar nerve a little above the wrist.
   a. It runs downwards and backwards round the medial side of the forearm to reach the back of the wrist and hand.
   b. It supplies the skin of the medial part of the dorsum of the hand and gives two or three ***dorsal digital branches***.
   c. The most medial digital branch supplies the medial side of the little finger.
   d. The next supplies the adjoining sides of the little and ring fingers.

e. A third branch is present occasionally: when present it supplies the adjacent sides of the ring and middle fingers.
f. The area of skin supplied by the dorsal digital branches extends only up to the middle phalanx: the skin over the distal phalanx (and over part of the middle phalanx) is supplied by the ventral branches.

3. The ***superficial terminal branch*** of the ulnar nerve arises after the nerve enters the hand.
   a. It divides into two ***palmar digital branches***: one for the medial side of the little finger; and the other for the contiguous sides of the little and ring fingers.
   b. These nerves supply the skin on the palmar surfaces of the digits.
   c. They also supply the nail bed and the skin over the dorsal surface of the distal phalanx and part of the middle phalanx of the digit concerned.

### *Muscular Branches*

1. Two main branches arising directly from the ulnar nerve supply the ***flexor carpi ulnaris*** and the medial part of the ***flexor digitorum profundus***.
2. The ***deep terminal branch*** of the ulnar nerve arises in the hand. It supplies several muscles as follows (6.16):
   a. The proximal part of the nerve supplies the ***hypothenar muscles***, namely the abductor digiti minimi, the opponens digiti minimi and the flexor digiti minimi.
   After supplying the hypothenar muscles the nerve runs transversely across the palm deep to the flexor tendons, along the deep palmar arch. Here it supplies the following:
      i. All the palmar and dorsal ***interossei*** of the hand.
      ii. The third and fourth ***lumbrical muscles***.
      iii. The adductor pollicis, and frequently the flexor pollicis brevis.
3. The ***palmaris brevis*** is supplied either by the palmar cutaneous branch, or by the superficial terminal branch.

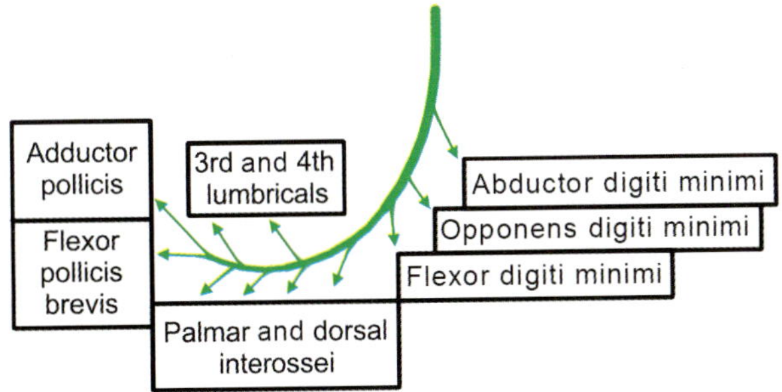


**6.16:** Distribution of the deep terminal branch of the ulnar nerve

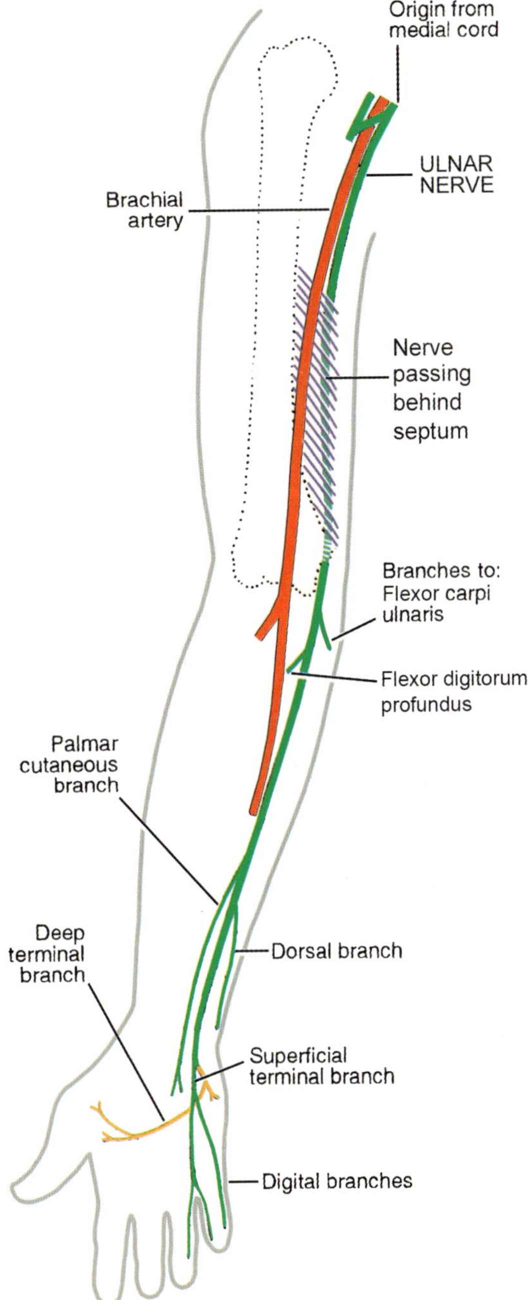


**6.15:** Scheme to show the course and branches of the ulnar nerve

### *Articular Branches*

Branches arising from the ulnar nerve or from its branches supply the elbow joint, the wrist joint, and various joints in the medial part of the hand.

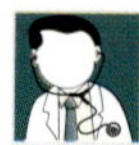

## CLINICAL CORRELATION

*Effects of Injury to the Ulnar Nerve*

1. The ulnar nerve is most often injured as it lies behind the medial epicondyle of the humerus. The ***muscles paralysed*** and the effects, thereof, are as follows:
   a. ***Flexor carpi ulnaris***: Flexion and adduction at the wrist are weak. The wrist is abducted by the flexor carpi radialis (median nerve) when flexion is attempted.
   b. Because of paralysis of the medial part of the ***flexor digitorum profundus,*** the terminal phalanges of the ring and little fingers cannot be flexed.
   c. ***Hypothenar muscles***: Movements of the little finger are affected. There is wasting of the hypothenar eminence.
   d. ***Interossei***:
      i. Abduction and adduction of the fingers is weak.
      ii. The force of adduction (palmar interossei) can be tested by asking the patient to try and hold a piece of paper forcibly between the fingers, while the examiner tries to pull it off.
      iii. The dorsal interossei can be tested by asking the patient to spread out the fingers against resistance.
      iv. Flexion of the metacarpophalangeal joints and extension of interphalangeal joints of the fingers is not possible: the metacarpophalangeal joints remain extended and the interphalangeal joints remain flexed resulting in a claw hand.
2. Ulnar nerve paralysis gives rise to a partial claw hand—the medial two digits being the most affected. Complete claw hand is seen in combined lesions of the ulnar and median nerves (6.17).
3. ***Sensations*** are impaired in the area of supply.

## The Radial Nerve

1. The radial nerve is the main continuation of the posterior cord of the brachial plexus. Its course and branches in the arm have been described in Chapter 5.
2. In the lower part of the arm, the nerve comes in the anterior compartment, lateral to the humerus. Here it descends between the brachialis (medially) and the brachioradialis and the extensor carpi radialis longus (laterally). It ends in front of the lateral epicondyle of the humerus by dividing into superficial and deep terminal branches.
3. The ***superficial terminal branch*** runs downwards in front of the lateral part of the forearm.
4. In the lower-third of the forearm the nerve passes backwards round the lateral side of the radius to reach the dorsum of the hand where it ends by dividing into four or five ***digital branches***.
5. The ***deep terminal branch*** is also called the ***posterior interosseous nerve***.
6. Soon after its origin it disappears from view by entering the substance of the supinator muscle: within the muscle it runs downwards winding round the lateral side of the radius.
7. It appears in the back of the forearm through the lower part of the supinator muscle and gives several branches that supply the muscles of this region.
8. The nerve first lies between the superficial and deep muscles of the back of the forearm, but its lowest part lies behind the interosseous membrane (where it is accompanied by the anterior interosseous artery). It ends by supplying the wrist joint.

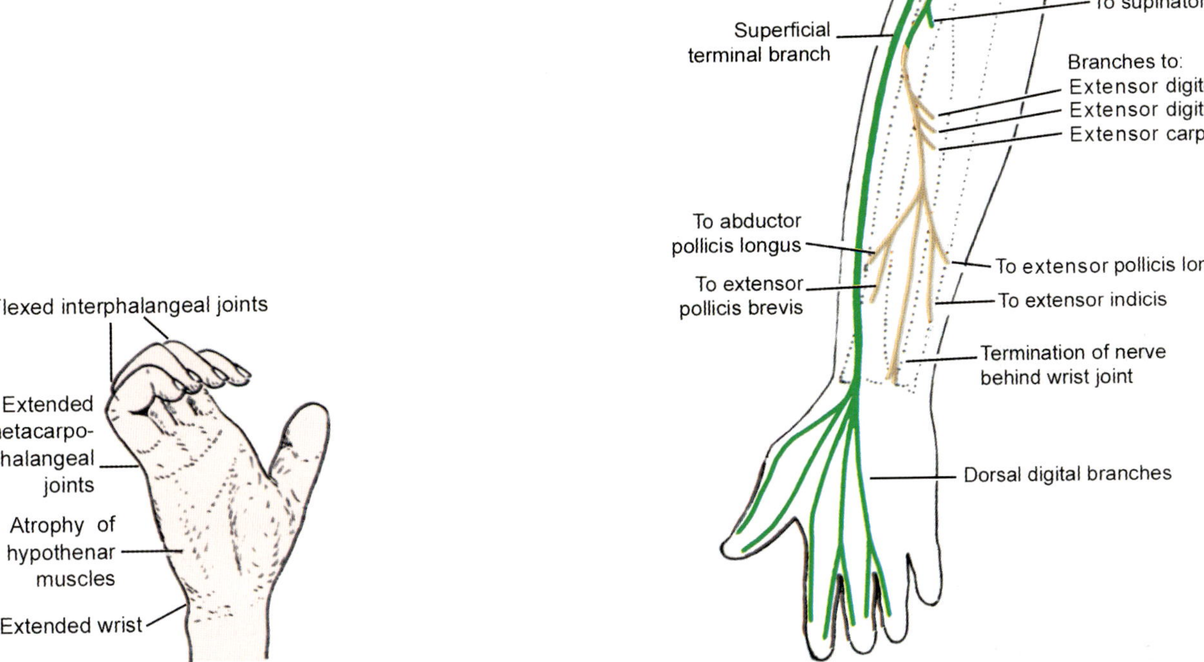


**6.17:** Complete claw hand (antero-lateral view) produced as a result of injury to both the median and ulnar nerves

**6.18:** Scheme to show the course and distribution of the radial nerve and its terminal branches in the lower part of the arm, the forearm and the hand as seen from the front. The parts of the nerve (and branches) shown in brown are placed on the dorsal aspect of the limb

9. Apart from its terminal branches the radial nerve gives off several branches: through its branches the nerve is widely distributed to skin, muscles and joints as follows. The course and distribution of the radial nerve and its terminal branches is illustrated in 6.18.

### *Muscular Branches to the Forearm and Hand*

1. One branch (arising from the nerve in the arm) descends through the medial head to reach the anconeus muscle.
2. Branches arising from the radial nerve after it has pierced the lateral intermuscular septum (i.e., as it lies in the lateral part of the front of the arm) supply:
   a. The brachialis (lateral part)
   b. The brachioradialis
   c. The extensor carpi radialis longus.

   Several muscles are supplied by branches from the deep terminal branch as follows:
3. The extensor carpi radialis brevis is supplied before the deep terminal branch enters the supinator (i.e., on the front of the forearm).
4. A branch is given off to the supinator before the nerve enters it: additional branches are given off as the nerve passes through the muscle.

5. On the back of the forearm branches are given off to the following muscles:
   a. Extensor digitorum
   b. Extensor digiti minimi
   c. Extensor carpi ulnaris
   d. Extensor pollicis longus
   e. Extensor indicis
   f. Abductor pollicis longus
   g. Extensor pollicis brevis (6.29).

   Note that in this way all extensor muscles of the arm and forearm are supplied by the radial nerve directly or through its deep terminal branch.

### *Cutaneous Branches to the Forearm and Hand*

These are as follows:

1. The ***posterior cutaneous nerve of the forearm*** arises from the radial nerve while the latter lies in the radial groove.
   a. It becomes superficial by piercing the lateral head of the triceps, and descends into the posterolateral part of the forearm reaching up to the wrist.
   b. It supplies an extensive area of skin on the back of the arm and on the back of the forearm.
2. Four to five ***dorsal digital branches*** arise from the superficial terminal branch of the radial nerve.
   a. The first of these (most lateral) supplies the skin of the lateral side of the thumb.
   b. The second branch supplies the medial side of the thumb.
   c. The third branch supplies the lateral side of the index finger.
   d. The fourth branch supplies the contiguous sides of the index and middle fingers; while
   e. The fifth (when present) supplies the contiguous sides of the middle and ring fingers which show the two variants.
3. The dorsal digital branches do not extend to the distal ends of the digits. As stated above the skin over the distal phalanges, and the whole or part of the middle phalanges is supplied by palmar digital branches of the median nerve.

### *Articular Branches*

1. Direct branches from the radial nerve help to supply the elbow joint.
2. Joints in the region of the wrist are supplied by branches from the lower end of the deep terminal branch.

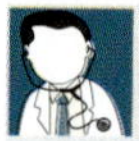

## CLINICAL CORRELATION

***Effects of Injury to the Radial Nerve***

1. The effects of injury to the radial nerve depend on the level of injury.
   a. All muscles supplied by it are affected in injuries to it in the axilla.
   b. It is, however, most frequently injured as it lies in the radial groove: in this case the triceps is spared as the nerves to it arise higher up.
2. The ***muscles paralysed*** in injury to the radial nerve, and the effects thereof are as follows:
   a. ***Triceps***: The elbow cannot be extended.
   b. ***Extensors of wrist and digits***: The wrist and proximal phalanges cannot be extended. The wrist remains flexed: this condition is called ***wrist drop*** (6.19).
   c. ***Supinator***: Supination is not possible with the forearm extended. However, if the forearm is flexed the biceps brachii produces this movement.

3. ***Sensory loss***: Although the radial nerve supplies an extensive area of skin, much of the area is also supplied by other nerves. Because of this fact sensations are lost only in a small area of skin on the lateral part of the dorsum of the hand.

## Summary of the Nerve Supply of Muscles of the Free Upper Limb

The nerve supply of muscles of the arm, forearm and hand is summarised in 6.20. Note that the brachialis, the flexor digitorum profundus and the flexor pollicis brevis have a double nerve supply. The lumbricals, considered as a group, also have a double supply.

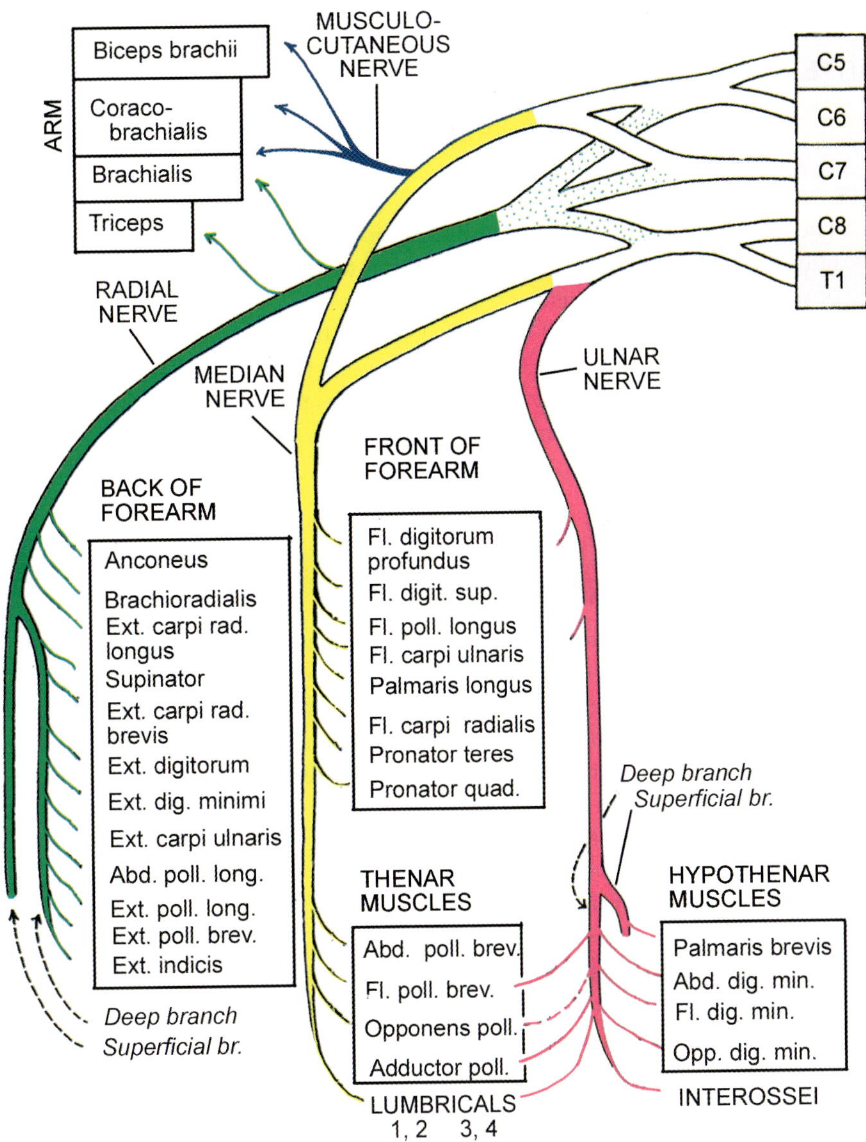


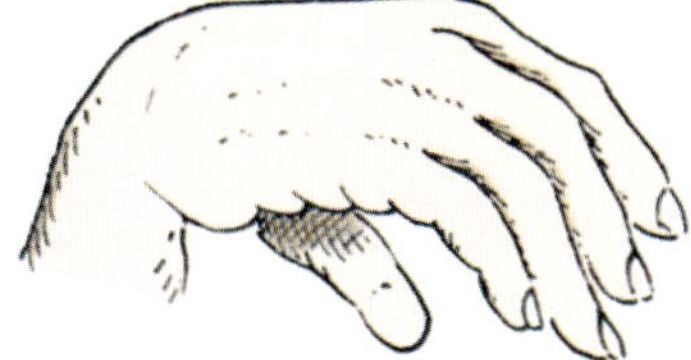

**6.19:** Wrist drop seen in radial nerve injury

**6.20:** Scheme to show the nerve supply of various muscles of the arm, forearm and hand

Ext. = Extensor; poll. = pollicis; Fl. = Flexor; brev. = brevis; Opp. = Opponens; long. = longus; rad. = radialis; br. = branch; min. = minimi; Abd. = Abductor; digit. = digitorum; dig. = digiti; quad. = quadratus

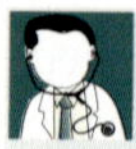

## CLINICAL CORRELATION

**Segmental Supply of Muscles of the Upper Limb**

From a clinical point of view it is important to know what muscles are supplied by each segment of the spinal cord.

a. Such information helps us to localise the level of a lesion involving the spinal cord, or of the roots of spinal nerves.
b. A simplified presentation of the muscles supplied through the various spinal segments contributing to the brachial plexus is given in 6.21.

## ARTERIES OF THE FOREARM

The main arteries of the forearm are the radial and ulnar branches of the brachial artery. They are described below.

### The Radial Artery

1. The radial artery begins in front of the elbow at the level of the neck of the radius. It first passes downwards and laterally reaching the lateral border of the forearm about its middle. It then descends along the lateral margin of the forearm to the wrist.
2. Thereafter, it winds round the lateral side of the carpus to reach the back of the hand (6.22).
3. It passes forwards through the space between the first and second metacarpal bones to reach the palm.
4. Finally, it runs transversely across the palm as the deep palmar arch, and ends by anastomosing with the deep palmar branch of the ulnar artery.

## WANT TO KNOW MORE?

**Relations of the Radial Artery**

1. In the forearm the artery is covered by skin and fascia. Near the apex of the cubital fossa the artery is related laterally to the brachioradialis and medially to the pronator teres: these muscles may overlap it.
2. Lower down, the artery continues to be related laterally to the brachioradialis, but medially it is related to the flexor carpi radialis. The tendon of the latter muscle lies medial to the artery at the wrist.
3. The superficial branch of the radial nerve is lateral to the artery in the middle-third of the forearm. Posteriorly, the artery rests (from above downwards) on:
   a. The biceps tendon
   b. The supinator
   c. The insertion of the pronator teres
   d. The flexor digitorum superficialis
   e. The flexor pollicis longus
   f. The pronator quadratus
   g. The anterior surface of the radius near its lower end.
4. At the wrist the artery runs backwards deep to the tendons of the abductor pollicis longus and the extensor pollicis brevis passing dorsal to the scaphoid bone and to the trapezium. Here it is crossed by the tendon of the extensor pollicis longus.
5. The artery reaches the interval between the first and second metacarpal bones where it passes between the two heads of the first dorsal interosseous muscle to enter the palm.
6. In the palm the artery forms the deep palmar arch. It runs medially deep to the oblique head of the adductor pollicis and then between the oblique and transverse heads. The artery ends by joining the deep branch of the ulnar artery.

<table>
<tr><th>C5</th><th>C6</th><th>C7</th><th>C8</th><th>T1</th></tr>
<tr><td colspan="2">Scapular muscles<br><br>Rhomboidei<br>Supraspinatus<br>Infraspinatus<br>Subscapularis<br>Teres major<br>Teres minor<br><br>Deltoid<br>Subclavius</td><td></td><td></td><td></td></tr>
<tr><td></td><td colspan="2">Large muscles connecting upper limb to trunk<br><br>Pectoralis major<br>Pectoralis minor<br>Latissimus dorsi<br>Serratus anterior<br><br>Muscles of front of arm<br><br>Biceps brachii<br>Coracobrachialis<br>Brachialis<br><br>Supinators<br><br>Biceps brachii<br>Supinator<br>Brachioradialis</td><td></td><td></td></tr>
<tr><td></td><td></td><td colspan="2">Muscles on back of arm<br><br>Triceps<br><br>Pronators<br><br>Pronator teres<br>Pronator quadratus<br><br>Other muscles of forearm<br><br>Flexor group<br>Extensor group</td><td></td></tr>
<tr><td></td><td></td><td></td><td colspan="2">Small muscles of hand<br><br>Thenar group<br>Hypothenar group<br>Interossei<br>Lumbricals</td></tr>
</table>

**6.21:** Simplified scheme to show muscles of upper extremity supplied by different spinal segments

### *Branches of Radial Artery*

Structures on the lateral side of wrist related to the radial artery are illustrated in 6.23 and branches of the radial artery in the hand are shown in 6.24.

1. The ***radial recurrent artery*** arises near the upper end of the radial artery. It ascends to anastomose with the radial collateral (anterior descending) branch of the profunda brachii artery.
   *All other branches of the radial artery arise near the wrist and hand.*

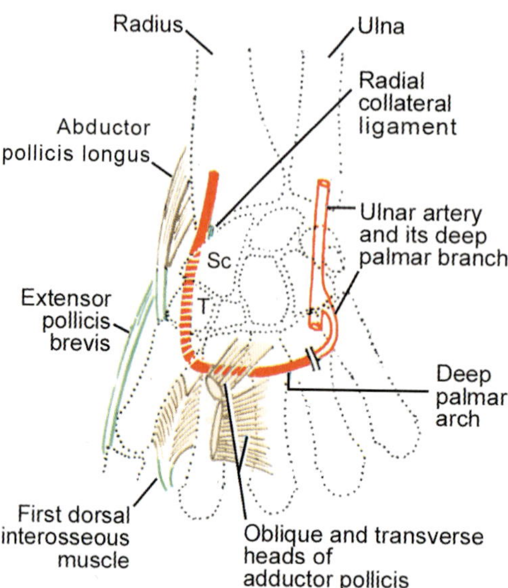


**6.22:** Course of radial artery at the wrist and in the hand

2. The ***palmar carpal branch*** passes medially in front of the carpus to anastomose with a corresponding branch from the ulnar artery to form the palmar carpal arch.
3. The ***dorsal carpal branch*** passes medially behind the carpus to anastomose with a corresponding branch from the ulnar artery to form the dorsal carpal arch.

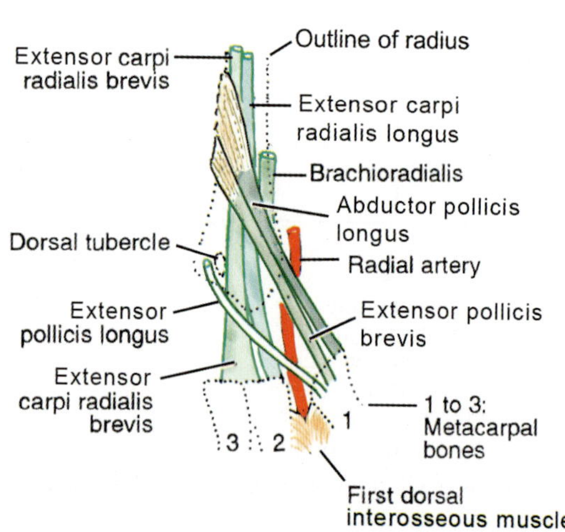


**6.23:** Structures on the lateral side of the wrist related to the radial artery

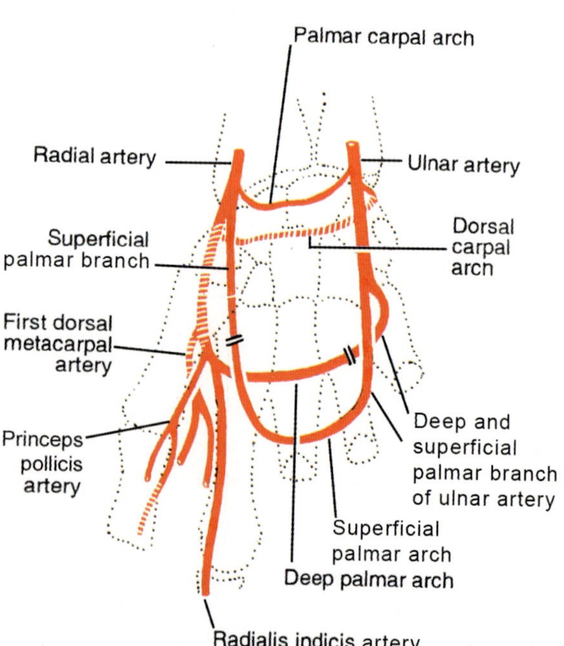


**6.24:** Schematic diagram to show branches of the radial artery in the hand. Some branches of the ulnar artery are also shown. The various arches are formed by corresponding branches of the radial and ulnar arteries

4. The ***superficial palmar branch*** arises before the radial artery turns backwards round the wrist. It runs distally into the palm in relation to the thenar muscles. It often joins the ulnar artery to complete the superficial palmar arch.
5. The ***first dorsal metacarpal*** artery arises from the radial on the dorsum of the hand as the latter reaches the interval between the first and second metacarpal bones. It divides into two branches, one for the medial side of the thumb and the other for the lateral side of the index finger.
6. The ***princeps pollicis*** artery arises just as the radial artery enters the palm after passing forwards between the first and second metacarpal bones. It supplies the lateral side of the thumb.
7. The ***radialis indicis*** artery arises near the princeps pollicis and runs along the lateral side of the index finger. Occasionally, these two arteries arise by a common stem that is then called the first palmar metacarpal artery.

The branches that arise from the deep palmar arch are considered on page 123.

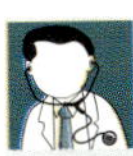

**CLINICAL CORRELATION**

1. The ***radial artery*** can be compressed where it lies over the anterior surface of the lower end of the radius.
2. The ***ulnar artery*** can be compressed immediately lateral to the pisiform bone.
3. However, it must be remembered that these two arteries anastomose freely through the superficial and deep palmar arches.

## The Ulnar Artery

1. The ulnar artery begins in front of the elbow, at the level of the neck of the radius. It passes downwards and medially to reach the medial margin of the forearm (at about its middle) and then runs vertically along this margin.
2. It runs across the wrist superficial to the flexor retinaculum.
3. Entering the palm it runs laterally across it as the superficial palmar arch. This arch is completed laterally by anastomosis with a branch of the radial artery which is usually the superficial palmar, but may be the princeps pollicis or the radialis indicis.

**WANT TO KNOW MORE?**

*Relations of the Ulnar Artery*

1. The upper half of the artery is deep, the lower half relatively superficial.
2. Posteriorly, the artery lies (from above downwards) on:
   a. The brachialis
   b. The flexor digitorum profundus
   c. The flexor retinaculum.
3. In the upper part of the forearm, it lies deep to the flexor digitorum superficialis which separates it from the pronator teres, the flexor carpi radialis and the palmaris longus.
4. In the middle-third of the forearm it is overlapped by the belly of the flexor carpi ulnaris while in the lower one-third of the forearm it is covered only by skin and fascia.
5. Here the tendon of the flexor carpi ulnaris is medial to it and the tendons of the flexor digitorum superficialis are lateral to it.

### Branches of Ulnar Artery

1. The ***anterior ulnar recurrent*** artery arises near the upper end of the ulnar artery. It passes upwards in front of the elbow to anastomose with the supratrochlear artery (6.25).
2. The ***posterior ulnar recurrent*** artery also arises near the upper end of the ulnar artery. It passes upwards behind the medial epicondyle and anastomoses with the superior ulnar collateral artery.
3. The ***common interosseous*** artery arises from the lateral side of the ulnar artery and very soon divides into anterior and posterior interosseous branches.
4. The ***anterior interosseous*** artery descends in front of the interosseous membrane. Near the upper border of the pronator quadratus it pierces the membrane and runs downward behind it to the back of the wrist. Here it joins the dorsal carpal arch.
   a. Before piercing the interosseous membrane, it gives off a branch that runs downwards anterior to the membrane and joins the palmar carpal arch.
   b. The anterior interosseous artery also gives off a median branch which accompanies the median nerve.
5. The ***posterior interosseous artery*** passes backwards above the upper margin of the interosseous membrane and then descends between muscles of the back of the forearm supplying them.
   a. Near its origin the posterior interosseous artery gives off an interosseous recurrent artery that runs upwards behind the elbow.
   b. It anastomoses with the posterior descending branch of the profunda brachii artery and with the supratrochlear artery.
6. The ***palmar and dorsal carpal branches*** of the ulnar artery arise at the wrist. They anastomose with the palmar and dorsal carpal branches of the radial artery to form the palmar and dorsal carpal arches.
7. The ***deep palmar branch*** of the ulnar artery arises just distal to the pisiform bone. It passes through the hypothenar muscles and ends by anastomosing with the radial artery to complete the deep palmar arch.
8. After giving off its deep branch the ulnar artery continues into the palm as the ***superficial palmar branch***.
   a. This branch runs transversely across the palm forming the superficial palmar arch: this arch lies distal to the deep palmar arch.
   b. The arch is completed laterally by a branch of the radial artery: usually the superficial palmar, but sometimes the radialis indicis or the princeps pollicis.
   c. Rarely the arch is formed by the ulnar artery alone.

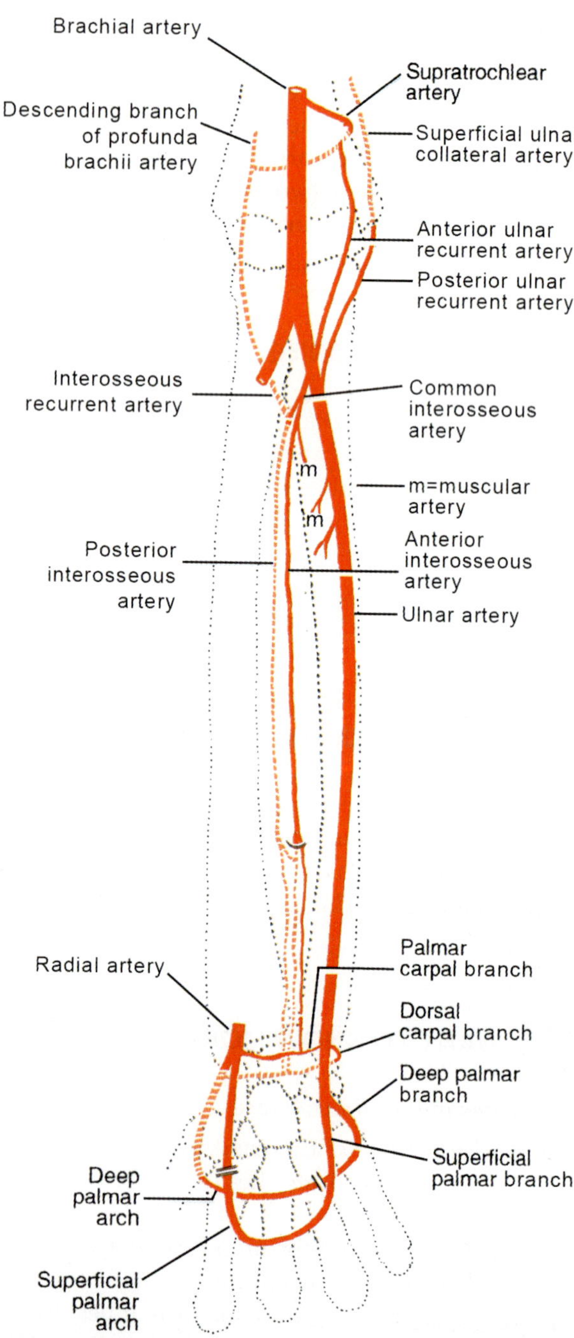


**6.25:** Scheme to show branches of the ulnar artery

## WANT TO KNOW MORE?

### Arteries of the Hand

The palm and digits receive a series of branches from the various arterial arches formed in the region. They are as follows:

1. There are four ***dorsal metacarpal arteries***.
   a. The first artery is a direct branch of the radial. It runs distally in the interval between the first and second metacarpal bones.
   b. The second, third and fourth arteries arise from the dorsal carpal arch.
   c. Each dorsal metacarpal artery ends by dividing into two dorsal digital arteries for continuous sides of two digits.
2. The ***palmar metacarpal arteries*** are also four in number.
   a. The first artery is represented by the common stem of the princeps pollicis and radialis indicis arteries: it is absent when these branches arise independently from the radial artery.
   b. The second, third and fourth arteries arise from the deep palmar arch: they end by joining the common palmar digital arteries (see below) of the corresponding intermetacarpal space.
3. The ***common palmar digital arteries*** arise from the superficial palmar arch.
   a. There are three of them, one lying in each space between the medial four metacarpal bones.
   b. Reaching the web between adjoining digits each artery divides into two branches that run along the adjoining sides of two digits.
4. The superficial palmar arch gives off a separate digital branch to the medial side of the little finger.
5. Each dorsal metacarpal artery is joined (near its origin) to the deep palmar arch by a ***proximal perforating artery***.
6. Just before its bifurcation, each common palmar digital artery is joined to the dorsal metacarpal artery of that space by a ***distal perforating artery***.

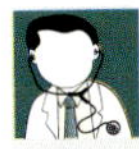

## CLINICAL CORRELATION

### *Arterial Anastomoses*

1. Numerous arterial anastomoses are present in the hand, the largest of these being between the radial and ulnar arteries through the superficial and deep palmar arches.
2. They serve as efficient communication channels in the event of blockage or ligature of one artery.

### *Gangrene and Ulceration*

1. Blockage of the arterial supply to the distal part of a limb can result in death of tissues within the part.
2. Such a part loses all function and gradually changes colour finally becoming black. This condition is called ***gangrene***. Such a part has to be removed by amputation.
3. Gangrene of the fingers can occur as a result of exposure to extreme cold. It can also be caused by some drugs.
4. Sometimes a gangrenous part may become infected. This makes the condition much more serious.
5. Ischaemia of a region can also lead to ***localised necrosis*** of tissue, and ulcers may form.

### *Raynaud's Disease (or phenomenon)*

1. In all persons, exposure to cold can cause ***vasoconstriction***. In some persons this response is abnormally high and vasoconstriction of arterioles in the distal part of the limb may seriously impair blood supply to the hands.
2. In such cases, a series of events may be observed.
   a. When the hand is cooled first there is a loss of colour (***blanching***) and the hand becomes pale.

   b. After an interval the arterioles dilate and blood starts flowing into the hand, but this blood is deoxygenated (because of stagnation in arteries). The hand becomes swollen and dark.
   c. As more blood flows into the hand the deoxygenated blood is washed off (with oxygenated blood) and the hand becomes red in colour.
3. Basically the condition is caused by abnormally active sympathetic nerves. It can be controlled with drugs.
4. In more severe cases ***sympathetic denervation*** of blood vessels of the limb is necessary. This can be achieved by surgical removal of the upper thoracic sympathetic ganglia (preganglionic cervico-dorsal sympathectomy).

***Injury to Palmar Arches***

1. A wound injuring one of the palmar arches causes severe bleeding and is difficult to treat.
2. As the arches receive blood from both the radial and ulnar arteries the injured arch bleeds from both ends.
3. Compression or ligation of the radial or ulnar artery cannot control bleeding.
4. Compression of the brachial artery may be necessary.

## INFECTIONS OF THE HAND

### Compartments and Spaces of the Hand

1. The ***palmar aponeurosis*** is a triangular sheet of dense fascia that covers the central part of the palm.
2. The lateral palmar septum passes from the lateral edge of the aponeurosis to the first metacarpal bone.
3. The medial edge of the palmar aponeurosis is connected to the fifth metacarpal bone by the medial palmar septum.
4. These septa divide the palm into three main compartments (6.26) as follows:
   a. The ***lateral compartment*** (lateral to the lateral septum) contains the thenar muscles (except the greater part of the adductor pollicis).
   b. The ***medial compartment*** (medial to the medial septum) contains the hypothenar muscles.
   c. The ***intermediate compartment***, lying deep to the palmar aponeurosis, is bounded medially and laterally by the corresponding palmar septa.
5. The intermediate compartment contains the following:
   a. Tendons of the flexor digitorum superficialis
   b. Tendon of the flexor digitorum profundus
   c. Tendon of the flexor pollicis longus
   d. The lumbrical muscles
   e. The superficial palmar arch and its digital branches
   f. The deep palmar arch
   g. Digital branches of the median and ulnar nerves.
6. The intermediate compartment is divided into two parts by an ***intermediate palmar septum***. (also called ***oblique palmar septum***). This septum passes from the deep surface of the lateral part of the palmar aponeurosis to the front of the third metacarpal bone (6.26).
7. The lateral and medial compartments are mainly of anatomical importance. The intermediate compartment is of surgical importance as described below.

### Midpalmar and Thenar Spaces

These are potential spaces of surgical importance as they can be infected. They lie within the intermediate compartment of the palm (see above), deep to the palmar aponeurosis and the flexor tendons.

1. The ***thenar space*** (not to be confused with the lateral compartment containing the thenar muscles) lies between the lateral and intermediate palmar septa.
2. The ***midpalmar space*** lies between the intermediate and medial palmar septa.

Both spaces are triangular: the base of each space lies distally, and the apex is directed proximally.

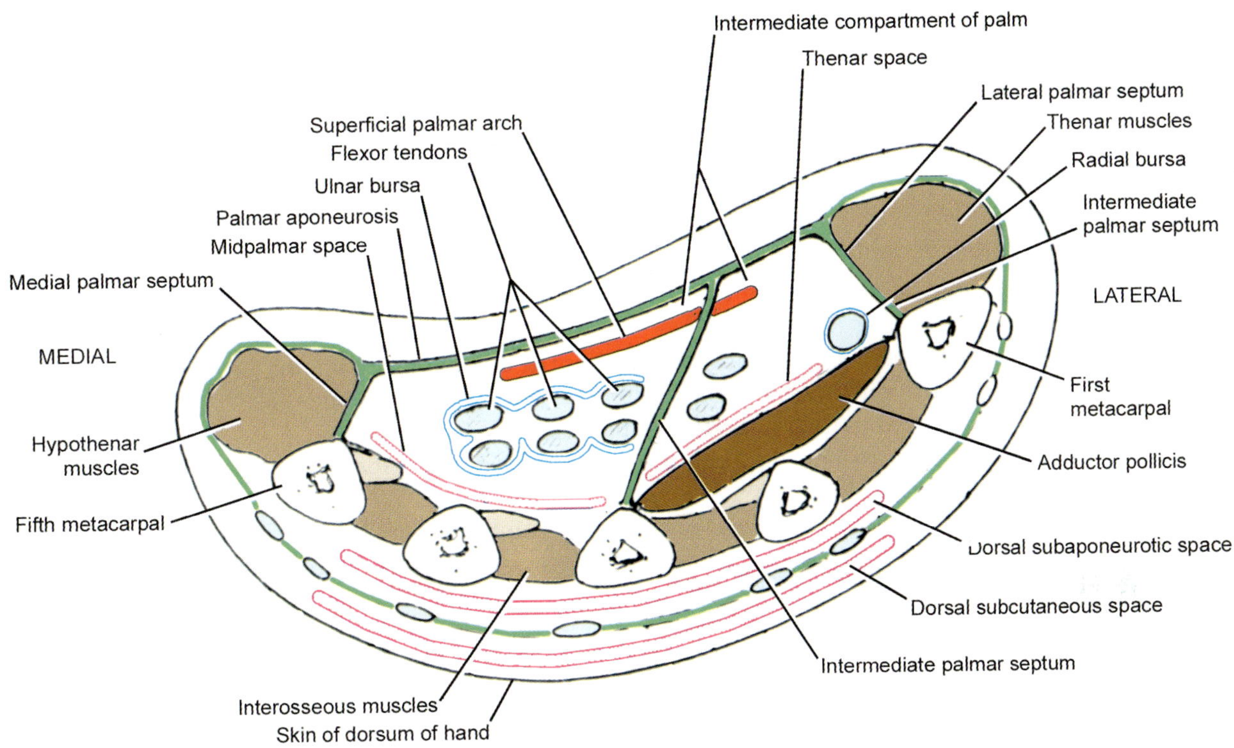


**6.26:** Transverse section across the hand to show its compartments, and the location of some spaces of surgical importance

### *Boundaries of Thenar Space*

1. Medially: Intermediate palmar septum.
2. Laterally: Lateral palmar septum.
3. Anteriorly: Lateral part of palmar aponeurosis, and flexor tendons to index finger.
4. Posteriorly: Adductor pollicis, transverse head.
   The tendon of the flexor pollicis longus lies in front of the lateral end of the space and is sometimes described as part of the lateral wall.

### *Boundaries of Midpalmar Space*

1. Medially: Medial palmar septum.
2. Laterally: Intermediate palmar septum.
3. Anteriorly: Medial part of palmar aponeurosis, and flexor tendons to medial three fingers.
4. Posteriorly: Fascia covering the medial three metacarpal bones and intervening interosseous muscles.

### *Proximal and Distal Extent of Spaces*

1. Proximally, the midpalmar and thenar spaces extend up to the distal margin of the flexor retinaculum.
2. Distally, the thenar space extends up to the proximal transverse crease of the palm, and the midpalmar space extends up to the distal transverse crease.
3. Incisions are made through these creases to drain the spaces.

### *Communications of Spaces*

1. The spaces are normally closed at the proximal end.
2. However, occasionally the midpalmar space may communicate with the forearm space (see later in the text) through the carpal tunnel.
3. The two spaces of the palm quite frequently communicate with each other, and infection can pass from one to the other.

### *Contents of the Thenar and Midpalmar Spaces*

1. The spaces are normally filled mainly with loose connective tissue. When infected they can be distended with pus.
2. These spaces are closely related to the lumbrical muscles. The thenar space contains the first lumbrical muscle, while the midpalmar space contains the second, third and fourth lumbrical muscles.
3. The tendon of each lumbrical muscle is surrounded by a ***lumbrical canal***.
   a. When traced distally, the thenar space becomes continuous with the lumbrical canal which surrounds the tendon of the first lumbrical muscle.
   b. The midpalmar space becomes continuous with the lumbrical canals of the second, third and fourth lumbrical muscles.

### *Variation in Spaces*

1. Occasionally, the intermediate palmar septum passes through the interval between the flexor tendons for the middle and ring fingers (instead of passing between the tendons of the index and middle fingers).
2. In that case the second lumbrical muscle, and its lumbrical canal, are related to the thenar space and not to the midpalmar space.

## Pulp Spaces of Fingers

1. Infections in the region of the fingertips (known as ***whitlow*** or ***felon***) are commonly caused through cuts or pin pricks.
2. Such infections cause much pain because the region of the tip of the finger is divided into a number of small compartments, and distension of any compartment with pus presses on nerve endings there.
3. The region of the fingertip is cut off from the proximal part of the digit by deep fascia which is adherent ventrally to skin at the distal digital crease, and dorsally to periosteum of the terminal phalanx just distal to insertion of the flexor digitorum profundus (6.27).
4. The pulp space, distal to the fascia, contains a number of septa that pass from skin to periosteum. Each compartment is normally occupied by fat.
5. The arterial supply to the shaft of the distal phalanx (diaphysis) passes through the pulp space and pressure on it can lead to necrosis of this part of the phalanx.
6. The base of the phalanx (epiphysis) is spared as the artery to it enters the bone proximal to the pulp space.
7. In the past, incisions along the lateral margin of the digit were advocated from draining collections of pus in the pulp space. At present most surgeons use short incisions directly over the point of maximum tenderness.

## Infection in Relation to Nails (Paronychia)

These infections are common. Initially the infection is subcuticular. When pus extends deep to the nail the affected part of the latter has to be removed.

## Digital Synovial Sheaths of the Hand

1. The flexor tendons to the digits are surrounded by synovial sheaths (6.5).
2. These include the digital synovial sheaths (over the digits), the ulnar bursa and the radial bursa.
3. Any of these can be the site of infection. The following points are worthy of note.
4. A digital sheath can be infected by any injury to a finger.
   a. In the case of the second, third and fourth digits infection remains confined to the digital sheath.

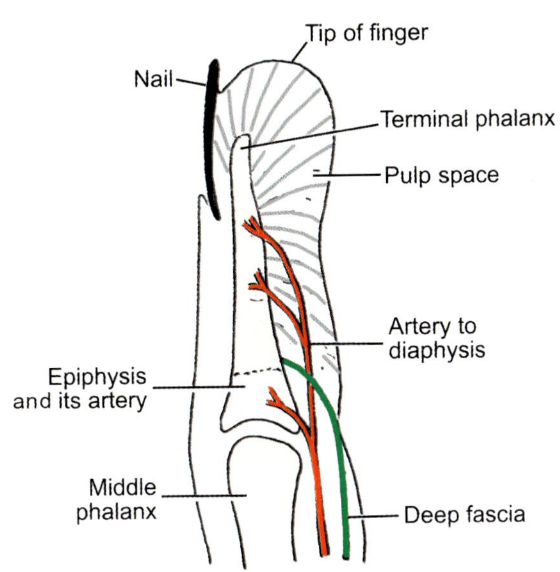


6.27: Pulp space of a digit. Note the position of arteries to the epiphysis and diaphysis of the terminal phalanx

b. However, as the digital sheath of the little finger communicates (proximally) with the ulnar bursa, infection from this finger can spread to the ulnar bursa (and reach right up to the lower part of the forearm).

c. The digital sheath for the thumb is continuous with the radial bursa, which also reaches the lower part of the forearm.

d. Infection from the ulnar or radial bursa can, therefore, travel to the forearm space of Parona (see below).

e. The radial and ulnar bursae may sometimes communicate with each other so that infection can pass from one to the other.

f. Surgical incisions for draining the tendon sheaths are made at the level of both ends of the space so that complete drainage is possible.

**Other Spaces in the Hand**

1. Infection may occur in a ***web space*** i.e., within the folds of skin connecting bases of the digits.
2. There are two spaces on the dorsum of the hand that are occasionally sites of infection.
   a. The ***subcutaneous space*** lies just under the skin.
   b. The ***subaponeurotic space*** lies deep to the extensor tendons (6.26).
3. Infections from the digits and palm can travel to these spaces through lymphatics.
4. Synovial sheaths are present in relation to tendons passing under cover of the extensor retinaculum.
   a. Infections of these sheaths are not common.
   b. However, repeated stress can lead to inflammation of one or more sheaths (***tenosynovitis***) in which there can be pain and restriction of movement.
5. The tendons of the abductor pollicis longus and the extensor pollicis brevis rub constantly against the styloid process of the radius. The common synovial sheath around them may undergo fibrosis (***stenosing tenosynovitis***) restricting movement, and may require incision of the sheath.

***Forearm Space (of Parona)***

This space does not lie in the hand, but it is convenient to consider it here.

1. It is located in the lower part of the anterior compartment of the forearm, deep to the flexor tendons and in front of the pronator quadratus.
2. Proximally, its upward extent is limited by the origin of the flexor digitorum superficialis.

3. Inferiorly (distally), it extends up to the upper border of the flexor retinaculum.
4. Occasionally, this space can be infected by spread of pus through the ulnar bursa. This results in an ***hour-glass swelling:*** one swelling in the forearm united to another in the palm through a constriction in the region of the flexor retinaculum.
5. The space is drained through incisions along the lateral and medial borders of the lower part of the forearm.

# BACK OF FOREARM AND HAND

## Superficial Structures

The cutaneous nerves and superficial veins present on the back of the forearm have been described in Chapter 5.

## MUSCLES OF THE BACK OF THE FOREARM

The muscles on the back of the forearm are present in two layers: superficial and deep.
*The superficial muscles are:*

1. Brachioradialis
2. Extensor carpi radialis longus
3. Extensor carpi radialis brevis
4. Extensor digitorum
5. Extensor digiti minimi
6. Extensor carpi ulnaris
7. Anconeus.

The main features of these muscles are presented in 6.28. Some further points of importance are given in notes that follow.

**6.28: Superficial muscles of the back of the forearm**

| *Muscle* | *Origin* | *Insertion* | *Action* | *Nerve Supply* |
|---|---|---|---|---|
| Brachioradialis | 1. Upper two-thirds of lateral supracondylar ridge of humerus<br>2. Lateral intermuscular septum | Lateral side of radius just above styloid process | 1. Flexes the forearm (especially in mid-prone position)<br>2. Supinates fully pronated arm and pronates fully supinated forearm (to midprone position) | Radial nerve (C5, 6, 7) |
| Extensor carpi radialis longus | 1. Lower one-third of lateral supracondylar ridge of humerus<br>2. Some fibres from lateral epicondyle<br>3. Some fibres from lateral intermuscular septum | Lateral side of base of second metacarpal bone (dorsal aspect) | Actions common to both muscles:<br>1. Extension of wrist (along with extensor carpi ulnaris)<br>2. Abduction of wrist (along with flexor carpi ulnaris<br>3. They fix the wrist and assist powerful movements of hand | Radial nerve (C6, 7) |

*Contd...*

*Contd...*

| *Muscle* | *Origin* | *Insertion* | *Action* | *Nerve Supply* |
|---|---|---|---|---|
| Extensor carpi radialis brevis | 1. Lateral epicondyle of humerus<br>2. Radial collateral ligament of elbow joint | Dorsal aspect of base of second and third metacarpal bones | Same as for extensor carpi radialis longus | Deep branch of radial nerve (C7, 8) |
| Extensor digitorum | Lateral epicondyle of humerus.<br>The tendon splits into four parts one for each digit other than the thumb. Over the proximal phalanx the tendon for each digit divides into three slips, one intermediate and two collateral | 1. Intermediate slip for each digit into base of middle phalanx (dorsal aspect)<br>2. Collateral slips reunite and are inserted into the base of the distal phalanx (dorsal aspect) | Extension at:<br>1. Interphalangeal joints<br>2. Metacarpophalangeal joints<br>3. Wrist joint | Deep branch of radial nerve (C7, 8) |
| Extensor digiti minimi | Lateral epicondyle of humerus<br>(The tendon is joined by the tendon of the extensor digitorum for fifth digit) | The tendon ends in the dorsal digital expansion of the little finger through which it is inserted into:<br>1. Dorsal aspect of the base of middle phalanx<br>2. Base of distal phalanx | Extension of little finger at:<br>1. Metacarpophalangeal joint<br>2. Interphalangeal joints | Deep branch of radial nerve (C7, 8) |
| Extensor carpi ulnaris | 1. Lateral epicondyle of humerus<br>2. Posterior border of ulna (by an aponeurosis common to it, the flexor carpi ulnaris and flexor digitorum profundus) | Medial side of the base of fifth metacarpal bone | 1. Extension of wrist (along with extensor carpi radialis longus and brevis)<br>2. Adduction of hand (with flexor carpi ulnaris)<br>3. Fixes the wrist during forceful movements of the hand (along with other muscles around the wrist) | Deep branch of radial nerve (C7, 8) |
| Anconeus | Lateral epicondyle of humerus (posterior aspect) | 1. Lateral aspect of olecranon process of ulna<br>2. Upper one-fourth of posterior surface of ulna | 1. Weak extensor of elbow<br>2. Moves ulna laterally during pronation | Branch from radial nerve (C7, 8, T1) given off in the arm and passing through medial head of triceps |

## WANT TO KNOW MORE?

**Notes on Brachioradialis**

1. The upper fleshy part of the brachioradialis forms the lateral boundary of the cubital fossa. Here the radial nerve is deep to it (between it and the brachialis).
2. Near its insertion its tendon is crossed by tendons of the abductor pollicis longus and the extensor pollicis brevis (6.23).
3. At the wrist the radial artery is medial to the tendon (between it and the tendon of the flexor carpi radialis).

**Notes on Extensor Carpi Radialis Longus and Extensor Carpi Radialis Brevis**

1. The extensor carpi radialis longus is superficial to the brevis.
2. The tendons of the two muscles run distally along the lateral side of the radius. They pass deep to the abductor pollicis longus and the extensor pollicis brevis muscles (6.23).
3. At the lower end of the radius the tendons occupy a groove just behind the styloid process (and lateral to the dorsal tubercle). The longus tendon lies lateral to the brevis tendon. Here the two tendons pass deep to the extensor retinaculum. They are surrounded by a common synovial sheath.
4. A little above their insertion, the tendons are crossed by the tendon of the extensor pollicis longus (6.23).

**Notes on Extensor Digitorum**

1. As the tendons of the muscle pass under cover of the extensor retinaculum, they are surrounded by a common synovial sheath. Distally the sheath extends for some distance beyond the retinaculum.
2. The tendon for the index finger is accompanied by the tendon of the extensor indicis.
3. The tendon for the little finger is joined by the tendon of the extensor digiti minimi.
4. Over the proximal phalanx the tendon (of that digit) becomes embedded in a triangular membrane called the dorsal digital expansion. This is described below.
5. Note that extension of the digits is accompanied by fanning out of the digits (i.e., abduction of the second, fourth and fifth digits). This is an indirect action of the extensor digitorum. (Flexion of digits – by flexor digitorum superficialis and profundus – is accompanied by adduction, as happens in closing the fist).

***Dorsal Digital Expansion and Insertion of the Extensor Digitorum***

1. The dorsal digital expansion is an aponeurosis present on the dorsal aspect of the proximal phalanx, and the metacarpophalangeal joint. The expansion is triangular (6.30). It has an apex directed distally, and a broad base that lies dorsal to the metacarpophalangeal joint.
2. The expansion may be regarded as an aponeurotic extension of the tendon of the extensor digitorum. This tendon joins the central part of the base of the expansion, and divides into its intermediate and collateral slips in the substance of the expansion.
3. For more details see 6.30.

*The deep muscles of the back of the forearm are:*

1. Supinator
2. Extensor pollicis longus
3. Abductor pollicis longus
4. Extensor indicis
5. Extensor pollicis brevis.

The main facts about these muscles are given in 6.31. Further facts of importance are given below.

**WANT TO KNOW MORE?**

**Notes on Supinator**

1. From 6.32 it will be seen that starting from their origin, the fibres of the supinator wind round the posterior, lateral and anterior aspects of the radius (in that order) to reach their insertion. The fibres thus have a spiral course that enables them to rotate the radius with ease.
2. The muscle has two layers: superficial and deep. The deep branch of radial nerve runs downwards between these layers.

**Notes on Abductor Pollicis Longus and Extensor Pollicis Brevis**

1. The abductor pollicis longus and the extensor pollicis brevis (see below) are deep to the superficial extensors in the upper part of the forearm.
2. They become superficial by emerging between the extensor carpi radialis brevis and the extensor digitorum.
3. For this reason they are referred to as the ***outcropping muscles of the forearm***.
4. They then run laterally and forwards across the tendons of the extensor carpi radialis brevis and longus.

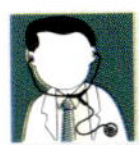

## CLINICAL CORRELATION

1. ***Tennis elbow***: Repeated strain on the extensor muscles of the forearm (as in a tennis player or a violinist) can cause tearing of tissue near the origin of these muscles from the common extensor origin (lateral epicondyle).
   a. Pain occurs over the lateral epicondyle and along the radial border of the forearm.
   b. The condition is called ***tennis elbow***.
2. A similar condition in relation to the medial epicondyle is called ***golfer's elbow***.
3. Sometimes, a strong force can pull a tendon off (evulsion) from its bony attachment.
   a. If the tendon of the extensor digitorum (for a digit) is evulsed from its insertion into the distal phalanx, complete extension of the phalanx is no longer possible.
   b. The distal phalanx remains in a state of partial flexion. This is called ***mallet finger*** (mallet = small hammer).

## Extensor Retinaculum

1. The extensor retinaculum is a thickened band of deep fascia that runs across the back (and sides) of the wrist (6.33). It is about 2.5 cm in width. It holds the extensor tendons in place and facilitates their action by acting as a pulley.
2. The space between the deep surface of the retinaculum and the underlying bones is divided into six compartments shown in 6.34.

## WANT TO KNOW MORE?

**Synovial Sheaths**

1. The tendons passing under the extensor retinaculum are surrounded by synovial sheaths (thick lines in 6.34 and 6.35).
2. Normally, there are six sheaths—one each for the tendons passing through each compartment under the extensor retinaculum.
3. However, the tendons of the first compartment (i.e., the abductor pollicis longus and the extensor pollicis brevis), and those of the second compartment, may have individual sheaths.
4. Proximally, the sheaths extend for a short distance proximal to the extensor retinaculum.
5. Distally, the sheaths of tendons that gain insertion into the bases of the metacarpal bones extend up to the insertion.
   a. The sheath for the extensor pollicis brevis extends to the base of the first metacarpal bone.
   b. The sheaths for the tendons going to the digits, and that for the extensor pollicis longus, extend to the level of the middle of the metacarpus.

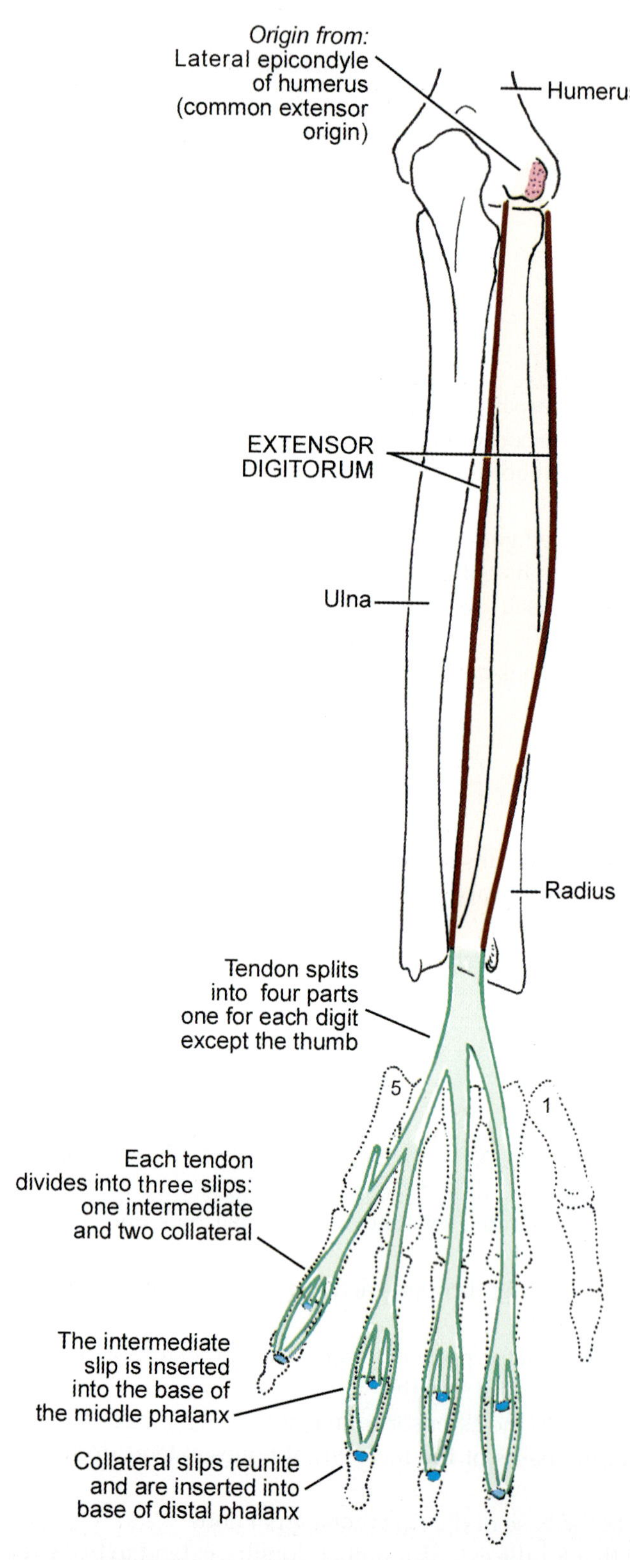


**6.29:** Attachments of the extensor digitorum

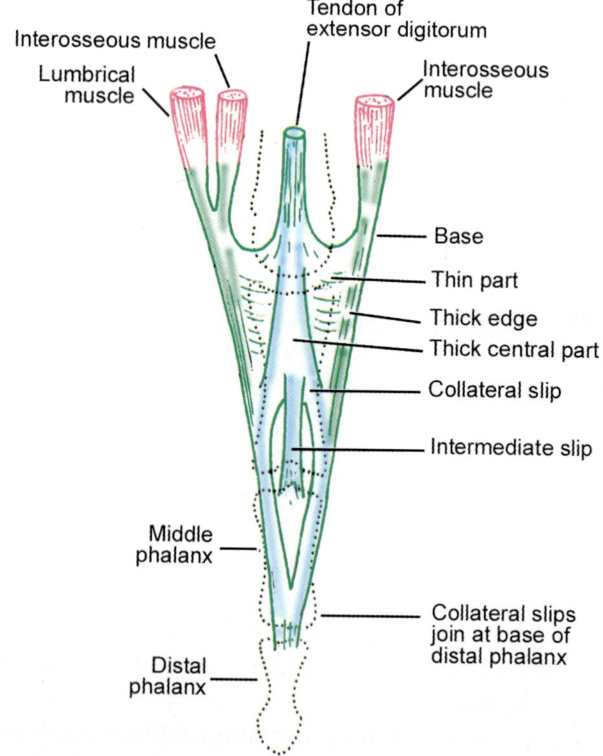


**6.30:** Dorsal digital expansion and insertion of the external digitorum

**6.31: Deep muscles of the back of the forearm**

| *Muscle* | *Origin* | *Insertion* | *Action* | *Nerve Supply* |
|---|---|---|---|---|
| Supinator | 1. Lateral epicondyle of humerus<br>2. Radial collateral ligament of elbow<br>3. Annular ligament<br>4. Supinator crest of ulna and posterior part of triangular area in front of it | Upper one-third of lateral surface of radius. (The area extends onto the anterior and posterior aspects of the upper part of the radius) | Supination of the arm | Deep branch of radial nerve (C7, 8) |
| Extensor pollicis longus | 1. Lateral part of posterior surface of ulna (below origin of abductor pollicis longus)<br>2. Interosseous membrane (adjoining part) | Base of distal phalanx of thumb (dorsal aspect) | 1. Extends distal phalanx of thumb<br>2. Extends proximal phalanx of thumb<br>3. Extends first metacarpal<br>4. Adduction and lateral rotation of thumb | Deep branch of radial nerve (C7, 8) |
| Abductor pollicis longus | 1. Lateral part of posterior surface of ulna. (below insertion of anconeus)<br>2. Interosseous membrane (adjoining part)<br>3. Posterior surface of radius (below insertion of supinator) | 1. Radial side of the base of first metacarpal<br>2. On trapezium | Abduction and extension of thumb (at carpometacarpal joint of thumb) | Deep branch of radial nerve (C7, 8) |
| Extensor indicis | 1. Posterior surface of ulna below origin of the extensor pollicis longus<br>2. Interosseous membrane (adjoining part) | Tendon ends by joining the ulnar side of the extensor digitorum tendon for the index finger (and is indirectly inserted into the middle and distal phalanges) | 1. Extends index finger<br>2. Helps to extend the wrist | Deep branch of radial nerve (C7, 8) |
| Extensor pollicis brevis | 1. Posterior surface of radius (below origin of abductor pollicis longus)<br>2. Interosseous membrane (adjoining part) | Dorsal surface of the base of the proximal phalanx of the thumb | Extends proximal phalanx and metacarpal bone of the thumb | Deep branch of radial nerve (C7, 8) |

## NERVES AND ARTERIES ON THE BACK OF THE FOREARM AND HAND

The arteries on the dorsum of the hand are branches of the radial and ulnar arteries. These have been described on pages 117 to 123.

The nerve supply to muscles on the back of the forearm is through the deep branch of the radial nerve. The dorsum of the hand is supplied by branches of the radial, ulnar and median nerves. These nerves have already been considered earlier in this chapter.

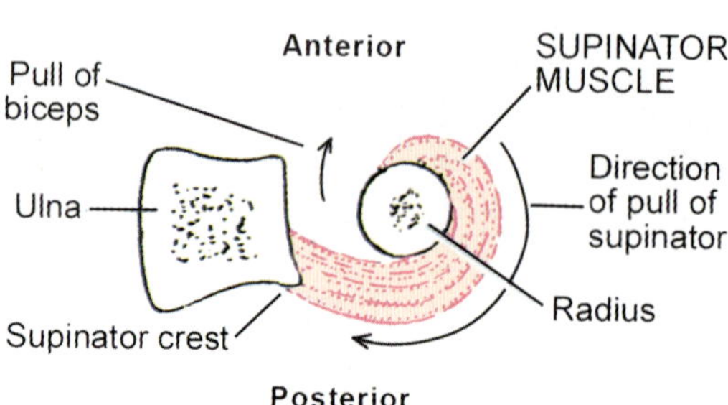


6.32: Arrangement of fibres of the supinator muscle

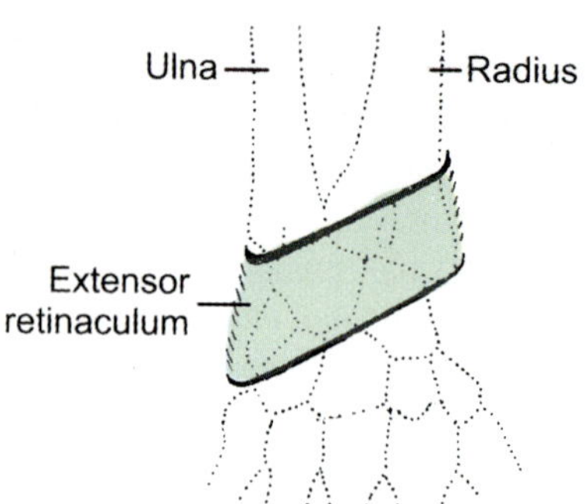


6.33: Attachments of the extensor retinaculum

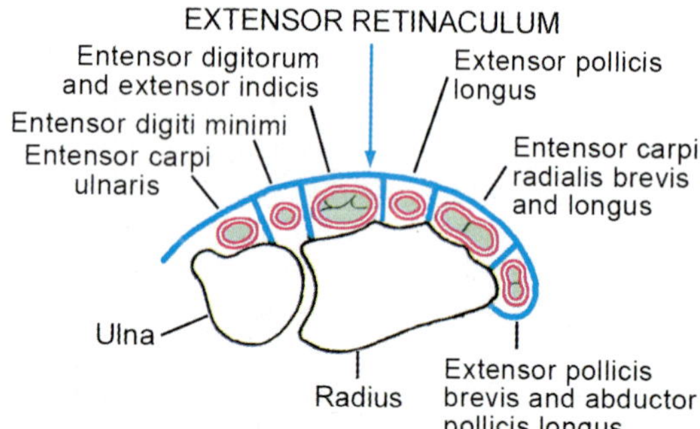


6.34: Tendons passing under cover of the extensor retinaculum

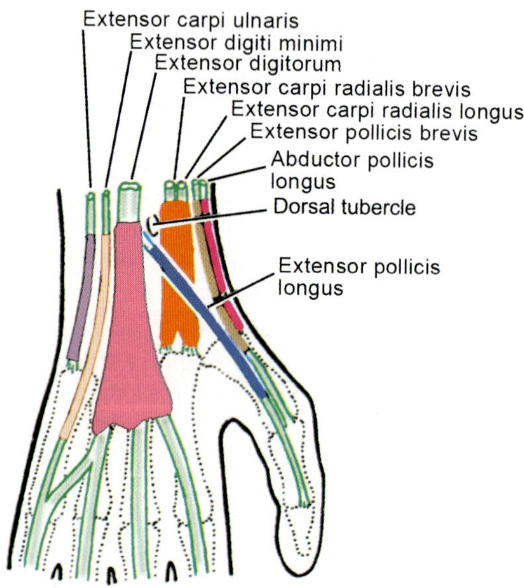


6.35: Synovial sheaths on the dorsum of the wrist and hand

7

CHAPTER

# General Features of Joints and Joints of the Upper Limb

## CLASSIFICATION OF JOINTS

In this chapter we will first discuss some general considerations that are essential for the understanding of the anatomy of joints in any part of the body. Thereafter, we will consider individual joints of the upper extremity.

1. A joint (or articulation) can be said to exist wherever two bones meet.
2. Joints can be classified into various types depending upon their structure and on the movements permitted by them.

## CLASSIFICATION OF JOINTS ON THE BASIS OF STRUCTURE

Joints can be divided into three main types on the basis of structure, namely:

1. Fibrous joints
2. Cartilaginous joints
3. Synovial joints.

### Fibrous Joints

Fibrous joints are of various types as follows:

1. The ***sutures*** of the skull are fibrous joints. The structure of a suture is shown in 7.1.
   a. The skull bones are lined on the outside by a membrane called the ***pericranium***, and on the inside by another membrane called the ***endocranium*** (which is the outer layer of duramater).
   b. These membranes pass across the suture from one bone to the other uniting them.
   c. Some fibrous tissue intervenes between the bone ends; on one side it is continuous with pericranium and on the other side with the endocranium. This tissue constitutes the ***sutural ligament***.
   d. The sutures start disappearing (by fusion of the bones) around the age of 30 years, the fusion starting first on the endocranial surface and gradually extending to the outer surface.
   e. Sutures are of various types depending on the shape of the bone ends as shown in 7.2 A to F.
2. The joints between the teeth and jaws are also fibrous joints, the cavity in the jaw and the root of the tooth being connected only by some fibrous tissue. These are ***peg and socket joints*** or ***gomphoses*** (7.2G).
3. The inferior ends of the tibia and fibula are directly united by fibrous tissue, which is in the form of a strong ligament (7.2H). Such a joint is called a ***syndesmosis***.

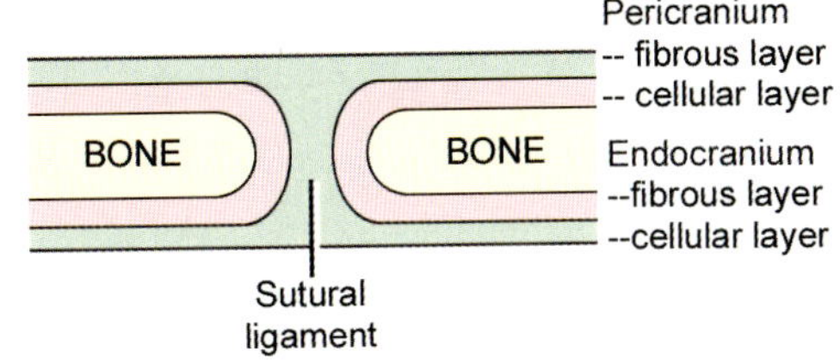


**7.1:** Section across a suture to show its structure

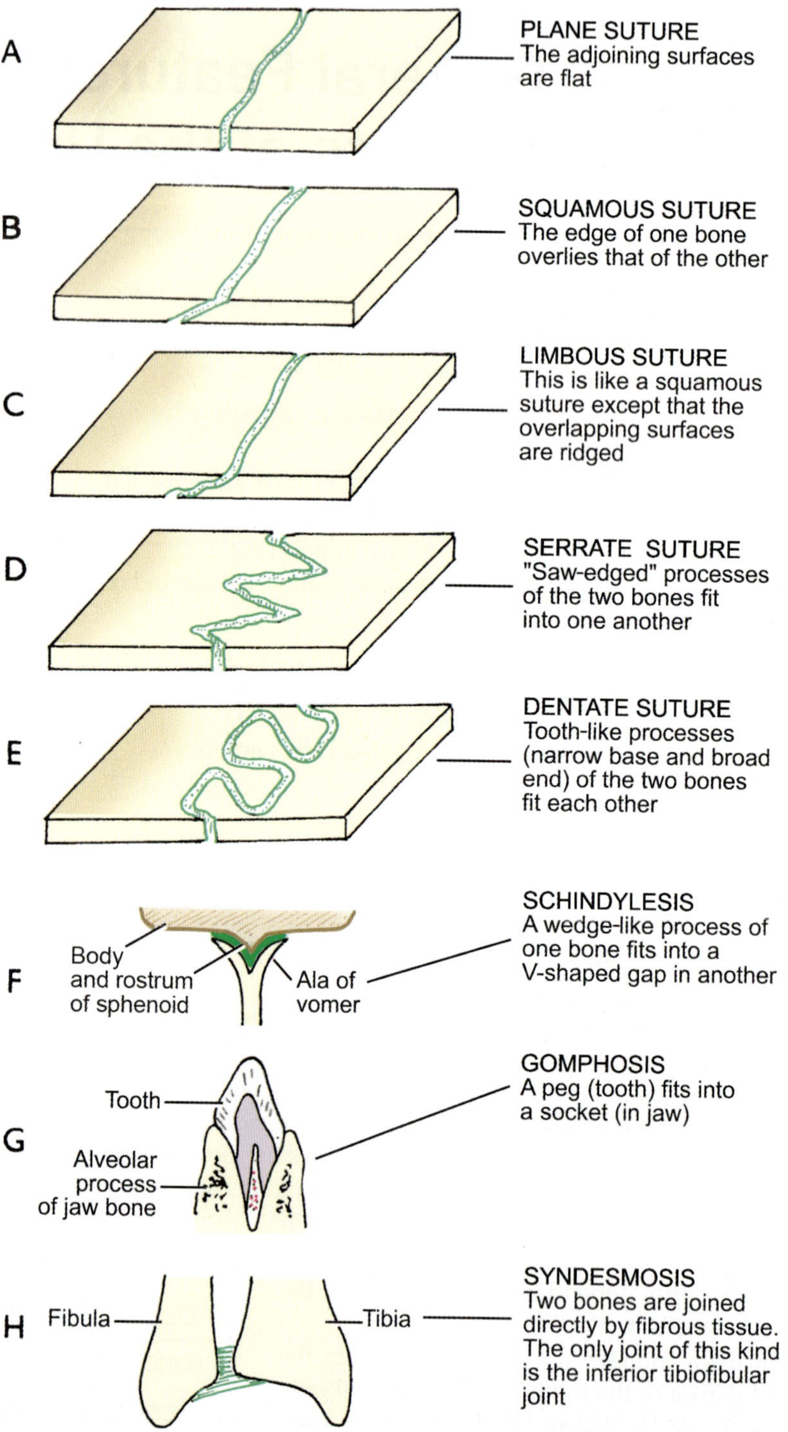


**7.2:** Various types of fibrous joints

## Cartilaginous Joints

1. In young individuals most long bones consist of a central part (corresponding to the shaft) called the ***diaphysis***, and of bony ends or ***epiphyses*** (7.3).
2. Each epiphysis is united to the diaphysis by a plate of hyaline cartilage called the ***epiphyseal plate***.
3. A joint may be said to exist between the epiphysis and the diaphysis through this plate. Such joints are called ***primary cartilaginous joints*** or ***synchondroses***.
4. The purpose of such a joint is to provide a region of growth. The joint is temporary. After full growth is attained (by the age of 18 years or so) the epiphyseal plates of various synchondroses disappear and the epiphyses and diaphyses fuse.

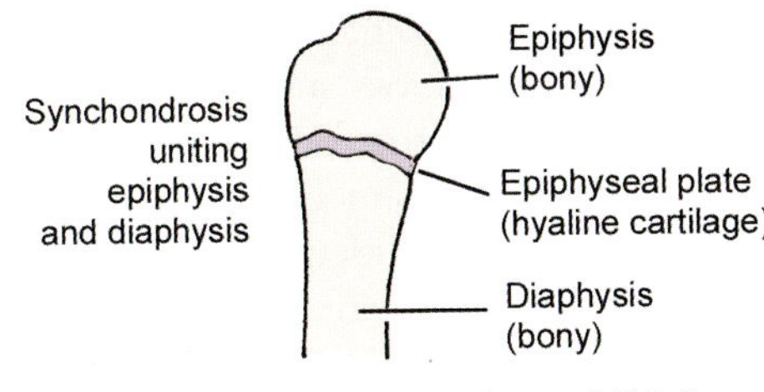


**7.3:** Diagram of a bone end in a child showing a synchondrosis

5. Synchondroses are located as follows:
   a. Long bones of limbs as described above.
   b. A synchondrosis is present between the bodies of the sphenoid and occipital bones.
   c. Another synchondrosis is located between the sphenoid and petrous temporal bones.
   d. The joint between the first costal cartilage and the manubrium sterni is a synchondrosis.
6. Some cartilaginous joints are permanent structures that do not disappear with age. They are called ***secondary cartilaginous joints*** or ***symphyses***.
7. The structure of such a joint is shown in 7.4.
   a. The bone ends forming the joint are covered by a thin layer of hyaline cartilage.
   b. The two layers of hyaline cartilage are united by an intervening layer of fibrocartilage.
   c. *It may be noted that all symphyses lie in the median plane.*
8. Examples of this type of joint are:
   a. Pubic symphysis.
   b. Joints between the vertebral bodies.
   c. Manubriosternal joint.
9. In the case of the joints between the vertebral bodies, the plate of fibrocartilage is represented by the intervertebral discs.
10. The so-called symphysis menti (joining the two halves of the mandible) is not a true symphysis as it disappears with age.

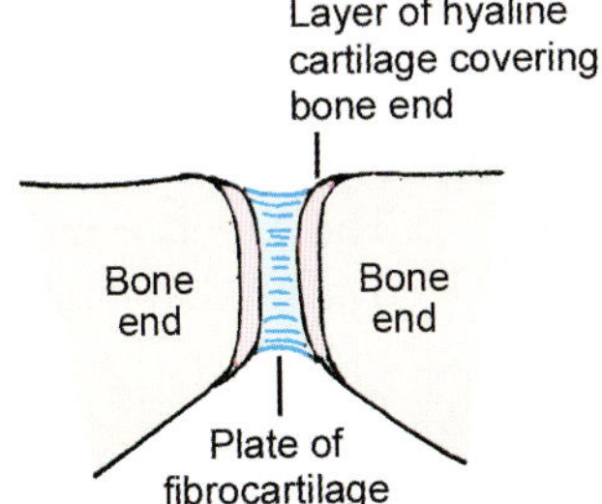


**7.4:** Structure of a symphysis (Secondary cartilaginous joint)

## Synovial Joints

The large majority of joints of the body are of the synovial type.

1. In this variety, the bone ends are not directly connected to one another by any tissue.
2. They have smooth articular surfaces that glide on each other.
3. To facilitate this movement the articular surfaces are covered by a layer of hyaline cartilage (***articular cartilage***).
4. The two bones are held together by a ***capsule*** made up of fibrous tissue. The capsule encloses the articular surfaces within a joint cavity (7.5).
5. The inside of the capsule is lined by ***synovial membrane***. This membrane secretes ***synovial fluid*** that has a lubricating and nutritive function.
6. Synovial joints may be classified on the basis of the shapes of the articular surfaces, as follows:
   a. A joint in which the articular surfaces are flat is called a ***plane joint*** (7.6). The intercarpal and intertarsal joints are mainly of this type.

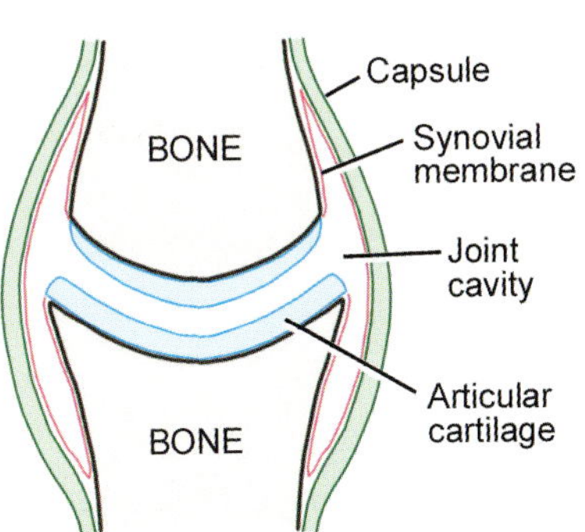


**7.5:** Structure of a typical synovial joint

b. In several joints of the body a convex articular surface on one bone fits into a concavity on the other bone (as shown in 7.5). When the convex surface is rounded (like part of a sphere) and the concave surface is cup shaped the joint is said to be of the ***ball and socket*** variety (7.7A).
If we cut across such a joint (along line ***xy*** in 7.7A) the appearance would be as seen in 7.7B. The point to note is that the convex element being spherical axis ***ab*** is approximately equal to ***cd***. As a result the sphere can rotate in any direction. Examples of ball and socket joints are:
   i. The shoulder joint
   ii. The hip joint.
c. In some cases, however, the two axes are not equal. In 7.8, axis ***a'b'*** is distinctly longer than ***c'd'***. The axis ***a'b'*** cannot rotate to the position of ***c'd'***. Such a joint is an ***ellipsoid joint***. Examples are:
   i. The wrist joint
   ii. The metacarpophalangeal joints.
d. In some cases, one bone end may have two convex surfaces (or ***condyles***) that fit two concavities on the opposite bone (7.9). Such joints are called ***condylar joints***.
   i. The two convexities may be continuous, being separated only by a ridge (as in ***interphalangeal joints***).
   ii. They may be separated by a non-articular area (as in the ***knee joint***).
   iii. An extreme example is the temporomandibular joint in which the two condyles lie in separate joint cavities (the right and left temporomandibular joints together constituting a condylar joint).
e. In some cases, one bone end may be convex in one direction and concave in another. The opposite bone shows a reciprocal convexity and concavity (7.10). The best example of such joint is the ***carpometacarpal joint of the thumb***. Such joints are called ***saddle joints***.
f. In a ***pivot joint***, one rod-like (or cylindrical) element fits into a ring formed partly by bone and partly by ligaments. Examples of such a joint are:
   i. The superior radioulnar joint
   ii. The median atlanto-axial joint (7.11).

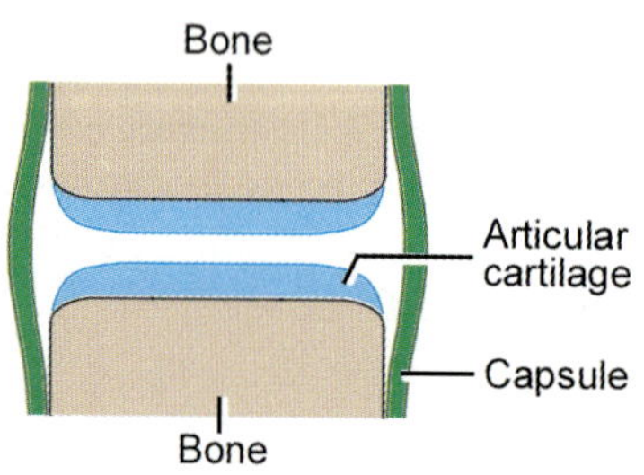


**7.6:** Structure of a plane joint

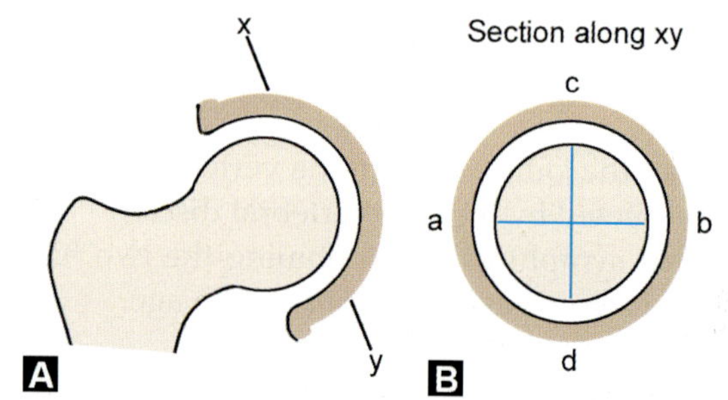


**7.7A and B:** Scheme to show the structure of a ball and socket joint

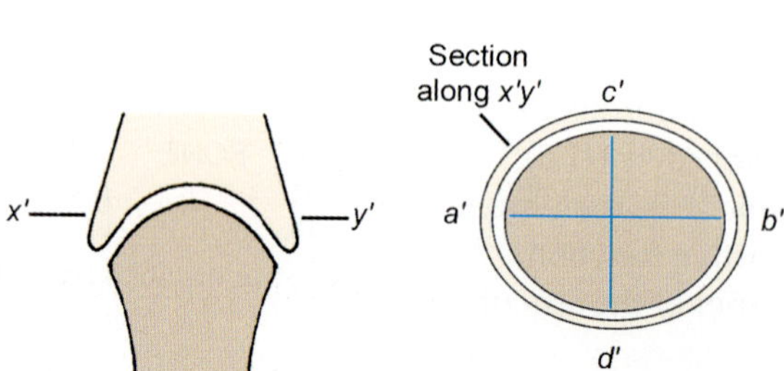


**7.8:** Scheme to show the features of an ellipsoid joint

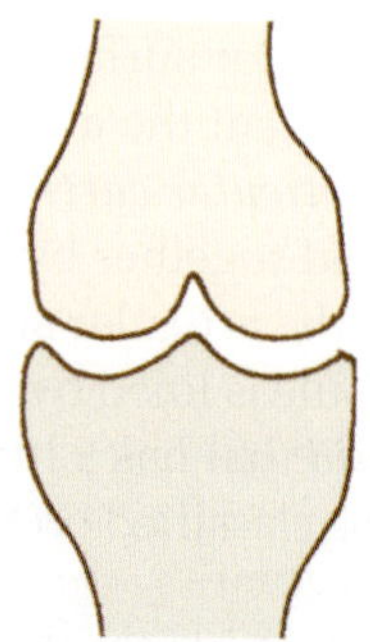

**7.9:** Scheme to show a condylar joint

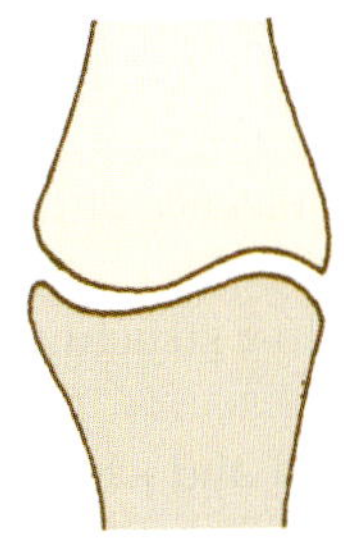

7.10: Scheme to show a saddle joint

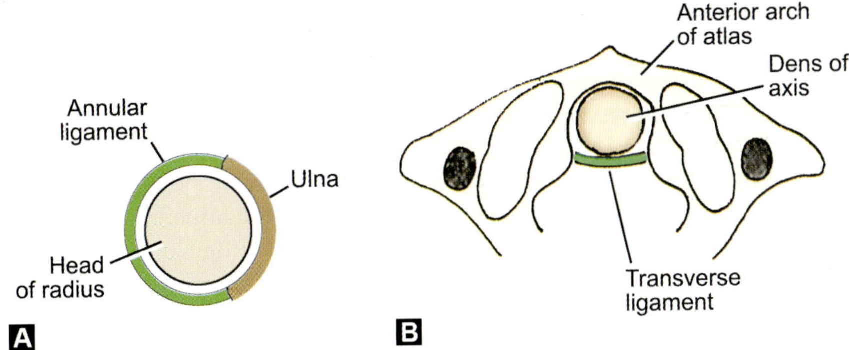


7.11A and B: Two examples of pivot joints. (A) Superior radioulnar joint; (B) Atlantoaxial joint

## CLASSIFICATION OF JOINTS ON THE BASIS OF MOVEMENTS

### Immovable Joints

1. Examples are:
   a. Synchondroses
   b. Sutures.
2. About sutures it may be noted that at the time of birth, the fibrous tissue of the sutural ligaments is sufficiently lax to permit over-riding of skull bones on one another.
3. This 'moulding' allows the head of the foetus to pass easily through the mother's pelvis.
4. In later life, sutures permit no movement.
5. Syndesmoses and gomphoses are usually included among immovable joints, but they do allow slight movement that affords resilience to these joints.

### *Joints Permitting Slight Movement*

1. Slight movement is possible at secondary cartilaginous joints. In the case of the vertebral column the movements between succeeding vertebrae get added together so that the total movement becomes considerable.
2. Synovial joints of the plane variety also permit slight gliding movements only. These joints provide resilience to regions like the wrist and ankle, and increase the total range of movement in these regions.

### *Joints Allowing Free Movement*

Free movement is possible only at synovial joints, but within these there is considerable variability in the type and range of movement permitted.

a. A ball and socket joint allows movement in almost any direction. Examples are the shoulder joint and the hip joint.
b. Ellipsoid joints allow flexion and extension, and also abduction and adduction. They do not allow rotation. Examples are:
   i. Wrist joint
   ii. Metacarpophalangeal joints.
c. A saddle joint permits flexion, extension, abduction and adduction like an ellipsoid joint. However, these movements are accompanied by a certain amount of rotation. (The rotation is automatic and is produced because of the shape of the articular surfaces: it cannot be performed independently).
d. In hinge joints the movements are like those of a door on a hinge. Flexion and extension are possible, but abduction and adduction or rotation are not possible.
   i. Typically, a hinge joint is of the condylar variety (7.9) that is seen in its pure form in the interphalangeal joints.

ii. The knee is also a hinge joint of the condylar variety, but because of differences in the size and shape of the medial and lateral femoral condyles the movements of the knee are associated with some rotation.
iii. The elbow is a hinge joint, but here instead of two condyles we have a pulley shaped trochlea. Functionally the two halves (medial and lateral) of the trochlea function as two condyles.
iv. Yet another example of a hinge joint is seen at the ankle where side-to-side movement and rotation are prevented partly by the pulley like shape of the upper surface of the talus, and partly by the presence of the medial and lateral malleoli on either side of the talus.
v. From the above it may be noted that the term hinge joint refers to a functional entity and not to a structural one.

e. From what has been said above it will be clear that ball and socket joints are ***multiaxial***, ellipsoid and saddle joints are ***biaxial***, and hinge joints are ***uniaxial***.
f. The pivot joint is another type of uniaxial joint (7.11). A pivot is a rod around which something else rotates.
   i. At the median atlantoaxial joint (7.11B) the dens of the axis vertebra represents the pivot around which the atlas vertebra rotates.
   ii. In the superior radioulnar joint the ring [formed by the radial notch of the ulna and the annular ligament (7.11A)] remains fixed, while the head of the radius (i.e., the pivot itself) moves within the ring.

## Compound and Complex Joints

1. A ***compound*** joint is one in which more than two bone ends are enclosed within a single capsule. For example, in the elbow we really have three separate joints within one capsule: the humeroulnar, the humeroradial, and the superior radioulnar.
2. A ***complex*** joint is one in which the cavity is divided completely or incompletely into two parts by an ***intra-articular disc*** of fibrocartilage.

Examples are (7.12):
   a. The temporomandibular joint
   b. The sternoclavicular joint
   c. The knee joint.

The ***intra-articular disc*** may perform various functions.
   a. It may help to provide better adaptation of articular surfaces to each other.
   b. The two halves of the joint may permit different types of movements. For example, the upper part of the temporomandibular joint permits forward and backward gliding; and its lower part acts like a hinge joint.
   c. The intra-articular disc may facilitate lubrication, and may act as a shock absorber.
   d. The discs of the sternoclavicular and inferior radioulnar joints act as important bonds of union between the bones concerned.

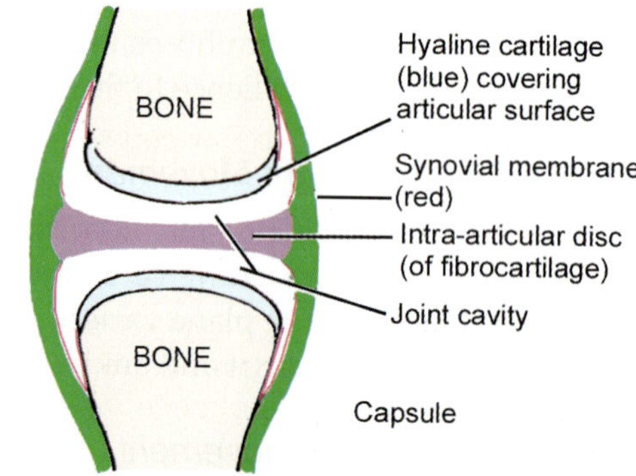


**7.12:** Diagram to show the structure of a typical complex joint

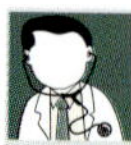

### CLINICAL CORRELATION (JOINTS IN GENERAL)

1. Severe injury can result in separation of the two bones taking part in a joint. This is called ***dislocation***.
   a. Dislocation is more likely to occur in joints which allow free movement e.g., the shoulder joint.
   b. Dislocation usually involves damage to the capsule and to some ligaments.
2. In some cases, the two articular surfaces are displaced from their normal position but retain some contact with each other. This condition is called ***subluxation***.
3. When dislocation at a joint is combined with fracture of one of the bones within the joint the condition is called ***fracture-dislocation***.

4. A force that strongly stretches a ligament can cause its rupture. This usually leads to displacement of the joint surfaces.
5. However, injury to a ligament short of rupture can be a cause of serious pain at a joint, especially during movements that tend to stretch the ligament. Such a condition is referred to as ***sprain*** or ***strain***.
6. Ligaments can also be damaged by prolonged mild stress and some authorities use the term strain only for such injury.
7. Wear and tear in joints is a common cause of joint pains in old persons. Abnormal outgrowths from bone ends can reduce mobility at joints and can also cause pain (***osteoarthritis***). In some cases, relief from pain can be obtained by replacing the joint with an artificial one.

# JOINTS OF THE UPPER LIMB

## JOINTS CONNECTING THE SCAPULA AND CLAVICLE

### The Acromioclavicular Joint

1. This is a plane synovial joint (7.13A and B). It is formed by articulation of small facets at:
   a. The lateral end of the clavicle.
   b. The medial margin of the acromion.
2. The cavity of the joint is occasionally subdivided by an articular disc.
3. Movements at this joint accompany those at the sternoclavicular joint. These movements are necessary for allowing various movements of the scapula associated with movements of the arm at the shoulder joint.

### The Coracoclavicular Ligament

1. The main bond of union between the scapula and clavicle is not through the acromioclavicular joint, but through the coracoclavicular ligament.
2. Though not usually so described it is really a syndesmosis connecting the clavicle to the coracoid process. The ligament consists of two parts: conoid and trapezoid.
   a. The trapezoid part is attached, below, to the upper surface of the coracoid process; and, above, to the trapezoid line on the inferior surface of the lateral part of the clavicle.
   b. The conoid part is attached, below, to the root of the coracoid process just lateral to the scapular notch. It is attached, above, to the inferior surface of the clavicle on the conoid tubercle.

### Coracoacromial Ligament

1. The coracoacromial ligament connects the coracoid and acromial processes of the scapula, and along with them forms the coracoacromial arch. It is triangular (7.14).
   a. Its apex is attached to the medial aspect of the tip of the acromion just in front of the clavicular facet.
   b. Its base is attached to the lateral border of the coracoid process.
2. The coracoacromial arch protects the head of the humerus and prevents its upward dislocation.

## THE STERNOCLAVICULAR JOINT

1. The sternoclavicular joint can be described in various ways which are as follows:
   a. It is a synovial joint.
   b. It is a compound joint as there are three elements taking part in it; namely the medial end of the clavicle, the clavicular notch of the manubrium sterni, and the upper surface of the first costal cartilage.
   c. It is a complex joint as its cavity is subdivided into two parts by an intra-articular disc.

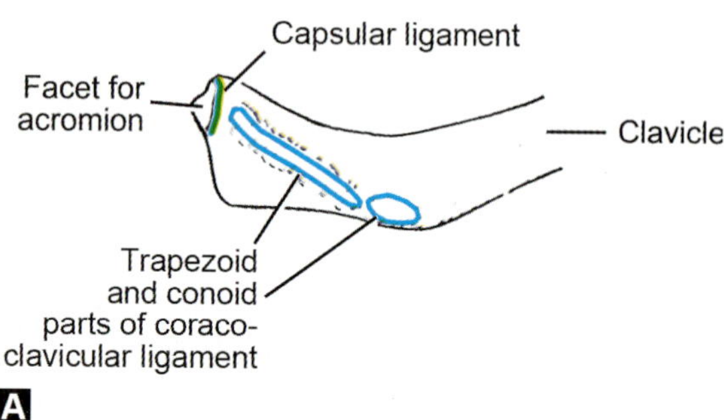

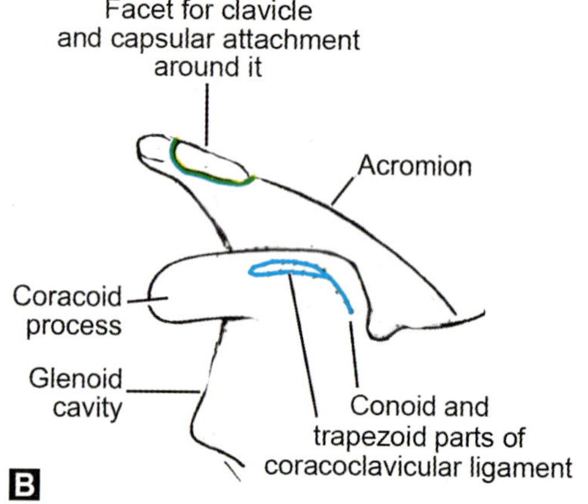


**7.13A and B:** Facets for acromioclavicular joint, and attachments of coracoclavicular ligament. (A) Lateral end of clavicle (seen from below); (B) Upper part of scapula (viewed from the front)

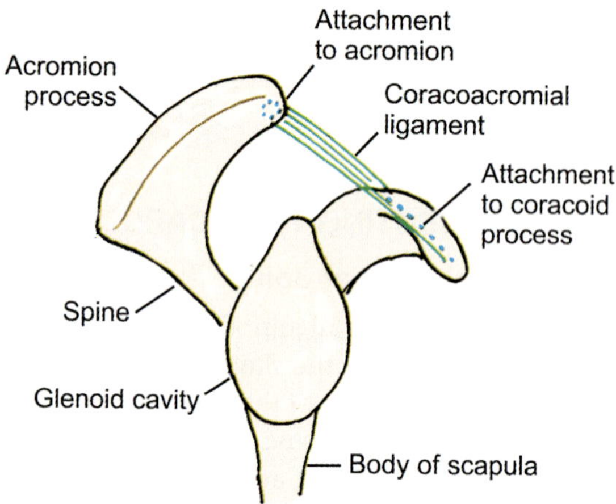


**7.14:** Upper part of scapula, lateral view, to show attachments of coracoacromial ligament

2. The articular surface of the clavicle is covered with fibrocartilage (not hyaline cartilage, as the clavicle is a membrane bone).
   a. The surface is convex from above downwards (7.15A) and slightly concave from front to back.
   b. The sternal surface is smaller than the clavicular surface (7.15A). It has reciprocal convexity and concavity. Because of the concavo-convex shape of the articular surfaces the joint can be classified as a saddle joint.
3. The structures holding the bones of the joint together are as follows:
   a. The capsular ligament is attached laterally to the margins of the clavicular articular surface; and medially to the margins of the articular areas on the sternum and on the first costal cartilage.
   b. It is strong anteriorly and posteriorly where it constitutes the anterior and posterior ***sternoclavicular ligaments***.
   c. However, the main bond of union at this joint is the ***articular disc***.
4. The articular disc is attached laterally to the clavicle on a rough area above and posterior to the area for the sternum (7.15B).
   a. Inferiorly, the disc is attached to the sternum and to the first costal cartilage at their junction.
   b. Anteriorly and posteriorly, the disc fuses with the capsule (7.15B).
5. There are two other ligaments associated with this joint.
6. The ***interclavicular ligament*** passes between the sternal ends of the right and left clavicles (7.15A), some of its fibres being attached to the upper border of the manubrium sterni.
7. The ***costoclavicular ligament*** is attached above to the rough area on the inferior aspect of the medial end of the clavicle (7.15A).
   a. Inferiorly, it is attached to the first costal cartilage and to the first rib.
   b. It consists of anterior and posterior laminae.

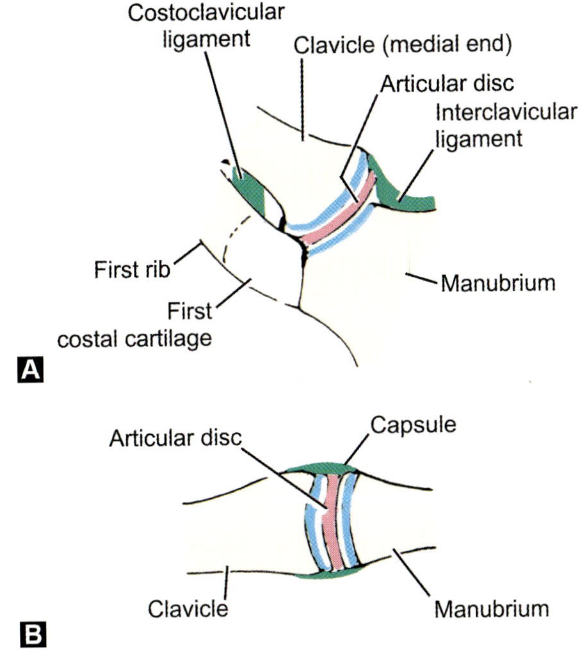


**7.15A and B:** (A) Sternoclavicular joint as seen in coronal section; (B) In transverse section

8. The precise movements occurring at this joint are complex.
   a. All that the student should know is that they are secondary to movements of the scapula, which are in turn secondary to movements of the arm.
   b. Simultaneous movements also occur at the acromioclavicular joint.

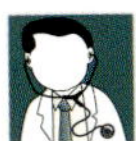

## CLINICAL CORRELATION

**Dislocation of sternoclavicular and acromioclavicular joints**

1. In the dislocation of the sternoclavicular joint the medial end of the clavicle is usually displaced forwards. Backward dislocation is much more serious as the bone may press on the trachea or one of the large vessels at the root of the neck.
2. Dislocation or subluxation of the acromioclavicular joint is more common than dislocation at the sternoclavicular joint, as the latter is a stronger joint.

## THE SHOULDER JOINT

The shoulder joint is a synovial joint of the ball and socket variety. The joint is formed by the head of the humerus and the glenoid cavity of the scapula.

1. The articular surface of the head of the humerus is rounded like a hemisphere (7.16, 7.17A and B).
   a. It is directed medially, backwards and upwards.
   b. It is covered by a layer of hyaline articular cartilage which is thickest in the centre and thinnest at the periphery, thus increasing the convexity.

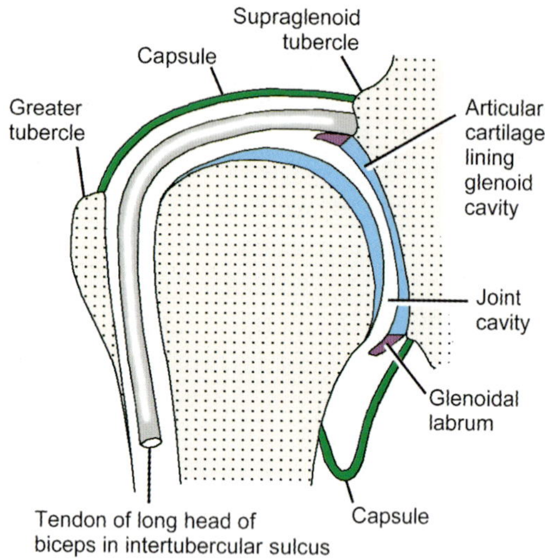


**7.16:** Schematic coronal section through the shoulder joint

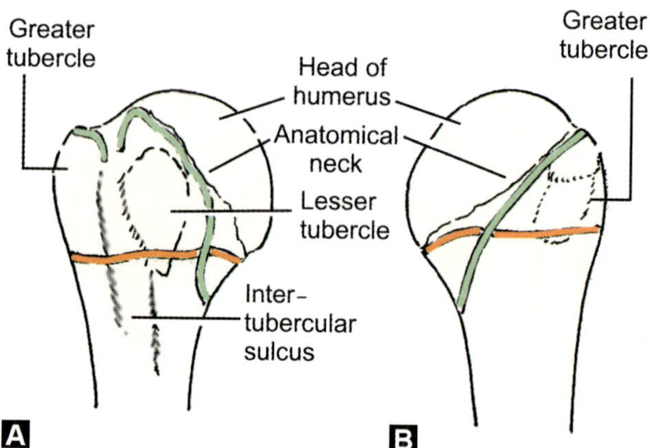


**7.17A and B:** Upper end of humerus seen from: (A) The front; (B) From behind. The attachment of the capsular ligament is shown in green line. Note its relationship to the epiphyseal lines (orange)

2. The glenoid cavity is directed laterally and forwards (7.18). It is much smaller than the head of the humerus (7.16). The cavity is shallow. The factors that compensate for the shallowness of the cavity are as folows:
   a. The depth of the cavity is increased somewhat by the articular cartilage lining it; the cartilage is thinnest in the centre and thickest at the periphery.
   b. The depth of the cavity is also increased by the presence of a rim of fibrocartilage attached to the margin of the glenoid cavity: this is the ***glenoidal labrum*** (7.16).

## Orientation of the Joint

Because of the orientation of the bones forming the joint, it lies in a plane set obliquely to the transverse plane of the body. This has an important bearing on the movements at the joint.

## Attachments of Capsule

1. The fibrous capsule is attached, medially, to the margins of the glenoid cavity beyond the glenoidal labrum (7.17A and B, 7.18). Superiorly, the line of attachment extends above the origin of the long head of the biceps from the supraglenoid tubercle.
2. On the lateral side, the capsule is attached to the head of the humerus just beyond the articular surface i.e., to the anatomical neck; however, on the medial side the line of attachment extends downwards onto the shaft so that part of it is within the joint cavity.
3. The capsule is strengthened by the following ligaments:
   a. The ***glenohumeral ligaments***: superior, middle and inferior, are attached medially to the upper part of the anteromedial margin of the glenoid cavity (7.19) and are fused with the glenoidal labrum.
      i. Laterally they fan out, the superior ligament passing along the medial side of the tendon of the long head of the biceps to reach the upper part of the lesser tubercle of the humerus.
      ii. The middle ligament is attached to the lower part of the lesser tubercle, and the inferior ligament still lower down on the anatomical neck (7.19).
   b. The ***coracohumeral ligament*** represents a thickening of the upper part of the capsule. Medially it is attached to the root of the coracoid process (above the supraglenoid tubercle) and laterally to the greater tubercle of the humerus.

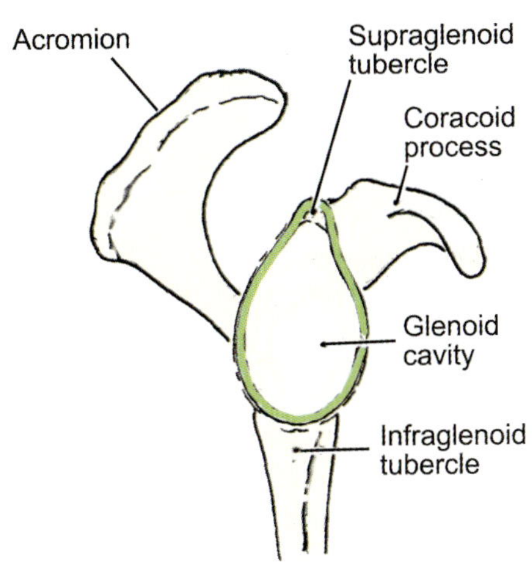


**7.18:** Attachment of the capsule of the shoulder joint to the scapula (viewed from the lateral side). Note the relationship of the capsular ligament to the supraglenoid tubercle

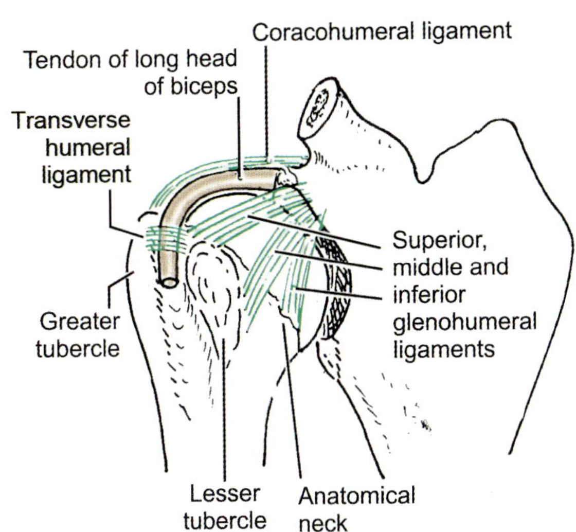


**7.19:** Some ligaments of the shoulder joint

c. Between the greater and lesser tubercles of the humerus there is a gap in the bony attachment of the capsule.
   i. Here the capsule is attached to the ***transverse humeral ligament*** which stretches between the two tubercles.
   ii. It converts the intertubercular sulcus into a canal through which the tendon of the long head of the biceps leaves the joint cavity.

## Factors Strengthening the Joint

1. The capsule of the shoulder joint and the ligaments mentioned above are not very strong. Stability of the joint depends upon muscles that surround it. These are as follows (7.20):
   a. The supraspinatus (superiorly).
   b. The subscapularis (in front).
   c. The infraspinatus and teres minor (behind).
   d. The long head of the triceps (below).
2. With the exception of the long head of the triceps, the tendons of these muscles blend with the capsule forming what is called the ***rotator cuff***.
3. The long head of the triceps is some distance away from the capsule: as a result the inferior part of the capsule is least supported and is the weakest part.

## Bursae around the Joint

The joint is surrounded by a number of bursae. They facilitate movements between structures surrounding the joint. They are shown in 7.20.

## Synovial Membrane

1. The synovial membrane lines the inside of the capsular ligament, both sides of the glenoidal labrum and the non-articular parts of the humerus enclosed within the capsule.
2. The tendon of the long head of the biceps is enclosed in a tubular sheath of synovial membrane: this sheath is prolonged, for some distance, into the intertubercular sulcus.

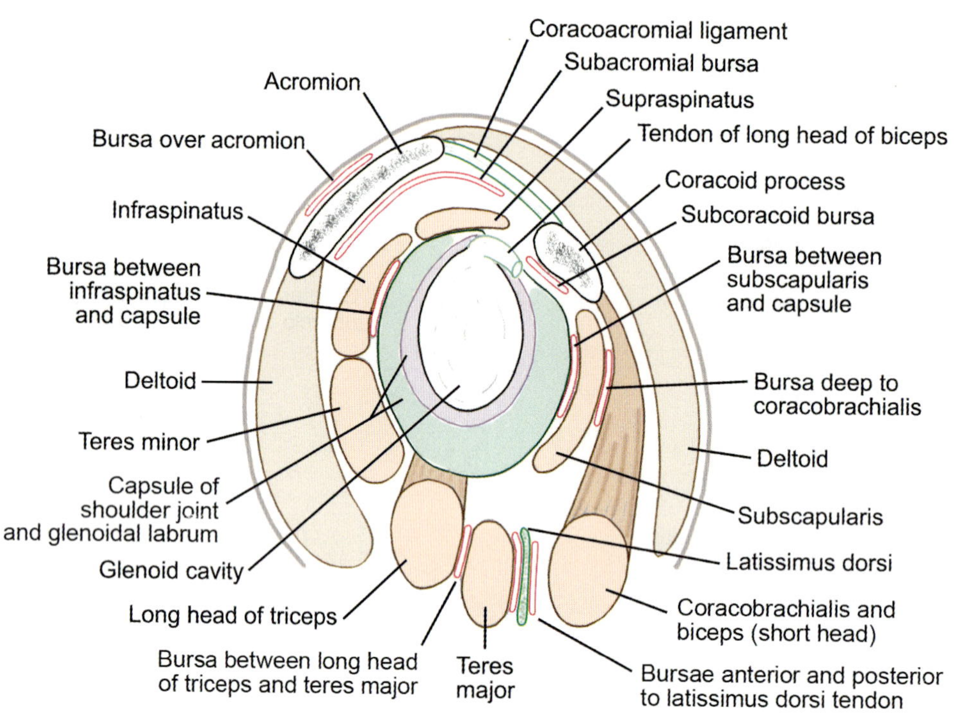


**7.20:** Schematic diagram to show muscles and bursae around the shoulder joint

## Blood Supply and Nerve Supply

The shoulder joint is supplied by the anterior and posterior circumflex humeral, and the suprascapular arteries; and by the suprascapular, axillary and lateral pectoral nerves.

## Movements at Shoulder Joint

1. To understand the movements at the shoulder joint we have to know that the scapula is placed obliquely (in relation to the wall of the thorax) so that its costal surface faces forwards ***and medially***, while the dorsal surface faces backwards ***and laterally***. Because of this orientation the glenoid cavity does not face directly laterally, but faces ***forwards and laterally***.
2. As movements of the arm are described with reference to the plane of the scapula (and not in relation to the trunk) the definition of some movements is somewhat different from that for other joints as follows:
   a. In the neutral position the arm hangs vertically by the side of the trunk.
      i. Flexion and extension take place in a plane ***at right angles to the plane of the scapula***.
      ii. In ***flexion*** the arm moves forwards ***and somewhat medially*** (7.21).
      iii. Reversal of this movement (i.e., bringing it back to the side of the trunk) is ***extension***.
      iv. Continuation of extension beyond the vertical position of the arm is called ***hyperextension***.
   b. The movements of abduction and adduction take place ***in the plane of the scapula***.
      i. In this movement the arm moves laterally, and somewhat forwards (7.22).
      ii. After reaching the horizontal position (i.e., from 1 to 2 in 7.22) the movement can be continued to raise the arm to a vertical position (3 in 7.22): this is referred to as ***overhead abduction***.
      iii. Bringing the arm back to the neutral position (i.e., back to 1 in 7.22) is called ***adduction***. Further adduction brings the arm in front of the chest (4 in 7.22).
      iv. Abduction and adduction take place partly at the shoulder joint, and partly by rotation of the scapula.

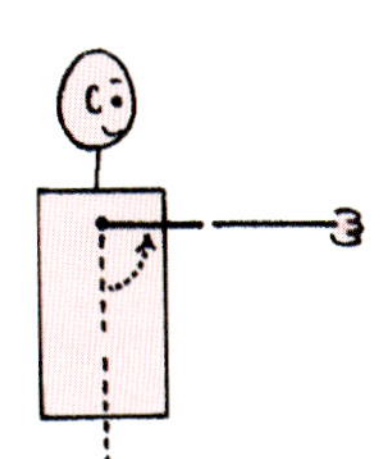

7.21: Scheme to explain flexion at the shoulder joint

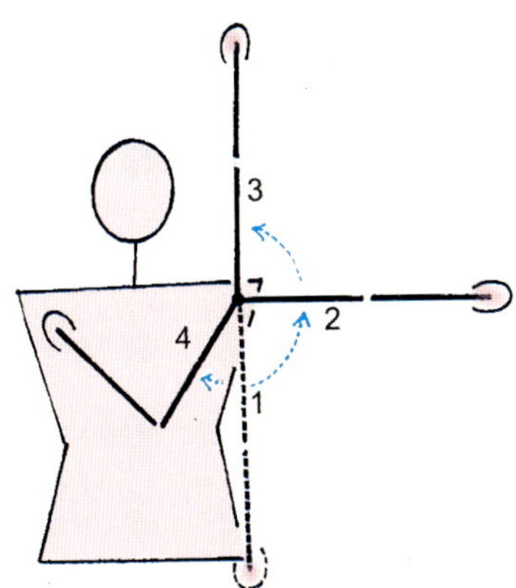


7.22: Scheme to explain abduction at the shoulder joint

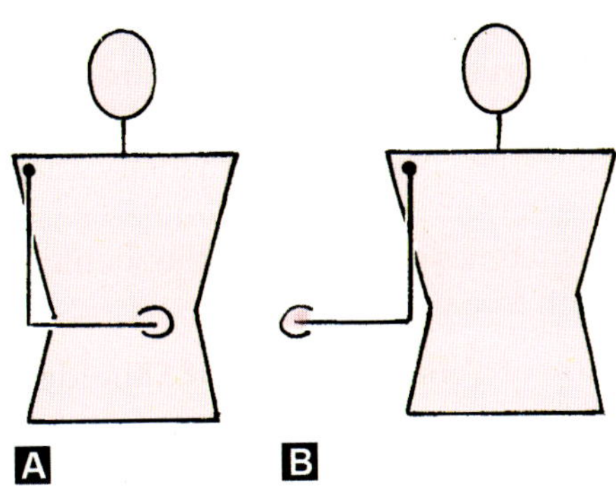


7.23A and B: Scheme to explain (A) Medial rotation and (B) Lateral rotation at the shoulder joint

c. The rotatory movements of the arm are ***medial rotation*** and ***lateral rotation*** (7.23).
   i. A rotation of the humerus that carries the flexed forearm medially is medial rotation.
   ii. The opposite movement in which the forearm is carried laterally is lateral rotation.
   iii. Note further that rotation is named with reference to the ***front*** of the humerus. It follows that any muscle passing from the trunk (or scapula) to the front of the humerus will be a medial rotator. A muscle passing to the back of the humerus will be a lateral rotator.

3. The shallowness of the glenoid cavity and the laxity of the capsule give the shoulder joint great freedom of movement, but this is at the expense of stability. Of all joints of the body the shoulder joint is most liable to dislocation (See below).
4. The muscles responsible for movements of the joint are shown in 7.24.

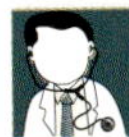

## CLINICAL CORRELATION

1. The tendon (of origin) of the long head of the biceps brachii lies within the capsule of the shoulder joint. In osteoarthritis of this joint abnormal irregular projections develop from the bones concerned and friction against them can lead to damage to the tendon ending in rupture.
2. The ***subacromial bursa*** lies deep to the coracoacromial arch and the adjoining part of the deltoid muscle. This bursa facilitates abduction at the shoulder joint.
   a. During over-head abduction the greater tuberosity slips below the bursa and comes to lie deep to the acromion.
   b. When the bursa is inflamed (***subacromial bursitus***) pressure over the deltoid, just below the acromion elicits pain, but pain cannot be elicited after abduction (as the bursa is now under the acromion).
   c. This is called ***Dawbarn's sign***.
   d. ***Subacromial bursitis*** is usually associated with inflammation of the supraspinatus tendon.

### Dislocation of the Shoulder Joint

a. Typically the head of the humerus is displaced forwards and comes to lie in the infraclavicular fossa just below the coracoid process. This condition is called ***anterior or subcoracoid*** dislocation.
b. Less commonly the head of the humerus may be displaced backwards. When this happens the arm is fixed in a medially rotated position.

c. It will be recalled that the capsule of the shoulder joint is least supported inferiorly. Hence the head of the humerus first passes downwards and then moves anteriorly or posteriorly.
d. Dislocations at the shoulder carry the risk of injury to the axillary nerve, to the brachial plexus (especially the posterior cord), or to the axillary artery. These dislocations may sometimes be accompanied by fracture of the greater tuberosity of the humerus.
e. Sometimes dislocation of the shoulder joint may occur repeatedly (***recurrent dislocation***), and may occur even with trivial force.

**Rupture of Tendinous Cuff of Shoulder**

1. Rupture of the ***tendinous cuff (rotator cuff)*** involves injury mainly to the tendon of the supraspinatus muscle.
2. It is more likely in old persons because of ***degeneration with age***.
3. The patient is unable to initiate abduction at the shoulder joint, but can maintain it once the arm is partially abducted.
4. Strain of the supraspinatus is common in persons who have to work for long periods with the arms in slight abduction (e.g., typists). It can cause distressing pain.

**Sprengel's Shoulder**

A condition in which the scapula (and therefore the shoulder joint) is placed higher than normal is called ***Sprengel's shoulder***.

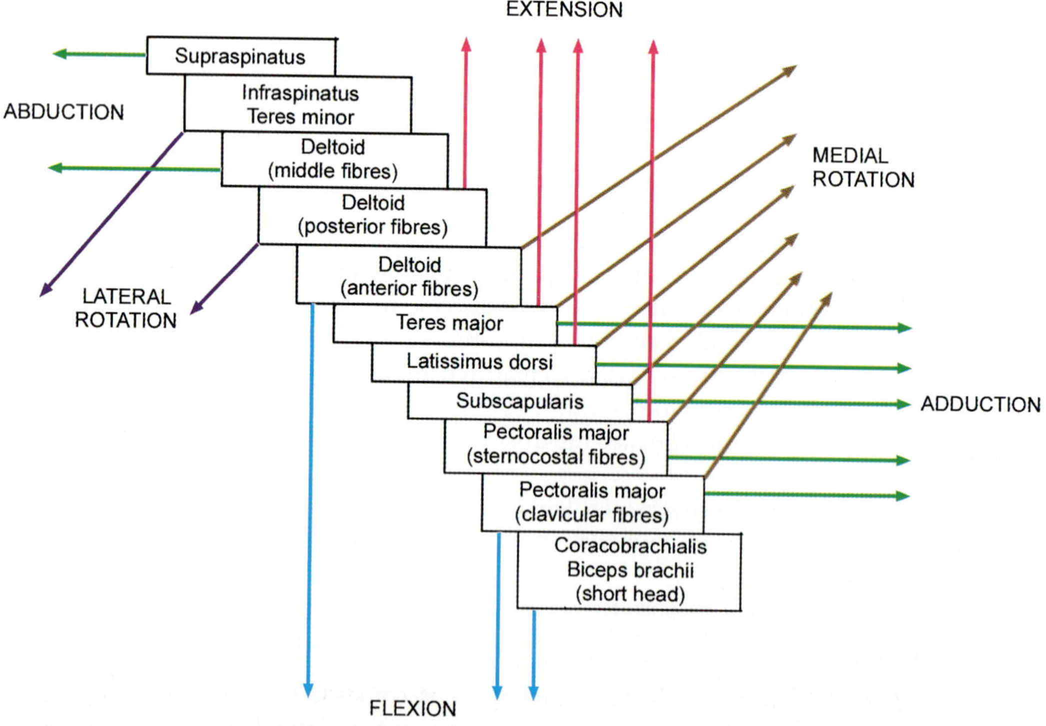


**7.24:** Scheme to show muscles producing movements at the shoulder joint

## THE ELBOW JOINT

1. This is a synovial joint of the hinge variety.
2. It is a compound joint as more than two bones take part in forming it.
   a. These are the lower end of the humerus and the upper ends of the radius and ulna (7.25A and B).
   b. The capitulum of the humerus articulates with the concave upper surface of the head of the radius (***humero-radial joint***); and the trochlear of the humerus articulates with the trochlear notch at the upper end of the ulna (***humero-ulnar joint***).
3. The cavity of the joint is continuous with that of the ***superior radio-ulnar joint***, the two sharing a common synovial membrane. All the three joints mentioned above are collectively referred to as the ***cubital articulation***.
4. The trochlea of the humerus is not symmetrical.
   a. Its medial flange is larger than the lateral and projects downwards to a lower level (7.25A and B).
   b. As a result the lower edge of the trochlea is not horizontal, but passes downwards and medially.
5. The trochlear notch on the ulna consists of an upper part present on the anterior surface of the olecranon and a lower part present on the upper surface of the coronoid process.
   a. The plane of the latter is directed downwards and medially, as in the trochlea.
   b. The upper and lower parts of the trochlear notch may be separated by a non-articular area.
   c. The articular surface of the trochlear notch is divided into medial and lateral parts by a ridge that projects forwards.
6. The attachment of the articular capsule to the lower end of the humerus is shown in 7.25A and B.
   a. It will be seen that considerable non-articular areas of the humerus are included within the joint cavity.
   b. These include the coronoid and radial fossae in front, the olecranon fossa behind, and the flat medial surface of the trochlea (7.20B).
   c. Inferiorly, the capsule is attached to the coronoid and olecranon processes of the ulna around the margins of the articular surface.
   d. On the lateral side it is not attached directly to the radius, but to the annular ligament of the superior radioulnar joint, which encircles the head of the bone.
7. The ***capsular ligament*** is thin anteriorly and posteriorly, but is thickened on the medial and lateral sides to form the ulnar and radial collateral ligaments.
8. The ***ulnar collateral ligament*** is triangular in form (7.26).
   a. Its apex is attached to the medial epicondyle of the humerus, and its base to the ulna.
   b. The ligament has thick anterior and posterior parts, and a thinner intervening part.
   c. The anterior band is attached below to the medial margin of the coronoid process; and the posterior band to the medial side of the olecranon.

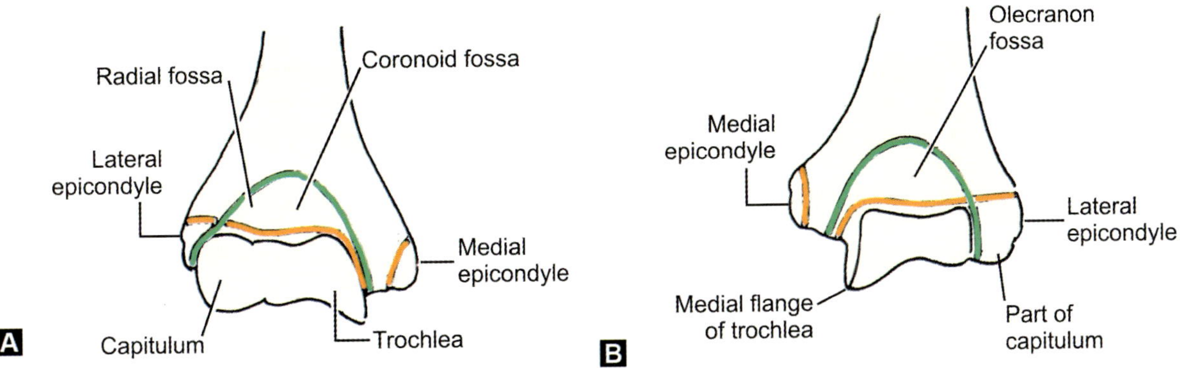


**7.25A and B:** Attachment of the capsular ligament (thick green line) of the elbow joint to the humerus. (A) Anterior aspect; (B) Posterior aspect. Epiphyseal lines are shown in thick orange line

d. These two parts are connected by an oblique band to which the thin intermediate part of the ligament is attached.

e. A space exists between the oblique band and the bone, and synovial membrane may bulge out through this gap in the attachment of the capsule.

9. The ***radial collateral ligament*** (7.27) is attached at its upper end to the lateral epicondyle of the humerus and below to the annular ligament of the superior radioulnar joint.

10. The ***synovial membrane*** of the joint is extensive and covers all non-articular areas of bone enclosed within the capsule.
    a. These include the radial, coronoid and olecranon fossae.
    b. Over these fossae, and in some other regions, the synovial membrane is separated from the capsular ligament by pads of fat. These pads fit into empty spaces in the joint at different phases in its movements.

11. The elbow joint receives its ***blood supply*** from the arterial anastomoses around it. It receives its ***nerve supply*** from nerves that cross it: mainly the musculocutaneous and the radial, but also from the ulnar, the median and the anterior interosseous nerves.

12. The elbow joint being a hinge joint, only allows flexion and extension.
    a. Bending the elbow so that the front of the forearm tends to touch the front of the arm is flexion. Straightening the limb at the elbow is extension.
    b. These ***movements*** are complicated by the fact that the line of the joint is not at right angles to the long axes of the arm and forearm, but (as seen above) it runs downwards and medially.
    c. When the joint is fully flexed, the forearm lies over the arm, but when the joint is extended the supinated forearm passes somewhat laterally (relative to the arm).
    d. The lateral angle between the arm and forearm is about 160 degrees and is called the ***carrying angle***.
    e. This angle disappears when the forearm is pronated and in this position the arm and forearm come to lie in line with each other.
    f. This may be correlated with the fact that most acts calling for precision and strength are performed with the forearm pronated and the obliquity in the line of the elbow joint may be regarded as a device to ensure that the arm and forearm are in line in this position.

13. The muscles responsible for producing flexion at the elbow joint are the brachialis, the biceps brachii and the brachioradialis. Extension is produced by the triceps. The anconeus plays a minor role in extension.

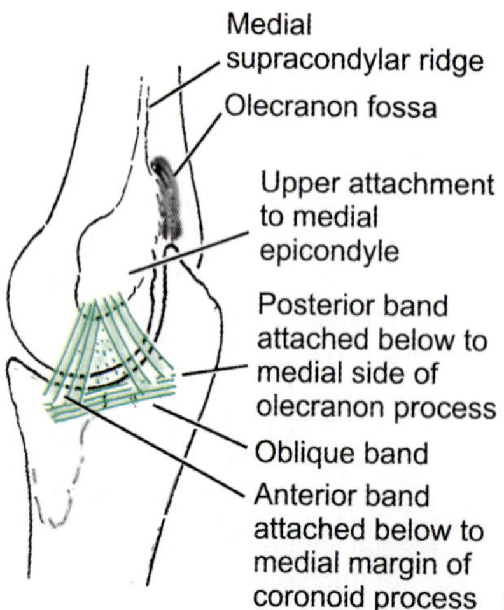


**7.26:** Attachments of the ulnar collateral ligament of the elbow joint

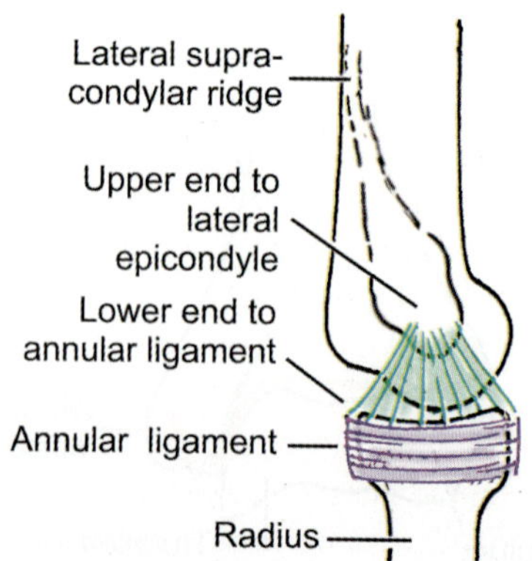


**7.27:** Attachments of the radial collateral ligament of the elbow joint

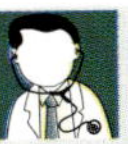

## CLINICAL CORRELATION

**Dislocation of the Elbow Joint**

1. In this dislocation, the radius and ulna are usually displaced backwards and laterally.
2. This dislocation may be associated with fracture of the bone in the region (coronoid process of ulna, head of radius, capitulum or medial epicondyle of humerus).
3. There is danger of injury to the brachial artery or to any of the nerves crossing the elbow.

**Bursitis and Student's Elbow**

Repeated pressure over the olecranon process can cause inflammation of the ***olecranon bursa***. The condition is called ***student's elbow*** or ***miner's elbow***.

**Tennis Elbow**

This is a painful condition caused by strain on the common extensor origin by repeated contraction of extensor muscles. Pain is felt over the lateral epicondyle and the posterior aspect of the forearm.

## THE RADIOULNAR JOINTS

1. The upper and lower ends of the radius and ulna are joined to each other at the superior and inferior radioulnar joints.
2. The shafts of the two bones are united by the interosseous membrane (sometimes called the middle radioulnar joint).
3. The superior and inferior joints are both synovial and of the pivot variety.
4. At the ***superior radioulnar joint,*** the head of the radius rotates within a ring formed by the radial notch of the ulna and the annular ligament (7.25).
   a. The annular ligament surrounds the circumference of the head of the radius and is attached anteriorly and posteriorly to margins of the radial notch of the ulna (7.28A).
   b. The annular ligament is continuous above with the capsular ligament of the elbow joint.
   c. The cavity of the superior radioulnar joint is continuous with that of the elbow joint.
5. The ***inferior radioulnar joint*** is formed by articulation of the convex articular surface on the lateral side of the head of the ulna (7.29A) with the ulnar notch of the radius (7.29B).
   a. The chief bond of union between the two bones is through an ***articular disc***.
   b. The disc is triangular.
   c. Its apex (directed medially) is attached to the ulna on a depression just lateral to the styloid process (7.29B).
   d. Its base is attached to the radius on the lower margin of the ulnar notch.
   e. Its upper surface forms part of the inferior radioulnar joint and articulates with the inferior surface of the head of the ulna.
   f. Its lower surface forms part of the proximal articular surface of the wrist joint.
   g. The cavities of these two joints are completely separated by the disc.
6. The movements taking place at the radioulnar joints are those of pronation and supination. These are described below.
   a. The muscles responsible for supination are the supinator and the biceps brachii. The latter can act only after the forearm has been semi-flexed.
   b. Pronation is produced by the pronator quadratus and the pronator teres.
   c. In the past, the brachioradialis has been said to bring the fully supinated or fully pronated forearm to the midprone position, but this action is controversial.
7. For relationship of supination and pronation to the carrying angle, see under elbow joint.

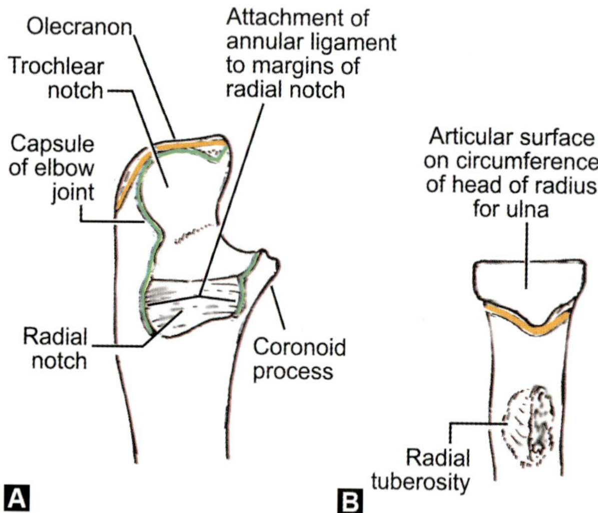


**7.28A and B:** Articular surfaces of the superior radioulnar joint. (A) Upper end of ulna, lateral aspect; (B) Upper end of radius, medial aspect

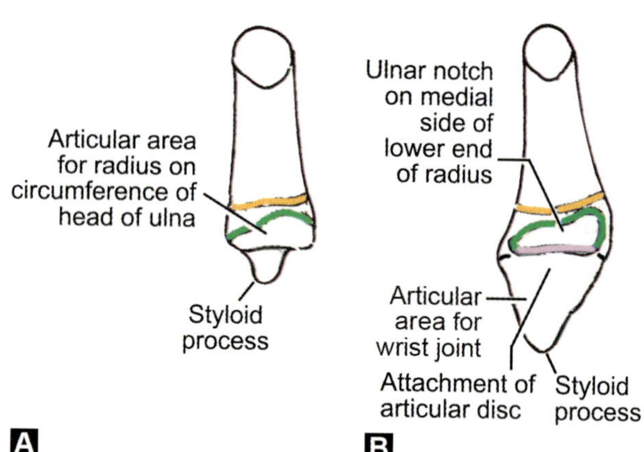


**7.29A and B:** Articular surfaces and capsular attachments of inferior radioulnar joint. (A) Lower end of ulna, lateral aspect; (B) Lower end of ulna, inferior aspect

## Supination and Pronation of Forearm

1. These are rotatory movements that take place at the superior and inferior radioulnar joints. When the forearm is held so that the palm faces forwards, the radius and ulna lie parallel to each other: this is the position of supination.
2. In pronation, the forearm rotates (along with the hand) so that the radius crosses in front of the ulna and its lower end comes to lie medial to that of the ulna (7.30B).
3. Note that, with the forearm extended at the elbow, the hand can rotate either as a result of rotation of the humerus, or as a result of supination and pronation.
4. However, with the elbow flexed to a right angle, such rotation occurs only as a result of supination and pronation: rotation of the humerus carries the forearm medially or laterally.

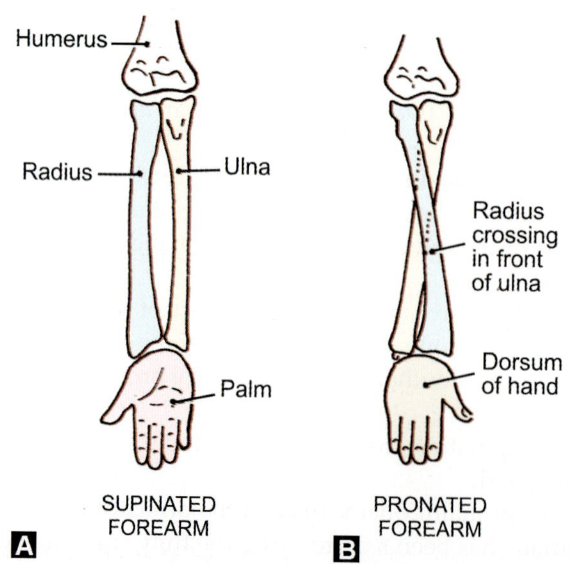


**7.30:** Diagrams illustrating supination and pronation of the forearm. The hand moves with the forearm

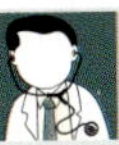

## CLINICAL CORRELATION

### Dislocation of Radioulnar Joints

1. Dislocation of the head of the radius is usually associated with fracture of the upper part of the shaft of the ulna (***Monteggia fracture-dislocation***).
2. In children, a sudden powerful jerk of the hand may pull the head of the radius out of its normal position within the ring of the annular ligament. This is called ***subluxation of the head of the radius*** (or ***pulled elbow***).
3. The condition can also occur by lifting a child by the wrist.
4. The displacement can be reduced by pushing the forearm upwards and then alternately pronating and supinating the forearm.
5. Dislocation of the inferior radio-ulnar joint is usually accompanied by a fracture of the shaft of the radius (***Galeazzi fracture-dislocation***).

## THE WRIST JOINT

The wrist joint is a synovial joint of the ellipsoid variety.

1. It has a concave proximal articular surface formed by the distal end of the radius, and by the inferior surface of the articular disc of the inferior radioulnar joint (7.31).
2. The distal articular surface is convex. It is formed by the proximal surfaces of the scaphoid, lunate and triquetral bones.
3. The ***articular capsule*** is attached to the margins of the proximal and distal articular surfaces. Parts of it are thickened to form several ligaments.
   a. The anterior part of the capsule is thickened in its lateral part to form the ***palmar radiocarpal ligament***; and in its medial part to form the ***palmar ulnocarpal ligament***.
   b. The posterior part of the capsule is thickened in its lateral part to form the ***dorsal radiocarpal ligament***.
   c. The strongest bonds of union are, however, the ulnar and radial collateral ligaments.
4. The ***ulnar collateral ligament*** is attached proximally to the styloid process of the ulna; and distally to the medial side of the triquetral and pisiform bones (7.31).

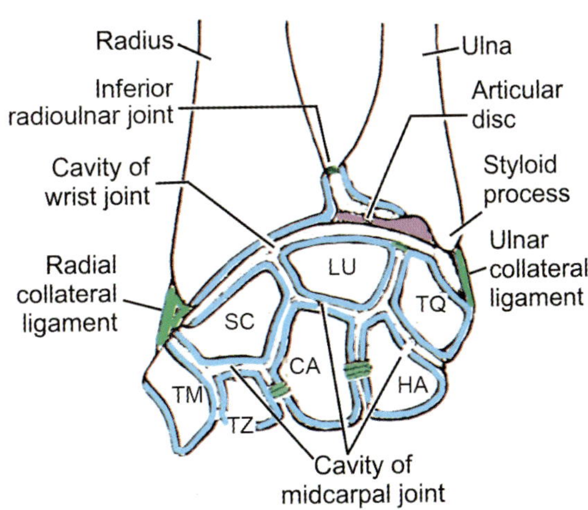


**7.31:** Schematic coronal section through the wrist to show the formation of the articular surfaces of the inferior radio-ulnar, wrist and midcarpal joints

5. The ***radial collateral ligament*** is attached proximally to the styloid process of the radius and distally to the lateral side of the scaphoid bone.
   a. The radial collateral ligament is crossed by the radial artery.
   b. It is also crossed by the tendons of the abductor pollicis longus and the extensor pollicis brevis.
6. The wrist joint is supplied by branches from various arteries present in its neighbourhood including the radial, ulnar, and anterior interosseous arteries, and the deep palmar arch. It is supplied by the anterior and posterior interosseous nerves.
7. The movements allowed at the wrist joint are those of flexion, extension, adduction and abduction.
   a. Flexion at the wrist joint tends to bring the palm and forearm together.
   b. Straightening the wrist and fingers is called extension.
   c. Hyperextension is possible at the wrist.
   d. Adduction and abduction are described with reference to the long axis of the forearm. Lateral movement is abduction, and movement medially is adduction.
   e. Similar movements take place at the joints between the proximal and distal rows of carpal bones (collectively called the ***midcarpal joint***), and add considerably to the range of these movements.
8. The muscles responsible for the movements are shown in 7.32.

## OTHER JOINTS OF THE UPPER LIMB

1. As stated above the ***midcarpal joint*** is present between the proximal and distal row of carpal bones. It is an ellipsoid joint and allows the same movements as the wrist joint, extending their range considerably.
2. The ***carpometacarpal joint of the thumb*** is a synovial joint. It is a typical example of a saddle joint.
   a. The bones taking part are the distal surface of the trapezium, and the proximal surface of the first metacarpal.
   b. The surface of the metacarpal is convex from side-to-side and concave from front to back. The surface on the trapezium shows reciprocal curvatures.
   c. Compared to other carpometacarpal joints this joint has considerable mobility.
   d. The movements are different from those of other digits of the hand because the thumb is rotated by ninety degrees relative to the other digits.

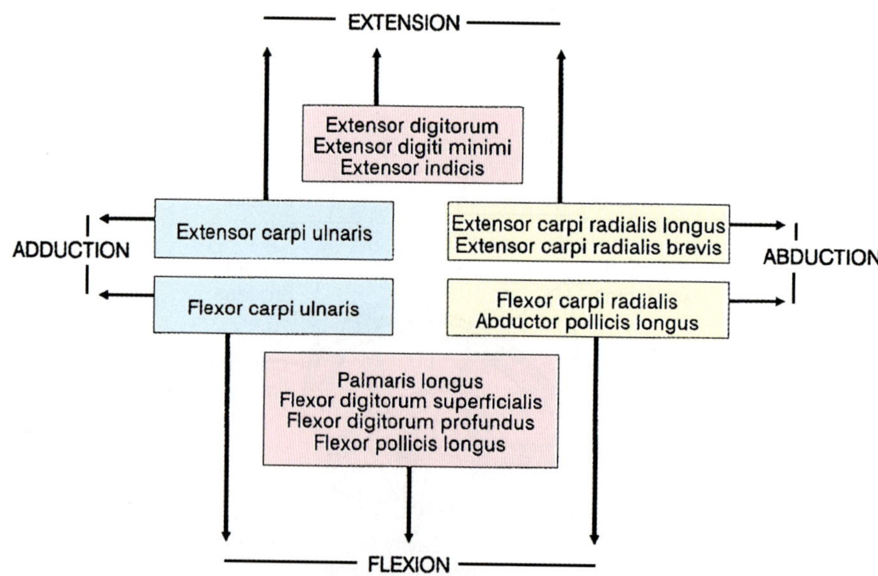


**7.32:** Scheme to show the muscles responsible for movements at the wrist joint

   e. As a result its ventral surface faces medially (not anteriorly) and its dorsal surface faces laterally (not posteriorly as in other digits). Therefore, flexion and extension of the thumb take place in a plane parallel to that of the palm, while the corresponding movements of other digits take place in planes at right angles to the palm.
   f. The muscles producing the movements are shown in 7.33.
3. The remaining ***intercarpal***, ***carpometacarpal***, and ***intermetacarpal*** joints are all plane joints and permit slight gliding movements only. These movements confer considerable resilience to the region of the wrist.
4. The ***metacarpophalangeal joints*** (7.34) are typical ellipsoid joints allowing flexion, extension, abduction and adduction of the fingers. Rotation is not permitted.
5. The ***interphalangeal joints*** (7.34) are typical hinge joints of the condylar type. The thumb has only one such joint. Each finger has two joints: proximal and distal.
   a. Movements at these joints are important in gripping and in all manipulative activity of the fingers.
   b. Abduction and adduction of the digits take place at the metacarpo-phalangeal joints. They are described with reference to the axis of the third digit.
   c. In abduction the index finger moves laterally, whereas the ring finger and the little finger move medially. Movement of third digit (middle finger) either medially or laterally is described as abduction.
   d. The opposite movements of the digits are referred to as adduction.
   e. The muscles producing the movements are as follows:
      i. Flexion at the proximal interphalangeal joint is produced by the flexor digitorum superficialis and flexor digitorum profundus; and at the distal joint by the profundus alone.
      ii. Extension of both proximal and distal interphalangeal joints is produced by the extensor digitorum, lumbricals and interossei. The extensor indicis helps in extension of the index finger, and the extensor digiti minimi in that of the little finger.
      iii. Flexion of the interphalangeal joint of the thumb is produced by the flexor pollicis longus, and extension by the extensor pollicis longus.

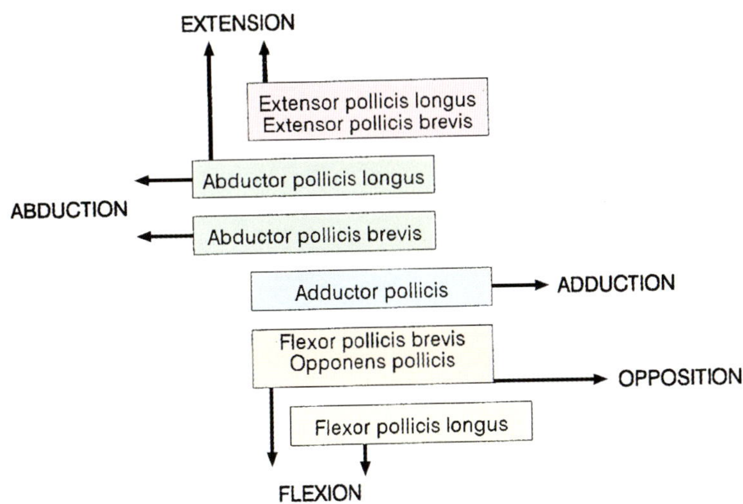


**7.33:** Scheme to show the muscles responsible for movements at the carpometacarpal joint of the thumb. Note that flexion is associated with a certain amount of medial rotation, and extension with lateral rotation. Flexion, abduction, extension and adduction occurring in sequence constitute circumduction

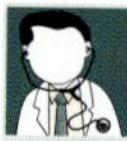

## CLINICAL CORRELATION

Dislocation can take place at any of these joints but this is not common.

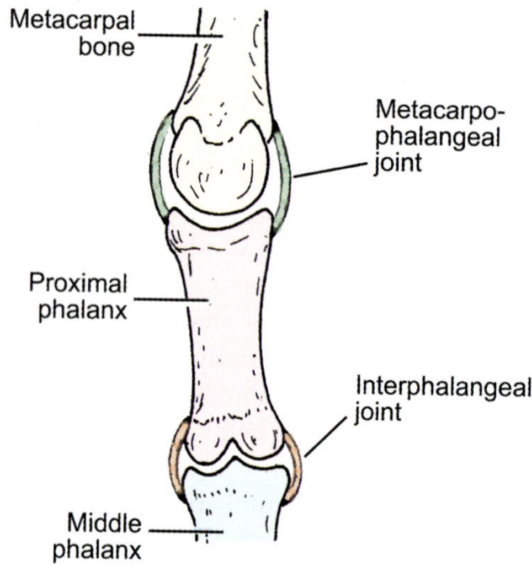


**7.34:** Metacarpophalangeal and proximal interphalangeal joints

# 8 CHAPTER Surface Marking and Radiological Anatomy of Upper Limb

## SURFACE MARKING

### INTRODUCTION

1. In clinical work, a physician wanting to examine a structure, or a surgeon planning an operation, needs to have a fairly accurate idea of where the structure lies in a living person.
2. Arteries can be directly palpated where they are superficial.
3. Nerves can be palpated only in very few situations.
4. Hence, it becomes necessary to use other landmarks (seen or palpable from the surface) to judge the position of important structures.
5. The position of the structure in question can be drawn on the surface of the body using such landmarks. This is called *surface marking*.
6. In this chapter we will consider the surface marking of some important structures in the upper limb.
7. Surface marking should always be done on a living subject. You will be able to feel many of the landmarks described in your own body also.

### Axillary Artery

#### *First Point*

Middle of the clavicle. To mark this point palpate the medial and lateral ends of the clavicle and take the point midway between them.

#### *Second Point*

A point, at the level of the lower border of the posterior fold of the axilla, where the pulsations of the artery can be felt.

1. To mark the lower end of the artery ask the subject to abduct the arm and rotate it so that the palm faces upwards.
2. Place your fingers in the interval between the anterior and posterior folds of the axilla and apply gentle pressure laterally. By moving the fingers forwards or backwards you should be able to feel the pulsation of the axillary artery.
3. Mark the point of pulsation that corresponds to the lower border of the posterior axillary fold.
4. If you are unable to feel the pulsation take a point at the junction of the anterior two-thirds and posterior one-third of the lateral wall of the axilla.
5. The artery is marked by joining the two points. Remember that the artery has some thickness. Give the line appropriate thickness. (This holds true for all arteries and nerves).

## Brachial Artery

### First Point

This corresponds to the lower end of the axillary artery, and can be palpated as described for the axillary artery.

### Second Point

The lower end lies ***at the level of*** (but not opposite) the neck of the radius.

1. To locate this level, flex the elbow of the subject slightly. Place your hand over the elbow so that the thumb is in front and the fingers behind.
2. With the index finger locate the line of the elbow joint, near its lateral part, and slip the finger slightly below this level.
3. Now ask the subject to alternately supinate and pronate the forearm. By moving your finger you will be able to feel the head of the radius as it rotates. The neck of the radius lies just below the head.
4. Having determined this level now turn to the front of the elbow and feel for the tendon of the biceps brachii.
5. The lower point for marking the brachial artery lies just medial to this tendon, at the level of the neck of the radius. This is the point at which the brachial artery bifurcates into the radial and ulnar arteries.

## Radial Artery

### First Point

The upper end of the radial artery corresponds to the lower end of the brachial artery that can be found as described above.

### Second Point

1. To locate the artery at the lower end of the forearm, place two fingers in front of the lower end of the radius and apply gentle pressure.
2. Move the fingers from side-to-side until pulsations of the radial artery are felt. This is the situation at which doctors usually examine the ***radial pulse*** of a patient.
3. Just lateral to the artery you will feel the sharp anterior border of the radius.
4. Just medial to the artery you can feel the tendon of the flexor carpi radialis.
5. The radial artery ***in the forearm*** can be marked by joining the upper and lower ends determined as described above. The line should be drawn with a slight convexity to the lateral side.
6. To mark the ***artery in the hand*** remember that at the wrist the artery winds round the lateral border to reach the back of the hand.
7. First identify the following points. The styloid process of the radius can be located by following the anterior border of the radius downwards. Pulsation of the artery can be felt just in front of this process.
8. Now extend the thumb and you will see a hollow on the posterior and lateral side of the wrist bounded on either side by bulging tendons. This hollow is the ***anatomical snuff box***.
9. The bulge to its anterior and lateral side is formed by tendons of the abductor pollicis longus and the extensor pollicis brevis, while the bulge to the posterior and medial side is formed by the tendon of the extensor pollicis longus. The pulsation of the radial can be felt in the depth of the fossa.
10. Finally, examine the interval between the first and second metacarpal bones and note that its proximal end lies just below the anatomical snuff box.
11. The course of the radial artery in the hand can now be marked by joining the following points:
    a. Point where radial pulse is felt at lower end of radius.
    b. A point just below the styloid process.
    c. Point in the floor of the snuff box.
    d. Proximal end of first intermetacarpal space. Also see radial nerve described below.

## Ulnar Artery

### *First Point*

The point indicating the upper end of the ulnar artery corresponds to the lower end of the brachial artery, and may be found as described for that artery. From the first point, the artery passes downwards and medially to reach the second point given below.

### *Second Point*

Medial border of the forearm at the junction of its upper one-third with the lower two-thirds. From here the artery descends vertically to reach the wrist.

### *Third Point*

This lies just lateral to the pisiform bone. From here the ulnar artery enters the palm where it becomes the superficial palmar arch. Also see ulnar nerve described below.

## Superficial Palmar Arch

### *First Point*

A point just lateral to the pisiform bone.

### *Second Point*

Hook of the hamate.

1. The arch descends vertically from the first point to the second.
2. The rest of the arch is marked as a curved line that passes laterally across the palm with a marked convexity directed distally.

### *Third Point*

Point on the distal border of the thenar eminence, in line with the cleft between the index and middle fingers.

1. In drawing the curve make sure that the most distal point on it lies at the level of the distal border of the fully extended thumb.
2. Remember that the tip of the extended thumb points ***laterally***.

## Deep Palmar Arch

1. The deep palmar arch is a continuation of the radial artery.
2. It lies about 1 cm proximal to the superficial palmar arch and has a slight distal convexity.
3. It begins at the proximal end of the first intermetacarpal space (*first point*), and ends just distal to the hook of the hamate (*second point*).

## Axillary Nerve

1. The axillary nerve follows a horizontal course a short distance above the middle of the deltoid muscle.
2. It can be marked on the surface by a horizontal line about 2 cm above the midpoint between the tip of the acromion process and the deltoid tuberosity of the humerus (insertion of deltoid).

## Musculocutaneous Nerve

The upper end of this nerve lies in the axilla, lateral to the axillary artery.

1. First mark the axillary artery (as described above) and take a point just lateral to the artery 3 cm above the lower border of the posterior fold of the axilla.
2. The lower end of the nerve can be taken as the point where it becomes superficial and continues as the lateral cutaneous nerve of the forearm. This point lies 2 cm above the bend of the elbow, just lateral to the biceps tendon.

## Median Nerve

The median nerve begins in the lower part of the axilla and extends into the hand.

1. ***In the arm,*** the nerve is closely related to the brachial artery. First mark this artery (as described above).
2. The median nerve can be marked as a broad line that lies lateral to the upper half of the artery, crosses the artery near its middle, and then descends along the medial side of the artery to reach the elbow.
3. ***In the forearm,*** the nerve descends almost vertically approximately midway between the radial and ulnar borders, and reaches the front of the wrist at about its middle. Here, the nerve lies over the tendon of the palmaris longus, or about 1 cm medial to the tendon of the flexor carpi radialis.

## Radial Nerve

To mark this nerve remember that it begins in the axilla, where it lies just behind the third part of the axillary artery. The nerve then passes to the ***back*** of the arm where it lies in the radial groove. Having crossed behind the humerus it reappears on the front of the lower part of the arm, and then descends into the forearm.

1. To mark the nerve ***in the arm***, first locate the lower end of the axillary artery as already described. This is our first point.
2. Next draw a line (on the lateral side of the arm) joining the lateral epicondyle of the humerus with the deltoid tuberosity (i.e., the insertion of the deltoid).
3. Divide this line into three equal parts. The point at the lower end of the upper one-third of this line is our second point for marking the nerve.
4. The third point is to be taken on the front of the elbow, at the level of the lateral epicondyle of the humerus, a short distance (about 1 cm) lateral to the tendon of the biceps brachii.
5. As the upper part of the radial nerve lies on the back of the arm the upper two points should be joined by a line passing on this aspect of the arm. At the lateral border of the arm, the line should curve forwards to reach the front, and should be prolonged to the third point.
6. To mark the nerve ***in the forearm***, remember that in the cubital fossa the radial nerve divides into its superficial and deep terminal branches. The superficial terminal branch is regarded as the main continuation of the nerve and it is this branch we mark on the front of the forearm. The nerve descends to the lateral border of the forearm and then passes around this border to reach the back of the hand.
7. Take one point corresponding to the third point for the nerve in the arm (described above).
8. Take another point over the lateral border of the forearm, at the junction of the upper two-thirds and lower one-third of this border.
9. Draw a line joining these two points. Carry it downwards round the lateral border of the arm to reach the anatomical snuff box. Here the nerve divides into smaller branches.

   If you are asked to mark both the radial nerve and radial artery, remember that the nerve is lateral to the artery, and that the two lie side-by-side only over the middle one-third of the forearm.

## Ulnar Nerve

This nerve begins in the axilla and extends up to the hand. It descends into the arm where it lies immediately medial to the upper half of the brachial artery. It then turns somewhat medially and downwards to reach behind the medial epicondyle of the humerus.

1. To mark this artery ***in the arm*** our first point corresponds to the upper end of the brachial artery (see above).
2. Our second point corresponds to the middle of the brachial artery: it lies at the middle of the medial border of the arm.
3. The third point is the ***posterior aspect*** of the medial epicondyle of the humerus. In this situation, the nerve can sometimes be rolled under the fingers. Pressure over the nerve here can produce a tingling sensation.
4. To mark the ulnar nerve ***in the forearm,*** connect the point behind the medial epicondyle with a point in front of the wrist, just lateral to the pisiform bone.
5. If you are asked to mark both the ulnar nerve and artery, remember that the ulnar nerve lies immediately medial to the ulnar artery in the lower two-thirds of the forearm.

## Flexor Retinaculum

You can easily mark this structure if you know its attachments.

1. To draw its upper border, join the pisiform bone to the tubercle of the scaphoid bone. The upper border should be drawn with a slight concavity upwards.
2. The lower border corresponds to a line joining the hook of the hamate to the tubercle of the trapezium. The lower border should be drawn with a slight concavity downwards.
3. The medial and lateral margins can be drawn by connecting the ends of the upper and lower borders to one another.

## Extensor Retinaculum

The extensor retinaculum is shown in 6.33.

1. To mark its upper border draw a line starting from the anterior border of the radius 2 cm above its lower end, and passing round the lateral side and back of the wrist to reach the styloid process of the ulna.
2. The lower border starts from the lower end of the anterior border of the radius and runs parallel to the upper border to reach the triquetral bone. Tendons passing under cover of the extensor retinaculum are shown in 6.34.

## RADIOLOGICAL ANATOMY

Some aspects of the radiological anatomy of the upper limb are shown in 8.1 to 8.3.

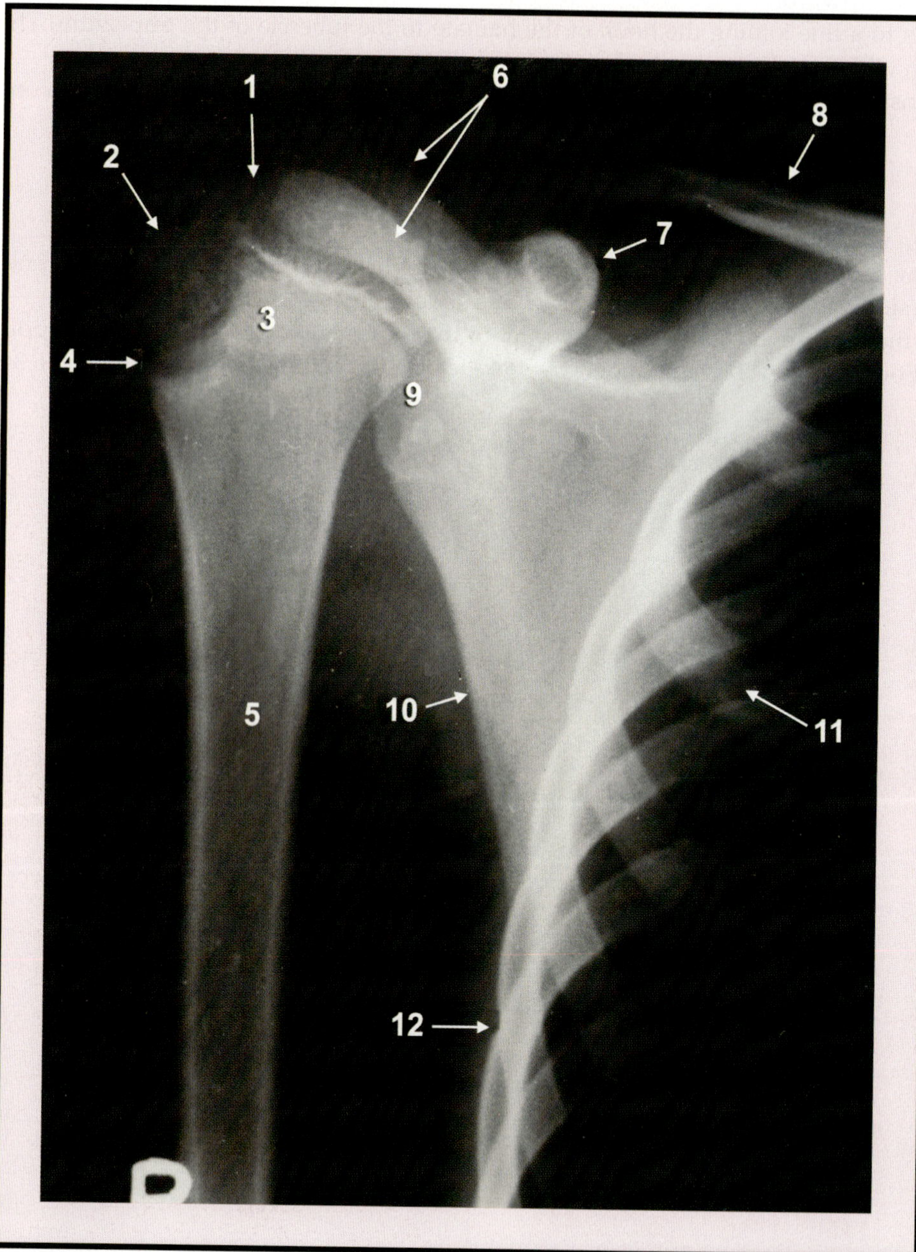


1. Head of humerus
2. Greater tubercle
3. Lesser tubercle
4. Epiphyseal plate of upper end of humerus
5. Shaft of humerus
6. Outline of acromion process (partially overlapping head of humerus)
7. Coracoid process
8. Clavicle
9. Glenoid cavity
10. Lateral border of body of scapula
11. Medial border of body of scapula
12. Ribs forming wall of thorax

**8.1:** Radiograph of the region of the shoulder in a child who is about 10 years old. Ossification of the upper end of the humerus is not complete. The centres for the head, the greater tubercle and the lesser tubercle are seen separately. The epiphyseal plate separating the upper end from the diaphysis is clearly seen. The shadow of the scapula is overlapped (in its medial part) by the thoracic cage (made up of ribs). The medial margin of the scapula can be made out (as the ribs appear lighter where they overlap the scapula). The acromion, the coracoid process, and the clavicle can be distinguished. The tip of the coracoid process is seen as a circular area as it is viewed head-on.

1. Shaft of humerus
2. Olecranon fossa
3. Epiphyseal plate of lower end of humerus
4. Conjoint epiphysis for capitulum and lateral epicondyle of humerus
5. Upper epiphysis of radius
6. Epiphysis for medial condyle
7. Olecranon, medial margin
8. Coronoid process
9. Radial tuberosity
10. Shaft of radius
11. Shaft of ulna

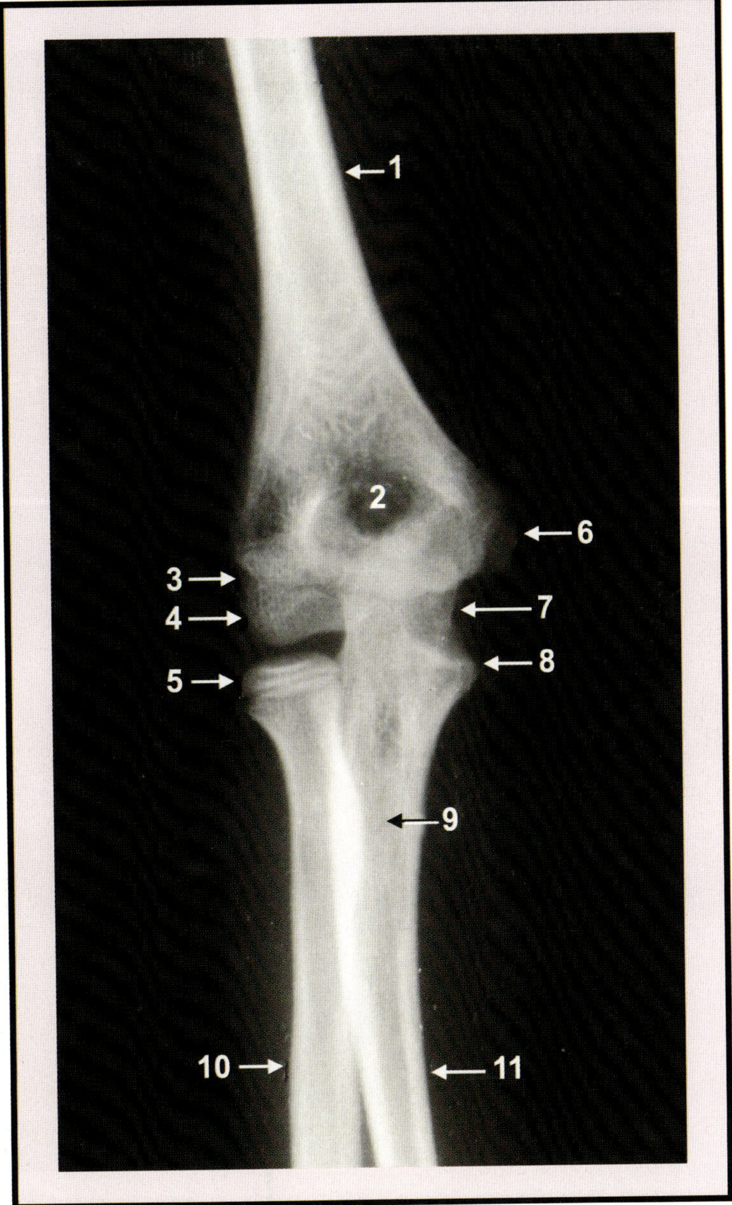


**8.2:** Radiograph of the region of the elbow in a child, about ten years old. At the lower end of the humerus the conjoined epiphysis for the capitulum and lateral epicondyle can be seen separated from the diaphysis by an epiphyseal plate. The medial epicondylar epiphysis is also separate from the shaft. The upper epiphysis of the radius (unfused with the shaft) is clearly seen

1. Distal phalanx
2. Epiphysis of distal phalanx
3. Middle phalanx
4. Epiphysis of middle phalanx
5. Proximal phalanx
6. Epiphysis of proximal phalanx
7. Epiphysis at distal end of second metacarpal bone
8. Second metacarpal
9. First metacarpal
10. Epiphysis at proximal end of first metacarpal bone
11. Trapezium
12. Scaphoid
13. Distal epiphysis of radius
14. Shaft of radius
15. Trapezoid
16. Capitate
17. Hamate
18. Triquetral bone
19. Lunate
20. Distal epiphysis of ulna
21. Shaft of ulna

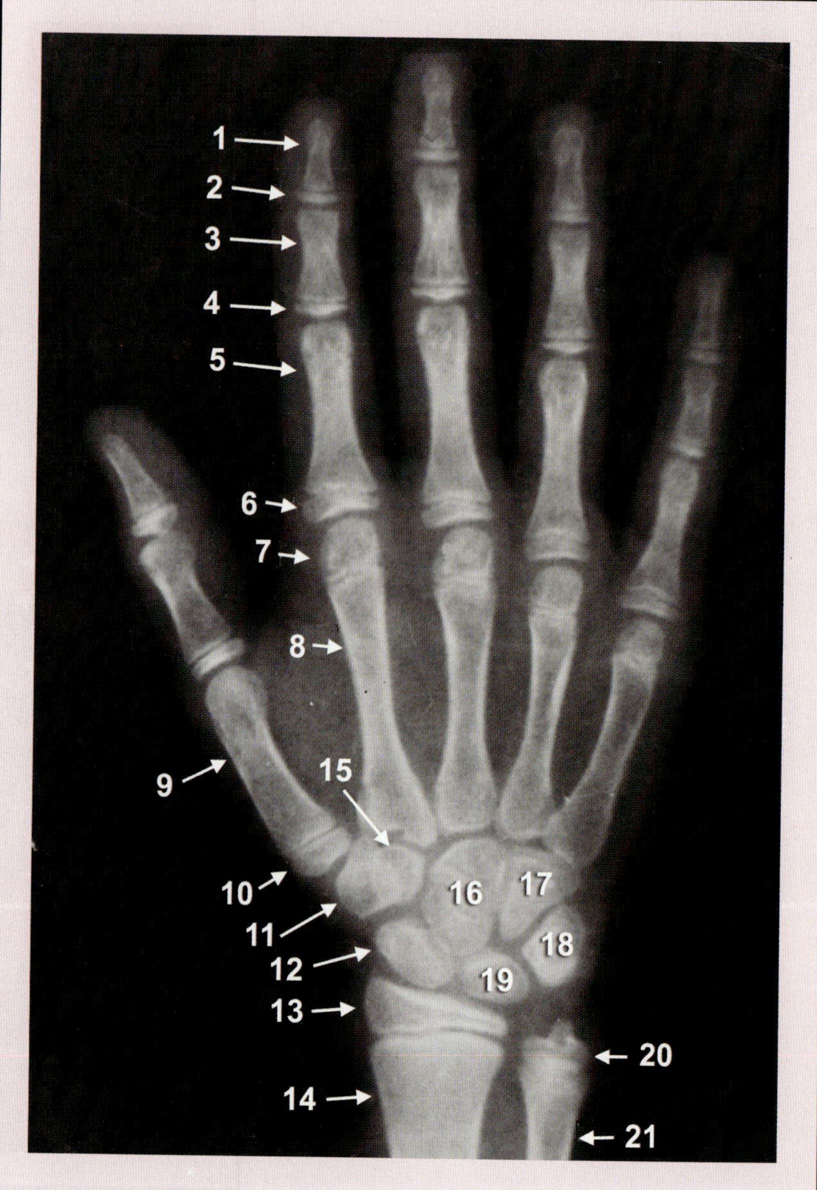


**8.3:** Radiograph of the hand and wrist in a child, about ten years old. Note that each phalanx (distal, middle and proximal in each digit other than the thumb; and only proximal and distal in the thumb) has an epiphysis at its proximal end. The second, third, fourth and fifth metacarpal bones have an epiphysis at their distal ends. The first metacarpal bone is different in that its epiphysis is at the proximal end (like a phalanx). Identify the various carpal bones. (The pisiform bone cannot be made out in this radiograph). Finally, note the unfused epiphyses at the lower ends of the radius and ulna.

# PART 2

## Lower Extremity

# 9 CHAPTER Bones of Lower Extremity

The bones of the lower limb are enumerated in 9.1 and shown in 9.2.

## THE HIP BONE

### Introductory Remarks

#### *Side Determination*

1. The hip bone (9.4 and 9.5) constitutes the pelvic girdle. Along with the sacrum and coccyx, the right and left hip bones form the bony pelvis (9.3).
2. The orientation of the hip bone in the body is best appreciated by viewing it in the intact pelvis.
3. Each hip bone consists of three parts.
   a. These are the ilium, the pubis, and the ischium.
   b. These three parts meet at the ***acetabulum*** which is a large deep cavity placed on the lateral aspect of the bone.
   c. The acetabulum takes part in forming the hip joint along with the head of the femur.
4. Below and medial to the acetabulum, the hip bone shows a large oval or triangular aperture called the ***obturator foramen.***
5. The ***ilium*** consists, in greater part, a large plate of bone that lies above and behind the acetabulum, and forms the side wall of the greater pelvis.
   a. Its upper border is in form of a broad ridge that is convex upwards and this ridge is called the ***iliac crest.***
   b. The posterior part of the ilium bears a large rough articular area on its medial side for articulation with the sacrum.

**9.1: Bones of lower extremity**

| | Name | Location |
|---|---|---|
| Bone attached to trunk forming pelvic girdle | Hip bone | Lowest part of trunk (pelvis) |
| Bones of free limb | Femur | Thigh |
| | Tibia | Leg (medially) |
| | Tarsal bones (7) | Posterior part of foot |
| | Metatarsal bones (5) | Anterior part of foot |
| | Phalanges | Toes or digits (3 in each toe and 2 in the big toe) |

6. The *pubis* lies in relation to the upper and medial part of the obturator foramen.
   a. It forms the most anterior part of the hip bone.
   b. The two pubic bones meet in the middle line, in front, to form the *pubic symphysis*.
7. The lowest part of the hip bone is formed by the *ischium* which lies below and behind the acetabulum and the obturator foramen. Using the information given above, a given hip bone can be correctly orientated and its side determined.
8. We will now consider the features of the ilium, the ischium and the pubis in detail. Features seen on the lateral aspect are shown in 9.4 and those seen on the medial aspect are shown in 9.5.

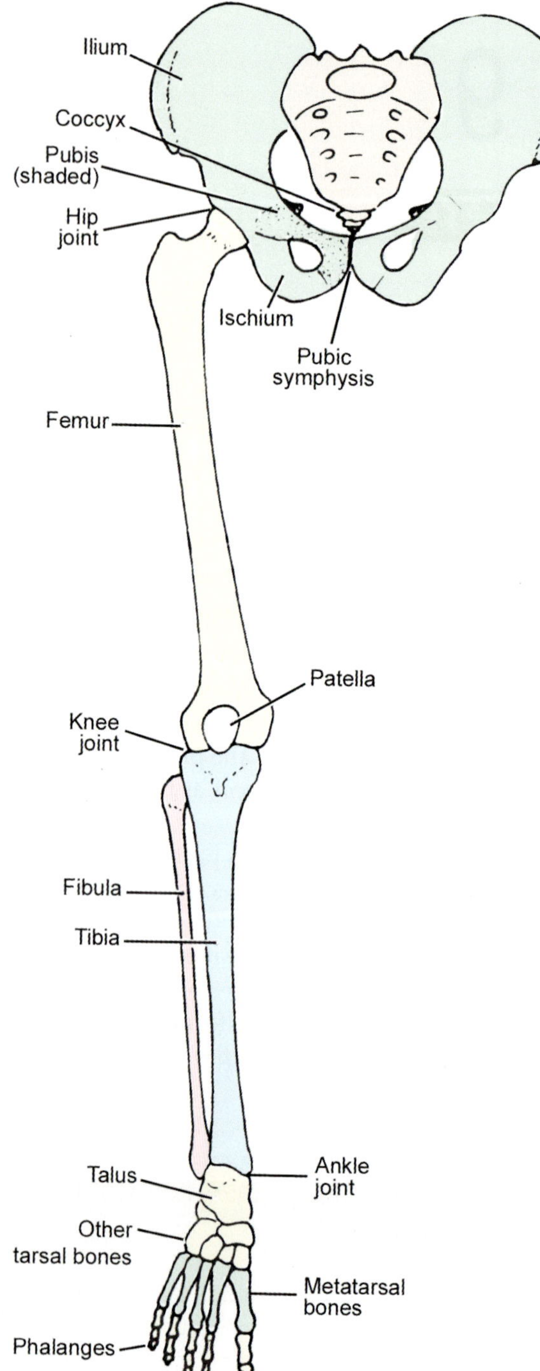

**9.2:** Bones and joints of the lower limb

## The Ilium

Note the following features in addition to the features already mentioned:

1. The anterior end of the iliac crest projects forwards as the *anterior superior iliac spine*.
2. The posterior end of the crest also forms a projection called the *posterior superior iliac spine*.
3. The iliac crest may be subdivided into a *ventral segment*, consisting of the anterior two-thirds of the crest, and a *dorsal segment* consisting of the posterior one-third.
4. The whole length of the ventral segment shows a broad intermediate area that is bounded by inner and outer lips.
   a. The outer lip of the iliac crest is most prominent about 5cm behind the anterior superior iliac spine. This prominence is called the *tubercle of the iliac crest*.
   b. The dorsal segment of the iliac crest has medial and lateral surfaces separated by a ridge.
5. The anterior border of the ilium extends from the anterior superior iliac spine to the acetabulum. Its lowest part presents a prominence called the *anterior inferior iliac spine*.
6. The posterior border of the ilium extends from the posterior superior iliac spine to the back of the acetabulum.
   a. A few centimetres below the posterior superior iliac spine the posterior border presents another prominence called the *posterior inferior iliac spine*.
   b. The lower part of the posterior border forms the upper boundary of a deep notch called the *greater sciatic notch*.
7. The lateral aspect of the ilium constitutes its *gluteal surface*. This surface is marked by three ridges called the anterior, posterior and inferior gluteal lines.
   a. The *posterior gluteal line* is vertical. It extends from the iliac crest, above, to the posterior inferior iliac spine below.
   b. The *anterior gluteal line* is convex upwards and backwards. Its anterior end meets the iliac crest in front of the tubercle; while its posterior end reaches the greater sciatic notch.

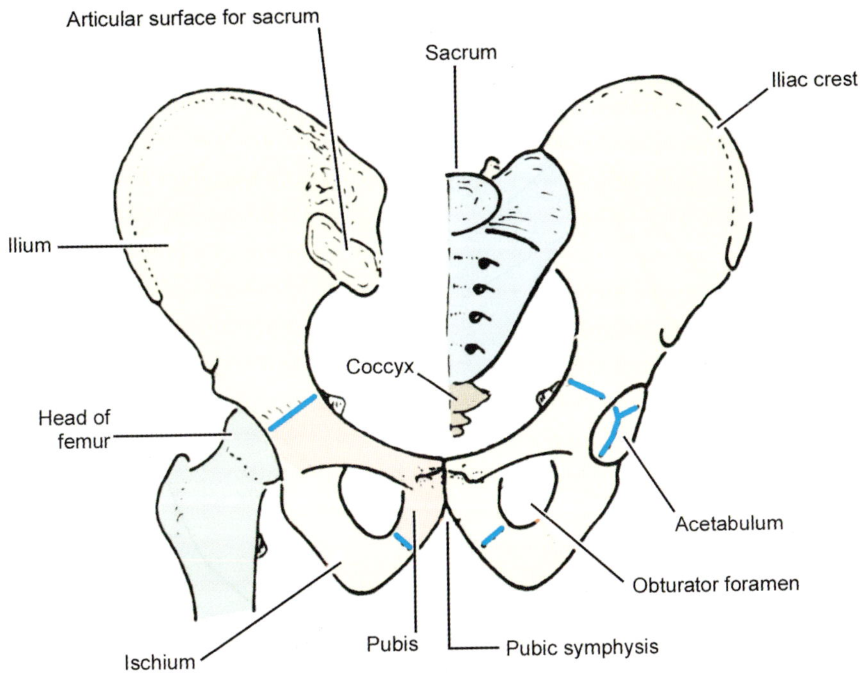


9.3: Pelvis viewed from the front: The sacrum is shown only in its left half, and the femur only on the right side

c. The ***inferior gluteal line*** is horizontal. Its anterior end lies just above the anterior inferior iliac spine; and its posterior end reaches the greater sciatic notch.

7a. Some other features on the gluteal surface are as follows:

i. The gluteal surface of the ilium bears a prominent groove just above the acetabulum.

ii. The lower part of the gluteal surface extends behind the acetabulum where it becomes continuous with the ischium.

iii. The lowest part of the ilium forms the upper two-fifths of the acetabulum.

8. The medial surface of the ilium is divisible into the following parts.

a. The ***iliac fossa*** is smooth and concave and forms the wall of the greater pelvis. It occupies the anterior part. of the medial surface.

b. The ***sacropelvic surface*** lies behind the iliac fossa. It can be subdivided into three parts.

i. The upper part is rough and constitutes the ***iliac tuberosity***.

ii. The middle part articulates with the lateral side of the sacrum. This part is called the ***auricular surface*** because of a resemblance to the pinna.

iii. The ***pelvic part*** of the medial surface lies below and in front of the auricular surface.

– It is smooth and takes part in forming the wall of the lesser pelvis.

– This surface is often marked (specially in the female) by a rough groove called the ***preauricular sulcus***.

c. The iliac fossa and the sacropelvic surface are separated by the medial border of the ilium.

i. This border is sharp in its upper part where it separates the iliac fossa from the auricular surface.

ii. Its lower part is rounded and forms the ***arcuate line***.

ii. The lower end of the arcuate line reaches the junction of the ilium and pubis.This junction shows an enlargement called the ***iliopubic eminence***.

## The Ischium

1. The ischium consists of a main part called the ***body***, and a projection called the ***ramus***. The upper end of the body forms the inferior and posterior part of the acetabulum.

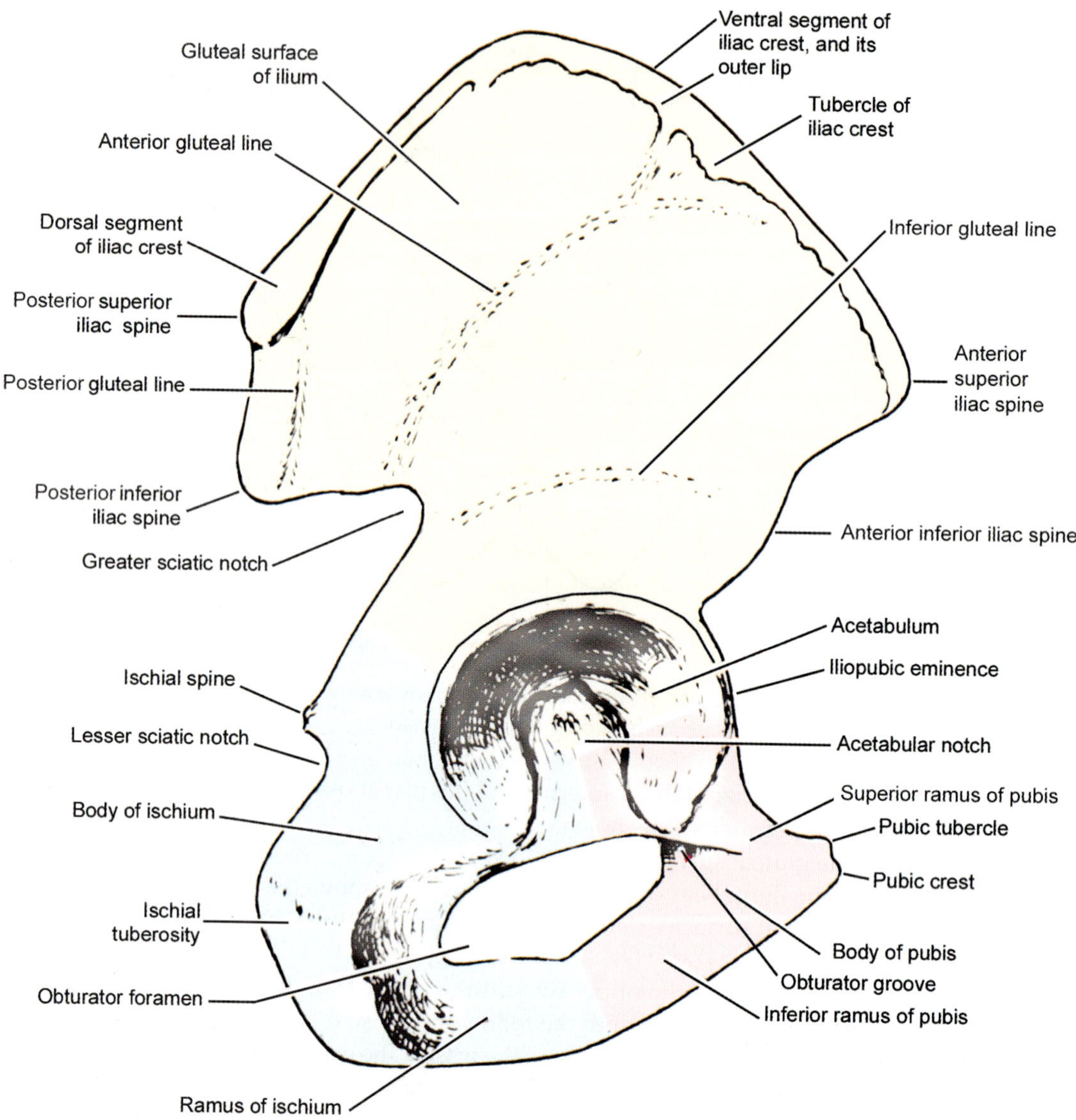


**9.4:** Right hip bone, external aspect

2. The lower part of the body has three surfaces namely dorsal, femoral and pelvic.
   a. The lower part of the dorsal surface has a large rough impression called the ***ischial tuberosity***.
   b. This tuberosity is divided into upper and lower parts by a transverse ridge.
   c. Each of these parts is again divided into medial and lateral parts.
3. The part of the dorsal surface above the ischial tuberosity shows a wide shallow groove. Above this, the dorsal surface becomes continuous with the gluteal surface of the ilium.
4. The posterior border of the dorsal surface of the ischium forms part of the lower margin of the greater sciatic notch.
   a. Just below this notch, the border projects backwards and medially as the ***ischial spine***.
   b. Between the ischial spine and the upper border of the ischial tuberosity we see a shallow ***lesser sciatic notch***.

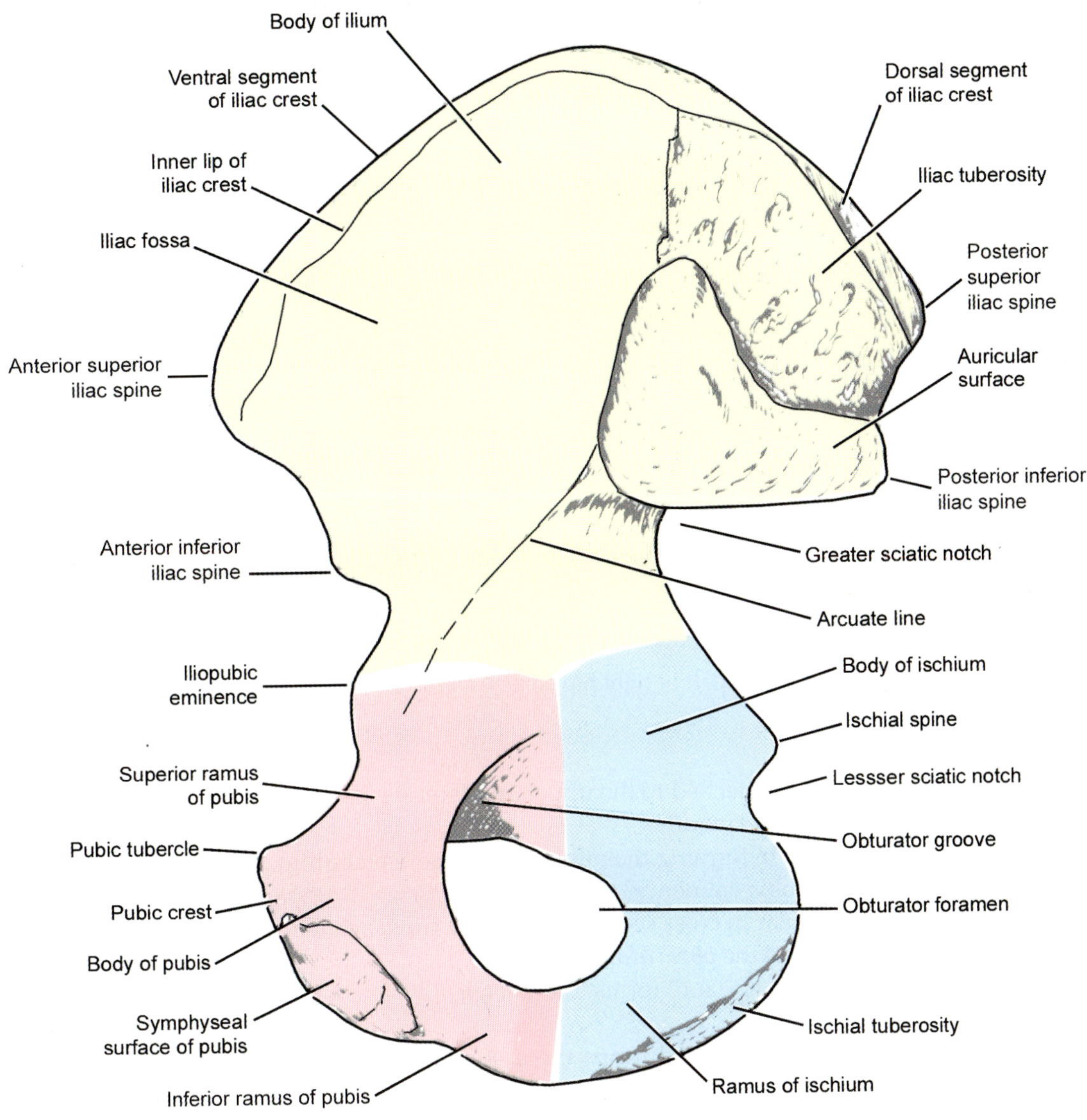


**9.5:** Right hip bone, internal aspect

5. The femoral surface of the ischium is directed downwards, forwards and laterally.
   a. It is continuous with the external surface of the ***ramus of the ischium*** that is attached to the medial side of the lower end of the body.
   b. The ramus has an anterior (external) surface and a posterior (internal) surface.

## The Pubis

1. The pubis consists of a body, a superior ramus and an inferior ramus.
2. The ***body*** (9.6) forms the anterior and most medial part of the hip bone.
   a. It has an anterior surface and a posterior surface.
   b. The upper border of the body forms a prominent ridge called the ***pubic crest***.
   c. The crest ends laterally in a projection called the ***pubic tubercle***.

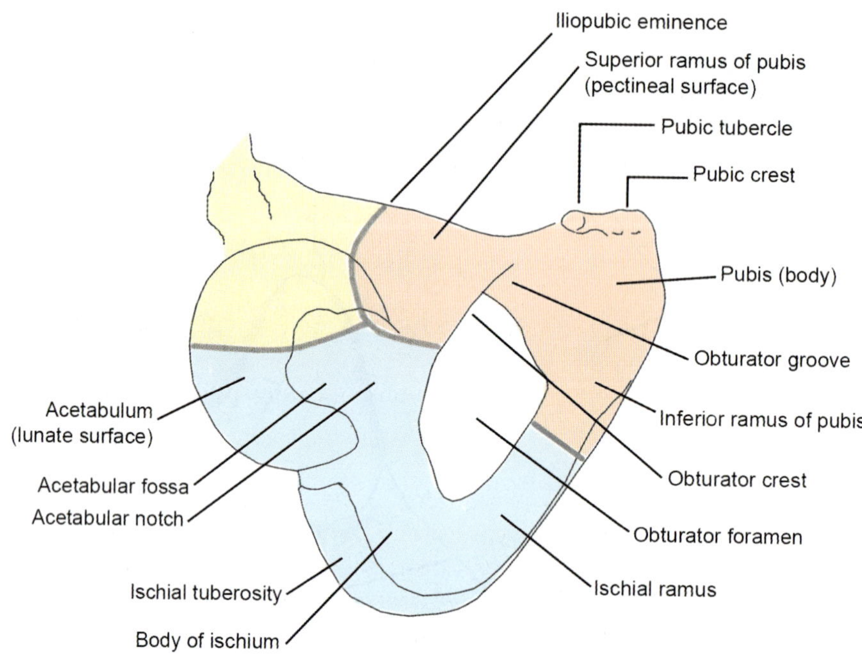


**9.6:** Medial part of right hip bone: Anterosuperior aspect

3. The ***superior ramus*** of the pubis is attached to the upper and lateral part of the body.
   a. It runs upwards, backwards and laterally.
   b. Its lateral extremity takes part in forming the pubic part of the acetabulum.
   c. It meets the ilium at the iliopubic eminence.
   d. The superior ramus is triangular in cross section (9.7). It has three borders and three surfaces.
      i. The anterior border is called the ***obturator crest***.
      ii. The posterior border is sharp and forms the ***pecten pubis*** or ***pectineal line***.
      iii. The inferior border is also sharp and forms the upper margin of the obturator foramen.
      iv. The surface between the obturator crest and the pecten pubis is the ***pectineal surface***.
      v. The pelvic surface lies between the pecten pubis and the inferior border.
      vi. The surface between the obturator crest and the inferior border is called the ***obturator surface***. A groove runs forwards and downwards across it and is called the ***obturator groove***.

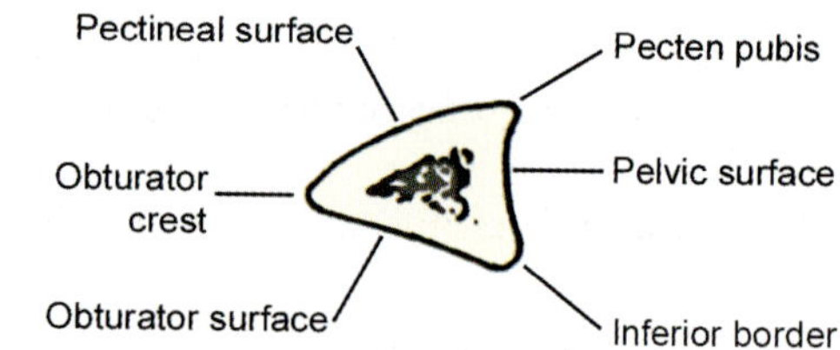


**9.7:** Section at right angles to the long axis of the superior ramus of the pubis

4. The ***inferior ramus*** is attached to the lower and lateral part of the body of the pubis.
   a. It passes downwards and laterally to meet the ramus of the ischium.
   b. These two rami form the medial boundary of the obturator foramen.
   c. In the intact pelvis (9.3) the conjoined rami of the pubis and ischium of the two sides form the boundaries of the ***pubic arch*** which lies below the pubic symphysis.
   d. The inferior ramus of the pubis has an anterior (or outer) surface, and a posterior (or inner) surface. These surfaces are continuous with corresponding surfaces of the ischial ramus.

## The Acetabulum

1. The acetabulum is a deep cup like cavity that lies on the lateral aspect of the hipbone.
2. It forms the hip joint with the head of the femur.
3. It is directed laterally and somewhat downwards and forwards.
4. The margin of the acetabulum is deficient in the anteroinferior part and the gap in the margin is called the ***acetabular notch***.
5. The floor of the acetabulum is partly articular and partly non-articular.
6. The articular area for the head of the femur is shaped like a horseshoe and is called the ***lunate surface***. This surface is widest superiorly.
7. The inner border of the lunate surface forms the margin of the non-articular part of the floor and that is called the ***acetabular fossa***.
8. The contributions to the acetabulum by the ilium, the ischium and the pubis are shown in 9.4 and in 9.6.

## The Obturator Foramen

1. The obturator foramen is bounded above by the superior ramus of the pubis; medially by the body of the pubis, by its inferior ramus and by the ramus of the ischium; and laterally by the body of the ischium.
2. In the intact body, the foramen is filled by a fibrous sheet called the ***obturator membrane***.
3. However, the membrane is deficient in the uppermost part of the foramen. Here the membrane has a free upper edge which is separated from the superior ramus of the pubis by a gap.

## WANT TO KNOW MORE?

### Attachments on the Hip Bone

The muscles attached to the iliac crest are as follows (See 9.8 and 9.9):

1. The ***internal oblique muscle of the abdomen*** arises from the intermediate area of the ventral segment of the iliac crest.
2. The ***external oblique muscle of the abdomen*** is inserted into the anterior two-thirds of the outer lip of the ventral segment of the iliac crest.
3. The lowest fibres of the ***latissimus dorsi*** take origin from the outer lip of the iliac crest just behind its highest point.
4. The ***tensor fasciae latae*** arises from the anterior part of the outer lip of the iliac crest.
5. The ***transversus abdominis*** arises from the anterior two-thirds of the inner lip of the ventral segment of the iliac crest.
6. The ***quadratus lumborum*** arises from the posterior one-third of the inner lip of the ventral segment of the iliac crest.
7. The ***gluteus maximus*** arises from the lateral surface of the dorsal segment of the iliac crest and from the gluteal surface of the ilium behind the posterior gluteal line.
8. The ***erector spinae*** arises from the medial surface of the dorsal segment of the iliac crest.

The muscles attached to the external aspect of the hip bone (excluding the iliac crest) are as follows (See 9.8):

1. See origin of gluteus maximus as described above.
2. The ***gluteus medius*** arises from the gluteal surface of the ilium between the anterior and posterior gluteal lines.
3. The ***gluteus minimus*** arises from the gluteal surface of the ilium between the anterior and inferior gluteal lines.
4. The ***sartorius*** arises from the anterior superior iliac spine and from a small area below the spine.
5. The straight head of the ***rectus femoris*** arises from the anterior inferior iliac spine; and its reflected head from the groove above the acetabulum.

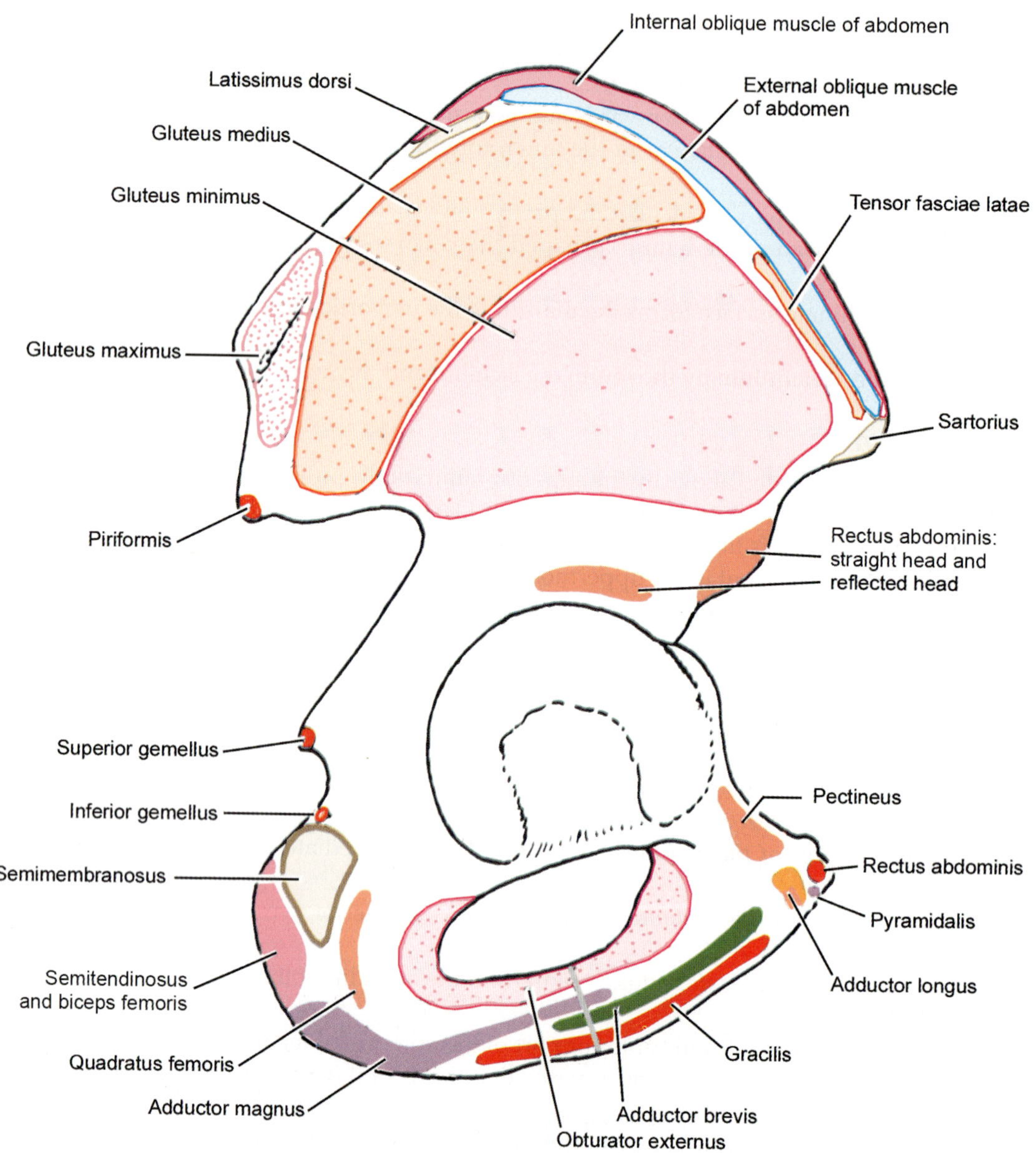


**9.8:** Right hip bone, showing attachments. External aspect

6. A few fibres of the ***piriformis*** arise from the upper border of the greater sciatic notch near the posterior inferior iliac spine.
7. The ***pectineus*** arises from the upper part of the pectineal surface of the superior ramus of the pubis.
8. The ***rectus abdominis*** (lateral head) arises from the pubic crest.

9,10. The ***pyramidalis*** and the ***adductor longus*** arise from the anterior surface of the body of the pubis.

11. The ***gracilis*** arises from the anterior surface of the body, and the inferior ramus, of the pubis; and from the ramus of the ischium.
12. The ***adductor brevis*** arises from the anterior surface of the body of the pubis and its inferior ramus, lateral to the origin of the gracilis.

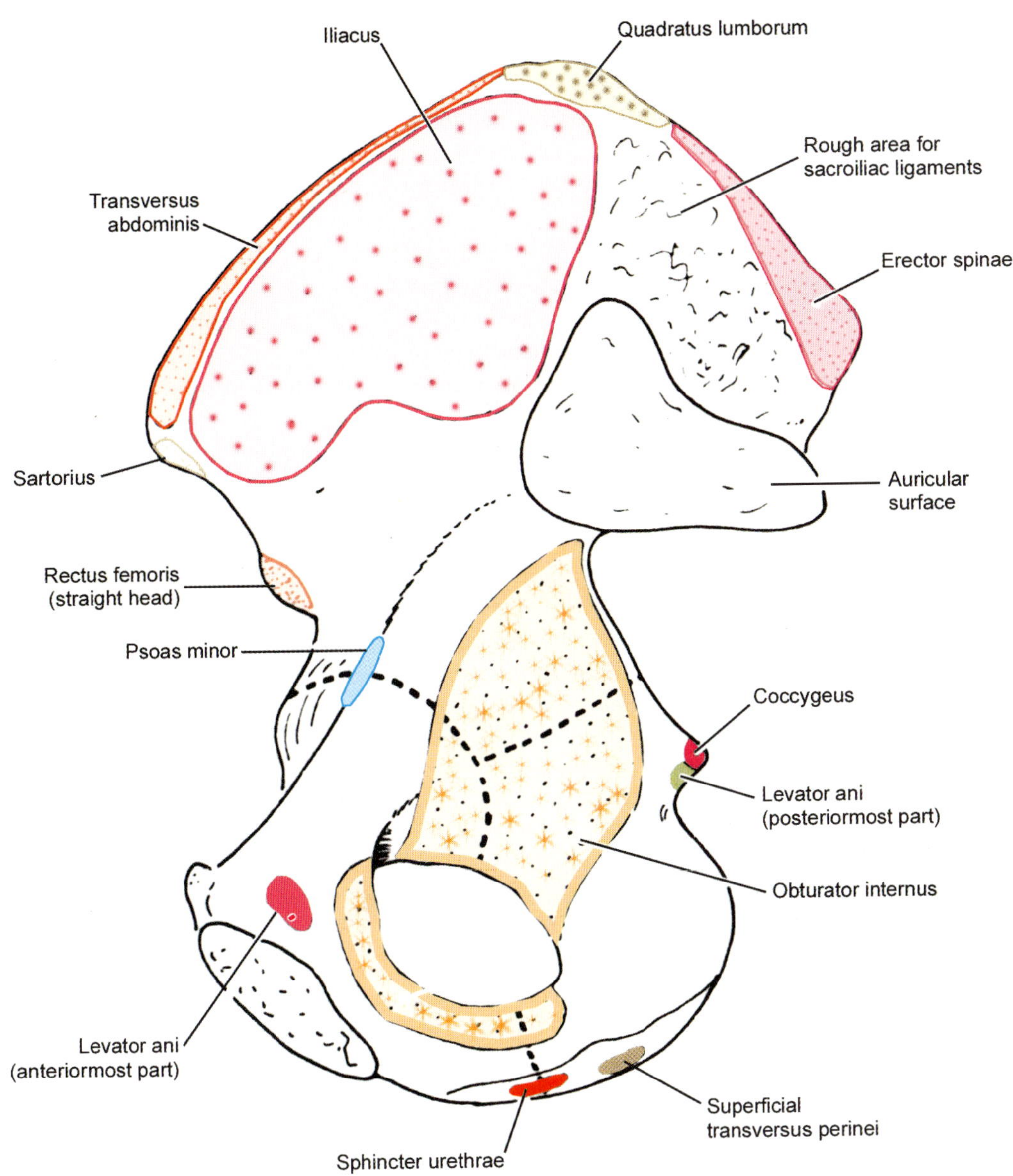


9.9: Right hip bone, showing attachments. Internal aspect

13. The ***obturator externus*** arises from the superior and inferior rami of the pubis, and from the ramus of the ischium, immediately around the obturator foramen.
14. The ***adductor magnus*** arises from the lower lateral part of the ischial tuberosity, and from the ramus of the ischium.

15,16. The ***semitendinosus*** and the ***biceps femoris*** (long head) arise from the upper medial part of the ischial tuberosity.

17. The ***semimembranosus*** arises from the upper lateral part of the ischial tuberosity.
18. The ***quadratus femoris*** arises from the femoral surface of the ischium just lateral to the ischial tuberosity.
19. The ***superior gemellus*** arises from the dorsal surface of the ischial spine.
20. The ***inferior gemellus*** arises from the ischium just above the ischial tuberosity.

*The muscles arising from the internal aspect of the hip bone are as follows:*
(See 9.9).

1. The ***iliacus*** arises from the upper two-thirds of the iliac fossa.
2. The ***obturator internus*** arises from the pelvic surfaces of the superior and inferior rami of the pubis, and the ramus of the ischium, immediately adjoining the obturator foramen and from the pelvic surfaces of the ischium and of the ilium.
3. The most posterior fibres of the ***levator ani*** arise from the pelvic surface of the ischial spine and its most anterior fibres from the posterior surface of the body of the pubis.
4. The ***psoas minor*** is inserted into the pecten pubis and into the iliopectineal eminence.
5. The ***coccygeus*** arises from the pelvic surface of the ischial spine.
6. The ***superficial transversus perinei*** and the ***ischiocavernosus*** arise from the posterior surface of the ramus of the ischium.
7. The ***sphincter urethrae*** arises from the posterior surfaces of the inferior pubic and ischial rami.

### *Some Other Attachments on the Hip Bone*

1. The ***inguinal ligament*** is attached medially to the pubic tubercle, and laterally to the anterior superior iliac spine.
2. The ***conjoint tendon*** is attached to the pubic crest and to the medial part of the pecten pubis.
3. The margin of the acetabulum gives attachment to the ***capsule of the hip joint***, and to the ***acetabular labrum***.
4. The ***capsule of the sacroiliac joint*** is attached around the margin of the auricular surface.
5. The upper end of the ***sacrotuberous ligament*** is attached to the posterior superior and posterior inferior iliac spines, and to the intervening part of the posterior border of the ilium. The lower end of the ligament is attached to the medial margin of the ischial tuberosity.
6. The ***sacrospinous ligament*** is attached to the apex of the ischial spine.

### Important Relations of Hip Bone

1. The posterior surface of the pubis is related to the ***urinary bladder***.
2. The right iliac fossa is related to the ***cecum*** and ***terminal ileum***. The left iliac fossa is related to the terminal part of the ***descending colon***.
3. The greater and lesser sciatic notches are converted into foramina by the sacrotuberous and sacrospinous ligaments.

   The ***greater sciatic foramen*** transmits the following structures:
   a. Piriformis
   b. The superior and inferior gluteal nerves and vessels
   c. The internal pudendal vessels
   d. The pudendal and sciatic nerves
   e. The posterior cutaneous nerve of the thigh
   f. The nerves to the obturator internus and to the quadratus femoris.
4. Having emerged from the greater sciatic foramen the pudendal nerve, the nerve to the obturator internus, and the internal pudendal vessels pass behind the ischial spine to enter the ***lesser sciatic foramen***.
5. The tendon of the obturator internus emerges from the pelvis through this foramen.

### Ossification of the Hip Bone

1. The hip bone has three primary centres, one each for the ilium, the ischium and the pubis. The centres appearing in intrauterine life are as follows:
   a. For the ilium in the 8th week
   b. For the ischium in the fourth month
   c. For the pubis in the fourth or fifth month.
2. At birth, the ilium, ischium and pubis are separated by a Y-shaped cartilage present in the region of the acetabulum. The three parts fuse completely only after the age of 18 years.

3. The inferior ramus of the pubis and the ramus of the ischium are at first separated by cartilage. They fuse with each other about the seventh year.
4. Several secondary centres appear in the hip bone.
   a. There are two in the iliac crest,
   b. two in the acetabular cartilage, and occasional centres
   c. in the anterior inferior iliac spine,
   d. the lower part of the acetabulum,
   e. the pubic tubercle and
   f. the pubic crest.
5. These centres appear at about the age of puberty or later and fuse with the rest of the bone between 20 and 25 years of age.

## PELVIS AS A WHOLE

1. We have seen that the bony pelvis is made up of the two hip bones, the sacrum and the coccyx (9.10). It may be subdivided into the ***greater (or false) pelvis*** and the ***lesser (or true) pelvis***.
2. The walls of the greater pelvis are formed by the broad upper parts of the two iliac bones (iliac fossae), and posteriorly by the base of the sacrum. Note that the greater pelvis has no bony ***anterior*** wall, and that it is merely the lower part of the abdomen.
3. The communication between the greater and lesser pelvis is called the ***superior pelvic aperture*** or ***pelvic inlet***. The margins of the aperture constitute the ***pelvic brim***. The pelvic brim is formed:
   a. Behind by the sacral promontory, and the ridge separating the superior and anterior surfaces of the sacrum
   b. On either side by the arcuate line of the ilium (also see 9.5)

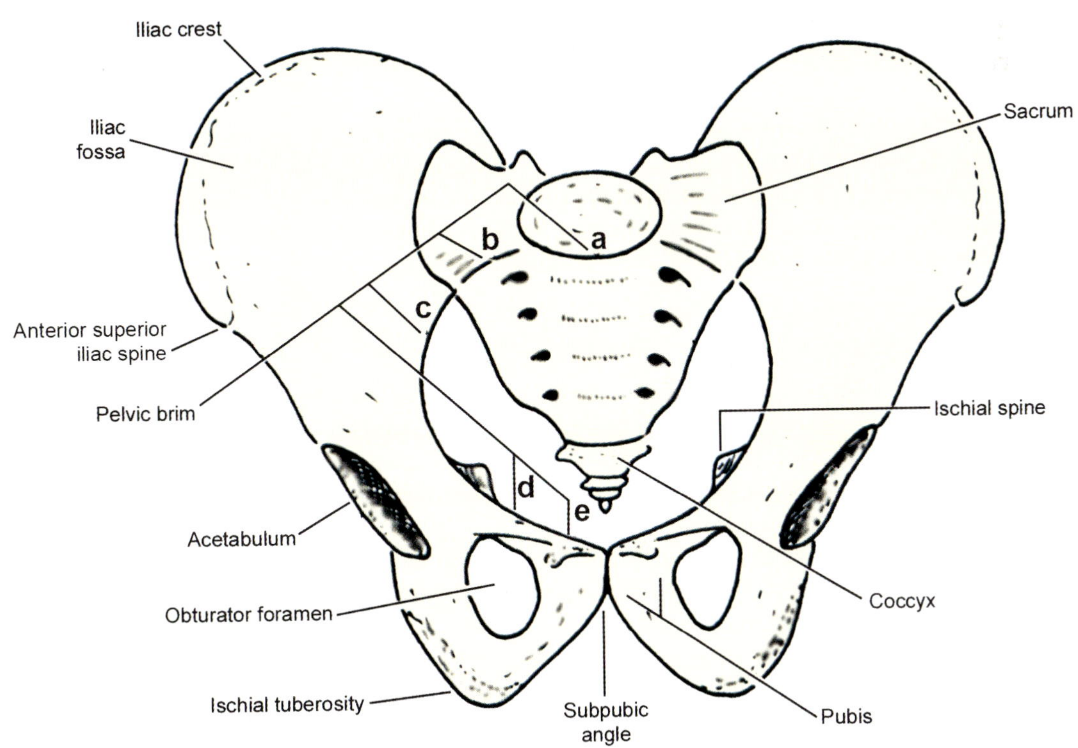


**9.10:** Pelvis seen from the front

   c. Anteriorly by the pecten pubis and by the pubic crest. The arcuate line, the pecten pubis and the pubic crest are collectively referred to as the ***linea terminalis***.
4. The ***cavity of the lesser pelvis*** is bounded:
   a. In front by the body and rami of the pubis
   b. On either side by the pelvic surfaces of the ilium and ischium below the arcuate line
   c. Behind by the anterior surfaces of the sacrum and coccyx.
5. The ***inferior pelvic aperture*** is highly irregular. It is bounded:
   a. Anteriorly by the pubic arch
   b. Laterally, in that order, by the ischial tuberosity, the lesser sciatic notch, the ischial spine and the greater sciatic notch.
   c. Posteriorly, it is formed by the lateral margin of the sacrum and coccyx.
   d. When the ligaments are intact the lateral margins are formed by the sacrotuberous ligaments (that stretch from the side of the sacrum and coccyx to the ischial tuberosity). The inferior aperture then appears to be rhomboidal (9.12).

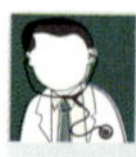

## CLINICAL CORRELATION

**Diameters of the bony pelvis**

The diameters of the pelvic inlet and outlet are important in obstetrics. Some of these are given below. All dimensions given are those in the female (9.11 to 9.13).

*INLET*

1. The ***anteroposterior diameter*** is measured from the upper border of the symphysis pubis to the sacral promontory. It is about 110 mm in the female (9.11).
2. The ***transverse diameter*** is measured across the widest part of the pelvic brim. It is about 130 mm.
3. The ***oblique diameter*** is measured from one iliopubic eminence to the opposite sacroiliac joint. It is about 125 mm.

*OUTLET*

1. The ***anteroposterior diameter*** is measured from the apex of the coccyx to the lower border of the symphysis pubis. It is about 125 mm (9.12).
2. The ***transverse diameter*** is measured between the two ischial tuberosities. It is about 110 mm.
3. The ***oblique diameter*** is measured from the midpoint of the sacrotuberous ligament of one side to the junction of the ischial and pubic rami on the other side. It is about 118 mm.

**Clinical Note**

*Sex Differences in the Pelvis*

It is significant in forensic medice

Of all the bones of the human skeleton sexual differences are most marked in the pelvis, and these are useful in deciding whether a given pelvis belongs to a male or a female individual.

1. As a rule, the male pelvis is more strongly built than in the female, and the bones have more prominent muscular markings.
2. All the articular areas including the acetabulum are larger in the male, for transmission of greater body weight.
3. In contrast, the female pelvis is adapted for the function of child bearing. For this purpose the true pelvis is broader and shallower than in the male.
4. Some points that are really useful in deciding the sex of a given pelvis are as follows. However, all the features have to be taken together, no one feature being decisive.
5. The ***subpubic angle*** (i.e., the angle between the right and left ischiopubic rami) is almost ninety degrees in the female, but is only fifty to sixty degrees in the male. The angle is sharp in the male, but tends to be rounded in the female.

6. The medial edges of the ***ischiopubic rami*** may be markedly everted in the male for attachment of the crura of the penis.
7. In the male, the distance from the pubic symphysis to the anterior margin of the acetabulum is equal to the total width of the acetabulum, but in the female distance from the pubic symphysis to the anterior margin of the acetabulum is distinctly more than the width of the acetabulum.
8. In the female ***sacrum,*** the width of the articular area for the body of the fifth lumbar vertebra is equal to the width of the lateral part (or ala). On the other hand, in the male the width of the body is distinctly more than the width of the lateral part.
9. The ***pelvic inlet*** is rounded in the female, but tends to be heart shaped in the male. The male inlet is smaller in all diameters.
10. The ***preauricular sulcus*** is deeper and more prominent in the female.

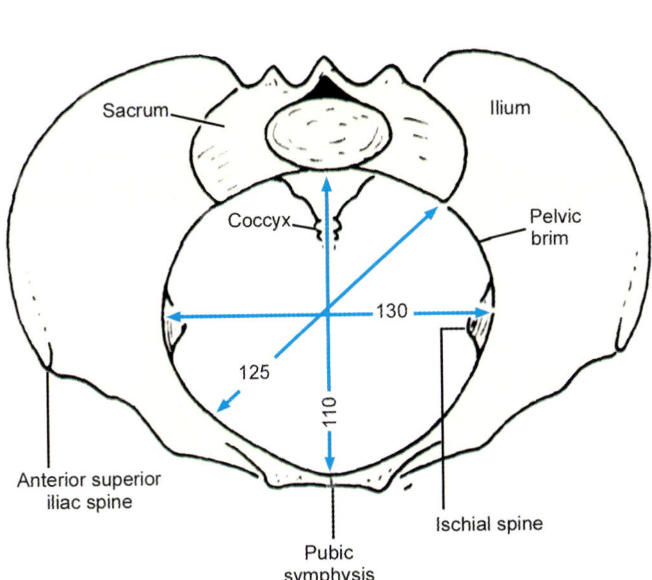


**9.11:** Anteroposterior view of the pelvis to show the diameters of the pelvic inlet (in mm)

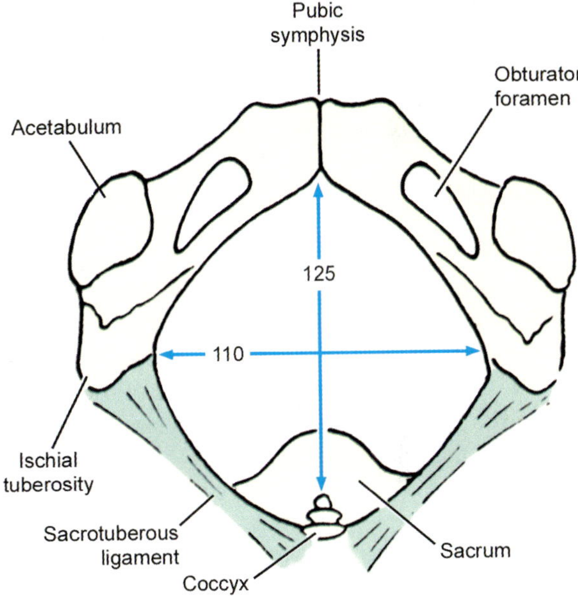


**9.12:** Pelvic outlet seen from below

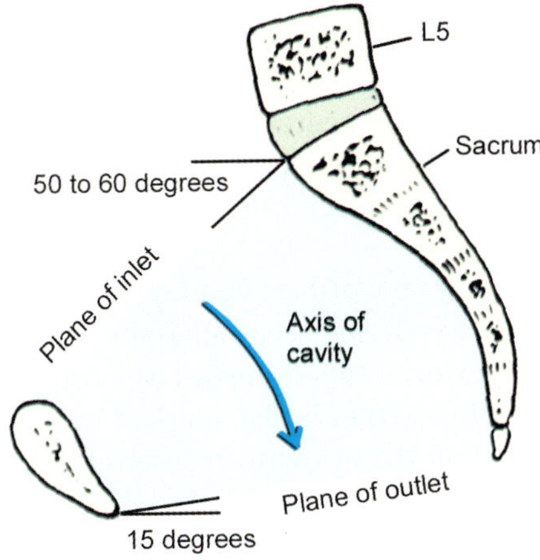


**9.13:** Schematic sagittal section of the pelvis to show orientation of the pelvic inlet and outlet

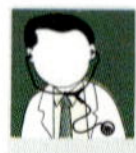

**CLINICAL CORRELATION**

**Fractures of the Pelvis**

1. These are not common. They may occur through the superior or inferior ischiopubic ramus, near the junction of the pubis and ischium (when they may involve the acetabulum), or the lateral part of the ilium.
2. Isolated fractures of one part of the pelvis are usually not serious as long as the ring formed by the two hip bones and sacrum is not disrupted.
3. Disruption of the ring occurs when it is broken (or dislocated) at two points (e.g., fracture of both ischiopubic rami combined with dislocation at the sacroiliac joint).
4. When disruption occurs, there can be injury to the urinary bladder, the urethra, the rectum, or the vagina.
5. Injury to a large artery in the pelvic wall can cause severe bleeding.
6. In serious disruption of the pelvis, there may be permanent damage to nerves of the lumbosacral plexus.
7. When a fracture of the pelvis involves the acetabulum, it can eventually lead to osteoarthritis at the hip joint.
8. Extremely strong contraction of muscles (in competitive sports) can tear off a tendon from its attachment along with a small piece of bone. The anterior superior and anterior inferior iliac spines can be torn off. These are called *avulsion fractures*.

## THE FEMUR

### Side Determination

1. The femur (9.14 and 9.15) is a long bone having a shaft, an upper end and a lower end.
2. The upper end is easily distinguished from the lower end by the presence of a rounded head that is joined to the shaft by an elongated neck. The head is directed medially to articulate with the acetabulum of the hip bone.
3. The anterior and posterior aspects of the bone can be distinguished by examining the shaft as it is convex forwards and the anterior aspect is smooth, while the posterior aspect is marked by a prominent vertical ridge called the linea aspera.
4. The information given above is sufficient to distinguish between a femur of the right or left side.

### The Upper End

Apart from the head and the neck, the upper end of the femur has two projections called the greater and lesser trochanters.

1. The ***head***, apart from being directed medially is also directed upwards and somewhat forwards.
    a. It is much more rounded than the head of the humerus and is slightly more than half a sphere.
    b. Near the centre of the head there is a pit or ***fovea***.
2. The ***neck*** connects the head to the shaft.
    a. It joins the shaft at an angle of about 125 degrees.
    b. The greater and lesser trochanters are situated near the junction of the neck with the shaft.
3. The ***greater trochanter*** forms a large quadrangular projection on the lateral aspect of the upper end of the femur.
    a. Its upper and posterior part projects upwards beyond the level of the neck and thus comes to have a medial surface. On this surface, we see a depressed area called the ***trochanteric fossa***.
    b. The anterior aspect of the greater trochanter shows a large rough area for muscle attachments.
    c. The lateral surface of the greater trochanter is also marked by an area for muscle attachments: the area is in the form of a ridge or a flat strip that runs downwards and forwards across the lateral surface.
4. The ***lesser trochanter*** is a conical projection attached to the shaft where the lower border of the neck meets the shaft. It points medially and backwards.
5. The posterior parts of the greater and lesser trochanters are joined together by a prominent ridge called the ***intertrochanteric crest***.

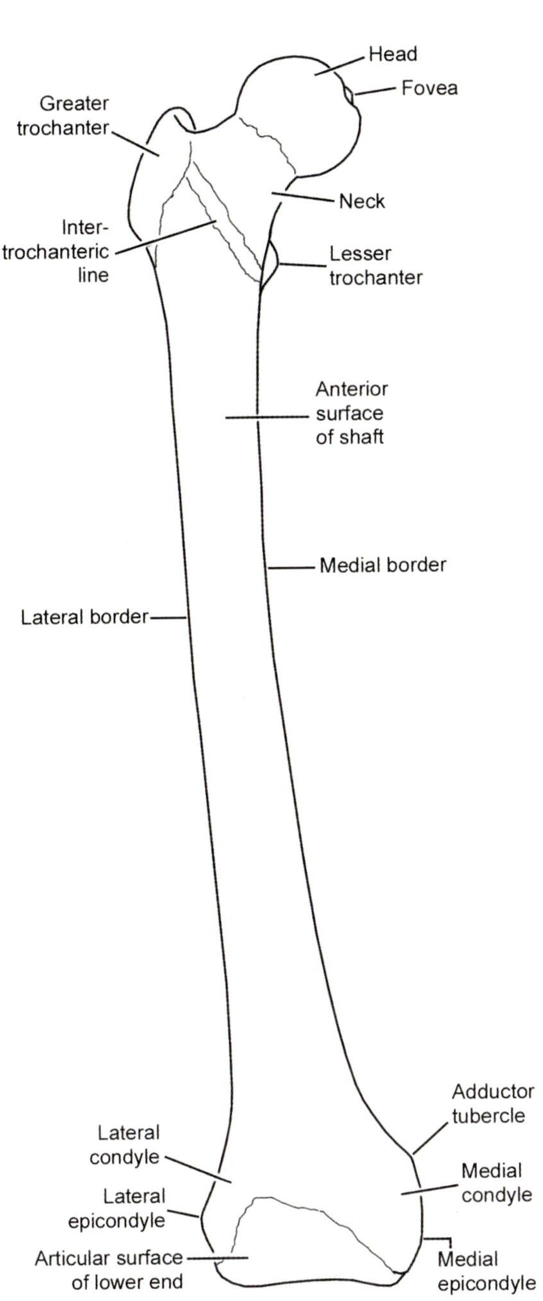


**9.14:** Right femur, anterior aspect

Neck
Head
Trochanteric fossa
Greater trochanter
Fovea
Quadrate tubercle
Inter-trochanteric crest
Lesser trochanter
Gluteal tuberosity
Spiral line
Medial and lateral lips of linea aspera
Medial border
Lateral border
Medial surface of shaft
Lateral surface of shaft
Lateral supracondylar line
Medial supracondylar line
Popliteal surface
Intercondylar line
Adductor tubercle
Lateral epicondyle
Medial epicondyle
Lateral condyle
Medial condyle
Intercondylar notch

**9.15:** Right femur, posterior aspect

6. A little above its middle, this crest bears a rounded elevation called the ***quadrate tubercle***.
7. Anteriorly, the junction of the neck and the shaft is marked by a much less prominent ***intertrochanteric line***. The upper end of this line reaches the anterior and upper part of the greater trochanter and its lower end lies a little in front of the lesser trochanter.
8. Here, it becomes continuous with the ***spiral line*** that runs downwards and backwards across the medial aspect of the shaft to reach its posterior aspect.

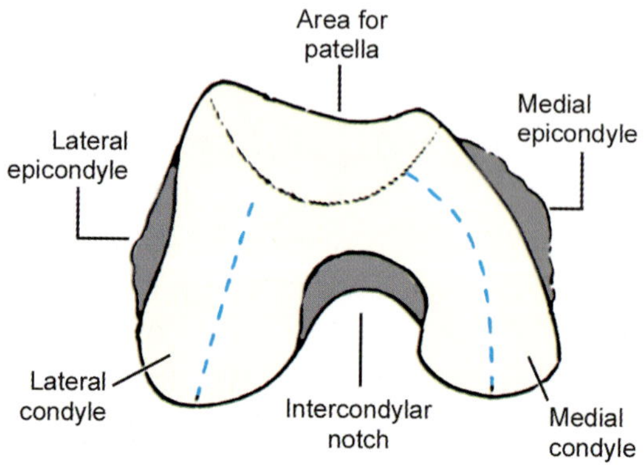


9.16: Right femur, lower end, viewed from below

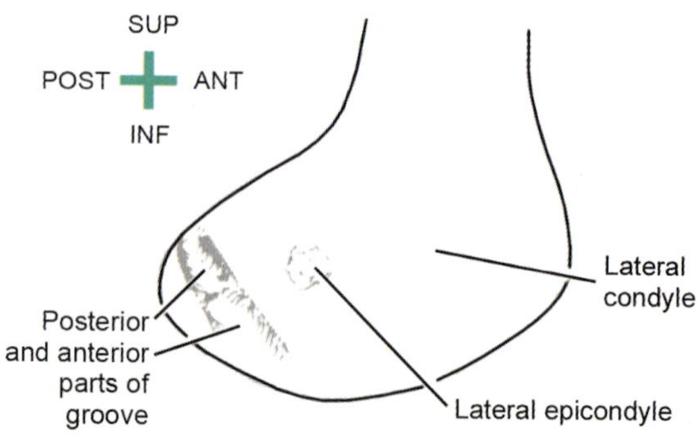


9.17: Right femur, lower end, seen from the lateral side

## The Shaft

1. The shaft of the femur has a forward convexity and is smooth anteriorly.
   a. Its posterior aspect is marked by a rough vertical ridge called the ***linea aspera***.
   b. The shaft is triangular having three borders (lateral, medial and posterior) and three surfaces (anterior, lateral and medial).
2. The lateral and medial borders are rounded. The posterior border corresponds to the linea aspera.
3. In addition to the directions indicated by their names, the medial and lateral surfaces also face backwards.
4. The linea aspera has distinct medial and lateral lips.
   a. When traced upwards to the upper one-third of the shaft, the lips diverge.
   b. The medial lip becomes continuous with the spiral line.
   c. The lateral lip of the linea aspera becomes continuous with a broad rough area called the ***gluteal tuberosity***. The upper end of the gluteal tuberosity reaches the greater trochanter.
5. The area between the gluteal tuberosity (laterally) and the spiral line (medially) constitutes a fourth surface (posterior) over the upper one-third of the shaft.
6. The two lips of the linea aspera diverge from each other over the lower one-third of the shaft to become continuous with ridges called the ***medial and lateral supracondylar lines***.
7. Here again, the shaft has an additional surface directed posteriorly. This surface is triangular and is called the ***popliteal surface***.

## The Lower End

1. The lower end of the femur consists of two large condyles namely medial and lateral.
   a. The two condyles are joined together anteriorly and, on this aspect, they lie in the same plane as the lower part of the shaft (9.16).
   b. Posteriorly, the two condyles project much beyond the plane of the shaft, and here they are separated by a deep ***intercondylar notch*** or fossa.
2. When viewed from the side the lower margin of each condyle is seen to form an arch that is convex downwards (9.17).
3. When seen from below (9.16) it is seen that the long axis of the lateral condyle is straight and is directed backwards and somewhat laterally. (In 9.16 the axis is indicated in interrupted line). In contrast, the medial condyle is slightly curved having a medial convexity.
4. The anterior aspect of the two condyles is marked by an articular area for the patella (9.16).
   a. The area is concave from side to side to accommodate the convex posterior surface of the patella.
   b. It is divided into medial and lateral parts. The lateral part is much larger. (Also see 9.14).

5. Inferiorly, the condyles articulate with the tibia to form the knee joint.
   a. For this purpose, each condyle bears a large convex articular surface that is continuous anteriorly with the patellar surface.
   b. The articular surface covers the inferior and posterior aspects of each condyle.
6. When seen from the lateral aspect, the lateral condyle of the femur is seen to be more or less flat (9.17).
   a. A little behind the middle it is marked by a prominence called the ***lateral epicondyle***.
   b. Behind and below the epicondyle, there is a prominent groove that is divided into an anterior deeper part and a shallower posterior part.
7. When seen from the medial aspect, the medial condyle is seen to be convex.
   a. The most prominent point on it is called the ***medial epicondyle*** (9.16).
   b. The uppermost part of the medial condyle is marked by a prominence called the ***adductor tubercle*** (9.15). This tubercle lies above and behind the medial epicondyle and is continuous with the lower end of the medial supracondylar line.

## WANT TO KNOW MORE?

### Attachments on the Femur

The muscles inserted into the femur are as follows:
(See 9.18 and 9.19) .

1. The ***gluteus minimus*** is inserted on the anterior aspect of the greater trochanter.
2. The ***gluteus medius*** is inserted into the oblique strip running downwards and forwards across the lateral surface of the greater trochanter.
3. The ***piriformis*** is inserted into the upper border of the greater trochanter.
4. The ***obturator internus*** and ***gemelli*** are inserted into the anterior part of the medial surface of the greater trochanter.
5. The ***obturator externus*** is inserted into the trochanteric fossa on the medial surface of the greater trochanter.
6. The ***psoas major*** is inserted into the medial part of the anterior surface of the lesser trochanter.
7. The ***iliacus*** is inserted into the medial side of the base of the lesser trochanter, and into a small area below the latter.
8. The ***pectineus*** is inserted along a line descending from the root of the lesser trochanter to the upper end of the linea aspera. The insertion lies between the gluteal tuberosity and the spiral line.
9. The ***quadratus femoris*** is inserted on the quadrate tubercle, and into a small area below the latter.
10. The deep fibres of the ***gluteus maximus*** are inserted into the gluteal tuberosity.
11. The upper part of the ***adductor brevis*** is inserted between the insertions of the pectineus (medially) and the adductor magnus (laterally) (see below). The lower part of the muscle is inserted into the linea aspera.
12. The ***adductor longus*** is inserted into the middle one-third of the linea aspera.
13. The ***adductor magnus*** is inserted into the medial margin of the gluteal tuberosity, the linea aspera, and the medial supracondylar line. The hamstring part of the muscle ends in a tendon that is attached to the adductor tubercle.

The muscles taking origin from the femur are as follows:

1. The ***vastus lateralis*** has a long linear origin.
   a. The line begins at the upper end of the intertrochanteric line. It passes along:
   b. The anterior and lower borders of the greater trochanter.
   c. The lateral margin of the gluteal tuberosity.
   d. The lateral lip of the linea aspera.
2. The ***vastus medialis*** also has a long linear origin from:
   a. The lower part of the intertrochanteric line
   b. The spiral line

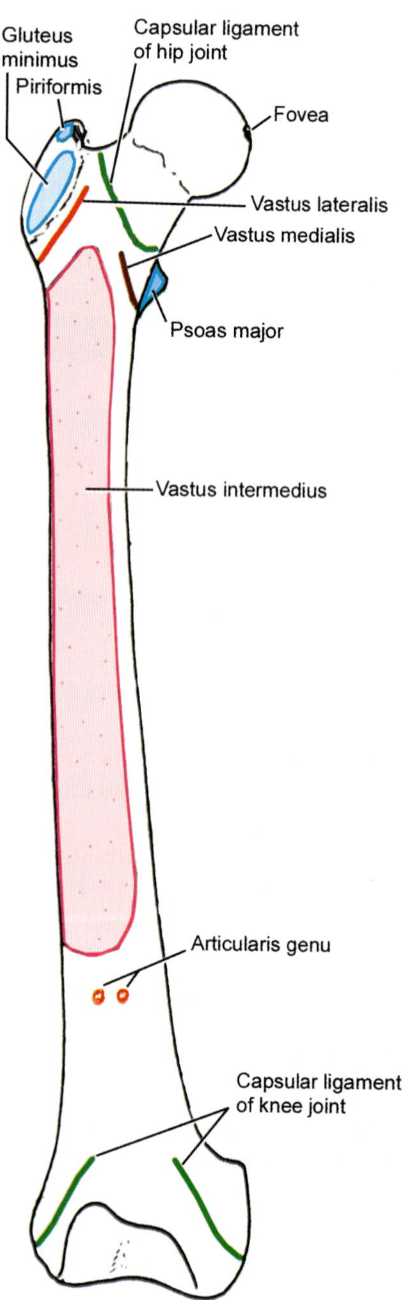


**9.18:** Right femur, showing attachments, seen from the front

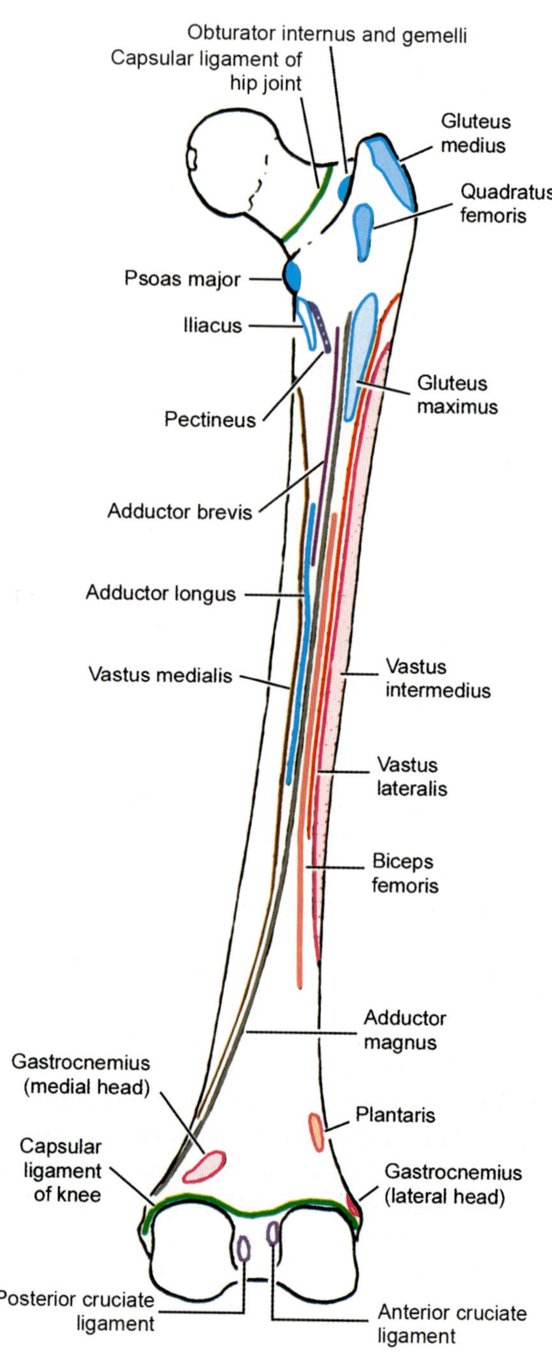


**9.19:** Right femur, showing attachments, seen from behind

   c. The medial lip of the linea aspera
   d. The medial supracondylar line right up to the adductor tubercle.
3. The ***vastus intermedius*** arises from the upper three-fourths of the anterior and lateral surfaces of the shaft. The medial surface of the shaft does not give origin to the muscle, but is covered by it.

4. The *articularis genu* arises from small areas on the anterior surface of the shaft below the origin of the vastus intermedius.
5. The short head of the *biceps femoris* arises from the linea aspera and from the upper part of the lateral supracondylar line.
6. a. The medial head of the *gastrocnemius* arises from the popliteal surface a little above the medial condyle.
   b. The lateral head of the muscle arises from the lateral surface of the lateral condyle.
7. The *plantaris* arises from the lower part of the lateral supracondylar line.
8. The *popliteus* arises (by a tendon) from the anterior part of the groove on the lateral aspect of the lateral condyle.

*Other Attachments on the Femur*

1. The *capsular ligament of the hip joint* is attached to the neck of the femur most of which is intracapsular.
   a. Anteriorly, the capsule is attached to the intertrochanteric line.
   b. But posteriorly the capsule is attached about 1cm medial to the intertrochanteric crest.
2. The *ligament of the head* is attached to the fovea on the head of the femur.
3. The *capsular ligament of the knee joint* is attached to the femoral condyles and to the posterior margin of the intercondylar fossa.
   a. On the lateral condyle it is attached above the origin of the popliteus.
   b. The capsule is deficient anteriorly, where it is replaced by the patella.
4. The *anterior cruciate ligament* is attached to the medial surface of the lateral condyle.
5. The *posterior cruciate ligament* is attached to the lateral surface of the medial condyle.

**Ossification of the Femur**

1. The femur is the second long bone in the body to start ossifying (the first being the clavicle).
2. The *primary centre* appears in the shaft during the 7th fetal week. It may be noted that the neck of the femur ossifies from the primary centre.
3. Three *secondary centres* appear at the upper end of the bone:
   a. One each for the head (first year),
   b. The greater trochanter (fourth year), and
   c. The lesser trochanter (around the twelfth year).
   d. Each of these centres fuses independently with the shaft in the reverse order of appearance:
      i. The lesser trochanter at about 13 years,
      ii. The greater trochanter at about 14 years, and the head around 16 years.
      iii. One centre appears for the distal end.
         - This centre appears before birth in the 9th month of fetal life.
         - It fuses with the shaft between the 16th and 18th years.

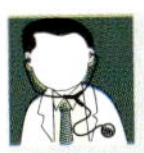

## CLINICAL CORRELATION

**Congenital Anomalies**

1. The angle between the neck and shaft of the femur may be less than normal (*coxa vera*) or more than normal (*coxa valga*).
2. *Absence* of the proximal part of the femur is a rare congenital anomaly.
3. The hip joint is a common site of *congenital dislocation* occurring as a result of imperfectly formed bone ends. Rarely, the knee may be similarly affected.

*Fractures of the Femur*

The femur may be fractured

1. Through the neck
2. Through the trochanteric region.
3. Through the shaft (at any level).
4. Just above the condyles (supracondylar fracture) or
5. Through a condyle.

*Fracture of the Neck of the Femur*

1. This fracture is common in old persons in whom the region has been weakened by osteoporosis. It can occur as a result of slight injury which is usually a rotational force. The fractured limb shows marked lateral rotation.
2. Fracture of the neck compromises ***blood supply*** to the head of the femur. Blood supply to the head is derived from three sources:
   a. Nutrient vessels passing through the neck to reach the head;
   b. Vessels entering the upper end of the femur along the attachment of capsule of the hip joint; and
   c. Vessels entering the head through the ligamentum teres.

2a. Following fracture of the neck of the femur the only remaining supply is that through the ligamentum teres.

3. Lack of adequate blood supply can be responsible for delayed union, or nonunion of the fracture.
   a. However, if blood supply of the head is insufficient to maintain its viability there is ***avascular necrosis*** of the head.
   b. When this happens bone of the head collapses and the hip joint becomes disorganised leaving the patient with a permanent limp.
   c. However, the joint can be repaired using artificial (metallic) components. This is called ***arthroplasty***.

*Other Fractures*

1. Fractures through the shaft of the femur are caused by severe injuries (like car accidents).
   a. Such injuries may also cause a simultaneous dislocation of the hip joint.
   b. The femoral artery or the sciatic nerve can be injured by the sharp edge of the fractured shaft.
2. A fracture through the femoral condyles may involve the knee joint. The popliteal artery or a nerve in the region may be injured.

## THE PATELLA

1. The tendons of some muscles have embedded in them, small bones that help them to glide over bony surfaces. Such bones are called ***sesamoid bones***.
2. The largest sesamoid bone in the body is to be seen in the tendon of the quadriceps femoris as it passes in front of the knee joint. This bone is called the patella.
3. The patella is shaped somewhat like a disc (9.20). It is roughly triangular in outline. It has anterior and posterior surfaces that are separated by three borders: superior, medial, and lateral.
4. The superior border is also called the ***base***. The inferior part of the bone shows a downward projection representing the ***apex*** of the triangle.
5. The ***anterior surface*** is rough and can be felt through the overlying skin.
6. The upper part of the ***posterior surface*** is articular.
   a. This part articulates with the patellar surface on the anterior aspect of the condyles of the femur.
   b. It consists of a larger lateral part and a smaller medial part, the two parts being separated by a ridge.
   c. The most medial part of the articular area may be recognisable as a separate area. This part articulates with the medial condyle of the femur only in extreme flexion of the knee joint.

6. The lower part of the posterior surface is nonarticular. It is rough for attachment of the ligamentum patellae.

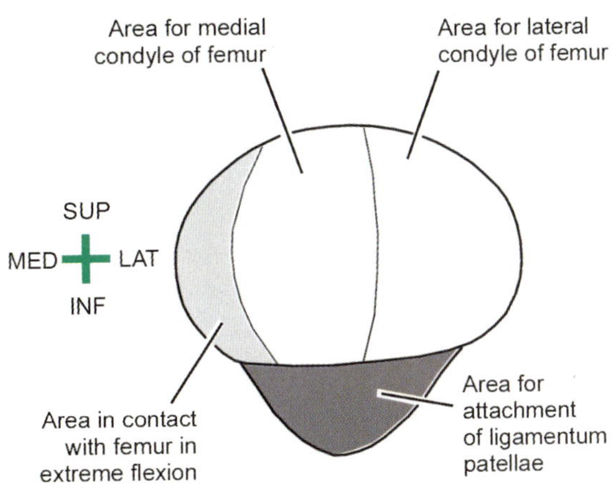


**9.20:** Right patella, posterior aspect

## WANT TO KNOW MORE?

### Some Attachments on the Patella

1. The superior border gives attachment to the ***rectus femoris*** and to the ***vastus intermedius***.
2. The apex gives attachment to the ***ligamentum patellae***.

### Ossification of the Patella

The patella ossifies from several centres that appear between the third and sixth years of life. The centres soon fuse with one another.

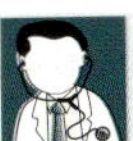

## CLINICAL CORRELATION

### Bipartite Patella

Sometimes the patella consists of two pieces, one main and one small piece in the upper lateral corner (***bipartite patella***). This is a congenital anomaly.

### Fractures of the Patella

1. The patella can be fractured by direct injury. This usually results in a comminuted fracture.
2. The patella can also be fractured by sudden violent contraction of the quadriceps femoris (as in a person trying to protect himself during a fall). In such cases, the fracture is usually clean cut.
3. Sudden contraction of the quadriceps can sometimes cause evulsion of the ligamentum patellae from the tibial tuberosity.
4. In a bad comminuted fracture, the entire patella may have to be removed. After this is done, the action of the quadriceps femoris become relatively weak as the angle of pull on the tibia is reduced.
5. A fractured patella needs to be distinguished carefully from a bipartite patella (see above). Pressure over a bipartite patella does not cause pain.

### Dislocation of the Patella

1. Injury may cause lateral dislocation of the patella.
2. The dislocation may become recurrent.

3. It should be noted that the patella has a natural tendency to be displaced laterally because of the direction of pull of the quadriceps (upwards and laterally).
4. This is prevented by the patellar retinacula and is counteracted, to some extent, by the fact that the vastus medialis tends to pull the patella medially.

## THE TIBIA

### Side Determination

1. The tibia is the medial bone of the leg. It has a shaft, an upper end and a lower end: (9.21 to 9.25).
2. The upper end can be distinguished from the lower end as it is much larger.
3. The medial and lateral sides of the bone can be distinguished by examining the lower end: This end has a prominent downward projection, the ***medial malleolus***, on its medial side.
4. The anterior and posterior aspects of the bone can be distinguished by examining the shaft. The shaft is triangular in section and has a sharp anterior border.

The side to which a tibia belongs can be determined from the information given above.

### The Upper End

1. The upper end of the tibia is expanded to form a mass that projects medially, laterally and posteriorly beyond the shaft.
   1a. When viewed from above, it is seen to consist of two parts called the ***medial and lateral condyles*** that are separated by an ***intercondylar area***.
2. The anterior aspect of the upper end of the tibia is marked by another projection called the ***tibial tuberosity***.
3. The upper surfaces of the medial and lateral condyles bear large, slightly concave, articular surfaces that take part in forming the knee joint.
   3a. The medial articular surface is oval, and is larger than the lateral surface which is rounded.
4. The articular surfaces are separated by the intercondylar area which is non-articular.
   a. The intercondylar area is raised in its central part to form the ***intercondylar eminence***.
   b. The medial and lateral parts of the eminence are more prominent than its central part and constitute the medial and lateral ***intercondylar tubercles***.
   c. The medial and lateral condylar articular surfaces extend on to the sides of the intercondylar tubercles.
5. In addition to its upper surface, the medial condyle has rough anterior, medial and posterior surfaces that are distinctly marked off from the shaft by a ridge (9.22). The posterior surface of the medial condyle is marked by a groove.
6. The lateral condyle has similar anterior, lateral and posterior surfaces.
   a. The posterolateral part of the lateral condyle bears an oval articular facet for the upper end of the fibula (9.22).
   b. The facet is directed backwards, downwards and laterally.
7. The anterior surfaces of the medial and lateral condyles merge to form a large rough triangular area.
   a. The apex of the triangle is placed inferiorly and is raised to form a large projection called the ***tibial tuberosity***.
   b. The tuberosity has an upper smooth part and a lower rough part (9.21).
   c. The lateral margin of the triangle mentioned above has a prominent impression (which is also triangular).

### The Shaft

1. If we cut a section across the shaft of the tibia we see that the shaft is triangular. It has anterior, medial and lateral (or interosseous) borders and medial, lateral and posterior surfaces.
2. The ***anterior border*** runs downwards from the tibial tuberosity. Its lower part turns medially and reaches the anterior margin of the medial malleolus.

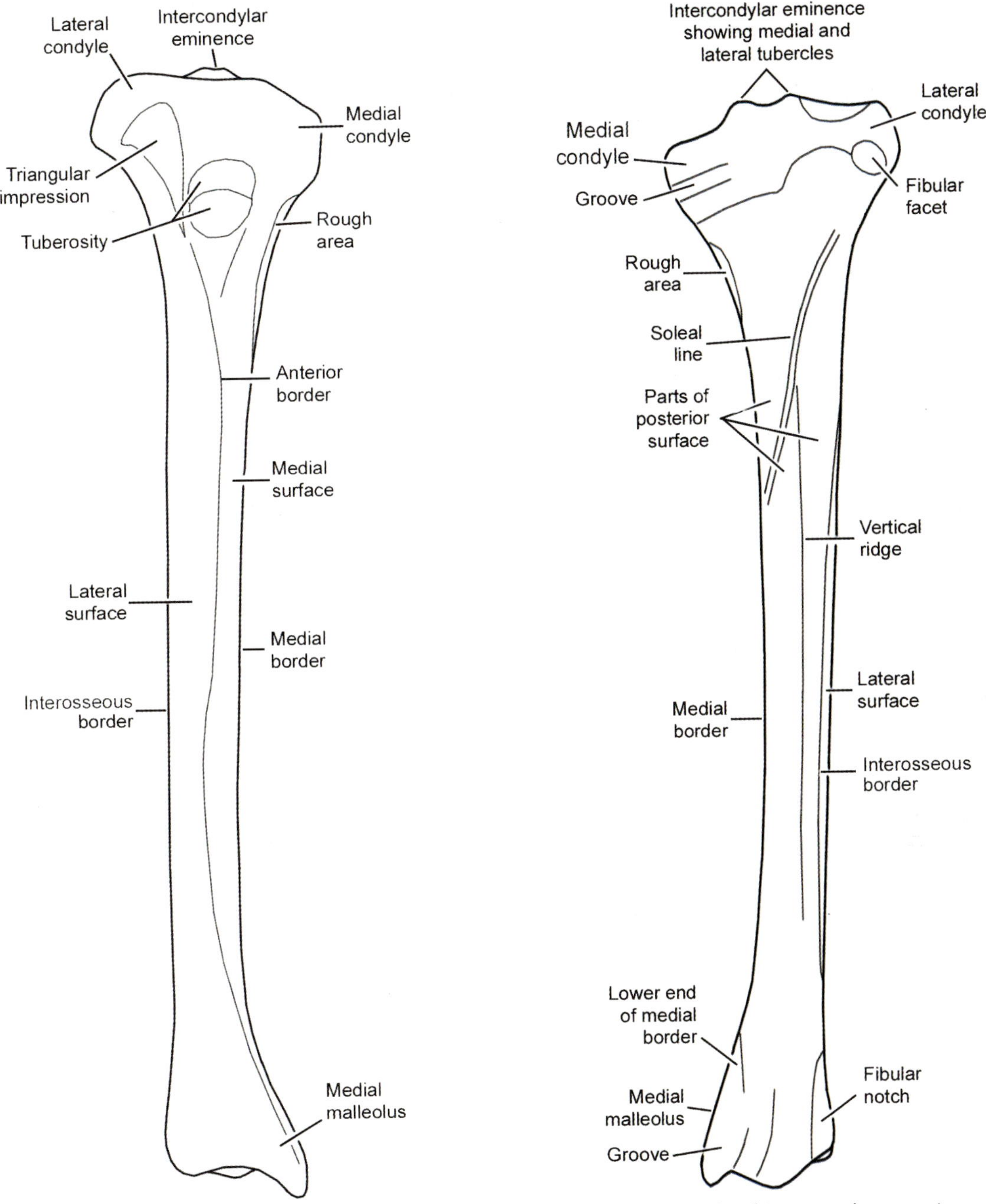


**9.21:** Right tibia, anterior aspect

**9.22:** Right tibia, posterior aspect

3. The ***interosseous*** or ***lateral border*** begins a little below and in front of the articular facet for the fibula.
   a. It descends along the lateral aspect of the shaft.
   b. Its lower end forms the anterior margin of a rough triangular area seen on the lateral aspect of the lower end.
4. The upper end of the ***medial border*** lies below the most medial part of the medial condyle. Its lower end becomes continuous with the posterior margin of the medial malleolus.
5. The ***medial surface*** lies between the anterior and medial borders. The upper end of the surface is rough just in front of the medial border. The rest of the surface is smooth and can be felt through the overlying skin.

6. The ***lateral surface*** lies between the anterior and interosseous borders. Because of the fact that the anterior border turns medially in its lower part, the lateral surface extends on to the anterior aspect of the lower part of the shaft.
7. The ***posterior surface*** (9.22) lies between the medial and interosseous borders.
   a Over the upper one-third of the shaft this surface is marked by a prominent ridge that runs downwards and medially across it.
   b This ridge is called the soleal line.
   c The part of the posterior surface above the soleal line is triangular.
   d The part below the soleal line is subdivided into medial and lateral parts by a faint vertical ridge.

## The Lower End

1. The lower end of the tibia is much less expanded than the upper end.
   a. Its medial part shows a downward projection called the ***medial malleolus***.
   b. The posterior aspect of the malleolus is marked by a prominent groove.
2. The lateral aspect of the lower end shows a triangular ***fibular notch*** for articulation with the fibula. It consists of an upper part that is rough and a lower part that is smooth.
3. The inferior surface of the lower end bears an articular area that articulates with the upper surface of the talus to form the ankle joint.
4. The area is continuous with another articular area on the lateral aspect of the medial malleolus that articulates with the medial side of the talus.

### WANT TO KNOW MORE?

**Attachments on the Tibia**

*The muscles inserted into the tibia are as follows (9.23 and 9.24):*

1. The pull of the ***quadriceps femoris*** is transmitted to the tibia through the ligamentum patellae that is attached to the smooth upper part of the tuberosity of the tibia. The attachment may extend to the rough lower part of the tuberosity also.
2. The ***sartorius***, the ***gracilis***, and the ***semitendinosus*** have linear vertical areas of insertion on the upper part of the medial surface.
   a. The area for the sartorius is most anterior.
   b. The area for semitendinosus is most posterior.
   c. The line for the gracilis is higher than that for the semitendinosus.
3. The ***semimembranosus*** is inserted into the posterior and medial aspects of the medial condyle.
4. The ***popliteus*** is inserted into the posterior surface of the shaft, on the triangular area above the soleal line.

*Muscles Taking Origin from the Tibia*

1. The ***tibialis anterior*** arises from the upper two-thirds of the lateral surface of the shaft.
2. The ***soleus*** arises from the soleal line, and from the middle one-third of the medial border of the shaft.
3. The ***tibialis posterior*** arises from the upper two-thirds of the lateral part of the posterior surface of the shaft, below the soleal line.
4. The ***flexor digitorum longus*** arises from the medial part of the posterior surface of the shaft below the soleal line.

*Some Other Attachments on the Tibia*

1. The ***capsular ligament of the knee joint*** is attached to the condyles of the tibia a little below the margins of the articular sufaces. In the region of the tuberosity, the attachment of the capsule is replaced by that of the ligamentum patellae.

2. The intercondylar area, on the superior aspect of the upper end of the tibia, has the following attachments (in anteroposterior sequence)(See 9.25).
   a. Anterior end of medial meniscus.
   b. Anterior cruciate ligament.
   c. Anterior end of lateral meniscus.
   d. Posterior end of lateral meniscus.
   e. Posterior end of medial meniscus.
   f. Posterior cruciate ligament.

***Some Relations of the Tibia***

1. The anterior aspect of the lower end of the tibia (which is continuous with the lateral surface of the shaft) is crossed by the tendons of the following muscles (from medial to lateral side).
   a. Tibialis anterior
   b. Extensor hallucis longus
   c. Extensor digitorum longus.
   d. Peroneus tertius.
2. The anterior tibial vessels and the deep peroneal nerve cross the anterior aspect of the lower end of the bone lying between the tendons of the extensor hallucis longus and the extensor digitorum longus.
3. The posterior aspect of the lower end of the tibia is crossed by tendons of the following muscles (from medial to lateral side).
   a. Tibialis posterior
   b. Flexor digitorum longus
   c. Flexor hallucis longus

3a. The tendon of the flexor digitorum longus crosses that of the tibialis posterior near the lower end of the bone.

4. The posterior tibial vessels and nerve cross the posterior aspect of the lower end of the bone lying between the tendons of the flexor digitorum longus and the flexor hallucis longus.

**Ossification of the Tibia**

The tibia has three centres of ossification.

1. The primary centre (for the shaft) appears in the 7th week of fetal life.
2. A secondary centre for the upper end appears towards the end of fetal life. It fuses with the shaft between the 16th and 18th years.
3. A secondary centre for the lower end appears during the first year, and fuses with the shaft between the 15th and 17th years.
4. A separate centre may exist for the tibial tuberosity.

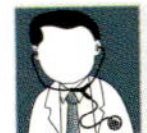

**CLINICAL CORRELATION**

1. Rarely the tibia may be absent.
2. The upper articular surfaces of the tibia may be poorly formed resulting in congenital dislocation of the knee.
3. Fractures of the tibia and fibula: See under fibula.

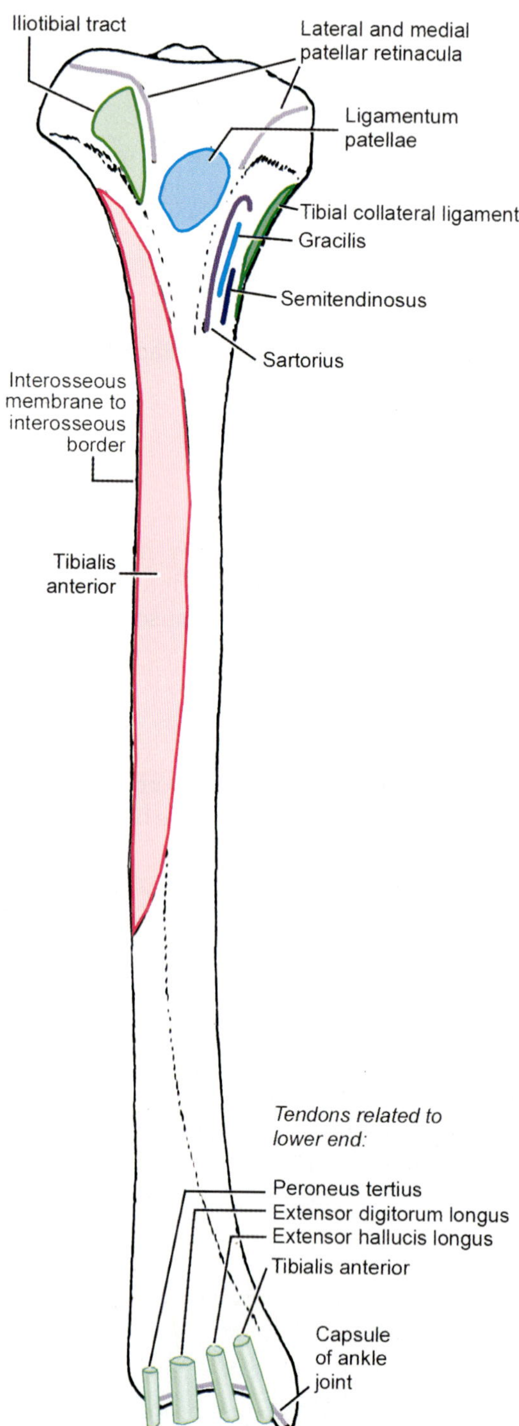


**9.23:** Right tibia, showing attachments, seen from the front

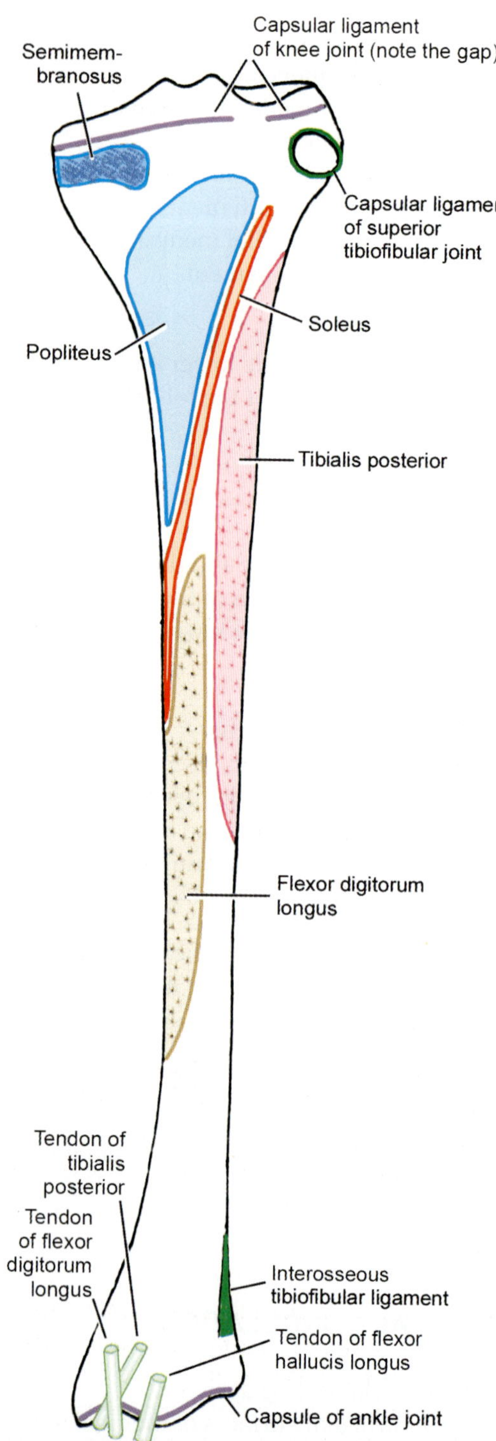


**9.24:** Right tibia, showing attachments, seen from behind

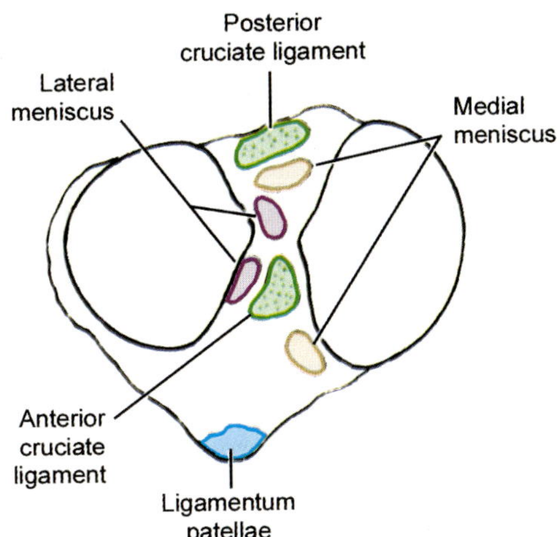


**9.25:** Right tibia, showing attachments, seen from above.

## THE FIBULA

### Side Determination

1. The fibula has a ***shaft***, an ***upper end*** and a ***lower end*** (9.26 to 9.29).
2. The upper end is irregularly expanded in all directions. In contrast, the lower end is flattened from side-to-side and forms the ***lateral malleolus***.
   a. The medial side of the malleolus bears a triangular articular surface (for the talus) (9.26).
3. Just behind this articular surface the malleolus shows a deep ***malleolar fossa*** and this fact enables the anterior and posterior aspects of the bone to be distinguished from one another.

The side to which a fibula belongs can be determined with the help of the information given above.

### The Upper End

1. The upper end of the fibula is also called the ***head***.
   a. Its posterior and lateral part shows an upward projection called the ***styloid process***.
2. In front of, and medial to, the styloid process the head shows a circular facet for articulation with the tibia (to form the superior tibiofibular joint). The facet is directed upwards and medially.
3. The part of the bone immediately below the head is called the ***neck***.

### The Lower End

1. The lower end of the fibula is called the ***lateral malleolus***. It has a convex lateral surface that can be felt through the overlying skin. This surface is continuous above with a triangular area on the shaft.
2. The medial surface of the malleolus bears a triangular facet, the apex of the triangle being directed downwards. This facet articulates with the lateral surface of the talus and forms part of the ankle joint.
3. Just above the facet, the lower part of the shaft shows a rough area. Behind the facet, the medial surface of the malleolus shows a deep ***malleolar fossa***.
4. The lower end also has a posterior surface which has a shallow groove on it.
5. It may be noted that the lateral malleolus projects to a lower level than the medial malleolus (of the tibia)

## The Shaft

The surfaces and borders of the shaft show considerable variation from bone to bone and may be difficult to identify. To trace them, it is important to first orientate the bone correctly by examining the lower end as described above.

1. The shaft has three borders: anterior, posterior and interosseous (or medial).
2. The ***anterior border*** is sharp (9.26).
   a. It begins just below the anterior aspect of the head.
   b. Near to its lower end, it turns laterally to join the apex of the triangular area of the shaft already identified above the lateral malleolus.
   c. The lowest part of the anterior border forms the posterior margin of the triangle.
3. The upper end of the ***posterior border*** lies in line with the styloid process (9.27). Its lower end reaches the medial part of the posterior surface of the lateral malleolus.
4. The ***interosseous border*** lies very near to the anterior border (9.26) and may be indistinguishable from the latter in the upper part of the shaft. When traced downwards it passes medially and merges with the upper part of the rough area above the talar facet of the lateral malleolus.
5. The ***lateral surface*** of the fibula lies between the anterior and posterior borders.
   5a. Because of the lateral inclination of the lower part of the anterior border, the lower part of the lateral surface faces backwards and becomes continuous with the posterior aspect of the lateral malleolus.
6. The ***medial surface*** lies between the anterior and interosseous borders.
   a. It is very narrow in the upper half of the shaft.
   b. Its lower broader part faces as much forwards as medially.
   c. This surface is, therefore, sometimes called the anterior surface.
7. The ***posterior surface*** lies between the interosseous and posterior borders.
   a. It occupies a very large area of the surface of the shaft.
   b. Over its upper three-fourths, it is divided into two distinct parts, medial and lateral, by a vertical ridge called the ***medial crest***. This ridge is more prominent than the interosseous or posterior borders.
8. The medial part of the posterior surface is deeply concave and faces forwards and medially.
   a. The lateral part of the posterior surface faces posteriorly in its upper part and medially in its lower part.
   b. The lowest part of the posterior surface lies just above the talar facet of the lateral malleolus.
   c. This part is roughened for attachment of a strong ligament that connects the fibula to the tibia.

### WANT TO KNOW MORE?

**Attachments on the Fibula**

The muscles attached to the fibula are as follows (9.28 to 9.29):

1. The ***biceps femoris*** is inserted into the head of the fibula. The attachment is through two separate slips that are separated by the fibular collateral ligament of the knee joint.
2. The narrow medial surface gives origin to the following.
   a. The ***extensor digitorum longus*** arises from the upper three-fourths of this surface.
   b. The ***peroneus tertius*** arises from an area on the medial surface below that for the extensor digitorum longus.
   c. The ***extensor hallucis longus*** arises from the middle two-fourths of the medial surface, medial to the origin of the extensor digitorum longus.
3. The lateral surface gives origin to the following.
   a. The ***peroneus longus*** arises from the upper two-thirds of the lateral surface. Part of the muscle also arises from the lateral aspect of the head of the fibula. The common peroneal nerve lies between the two areas of origin.
   b. The ***peroneus brevis*** arises from the lower two-thirds of the lateral surface.

4. The following muscles are attached to the posterior surface.
   a. The ***tibialis posterior*** arises from the upper two-third of the medial part of the posterior surface.
   b. The ***soleus*** arises from the posterior aspect of the head and from the upper one-fourth of the lateral part of the posterior surface.
   c. The ***flexor hallucis longus*** arises from the lower two-thirds of the lateral part of the posterior surface.

**Some Relations of the Fibula**

1. The common peroneal nerve winds round the lateral aspect of the neck of the fibula (9.29).
2. The tendons of the peroneus longus and the peroneus brevis pass downwards just behind the lateral malleolus.

**Ossification of the Fibula**

The fibula has three centres of ossification.

1. The primary centre, for the shaft, appears in the 8th fetal week.
2. A secondary centre for the upper end appears in the 3rd or 4th year and fuses with the shaft between the 17th and 19th years.
3. A secondary centre for the lower end appears in the first year; and fuses with the shaft between the 15th and 17th years.
4. Note that in most long bones, the secondary centre that appears first is the last to fuse. The fibula is an exception in that the centre that appears first (for the lower end) is also the first to fuse. Compare with the tibia.

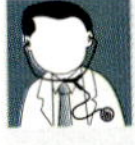

## CLINICAL CORRELATION

1. Rarely the fibula may be missing.
2. Part of the fibula may be taken by a surgeon for use as a graft at some other site.

**Fractures of the Tibia and Fibula**

1. Fractures of the bones of the leg are commonly seen in motorcycle accidents.
   a. The tibia may be fractured through a condyle (usually lateral), through the shaft, or through the medial malleolus.
   b. Fracture of the shaft of the tibia is usually accompanied by a corresponding fracture of the fibula.
   c. The fibula may also be fractured through the lateral malleolus.
2. Injuries to the tibia and fibula in the region of the ankle are referred to as ***Pott's fracture*** which can be of several types.
   a. Forceful abduction or lateral rotation of the foot can lead to a fracture of the lateral malleolus.
   b. Once this malleolus is broken, the injuring force acts on the medial ligament of the ankle joint leading to its rupture, or to its evulsion along with the tip of the medial malleolus (***evulsion fracture*** of the medial malleolus).
3. More severe injury can lead to disorganisation of the ankle joint as a result of rupture of the interosseus tibiofibular ligament, or as a result of fractures through both malleoli. In such injury, the fibula is sometimes fractured through the lower part of its shaft.
4. Forcible adduction and medial rotation of the foot can lead to fracture of the medial malleolus; and rupture of the lateral ligament or evulsion fracture of the lateral malleolus.
5. Blood supply to the tibia is poor at the junction of the upper two-thirds and lower one-third of the shaft. Fractures here may therefore show delayed union or non-union.

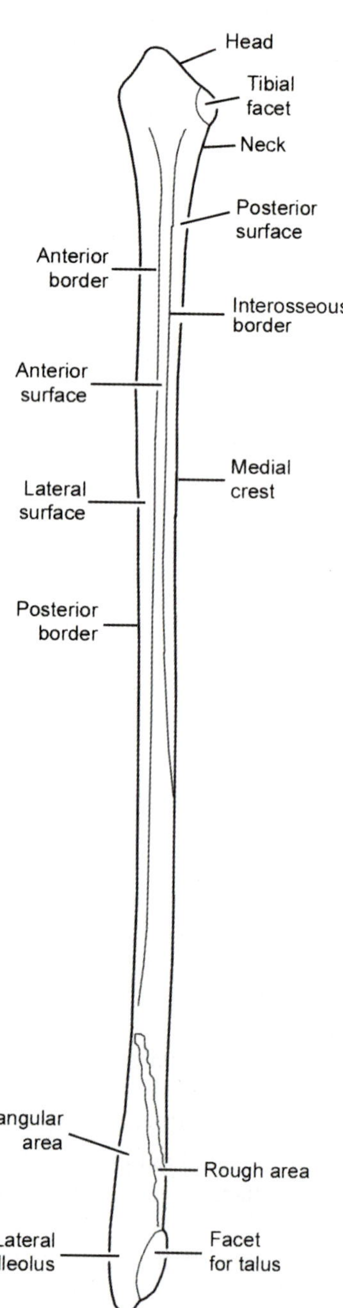


**9.26:** Right fibula seen from the front

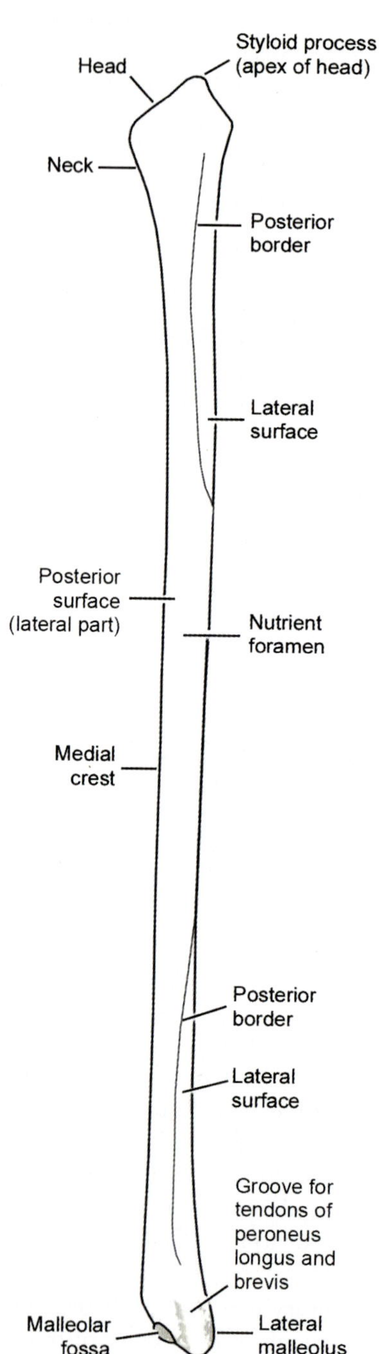


**9.27:** Right fibula seen from behind

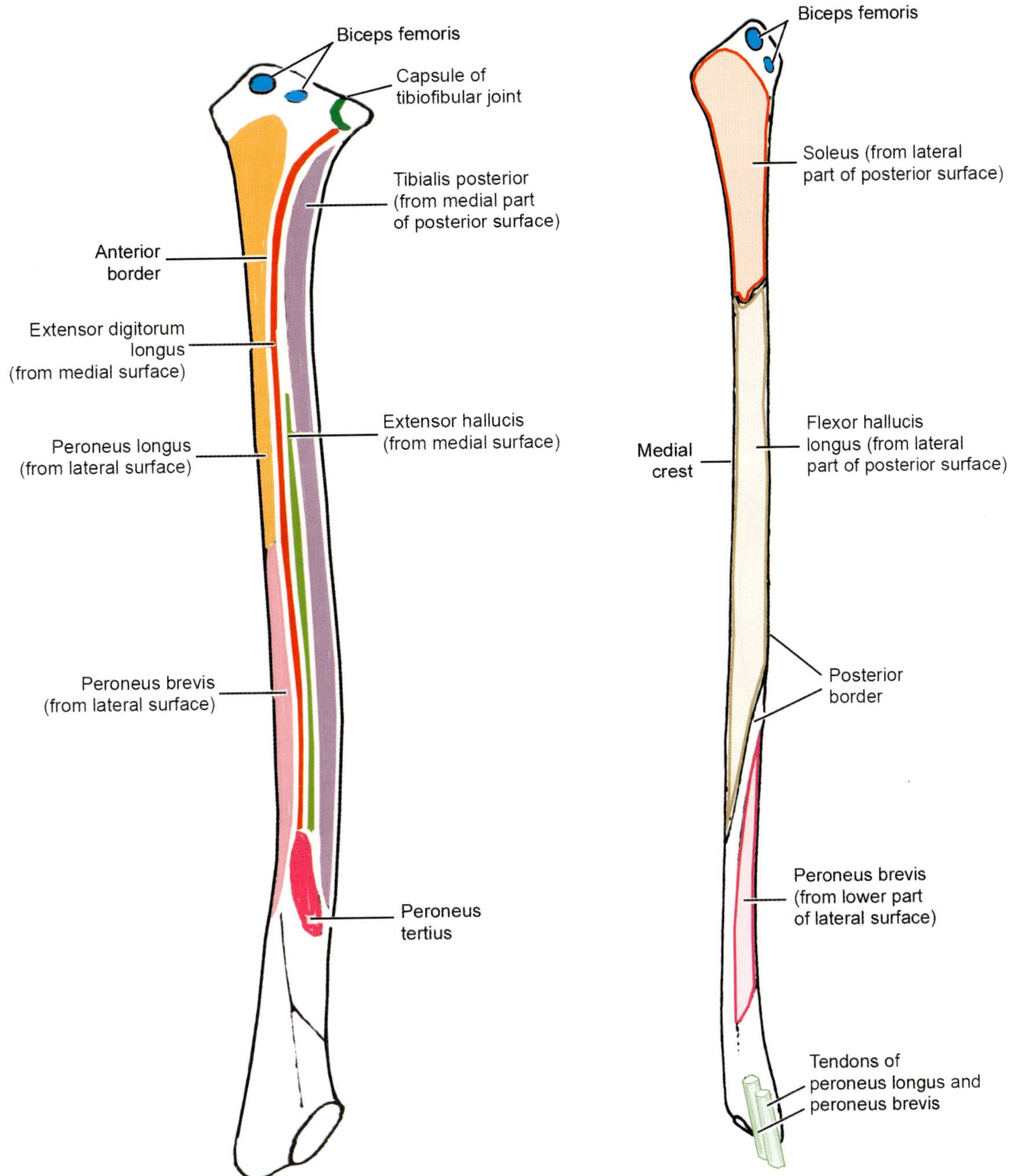


**9.28:** Right fibula, showing attachments, seen from the front

**9.29:** Right fibula, showing attachments, seen from behind

## THE SKELETON OF THE FOOT

The skeleton of the foot is seen from above (dorsal aspect) in 9.30, and from below (plantar aspect) in 9.31.

1. The posterior half (or so) of the foot is made up of seven ***tarsal bones***.
   a. The largest tarsal bone is called the ***calcaneus***: It is the bone that forms the heel.
   b. Placed above the calcaneus there is another large bone called the ***talus***. The talus articulates with the lower ends of the tibia and fibula to form the ***ankle joint***.

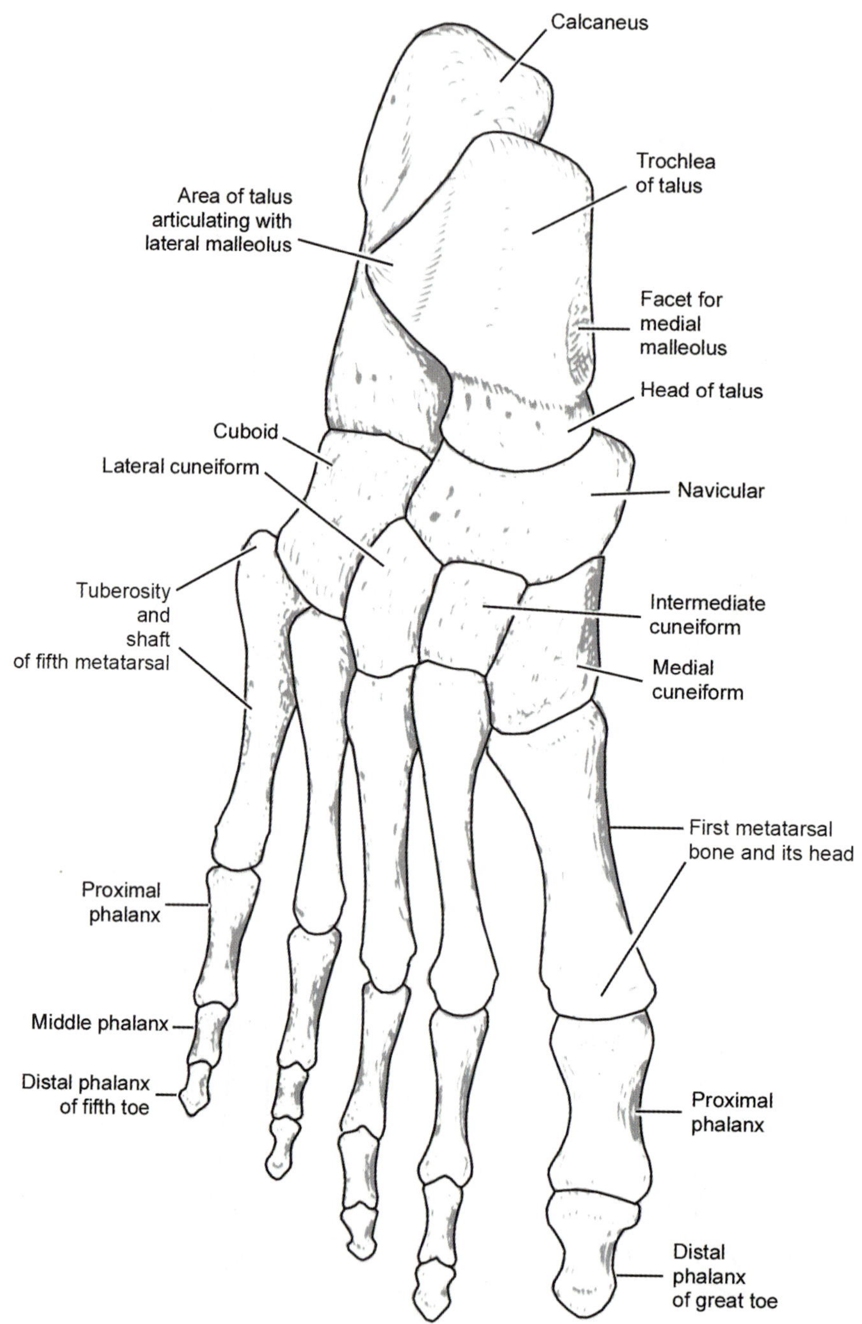


**9.30:** Skeleton of the foot seen from above (dorsal aspect)

2. Anterior (or distal) to the calcaneus and the talus, there are two bones of intermediate size.
   2a. These are the ***navicular bone*** placed medially, and the ***cuboid bone*** placed laterally.
3. Distal to the navicular bone there are three smaller bones.
   3a. These are the ***medial cuneiform***, the ***intermediate cuneiform***, and the ***lateral cuneiform*** bones.
4. Anterior to the tarsal bones we see five ***metatarsal bones***.
5. Distal to the metatarsal bones there are the ***phalanges***: three (proximal, middle, distal) for each digit except the great toe which has only two phalanges, proximal and distal.

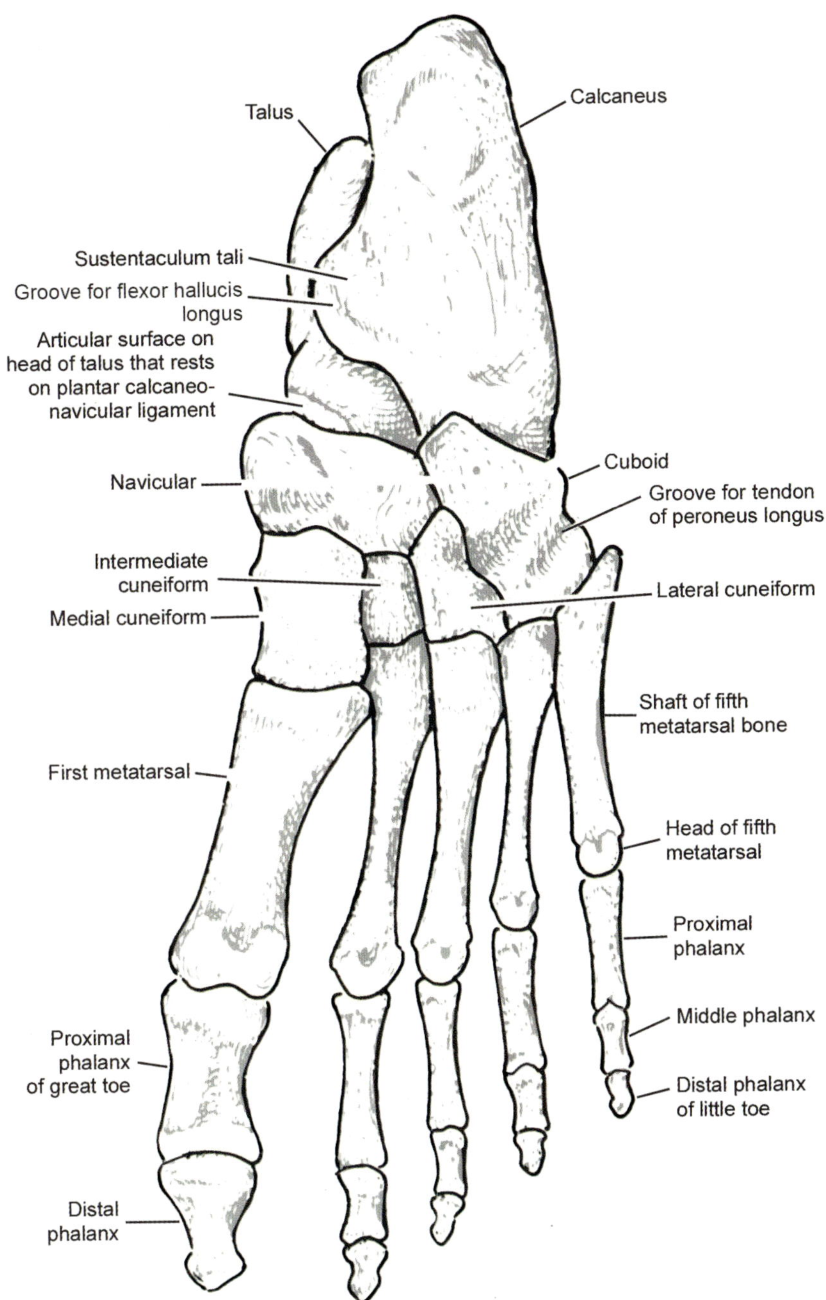


**9.31:** Skeleton of the foot seen from below (plantar aspect)

## The Calcaneus

### *Side Determination*

The calcaneus can be correctly orientated, and its side can be determined using the following information (9.30 to 9.33)

1. The bone is elongated anteroposteriorly. The anterior aspect is easily distinguished from the posterior as it is covered by a large articular facet, while the posterior aspect is non-articular.

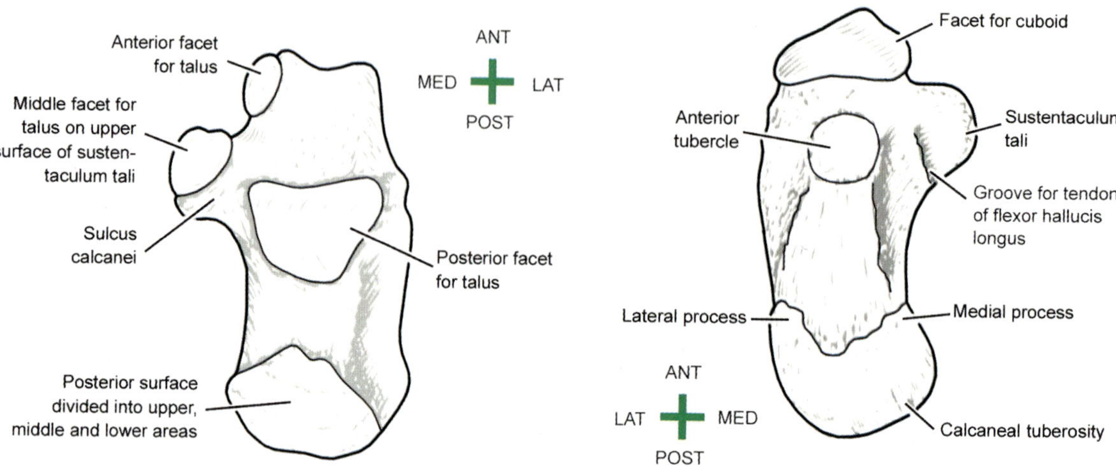


**9.32:** Right calcaneus seen from above

**9.33:** Right calcaneus seen from below

2. The superior aspect can be distinguished from the inferior as it bears three facets, while the inferior aspect is non-articular.
3. The medial aspect can be distinguished from the lateral aspect as it bears a prominent projection.

Having orientated the bone correctly, the following facts can now be appreciated.

1. The calcaneus has anterior, posterior, superior, inferior, medial and lateral surfaces. The ***anterior surface*** is fully covered by a large articular facet for the cuboid bone.
2. The ***posterior surface*** is non-articular. It is divisible into upper, middle and inferior parts.
3. The ***lateral surface*** is more or less flat. Its anterior part shows a small elevation called the ***peroneal trochlea*** (or ***tubercle***). The anterosuperior and the posteroinferior aspects of the tubercle are grooved.
4. The ***medial surface*** is easily distinguished, as it bears a large projection called the ***sustentaculum tali*** that projects medially from its anterior and upper part.
   a. The inferior aspect of the sustentaculum tali is marked by a groove.
5. The ***superior or dorsal surface*** bears three facets: anterior, middle and posterior that articulate with corresponding facets on the talus.
   a. The middle facet lies on the upper surface of the sustentaculum tali. It is separated from the posterior facet by a deep groove called the ***sulcus calcanei***.
   b. In the articulated foot, the sulcus calcanei comes into apposition with a similar groove on the talus (called the sulcus tali), to form the ***sinus tarsi***.
6. The ***plantar (or inferior) surface*** of the calcaneus shows a prominence in its posterior part called the ***calcaneal tuberosity***.
   a. The lateral and medial parts of the tuberosity extend further forwards than its central part and are called the ***lateral and medial processes*** respectively, of the tuberosity.
   b. The anterior part of the plantar surface shows another elevation called the ***anterior tubercle***.

## The Talus

### *Side Determination*

The talus can be orientated correctly, and its side determined using the following information (9.30, 9.31, 9.34 and 9.35).

1. The bone is elongated anteroposteriorly. The anterior end (or head) can be distinguished from the posterior end as it is rounded and has a large convex articular surface.
2. The superior aspect of the bone bears a large pulley shaped surface that is convex upwards. The inferior aspect bears three facets.

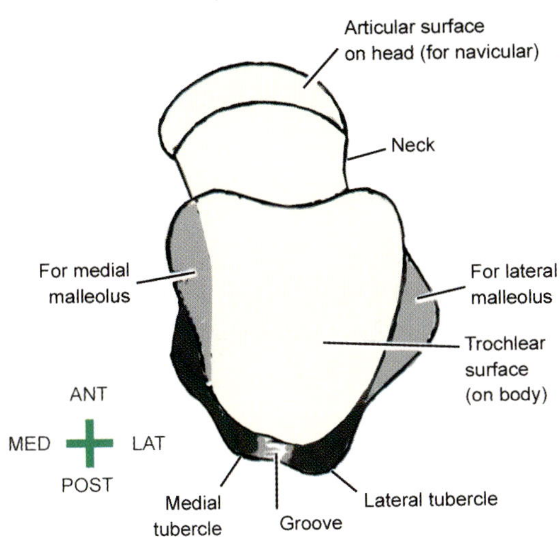


**9.34:** Right talus, seen from above

**9.35:** Right talus seen from below

3. The lateral surface bears a large triangular facet, while the medial side shows a 'comma' shaped facet. The talus is seen from above in 9.34. In this figure, we see that the bone has a ***head***, a neck and a ***body.***
4. The distal surface of the head has a large convex surface that articulates with the navicular bone.
5. The upper surface of the body is covered by a large ***trochlear articular surface*** which articulates with the lower end of the tibia. This surface is convex from front to back, and concave from side to side.
6. The ***lateral surface*** bears a large triangular facet for articulation with the lateral malleolus of the fibula, while the ***medial surface*** bears a 'comma' shaped facet that is broad anteriorly and tapers off posteriorly. This facet articulates with the medial malleolus of the tibia.
7. The lower and posterior part of the body of the talus projects backwards. This projection is called the ***posterior process***. A groove divides this process into ***medial and lateral tubercles.***
8. When the talus is viewed from below (9.35), we see the following:
   a. The articular area on the head, for the navicular bone, extends on to the inferior aspect of the head.
   b. Behind this there are three facets, anterior, middle and posterior, that articulate with corresponding facets on the upper surface of the calcaneus.
   c. The middle and posterior facets are separated by a deep groove called the sulcus tali. We have already seen that, along with the sulcus calcanei, the sulcus tali forms the sinus tarsi.
   d. Medial to the anterior calcaneal facet the lower aspect of the head of the talus has an area that rests on the plantar calcaneonavicular ligament.

## The Navicular Bone

1. The navicular bone articulates proximally with the head of the talus, distally with the three cuneiform bones, and laterally with the cuboid (9.30).
2. The medial part of the bone has a projection called the ***tuberosity***.

### WANT TO KNOW MORE?

3. The side to which a navicular bone belongs can be determined as follows.
   a. The proximal surface is covered by a single large concave articular facet for the head of the talus. The distal surface has an articular surface that is subdivided by ridges into three triangular areas for the three cuneiform bones.

b. The dorsal surface is convex, while the plantar surface is concave. Both surfaces are rough.
c. The medial and lateral aspects of the bone can be distinguished by the fact that the tuberosity is directed downwards and medially, and by the fact that the lateral surface usually has a facet for the cuboid bone.

### The Cuboid Bone

1. The cuboid bone articulates proximally with the calcaneus; distally with the fourth and fifth metatarsal bones, and medially with the navicular and lateral cuneiform bones (9.30 and 9.31).
2. The lateral and plantar aspects of the bone show a groove that is limited posteriorly by a ridge. The lateral end of this ridge forms a projection called the ***tuberosity***.

**WANT TO KNOW MORE?**

3. The side to which a given cuboid bone belongs can be determined by the following:
   a. The proximal end bears a large concavoconvex facet for the calcaneus, while the distal end bears an articular surface that is divided into two parts for the 4th and 5th metatarsal bones.
   b. The plantar or inferior surface can be distinguished from the dorsal surface as it bears a deep groove that is limited posteriorly by a ridge.
   c. The lateral aspect of the bone can be identified by the fact that the groove on the plantar surface extends onto the lateral surface also.
   d. Further, the lateral end of the ridge is enlarged to form the tuberosity.
   e. The medial surface bears a facet for the lateral cuneiform bone, and occasionally one for the navicular bone.

### The Medial Cuneiform Bone

1. The medial cuneiform bone is the largest of the cuneiform bones (9.30 and 9.31).
2. It can be distinguished by the fact that it bears a large kidney-shaped facet on one side.
3. It articulates proximally with the navicular bone, distally with the first metatarsal bone, and laterally with the intermediate cuneiform and second metatarsal bones.

**WANT TO KNOW MORE?**

4. The side to which a given medial cuneiform bone belongs can be determined as follows:
   a. The dorsal surface is narrower than the plantar surface. Both are non-articular.
   b. The proximal end bears a piriform facet (for the navicular bone), while the distal surface bears a kidney shaped facet (for the first metatarsal).
   c. The medial surface is non-articular, while the lateral surface bears articular areas for the intermediate cuneiform and second metatarsal bones.

### The Intermediate Cuneiform Bone

1. The intermediate cuneiform bone is the smallest of the cuneiform bones.
2. It is shaped like a typical wedge (9.30 and 9.31).
3. It articulates proximally with the navicular bone, distally with the second metatarsal bone, medially with the medial cuneiform bone, and laterally with the lateral cuneiform bone.

**WANT TO KNOW MORE?**

4. The side to which an intermediate cuneiform bone belongs can be determined as follows:
   a. The dorsal surface is wide, while the plantar surface is narrow.
   b. The medial surface bears an L-shaped facet (for the medial cuneiform), while the lateral side bears a vertical facet (for the lateral cuneiform).
   c. The proximal and distal aspects are both fully covered by triangular facets.
   d. The proximal aspect can be distinguished from the distal by looking at the lateral surface. The vertical facet for the lateral cuneiform is placed along the proximal margin of this surface. The distal part of the lateral surface is non-articular.

## The Lateral Cuneiform Bone

1. The lateral cuneiform bone articulates proximally with the navicular bone, distally with the third metatarsal bone, medially with the intermediate cuneiform and second metatarsal bones; and laterally with the cuboid and fourth metatarsal bones (9.30 and 9.31).

**WANT TO KNOW MORE?**

2. The side to which a particular lateral cuneiform bone belongs can be determined as follows:
   a. The dorsal surface is wider than the plantar surface.
   b. The proximal and distal surfaces can be distinguished by the fact that the entire distal surface is covered by a triangular facet (for the 3rd metatarsal); but the proximal surface is covered by a smaller facet (for the navicular) which is confined to the dorsal two-thirds of the surface.
   c. Both the medial and lateral surfaces bear facets, but these are larger and more prominent on the medial aspect.

## The Metatarsal Bones

The metatarsal bones are five in number (9.30, 9.31, 9.36 to 9.38).

1. They are numbered from medial to lateral side (in contrast to the metacarpal bones which are numbered from lateral to medial side).
2. The metatarsal bones are similar in structure to the metacarpal bones. Each bone has a distal end or head; a proximal end or base and an intervening shaft.
3. The head is rounded. The base is enlarged and has proximal, dorsal, plantar, medial and lateral surfaces.
4. The shaft is slightly convex on its dorsal side and concave on the plantar side.

**WANT TO KNOW MORE?**

**Articulations of the Metatarsal Bones**

The head of each metatarsal bone articulates with the proximal phalanx of the digit concerned. The articulations of the bases of the metatarsal bones are as follows (9.37):

1. The first metatarsal bone has a large kidney shaped facet on the proximal surface of its base. This facet articulates with the medial cuneiform bone.
2. The base of the second metatarsal bone articulates:
   a. Proximally with the intermediate cuneiform bone.
   b. Medially with the medial cuneiform bone.
   c. Laterally with the lateral cuneiform bone and with the base of the third metatarsal bone.

3. The base of the third metatarsal bone articulates:
   a. Proximally with the lateral cuneiform bone.
   b. Medially with the second metatarsal bone.
   c. Laterally with the fourth metatarsal bone.
4. The base of the fourth metatarsal bone articulates:
   a. Proximally with the cuboid bone
   b. Medially with the lateral cuneiform bone and with the base of the third metatarsal
   c. Laterally with the base of the fifth metatarsal bone.
5. The fifth metatarsal bone articulates proximally with the cuboid bone and medially with the fourth metatarsal bone.

### The Phalanges of the Foot

1. The phalanges of the foot are arranged on a pattern similar to that in the hand (9.30 and 9.31).
2. There are three phalanges in each toe except the great toe: proximal, middle and distal.
3. The great toe has only two phalanges, proximal and distal.
4. The phalanges of the foot are similar in shape to those of the hand, but are much shorter and thinner than the latter.

#### WANT TO KNOW MORE?

**Attachments on the Skeleton of the Foot**

Some attachments on the bones of the foot are shown in 9.39 and 9.40.

**Ossification of the Bones of the Foot**

1. The calcaneus has one main centre of ossification that appears in the third fetal month; and a secondary centre (for a scale like epiphysis that covers its posterior part) that appears in the 6th to 8th year.
2. All other tarsal bones normally have one centre each that appears as follows:

| | |
|---|---|
| Talus | 6th fetal month |
| Cuboid | Just before or after birth |
| Medial cuneiform | 3rd year |
| Intermediate cuneiform | 1st year |
| Lateral cuneiform | 1st year |
| Navicular | 3rd year |

3. Each metatarsal bone has a primary centre for the shaft appearing in the 9th or 10th fetal week.
   a. The first metatarsal has a secondary centre for its base appearing in the 3rd year.
   b. The other metatarsals have secondary centres for their heads (not bases) appearing in the 3rd or 4th year (Compare with metacarpal bones).
   c. The secondary centres unite with the shafts between the 17th and 20th years.
4. Each phalanx has a primary centre for the shaft (appearing in the 7th to 15th fetal weeks); and a secondary centre for the base (appearing between the 2nd to 8th years) which unites with the shaft by the 18th year.

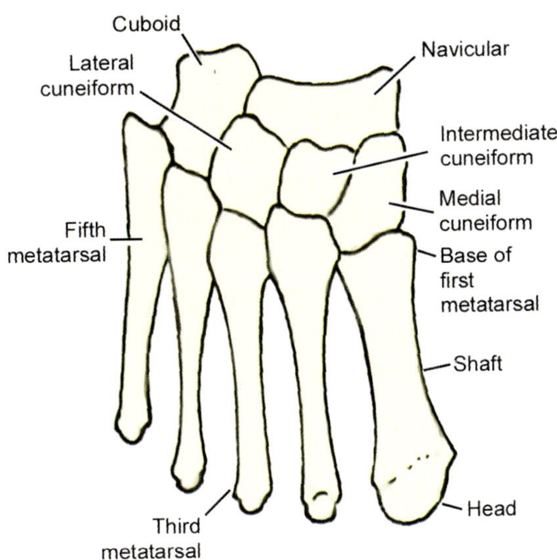


**9.36:** Scheme to show the articulations of the metatarsal bones

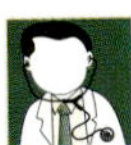

## CLINICAL CORRELATION

### Congenital Deformities

Congenital deformities are frequently seen in the region of the ankle and foot, and are of various types. The general term ***talipes*** is applied to them.

1. In the most common variety of deformity, the foot shows marked plantar flexion (= ***equinus***: like the foot of a horse), and inversion (= varus: inward bend).
   a. Hence this condition is called ***talipes equinovarus***.
   b. In layman's parlance, it is called ***club foot***.
   c. The condition may be unilateral or bilateral.
2. The medial longitudinal arch of the foot may be poorly developed (***pes planus*** or ***flat foot***). A flat footed person may have difficulty in walking long distances, or in running.
3. Conversely, the foot may be too highly arched (***pes cavus***). This condition is often associated with neurological disorders.

### Fractures of the Bones of the Foot

1. These are not common.
   a. Occasionally the calcaneus and, less commonly, the talus may be fractured.
   b. In a fracture of the neck of the talus, there may be avascular necrosis of the head.
   c. Calcaneal fractures are often caused when a person falls on the heel. The bone may break up into small pieces (comminuted fracture).
2. Metatarsal bones and phalanges of the foot can be fractured by dropping of a heavy object on the foot.
3. The fifth metatarsal bone can be fractured through its base as a result of a twisting injury of the foot.
4. Metacarpal bones can also be fractured by the stress of prolonged walking or running (***fatigue fracture, stress fracture, or March fracture***).
5. Metacarpal bones sometimes fracture when a dancer loses balance and the weight of the body falls on these bones.

| FACETS SEEN ON BASES OF METATARSAL BONES (RIGHT) | | |
|---|---|---|
| | MEDIAL SIDE | LATERAL SIDE |
| ORIENTATION | DIST<br>VENT + DORS<br>PROX | DIST<br>DORS + VENT<br>PROX |
| FIRST METATARSAL | None | None |
| SECOND METATARSAL | Rough area in contact with first metatarsal<br>For medial cuneiform<br>For intermediate cuneiform | For 3rd metatarsal<br>For lateral cuneiform |
| THIRD METATARSAL | For 2nd metatarsal<br>For lateral cuneiform | For 4th metatarsal |
| FOURTH METATARSAL | For 3rd metatarsal<br>For lateral cuneiform<br>For cuboid | For 5th metatarsal |
| FIFTH METATARSAL | For 4th metatarsal<br>For cuboid<br>Tuberosity | Tuberosity |

**9.37:** Facets seen on bases of metatarsal bone

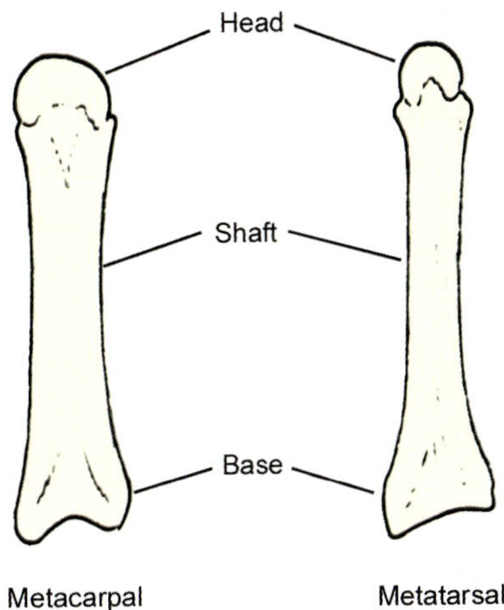


**9.38:** Comparison between metacarpal and metatarsal bone

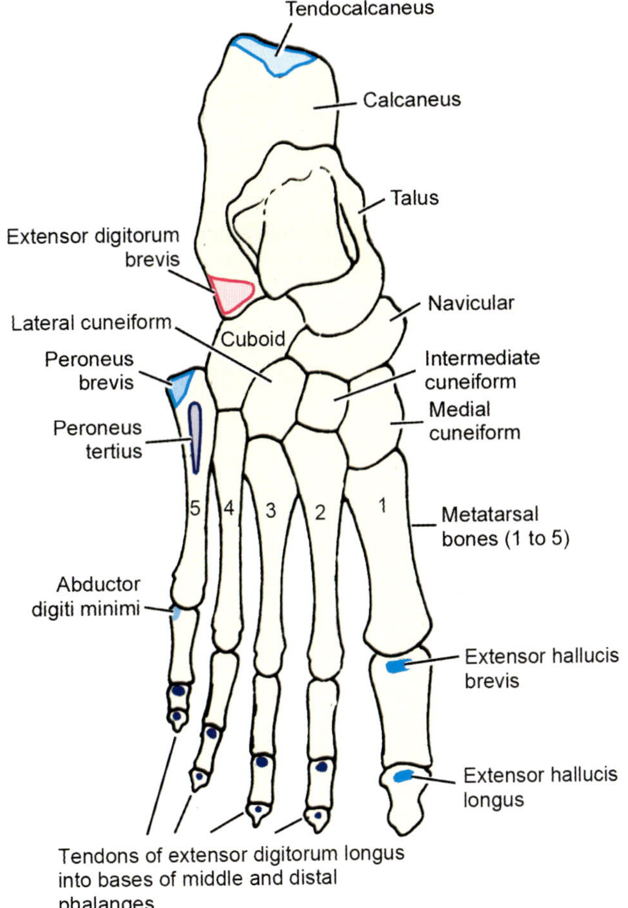


**9.39:** Skeleton of the right foot, showing attachments, seen from the dorsal aspect

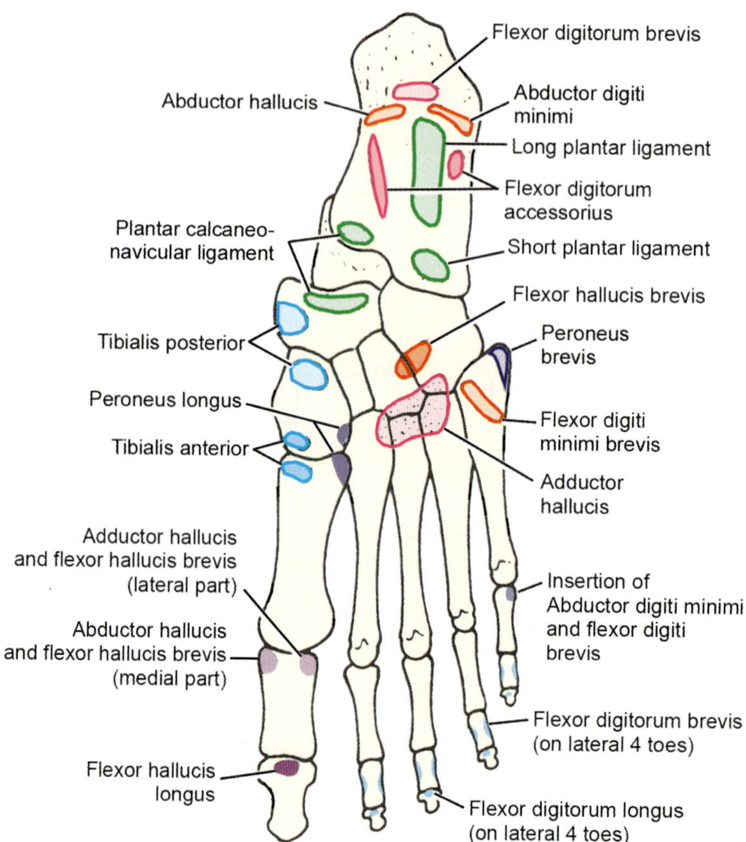


**9.40:**Skeleton of right foot, showing attachments, seen from the ventral aspect

CHAPTER 10

# Cutaneous Nerves, Veins and Lymphatic Drainage: Front and Medial Side of Thigh

## CUTANEOUS INNERVATION OF THE LOWER LIMB

### Front of Thigh

1. The areas supplied by cutaneous nerves to be seen on the front of thigh are shown in 10.1. Four longitudinal strips of skin are supplied (from lateral to medial side) by:
   a. The lateral cutaneous nerve of the thigh.
   b. The intermediate cutaneous nerve of the thigh.
   c. The medial cutaneous nerve of the thigh.
   d. Cutaneous branches of the obturator nerve.
2. Three areas just below the inguinal ligament are supplied (from lateral to medial side) by:
   a. The subcostal and iliohypogastric nerves.
   b. The femoral branch of the genitofemoral nerve.
   c. The ilioinguinal nerve.
3. In the region of the knee, small areas are innervated by the ***lateral cutaneous nerve of the calf***, laterally, and by the ***saphenous nerve***, medially.
4. In front of the knee, a number of cutaneous nerves join to form the ***patellar plexus***.



**10.1:** Cutaneous nerves supplying the front of the thigh

### Front of Leg and Dorsum of Foot

1. The cutaneous nerve supply of the front of the leg is shown in 10.2.
2. The medial side of the front of the leg is supplied by the ***saphenous nerve***.
3. The lateral side of the leg is supplied, in its upper part, by the ***lateral cutaneous nerve of the calf*** and, lower down, by the ***superficial peroneal nerve***.
4. The greater part of the dorsum of the foot, including most of the toes, is supplied by the ***superficial peroneal nerve***.
5. A triangular area of skin covering the adjoining sides of the big toe and the second toe is supplied by the ***deep peroneal nerve***.
6. A strip along the medial side of the foot is supplied by the ***saphenous nerve***, but the area supplied does not reach the big toe.
7. A strip along the lateral side of the foot is supplied by the ***sural nerve***: the area reaches the little toe.
8. With regard to the nerve supply of the digits note that the terminal part of the digit (including the nail bed) is through nerves that curve round from the plantar aspect (Compare with hand).

## Gluteal Region

1. The cutaneous nerves supplying the gluteal region are shown in 10.3.
2. The first point to note is that whereas the predominant nerve supply of the entire lower limb is through ***ventral rami*** of spinal nerves, some areas of skin over the gluteal region are supplied by ***dorsal rami***.
   a. An area over the sacrum is innervated by dorsal rami of spinal nerves S1, 2, 3.
   b. More laterally a wide area is innervated by dorsal rami of nerves L1, 2, 3.
   c. All other areas are innervated by nerves derived from ventral rami.
3. The upper and lateral part of the gluteal region is supplied by lateral cutaneous branches of the ***subcostal nerve***, and of the ***iliohypogastric nerve***.
4. The lower lateral part of the gluteal region receives a branch from the ***lateral cutaneous nerve of the thigh***.
5. Areas just above the fold of the buttock are supplied by the ***perforating cutaneous nerve***, near the midline, and by the gluteal branch of the ***posterior cutaneous nerve of the thigh***, more laterally.

## Back of Thigh

1. The cutaneous nerve supply of the back of the thigh is shown in 10.4.
2. Most of this aspect of the thigh is innervated by the ***posterior cutaneous nerve of the thigh***. Note that, this nerve also supplies the upper part of the back of the leg.
3. Laterally and medially, we can see some areas supplied by the same nerves that have already been seen from the front. These are:
   a. The obturator nerve,
   b. The medial cutaneous nerve of the thigh, on the medial side; and
   c. The lateral cutaneous nerve of the thigh on the lateral side.

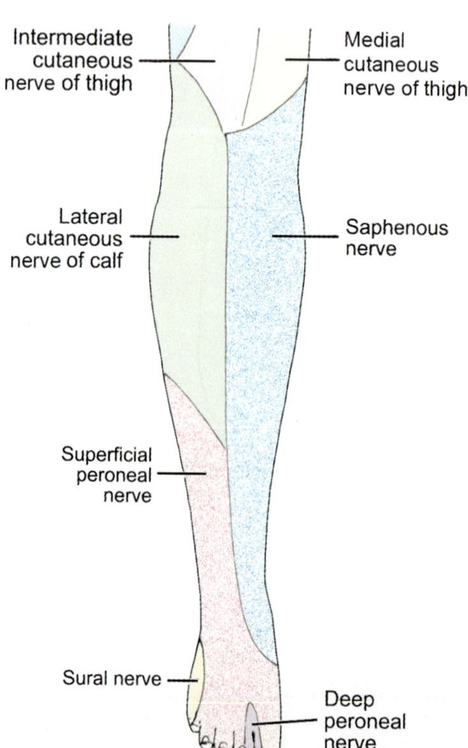


**10.2:** Cutaneous nerves on the front of the leg and dorsum of the foot

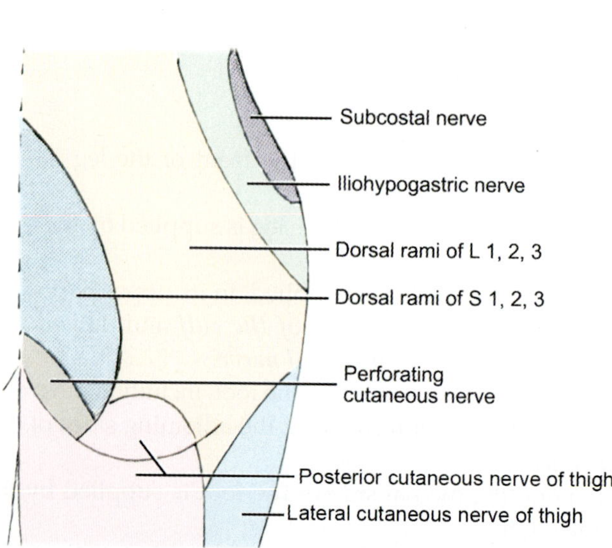


**10.3:** Cutaneous nerves in the gluteal region

4. Near the knee, the lower part of the back of the thigh receives some branches from the ***saphenous nerve*** (medially), and from the ***lateral cutaneous nerve of the calf*** (laterally).

## Back of Leg

1. The cutaneous nerve supply of the back of the leg is shown in 10.5.
2. On the medial and lateral sides, we see the same nerves as seen from the front viz.,
   a. The ***saphenous nerve*** medially.
   b. The ***lateral cutaneous nerve of the calf*** laterally.
3. A strip along the middle of the back of the leg is innervated, in its upper part, by the ***posterior cutaneous nerve of the thigh***, and in its lower part by the ***sural nerve***.
4. The skin over the heel is supplied by ***medial calcaneal branches*** of the tibial nerve.

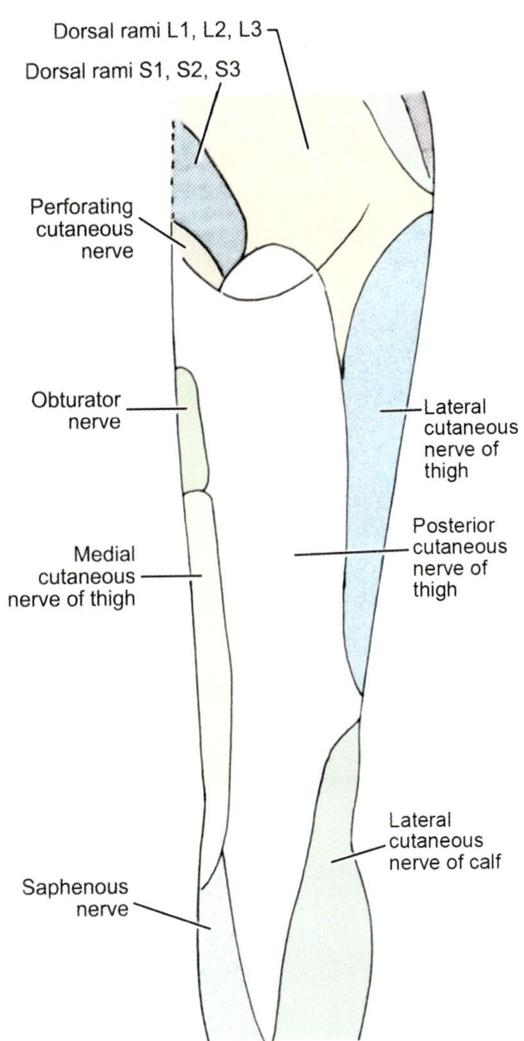


**10.4:** Cutaneous nerves on the back of the thigh

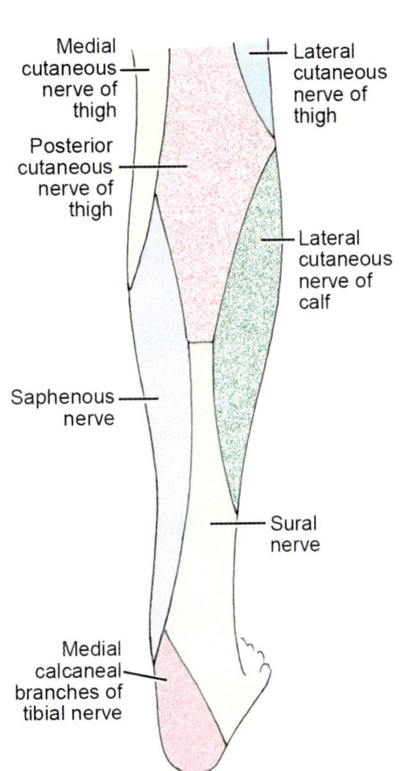


**10.5:** Cutaneous nerves on the back of the leg

## Sole

1. The cutaneous innervation of the skin of the sole is shown in 10.6.
2. The anterior part of the sole, including the medial 3½ digits, is supplied by the ***medial plantar nerve***.
3. The lateral part (including the lateral 1½ digits) is supplied through the ***lateral plantar nerve***.
4. As mentioned above, branches from these nerves also supply the dorsal aspect of the terminal parts of the toes including the nail beds.
5. A strip of skin along the lateral margin of the sole (reaching up to the lateral surface of the little toe) is supplied by the sural nerve.
6. On the medial side, a strip is supplied by the saphenous nerve. This strip does not reach the big toe. Skin over the heel is supplied by medial calcaneal branches of the tibial nerve.

The various nerves involved in supplying the skin of the lower extremity are briefly described below:

1. The ***subcostal nerve*** is formed by the ventral ramus of the 12th thoracic nerve. It is the only thoracic nerve taking part in supply of the lower limb.
2. The ***iliohypogastric nerve*** arises from root L1 of the lumbar plexus.
   a. It runs forwards within the layers of the abdominal wall.
   b. The nerve gives off a lateral cutaneous branch that becomes superficial a little above the iliac crest. While crossing the crest, it supplies the skin in the anterior part of the gluteal region.
   c. The nerve ends as the anterior cutaneous branch. This becomes superficial a little above the superficial inguinal ring, and ends by supplying the skin above the pubis.
3. ***The ilioinguinal nerve*** (L1) arises in common with the iliohypogastric nerve and has a similar course.
   a. It runs through the abdominal wall. It enters the inguinal canal and emerges through the superficial inguinal ring.
   b. It ends by supplying the skin of the upper and medial part of the thigh, over the pubis and the adjoining part of the genitalia. (Note that the ilioinguinal nerve does not give off a lateral cutaneous branch).
4. The ***genitofemoral nerve*** is a branch of the lumbar plexus (L1, L2). It runs through the layers of the abdominal wall. It ends up by dividing into genital and femoral branches.
   a. The ***genital branch*** passes through the inguinal canal. It gives some branches to the skin of the scrotum or of the labium majus.
   b. The ***femoral branch*** passes deep to the inguinal ligament and comes to lie lateral to the femoral artery. Here it lies within the femoral sheath. It becomes superficial by piercing the anterior wall of the sheath, and the deep fascia, and supplies an area of skin over the upper part of the femoral triangle.

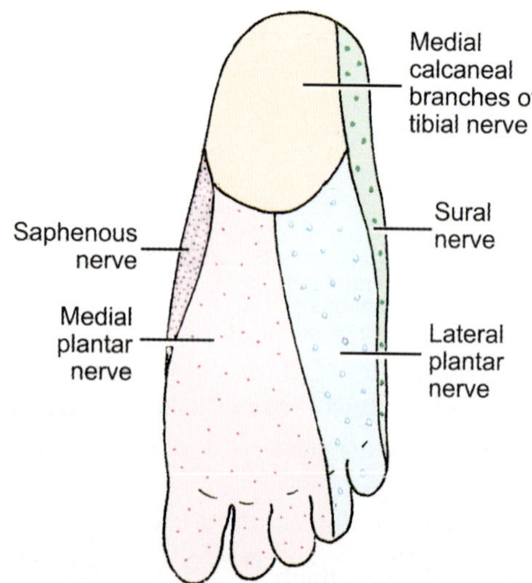


**10.6:** Cutaneous nerve supply of the sole

5. The ***lateral cutaneous nerve of the thigh*** is a branch of the lumbar plexus ((L2 and L3). Its initial part lies within the psoas major.
   a. Emerging from the lateral border of the muscle, the nerve runs downwards over the iliacus muscle to reach the anterior superior iliac spine.
   b. It enters the thigh by passing behind the lateral end of the inguinal ligament. It divides into anterior and posterior branches through which it supplies the skin on the anterolateral part of the thigh right up to the knee.
6. The ***obturator nerve*** is a branch of the lumbar plexus. It is formed by union of roots arising from L2, L3, and L4.
   a. The obturator nerve gives branches that supply the skin of the lower medial part of the thigh.
   b. These fibres may reach the skin through a branch that joins the medial cutaneous and saphenous branches of the femoral nerve to form the ***subsartorial plexus.***
7. The ***intermediate cutaneous nerve of the thigh*** arises from the anterior division of the femoral nerve. It supplies a long strip of skin on the front of the thigh. Its lowest part supplies skin over the front of the knee.
8. The ***medial cutaneous nerve of the thigh*** is a branch of the anterior division of the femoral nerve. It runs part of its course along the lateral side of the femoral artery.
   a. It crosses the artery near the apex of the femoral triangle.
   b. It divides into branches that supply the skin of the medial side of the thigh. The area of skin supplied is shown in 10.1.
   c. The nerve takes part in forming the ***subsartorial plexus*** (along with branches of the saphenous and obturator nerves).
9. The ***saphenous nerve*** arises from the posterior division of the femoral nerve.
   a. It descends along the lateral side of the femoral artery.
   b. It passess through the adductor canal.
   c. It leaves the adductor canal at its lower end and runs down along the medial side of the knee. Here, it pierces the deep fascia and becomes subcutaneous.
   d. It then runs down the medial side of the leg (alongside the long saphenous vein).
   e. A branch extends along the medial side of the foot (but ends short of the great toe). The area of skin supplied by the nerve is shown in 10.2.
   f. The saphenous nerve takes part in forming the ***subsartorial plexus*** and the ***patellar plexus.***
10. The ***posterior cutaneous nerve of the thigh*** is a branch of the sacral plexus. It is derived from segments S1, and S2 and S3.
    a. It passes from the pelvis to the gluteal region through the greater sciatic foramen.
    b. It passes downward through the gluteal region (deep to the gluteus maximus) to enter the back of the thigh.
    c. Its lowest part extends into the upper part of the leg.
    d. It supplies an extensive area of skin including that over the lower part of the gluteal region, the perineum, the back of the thigh, and the back of the upper part of the leg.
11. The ***perforating cutaneous nerve*** is a branch of the sacral plexus. It is derived from segments S2 and S3.
    a. It bears this name because it pierces through the sacrotuberous ligament. This is how it passes from within the pelvis to the gluteal region.
    b. Finally, it winds round the inferior edge of the gluteus maximus and supplies the skin over the inferomedial part of the muscle.
12. The ***sural nerve*** is the main cutaneous branch of the tibial nerve.
    a. It arises in the lower part of the popliteal fossa. It runs down the back of the leg.
    b. In its lower part, the nerve inclines laterally and passes forwards below the lateral malleolus.
    c. The terminal part of the nerve runs forwards along the lateral margin of the foot reaching right up to the lateral side of the little toe.
    d. The nerve supplies skin on the posterolateral part of the leg and along the lateral margin of the foot.
13. The ***medial calcaneal branches*** arise from the tibial nerve in the lower part of the leg. They pass medially, become superficial by piercing the flexor retinaculum and supply the skin over the heel.

14. The ***medial plantar nerve*** is a terminal branch of the tibial nerve. It ends by dividing into one ***proper digital branch*** for the great toe, and three ***common plantar digital branches***.
    a. Branches arising from the ***trunk*** of the medial plantar nerve supply the skin of the medial part of the sole.
    b. The skin on the medial side of the great toe is supplied by the proper digital branch to this digit.
    c. Each common plantar digital nerve divides into two ***proper digital nerves***.
    d. The first (most medial) common plantar digital nerve divides into the proper digital nerves that supply the skin on the adjacent sides of the great toe and second toe.
    e. The second into branches that supply the second and third toes.
    f. The third into branches that supply the third and fourth toes.
    g. Each digital nerve gives a dorsal branch that supplies the nail bed.
15. The ***lateral plantar nerve*** is a terminal branch of the tibial nerve.
    1. It divides into superficial and deep branches.
        a. The ***superficial branch*** runs distally and ends by dividing into two ***plantar digital nerves***.
        b. The lateral of these runs along the lateral side of the fifth digit.
        c. The medial one divides into two branches that supply the adjacent sides of the fourth and fifth digits.
    2. Some branches arising from the trunk of the nerve supply the skin of the lateral part of the sole.
    3. The skin on the lateral side of the little toe and the contiguous sides of the fourth and fifth toes is supplied by the corresponding digital branches.
16. The ***lateral cutaneous nerve of the calf*** is a branch of the common peroneal nerve.
    a. It supplies the skin over the upper two-thirds of the lateral side of the leg.
    b. The area of supply also extends on to the anterior and posterior aspects of the leg.
17. The ***deep peroneal nerve*** supplies skin as follows:
    a. The skin of part of the dorsum of the foot is supplied by the deep peroneal nerve through its medial terminal branch.
    b. This branch runs forwards on the dorsum of the foot along with the dorsalis pedis artery.
    c. It divides into two ***dorsal digital nerves*** which supply the adjacent sides of the great toe and the second toe.
18. The ***superficial peroneal nerve*** becomes superficial in the lower part of the leg. It supplies the skin on its lateral side. It then divides into medial and lateral terminal branches that descend across the ankle to reach the dorsum of the foot.
    a. Each terminal branch divides into two ***dorsal digital nerves***.
    b. The medial branch gives one dorsal digital nerve to the medial side of the great toe and another to the adjacent sides of the second and third toes.
    c. The lateral branch gives one dorsal digital nerve to the contiguous sides of the third and fourth toes and another to the adjacent sides of the fourth and fifth toes.
    d. The lateral terminal branch also supplies the skin on the lateral side of the ankle.

## VEINS OF THE LOWER LIMB

1. The veins of the lower limbs can be divided into ***deep*** and ***superficial*** veins (like those of the upper limbs).
2. The deep veins are placed subjacent to the deep fascia, and run along arteries.
3. The superficial veins lie in the superficial fascia and many of them can be seen through the skin.
4. The superficial veins drain into deep veins at their termination. They are also connected to deep veins through ***perforating*** veins that pass through deep fascia.

### Deep Veins of Lower Limb

The deep veins of the lower limb are:

1. The femoral vein
2. The popliteal vein
3. The anterior and posterior tibial veins

4. The medial and lateral plantar veins
5. The plantar venous arch
6. The metatarsal veins
7. The digital veins.

These veins accompany the corresponding arteries and (by and large) have tributaries corresponding to the branches of the arteries. The femoral and poptileal veins are large. The veins accompanying the other arteries of the lower limb are in the nature of venae comitantes. They are small veins lying in intimate relationship to the arteries. They may be double and may form plexuses over the arteries.

## Superficial Veins of the Lower Limb

1. The dorsal and plantar surfaces of the foot are covered by subcutaneous venous plexuses.
2. On the dorsum of the foot, a ***dorsal venous arch*** can be recognised (10.7). Dorsal digital and dorsal metatarsal veins drain into this arch.
3. Along the sides of the foot, there are ***medial and lateral marginal veins*** that communicate with both the plantar and dorsal venous networks. These veins are continued into two large superficial veins, the ***great (or long) saphenous vein***; and the ***small (or short) saphenous vein*** respectively.

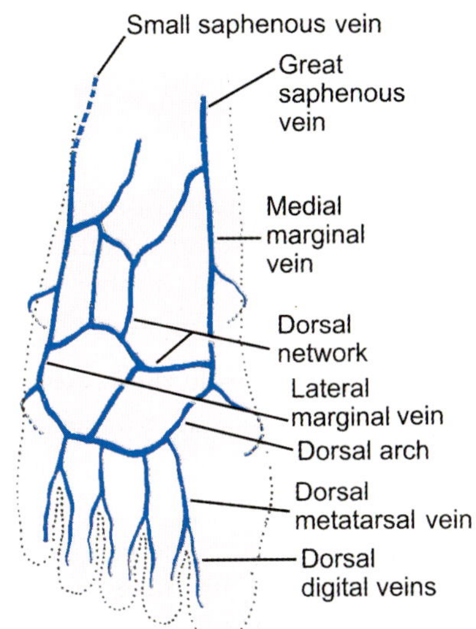


**10.7:** Veins on the dorsum of the foot

### *Great Saphenous Vein*

1. The ***great (or long) saphenous vein*** is a continuation of the medial marginal vein of the foot.
2. It ascends into the leg, a little in front of the medial malleolus and lies for some distance on the medial surface of the tibia.
3. Ascending on the medial side of the leg, it crosses the medial side of the knee joint, and ascends on the medial side of the thigh.
4. In the upper part of the thigh, it passes somewhat laterally and passes through an aperture in the deep fascia (saphenous opening) to end in the femoral vein (10.8).
5. The great saphenous vein receives numerous tributaries from the front and back of the leg, and from the front of the thigh.
   a. Just before it pierces the deep fascia, it receives the superficial epigastric, superficial circumflex iliac and external pudendal veins. These veins accompany the corresponding arteries.
   b. It also receives the ***anterior cutaneous vein of the thigh*** which drains the lower part of the front of the thigh.
   c. Just below the knee it receives the ***anterior vein of the leg***, and the ***posterior arch vein***.
   d. Over the dorsum of the foot the great saphenous vein receives the ***medial marginal vein*** of the foot.
   e. The great saphenous vein is connected to the deep veins of the leg and thigh through a number of ***perforating veins*** that are mentioned below.

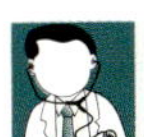

## CLINICAL CORRELATION

**Some Additional Facts about the Long Saphenous Vein**

1. In emergencies (requiring transfusions), when the vein cannot be seen, it is useful to remember that this vein is constantly located immediately in front of the medial malleolus. An incision at this site (termed ***saphenous cut-down***) exposes the vein.
2. Segments taken from this vein are used as grafts in coronary bypass surgery (i.e., for replacing a blocked segment of a coronary artery). Segments can also be used for bypass operations at other sites. In such operations the direction of the segment is reversed, so that valves do not interfere with blood flow.

### Small (or short) Saphenous Vein

1. The ***small (or short) saphenous vein*** is a continuation of the lateral marginal vein of the foot.
2. It ascends behind the lateral malleolus, and runs upwards along the middle of the back of the leg.
3. Over the lower part of the popliteal fossa, it perforates the deep fascia and ends in the popliteal vein, a few centimeters above the knee joint (10.8).

### Perforating Veins

1. The perforating veins (or perforators) are so called, as they perforate through the deep fascia.
2. They connect the superficial veins to deep veins.
3. Valves in them allow blood flow from superficial to deep veins, but not in the reverse direction (10.9).
4. Similar communications with deep veins exist where the great and small saphenous veins end in deep veins.
5. The sites at which perforators are present are variable.
6. Some common sites of perforators are as follows. (Numbers below correspond to numbered arrows in 10.8).
    a. A perforator that connects the great saphenous vein to the femoral vein is present in the lower part of the adductor canal (Number 1).
    b. A perforator present just below the knee connects the great saphenous vein, or the posterior arch vein, with the posterior tibial vein (Number 2).
    c. On the lateral side there is one lateral perforator. On the medial side there are upper, middle and lower perforators (Number 3).
    d. There are a number of perforators in the lower one third of the leg (number 4, 5, 6).

### Venous Return from the Lower Limb

Venous blood from the lower limbs has to ascend to the heart against gravity. This ascent depends on the following factors.

1. The atmospheric pressure within the thoracic cavity is negative and this tends to suck blood in the venous system towards the heart.
2. The veins of the lower limb are provided with numerous valves along their course. The valves, when competent, allow blood flow only towards the heart.
3. The leg and thigh are enclosed in a tight sleeve of deep fascia.
    a. The deep veins lie within the sleeve, along with arteries and muscles. The superficial veins lie outside the sleeve. Perforators penetrate the sleeve.
    b. When muscles contract, they increase in thickness raising the pressure within the sleeve.
    c. This pressure compresses the deep veins and, because of the presence of valves, blood is pushed towards the heart.
    d. In this way, muscular contraction acts as a pump that helps in venous return from the lower limbs. The muscles of the calf are specially important in this regard.
4. Venous return through deep veins is also aided by pulsations of adjoining arteries.

## LYMPH NODES AND LYMPHATIC DRAINAGE OF THE LOWER LIMB

### Lymph Nodes of the Lower Limb

With the exception of a few small nodes in the popliteal fossa, all the lymph nodes of the lower limb lie in the inguinal region. These ***inguinal lymph nodes*** are present in two groups, superficial and deep, that are separated by the deep fascia. The superficial nodes are further divided into upper and lower groups (10.10).

1. The ***upper superficial inguinal lymph nodes*** lie along the inguinal ligament, immediately below the latter. They are divisible into medial and lateral subgroups.
2. The ***lower superficial inguinal lymph nodes*** lie along the great saphenous vein.

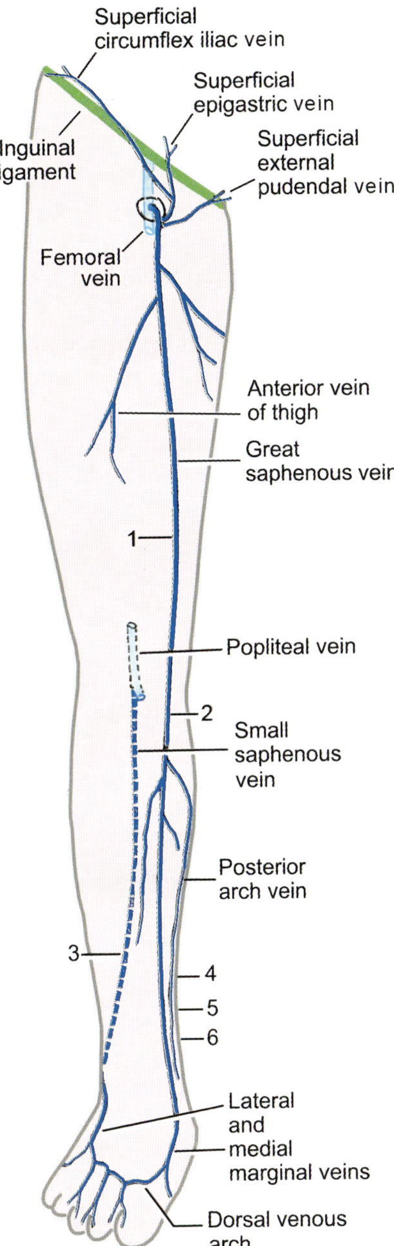


**10.8:** Superficial veins of lower limb. Numbered arrows indicate the position of perforating veins

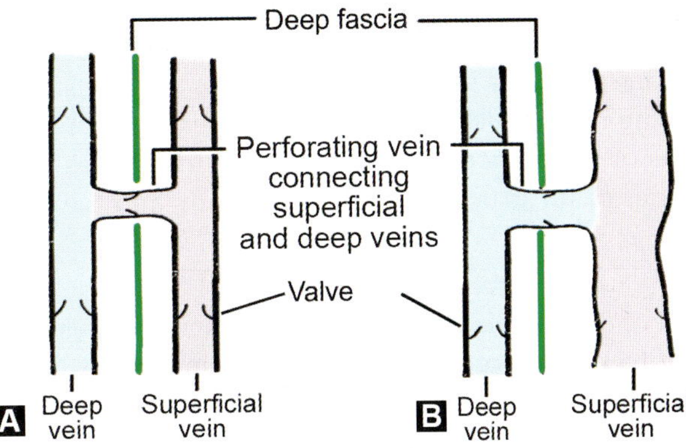


**10.9A and B:** Scheme to show the role of perforating veins. (A) Normally blood flows only from superficial to deep veins; (B) When the valves in perforating veins become incompetent, blood flows from deep to superficial veins leading to distension of the latter

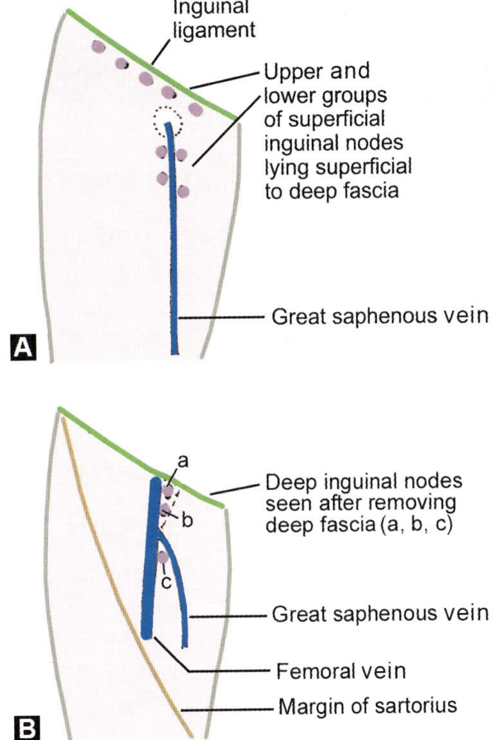


**10.10A and B:** Superficial and deep inguinal lymph nodes

3. The ***deep group of inguinal nodes*** lies along the medial side of the femoral vein. There are usually three nodes.
   a. The highest of these lies in the femoral ring.
   b. One node lies in the femoral canal.
   c. The third node lies just below the termination of the great saphenous vein.

The areas of the body drained by the inguinal nodes are shown in 10.11. Note that in addition to the lower limb these nodes drain structures in the perineum, and the abdominal wall below the level of the umbilicus.

### Lymphatic Drainage of the Lower Limb

1. Most of the vessels draining the superficial tissues of the limb travel along the great saphenous vein and end in the lower group of the superficial inguinal nodes.
2. The skin of the lateral side and back of the leg is drained by vessels which run along the short saphenous vein and end in the popliteal lymph nodes, from where the lymph passes through deeply placed lymph vessels to the deep inguinal nodes.
3. The deep lymph vessels of the limb run along the main blood vessels. They end in the deep inguinal nodes.
4. Some deep vessels of the gluteal region run along the superior and inferior gluteal vessels to end in nodes along the internal iliac vessels.

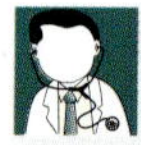

### CLINICAL CORRELATION

**Lymphadenitis**

1. Infection in any part of the lower limb can result in enlargement and tenderness of the inguinal lymph nodes.
2. These nodes can also be enlarged in carcinoma in the area of drainage. It has to be remembered that in addition to the lower limb, the inguinal nodes drain the lower part of the abdominal wall (up to the level of the umbilicus). They also drain the perineum including the lower parts of the anal canal, the vagina, and the urethra.
3. In syphilitic infection, the inguinal lymph nodes are palpable and have a firm feel, but they are painless.

## GENERAL REVIEW OF THE FRONT AND MEDIAL SIDE OF THIGH

### Some Superficial Structures in the Thigh

1. At the upper end of the front of the thigh i.e., at its junction with the anterior abdominal wall we see the ***inguinal ligament***.
   a. The ligament is attached at its lateral end to the anterior superior iliac spine, and at its medial end to the pubic tubercle.
   b. The ligament is really the folded lower edge of the aponeurosis of a muscle of the abdominal wall called the external oblique muscle.
   c. The deep fascia of the thigh is attached to the ligament, and because of the pull of this fascia the ligament has a gentle downward convexity.

   (The inguinal ligament also has some deeper parts that will be considered later).
2. Near the medial end of the inguinal ligament, we see the ***spermatic cord*** . It is seen to emerge through an aperture in the abdominal wall located just above the medial end of the inguinal ligament. This aperture is called the ***superficial inguinal ring***. The spermatic cord and the superficial inguinal ring will be studied in the abdomen.
3. A little below the medial end of the inguinal ligament, we see the ***saphenous opening***. This is an oval aperture in the deep fascia of the thigh. The lateral and inferior margins of the opening are sharp. This sharp margin is called the ***falciform margin***.
4. On the medial side, the fascia forming the boundary of the saphenous opening merges with the fascia over a muscle called the pectineus.

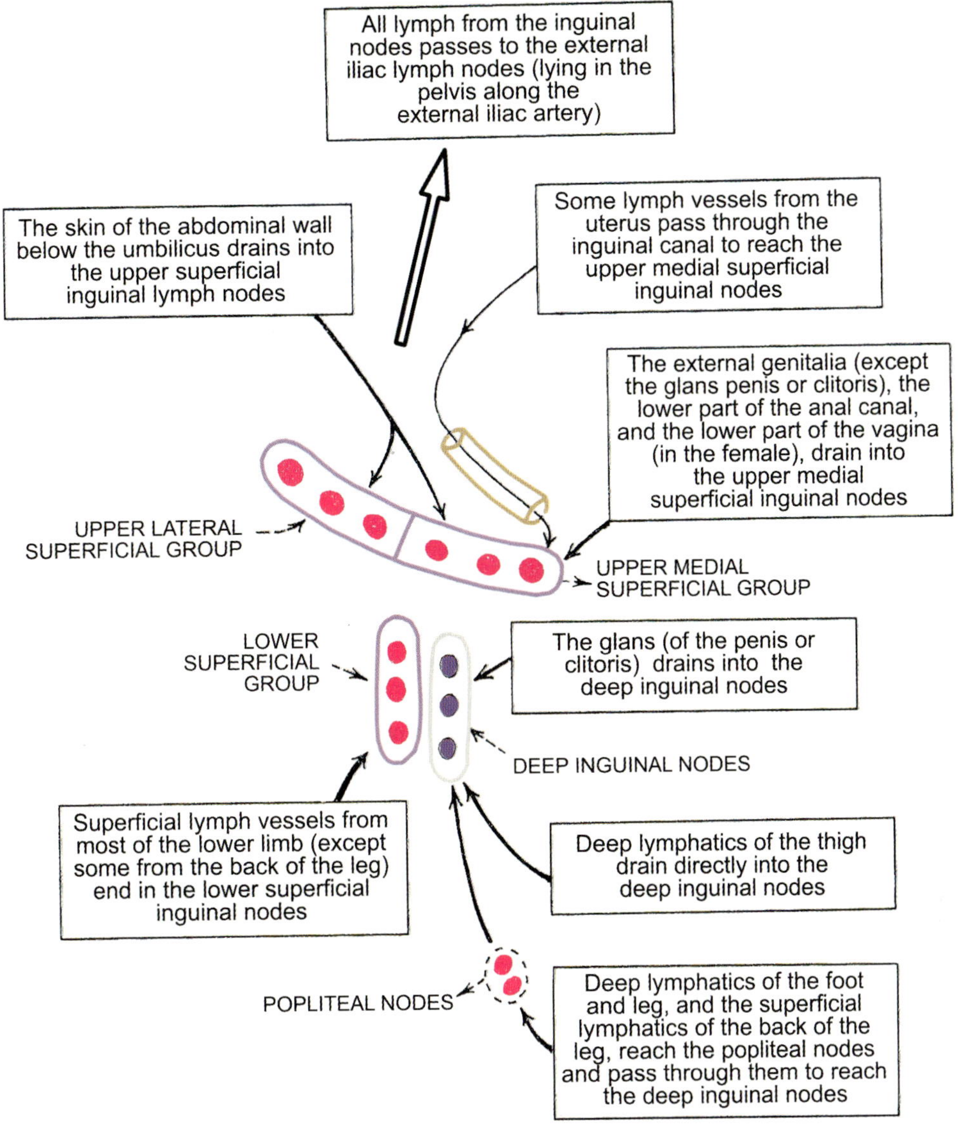


**10.11:** Scheme to show areas drained by the inguinal lymph nodes

5. The saphenous opening is closed by a sheet of fascia which has many small holes in it. This is the ***cribriform fascia***. The saphenous vein curves round the lower margin of the saphenous opening, and pierces the cribriform fascia to end by joining the femoral vein.
6. The cribriform fascia is also penetrated by three small branches of the femoral artery. These are the ***superficial circumflex iliac artery*** (laterally), the ***superficial epigastric artery*** (in the middle) and the ***superficial external pudendal artery*** (on the medial side). Veins accompanying these three arteries usually end in the terminal part of the saphenous vein before the latter pierces the cribriform fascia.
7. The superficial fascia in the upper part of the front of the thigh is different from fascia over the greater part of the body in that it consists of two layers. There is a superficial fatty layer, and a deep membranous layer (a similar arrangement of superficial fascia is seen over the anterior abdominal wall, and over the perineum).

8. The membranous layer of superficial fascia is loosely attached to the deep fascia of the thigh. However, the two fasciae are firmly adherent to each other along a horizontal line starting at the pubic tubercle and passing laterally for about 8 cm. This horizontal line is referred to as ***Holden's line***.

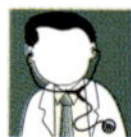

**CLINICAL CORRELATION**

9. The importance of this line is as follows:
   a. Sometimes the urethra may rupture in the perineum as a result of injury.
   b. Urine may flow out of the ruptured urethra and enter the space deep to the membranous layer of superficial fascia (This is called ***extravasation*** of urine).
   c. The fascia in the perineum is directly continuous (over the pubic symphysis) with the corresponding fascia over the abdominal wall. Therefore, the extravasated urine can pass upwards on to the abdominal wall. It can then pass laterally and flow across the inguinal ligament into the thigh.
   d. However, the firm attachment of fascial layers along Holden's line prevents this urine from descending lower into the thigh.

10. The deep fascia of the thigh is called the ***fascia lata***. When traced superiorly, its gains attachment to bones and ligaments that lie at the upper limit of the upper limb. These include the inguinal ligament as already mentioned. Traced inferiorly it becomes continuous with the fascia of the leg, but it also gains attachment to various bony prominences that are superficial.
11. Along the lateral margin of the thigh, the fascia lata is thickened and forms a strong band passing from the anterior part of the iliac crest to the upper end of the tibia (front of lateral condyle).
    a. This band is, therefore, called the ***iliotibial tract***.
    b. At its upper end, the tract splits to enclose a muscle called the ***tensor fasciae latae***.
    c. Posteriorly, the iliotibial tract receives the insertion of many fibres of the ***gluteus maximus*** (a large muscle of the gluteal region).
    d. The thickness of the deep fascia in the region of the iliotibial tract is due to the pull of these muscles. The iliotibial tract helps to transmit the pull of these muscles to the tibia and helps to stabilize the knee.
    e. The area of attachment of the iliotibial tract to the tibia forms a prominent triangular impression on the bone (9.21 and 9.23).
12. ***Intermuscular septa*** (lateral, medial and posterior) passing from deep fascia to the femur help to divide the thigh into anterior, medial and posterior compartments.

## Preliminary Identification of Muscles seen on the Front and Medial Side of the Thigh

The muscles to be seen on the front and medial side of the thigh after removal of deep fascia are shown in 10.12.

1. Running diagonally across the thigh, there is a long thin muscle called the ***sartorius***. Its upper end is attached to the anterior superior iliac spine, while its lower end (insertion) reaches the medial side of the upper end of the tibia.
2. Running downwards along the lateral margin of the upper part of the thigh we see the ***tensor fasciae latae*** and the ***iliotibial tract*** (already mentioned above).
3. Between the sartorius and the tensor fasciae latae we see parts of a large muscle, the ***quadriceps femoris***. This is the main muscle of the front of the thigh. It is so called as it consists of four parts. Three of these are seen in 10.12.
   a. Running more or less vertically down the centre of the thigh there is the ***rectus femoris*** (rectus = straight). Its lower end is attached to the upper border of the patella.
   b. To the lateral side of the rectus femoris, we see the ***vastus lateralis***.
   c. To the medial side of the rectus femoris, we see the ***vastus medialis***.
   d. The fourth part is called the ***vastus intermedius***. It lies deep to the other muscles.
   e. The three vasti are large muscles wrapped around the shaft of the femur.

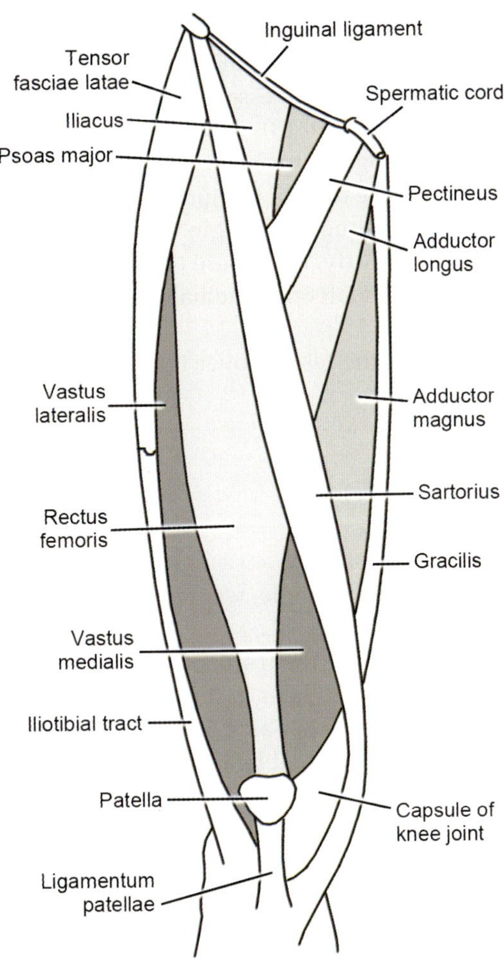


**10.12:** Muscles seen on the front and medial side of thigh

   f. All the four parts of the quadriceps femoris are inserted into the patella. Their pull is transmitted to the tibia through the ***ligamentum patellae*** that passes from the lower end of the patella to the tibia.
   g. The quadriceps femoris is an extensor of the knee joint.
4. Medial to the upper part of the sartorius, we see two muscles: the ***iliacus*** laterally, and the ***psoas major*** medially. These two muscles are often referred to collectively as the ***iliopsoas***.
   a. Both these muscles have their origin within the abdominal cavity.
   b. They enter the thigh by passing deep to the inguinal ligament and are inserted into the upper part of the femur.
   c. These muscles are flexors of the hip joint.
5. The area medial to the sartorius, and below the level of the psoas major is occupied by a number of muscle belonging to the medial compartment of the thigh. From above downwards, these are:
   a. The ***pectineus***
   b. The ***adductor longus***
   c. The ***adductor magnus***
   d. The ***gracilis***.
6. All these are adductors of the femur.
7. Deep to the adductor longus there is another muscle, the ***adductor brevis***.

## Femoral Triangle

1. The region on the front of thigh medial to the upper part of the sartorius is called the femoral triangle.
2. The region is of importance, as it contains several vessels and nerves.
3. The ***boundaries*** of the triangle are as follows (10.13).
   a. The ***upper boundary*** or ***base*** of the triangle is formed by the inguinal ligament.
   b. The triangle is bounded ***laterally***, by the medial margin of the sartorius.
   c. The triangle is bounded medially by the medial margin of the adductor longus.
   d. The apex of the triangle, directed inferiorly, lies where the medial and lateral borders meet.
   e. The ***floor*** of the triangle is formed (from lateral to medial side) by the iliacus, the psoas major, the pectineus and the adductor longus.
   f. The ***roof*** of the triangle is formed by the fasciae over the region, and superficial structures within them. These include:
      1. The saphenous opening
      2. The cribriform fascia
      3. The terminal part of the saphenous vein
      4. The superficial inguinal lymph nodes.
4. The contents of the femoral triangle are as follows:
   a. Running down the middle of the femoral triangle, we see the ***femoral artery***.
   b. Medial to the artery, we see the ***femoral vein***.
   c. A short distance lateral to the artery, we see the trunk of the ***femoral nerve***.

   The femoral vessels and nerve will be described later in this chapter.
5. The femoral artery gives off the following branches as it lies in the femoral triangle.
6. Three branches are given off just below the inguinal ligament. These are:
   a. The superficial circumflex iliac artery
   b. The superficial epigastric artery
   c. The superficial external pudendal artery.

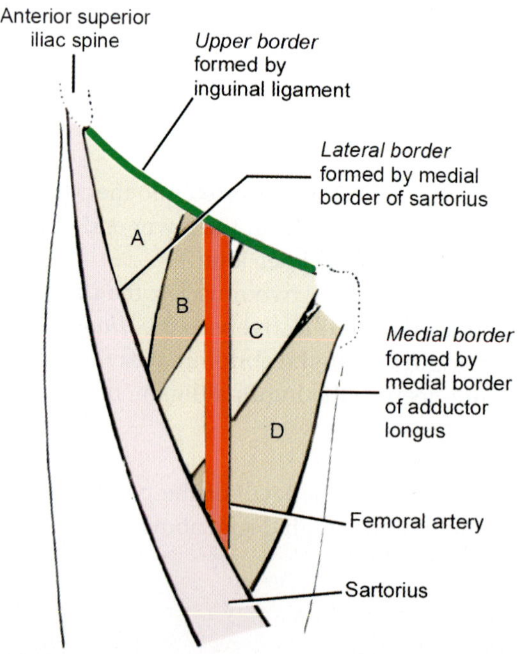


**10.13:** Femoral artery in femoral triangle: The boundaries of the triangle are shown. (A) Iliacus; (B) Psoas major; (C) Pectineus; (D) Adductor longus

They pass through the cribriform fascia to become superficial.

7. A short distance below the inguinal ligament, the femoral artery gives off two branches.
   a. The ***deep external pudendal artery*** arises from the medial side of the femoral artery and runs medially over the floor of the triangle.
   b. The largest branch of the femoral artery is the ***profunda femoris artery*** (literally, deep artery of the thigh). It arises from the posterolateral aspect of the femoral artery, and runs downwards lateral to the femoral artery. The profunda femoris artery is seen giving off two major branches. These are the ***medial and lateral circumflex femoral arteries***.
8. The upper end of the femoral vein lies medial to the femoral artery. However, at the apex of the femoral triangle the vein lies behind the artery. The great saphenous vein joins the femoral vein. Other tributaries of the femoral vein correspond to branches of the femoral artery.
9. After a short course, the femoral nerve divides into anterior and posterior divisions, each of which divides into a number of branches.
   The posterior division gives off several muscular branches. These are:
   a. Branch to the rectus femoris
   b. Branch to vastus lateralis
   c. Branch to vastus intermedius
   d. Branch to vastus medialis.
   e. The ***saphenous nerve*** is a large sensory branch. It runs downwards lateral to the profunda femoris artery. Near the apex of the femoral triangle, it disappears under the cover of the sartorius.
   f. The anterior division of the femoral nerve gives off a stem that supplies the sartorius muscle and then continues as the ***intermediate cutaneous nerve of the thigh***.
   g. It also gives off the ***medial cutaneous nerve of the thigh***. This nerve crosses anterior to the femoral vessels in the lower part of the femoral triangle.
10. Some smaller structures present in the femoral triangle are as follows.
   a. Just medial to the femoral nerve, we see the ***nerve to the pectineus***. This nerve arises from the femoral nerve within the pelvis and enters the thigh by passing deep to the inguinal ligament. It passes medially deep to the femoral artery to reach the pectineus.
   b. The ***femoral branch of the genitofemoral nerve*** is seen running downwards anterior to the femoral artery. This nerve supplies an area of skin over the femoral triangle.
   c. The ***lateral cutaneous nerve of the thigh*** is seen near the lateral angle of the femoral triangle.

## Adductor Canal

1. The space deep to the sartorius, over the middle one-third of the thigh, is called the ***adductor canal***. It is also called the ***subsartorial canal***.
2. The boundaries of the canal can be visualised by examining a transverse section (10.14).
   a. The canal is bounded ***anteriorly*** by the vastus medialis.
   b. It is bounded ***posteriorly***, by the adductor longus (above) and the adductor magnus (below).
   c. It is bounded ***medially***, by a strong fibrous membrane lying deep to the sartorius.
3. The contents of the canal are:
   a. The femoral artery and vein where the vein lies posterior to the femoral artery in the upper part of the canal, and lateral (deep) to it in the lower part.
   b. At the lower end of the canal the femoral vessels pass through a large aperture in the aponeurosis of the adductor magnus (to reach the popliteal fossa).
   c. The ***saphenous nerve*** runs along the femoral artery gradually crossing it from lateral to medial side. At the lower end of the canal the nerve pierces the fibrous roof to become superficial.
   d. The branch of the femoral nerve to the vastus medialis runs downwards lateral to the femoral artery.
   e. Some branches of the obturator nerve descend along the femoral artery.
   f. The ***subsartorial plexus of nerves*** lies over the fascia forming the roof of the adductor canal. The plexus receives contributions from the medial cutaneous nerve of the thigh, the saphenous nerve, and the anterior division of the obturator nerve.

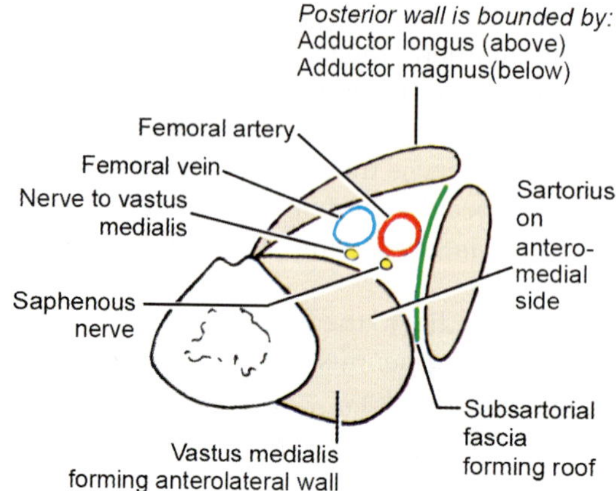


**10.14:** Femoral vessels and boundaries in adductor canal

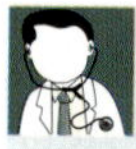

## CLINICAL CORRELATION

The adductor canal is a region of surgical importance. The femoral artery can be easily approached here.

## MUSCLES OF FRONT OF THIGH

These are:

1. Psoas major (10.15B and 10.16)
2. Psoas minor (10.15B and 10.16)
3. Iliacus (10.15B and 10.16)
4. Tensor fasciae latae (10.15B and 10.17)
5. Sartorius (10.15B)
6. Rectus femoris (10.15A and 10.18)
7. Articularis genu.

All these, except the articularis genu are described in 10.15.

Some points to note are:

a. The psoas minor is not always present. The muscle lies within the abdomen. It is described here because it is closely associated with the psoas major.
b. The length of the tensor fasciae latae is variable.
c. The quadriceps femoris is not active during standing upright because the knee is locked when it is fully extended.

## WANT TO KNOW MORE?

### Articularis Genu

1. The articularis genu consists of a few fascicles of muscle fibres ***arising from*** the anterior surface of the shaft of the femur, below the origin of the vastus intermedius (of which they may be considered a separated part).
2. The fibres are ***inserted into*** the synovial membrane of the knee joint.
3. The fibres pull the synovial membrane up during extension of the knee, and thus prevent it from being pinched between the femur and the patella. The muscle is supplied through the femoral nerve.

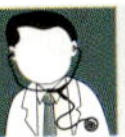

## CLINICAL CORRELATION

1. There are bursae in relation to the patella (prepatellar or suprapatellar bursa). They can get inflamned (bursitis) in persons who support their weight on the knees for long periods. The condition is called ***housemaids knee***.
2. Pain deep to the patella can occur in persons doing a lot of running (e.g., long distance runners).
3. When a person is sitting with the legs hanging free, striking the ligamentum patellae with a rubber hammer causes reflex extension of the knee.
   a. This is the ***knee jerk*** or ***patellar tendon reflex***.
   b. Any condition that causes paralysis of the quadriceps femoris (e.g., injury to the femoral nerve) abolishes the reflex.
   c. The reflex is exaggerated in upper motor neuron paralysis (e.g., hemiplegia).

**10.15A: Quadriceps femoris**

| *Attachments of Individual Parts* | | | *Ultimate Insertion of Quadriceps Femoris* |
|---|---|---|---|
| *Part* | *Origin* | *Insertion* | 1. All the four parts of the muscle are inserted into the patella<br>2. The patella transmits their pull to the ligamentum patellae<br>3. The lower end of the ligametum patellae is attached to the tibial tuberosity (smooth upper part)<br>4. Thus the quadriceps femoris is utimately inserted into the tibia |
| Rectus Femoris | Tendinous origin from hip bone by two heads<br>1. Straight head: From anterior inferior iliac spine<br>2. Reflected head: From ilium just above acetabulum | Upper border of patella | |
| Vastus medialis | From following parts of shaft of femur:<br>1. Intertrochanteric line, lower part<br>2. Spiral line<br>3. Medial lip of linea aspera<br>4. Medial supracondylar line | 1. Medial border of patella<br>2. Through medial patellar retinaculum into medial condyle of tibia | |
| Vastus intermedius | From shaft of femur:<br>1. Anterior surface<br>2. Lateral surface | Upper border of patella (deep to rectus femoris) | *Nerve Supply and Actions of Quadriceps Femoris*<br>Nerve supply: Femoral nerve (L2, 3, 4) |
| Vastus lateralis | From following parts of femur:<br>1. Upper end of intertrochanteric line<br>2. Anterior border of greater trochanter<br>3. Lower border of greater trochanter<br>4. Lateral margin of gluteal tuberosity<br>5. Lateral lip of linea aspera | 1. Lateral border of patella<br>2. Through lateral patellar retinaculum into lateral condyle of tibia | Actions of quadriceps femoris:<br>1. The muscle straightens the lower extremity at the knee (as in standing up from a sitting position)<br>2. When sitting down, the muscle relaxes gradually and ensures proper control<br>3. The rectus femoris can flex the thigh. It can rotate the pelvis on the head of the femur<br>4. The vastus medialis prevents lateral displacement of the patella |

**10.15B: Various other muscles of front of thigh**

| *Muscle* | *Psoas Major* | *Psoas Minor* | *Iliacus* |
|---|---|---|---|
| Origin | Through several slips from the following:<br>1. Transverse process of each lumbar vertebra (anterior surface)<br>2. Intervertebral discs and bodies of vertebrae (lateral parts). Five slips highest between T12 and L1, lowest between L4 and L5<br>3. Tendinous arches along sides of upper four lumbar vertebrae | 1. Intervertebral disc between T12 and L1<br>2. Adjoining parts of bodies of vertebrae | 1. Iliac fossa (on inner side of hip bone)<br>2. Iliac crest, inner lip<br>3. Iliolumbar ligament<br>4. Anterior sacroiliac ligament<br>5. Sacrum: Lateral part of upper surface |
| Insertion | Lesser trochanter of femur. | 1. Iliopectineal eminence<br>2. Pecten pubis | 1. Tendon of psoas major<br>2. Lesser trochanter of femur<br>3. Small area below lesser trochanter |
| Nerve supply | Ventral rami of spinal nerves L1, L2, L3 | Branch from spinal nerve L1 | Femoral nerve |
| Action | 1. Flexion of thigh at hip joint<br>2. Flexion of lumbar part of vertebral column<br>3. Balances trunk in standing | Weak flexor of lumbar vertebral column | 1. Flexion of thigh (hip joint)<br>2. Flexion of lumbar part of vertebral column |

| *Muscle* | *Tensor Fasciae Latae* | *Sartorius* |
|---|---|---|
| Origin | 1. Anterior part of outer lip of iliac crest<br>2. Outer aspect of anterior superior iliac spine | 1. Anterior superior iliac spine<br>2. Small area below the spine |
| Insertion | Upper end of iliotibial tract. Through this tract, it pulls on the lateral condyle of the tibia (triangular area on front of condyle) | Upper end of tibia (on a vertical line on the upper part of medial surface). Insertion is anterior to that of the gracilis and of semitendinosus |
| Nerve supply | Superior gluteal nerve (L4, 5, S1) | Femoral nerve (L2, 3) |
| Action | 1. Helps to maintain erect posture. It stablises the pelvis on head of femur, and the femur on the tibia<br>2. Helps to extend the leg<br>3. Helps in medial rotation of thigh<br>4. May abduct the thigh | Helps in:<br>1. Flexion of leg (at knee joint)<br>2. Flexion of thigh (at hip joint)<br>3. Abduction of thigh<br>4. Lateral rotation of thigh |
| Note | Length of the muscle is variable | 1. The medial border of the upper part of the sartorius forms the lateral boundary of the femoral triangle<br>2. Forms roof of adductor canal (in middle one-third of thigh) |

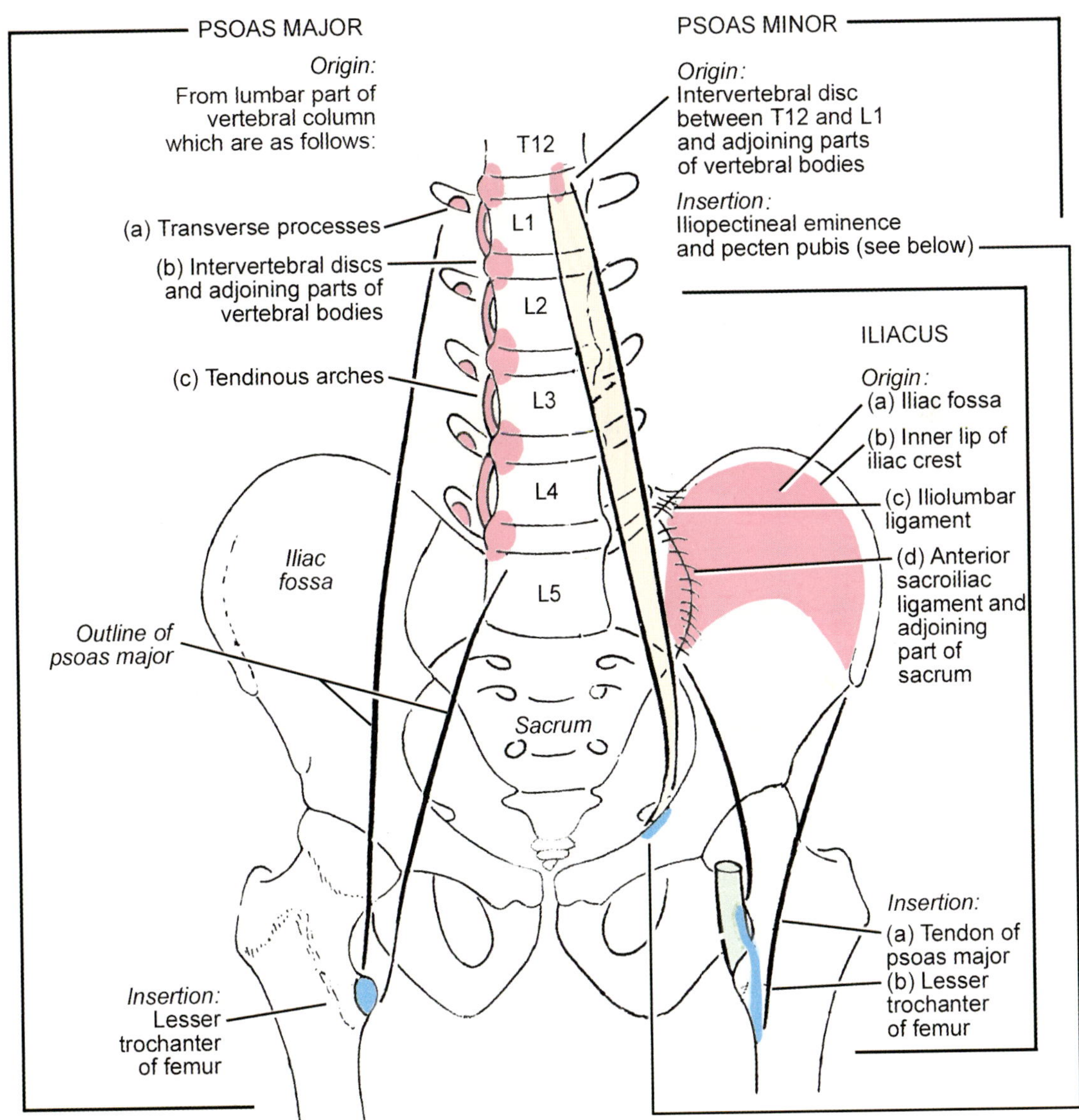


**10.16:** Scheme to show attachments of psoas major, psoas minor and iliacus

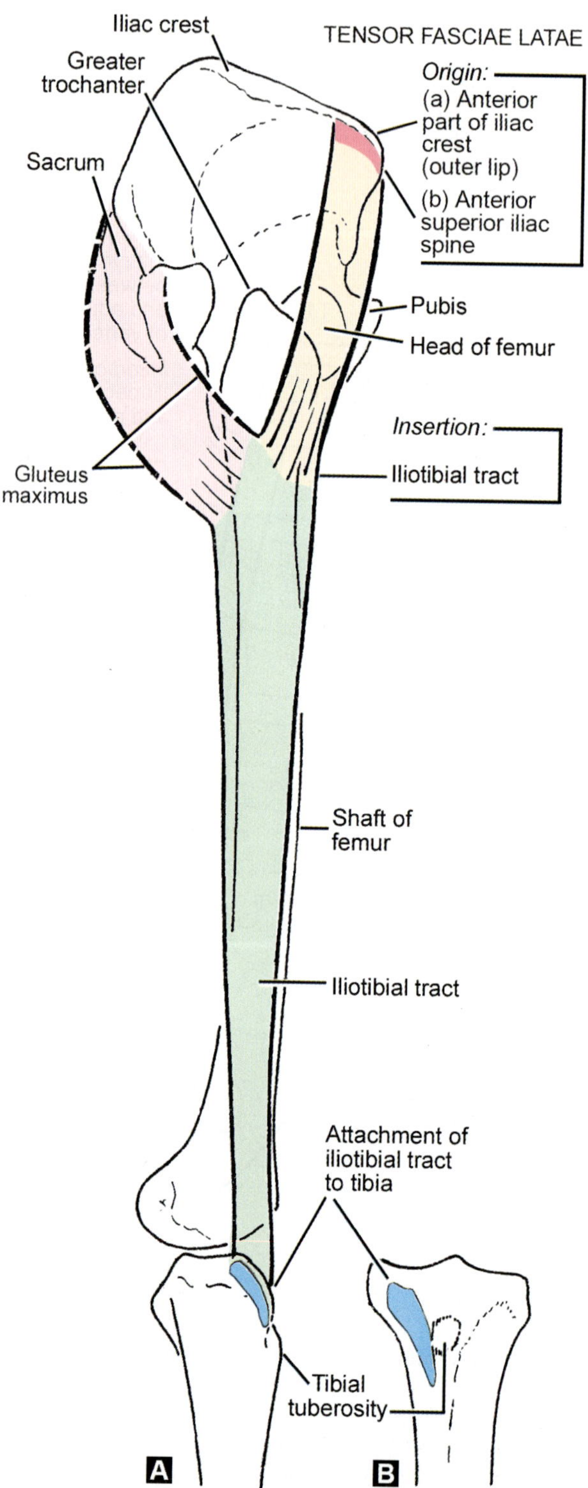


**10.17A and B:** Scheme to show the attachments of the tensor fasciae latae and the iliotibial tract

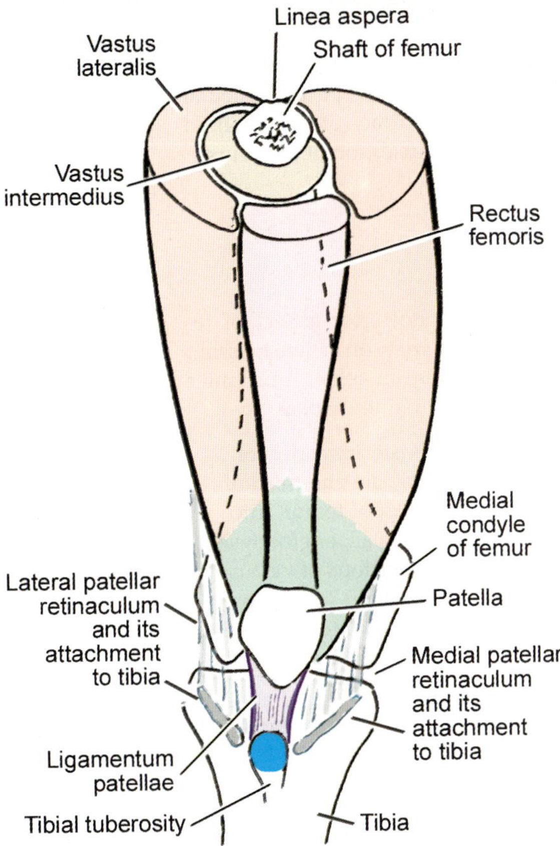


**10.18:** Scheme to show the arrangement of the parts of the quadriceps femoris. The muscle and femur have been cut across in the lower part of the thigh

## MUSCLES OF MEDIAL SIDE OF THIGH

These are:

1. The gracilis (10.19)
2. The pectineus (10.19)
3. The adductor longus (10.19)
4. The adductor brevis (10.19)
5. The adductor magnus (10.20 and 10.21)

Their attachments are given in 10.19.

### Notes on Pectineus

1. It forms part of the floor of the femoral triangle. Here the ilio psoas lies lateral to it and the adductor longus lies medial to it.
2. The femoral vessels and the great saphenous vein lie in front of this muscle.

### Notes on Adductor Longus

1. The muscle helps to form the floor of the femoral triangle. The medial border of this muscle forms the medial border of the triangle.

| 10.19: Muscles of medial side of thigh | | | | |
|---|---|---|---|---|
| *Muscle* | *Origin* | *Insertion* | *Action* | *Nerve Supply* |
| Gracilis | Medial margin of pubic arch. The area includes parts of:<br>1. Body of pubis<br>2. Inferior ramus of pubis<br>3. Ramus of ischium | Upper part of medial surface of tibia (behind insertion of sartorius) | 1. Flexion of leg<br>2. Medial rotation of thigh<br>3. Adduction of thigh | Obturator nerve (L2, 3) |
| Pectineus | Superior ramus of pubis (pecten pubis and part of pectineal surface) | Posterior aspect of femur on a line passing from lesser trochanter to linea aspera | 1. Adduction of thigh<br>2. Flexion of thigh | 1. Femoral nerve<br>2. Obturator nerve (or accessory obturator nerve). (L2, 3) |
| Adductor longus | Front of body of pubis | Posterior aspect of middle one-third of shaft of femur, into linea aspera (between insertions of vastus medialis (medially) and of adductor brevis and adductor magnus (laterally) | 1. Adduction of thigh<br>2. Flexion of thigh | Obturator nerve (anterior division) (L2, 3, 4) |
| Adductor brevis | From following parts of pubis:<br>a. Lower part of body<br>b. Inferior ramus<br>(The origin is lateral to that of the gracilis and below that of adductor longus) | Posterior aspect of femur:<br>1. Along a line running from lesser trochanter to linea aspera<br>2. Upper part of linea aspera | 1. Adduction of thigh<br>2. Flexion of thigh<br>3. Role in rotation of thigh is controversial | Obturator nerve (L2, 3, 4) |
| Adductor magnus<br>Adductor part | Mainly from ramus of ischium. Upper end of origin from ramus of pubis | 1. Medial margin of gluteal tuberosity<br>2. Linea aspera<br>3. Medial supracondylar line | Adduction of thigh | Obturator nerve (L2, 3, 4) |
| Hamstring part | Inferior and lateral part of ischial tuberosity | Adductor tubercle on medial condyle of tibia | Adduction of thigh May produce extension of thigh. Role in rotation of thigh is controversial | Sciatic nerve (tibial part) (L4) |

2. Its lower part forms the posterior wall of the adductor canal.
3. Deep to it, there are adductor brevis and a small part of the adductor magnus.
4. The femoral vessels and the great saphenous vein lie in front of this muscle. The spermatic cord crosses it near its origin.
5. The profunda femoris vessels, and the anterior division of the obturator nerve, lie deep to it.

## Notes on Adductor Brevis

1. This muscle lies deep to the pectineus and adductor longus.
2. It is superficial to the adductor magnus.

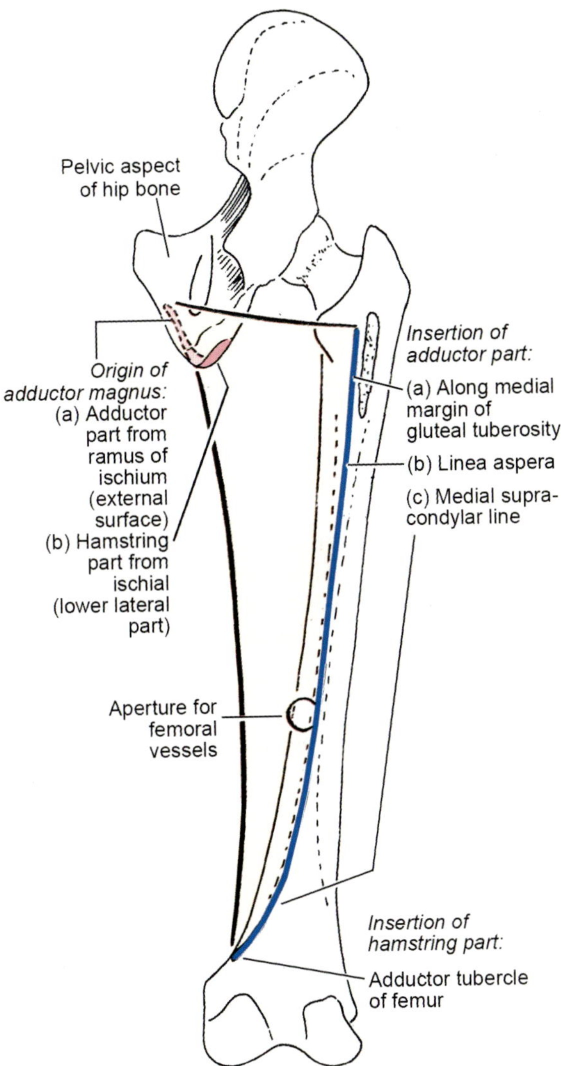


**10.20:** Scheme to show the attachments of the adductor magnus muscle

3. The profunda femoris vessels and the anterior division of the obturator nerve lie in front of it.
4. The posterior division of the obturator nerve is deep to it.

## Notes on Adductor Magnus

1. The muscle forms a partition separating structures on the front and medial side of the thigh from those on the back of the thigh.
2. Structures anterior to it are:
   a. Femoral vessels
   b. Profunda femoris vessels
   c. Obturator nerve
   d. Pectineus, adductor longus and adductor brevis muscles.

3. The sciatic nerve and the hamstring muscles are posterior to it.
4. Near the insertion of the muscle, there are a series of apertures for passage of blood vessels. The largest (and lowest) of these is for the femoral vessels. The others are for the profunda femoris and perforating arteries.

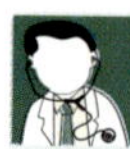

## CLINICAL CORRELATION

1. In certain neurological disorders, the adductor muscles of the thigh go into painful spasm. The spasm can be relieved by cutting the tendon of the adductor longus (adductor tenotomy) or by crushing the obturator nerve.
2. The gracilis is sometimes used to replace a damaged muscle at some other site. This can be done because removal of the gracilis does not make much difference to movements of the thigh.

## THE FEMORAL ARTERY

1. The femoral artery is the continuation of the external iliac artery into the thigh (10.21).
2. It begins at the midinguinal point (i.e., midway between the pubic symphysis and the anterior superior iliac spine). It descends first on the front of the thigh (upper third), and then on its medial side (middle third).
3. It ends at the junction of the middle, and lower, thirds of the thigh. Here, it passes through an aperture in the adductor magnus muscle to reach the back of the thigh, where it becomes the ***popliteal artery.***
4. The upper part of the femoral artery lies in the femoral triangle (10.13). Within the triangle the femoral artery lies successively over:
   a. The psoas major
   b. The pectineus
   c. The adductor longus.
5. Within the femoral triangle, the artery is covered by skin, superficial and deep fascia (Also see femoral sheath below).
6. At the apex of the femoral triangle, the artery passes into the adductor canal. Within the canal the artery lies first on the adductor longus and then on the adductor magnus (10.14). It is surrounded by muscles that are shown in 10.14.

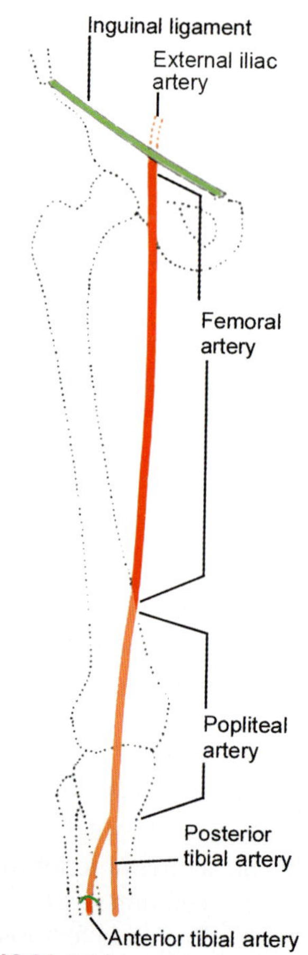


**10.21:** Main arteries in the thigh and upper part of leg

### Other Relations of Femoral Artery

1. The femoral artery is accompanied by the femoral vein. Just below the inguinal ligament, the vein is medial to the artery (10.22. However, the vein gradually crosses to the lateral side posterior to artery. It is directly behind the artery at the apex of the femoral triangle, and lateral to the lower end of the artery.
2. The femoral nerve is lateral to the upper part of the artery (10.23). Lower down, the artery is related to the branches of the nerve, some of which cross it.
   a. The branch to the pectineus crosses behind the upper part of the artery.
   b. The medial cutaneous nerve of the thigh crosses the artery from lateral to medial side near the apex of the femoral triangle.
   c. The saphenous branch crosses the artery within the adductor canal.
3. The nerve to the vastus medialis is lateral to the artery in the adductor canal.
4. The femoral branch of the genitofemoral nerve is also lateral to the upper part of the femoral artery (within the femoral sheath), but lower down it passes to the front of the artery (10.23).
5. The profunda femoris artery (a branch of the femoral artery itself) and its com-

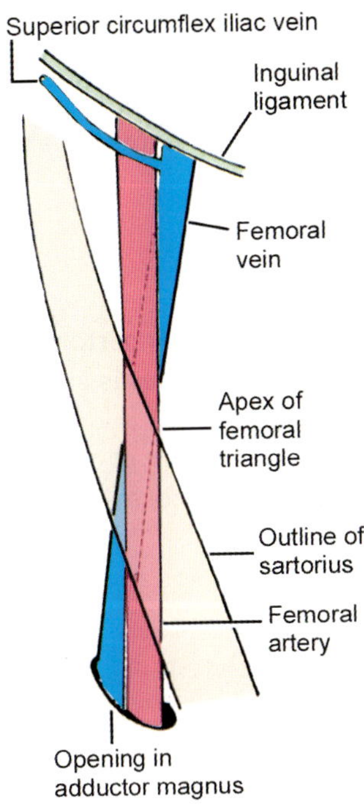


**10.22:** Relationship of femoral artery to femoral vein

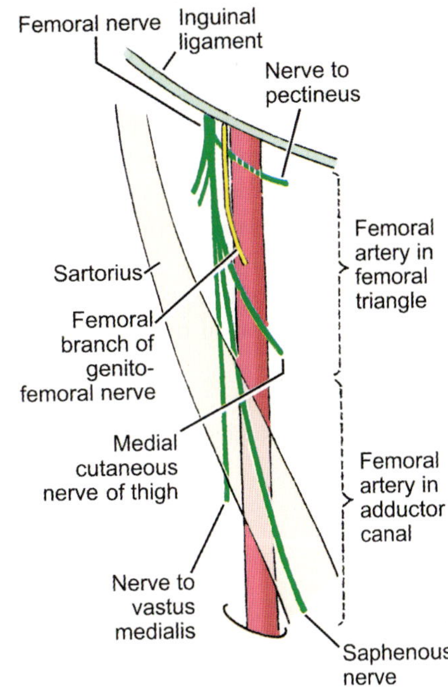


**10.23:** Relationship of femoral artery to femoral nerve and its branches

panion vein, lie behind the upper part of the femoral artery (where it lies on the pectineus). Lower down, however, the femoral and profunda femoris arteries are separated by the adductor longus.

6. In the upper part of the femoral triangle, the femoral artery and vein are enclosed in a funnel-like covering of fascia which is called the ***femoral sheath.*** The cavity within the femoral sheath is divisible into three parts.
   a. The lateral part contains the femoral artery (10.28).
   b. The middle part contains the femoral vein.
   c. The medial part is occupied only by some lymph nodes and some areolar tissue: and this part is called the ***femoral canal.***

## Branches of the Femoral Artery

1. These are shown in 10.24. The first three branches are superficial and the remaining are deep.
2. The superficial branches arise from the femoral artery just below the inguinal ligament and piercing the femoral sheath and the cribriform fascia they become subcutaneous. Their further course is given below.
   a. The ***superficial epigastric*** artery ascends across the inguinal ligament and then runs upwards and medially towards the umbilicus.
   b. The ***superficial external pudendal*** artery runs medially to supply the skin over the external genitalia and on the lower part of the abdomen.
   c. The ***deep external pudendal*** artery runs medially deep to the fascia lata. It becomes superficial after crossing the adductor longus and supplies the external genitalia.
   d. The ***descending genicular*** artery arises from the femoral artery near its lower end. It gives:
      i. Numerous muscular branches
      ii. Articular branches to the knee joint
      iii. A saphenous branch that accompanies the saphenous nerve (through the adductor canal) and supplies the skin over the upper and medial part of the leg.

e. The ***profunda femoris*** artery is the largest branch of the femoral artery (10.25). It is the main artery of supply for the muscles of the thigh.
   i. It arises from the lateral side of the femoral artery, 3 to 4 cm below the inguinal ligament.
   ii. It descends first lateral to the femoral vessels and then behind them. In the lower part of its course, it is separated from the femoral artery by the adductor longus.
   iii. It gives off several branches that are shown in 10.25. These are:
      - The medial and lateral circumflex femoral arteries
      - Three perforating arteries
      - The terminal part of the profunda femoris artery itself is called the fourth perforating artery.
   iv. The further distribution of the medial and lateral circumflex femoral arteries is shown in 10.25, and is given below.
   v. The perforating branches pass through several muscles attached to the femur, at or near the linea aspera.
      - The perforating arteries are connected to each other by vertical anastomoses.

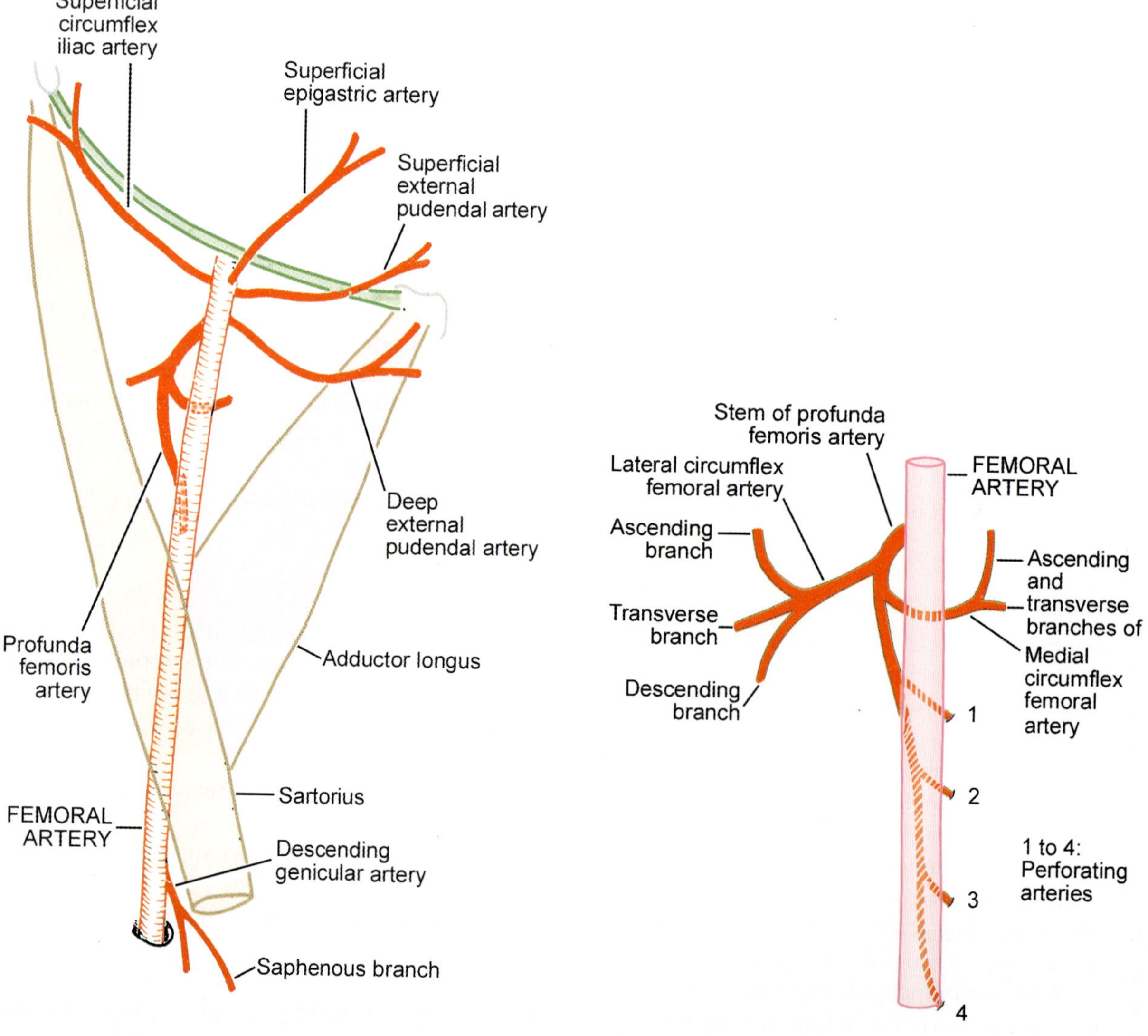


**10.24:** Branches of femoral artery

**10.25:** Branches of the profunda femoris artery

- The first perforating artery anastomoses above with the inferior gluteal artery.
- The fourth perforating artery anastomoses with branches of the popliteal artery.

vi. These anastomoses provide an important collateral circulation, if the femoral artery is blocked.

## Lateral Circumflex Artery

1. Its ***ascending branch*** passes laterally to the lateral side of the hip joint (10.25).
2. The ***transverse branch*** winds round the lateral side of the femur (passing through muscles) and takes part in forming the cruciate anastomosis.
3. The ***descending branch*** runs downwards behind the rectus femoris and along the vastus lateralis. Some of its branches reach the knee.

## Medial Circumflex Artery

1. This artery winds round the medial side of the femur passing through muscles. It emerges on the back of the thigh between the upper border of the adductor magnus and the quadratus femoris.
2. It then divides into transverse and ascending branches.

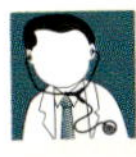

## CLINICAL CORRELATION

1. Pulsations of the femoral artery can be felt just below the midinguinal point.
2. Here the artery can be pressed against the superior ischiopubic ramus to stop bleeding.

**Use of Femoral Artery for Arteriography**

1. The femoral artery is used for inserting a catheter that is passed through the external iliac and common iliac arteries into the aorta.
   a. It can then be passed into one of the branches of the aorta.
   b. The catheter can be used for injecting a suitable contrast medium into the artery.
   c. A radiograph taken immediately after the injection displays the branches of the artery into which the dye is injected.
   d. The procedure is called angiography. Points of narrowing of the artery can be detected.
2. A suitable catheter passed through the aorta can reach the opening of a coronary artery. Dye injected can outline the coronary artery and any points of narrowing can be seen (***left cardiac angiography***).
3. Catheters introduced into an artery can also be used for recording pressures within the vessel, and for obtaining samples for analysis of blood gases.

3. The ***transverse branch*** takes part in forming the cruciate anastomosis.
4. The ***ascending branch*** ascends to reach the trochanteric fossa.
5. The medial circumflex artery also gives an ***acetabular branch*** to the hip joint.

## FEMORAL VEIN

1. The course and relations of the femoral vein correspond to those of the femoral artery. These have been considered above.
2. The relationship of the femoral vein to the femoral artery is shown in 10.22 and has been described while describing the femoral artery.
3. The chief tributaries of the femoral vein are shown in 10.26. They are:
   a. The great saphenous vein
   b. The profunda femoris vein
   c. The medial and lateral circumflex femoral veins
   d. A number of muscular branches.
4. Note that the medial and lateral circumflex veins generally open directly into the femoral vein and not through the profunda femoris vein.

5. The veins accompanying the superficial branches of the femoral artery (viz. the superficial circumflex iliac, the superficial epigastric and the superficial external pudendal) end in the great saphenous vein and not directly into the femoral vein.

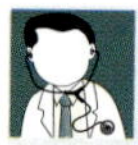

## CLINICAL CORRELATION

**Canulation of Femoral Vein**

A canula passes into the femoral vein can go right up to the right side of the heart. It can be used for taking blood samples and for recording pressures. The femoral vein is canulated as it lies in the femoral triangle.

## WANT TO KNOW MORE?

**Femoral Sheath**

1. In the upper part of the femoral triangle, the femoral artery and vein are enclosed in a funnel-like covering of fascia which is called as femoral sheath.
2. The sheath is formed by prolongations of fascia from within the abdomen.
   a. The anterior wall is formed by the fascia transversalis (which lines the inner aspect of the anterior abdominal wall).
   b. The posterior wall is formed by the fascia iliaca (fascia covering the iliopsoas muscle)(10.27).
   c. The two fasciae fuse with each other on the medial and lateral sides.
   d. They blend with the femoral vessels about 3 cm below the inguinal ligament (10.28).
3. The cavity within the femoral sheath is divisible into three parts:
   a. The lateral part contains the femoral artery (10.28). (It also contains the femoral branch of the genitofemoral nerve).
   b. The middle part contains the femoral vein.
   c. The medial part is occupied only by some lymph nodes and some areolar tissue and this part is called the femoral canal.

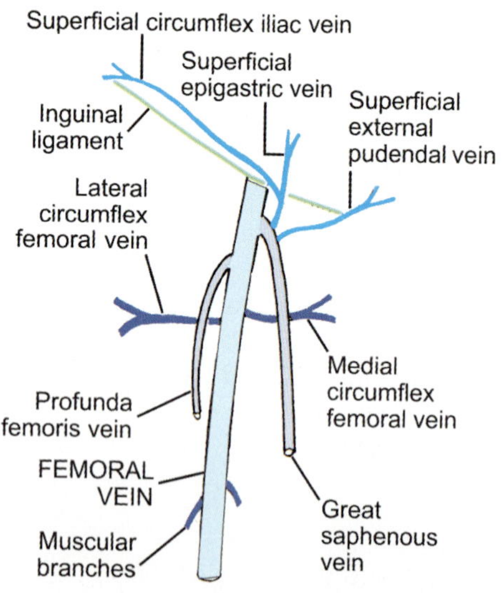


**10.26:** Tributaries of the femoral vein

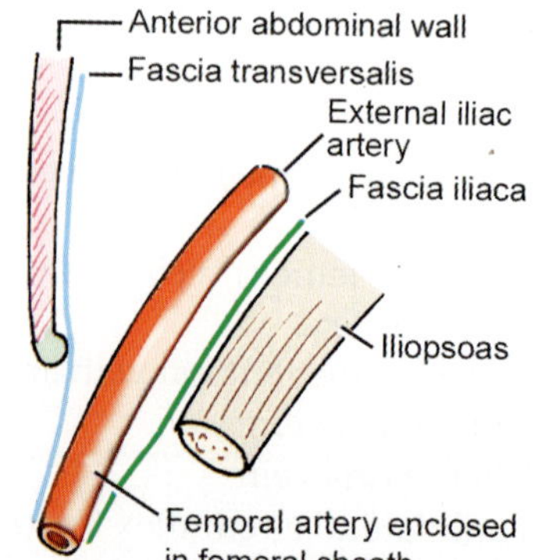


**10.27:** Scheme to show formation of the femoral sheath

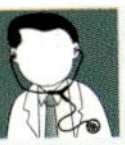

## CLINICAL CORRELATION

### Femoral Canal

1. The upper end of the femoral canal is called the ***femoral ring***. The ring is bounded as follows:
   a. Anteriorly by the inguinal ligament.
   b. Medially by the free margin of the lacunar ligament.
   c. Laterally by the femoral vein.
   d. Posteriorly by the pectineus and its fascia (10.28).
2. The extraperitoneal tissue filling the femoral ring is called the ***femoral septum***.
3. Lymph nodes lying within the canal drain the glans penis in the male and the clitoris in the female. The importance of the femoral canal is that, it can be the site of hernia.

### Hernia

1. The term hernia is applied to a protrusion of structures lying within a cavity through an area of weakness in the wall of the cavity.
   a. For example abdominal contents (like coils of intestine) can press upon an area of weakness in the abdominal wall.
   b. The pressure gradually creates a sac like protrusion of peritoneum that passes through the abdominal wall. Loops of intestine (or other contents) pass into the peritoneal protrusion and create a swelling.
2. The process of passage of contents out of the abdominal wall is ***herniation*** and the swelling is a ***hernia***. The peritoneal protrusion is the ***sac*** of the hernia, and the coils of intestine are the ***contents*** of the hernia.
3. Pressure on the swelling can push the contents back into the abdominal cavity. This is referred to as ***reduction*** of hernia.
4. Sometimes, the opening in the abdominal wall through which herniation takes place is narrow and reduction of the hernia may not be possible. Pressure on the loops of intestine (or other contents) by the narrow opening may occlude blood supply to the coils. The hernia is then said to be ***strangulated***. Such a hernia needs to be operated upon urgently to prevent the coils of intestine from undergoing necrosis.

### *Femoral Hernia*

1. A ***femoral hernia*** is one in which abdominal contents pass into the femoral canal (which represents the area of weakness).
   a. As the hernia enlarges the contents first pass downwards into the femoral canal.
   b. They then pass forwards through the saphenous opening.
   c. Finally they pass upwards to lie just below the inguinal ligament.
2. Femoral hernia is more common in the female because the pelvis (and as a result, the femoral canal) is wider in this sex.
3. In case of strangulation of a femoral hernia, the surgeon has to enlarge the femoral ring.
   a. This enlargement can only be done into the medial wall (lacunar ligament).
   b. Cutting of the lacunar ligament can sometimes result in serious bleeding caused by an abnormal obturator artery.

### Abnormal Obturator Artery and Femoral Canal

1. The obturator artery lies within the pelvis and is a branch of the internal iliac artery. It gives off a pubic branch that anastomoses with the pubic branch of the inferior epigastric artery (a branch of the external iliac artery).
2. Sometimes, this anastomosis is very large and blood flowing into the obturator artery is mainly through this anastomosis. This is referred to as abnormal obturator artery.
3. This abnormal artery is closely related to the femoral ring.
   a. Usually it lies in the lateral wall of the ring, near the femoral vein.
   b. Sometimes, however, it lies medial to the ring, along the edge of the lacunar ligament (10.31). When the abnormal artery is in this position it is likely to be cut when the ring is enlarged medially to relieve a strangulated femoral hernia.

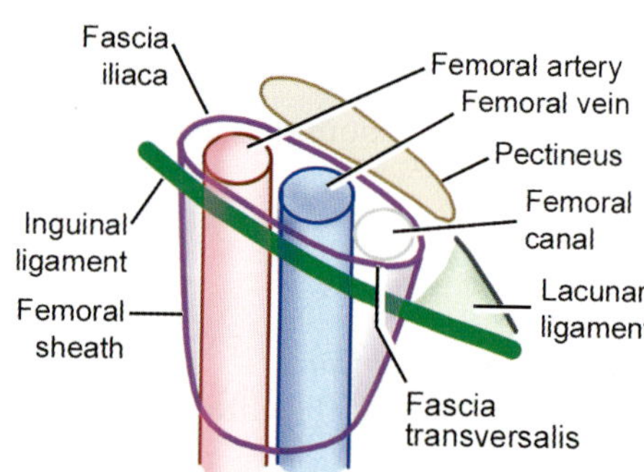


10.28: Scheme to show the formation of the femoral canal

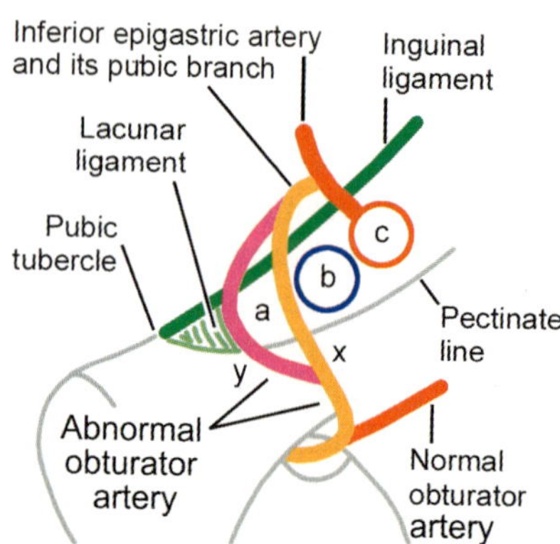


10.29: Pubic region seen from behind to show the course of an abnormal obturator artery in relation to the femoral canal. The usual position of this artery is shown at x. When the artery is at position y it can be damaged if the femoral canal (a) is widened by incision into the medial wall. Here, (b) refers to femoral vein and (c) refers to junction of external iliac artery with femoral artery

## NERVES ON FRONT AND MEDIAL SIDE OF THIGH

The nerves to be seen on the front and medial side of the thigh are branches of the lumbar plexus. As a preliminary to a study of the nerves we will first study the formation and branches of the lumbar plexus.

### Lumbar Nerves and Lumbar Plexus

1. The lumbar plexus is formed by the upper four lumbar nerves. After emerging from the intervertebral foramina each nerve divides into a dorsal ramus and a ventral ramus.
2. The ***dorsal rami*** are distributed as described in Chapter 4 (page 56). In 10.3, note that the dorsal rami of lumbar and sacral nerves contribute to the cutaneous nerve supply of the gluteal region.
3. The ***ventral rami*** enter the substance of the psoas major muscle. Within the muscle, the rami from the upper four lumbar nerves join each other to form the ***lumbar plexus*** which is shown in 10.30. Note that part of the fourth lumbar nerve joins the fifth lumbar to form the lumbosacral trunk which takes part in forming the sacral plexus.
4. The greater part of the first lumbar nerve is continued into a nerve trunk that divides into the ***iliohypogastric*** and ***ilioinguinal*** nerves.
5. The rest of the first lumbar nerve is joined by a branch from the second lumbar to form the ***genitofemoral*** nerve.
6. The second, third and the greater part of the fourth lumbar nerve divide into ***anterior*** and ***posterior divisions***.
7. The posterior divisions (which are large) form the ***femoral nerve***. The posterior divisions of L2 and L3 also give rise to the ***lateral cutaneous nerve of the thigh***.
8. The anterior divisions unite to form the ***obturator nerve***.

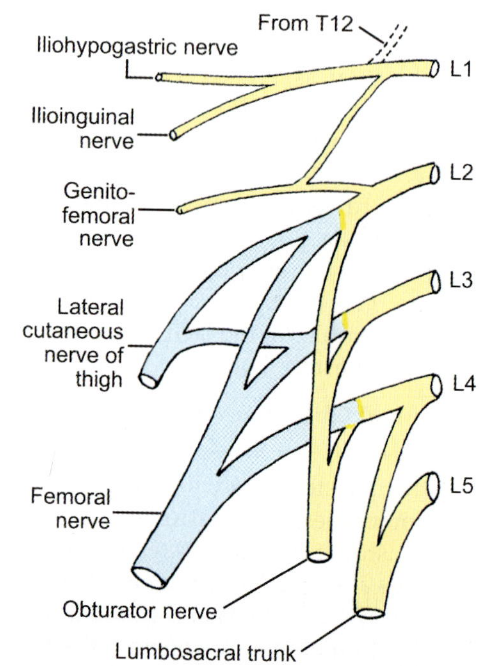


10.30: Scheme to show the lumbar plexus and its branches

9. In addition to the above named branches others are given off to the psoas major (L2, L3), the quadratus lumborum (T12, L1, L2, L3), the psoas minor (L1) and the iliacus (L2, L3).
We will now consider the branches of the plexus one by one. Some of the points will be understood only after the abdomen has been studied, but it is useful to give a complete description here.

## Iliohypogastric Nerve

1. The iliohypogastric nerve (L1) runs a short course within the substance of the psoas major and emerges from the muscle at its lateral margin.
2. The nerve then runs downwards and laterally over the quadratus lumborum. Here, it lies behind the corresponding kidney (10.31). At the lateral margin of the quadratus lumborum, the nerve enters the interval between the internal oblique and transversus muscles (10.32).
3. It runs downwards, forwards and medially between these muscles.
4. The nerve gives off a lateral cutaneous branch that becomes superficial by piercing the internal and external oblique muscles a little above the iliac crest. It crosses the crest and supplies the skin in the anterior part of the gluteal region.

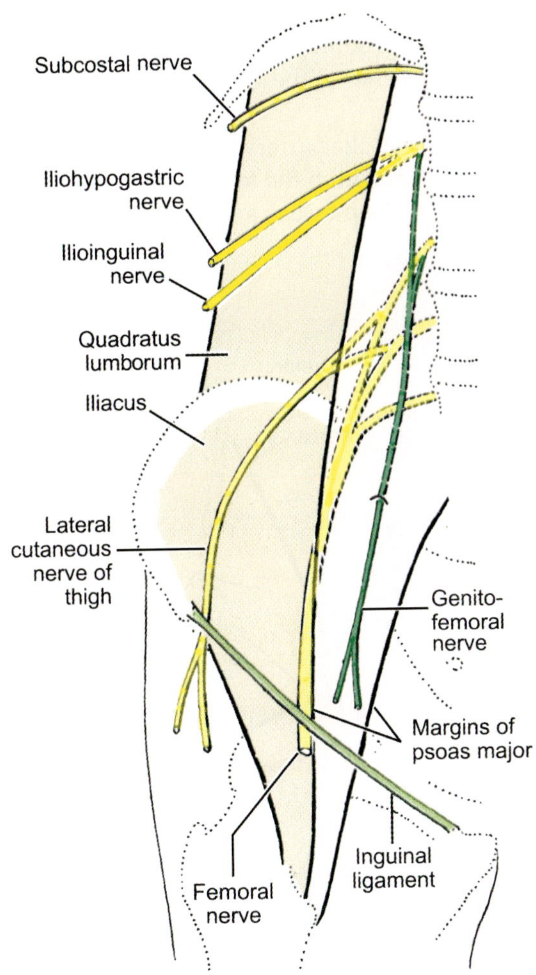


**10.31:** Scheme to show some branches of the lumbar plexus as they lie on the posterior abdominal wall

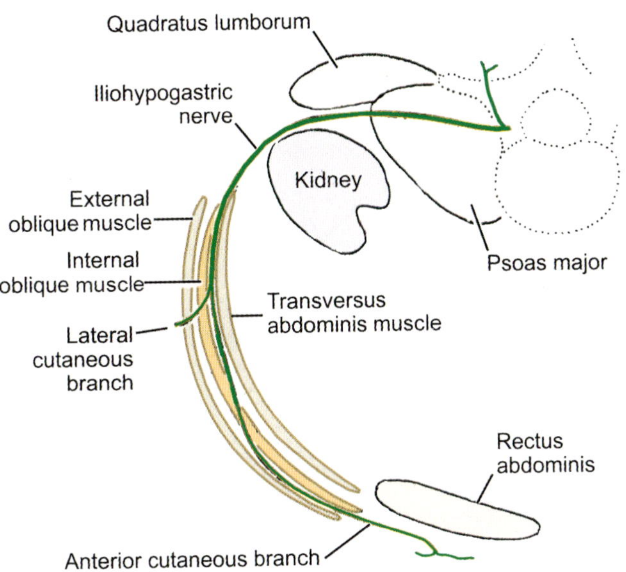


**10.32:** Scheme to show the course of the iliohypogastric nerve

5. The rest of the iliohypogastric nerve is called the ***anterior cutaneous branch***. It runs medially and becomes superficial by piercing the internal oblique muscle and the aponeurosis of the external oblique muscle. It emerges from the latter a little above the superficial inguinal ring, and ends by supplying the skin above the pubis.

## Ilioinguinal Nerve

1. The ilioinguinal nerve (L1) arises in common with the iliohypogastric nerve and has a similar course first through the psoas major, next in front of the quadratus lumborum (behind the kidney), and then between the transversus abdominis and the internal oblique muscles (10.31).
2. It pierces the internal oblique a little above the lateral part of the inguinal ligament to enter the inguinal canal. (Note that the nerve does not pass through the deep inguinal ring).
3. It leaves the inguinal canal by passing through the superficial inguinal ring.
4. It ends by supplying the skin of the upper and medial part of the thigh (10.33), over the pubis and the adjoining part of the genitalia. (Note that the ilioinguinal nerve does not give off a lateral cutaneous branch).

## Genitofemoral Nerve

1. The genitofemoral nerve (L1, L2) runs downwards first in the substance of the psoas major and then on its anterior surface (10.31). The nerve passes deep to the ureter. It ends by dividing into genital and femoral branches.
2. The ***genital branch*** comes into relationship with the lateral side of the external iliac artery. It crosses in front of the lower part of the artery and enters the inguinal canal through the deep inguinal ring (10.34).
3. The nerve supplies the ***cremaster and dartos muscles,*** and gives some branches to the skin of the scrotum or of the labium majus.
4. The ***femoral branch*** continues to descend on the lateral side of the external iliac artery. It passes deep to the inguinal ligament and comes to lie lateral to the femoral artery. Here, it lies within the femoral sheath.
5. It becomes superficial by piercing the anterior wall of the sheath, and the deep fascia, and supplies an area of skin over the upper part of the femoral triangle (10.34).

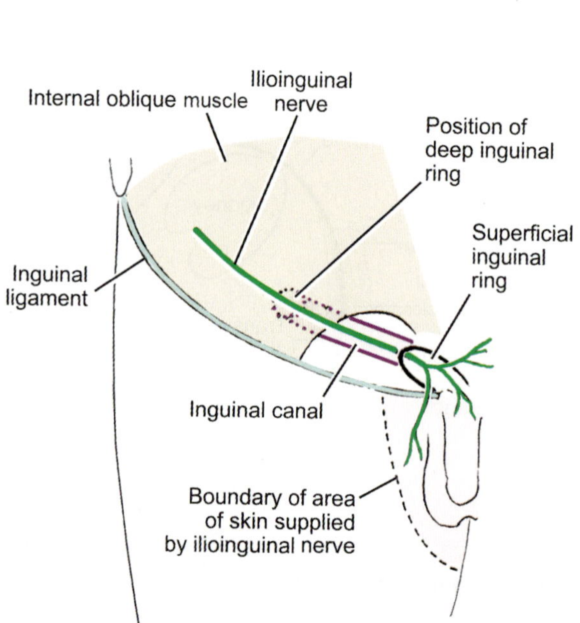


**10.33:** Scheme to show the course of the anterior part of the ilioinguinal nerve

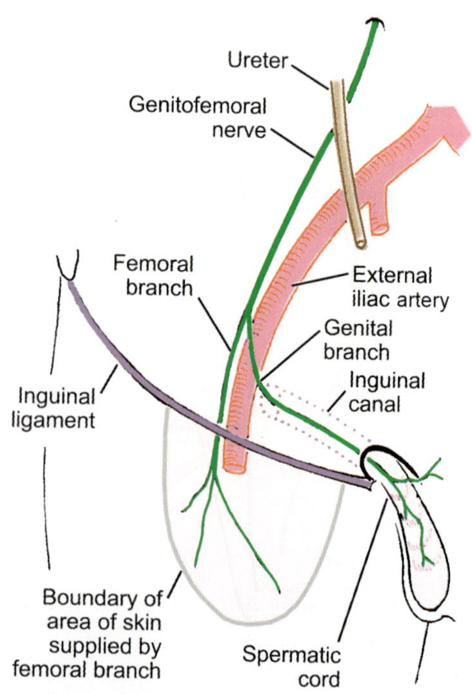


**10.34:** Scheme to show the course of the genitofemoral nerve

## Lateral Cutaneous Nerve of Thigh

1. The lateral cutaneous nerve of the thigh is derived from the dorsal divisions of L2 and L3. Its initial part lies within the psoas major. Emerging from the lateral border of the muscle the nerve runs downwards, laterally and forwards over the iliacus muscle to reach the anterior superior iliac spine (10.31).
2. It enters the thigh by passing behind the lateral end of the inguinal ligament. It divides into anterior and posterior branches through which it supplies the skin on the anterolateral part of the thigh right up to the knee.
3. While the nerve is over the iliacus muscle, it is related to the caecum on the right side, and to the part of the descending colon on the left side.

## The Obturator Nerve

1. This nerve is formed by union of roots arising from L2, L3, and L4 (10.30 and 10.35). For convenience of description its course can be considered in three parts.
2. The first part runs downwards in the substance of the psoas major.
3. The second part of the nerve lies in the lateral wall of the true pelvis (10.36). It runs downwards and forwards lying over the obturator internus muscle.
   a. This part of the nerve is crossed by the internal iliac artery and vein.
   b. It is accompanied by the obturator vessels which lie below and behind it.
4. It leaves the lateral wall of the pelvis by passing through the upper part of the obturator foramen to enter the thigh.
5. The third part of the nerve lies in the thigh. As it passes through the obturator foramen, it divides into anterior and posterior divisions (10.35).
6. The anterior division lies in front of the obturator externus (above) and the adductor brevis (below): It lies behind the pectineus (above) and the adductor longus (below).
7. The posterior division lies in front of the obturator externus (above) and the adductor magnus (below). It is behind the pectineus (above) and the adductor brevis (below).

   The obturator nerve is distributed as follows (10.35):

***Muscular Branches***

Branches arising from the anterior division supply:

a. Obturator externus
b. Adductor longus
c. Gracilis
d. Pectineus and the adductor brevis (sometimes).

Branches of the posterior division supply:

a. Obturator externus
b. Adductor brevis
c. Adductor magnus.

### *Cutaneous Branches*

After supplying the muscles named above the anterior division supplies the skin of the lower medial part of the thigh. (These fibres may reach the skin through a branch that joins the medial cutaneous and saphenous branches of the femoral nerve to form the ***subsartorial plexus***).

### *Articular Branches*

These are given off to the hip joint and to the knee joint. The latter is a continuation of the posterior division and travels along the femoral artery.

### *Vascular Branches*

The anterior division ends by supplying the femoral artery.

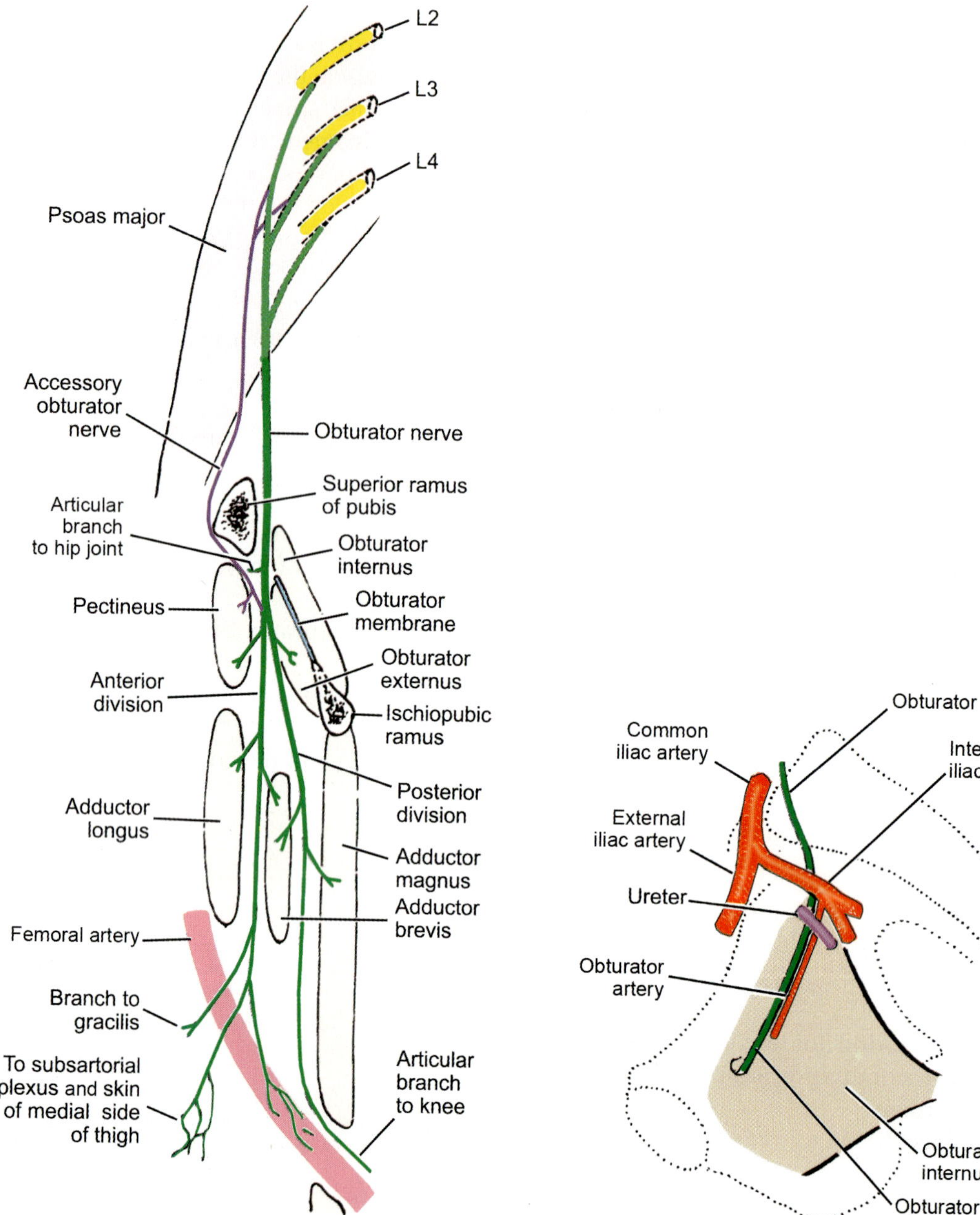


**10.35:** Scheme to show the course and distribution of the obturator nerve

**10.36:** Lateral wall of true pelvis showing the obturator nerve and some related structures

## Accessory Obturator Nerve

1. Occasionally, some fibres of the obturator nerve follow a separate course and are termed the ***accessory obturator nerve*** (10.35).
2. Arising from L2 and L3 this nerve runs downwards along the medial margin of the psoas major in company with the external iliac vessels.
3. It does not enter the true pelvis, but passes behind the inguinal ligament (deep to the pectineus) to reach the thigh.

4. The nerve ends by supplying the pectineus and the hip joint and communicates with the anterior division of the obturator nerve.

## The Femoral Nerve

1. The femoral nerve arises from the ventral rami of spinal nerves L2, L3 and L4 within the substance of the psoas major. It descends through this muscle and emerges from its lateral border a few centimetres above the inguinal ligament (10.31).
2. It now comes to lie in the groove between the iliacus (laterally) and the psoas (medially). In this position, it passes behind the inguinal ligament to enter the thigh. Here, it lies lateral to the femoral artery. After a short course it ends by dividing into anterior and posterior divisions. The distribution of the femoral nerve is as follows:

### *Muscular Branches*

1. While still in the abdomen, the femoral nerve gives branches to the iliacus (10.37).
2. A little above the inguinal ligament, the femoral nerve gives off the ***nerve to the pectineus***. The nerve passes downwards and medially ***behind*** the femoral vessels to reach the pectineus.
3. The sartorius receives a branch from the anterior division of the femoral nerve. This branch arises in common with the intermediate cutaneous nerve of the thigh (see below).
4. The posterior division of the femoral nerve supplies:
   a. The rectus femoris
   b. The vastus lateralis

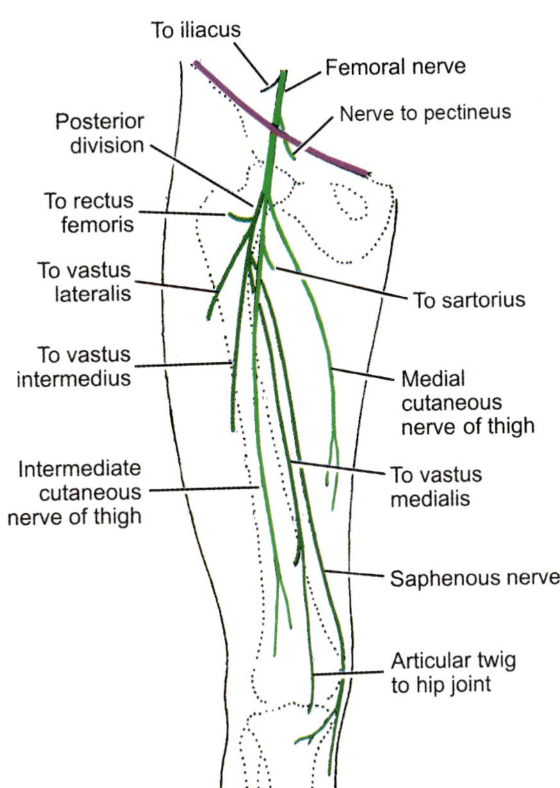


**10.37:** Scheme to show the distribution of the femoral nerve in the thigh

c. The vastus medialis
d. The vastus intermedius.

### Cutaneous Branches

1. The ***intermediate cutaneous nerve of the thigh*** arises from the anterior division of the femoral nerve (10.37).
   a. It supplies a broad strip of skin on the front of thigh.
   b. The lower end of the area reaches the front of the knee (10.1).
2. The ***medial cutaneous nerve of the thigh*** is a branch of the anterior division of the femoral nerve.
   a. It first lies along the lateral side of the femoral artery which it crosses near the apex of the femoral triangle.
   b. It divides into branches that supply the skin of the medial side of the thigh. The area of skin supplied is shown in 10.1.
   c. The nerve takes part in forming the ***subsartorial plexus*** (along with branches of the saphenous and obturator nerves).
3. The ***saphenous nerve*** arises from the posterior division of the femoral nerve.
   a. It descends along the lateral side of the femoral artery.
   b. In the adductor canal, the nerve crosses the artery from lateral to medial side (10.23).
   c. It leaves the adductor canal at its lower end and runs down along the medial side of the knee. Here, it pierces the deep fascia and becomes subcutaneous.
   d. It then runs down the medial side of the leg (alongside the long saphenous vein). A branch extends along the medial side of the foot (but ends short of the great toe). The area of skin supplied by the nerve is shown in 10.2.
   e. The saphenous nerve takes part in forming the subsartorial plexus and the ***patellar plexus***.

### Articular Branches

1. The posterior division of the femoral nerve sends fibres to the knee joint through the nerve to the vastus medialis.
2. Some fibres reach the hip joint through the nerve to the rectus femoris.

### Vascular Branches of Femoral Nerve

These reach the femoral artery and its branches.

# Gluteal Region, Back of Thigh and Popliteal Fossa

## GLUTEAL REGION

### Superficial Structures

1. The cutaneous nerve supply has been described in Chapter 10 and is shown in 10.3.
2. The superficial fascia over the gluteal region usually contains abundant fat. This fat serves as a cushion while sitting.
3. Lymphatics of the region drain into the lateral group of superficial inguinal lymph nodes.

## MUSCLES OF THE GLUTEAL REGION

The muscles of the gluteal region are:

1. Gluteus maximus
2. Gluteus medius
3. Gluteus minimus
4. Piriformis
5. Obturator internus
6. Gemelli
7. Quadratus femoris
8. Obturator externus.

The attachments of the muscles are given in 11.1 (Also see 11.2).

### Note on Gluteus Maximus

1. Through a combination of all the actions described in 11.1, this muscle plays a very important role in maintaining the upright position of the body.
2. Several bones, ligaments, muscles, nerves and vessels lie under cover of the gluteus maximus.

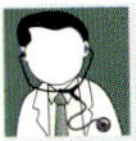

### CLINICAL CORRELATION

**Trendelenberg sign**

1. With the femur fixed (as in standing), the gluteus medius and minimus pulls the corresponding side of the pelvis downwards by rotating it over the head of the femur.
2. As a result, the opposite side of the pelvis is raised. In this way, the muscles of one side prevent the opposite side of the pelvis from sinking downwards, when the limb of that side is off the ground. In fact, the pelvis on the unsupported side is somewhat higher than on the supported side.
3. In paralysis of the medius and minimus, the unsupported side becomes lower than the supported side. This is referred to as the ***Trendelenberg sign***.
4. A positive Trendelenberg sign can also be seen in dislocation of the hip joint or fracture of the neck of the femur.

**11.1: Muscles of the gluteal region**

| *Muscle* | *Origin* | *Insertion* | *Action* | *Nerve supply* |
|---|---|---|---|---|
| Gluteus Maximus | 1. External surface of ilium (posterior gluteal line and area behind it)<br>2. Sacrotuberous ligament<br>3. Aponeurosis covering erector spinae<br>4. Posterior surface of sacrum (lower lateral part)<br>5. Posterior surface of coccyx (lateral part) | 1. Iliotibial tract. (Pulls on lateral condyle of tibia)<br>2. Gluteal tuberosity of femur (deep fibres) | 1. Extension of thigh (as in standing up from sitting position or climbing)<br>2. When the femur and tibia are fixed as in standing:<br>a. Straightens the trunk, after stooping<br>b. Maintains upright position of trunk<br>3. Through iliotibial tract, it steadies femur on tibia (in standing) | Inferior gluteal nerve (L5, S1, 2) |
| Gluteus Medius | External surface of ilium. The area is bounded, by the iliac crest (above), posterior gluteal line (behind), and anterior gluteal line (in front) | Lateral surface of greater trochanter of femur (on ridge running downward and forward) | Action common for both the muscles:<br>1. Both muscles are abductors of the thigh<br>2. The minimus and anterior fibres of medius can act as flexors and medial rotators<br>3. Posterior fibres of medius act as extensors and lateral rotators of thigh<br>4. When the femur is fixed (as in standing), the medius and minimus pull their own side of the pelvis downward (by rotating it over the head of the femur). The opposite side of the pelvis is raised | Superior gluteal nerve (L5, S1) |
| Gluteus Minimus | External surface of ilium, between the anterior and inferior gluteal lines | Anterior aspect of greater trochanter of femur | | Superior gluteal nerve (L5, S1) |
| Piriformis | Anterior (pelvic) surface of sacrum (by three digitations) | Upper border of greater trochanter of femur | Lateral rotator of femur | Direct branches from nerves (L5, S1, S2) |
| Obturator internus | 1. From pelvic surface of hip bone including the following:<br>a. Body, superior ramus, and inferior ramus of pubis<br>b. Ramus and body of ischium<br>c. Part of ilium<br>2. Obturator membrane | 1. Tendon leaves the pelvis through the lesser sciatic foramen to appear in the gluteal region<br>2. Tendon then runs laterally behind the hip joint to reach the medial surface of greater trochanter of femur (in front of trochanteric fossa) | Lateral rotator of femur | Nerve to obturator internus (L5, S1) |

*Contd...*

*Contd...*

| *Muscle* | *Origin* | *Insertion* | *Action* | *Nerve supply* |
|---|---|---|---|---|
| Superior gemellus | Posterior aspect of ischial spine | Tendon of obturator internus (thus indirectly into greater trochanter of femur) | Lateral rotator of femur | Nerve to obturator internus (L5, S1) |
| Inferior gemellus | Uppermost part of ischial tuberosity | | | Nerve to quadratus femoris (L5, S1) |
| Quadratus femoris | Lateral border of ischial tuberosity | Quadrate tubercle (on upper part of trochanteric crest of femur) | Lateral rotator of femur | Nerve to quadratus femoris (L4, 5, S1) |
| Obturator externus | External surface of anterior part of pelvis including parts of:<br>a. Ramus of ischium<br>b. Ramus of pubis<br>c. Obturator membrane (medial two-thirds) | Tendon runs laterally behind neck of femur to be inserted into trochanteric fossa (on medial surface of greater trochanter) | Lateral rotator of femur | Obturator nerve (L3, 4) |

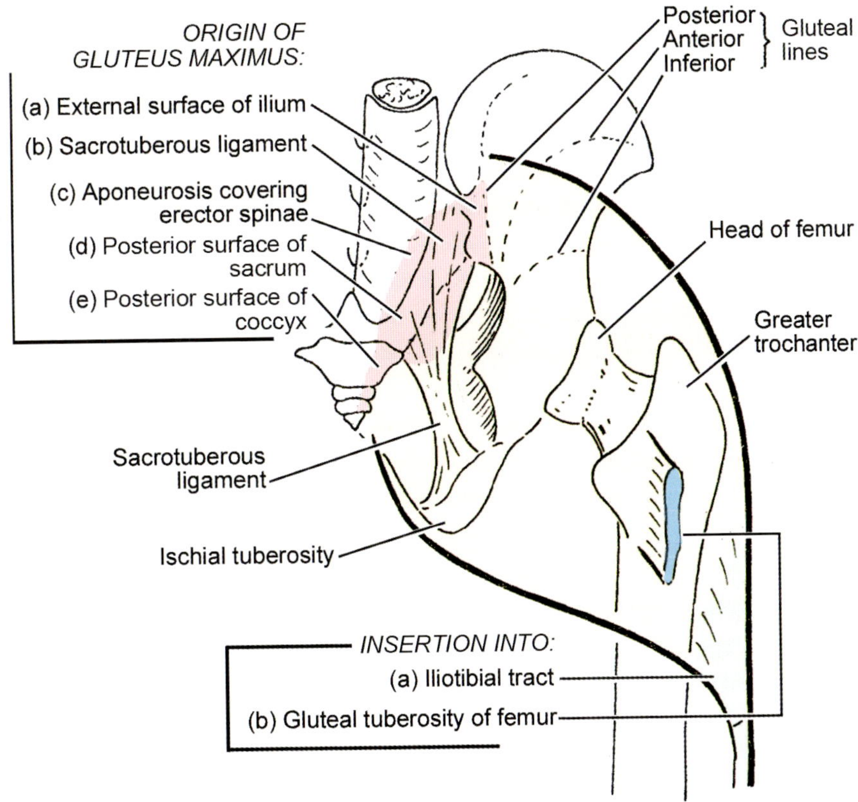


**11.2:** Scheme to show the attachments of the gluteus maximus

## Note on Piriformis

The pelvic part of the piriformis is related anteriorly to:

1. Rectum
2. Branches of sacral plexus
3. Branches of internal iliac vessels
4. Posterior aspect of ischium.

## Note on Obturator Internus

1. This muscle arises from the inner (pelvic) surface of the hip bone and from the pelvic surface of the obturator membrane.
   a. The fibres of the muscle converge towards a tendon, that leaves the pelvis through the lesser sciatic foramen to enter the gluteal region.
   b. The tendon turns through 90 degrees and runs laterally behind the hip joint to reach its insertion.
2. The muscle is covered by a thick ***obturator fascia.***
   a. The levator ani muscle (present in the true pelvis) has a linear origin from this fascia (11.3).
   b. The part of the fascia below the origin of the levator ani forms the lateral wall of the ***ischiorectal fossa*** and is closely related to the ***pudendal canal*** (through which the pudendal nerve and internal pudendal vessels pass) (This region will be studied when we deal with the pelvis in volume 2).

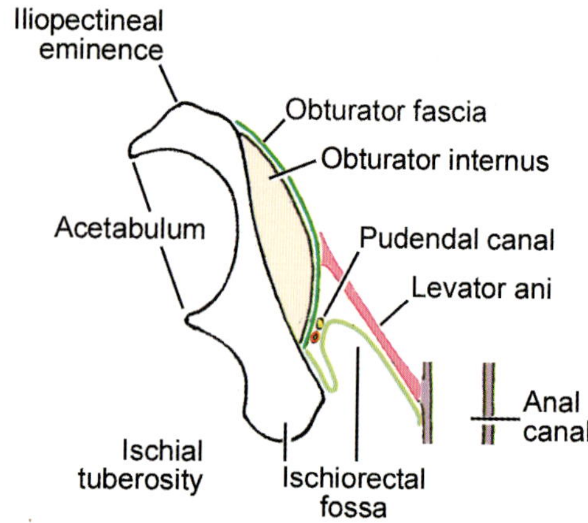


**11.3:** Vertical section through the anterior and inferior parts of the pelvis to show some relations of the obturator internus muscle

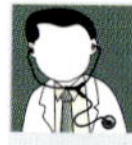

### CLINICAL CORRELATION

**Note on Actions of Small Muscles around the Hip Joint**

1. Although, the various small muscles related to the hip joint are described as medial or lateral rotators, their main action is to stabilise the joint.
2. In performing this action, they have an advantage over ligaments in that they can fix the joint in any position, whereas a ligament can do so only when fully stretched. Such muscles are, therefore, sometimes referred to as ***extensible*** or ***adjustable ligaments***.

**Gluteal Muscles**

Intramuscular injections are commonly given into the gluteal region. Injury to the sciatic nerve can be avoided by giving injections only in the ***upper and anterior quadrant of the gluteal region***.

**Bursitis and Sores**

1. The bursa over the ischial tuberosity may get inflamed. This condition, is called ***Weaver's bottom***.
2. The ischial tuberosities bear body weight while sitting. In old people, in whom tissues have lost some vitality, the pressure can cause discomfort while sitting. In people who are paralysed (and cannot change position periodically) pressure on skin can lead to formation of sores.
3. Inflammation of a bursa overlying the greater trochanter (***trochanteric bursitis***) can lead to pain over the trochanter.

## ARTERIES OF GLUTEAL REGION

1. Most of the arteries to be seen in the gluteal region are branches of the internal iliac artery.
2. The internal iliac artery is a terminal branch of the common iliac artery, and lies within the pelvis.
3. It divides into anterior and posterior divisions, both of which give several further branches.

### Inferior Gluteal Artery

1. The inferior gluteal artery is a branch of the anterior division of the internal iliac artery.
2. It begins within the pelvis, where it lies anterior to the piriformis.

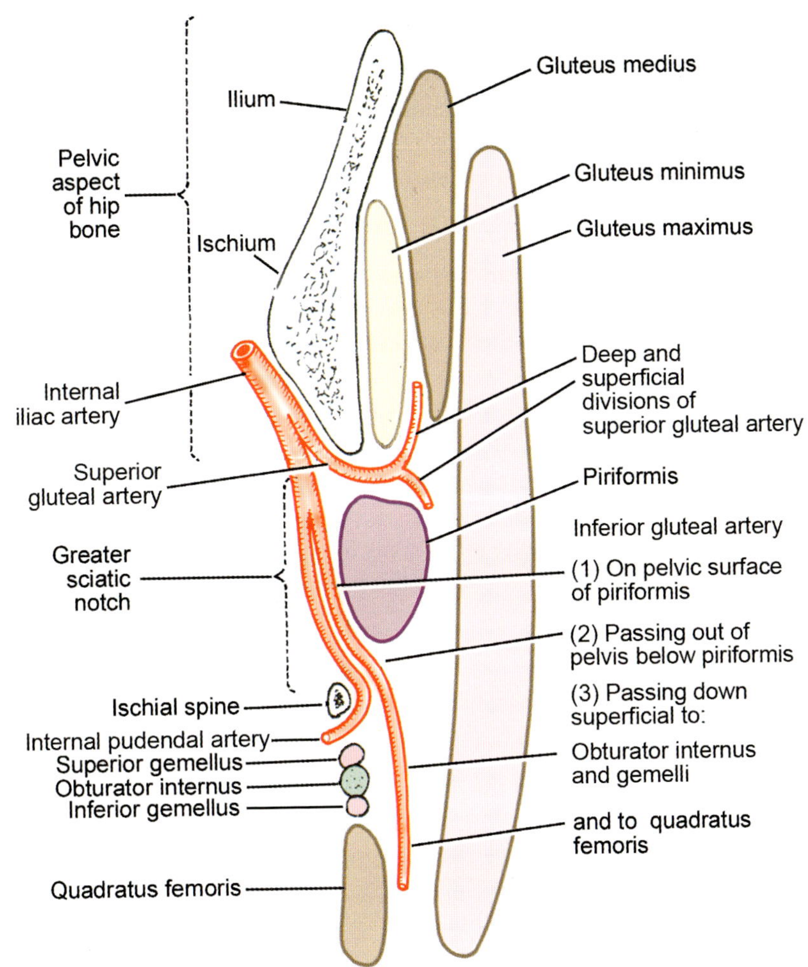


**11.4:** Schematic vertical section of the gluteal region to show the course of some arteries

3. It passes through the greater sciatic foramen, below the piriformis to enter the gluteal region (See 11.4).
4. It then descends deep to the gluteus maximus muscle, over the obturator internus (and gemelli) and the quadratus femoris and extends into the upper part of the thigh. Branches from the artery are meant mainly for supply of the muscles mentioned above.

## WANT TO KNOW MORE?

Other branches are as follows:

1. A fine branch, the ***artery of the sciatic nerve,*** descends along this nerve into the thigh.
2. An ***anastomotic branch*** takes part in forming the cruciate anastomosis.
3. A ***coccygeal branch*** runs towards the coccyx.
4. Some branches are also given to the hip joint and to the skin of the gluteal region.

### Superior Gluteal Artery

1. The superior gluteal artery is the main continuation of the posterior trunk of the internal iliac artery.
2. It leaves the pelvic cavity by passing through the greater sciatic foramen, above the piriformis muscle (11.5). The artery divides into superficial and deep branches.
3. The ***superficial branch*** ramifies deep to the gluteus maximus and supplies it.
4. The ***deep branch*** passes upwards over the gluteal surface of the ilium. It divides into superior and inferior divisions both of which lie deep to the gluteus medius.
5. The superior division runs along the upper border of the gluteus minimus, while the inferior division crosses the lower part of the same muscle. These branches supply the gluteus medius and gluteus minimus, and also send twigs to the hip joint.
6. The inferior division also sends a branch to the trochanteric anastomosis described below.

### Internal Pudendal Artery

1. This artery is a branch of the anterior trunk of the internal iliac artery.
2. The artery passes out of the pelvic cavity through the greater sciatic foramen to enter the gluteal region (11.4). Here, it lies inferior to the piriformis muscle.
3. It descends across the back of the ischial spine and leaves the gluteal region through the lesser sciatic foramen. Its further course will be considered, when we study the perineum.

**WANT TO KNOW MORE?**

**Cruciate Anastomosis**

This anastomosis (shaped like a cross) is seen in the lower part of the gluteal region.
The arteries taking part are:

1. The anastomotic branch of the inferior gluteal artery (from above).
2. The first perforating artery (from below).
3. Transverse branches of the medial and lateral circumflex femoral arteries (on the medial and lateral sides respectively).

**Trochanteric Anastomosis**

This anastomosis is seen in relation to the greater trochanter of the femur. The arteries taking part are:

1. The descending branch of the superior gluteal artery.
2. The ascending branches of the medial and lateral circumflex femoral arteries.
3. Sometimes a branch from the inferior gluteal artery also joins the anastomosis.

In the gluteal region, we also see the terminal part of the medial circumflex femoral artery.
The nerves of the gluteal region are described later in this chapter.

## BACK OF THIGH AND POPLITEAL FOSSA

## MUSCLES OF THE BACK OF THE THIGH

The muscles of the back of the thigh are:

1. Semitendinosus
2. Semimembranosus
3. Biceps femoris.

These are called the hamstring muscles. Their attachments are given in 11.5. (Also see 11.6 and 11.7).

**11.5: Muscles of the back of the thigh**

| | *Semitendinosus* | *Semimembranosus* | *Biceps Femoris* |
|---|---|---|---|
| Origin | Upper medial part of ischial tuberosity | Upper lateral part of ischial tuberosity | Long head from:<br>1. Upper medial part of ischial tuberosity<br>2. Sacrotuberous ligament.<br>Short head from linea aspera of femur |
| Insertion | Upper part of medial surface of tibia (behind sartorius, below and behind gracilis) | Medial condyle of tibia | Both heads end in a common tendon that is attached to the head of the fibula. |
| Nerve supply | Sciatic nerve (tibial part) (L5, S1, 2) | Sciatic nerve (tibial part) (L5, S1, 2) | Long head by sciatic nerve, tibial part (L5, S1, S2, S3)<br>Short head by peroneal part of sciatic nerve (L5, S1, 2) |
| Action | These are common to all hamstring muscles.<br>1. Flexion of leg at knee joint (when pelvis is fixed)<br>2. When the knee is fixed (as in standing) the ischial tuberosity is pulled downwards. This is useful in:<br>a. Preventing the pelvis from rolling forwards on the head of the femur<br>b. Straightening the trunk after bending forwards | | |

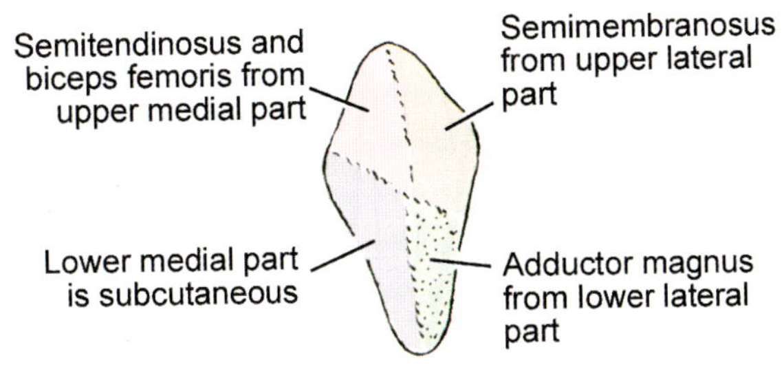


**11.6:** Ischial tuberosity seen from below and behind to show muscular attachments on it

## WANT TO KNOW MORE?

**Note on Semitendinosus**

1. The muscle is so called because its lower half is tendinous.
2. On reaching the knee, the tendon of the semitendinosus runs forwards across the tibial collateral ligament to reach its insertion.

**Note on Semimembranosus**

1. The muscle is so called because its upper part is membranous. The membranous part of the muscle lies under cover of the biceps femoris.
2. The origin of the muscle is tendinous. The lower part is fleshy. The fleshy fibres of the muscle end in a tendon which is placed along the medial edge of the muscle.

*Contd...*

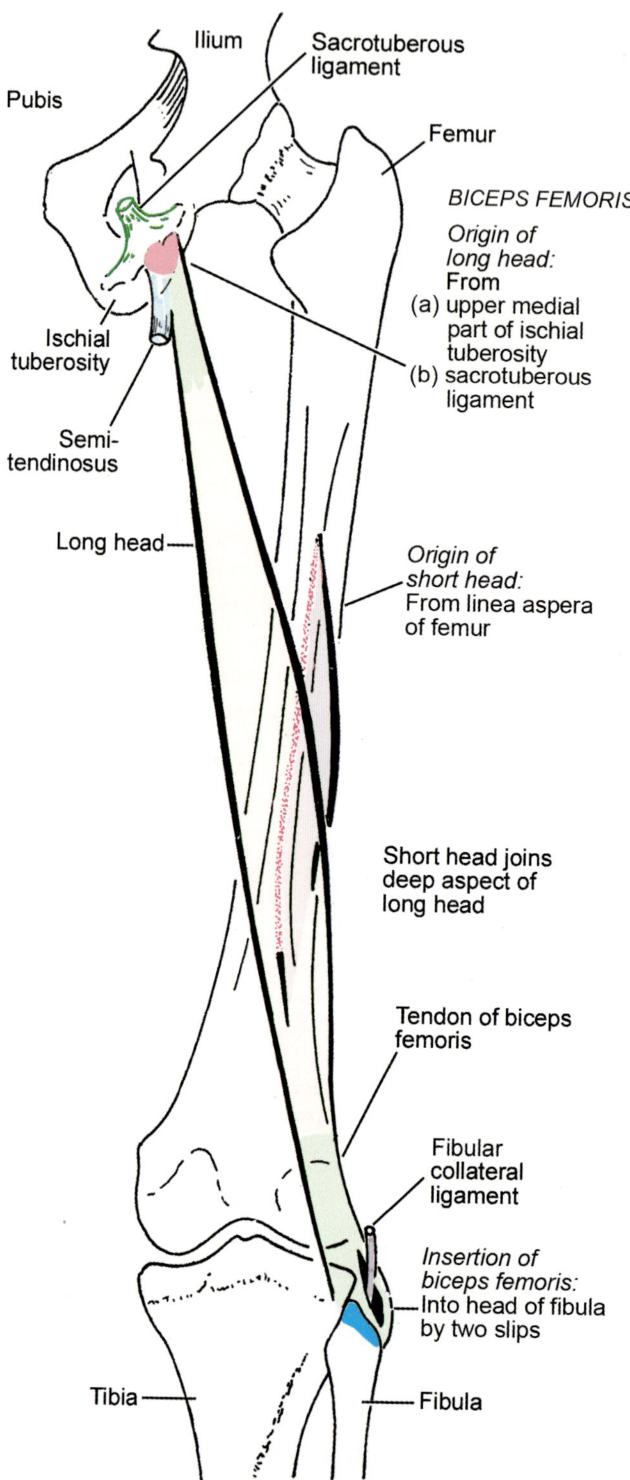


**11.7:** Scheme to show attachments of the biceps femoris muscle

*Contd...*

The following points should be noted about the insertion:

1. The posterior aspect of the medial condyle of the tibia is marked by a groove, at the lateral end of which there is a tubercle. The main insertion is into this tubercle.
2. Some fibres are inserted into the groove itself, and extend onto the medial aspect of the condyle as well.
3. Some fibres of the tendon pass upwards and laterally (forming the *oblique popliteal ligament* of the knee joint) and get attached to the lateral condyle of the femur.
4. Some fibres become continuous with the fascia covering the popliteus.
5. Some fibres descend to be attached to the medial margin of the shaft of the tibia behind the tibial collateral ligament.

**Note on Biceps Femoris**

1. The origin of the short head from the linea aspera lies between the insertion of the adductor magnus, medially, and the origin of the vastus lateralis, laterally.
2. The short head ends by joining the deep aspect of the long head. The two heads end in a common tendon which is inserted into the head of the fibula.
3. Just above the insertion, the tendon splits into two parts that embrace the fibular collateral ligament.

## POPLITEAL FOSSA

1. The popliteal fossa is a quadrilateral depression present on the back of the knee.
2. Its upper boundaries (medial and lateral) are formed by the hamstring muscles (11.8).
3. Its lower boundaries (medial and lateral) are formed by a large muscle, the gastrocnemius that will be studied in the leg.
4. A small muscle of the leg, the plantaris also appears in the lower lateral wall. Another muscle of the leg, the popliteus is seen in the floor of the fossa. The boundaries are:
   a. Above and laterally: Biceps femoris.
   b. Above and medially: Semitendinosus, and semimembranosus.
   c. Below and laterally: Lateral head of gastrocnemius, and plantaris.
   d. Below and medially: Medial head of gastrocnemius.
   e. Roof: Fascia over the fossa.
   f. Floor: Popliteal surface of femur, capsule of knee joint (including the oblique popliteal ligament), and fascia over the popliteus muscle (11.8).

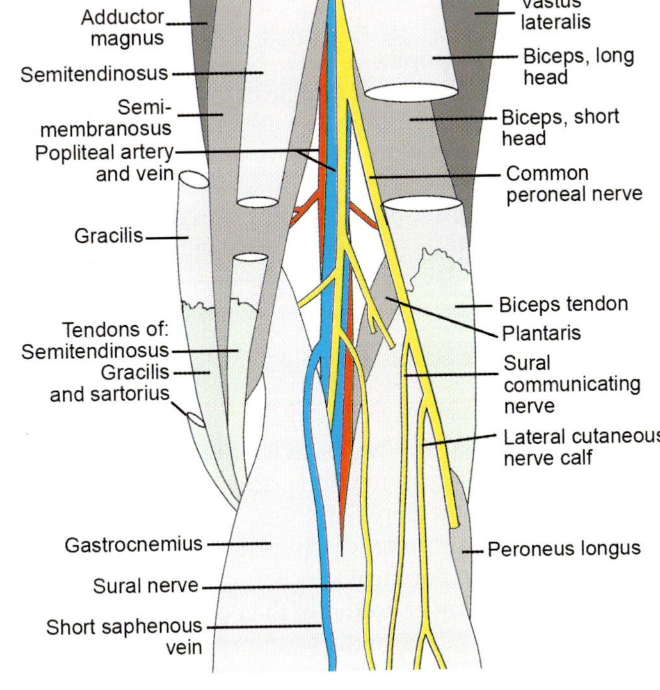


**11.8:** Popliteal fossa

**The structures encountered in the fossa are:**

1. The popliteal artery runs vertically down the middle of the popliteal fossa (11.10). It gives off a number of branches that are shown in 11.11.
2. The popliteal vein partially overlaps the popliteal artery.
3. The tibial nerve lies superficial to the popliteal vein (11.11). This nerve is a terminal branch of the sciatic nerve. In the fossa, this nerve gives branches to:
   a. Both heads of the gastrocnemius
   b. The plantaris

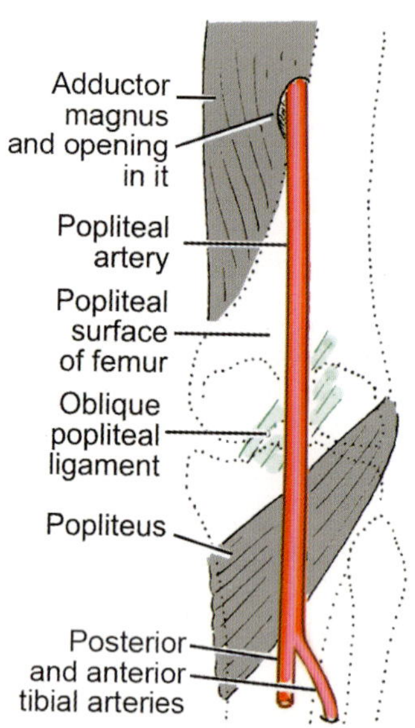


**11.9:** Diagram to show the course of the popliteal artery

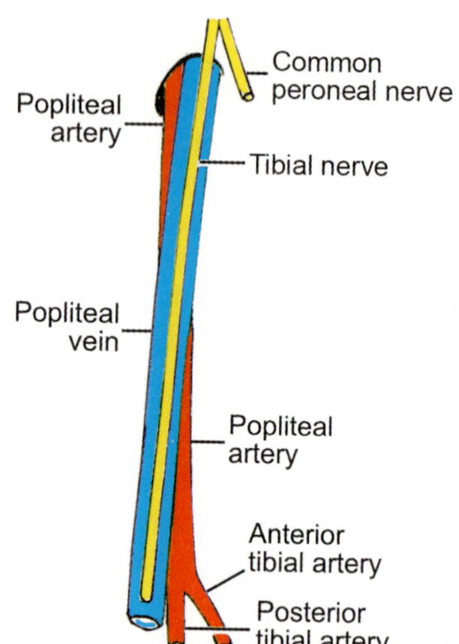


**11.10:** Relationship of popliteal artery to popliteal vein and tibial nerve

   c. The popliteus
   d. The soleus, a muscle of the leg lying deep to the gastrocnemius
   e. Genicular branches are given to the knee joint.
4. The common peroneal nerve is also a terminal branch of the sciatic nerve. It runs downwards and laterally along the biceps femoris. In the fossa, it gives off some branches. These are:
   a. The sural communicating nerve (that joins the sural nerve).
   b. The lateral cutaneous nerve of the calf that supplies skin on the lateral side of the back of the leg.
   c. Genicular branches to the knee joint.

## POPLITEAL VESSELS

### The Popliteal Artery

1. The popliteal artery begins at the junction of the middle-and lower-thirds of the thigh, being continuous with the lower end of the femoral artery through the opening in the adductor magnus.
2. It lies deep in the popliteal fossa, on the back of the knee joint (11.9). The artery runs downwards and laterally lying successively on the popliteal surface of the femur, the capsule of the knee joint and the popliteus (i.e., over the floor of the popliteal fossa).
3. It ends at the lower border of the popliteus by dividing into the ***anterior*** and ***posterior tibial arteries.***
4. Superficially (i.e., posteriorly) the artery is partly overlapped by muscles forming the medial margin of the popliteal fossa. These are the semimembranosus (over the upper part) and the medial head of the gastrocnemius (over the lower part). It is also covered by skin and fascia.
5. The artery is accompanied by the popliteal vein. The vein is posterior (i.e., superficial) to the artery. At the upper end of the artery, the vein is on its lateral side. The vein gradually crosses the artery so that it comes to lie medial to the lower end of the artery (11.10).
6. The artery is also related to the tibial nerve that is separated from it by the popliteal vein. Like the vein the nerve crosses the artery from lateral to medial side (11.10).
7. The branches of the popliteal artery are shown in 11.11.

### Anastomoses Around the Knee Joint

The knee is surrounded by complex arterial anastomoses as shown in 11.12

## WANT TO KNOW MORE?

1. The two superior genicular branches of the popliteal artery anastomose with each other in front of the femur.
2. The two inferior genicular arteries anastomose in front of the tibia.
3. The two medial arteries and the two lateral arteries are joined by vertical anastomoses.
4. Superiorly, these anastomoses are joined by the descending genicular branch of the femoral artery and by the descending branch of the lateral circumflex femoral artery.
5. Inferiorly, the recurrent branch of the anterior tibial artery and the circumflex fibular branch of the posterior tibial artery join the anastomoses.

**Anastomoses on the Back of the Thigh**

The arteries in the back of the thigh join each other to form one or more vertical chains that can help to maintain circulation in case of blockage or insufficiency of the main arterial trunk. The arteries taking part in these anastomoses are (from above downwards):

1. The superior and inferior gluteal arteries.
2. The medial and lateral circumflex femoral arteries.
3. Perforating branches of the profunda femoris artery.
4. Muscular branches of the popliteal artery.

Through these anastomoses, links are established between the internal iliac, femoral and popliteal arteries.

## The Popliteal Vein

1. The course and relations of the popliteal vein are similar to those of the popliteal artery described above. The relationship of the vein to the artery is shown in 11.10.
2. The tributiaries of the popliteal vein correspond to the branches of the popliteal artery. In addition, the popliteal vein receives the short saphenous vein (11.8).

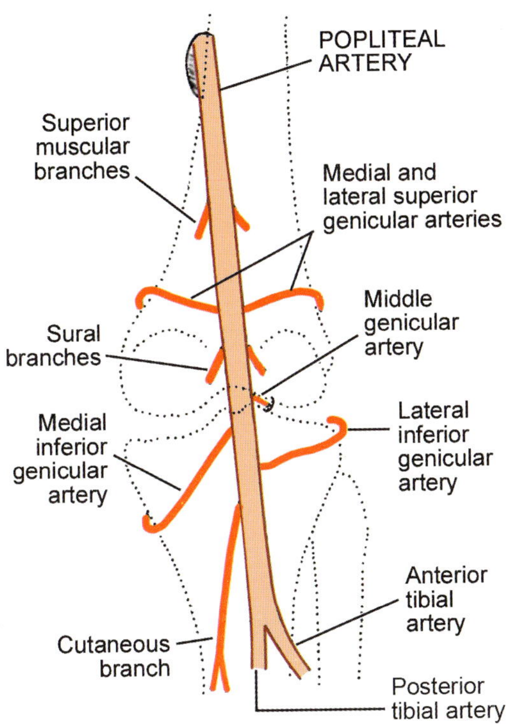


11.11: Branches of popliteal artery

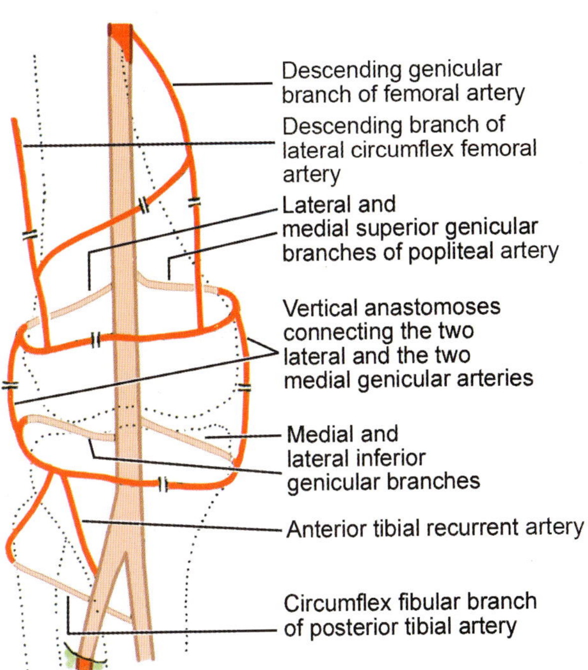


11.12: Anastomoses around the knee joint

# NERVES IN THE GLUTEAL REGION AND BACK OF THIGH

These are branches arising from the sacral plexus. We will, therefore study this plexus first.

## SACRAL VENTRAL RAMI AND SACRAL PLEXUS

### Sacral Ventral Rami

1. The ventral rami of sacral nerves (referred to below simply as sacral nerves) leave the vertebral canal by passing through the anterior sacral foramina.
2. They take part in forming the sacral plexus and the coccygeal plexus.
3. The sacral nerves also have important connections with the autonomic nervous system.

### Sacral Plexus

1. The sacral plexus is formed by the upper four sacral nerves along with the lumbosacral trunk (derived from L4 and L5).
2. Nerves L4, L5, S1 and S2 each divide into anterior and posterior divisions.
   a. The posterior divisions of these nerves unite to form the common peroneal part of the sciatic nerve.
   b. The anterior divisions of these nerves, and S3 (which does not divide into anterior and posterior divisions) unite to form the tibial part of the sciatic nerve.
3. Part of nerve S4 joins branches from the ventral divisions of S2 and S3 to form the pudendal nerve.
4. Apart from the sciatic and pudendal nerves and sacral plexus gives off several branches that are shown in 11.13.
5. The branches arising from the posterior divisions (shown in blue in 11.13) are:
   a. The superior gluteal (L4, L5, S1)
   b. The inferior gluteal (L5, S1, S2)
   c. The nerve to the piriformis (S1, S2)
   d. The perforating cutaneous nerve (S2, S3)

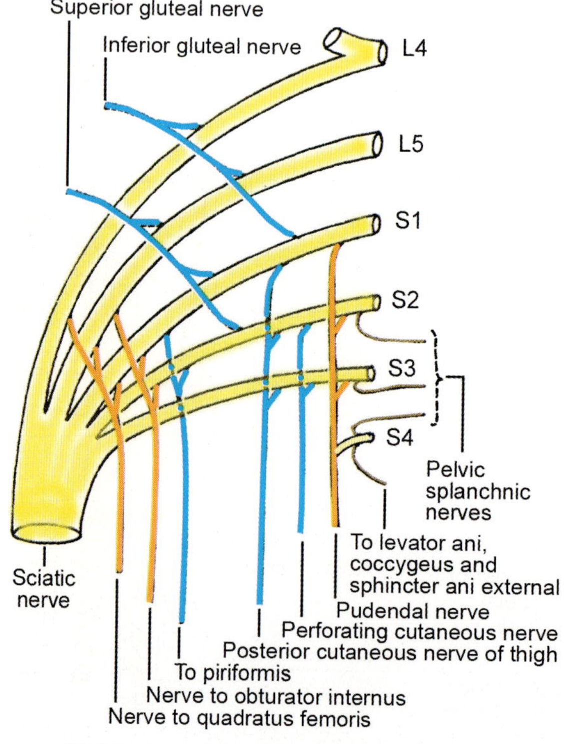


**11.13:** Simplified plan of the sacral plexus

e. The posterior cutaneous nerve of the thigh receives contributions from both the posterior divisions (S2, S3) and anterior divisions (S1, S2).

6. The branches arising from the anterior divisions (shown in 11.13) are:
   a. The nerve to the quadratus femoris (L4, L5, S1).
   b. The nerve to the obturator internus (L5, S1, S2).
7. Nerve S4 gives branches to the levator ani, the coccygeus and the sphincter ani externus.
8. Branches to pelvic viscera (***pelvic splanchnic nerves***) arise from S2, S3 and S4.

We will now consider these branches one by one.

## Superior Gluteal Nerve

1. The superior gluteal nerve is derived from spinal nerves L4, L5 and S1.
2. It passes from the pelvis to the gluteal region through the greater sciatic foramen, above the piriformis.
3. It divides into superior and inferior branches.
4. Both these branches run forwards deep to the gluteus medius.
5. The superior branch supplies the gluteus medius, and (occasionally) the gluteus minimus.
6. The inferior branch also supplies these two muscles. It ends by supplying the tensor fasciae latae (11.14).

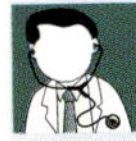

### CLINICAL CORRELATION

In injury to the superior gluteal nerve, the gluteus medius and minimus are paralysed. The Trendelenberg test is positive.

## Inferior Gluteal Nerve

1. The inferior gluteal nerve is derived from spinal nerves L5, S1 and S2.
2. It passes from the pelvis to the gluteal region through the greater sciatic foramen, below the piriformis.
3. It supplies the gluteus maximus (11.14).

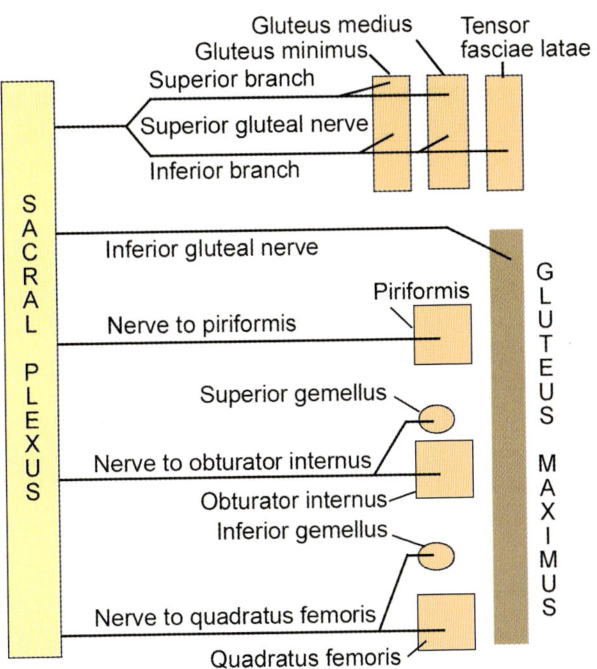


**11.14:** Scheme to show the nerve supply of muscles in the gluteal region

### Nerve to Quadratus Femoris

1. The nerve to the quadratus femoris is derived from spinal nerves L4, L5 and S1.
2. It passes from the pelvis to the gluteal region through the greater sciatic foramen, below the piriformis.
3. It runs downwards deep to the superior gemellus, the tendon of the obturator internus, and the inferior gemellus.
4. After giving a branch to the inferior gemellus, it reaches the anterior (or deep) surface of the quadratus femoris and enters it to supply the muscle.

### Nerve to Obturator Internus

1. The nerve to the obturator internus is derived from L5, S1 and S2.
2. It passes from the pelvis to the gluteal region through the greater sciatic foramen passing below the piriformis.
3. It runs down posterior to the ischial spine and again enters the pelvis by passing through the lesser sciatic foramen.
4. The nerve ends by supplying the obturator internus.
5. Before passing through the lesser sciatic foramen, it gives a branch to the superior gemellus (11.14).

### Nerve to Piriformis

1. The nerve to the piriformis arises from S1 and S2.
2. It is confined to the pelvis and ends by entering the anterior surface of the piriformis (11.14).

### Posterior Cutaneous Nerve of Thigh

1. The posterior cutaneous nerve of the thigh is derived from S1, S2, and S3.
2. It passes from the pelvis to the gluteal region through the greater sciatic foramen, below the piriformis.
3. It passes downwards through the gluteal region (deep to the gluteus maximus) to enter the back of the thigh.
4. Its lowest part extends into the upper part of the leg. It supplies an extensive area of skin including that over the lower part of the gluteal region, the perineum, the back of the thigh, and the back of the upper part of the leg.

### Perforating Cutaneous Nerve

1. The perforating cutaneous nerve is derived from S2 and S3.
2. It bears this name because it pierces through the sacrotuberous ligament (below the lesser sciatic foramen). This is how, it passes from within the pelvis to the gluteal region.
3. Finally, it winds round the inferior edge of the gluteus maximus and supplies the skin over the inferomedial part of the muscle.

## THE SCIATIC NERVE

1. The sciatic nerve is the main continuation of the sacral plexus. It is also the thickest nerve of the body.
2. It receives fibres from spinal nerves L4 to S3. It passes from the pelvis to the gluteal region through the greater sciatic foramen, below the piriformis.
3. It descends through the gluteal region into the back of the thigh. At the junction of the middle-and lower-thirds of the thigh, the sciatic nerve ends by dividing into the tibial and common peroneal nerves. The level of division is variable (11.8).
4. In its course through the gluteal region, the nerve lies deep (or anterior) to the gluteus maximus. It lies successively on:
   a. The posterior surface of the ischium
   b. The superior gemellus
   c. The obturator internus (tendon)
   d. The inferior gemellus
   e. The quadratus femoris.

5. In the thigh the nerve lies upon the adductor magnus, and is crossed superficially (i.e., posteriorly) by the long head of the biceps femoris.
6. Apart from its terminal branches the sciatic nerve gives the following branches.
   a. Branches arising from the tibial part of the nerve supply the hamstrings viz., the long head of the biceps femoris, the semitendinosus, the semimembranosus and the adductor magnus (part arising from the ischial tuberosity).
   b. The common peroneal part of the sciatic nerve gives a branch to the short head of the biceps femoris muscle.
   c. Articular branches are given off to the hip joint.

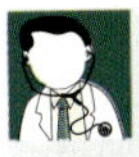

## CLINICAL CORRELATION

**Sciatic Nerve**

1. The sciatic nerve can be injured by carelessly given intramuscular injections in the gluteal region. (This can be avoided by giving injections only in the upper and lateral part of the gluteal region). The nerve can also be injured in fractures of the pelvis and dislocations of the hip joint.
2. Injury to the nerve paralyses muscles of the back of the thigh (hamstrings), and all muscles of the leg and foot.
3. The foot hangs downwards (by its own weight): the condition is called foot drop. Foot drop is also caused by injury to the common peroneal nerve as described below. There is sensory loss over the greater part of the leg and foot, but the area supplied by the saphenous branch of the femoral nerve is spared.

## THE TIBIAL NERVE

The nerve has an extensive course and distribution. Here, we will consider only the part seen in the popliteal fossa.

1. The fibres of the tibial nerve are derived from ventral rami of spinal nerves L4 to S3.
2. Separating from the common peroneal at the junction of the middle-and lower-thirds of the thigh, it descends through the popliteal fossa, and passes into the back of the leg.

### Important Relations of the Tibial Nerve in the Popliteal Fossa

1. In the upper part of the popliteal fossa the nerve lies lateral to the popliteal artery and vein (11.8). It crosses superficial (i.e., posterior) to these vessels at the level of the knee joint and, thereafter, lies medial to them.
2. In the popliteal fossa the structures that lie anterior (or deep) to the nerve are (from above downwards):
   a. The popliteal surface of the femur
   b. The knee joint
   c. The popliteus.
3. The superficial relations of the nerve are as follows.
   a. At the upper angle of the popliteal fossa the nerve is covered by the semimembranosus medially, and by the biceps femoris laterally (11.8).
   b. In the middle of the fossa, the nerve is covered only by skin and, fasciae.
   c. At the lower end of the fossa, the nerve is covered by the overlapping margins of the medial and lateral heads of the gastrocnemius.

### Branches Given off in Popliteal Fossa

*Muscular Branches*

1. Branches given off in the lower part of the popliteal fossa supply the two heads of the gastrocnemius, the plantaris, the soleus and the popliteus.
2. The ***nerve to the popliteus*** has an interesting course. After running down superficial (posterior) to this muscle, the nerve turns round its lower border to reach its anterior surface that it enters.

### *Cutaneous Branches*

The *sural nerve* is the main cutaneous branch. It arises in the lower part of the popliteal fossa and passes backwards between the two heads of the gastrocnemius. It then runs down the back of the leg.

### *Articular Branches*

The upper part of the tibial nerve gives three branches to the knee joint. They accompany the superior medial genicular, the middle genicular, and the inferior medial genicular arteries.

## THE COMMON PERONEAL NERVE

This is also called the ***common fibular nerve***.

1. It is derived from the sacral plexus through roots L4, L5, S1 and S2.
2. Starting at the bifurcation of the sciatic nerve, it runs downwards and laterally along the lower part of the biceps femoris muscle to reach the head of the fibula.
3. It winds round the lateral side of the neck of the fibula. The nerve ends here by dividing into its superficial and deep peroneal branches.

The further course and distribution of the tibial and comon peroneal nerve will be studied in the leg.

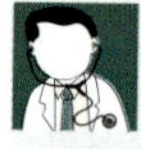

## CLINICAL CORRELATION

**Segmental Innervation of the Lower Limb**

1. From a clinical point of view, it is important to know the muscles and areas of skin supplied by individual segments of the spinal cord.
2. Pressure on the spinal cord, or on the lumbar and sacral nerve roots can give rise to symptoms in the region supplied by nerves arising from the lumbar and sacral plexuses.
3. In such cases, it is important to localise the particular spinal segments involved.
4. A simplified scheme of the root values of nerves that supply muscles of the lower limb is given in 11.15. The dermatomes of the limb are shown in 11.16.
5. Pressure on the lumbosacral nerve roots is often produced by prolapse of an intervertebral disc. Typically, the condition causes severe pain that begins in the gluteal region and radiates down the back of the leg to reach the foot. The condition is called ***sciatica***.

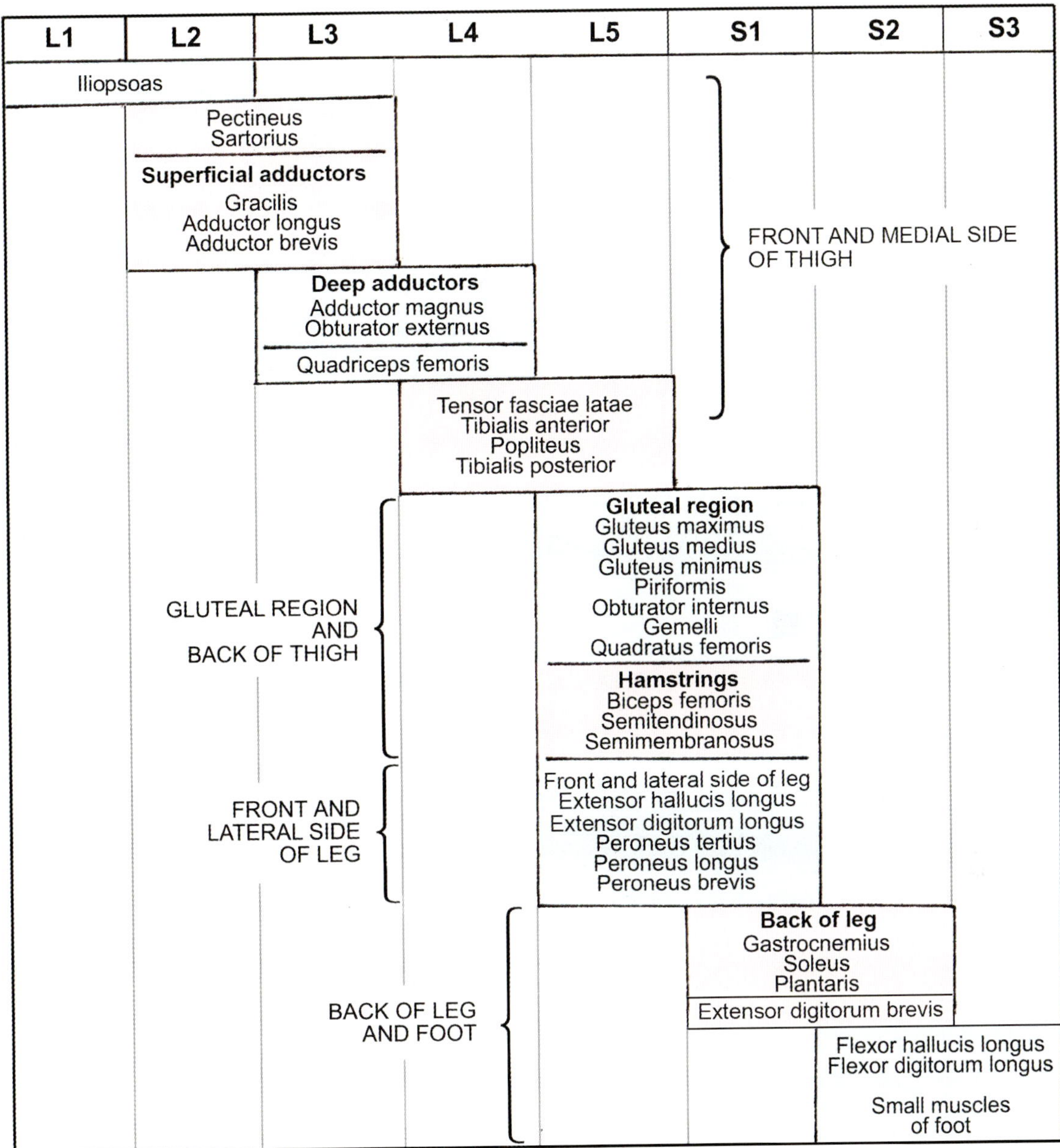


**11.15:** Simplified scheme to show segmental nerve supply of muscles of the lower limb

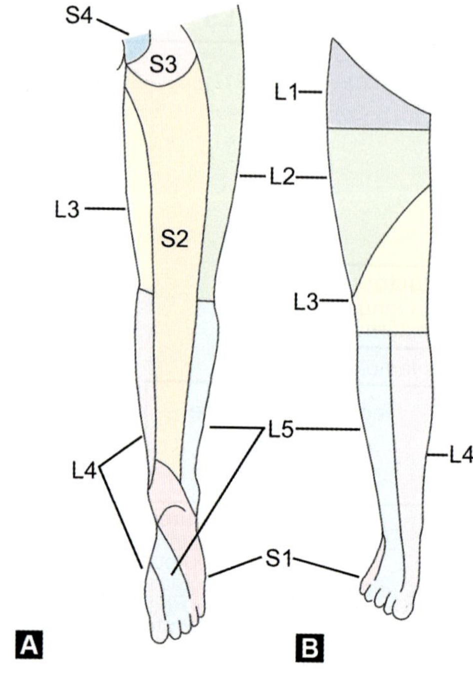


**11.16A and B:** Dermatomes of the lower limb

12

CHAPTER

# Front and Lateral Side of Leg and the Dorsum of Foot

## COMPARTMENTS OF THE LEG

The leg is divided into anterior, lateral and posterior compartments by intermuscular septa (12.1). These septa may be regarded as extensions of deep fascia.

1. The ***anterior intermuscular septum*** passes from deep fascia to the anterior border of the fibula. It separates the anterior and lateral compartments.
2. The ***posterior intermuscular septum*** passes from deep fascia to the posterior border of the fibula. It separates the lateral and posterior compartments.
3. The anterior and posterior compartments are separated from each other by the ***interosseous membrane*** (that stretches between the interosseous borders of the tibia and fibula).
4. The posterior compartment of the leg is divided into superficial, middle and deep parts by ***superficial*** and ***deep transverse septa***.

## MUSCLES OF ANTERIOR COMPARTMENT OF LEG

The muscles to be seen on the front of the leg and the dorsum of the foot are the following:

1. Tibialis anterior (12.2)
2. Extensor hallucis longus (12.2)
3. Extensor digitorum longus (12.2, 12.3 and 12.4)
4. Extensor digitorum brevis (12.2)
5. Peroneus tertius (or Fibularis tertius) (12.2)

These are described in 12.2 and illustrated in figures cited above. Some details are given below.

### Note on Tibialis Anterior

1. The muscle ends in a tendon that runs across the front of the ankle.
2. In the living person the tendon of the tibialis anterior can be felt just lateral to the anterior border of the tibia. Its relationship to the extensor retinacula is described below.

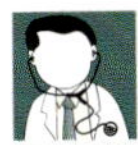

### CLINICAL CORRELATION

Excessive strain on the tibialis anterior muscle (in atheletes) produces small tears near its attachments. There is pain and edema over the lower two-thirds of the tibia.

### Note on Extensor Hallucis Longus

The muscle ends in a tendon which runs downwards across the ankle. Here it can be felt just lateral to the tendon of the tibialis anterior.

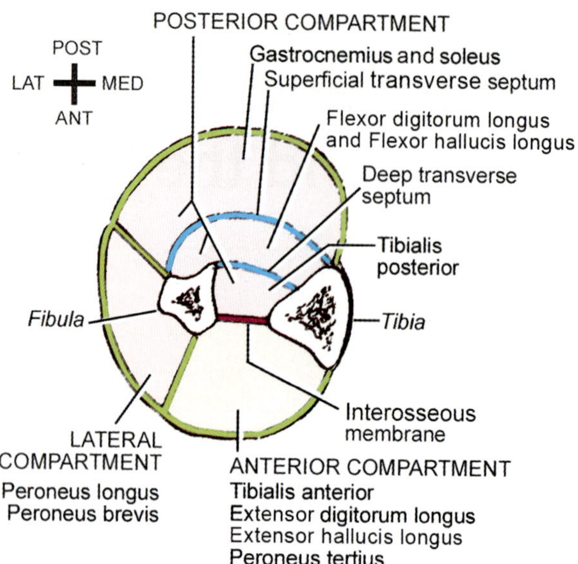


**12.1:** Intermuscular septa and compartments of the leg

**12.2: Muscles of anterior compartment of leg**

| *Muscle* | *Origin* | *Insertion* | *Action* | *Nerve supply* |
|---|---|---|---|---|
| Tibialis anterior | 1. Lateral surface of shaft of tibia (upper 1/2 to 2/3)<br>2. Interosseous membrane (adjoining) | 1. Medial cuneiform bone (medial and plantar aspect)<br>2. First metatarsal bone (medial side of base) | 1. Dorsiflexion of foot<br>2. Inversion of foot<br>3. Helps to maintain arches of foot | Deep peroneal nerve (L4, 5) |
| Extensor hallucis longus | 1. Medial surface of fibula (middle two-fourths)<br>2. Interosseous membrane (adjoining) | Base of distal phalanx of great toe (dorsal aspect) | 1. Extends phalanges of great toe<br>2. Helps dorsiflexion of foot | Deep peroneal nerve (L5, S1) |
| Extensor digitorum longus | 1. Fibula (upper 3/4 of medial surface)<br>2. Interosseous membrane (for upper part of muscle only)<br>3. Uppermost part from lateral condyle of tibia | 1. Tendon divides into four slips one each for 2nd, 3rd, 4th and 5th toes<br>2. Over the proximal phalanx the tendon (for that digit) divides into three slips, one intermediate and two collateral<br>3. The intermediate slip is inserted into the base of the middle phalanx<br>4. The collateral slips reunite and are inserted into the base of the distal phalanx | 1. Extension of toes<br>2. Dorsiflexion of foot | Deep peroneal nerve (L5, S1) |

*Contd...*

*Contd...*

| *Muscle* | *Origin* | *Insertion* | *Action* | *Nerve supply* |
|---|---|---|---|---|
| Extensor digitorum brevis | Anterior part of calcaneus (on superior and lateral aspect) | 1. Muscle ends in four tendons (for first, second, third and fourth digits)<br>2. Tendons for 2nd to 4th digits joins the corresponding tendon of extensor digitorum longus<br>3. The tendon for the first digit is inserted into the dorsal surface of the base of the proximal phalanx of the great toe | 1. Helps extensor digitorum longus in extension of 2nd, 3rd, and 4th toes<br>2. Extension of proximal phalanx of great toe | Deep peroneal nerve (S1, 2) |
| Peroneus tertius | 1. Medial surface of shaft of fibula (below origin of extensor digitorum longus)<br>2. Interosseous membrane (adjoining) | Fifth metatarsal bone (dorsal surface of base) | 1. Dorsiflexion of foot<br>2. Eversion of foot | Deep peroneal nerve (L5, S1) |

### Note on Extensor Digitorum Longus

1. In the middle two-fourths of the fibula, the area of origin of this muscle is lateral to that of the extensor hallucis longus. It can, therefore, not extend to the interosseous membrane here.
2. At the ankle, the tendon passes deep to the extensor retinacula (12.6).
3. Over the proximal phalanx, the tendon for each digit is expanded into a triangular ***dorsal digital expansion***, which receives the insertions of interosseous and lumbrical muscles (12.4).

### Note on Peroneus Tertius

1. This muscle may be regarded as the lower separated part of the extensor digitorum longus.
2. It is also called the fibularis tertius. (This applies to all peroneus muscles).
3. The tendon passes deep to the extensor retinacula.

## EXTENSOR AND PERONEAL RETINACULA

1. Around the ankle, the deep fascia forms a number of thickened bands that hold underlying tendons in place. These bands are called ***retinacula***.
2. These bands also act as pulleys allowing the tendon to change direction.
3. On the front of the ankle there are ***superior*** and ***inferior extensor retinacula***.
4. On the lateral side there are (much less prominent) ***superior*** and ***inferior peroneal retinacula***.
5. On the medial side of the ankle there is the ***flexor retinaculum***.

### Extensor Retinacula

1. The ***superior extensor retinaculum*** is attached:
   a. Medially to the anterior border of the tibia.
   b. Laterally to the anterior aspect of the fibula (12.5).

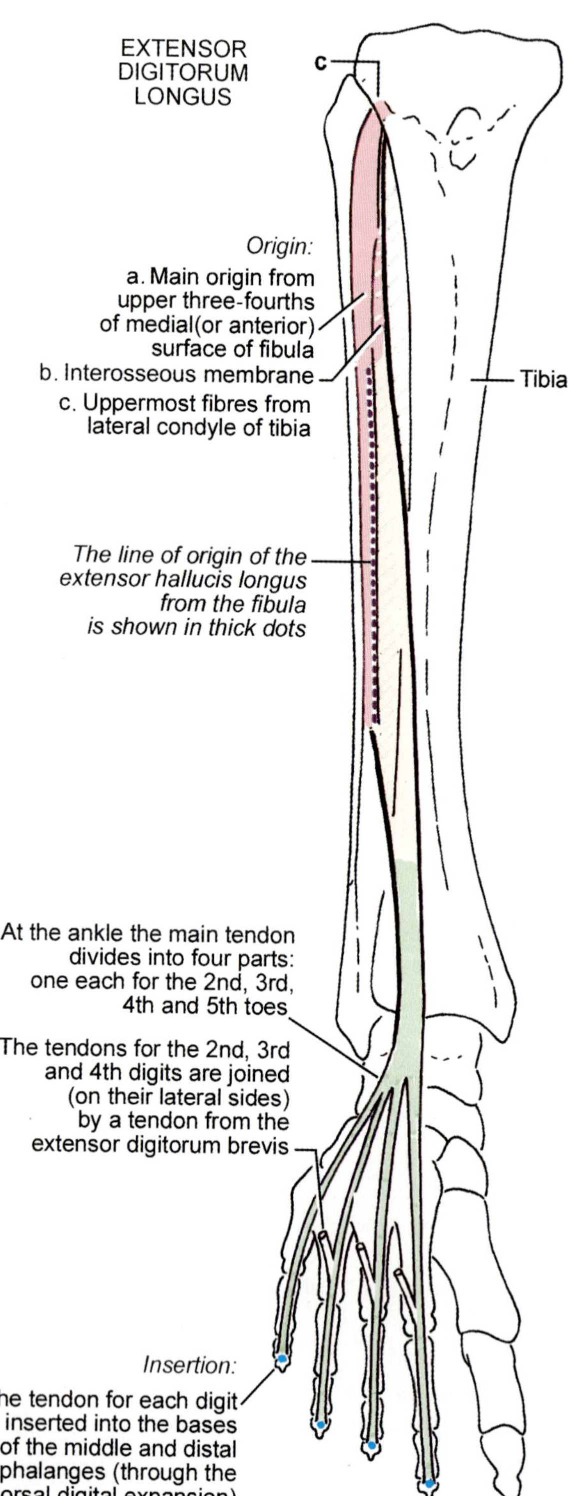


**12.3:** Scheme to show the attachments of the extensor digitorum longus

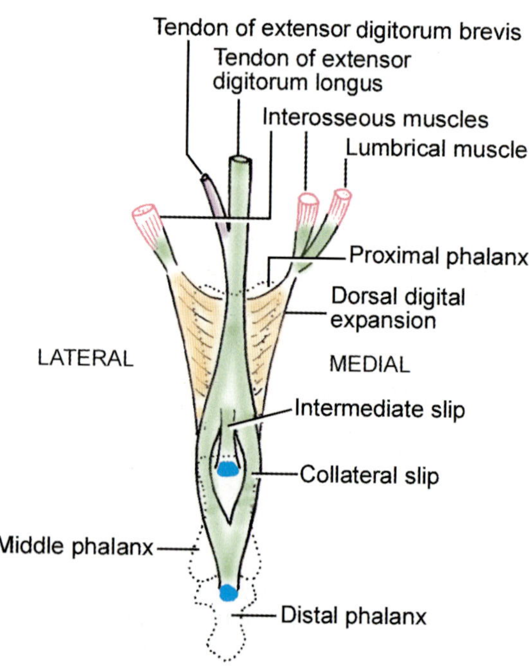


**12.4:** Dorsal aspect of a digit to show the dorsal digital expansion, and details of insertion of the extensor digitorum longus

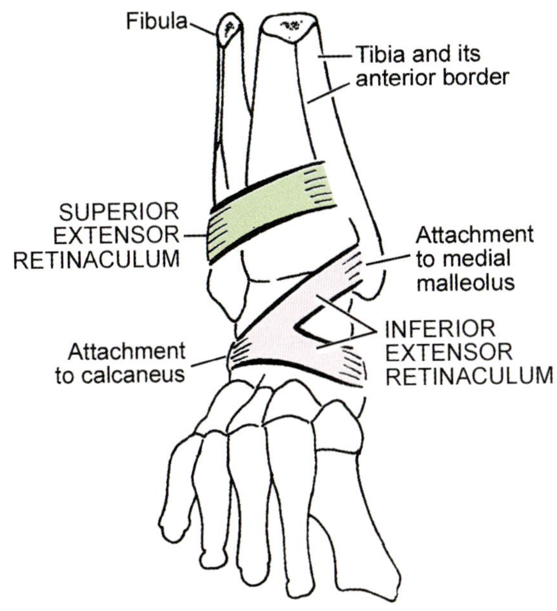


**12.5:** Attachments of superior and inferior extensor retinacula

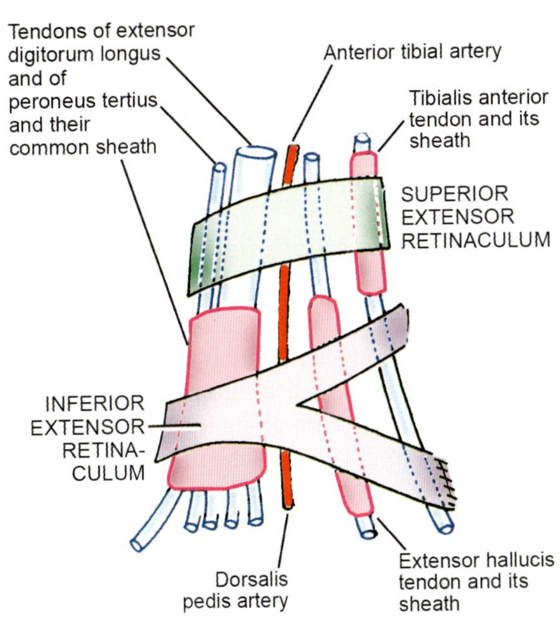


**12.6:** Tendons on the front of the ankle, their synovial sheaths, and relationship to the extensor retinacula

2. The ***inferior extensor retinaculum*** is shaped like the letter 'Y' placed on its side; the stem of the 'Y' is directed laterally and the two limbs pass medially.
   a. The stem of the 'Y' is attached to the upper surface of the calcaneus.
   b. The upper limb of the 'Y' is attached to the medial malleolus.
   c. The lower limb of the 'Y' winds round the medial side of the foot to become continuous with the plantar aponeurosis.

### *Tendons Passing Under Cover of Extensor Retinacula*

1. The tendons passing under cover of the extensor retinacula are (from medial to lateral side in 12.6) those of:
   a. The tibialis anterior
   b. The extensor hallucis longus
   c. The extensor digitorum longus
   d. The peroneus tertius.
2. The superior extensor retinaculum is superficial to all the tendons.
3. The relationship of the inferior extensor retinaculum to the tendons is as follows:
   a. The stem is in the form of a loop through which the tendons of the extensor digitorum and peroneus tertius pass.
   b. The superior limb has two layers one passing superficial to the extensor hallucis and the tibialis anterior, and the other deep to them.
   c. The inferior limb is superficial to these tendons; it may sometimes have an additional layer deep to the tendons.
4. As they pass under the retinacula, the extensor tendons are surrounded by synovial sheaths (12.6).
   a. There is one sheath each for the tibialis anterior and for the extensor hallucis.
   b. The extensor digitorum and the peroneus tertius have a common sheath.

## MUSCLES OF LATERAL COMPARTMENT OF LEG

These are:

1. Peroneus longus (12.7, 12.8 A and B)
2. Peroneus brevis (12.7).

Some details are given below.

### Note on Peroneus Longus

1. There is a gap between the areas of origin of this muscle from the head of the fibula and from the shaft. The common peroneal nerve passes through this gap.
2. The muscle ends in a tendon that passes along a groove behind the lateral malleolus; here it is covered by the superior peroneal retinaculum.
3. The tendon then runs along the lateral aspect of the calcaneus. It passes just below the peroneal trochlea, where the tendon is covered by the inferior peroneal retinaculum.
4. Thereafter, the tendon winds round the lateral side of the cuboid bone to reach its plantar aspect (12.8B). This aspect of the cuboid bone bears a groove for the tendon (which is converted into a canal by the long plantar ligament).
5. The muscle helps to maintain the arches of the foot (both longitudinal and transverse).

**12.7: Muscles of lateral compartment of leg (Peroneal or fibular muscles)**

| *Muscle* | *Origin* | *Insertion* | *Action* | *Nerve supply* |
|---|---|---|---|---|
| Peroneus longus (Fibularis longus) | 1. Head of fibula<br>2. Lateral surface of fibula (upper two-thirds) | The tendon passes:<br>1. Behind lateral malleolus<br>2. Across lateral surface of calcaneus<br>3. Round cuboid bone to enter the sole. It runs medially across the sole<br>4. The tendon is attached to:<br>a. First metatarsal bone (lateral side of base)<br>b. Medial cuneiform bone (lateral side) | 1. Eversion of foot<br>2. Steadies the leg on the foot<br>3. Maintains arches of foot | Superficial peroneal nerve (L5, S1, S2) |
| Peroneus brevis (Fibularis brevis) | Shaft of fibula (lower two-thirds of lateral surface) | 1. Tendon passes behind lateral malleolus, (lying anterior to that of peroneus longus)<br>2. Runs forward on lateral. side of calcaneus<br>3. Tendon gets inserted into fifth metatarsal bone (lateral side of base) | 1. Eversion of foot<br>2. Steadies the leg on the foot | Superficial peroneal nerve (L5, S1, S2) |

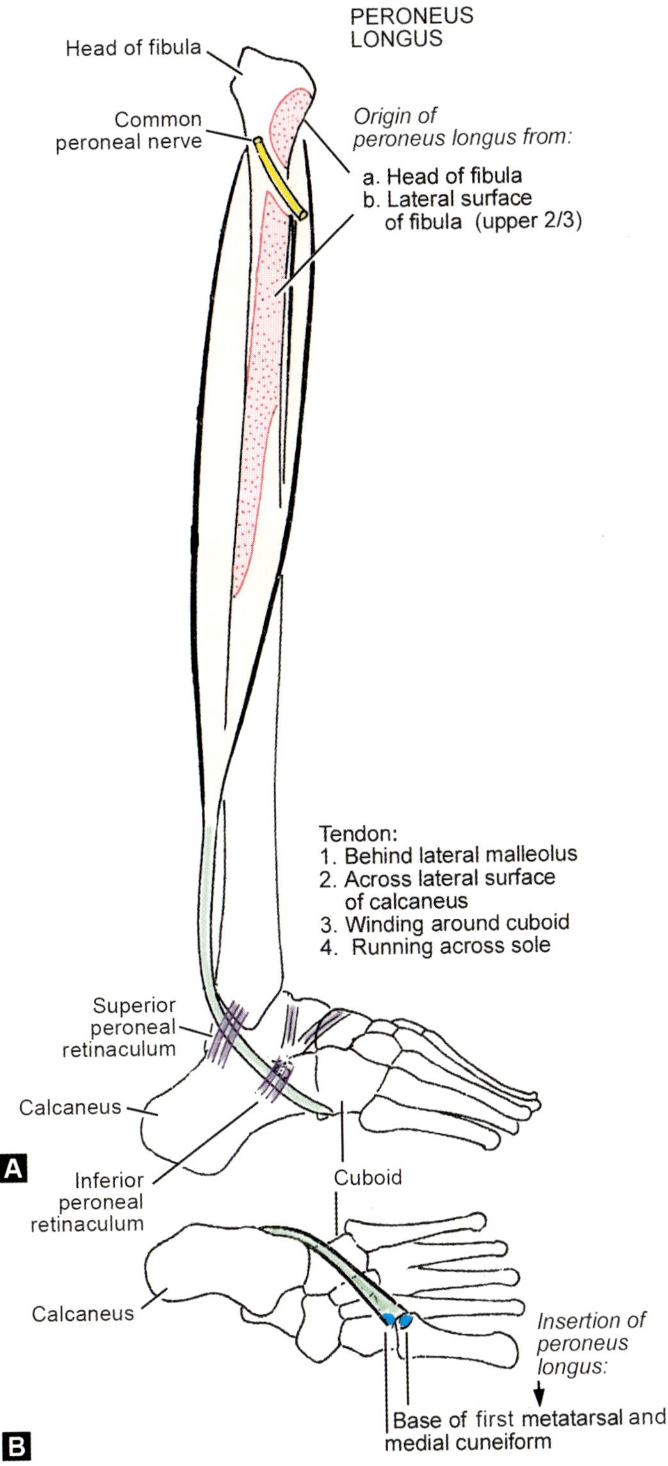


**12.8A and B:** Attachments of peroneus longus as seen from (A) The lateral side; (B) From below

### Note on Peroneus Brevis

1. Because of the fact that the posterior border of the fibula turns medially in its lower part, the area of origin of the peroneus brevis (on the lateral surface) extends onto the posterior aspect of the bone.
2. At the ankle the tendon passes behind the lateral malleolus: here it lies anterior to the tendon of the peroneus longus.
3. It then runs forwards on the lateral surface of the calcaneus; here it lies above the longus tendon, the two being separated by the peroneal trochlea.

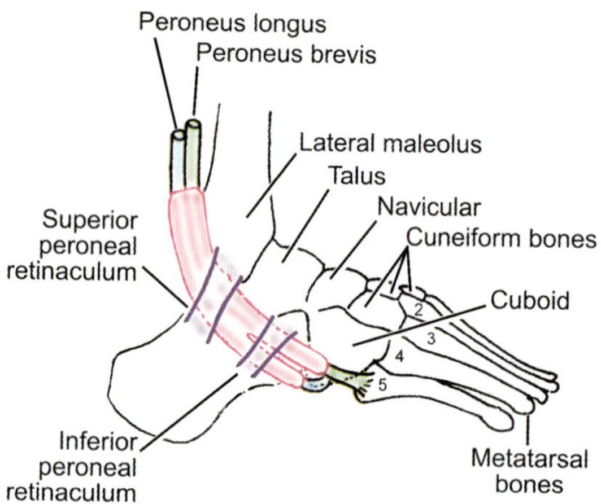


12.9: Lateral side of ankle and foot to show the peroneal retinacula, and synovial sheaths of peroneal tendons

### Peroneal Retinacula

The peroneal retinacula (12.8 and 12.9) are present on the lateral aspect of the ankle. They keep the peroneal tendons in place.

1. The ***superior peroneal retinaculum*** is attached above to the lateral malleolus and below to the lateral surface of the calcaneus.
2. The ***inferior peroneal retinaculum*** is attached below to the lateral surface of the calcaneus. Above it becomes continuous with the inferior extensor retinaculum.

#### *Synovial Sheath of Peroneal Tendons*

1. As the tendons of the peroneus longus and brevis run downwards and forwards on the lateral side of the ankle, they are held in place by the superior and inferior peroneal retinacula.
2. They are enclosed in a synovial sheath that is common to the two tendons above, but bifurcates below (12.9).

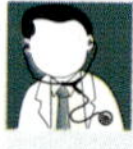

### CLINICAL CORRELATION

1. The synovial tendon sheaths around the tendons of the peroneus longus and peroneus brevis may be inflamed.
2. Occasionally, these tendons can be dislocated from their position behind the lateral malleolus.

## BLOOD VESSELS OF THE REGION

### The Anterior Tibial Artery

1. The anterior tibial artery begins as a terminal branch of the popliteal artery near the lower border of the popliteus muscle (12.11). Its origin is, therefore, situated in the upper part of the back of the leg.
2. Almost immediately, the artery turns forwards through the upper part of the interosseous membrane to enter the anterior compartment of the leg.
3. It now descends over the anterior surface of the interosseous membrane (12.10). It gradually passes medially so that in the lower part of the leg it comes to lie in front of the tibia.
4. It terminates in front of the ankle joint, midway between the medial and lateral malleoli, by becoming continuous with the ***dorsalis pedis*** artery.
5. In the upper part of the leg, the artery lies deep in the interval between the tibialis anterior (medially) and the extensor digitorum longus (laterally).
6. In the middle of the leg, it is related laterally to the extensor hallucis longus. The tendon of this muscle crosses the artery from lateral to medial side above the ankle.

7. For a short distance above the ankle the artery is covered only by skin, superficial fascia and deep fascia including the retinacula. Here it lies between the tendons of the extensor hallucis longus (medially) and the extensor digitorum longus (laterally).
8. The artery is accompanied by the deep peroneal (anterior tibial) nerve which lies lateral to the artery.

The ***branches of the anterior tibial artery*** are shown in 12.11. They are as follows:

1. The ***anterior tibial recurrent artery*** ascends to take part in the anastomoses around the knee.
2. The ***posterior tibial recurrent artery*** arises from the uppermost part of the anterior tibial artery in the back of the leg. It supplies the superior tibiofibular joint.

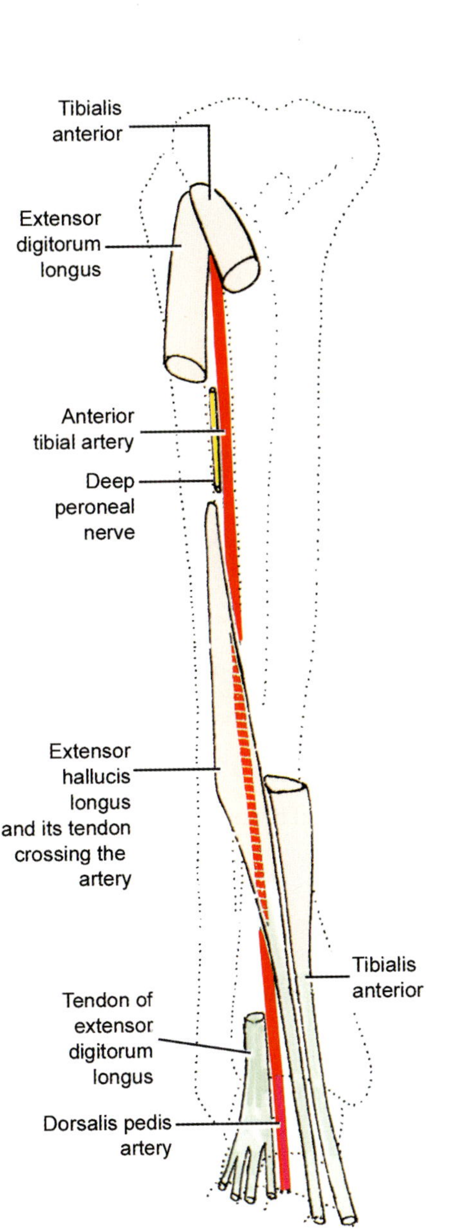


**12.10:** Scheme to show course and some relations of the anterior tibial artery

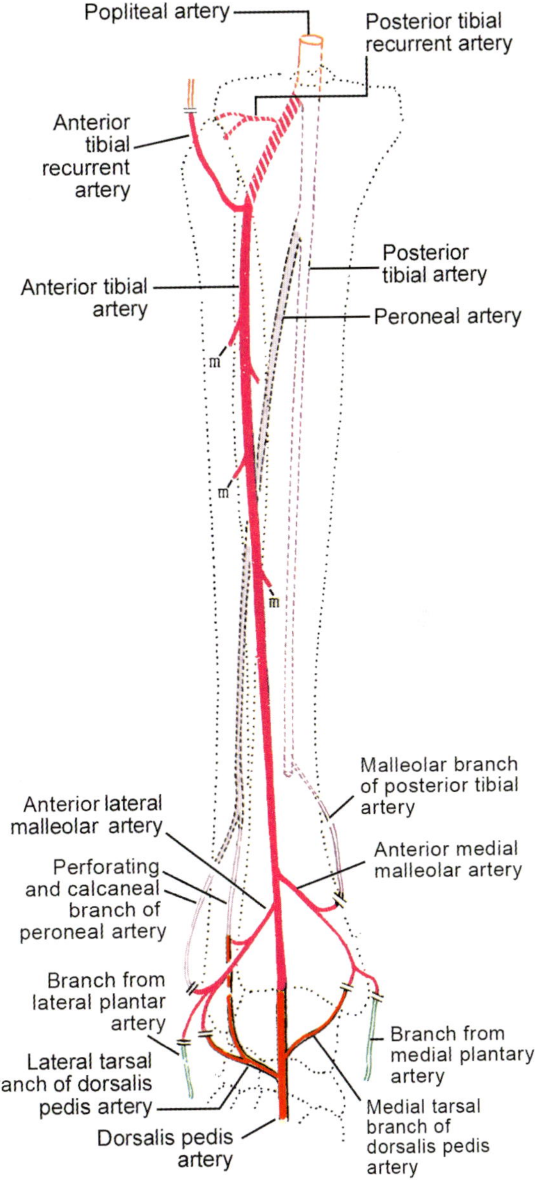


**12.11:** Branches of the anterior tibial artery. m=muscular branches. Anastomoses around the ankle are also shown

3. Numerous ***muscular branches (m)*** supply muscles of the anterior compartment of the leg.
4. The ***anterior lateral malleolar artery*** arises near the ankle and runs to the lateral malleolus.
5. The ***anterior medial malleolar artery*** arises near the ankle and runs to the medial malleolus.

The malleolar arteries anastomose with other arteries in the region.

## The Dorsalis Pedis Artery

1. This artery is also called the ***dorsal artery of the foot***. It is the continuation of the anterior tibial artery.
2. Beginning in front of the ankle it runs forwards, downwards and medially on the dorsum of the foot to reach the space between the first and second metatarsal bones (12.12).
3. Here it turns downwards through the space (between the two heads of the first dorsal interosseous muscle) to enter the sole of the foot.
4. The artery is relatively superficial being covered only by skin and fascia. Its proximal part passes under cover of the inferior extensor retinaculum.
5. Medial to the artery there is the tendon of the extensor digitorum longus, and the medial terminal branch of the deep peroneal nerve.
6. The artery is crossed by the tendon of the extensor hallucis brevis.
7. The ***branches of the dorsalis pedis artery*** are shown in 12.13.

### WANT TO KNOW MORE?

They are as follows:

1. The ***lateral tarsal branch*** goes to the lateral side of the tarsus.
2. The ***medial tarsal branch*** goes to the medial side of the foot and ankle (Also see 12.10).
3. The ***arcuate artery*** runs laterally over the bases of the metatarsal bones.
4. The ***dorsal metatarsal arteries*** are four in number.
   a. The first artery ('a' in 12.13) arises directly from the dorsalis pedis artery.
   b. the second ('b'), third ('c'), and fourth ('d') arise from the arcuate artery.
   c. Each dorsal metatarsal artery divides into two ***dorsal digital arteries*** ('e').
   d. The first artery also gives a branch ('f') to the medial side of the great toe.
   e. The fourth artery also gives a branch ('g') to the lateral side of the little toe.
   f. The dorsal metatarsal arteries are connected to the arteries of the sole by two sets of perforating arteries: proximal and distal.
   g. The ***proximal perforating arteries*** connect them to the plantar arch.
   h. The ***distal perforating arteries*** connect them to the plantar metatarsal branches of the plantar arch.

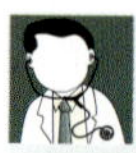

### CLINICAL CORRELATION

1. The ***dorsalis pedis artery*** lies in front of the ankle where it can be palpated and pressed upon to stop bleeding.
2. Palpation of the pulse can be facilitated by slight dorsiflexion of the foot.
3. If the dorsalis pedis pulse is absent, the reason may be:
   a. Congenital replacement of dorsalis pedis by a branch from the peroneal artery.
   b. Blockage due to arterial disease.

**Veins of the Front of the Leg**

Superficial veins over the dorsum of the foot and the front of the leg have been described in Chapter 10. The anterior tibial artery is accompanied by venae comitantes that end in the popliteal vein.

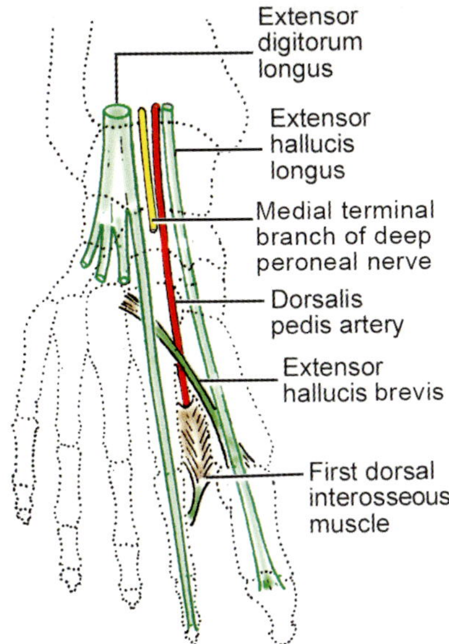


**12.12:** Course and some relations of dorsalis pedis artery

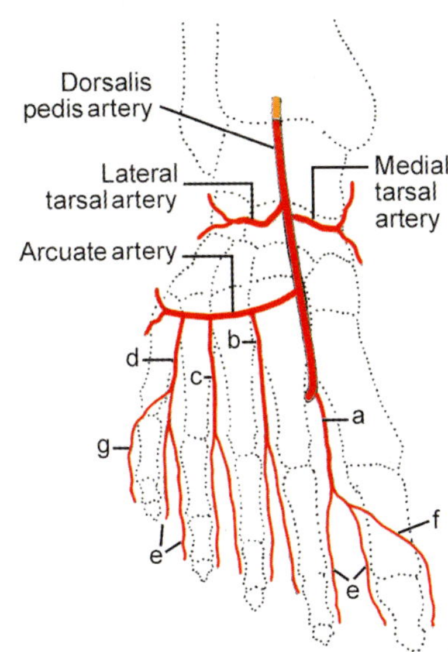


**12.13:** Branches of dorsalis pedis artery. a–d=dorsal metatarsal arteries. e–g=dorsal digital arteries

## THE TIBIAL NERVE (IN POPLITEAL FOSSA)

1. The fibres of this nerve are derived from ventral rami of spinal nerves: L4 to S3.
2. Separating from the common peroneal at the junction of the middle and lower-thirds of the thigh it descends through the popliteal fossa, and passes into the back of the leg.

The relations and branches of the tibial nerve in the leg will be described in Chapter 13.

*Important relations of the tibial nerve (in popliteal fossa)*

1. In the upper part of the popliteal fossa the nerve lies lateral to the popliteal artery and vein. It crosses superficial (i.e., posterior) to these vessels at the level of the knee joint and, thereafter, lies medial to them.
2. Anterior (or deep) to the nerve there are (from above downwards):
   a. The popliteal surface of the femur
   b. The knee joint
   c. The popliteus.
3. The posterior (or superficial) relations of the nerve are as follows.
   a. At the upper angle of the popliteal fossa the nerve is covered by the semimembranosus medially, and by the biceps femoris (laterally).
   b. In the middle of the fossa the nerve is covered only by skin and fasciae.
   c. At the lower end of the fossa the nerve is covered by the overlapping margins of the medial and lateral heads of the gastrocnemius.

*The branches of the tibial nerve (in popliteal fossa) are as follows*

1. Muscular branches given off in the lower part of the popliteal fossa supply the two heads of the gastrocnemius, the plantaris, the soleus and the popliteus (12.14).
   The ***nerve to the popliteus*** has an interesting course. After running down superficial (posterior) to this muscle the nerve turns round its lower border to reach its anterior surface that it enters.

2. The *sural nerve* is the main cutaneous branch. It arises in the lower part of the popliteal fossa and passes backwards between the two heads of the gastrocnemius. It will be seen again in the leg.
3. The upper part of the tibial nerve gives three branches to the knee joint: They accompany the superior medial genicular, the middle genicular, and the inferior medial genicular arteries.

## THE COMMON PERONEAL NERVE

This is also called the ***common fibular nerve***.

1. It is derived from the sacral plexus through roots L4, L5, S1 and S2.
2. Starting at the bifurcation of the sciatic nerve, it runs downwards and laterally along the lower part of the biceps femoris muscle to reach the head of the fibula.
3. It winds round the lateral side of the neck of the fibula: as it does so it lies deep to the peroneus longus. The nerve ends here by dividing into its superficial and deep peroneal branches.
4. Apart from these terminal branches the common peroneal nerve gives off the following branches:
   a. The ***lateral cutaneous nerve of the calf*** supplies the skin over the upper two-thirds of the lateral side of the leg. The area of supply also extends onto the anterior and posterior aspects of the leg.
   b. The ***sural communicating branch*** arises near the upper end of the fibula. It runs downwards and medially across the lateral head of the gastrocnemius muscle to join the sural nerve along with which it is distributed.

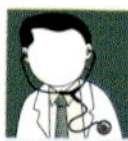

### CLINICAL CORRELATION

**Common peroneal (fibular) nerve**

1. This nerve is commonly injured as it is superficially placed. It can be involved in fractures of the upper end of the fibula.
2. Muscles of the anterior and lateral compartments of the leg are paralysed.
3. The foot is plantar flexed (as the dorsi flexors are paralysed, but the plantar flexors are not). As a result there is foot drop.
4. Because of paralysis of the peronei (which are evertors) the foot may be inverted.
5. There is loss of sensation in the areas of skin supplied by the deep peroneal and superficial peroneal nerves.

## THE DEEP PERONEAL (FIBULAR) NERVE

1. This is also called the anterior tibial nerve, or the deep fibular nerve.
2. It begins on the lateral side of the neck of the fibula, deep to the peroneus longus.
3. It passes downwards and medially, enters the anterior compartment of the leg and descends in front of the interosseous membrane, and lower down on the anterior aspect of the shaft of the tibia.
4. Accompanied by the anterior tibial artery it reaches the front of the ankle joint. It ends here by dividing into lateral and medial terminal branches.

The distribution of the deep peroneal nerve is as follows (12.15):

### *Muscular Branches*

a. In the leg the nerve gives branches to muscles of the anterior compartment: These are the tibialis anterior, the extensor hallucis longus, the extensor digitorum longus, and the peroneus tertius.
b. The lateral terminal branch supplies the extensor digitorum brevis.

### *Cutaneous Branches*

a. The skin of part of the dorsum of the foot is supplied by the deep peroneal nerve through its medial terminal branch.

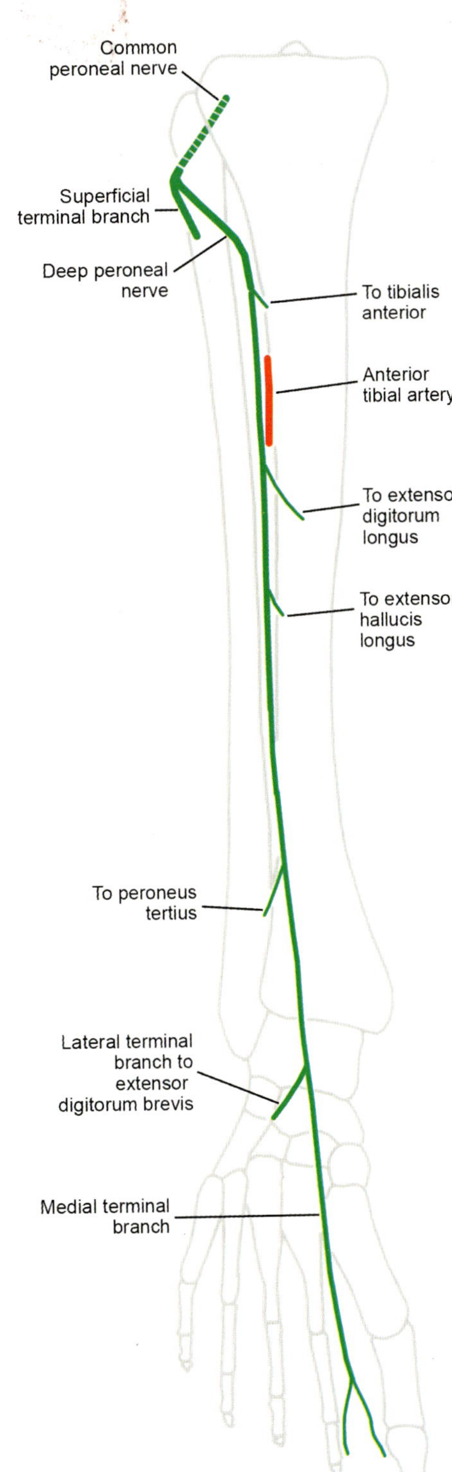


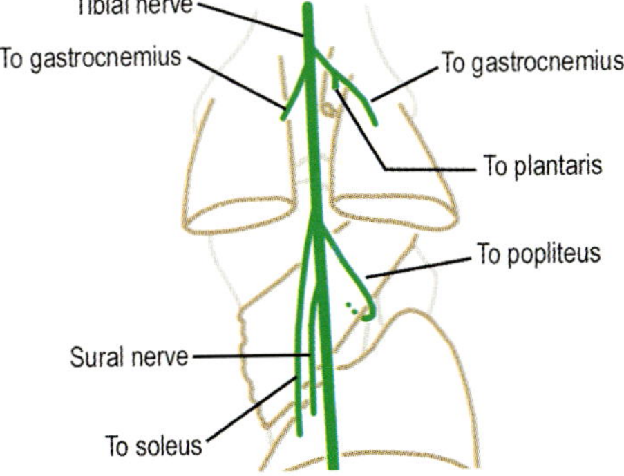


**12.14:** Scheme to show the branches of the tibial nerve in the popliteal fossa

**12.15:** Distribution of deep peroneal nerve

b. This branch runs forwards on the dorsum of the foot along with the dorsalis pedis artery.
c. It divides into two dorsal digital nerves that supply the adjacent sides of the great toe and the second toe.

### *Articular Branches*

a. The ankle joint receives a branch from the lower end of the deep peroneal nerve.
b. The lateral terminal branch gives branches to some tarsal and metatarsal joints.
c. The metatarsophalangeal joint of the great toe receives a branch from the medial terminal branch.

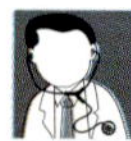

### CLINICAL CORRELATION

1. Excessive (or unaccustomed) use of muscles of the anterior compartment can lead to oedema in the compartment and pressure on the deep peroneal nerve. There is pain in the front of the leg.
2. This nerve can also be compressed as it passes under the inferior extensor retinaculum in persons wearing tight boots. There is pain over the dorsum of the foot.

## THE SUPERFICIAL PERONEAL (FIBULAR) NERVE

1. This nerve is also called the ***superficial fibular nerve***. It begins at the neck of the fibula deep to the peroneus longus (12.16).
2. It is the nerve to muscles of the lateral compartment of the leg: These are the peroneus longus and the peroneus brevis.
3. Reaching the lower part of the leg the nerve becomes superficial and supplies the skin on its lateral side. It then divides into medial and lateral terminal branches that descend across the ankle to reach the dorsum of the foot.
4. Each terminal branch divides into two dorsal digital nerves.
   a. The medial branch gives one dorsal digital nerve to the medial side of the great toe; and another to the adjacent sides of the second and third toes.
   b. The lateral branch gives one dorsal digital nerve to the contiguous sides of the third and fourth toes and another to the adjacent sides of the fourth and fifth toes.
   c. The lateral terminal branch also supplies the skin on the lateral side of the ankle.

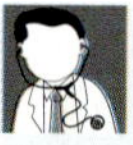

### CLINICAL CORRELATION

**Superficial Peroneal Nerve**

The nerve can be stretched in atheletes. This is associated with sprains of the ankle. There is pain along the lateral side of the leg and dorsum of the foot.

**Ingrowing Toe Nail**

In this condition, seen in the big toe, one end of the distal edge of the nail grows into soft tissue causing pain and setting up inflammation. The condition can be prevented by trimming the nail straight (not curved) and making sure that it does not grow into soft tissue. In serious cases, part of the nail may need removal.

**Paronychia**

This is infection of soft tissue in relation to a nail bed similar to that seen in the hand.

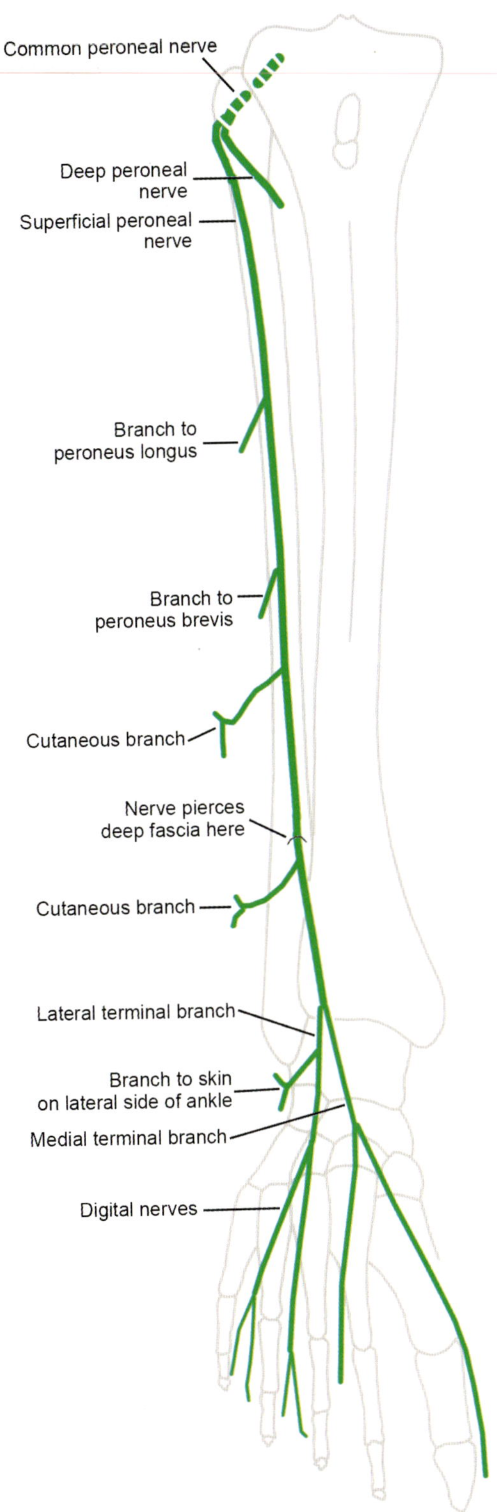


**12.16:** Distribution of superficial peroneal nerve

13

CHAPTER

# Back of Leg, and Sole

## Some Facts About Veins of the Lower Limb

The superficial veins of the lower limb have been described in Chapter 10. Some additional facts about the veins of the limb are given below.

*Venous return from the lower limbs*

1. The veins of the lower limbs can be classified into superficial and deep. The superficial veins drain into the deep veins at their terminations, and are also connected to them through a series of perforators.
2. Valves in the perforators prevent reverse flow (i.e., from deep to superficial veins).
3. Venous blood from the lower limbs has to ascend to the heart against gravity. This ascent depends on the following factors:
   a. The atmospheric pressure within the thoracic cavity is negative and this tends to suck blood in the venous system towards the heart.
   b. The veins of the lower limb are provided with numerous valves along their course. The valves, when competent, allow blood flow only towards the heart.
   c. The leg and thigh are enclosed in a tight sleeve of deep fascia.
      i. The deep veins lie within the sleeve, along with arteries and muscles.
      ii. The superficial veins lie outside the sleeve.
      iii. Perforators penetrate the sleeve.
      iv. When muscles contract they increase in thickness raising the pressure within the sleeve. This pressure compresses the deep veins and, because of the presence of valves, blood is pushed towards the heart.
      v. In this way muscular contraction acts as a pump that helps venous return from the lower limbs. The muscles of the calf are especially important in this regard.
   d. Venous return through deep veins is also aided by pulsations of adjoining arteries.

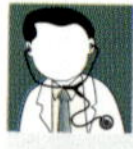

### CLINICAL CORRELATION

**Varicose Veins**

1. In some persons veins over the calf (or sometimes over other regions) become dilated and tortuous. These are called ***varicose veins***.
2. The basic cause of the development of varicose veins is incompetence of valves at the termination of superficial veins and in perforators. Once one of these valves becomes incompetent the perforator serves as a leak through which high pressure within the deep veins is transmitted to superficial veins leading to their dilatation.
3. Incompetence of valves may be congenital. It can also be a result of increased resistance to flow of blood through deep veins. Such resistance dilates the veins and dilatation in the region of a valve makes the latter incompetent.

4. Increased resistance to blood flow may be a result of blockage of deep veins by thrombophlebitis.
5. It can also be secondary to increased intra-abdominal pressure because of pregnancy or tumour.
6. The site of the high pressure leak can be determined using the ***Trendelenburg test*** as follows:
   a. The patient is asked to lie down on his back and raise the leg. This empties the superficial veins. Emptying can be facilitated by stroking the varicose veins in a proximal direction.
   b. The spheno-femoral junction is closed either by a tourniquet (an elastic band) or by pressure of the thumb. The patient is now made to stand up.
   c. If the veins are normal the veins should not refill until the pressure is released.
   d. Immediate filling of the veins from above indicates that the valve at the spheno-femoral junction is not competent.
   e. Slow filling from below indicates the presence of an incompetent perforator below the level of the tourniquet.
   f. The exact level of the incompetent perforator can be determined by repeating the test by applying the tourniquet at progressively lower levels.
7. Sophisticated techniques are now available for detailed assessment of the venous system (in the limbs and elsewhere).
   a. The veins of a region can be visualised radiographically after injecting a suitable contrast medium: this is called ***venography***.
   b. With functional venography, the functioning of veins and their valves can be seen.
   c. Movement of blood within veins can be investigated using a technique called ***Doppler ultrasound blood flow detection***. With this method the patency of a vein can be established and the presence of flow in reverse direction can also be determined.

***Some Additional Facts about the Long Saphenous Vein***

**a.** In emergencies (when the blood pressure is very low and a transfusion is required) it may be difficult to see this vein. It is useful to remember that this vein is constantly located immediately in front of the medial malleolus.

**b.** Segments taken from this vein are used as grafts in coronary bypass surgery (i.e., for replacing a blocked segment of a coronary artery). Segments can also be used for bypass operations at other sites. In such operations the direction of the vein segment is reversed so that valves do not interfere with blood flow.

## MUSCLES OF THE BACK OF THE LEG

The muscles to be seen on the back of the leg are the following:

1. Gastrocnemius
2. Soleus
3. Plantaris
4. Popliteus
5. Flexor hallucis longus
6. Flexor digitorum longus
7. Tibialis posterior.

The attachments of the muscles are given in 13.1. Also see 13.2 to 13.5.

### Note on Gastrocnemius and Soleus

1. The gastrocnemius and the soleus are together called the ***triceps surae***. They are amongst the most powerful muscles of the body. By pulling on the calcaneus they produce plantar flexion of the foot, and provide the propulsive force for walking, running and jumping.

**13.1: Muscles of the back of the leg**

| *Muscle* | *Origin* | *Insertion* | *Action* | *Nerve supply* |
|---|---|---|---|---|
| Gastrocnemius | 1. Medial head:<br>a. Posterior aspect of medial condyle of femur<br>b. Adjoining part of posterior surface<br>2. Lateral head: Lateral surface of lateral condyle of femur | Through tendocalcaneus into middle of posterior surface of calcaneus | 1. Strong plantar flexion of foot (in walking, running, jumping)<br>2. Helps in flexion of knee joint.<br>3. Steadies leg on foot | Tibial nerve (S1, 2) |
| Plantaris | Lower part of lateral supracondylar line of femur | Long thin tendon which is attached to medial margin of tendocalcaneus | Similar to above but action is very weak | Tibial nerve (S1, 2) |
| Soleus | 1. Posterior aspect of head of fibula<br>2. Posterior surface of fibula (upper 1/4)<br>3. Fibrous band connecting tibia and fibula<br>4. Soleal line of tibia<br>5. Middle one-third of medial border of tibia | Through tendocalcaneus into middle of posterior surface of calcaneus | Same as gastrocnemius | Tibial nerve (S1, 2) |
| Popliteus | 1. Lateral condyle of tibia (from anterior part of groove)<br>2. Some fibres arise from the lateral meniscus of the knee joint | Posterior surface of shaft of tibia (triangular area) | 1. Rotates the tibia medially on the femur (when the leg is off the ground)<br>2. When the leg is on the ground (fixing the tibia) it rotates the femur laterally on the tibia. This unlocks the knee joint (at beginning of flexion)<br>3. It pulls the lateral meniscus backwards during lateral rotation of the femur (preventing injury to the meniscus | Tibial nerve (L4, 5, S1) |
| Flexor hallucis longus | 1. Posterior surface of fibula<br>2. Lowest part of interosseous membrane | 1. Tendon runs down over lower part of tibia, and behind talus<br>2. It turns forwards below the sustentaculum tali (on calcaneus) into the sole<br>3. Attached to base of distal phalanx of great toe (plantar aspect) | 1. Flexion of distal phalanx of great toe<br>2. Plantar flexion of foot.<br>3. Maintains longitudinal arch of foot | Tibial nerve (S2, 3) |

*Contd...*

*Contd...*

| *Muscle* | *Origin* | *Insertion* | *Action* | *Nerve supply* |
|---|---|---|---|---|
| Flexor digitorum longus | Posterior surface of shaft of tibia | 1. Tendon passes behind medial malleolus and then on medial side of talus<br>2. In the sole the tendon divides into four slips one each for 2nd, 3rd, 4th and 5th digits<br>3. Each slip is attached to base of distal phalanx of the digit concerned (plantar aspect) | 1. Plantar flexion of distal phalanges<br>2. Continued action causes plantar flexion of other phalanges, and of the foot<br>3. Helps to maintain longitudinal arch of foot | Tibial nerve (S2, 3) |
| Tibialis posterior | 1. Posterior surface of shaft of tibia (upper two-thirds, below soleal line)<br>2. Posterior surface of fibula (upper two-thirds of medial part)<br>3. Interosseous membrane | 1. Main insertion into tuberosity of navicular bone<br>2. Slips to various tarsal and metatarsal bones (bases) | 1. Inversion of foot<br>2. Helps to maintain longitudinal arch of foot | Tibial nerve (L4, 5) |

2. The ***tendocalcaneus*** (or calcaneal tendon) is the common tendon of insertion of both the gastrocnemius and the soleus. It is the strongest tendon in the body. The integrity of the tendon is very important in walking.
3. The uppermost parts of the medial and lateral heads of the gastrocnemius form the boundaries of the lower part of the popliteal fossa.
4. The popliteal vessels and the tibial nerve pass deep to the fibrous band (between the fibula and the tibia) from which the soleus takes origin.

## Note on Plantaris

1. The muscle belly, which is only a few centimetres long, ends in a long thin tendon that runs downwards between the gastrocnemius and the soleus.
2. The plantaris is a vestigial remnant of a large muscle that was originally attached, below, to the plantar aponeurosis (Compare with the palmaris longus).
3. Because of its small size it is of little functional importance.

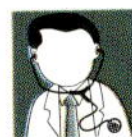

## CLINICAL CORRELATION

1. A bursa between the tendocalcaneus and the upper part of the calcaneus may get inflamed (***bursitis***) due to repeated irritation (e.g., in long-distance runners).
2. Apart from enlargement of the naturally occurring bursa, constant friction can give rise to the formation of ***adventitial bursae***. Such a bursa may form over the tendocalcaneus in a person wearing badly fitting shoes.
3. Repeated irritation can cause ***tendinitis***.
4. ***Rupture*** of the tendocalcaneus leads to loss of plantar flexion of the foot, and consequent inablity to walk.

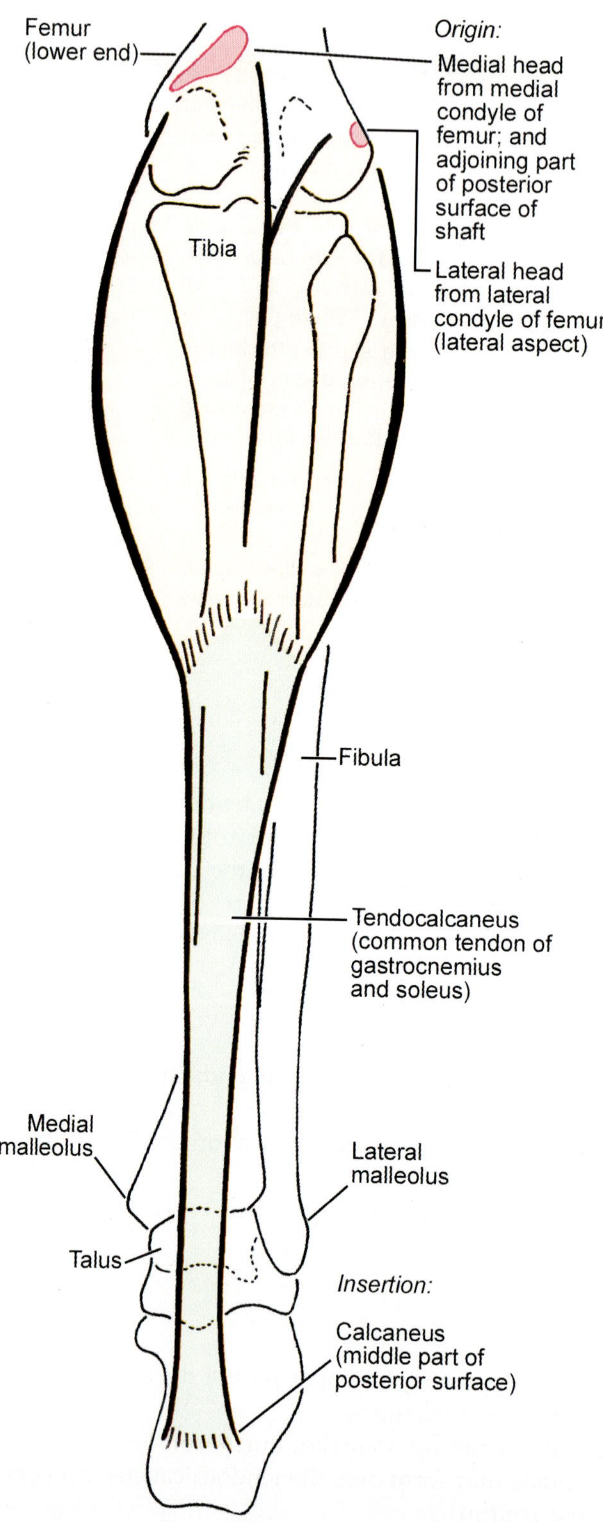


**13.2:** Scheme to show attachments of the gastrocnemius

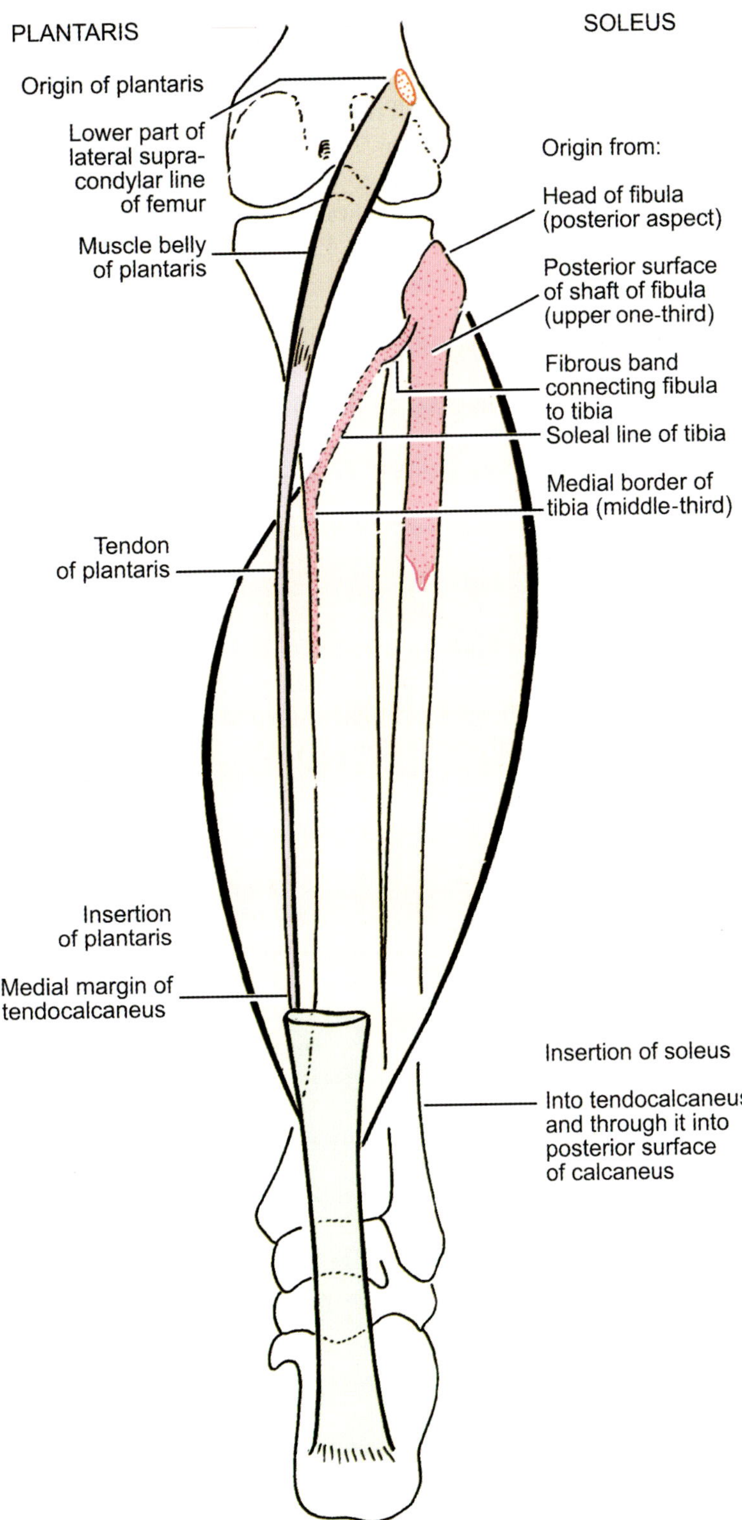


**13.3:** Scheme showing attachments of the soleus and of the plantaris

## Note on Popliteus

1. The muscle arises, by a tendon, from the lateral aspect of the lateral condyle of the femur. In this situation there is a prominent groove: the popliteus takes origin from the anterior part of the groove. The posterior part of the groove is occupied by the popliteus tendon in full flexion at the knee.
2. The origin lies within the capsule of the knee joint. It is covered by the fibular collateral ligament and by the biceps tendon.
3. The muscle emerges from the knee joint through an aperture in the capsule. The superficial margin of this aperture is formed by the ***arcuate popliteal ligament*** (13.4), which also gives origin to some fibres of the muscle.

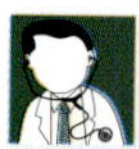

### CLINICAL CORRELATION

1. The lateral meniscus of the knee joint lies deep to the tendon of origin of the popliteus. Some fibres of the muscle take origin from this meniscus.
2. Because of its attachment to the lateral meniscus the popliteus pulls the meniscus backwards during lateral rotation of the femur.
3. This prevents injury to the meniscus.

## Note on Flexor Hallucis Longus

The tendon turns forwards below the sustentaculum tali that serves as a pulley for it. As the tendon lies on the medial side of the calcaneus it runs deep to the flexor retinaculum and is surrounded by a synovial sheath. It passes above (i.e., deep to) the tendon of the flexor digitorum longus (13.5).

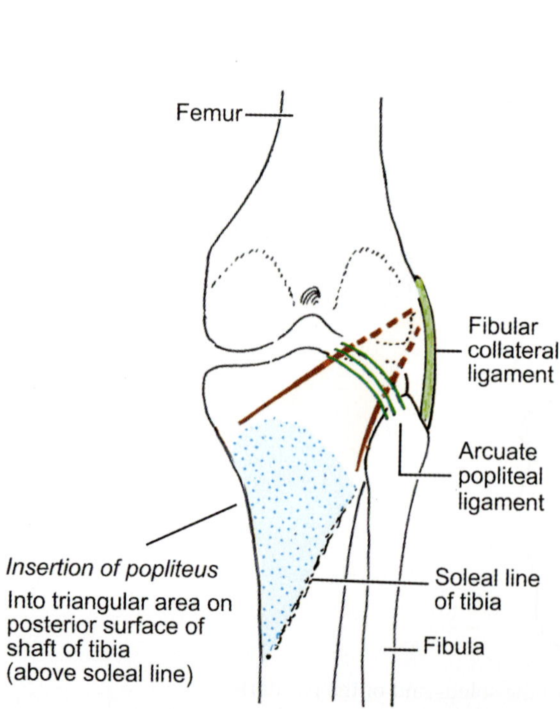


**13.4:** Posterior aspect of the bones of the popliteal region showing the insertion of the popliteus

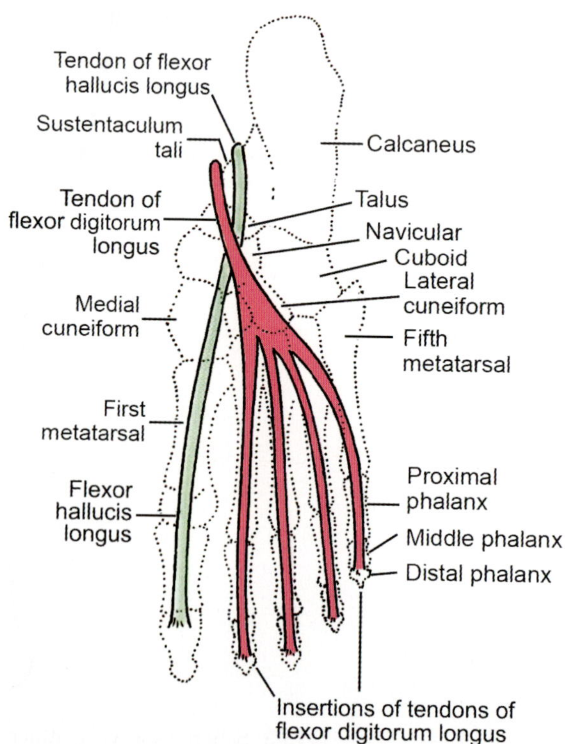


**13.5:** Course and attachments of tendons of flexor hallucis longus and flexor digitorum longus in the sole

## Note on Flexor Digitorum Longus

1. The muscle ends in a tendon that passes behind the medial malleolus.
2. Here it is covered by the flexor retinaculum (13.6), and is surrounded by a synovial sheath.
3. The tendon runs down the lateral side of the talus and passes above the sustentaculum tali.
4. It then turns laterally to enter the sole of the foot.
5. As it does so it crosses below (i.e., superficial to) the tendon of the flexor hallucis longus.

## Note on Tibialis Posterior

1. The muscle ends in a tendon that passes behind the medial malleolus; and then deep to the flexor retinaculum (13.6) to reach the sole of the foot.
2. The tendon divides into a number of slips.
   a. The main slip is inserted into the tuberosity of the navicular bone.
   b. Into the medial cuneiform bone. Other slips are inserted into:
   c. The sustentaculum tali of the calcaneus.
   d. The intermediate cuneiform.
   e. The bases of the 2nd, 3rd and 4th metatarsals.
   f. Occasionally, some slips may reach the lateral cuneiform and cuboid bones.

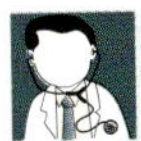

### CLINICAL CORRELATION

The calf muscles are frequently injured during violent exercise (as in atheletes).

1. The tendocalcaneus might rupture, or may undergo inflammation (***Achilles tendonitis***).
2. The plantaris tendon is sometimes ruptured.
3. The gastrocnemius can be strained during sports involving repeated strong plantar flexion (e.g., tennis). The damage is usually at the origin of the medial head. There is pain in the calf. The condition is referred to as ***tennis leg*** but it can happen in other sports as well.
4. Tapping the tendocalcaneus leads to reflex contraction of the calf muscles, and plantar flexion of the foot. This is referred to as the ***ankle jerk*** (or the ***Achilles tendon reflex***).
5. The importance of muscles of the calf in promoting venous return from the lower limbs has been explained above.

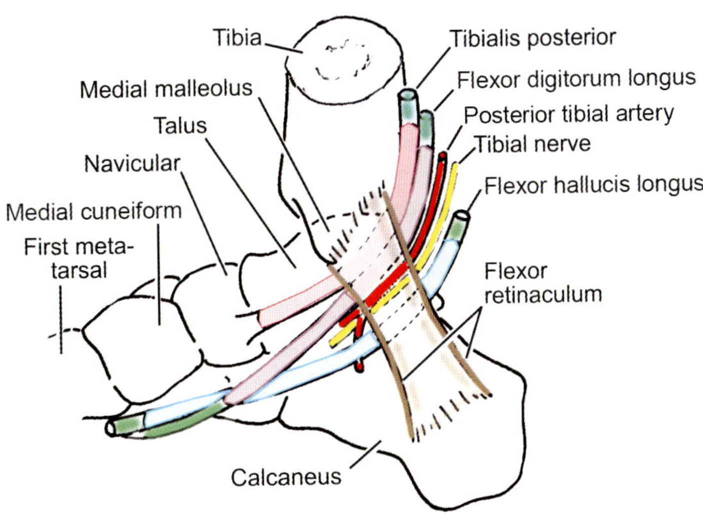


**13.6:** Flexor retinaculum and structures passing deep to it. Note the extent of the tendon sheaths

## Flexor Retinaculum

1. The flexor retinaculum is a thickened band of deep fascia present on the medial side of the ankle (13.6).
2. It is attached above to the medial malleolus, and below to the medial surface of the calcaneus.
3. It is directed downwards, backwards and laterally.
4. The structures passing under cover of it are as follows (from above downwards, and also from medial to lateral side):
   a. Tendon of the tibialis posterior.
   b. Tendon of the flexor digitorum longus.
   c. The posterior tibial vessels.
   d. The tibial nerve.
   e. The tendon of the flexor hallucis longus.

### *Synovial Sheaths*

1. The three tendons passing deep to the flexor retinaculum are surrounded by synovial sheaths which extend for some distance proximal to the retinaculum (13.7). Their distal extent is variable.
2. The sheath for the tibialis posterior extends almost to the insertion of the muscle.
3. The sheath for the flexor hallucis longus may end near the base of the first metatarsal, or may extend right up to the insertion into the terminal phalanx.
4. The sheath for the flexor digitorum longus may end near the navicular bone; or may expand to enclose the proximal parts of the tendons for the digits.
5. The distal parts of the tendons for the 2nd, 3rd and 4th digits have independent synovial sheaths, which facilitate their movement through osseo-aponeurotic canals.
6. The 5th digit has a similar sheath that is continuous proximally with the sheath for the tendon of the flexor digitorum longus.

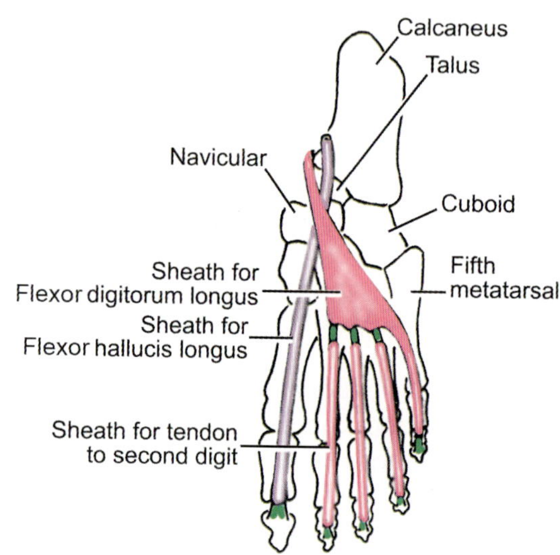


**13.7:** Synovial sheaths related to tendons of flexor muscles of the back of the leg as seen in the sole

## ARTERIES OF THE BACK OF THE LEG

## The Posterior Tibial Artery

1. The posterior tibial artery is a terminal branch of the popliteal artery (13.8). It, therefore, begins in the upper part of the back of the leg, at the lower border of the popliteus muscle.
2. The artery descends in the back of the leg, passing medially as it does so.
3. It terminates by dividing into the medial and lateral plantar arteries (on the posteromedial side of the ankle, midway between the medial malleolus and the medial tubercle of the calcaneus).
4. Superficially, the structures covering the artery (or posterior to it) are:
   a. The gastrocnemius
   b. Soleus muscles, in it upper part
   c. Only skin and fascia, in its lower part.
5. Anterior to the artery (or deep to it) there are (from above downwards):
   a. The tibialis posterior
   b. The flexor digitorum longus
   c. The posterior aspect of the tibia
   d. The ankle joint.
6. The artery is accompanied by the tibial nerve. The nerve is at first medial to the upper end of the artery, but it soon crosses behind the artery and comes to lie on its lateral side.

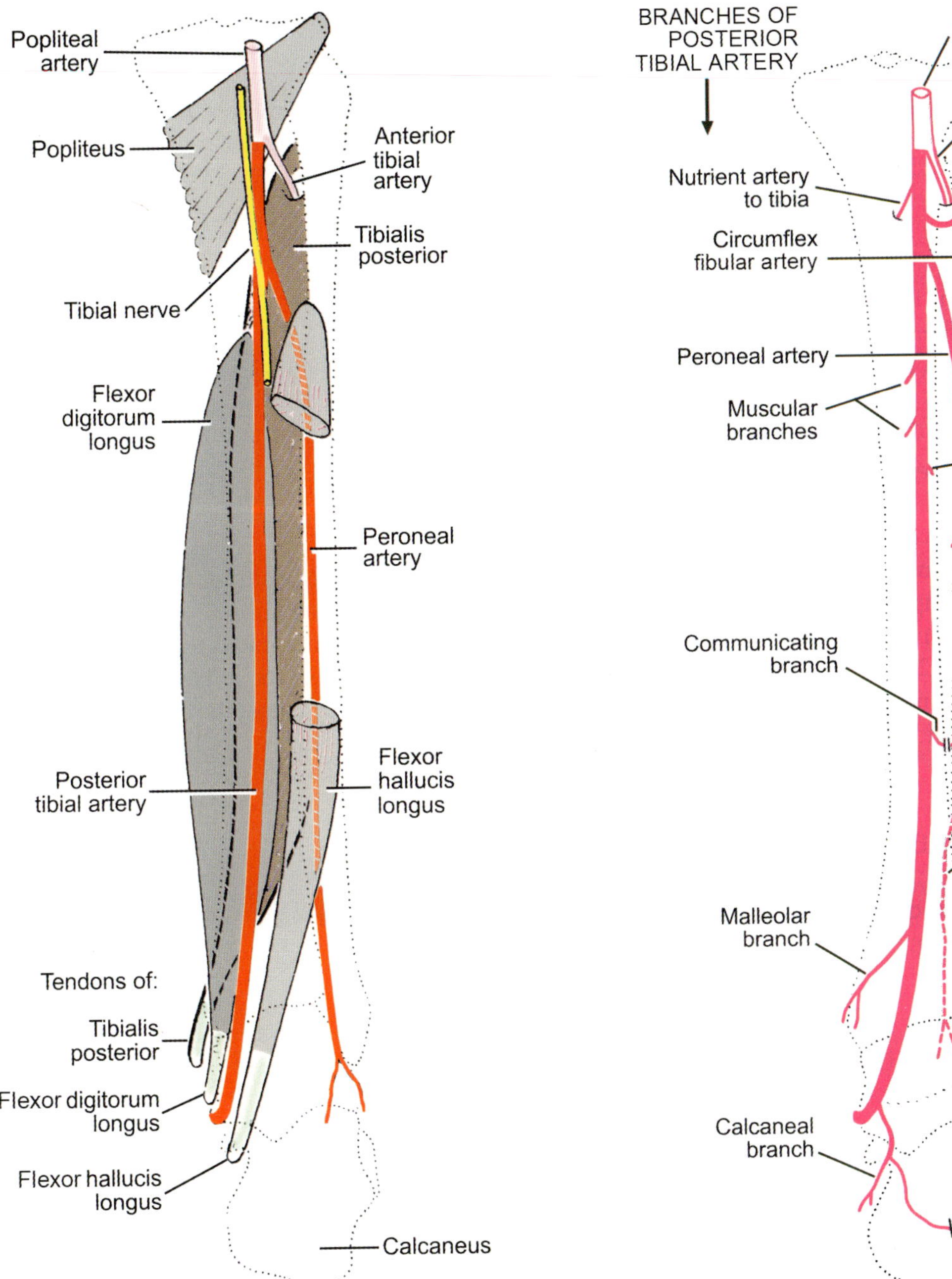


**13.8:** Course and relations of posterior tibial and peroneal arteries

**13.9:** Branches of posterior tibial and peroneal arteries

### *Branches of Posterior Tibial Artery*

The branches of the posterior tibial artery are shown in 13.9.

1. A ***nutrient*** artery is given off to the tibia.
2. The ***circumflex fibular*** branch winds round the lateral side of the neck of the fibula to reach the front of the knee (12.16).
3. ***Peroneal*** artery is described below.
4. Several ***muscular*** branches supply muscles of the region.
5. A ***communicating*** branch forms an arch with a similar branch of the peroneal artery.
6. A ***malleolar*** branch anastomoses with other arteries on the medial malleolus.
7. ***Calcaneal*** branches arise near the lower end of the artery and supply tissues of the heel.

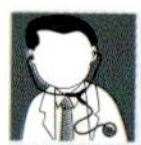

**CLINICAL CORRELATION**

1. Palpation of the posterior tibial pulse is facilitated by inversion of the foot (that relaxes the flexor retinaculum).
2. Failure to feel the pulse can occur in some normal persons, but is usually the effect of arterial obstruction. Such a person may have intermittent claudication (intermittent pain on trying to walk).

### Peroneal Artery

1. The peroneal artery is the largest branch of the posterior tibial.
2. It is given off from the posterior tibial near the upper end of the latter (13.9).
3. It runs downwards on the back of the fibula lying deep to the flexor hallucis longus (13.8).

#### *Branches of Peroneal Artery*

The branches of the peroneal artery are shown in 13.9, and are as follows:

1. ***Muscular*** branches are given off to the muscles of the region.
2. A ***nutrient*** artery is given off to the fibula.
3. A ***communicating*** branch anastomoses with a corresponding branch from the posterior tibial artery.
4. ***Calcaneal*** branches supply the heel and anastomose with other arteries in the region.
5. A ***perforating*** branch passes through the lower part of the interosseous membrane to reach the anterior compartment of the leg (12.11). Here it anastomoses with other arteries in front of the ankle including the lateral tarsal branch of the dorsalis pedis artery. Sometimes, this anastomosis is so large that the dorsalis pedis appears to be a continuation of the peroneal artery.

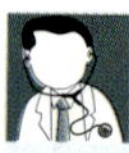

**CLINICAL CORRELATION**

In the condition when the dorsalis pedis is seen as a branch of the peroneal artery, the pulse of the dorsalis pedis cannot be felt in the normal position.

## MUSCLES AND RELATED STRUCTURES IN THE SOLE

### Plantar Aponeurosis

1. Underlying the skin of the sole there is a thick layer of deep fascia that is called the ***plantar aponeurosis***.
2. It consists of central, medial and lateral parts.
   a. The medial and lateral parts of the aponeurosis are relatively thin. They cover the abductor hallucis and the abductor digiti minimi respectively.
   b. The central part is thick and strong (13.10). It overlies the flexor digitorum brevis. (Some authors describe this part alone as the plantar aponeurosis).
3. The central part of the aponeurosis is made up of longitudinal fibres that are attached posteriorly to the medial process of the calcaneal tuberosity. Traced distally the aponeurosis broadens and divides into five processes, one for each digit.
4. Near the head of the corresponding metatarsal bone, each process divides into two slips.
5. The slips pass round the sides of the flexor tendons of the digit concerned and get attached to the deep transverse metatarsal ligaments (which stretch between the heads of the metatarsals).
6. Distally, the two slips of each process become continuous with the proximal end of the fibrous flexor sheath of the digit.

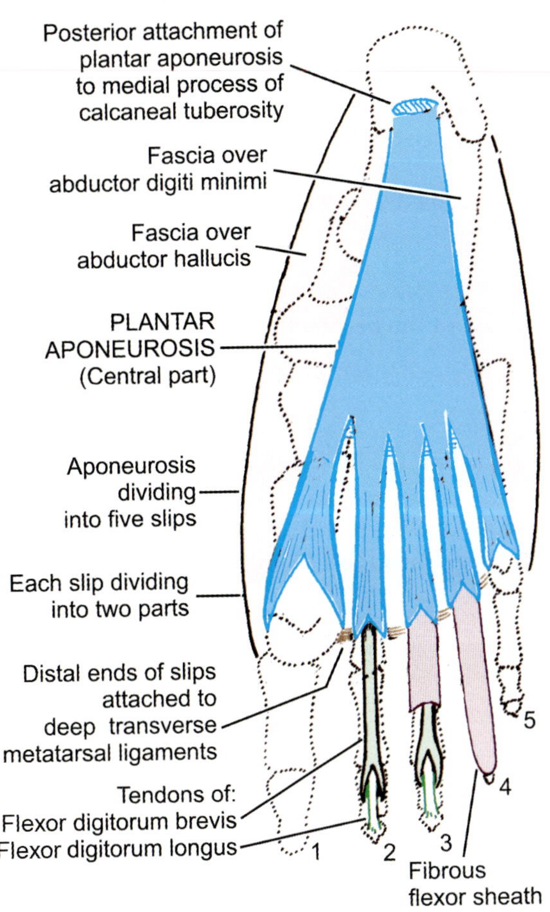


**13.10:** Scheme to show arrangement of the plantar aponeurosis

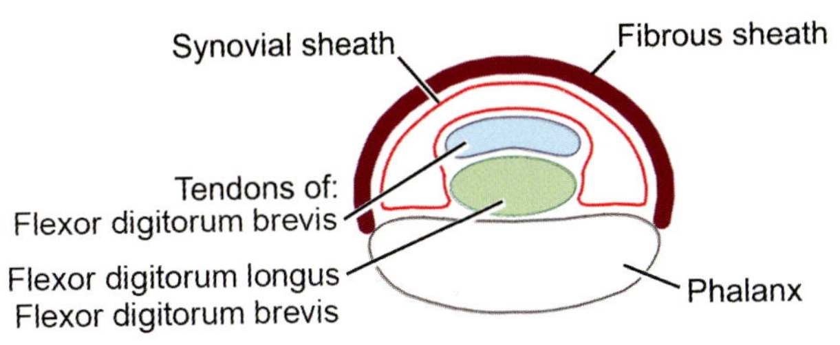


**13.11:** Transverse section across a digit to show the fibrous flexor sheath and the synovial sheath for flexor tendons

### *Fibrous Flexor Sheaths*

1. Over each toe the deep fascia (which is thick) winds round the sides of the flexor tendons of the digit to get attached to the lateral margins of the phalanges. The fascia constitutes the ***fibrous flexor sheath***.
2. The tendons are thus enclosed in an osseo-aponeurotic canal (13.11). This canal is lined by a synovial sheath to permit smooth movement of the tendons.
3. The fibrous sheath is closed distally by attachment to the base of the terminal phalanx. Proximally, the fibrous sheath is continuous with the distal margins of the slips of the plantar aponeurosis (as described above).

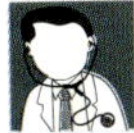

## CLINICAL CORRELATION

**Plantar Fasciitis**

1. In persons who have to do a lot of standing or walking pain over the sole of the foot may be caused by inflammation or injury to the ***plantar aponeurosis***.
2. Inflammation of the calcaneal attachment of the aponeurosis can cause considerable pain on putting the heel on the ground.

3. Ossification of the posterior end of the aponeurosis leads to the formation of a projection from the calcaneus (***calcaneal spur***). These spurs have been regarded as the cause of pain, but the recent view is that the pain is of fascial origin.

**Deep plantar abscess**

The space deep to the plantar aponeurosis may be infected. Infection can be drained by an incision parallel to the medial border of the foot.

**Bunion**

The term ***bunion*** is used for an inflamed adventitial bursa over the head of the first metatarsal bone.

### *Layers of the Sole*

1. The muscles and tendons seen in the sole lie in four layers that are separated by fascia.
2. The structures in each layer are shown in 13.12A.
3. The muscles present in the first layer are described in 13.12B, those of the second layer in 13.14, those of the third layer in 13.16 and of the fourth layer in 13.17. For more details go through 13.5 to 13.15.

**13.12A: Layers of the sole**

| | *Muscles* | *Tendons of* |
|---|---|---|
| First Layer | 1. Flexor digitorum brevis<br>2. Abductor hallucis<br>3. Abductor digiti minimi | |
| Second Layer | 1. Flexor digitorum accesorius (Quadratus plantae)<br>2. Lumbrical muscles | 1. Flexor hallucis longus<br>2. Flexor digitorum longus |
| Third layer | 1. Flexor hallucis brevis<br>2. Flexor digiti minimi brevis<br>3. Adductor hallucis | |
| Fourth Layer | 1. Plantar interossei<br>2. Dorsal interossei | 1. Tibialis posterior<br>2. Peroneus longus |

**13.12B: Muscles of the first layer of the sole**

| | *Flexor Digitorum Brevis* | *Abductor Hallucis* | *Abductor Digiti Minimi* |
|---|---|---|---|
| Origin | Tuberosity of calcaneus (medial process) | 1. Tuberosity of calcaneus (medial process)<br>2. Flexor retinaculum<br>3. Some fibres from plantar aponeurosis (deep aspect) | 1. Tuberosity of calcaneus (both processes)<br>2. Some fibres from plantar aponeurosis (deep aspect) |
| Insertion | 1. Muscle ends in four tendons (for 2nd to 5th digits)<br>2. Each digit divides into two slips<br>3. The slips reunite and again separate to be inserted into the sides of the shaft of the middle phalanx | Medial side of base of proximal phalanx of great toe | Lateral side of proximal phalanx of fifth toe |

*Contd...*

*Contd...*

| | | | |
|---|---|---|---|
| Nerve supply | Medial plantar nerve (S2, 3) | Medial plantar nerve (S2, 3) | Lateral plantar nerve (S2, 3) |
| Action | 1. Flexion of middle and proximal phalanges<br>2. Steadies toes during walking<br>3. Helps to maintain arches of the foot | 1. Abduction of great toe<br>2. Flexion of great toe<br>3. Stabilises toes during walking<br>4. Helps to maintain arches of foot | 1. Abducts fifth toe<br>2 Stabilises toes during walking<br>3. Helps to maintain arches of foot |
| Note | The two slips of the tendon for each digit form a tunnel through which the tendon of the flexor digitorum longus passes to reach its insertion into the distal phalanx | | |

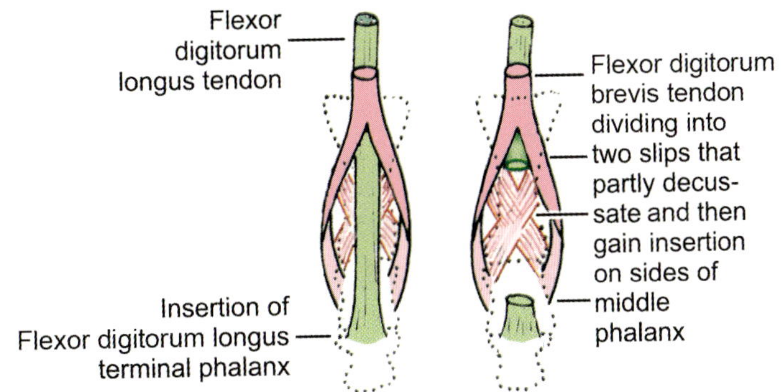


**13.13:** Arrangement of tendons of flexor digitorum longus and brevis over a digit

| **13.14: Muscles of the second layer of sole<br>Flexor digitorum accessorius (Quadratus plantae)** | |
|---|---|
| Origin | By two heads:<br>Medial head from medial surface of calcaneus<br>Lateral head from tuberosity of calcaneus (lateral process) |
| Insertion | Lateral border of tendon of flexor digitorum longus |
| Nerve supply | Lateral plantar nerve (S2, 3) |
| Actions | 1. Straightens oblique pull of flexor digitorum longus<br>2. It can flex the toes (through the tendon of the flexor digitorum longus |
| **LUMBRICALS OF FOOT** | |
| These are four small muscles that take origin from the tendons of the flexor digitorum longus | |
| Origin | 1. 1st lumbrical from medial side of tendon for 2nd toe<br>2. 2nd lumbrical from contiguous sides of tendons for 2nd and 3rd toes<br>3. 3rd lumbrical from contiguous sides of tendons for 3rd and 4th toes<br>4. 4th lumbrical from contiguous sides of tendons for 4th and 5th toes |

*Contd...*

*Contd...*

| | Flexor digitorum accessorius (Quadratus plantae) |
|---|---|
| Insertion | Each muscle ends in a tendon that passes backwards on the medial side of one metatarsophalangeal joint and is inserted into the medial basal angle of the extensor expansion for that digit in the following order:<br>1. Tendon of first lumbrical into second digit<br>2. Tendon of second lumbrical into third digit<br>3. Tendon of third lumbrical into fourth digit<br>4. Tendon of fourth lumbrical into fifth digit |
| Nerve supply | 1. First lumbrical by medial plantar nerve (S2, 3)<br>2. Other lumbricals by lateral plantar nerve (S2, 3) |
| Action | They maintain extension of interphalangeal joints of toes |

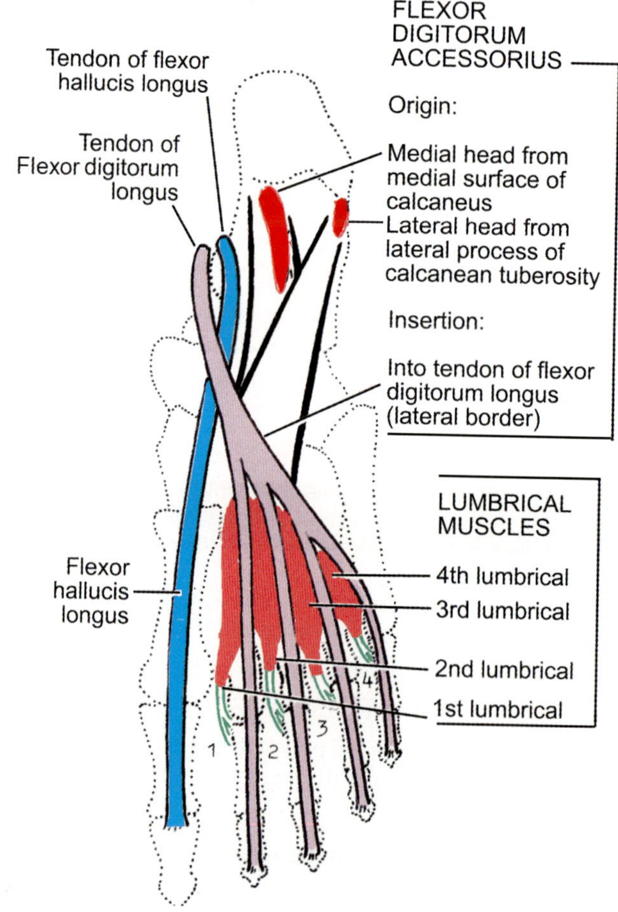


**13.15:** Scheme to show the attachments of the flexor digitorum accessorius and the lumbrical muscles

**13.16: Muscles of the third layer of the sole**

| | *Flexor Hallucis Brevis* | *Flexor Digiti Minimi Brevis* | *Adductor Hallucis* |
|---|---|---|---|
| Origin | 1. Cuboid bone, plantar surface.<br>2. Lateral cuneiform bone (some fibres)<br>3. Some fibres from slips of tendon of tibialis posterior | 1. Base of fifth metatarsal bone (plantar surface)<br>2. Some fibres from sheath covering the tendon of peroneus longus | Oblique head:<br>1. Bases of 2nd, 3rd, 4th metatarsal bones<br>2. Sheath covering tendon of peroneus longus.<br>Transverse head: Ligaments on plantar aspect of metatarsophalangeal joints of 3rd, 4th and 5th toes |
| Insertion | Muscle divides into two parts. Each part is inserted into corresponding side of base of proximal phalanx of great toe | Proximal phalanx of little toe (on lateral side of base) | The two heads end in a common tendon. It is attached to the proximal phalanx of the great toe (lateral side of base) |
| Nerve supply | Medial plantar nerve (S2, 3) | Lateral plantar nerve (S1, 2) | Lateral plantar nerve (S2, 3) |
| Action | 1. Flexion of great toe<br>2. Stabilises the toe (by preventing extension during walking)<br>3. Helps in maintaining arches of foot | 1. Flexion of little toe<br>2. Stabilises the toe (by preventing extension during walking)<br>3. Helps in maintaining arches of foot | 1. Adduction of great toe<br>2. Stabilises the toe (by preventing extension during walking)<br>3. Helps in maintaining arches of foot |

**13.17: Plantar and dorsal interosseous muscles of foot compared**

| | *Plantar Interossei* | *Dorsal Interossei* |
|---|---|---|
| FEATURES COMMON TO BOTH | 1. Numbered from medial to lateral side<br>2. Movements described with reference to the second digit<br>3. A palmar interosseous muscle is inserted into the base of the proximal phalanx of the digit concerned and into the dorsal digital expansion<br>4. Nerve supply from lateral plantar nerve (S2, 3).<br>5. They flex the metatarsophalangeal joint and extend the interphalangeal joints of the digit concerned | 1. Numbered from medial to lateral side<br>2. Movements described with reference to the second digit<br>3. A dorsal interosseous muscle is inserted into the base of the proximal phalanx of the digit concerned and into the dorsal digital expansion<br>4. Nerve supply from lateral plantar nerve (S2, 3)<br>5. They flex the metatarso-phalangeal joint and extend the interphalangeal joints of the digit concerned |
| FEATURES DIFFERENT IN THE TWO | 1. Three plantar interossei<br>2. Each muscle arises fron one metatarsal<br>3. The second digit does not give origin to, or receive the insertion of any plantar interosseous muscle<br>4. These are ADDUCTORS of the digit towards the line of the second toe<br>5. Plantar interossei take origin from, and are inserted into the third, fourth, and fifth digits (not the second)<br>6. Insertion of each muscle into medial side of one digit, third, fourth and fifth | 1. Four dorsal interossei<br>2. Each muscle arises from two adjoining metatarsals<br>3. The second digit gives origin to, and receives insertions of two muscles (one on each side: medial and lateral)<br>4. These are ABDUCTORS of digits away from the line of the second toe<br>5. Dorsal interossei take origin from all five metatarsals and are inserted into the second, third and fourth digits (not first and fifth)<br>6. Insertion of first and second muscles into medial and lateral sides of second digit and of 3rd and 4th muscles into lateral side of corresponding digit |

*Contd....*

### Main Function of Muscles in the Sole

1. The various muscles in the sole perform the movements described in the relevant tables. However, their main function is to stabilise the toes while walking. This is necessary as the propulsive force is transmitted to the ground through the toes.
2. Some phases of walking are as follows:
   a. When a foot touches the ground (during walking) it first lands on the calcaneus.
   b. In the next phase both the anterior and posterior parts of the foot touch the ground.
   c. In the third phase, the calcaneus is lifted off the ground and the anterior part of the foot exerts strong propulsive pressure on the ground.
3. The propulsive pressure (created by the gastrocnemius and soleus) reaches the foot through the tendocalcaneus.
   a. It is transmitted to the anterior part of the foot through the longitudinal arch.
   b. The integrity of the arch is essential for transmitting propulsive force to the ground.
   c. The arch is maintained by all structures connecting the anterior and posterior parts of the foot.

### Note on Interosseous Muscles of the Foot

Details of the attachments of individual interosseous muscles are easily remembered if their actions are first understood.

*Actions of interossei*

1. The interossei adduct or abduct the toes with reference to an axis passing through the ***second*** digit.
2. The plantar interossei are adductors. They pull the 3rd, 4th and 5th toes towards the second toe.
3. The dorsal interossei are abductors.
   a. To understand their action note that as the axis of the second digit is the line of reference for defining abduction: movement of this digit to either the medial or lateral side is described as abduction.
   b. The first dorsal interosseous muscle pulls the second toe medially.
   c. The second dorsal interosseous muscle pulls the same (2nd) digit laterally.
   d. The 3rd muscle pulls the 3rd digit, and the 4th muscle pulls the 4th digit laterally (i.e., away from the second digit).
4. In addition to abduction and adduction, the interossei flex the metatarsophalangeal joints and extend the interphalangeal joints by virtue of their insertion into the dorsal digital expansions (See below).

#### *Differences from Interosseous Muscles of the Hand*

Note the following differences between the interossei of the hand and those of the foot.

1. There are ***four*** palmar interossei, but only ***three*** plantar interossei.

to which the interossei produce adduction and abduction is the ***third*** digit in the hand; in the foot it is the ***second*** digit.

## ARTERIES OF THE SOLE

### Medial Plantar Artery

1. The medial plantar artery is a terminal branch of the posterior tibial artery.
2. It begins behind the medial malleolus, deep to the flexor retinaculum, and runs distally along the medial border of the sole of the foot.
3. At first, it is deep to the abductor hallucis muscle. Thereafter, it lies in the interval between the abductor hallucis medially and the flexor digitorum brevis laterally.

### *Branches of Medial Plantar Artery*

The branches of the artery are as follows (13.18):

1. Some muscular branches.
2. Three ***digital*** branches that end by joining the first, second and third plantar metatarsal arteries.
3. The main artery continues as a small branch to the medial side of the great toe.

## Lateral Plantar Artery

1. This is the other terminal branch of the posterior tibial artery.
2. It begins behind the medial malleolus deep to the flexor retinaculum.
3. At first it is deep to the abductor hallucis muscle. From here it runs obliquely across the sole in a lateral and distal direction to reach the base of the fifth metatarsal bone. This part of the artery is deep to the flexor digitorum brevis and lies over the flexor accessorius.
4. The artery now turns medially and runs deep in the sole across the bases of the metatarsal bones. This part of the artery is called the ***plantar arch***. It ends by joining the termination of the dorsalis pedis artery (in the interval between the bases of the first and second metatarsal bones).
5. The plantar arch is overlapped (apart from skin, fascia and plantar aponeurosis) by the flexor digitorum brevis, the tendons of the flexor digitorum longus and by the oblique head of the adductor hallucis muscle.

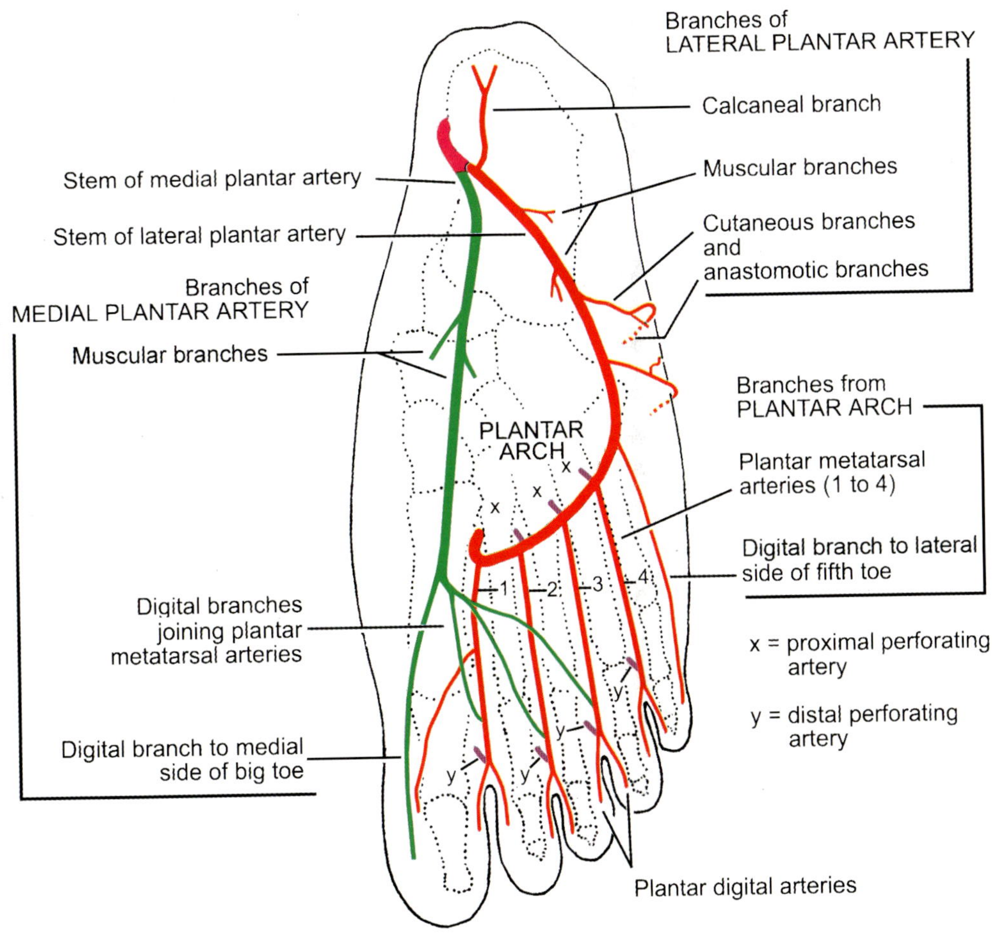


**13.18:** Scheme to show branches of medial and lateral plantar arteries

### Branches of Lateral Plantar Artery

The branches of the lateral plantar artery are shown in 13.18 and are described below.

1. A ***calcaneal*** branch arises near the beginning of the artery and supplies the skin of the heel.
2. Several ***muscular*** branches, and several ***cutaneous*** branches are given off. The latter supply the skin of the lateral part of the sole.
3. Some ***anastomotic*** branches reach the lateral border of the foot and anastomose with arteries of the dorsum of the foot.

### Branches of Plantar Arch

The branches arising from the plantar arch are as follows:

1. Four ***plantar metatarsal arteries*** ( 1 to 4) run distally, one in each intermetatarsal space.
   a. Each ends by dividing into two ***plantar digital branches*** for adjacent sides of two digits.
   b. The first artery also gives off a branch to the medial side of the great toe. The lateral side of the little toe gets a direct branch from the lateral plantar artery.
2. The plantar arch gives off three ***proximal perforating arteries*** (x) that pass through the second, third and fourth intermetatarsal spaces and communicate with the dorsal metatarsal arteries (branches of arcuate artery).
3. The distal end of each plantar metatarsal artery gives off a ***distal perforating artery*** (y) which joins the distal part of the corresponding dorsal metatarsal artery.

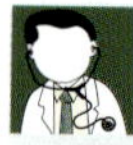

## CLINICAL CORRELATION

1. Pressure can be applied on the dorsalis pedis artery and the posterior tibial artery to stop bleeding from the foot. The dorsalis pedis artery lies in front of the ankle. The posterior tibial artery can be palpated just behind the medial malleolus. Pressure can be applied over them in these locations.
2. Arteries may be injured or pressed upon by fractured or dislocated bone ends.

*Arterial Insufficiency in the Lower Limb*

1. Arteries supplying the lower limb (like arteries elsewhere) become narrower with age and can sometimes be blocked. The level of blockage can be ascertained by feeling for the arterial pulse at different levels.
2. Bilateral absence or feebleness of the femoral pulse may be produced by narrowing of the aorta (coarctation) or by blockage.
3. Pulsation of the popliteal artery is absent in blockage of the femoral artery. The popliteal pulse is difficult to feel with the knee extended as this stretches the popliteal fascia. Flexion of the knee relaxes the fascia and overlying muscles, and makes it easier to feel the pulse.
4. In case pulsation of the dorsalis pedis artery cannot be felt it should be remembered that occasionally the artery is absent, and its area of supply is taken over by an enlarged perforating branch of the peroneal artery.
5. When an artery undergoes gradual narrowing, circulation is maintained through collateral channels.
   a. In blockage or narrowing of the proximal part of the femoral artery, circulation is maintained through the ***cruciate and trochanteric anastomoses***.
   b. When the femoral artery is blocked in the lower part of the thigh the lower part of the limb is supplied through the perforating branches of the profunda femoris artery and its anastomoses with branches of the popliteal artery.
6. Severe narrowing of arteries of the lower limb, with an inadequate collateral circulation, can lead to pain in muscles. The pain is brought on by walking and disappears with rest. As the pain appears every time the person takes a few steps it is called ***intermittent claudication*** (Claudication = limping).
   a. The pain is felt most commonly in calf muscles, but it can also occur in the thigh or in the gluteal region (depending on the level of blockage).
   b. With more serious narrowing of arteries there can be pain even at rest (rest pain); and the part becomes cold and numb.
   c. Complete blockage of supply leads to gangrene of the part.

7. In recent years there has been considerable advance in vascular surgery and various procedures are now available for relieving symptoms arising from blockage of larger arteries and for avoiding gangrene. These include the use of grafts that bypass the obstruction. Sometimes the obstruction in the vessel can be removed ***(angioplasty)***.
8. It may be remembered that apart from narrowing of vessels, insufficiency of blood supply can also be produced by spasm of smooth muscle in the walls of arteries. Spasm often coexists with physical narrowing, and relief can be obtained if spasm can be removed. This can be done by the use of drugs or by cutting off sympathetic nerve supply by lumbar sympathectomy. In this procedure the upper lumbar sympathetic ganglia are removed. However, all cases do not benefit from this operation.

***Thromboangitis obliterans (Buerger's disease)***

1. In this condition, arteries of the leg and foot are narrowed, and there is ***thrombophlebitis of veins***.
2. The condition is seen only in male smokers.
3. Localised inflammatory changes are present in the walls of arteries and veins.
4. Symptoms of arterial insufficiency are present. Gangrene of toes can occur.
5. The condition can sometimes be controlled by complete abstinence from smoking, and may benefit from lumbar sympathectomy.

## Nerves of the Back of Leg and Sole

The tibial nerve is the nerve of the back of the leg. The nerves of the sole are the medial and lateral plantar nerves.

### THE TIBIAL NERVE

This nerve has been seen in the popliteal fossa where it has been briefly described. A complete description is given below (13.19).

1. The fibres of the tibial nerve are derived from ventral rami of spinal nerves L4 to S3.
2. Separating from the common peroneal at the junction of the middle and lower thirds of the thigh it descends through the popliteal fossa, and passes into the back of the leg.
3. In the lower part of the leg it passes medially and ends midway between the medial malleolus and the tendocalcaneus by dividing into the medial and lateral plantar nerves.

*Important relations of the tibial nerve are as follows:*

1. In the upper part of the popliteal fossa, the nerve lies lateral to the popliteal artery and vein. It crosses superficial (i.e., posterior) to these vessels at the level of the knee joint and, thereafter, lies medial to them.
2. In the leg the nerve is at first medial to the posterior tibial vessels, but crosses behind these vessels to reach their lateral side.
3. Anterior (or deep) to the nerve there are (from above downwards):
   a. The popliteal surface of the femur
   b. The knee joint
   c. The popliteus
   d. The tibialis posterior
   e. The flexor digitorum longus
   f. The posterior aspect of the lower part of the tibia.
4. The posterior (or superficial) relations of the nerve are as follows:
   a. At the upper angle of the popliteal fossa the nerve is covered by the semimembranosus medially, and by the biceps femoris (laterally).
   b. In the middle of the fossa the nerve is covered only by skin and fasciae.
   c. At the lower end of the fossa the nerve is covered by the overlapping margins of the medial and lateral heads of the gastrocnemius.

d. In the upper two-thirds of the leg the nerve is overlapped by the gastrocnemius and soleus muscles. In the lower one-third of the leg (as it turns medially) the nerve is covered only by skin and fasciae.

The distribution of the tibial nerve (excluding that of its terminal branches) is as follows:

### *Muscular Branches*

1. Branches given off in the lower part of the popliteal fossa supply the two heads of the gastrocnemius, the plantaris, the soleus and the popliteus.
   The ***nerve to the popliteus*** has an interesting course. After running down superficial (posterior) to this muscle the nerve turns round its lower border to reach its anterior surface which it enters (13.19).
2. Branches arising in the leg supply the soleus, the tibialis posterior, the flexor digitorum longus and the flexor hallucis longus.

### *Cutaneous Branches*

1. The ***sural nerve*** is the main cutaneous branch.
   a. It arises in the lower part of the popliteal fossa and passes backwards between the two heads of the gastrocnemius.
   b. It then runs down the back of the leg. In its lower part the nerve inclines laterally and passes forwards below the lateral malleolus.
   c. The terminal part of the nerve runs forwards along the lateral margin of the foot reaching right up to the lateral side of the little toe.
   d. The nerve supplies skin on the posterolateral part of the leg and along the lateral margin of the foot.

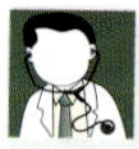

**CLINICAL CORRELATION**

The sural nerve is used as a source for nerve grafts.

2. The ***medial calcaneal branches*** arise from the tibial nerve in the lower part of the leg. They pass medially, become superficial by piercing the flexor retinaculum and supply the skin over the heel.

### *Articular Branches*

1. The upper part of the tibial nerve gives three branches to the knee joint: they accompany the superior medial genicular, the middle genicular, and the inferior medial genicular arteries.
2. The lower part of the tibial nerve gives a branch to the ankle joint.

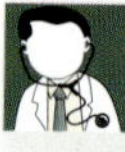

**CLINICAL CORRELATION**

1. Injury to the posterior tibial nerve is uncommon because the nerve lies deep.
2. Injury to the nerve can occur in posterior dislocation of the knee joint.
3. When the nerve is completely cut the power of plantar flexion is lost, and there is loss of sensation over part of the sole.

## MEDIAL PLANTAR NERVE

1. The medial plantar nerve is a terminal branch of the tibial nerve (13.20).
2. It begins on the posteromedial aspect of the ankle midway between the tendocalcaneus and the medial malleolus: here it lies under cover of the flexor retinaculum.

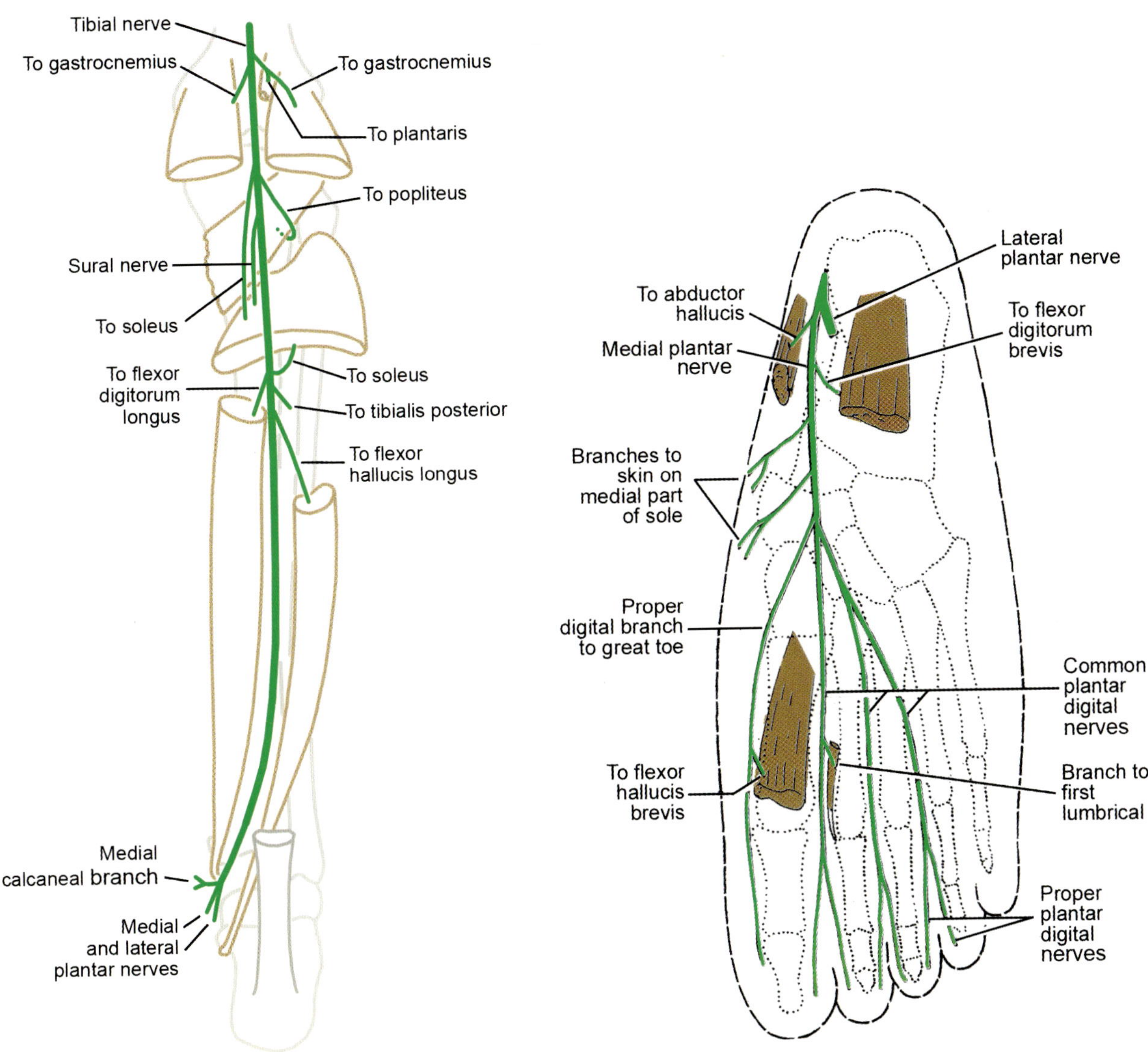


**13.19:** Scheme to show the distribution of the tibial nerve

**13.20:** Scheme to show the distribution of the medial plantar nerve

3. The nerve passes forwards for a short distance in the medial part of the sole. It is accompanied by the medial plantar artery that is medial to it.
   a. Here the nerve is at first deep to the abductor hallucis, and then lies between this muscle and the flexor digitorum brevis.
4. The nerve ends by dividing into one ***proper digital branch*** for the great toe, and three ***common plantar digital branches.*** The nerve is distributed as given below (13.20).

### Cutaneous Branches

1. Branches arising from the trunk of the nerve supply the skin of the medial part of the sole.
2. The skin on the medial side of the great toe is supplied by the proper digital branch to this digit.

3. Each common plantar digital nerve divides into two ***proper digital nerves***.
   a. The first (most medial) common plantar digital nerve divides into the proper digital nerves that supply the skin on the adjacent sides of the great toe and second toe.
   b. The second nerve divides into branches that supply the second and third toes.
   c. The third nerve divides into branches that supply the third and fourth toes.
   Each digital nerve gives a dorsal branch that supplies the nail bed.

### *Muscular Branches*

1. Branches arising from the trunk of the nerve supply the abductor hallucis, and the flexor digitorum brevis.
2. The flexor hallucis brevis receives a branch from the digital nerve to the great toe.
3. The first lumbrical muscle is supplied by a branch from the first plantar digital nerve.

### *Articular Branches*

Branches arising from the main trunk help to supply the tarsal and tarsometatarsal joints, while branches arising from the digital nerves supply metatarsophalangeal and interphalangeal joints.

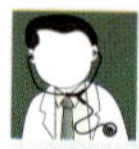

### CLINICAL CORRELATION

The medial plantar nerve may be compressed or irritated as it passes under the flexor retinaculum. There is pain on the medial side of the foot and in the heel. Sensations are abnormal. The condition is seen in long distance runners (***Jogger's foot***).

## THE LATERAL PLANTAR NERVE

1. The lateral plantar nerve is a terminal branch of the tibial nerve (13.21).
2. It begins on the posteromedial aspect of the ankle midway between the tendocalcaneus and the medial malleolus.
3. It passes forwards and laterally across the sole (13.21).
4. The nerve ends (near the tubercle of the fifth metatarsal bone) by dividing into superficial and deep branches.
5. The trunk of the lateral plantar nerve is accompanied by the lateral plantar artery, which lies lateral to it. (Note that the two nerves lie between the two arteries).
6. The nerve lies between the flexor digitorum brevis (superficial to it) and the flexor accessorius (deep to it).
7. At its termination, the trunk of the nerve lies between the flexor digitorum brevis and the abductor digiti minimi.
8. The ***superficial branch*** runs distally and ends by dividing into two plantar digital nerves.
   a. The lateral of these runs along the lateral side of the fifth digit.
   b. The medial one divides into two branches that supply the adjacent sides of the fourth and fifth digits (13.21).
9. The ***deep branch*** begins near the tubercle of the fifth metatarsal bone. From here it runs medially deep to the flexor tendons and the adductor hallucis.
   The distribution of the lateral plantar nerve and its terminal branches is as follows.

### *Muscular Branches*

1. Branches arising from the trunk supply the flexor digitorum accessorius and the abductor digiti minimi.
2. The flexor digiti minimi brevis is supplied by the digital branch for the lateral side of the fifth toe. This nerve also supplies the interosseous muscles that lie between the fourth and fifth metatarsal bones (i.e., the third plantar and the fourth dorsal interosseous muscles).

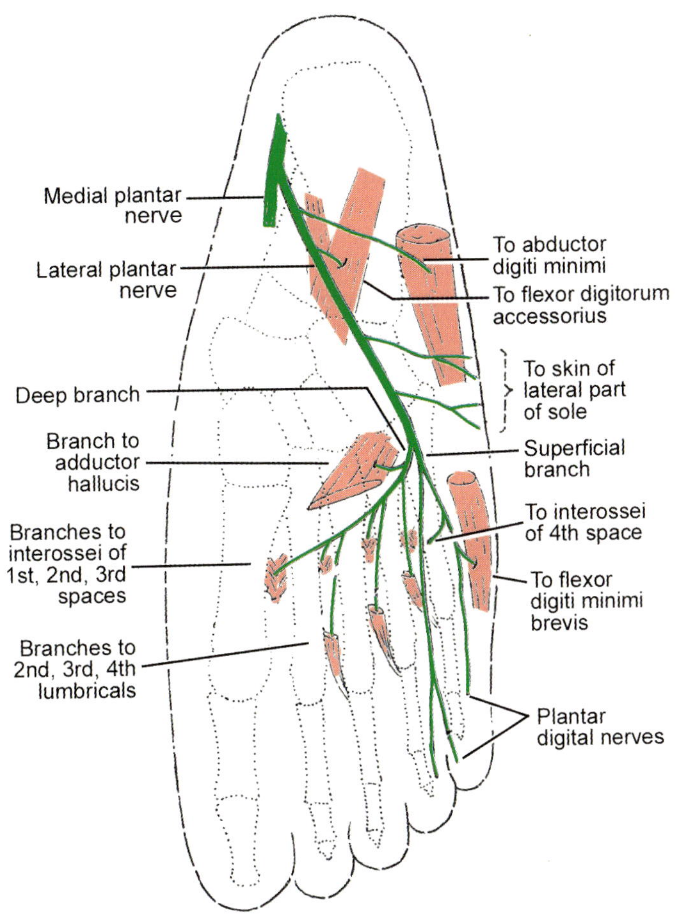


**13.21:** Scheme to show the distribution of the lateral plantar nerve

3. The deep branch supplies all interossei except those lying between the fourth and fifth metatarsals. It also supplies the 2nd, 3rd and 4th lumbrical muscles, and the adductor hallucis. (Compare the distribution of the deep branch with that of the deep branch of the ulnar nerve).

### *Cutaneous Branches*

1. Some branches arising from the trunk of the nerve supply the skin of the lateral part of the sole.
2. The skin on the lateral side of the little toe and the contiguous sides of the fourth and fifth toes is supplied by the corresponding digital branches.

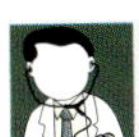

## CLINICAL CORRELATION

**The Plantar Reflex**

1. Stroking the lateral side of the sole of the foot (and carrying the stroke towards the base of the great toe) results in reflex flexion of the toes. This is the normal response.
2. In upper motor neuron paralysis (e.g., hemiplegia) there is an ***extensor response***. There is dorsiflexion (extension) of the great toe and fanning out of other toes. This is called the ***Babinski sign***.
3. In children up to the age of four years an extensor response is normal. This is because the pyramidal tracts are not fully myelinated.

*Segmental innervation*

See chapter 11.

*Sciatica*

Pressure on the lumbosacral nerve roots is often produced by prolapse of an intervertebral disc. Typically, the condition causes severe pain that begins in the gluteal region and radiates down the back of the thigh and leg to reach the foot (***sciatica***).

**Deformities of the Foot**

1. Congenital deformities are frequently seen in the region of the ankle and foot, and are of various types. The general term ***talipes*** is applied to them.
2. In the most common variety of deformity the foot shows marked plantar flexion (= ***equinus***: like the foot of a horse), and inversion (= varus: inward bend). Hence this condition is called ***talipes equino varus***. In layman's language it is called ***club foot***. The condition may be unilateral or bilateral.
3. The medial longitudinal arch of the foot may be poorly developed (***pes planus*** or ***flat foot***). A flat footed person may have difficulty in walking long distances, or in running.
4. Conversely, the foot may be too highly arched (***pes cavis***). This condition is often associated with neurological disorders (including poliomyelitis).
5. Deformities in the region of the toes can be produced by ill-fitting shoes.
   a. In ***hallux valgus,*** there is lateral deviation of the big toe that may come to lie below, or above, the second toe.
   b. In ***hallux rigidus,*** there is pain and limitation of movement of the big toe at the metacarpophalangeal joint.
   c. The deformity called ***hammer toe*** is usually seen in the 2nd, 3rd or 4th digits. The affected toe is hyperextended at the metacarpophalangeal joint, flexed at the proximal interphalangeal joint, and again hyperextended at the distal interphalangeal joint. Hammer toe can also be produced by paralysis of dorsiflexors of the foot.

**Some other Clinical Conditions in the Foot**

***Metatarsalgia*** is a condition in which there is pain in the forefoot on walking. The pain is usually located in the interspace between the 3rd and 4th toes and is caused by pressure on the digital nerve present here.

*Ingrowing Toe Nail*

In this condition, seen in the big toe, one end of the distal edge of the nail grows into soft tissue causing pain and setting up inflammation. The condition can be prevented by trimming the nail straight and making sure that it does not grow into soft tissue. In serious cases part of the nail may need removal.

*Paronychia*

This is infection of soft tissue in relation to a nail bed similar to that seen in the hand.

*Deep Plantar Abscess*

The space deep to the plantar aponeurosis may be infected. Infection can be drained by an incision parallel to the medial border of the foot.

# 14 CHAPTER Joints of the Lower Limb

## JOINTS AND LIGAMENTS OF THE PELVIS

### Pubic Symphysis

1. The two pubic bones are united in front at the ***pubic symphysis***.
2. This joint corresponds in structure to that of a secondary cartilaginous joint (See chapter 9).

### Sacroiliac Joints

1. The sacrum articulates on each side with the corresponding ilium forming the right and left sacroiliac joints. These are synovial joints.
2. The iliac and sacral surfaces are both shaped like the auricle (pinna) and are, therefore, called ***auricular surfaces***. The surfaces are covered by cartilage, but because of the presence of a number of raised and depressed areas the joint allows little movement.
3. The capsule of the joint is attached around the margins of the articular surfaces.
4. It is thickened in its anterior part to form the ***ventral sacroiliac ligament***.
5. The main bond of union between the sacrum and ilium is, however, the ***interosseous sacroiliac ligament*** that is attached to rough areas above and behind the auricular surfaces of the two bones.
6. The posterior aspects of the sacrum and ilium are connected by a strong ***dorsal sacroiliac ligament*** which covers the interosseous ligament from behind.
7. The stability of the sacroiliac joints is important as body weight is transmitted from the sacrum to the lower limbs through them.
   Two other ligaments that connect the sacrum to the hip bone are the sacrotuberous and the sacrospinous ligaments that have been encountered in the gluteal region (14.1).

#### *Sacrotuberous Ligament*

1. The sacrotuberous ligament is large and strong.
2. It has a broad upper medial end and a narrower lower lateral end.
3. The upper end is attached (from above downwards) to:
   a. The posterior superior and posterior inferior iliac spines.
   b. The lower part of the posterior surface of the sacrum (transverse tubercles).
   c. The lateral margin of the lower part of the sacrum and the upper part of the coccyx.
4. Its lower end is attached to:
   a. The medial margin of the ischial tuberosity.
   b. Some fibres that are continued onto the ramus of the ischium constitute the ***falciform process***.

#### *Sacrospinous Ligament*

The sacrospinous ligament is attached medially to the sacrum and coccyx and laterally to the ischial spine.

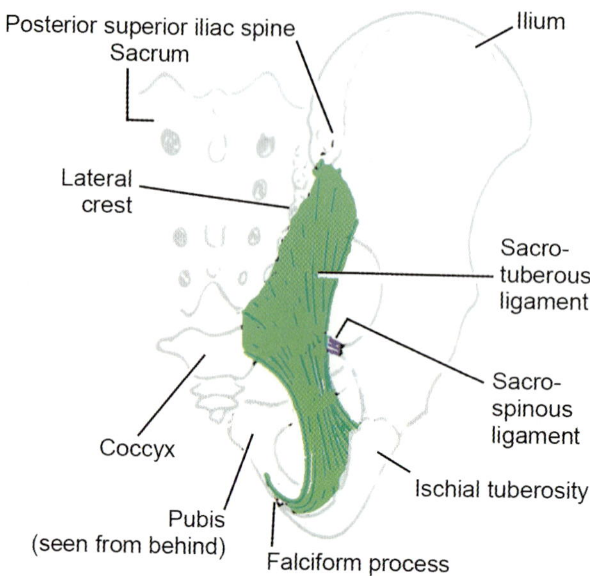


**14.1:** Posterior aspect of the pelvis showing the attachments of the sacrotuberous and sacrospinous ligaments

## THE HIP JOINT

1. This is a synovial joint of the ball and socket variety. The rounded head of the femur fits into the deep cavity provided by the acetabulum of the hip bone.
2. The hip joint has several similarities with the shoulder joint.
   a. The articular cartilage lining the head of the femur is thickest in the centre and thinnest at the periphery (14.2) having the effect of increasing the convexity of the head.
   b. The depth of the acetabulum is increased by the presence of a rim of fibrocartilage called the ***acetabular labrum***.
3. However, the difference between the two joints are more striking.
   a. The acetabulum is a much deeper cavity than the glenoid cavity.
   b. As a result the adaptation of the head of the femur with the acetabulum is far more intimate than that of the head of the humerus with the glenoid cavity.
   c. As a result the hip joint is much more stable, and much less mobile than the shoulder joint.
4. The cavity of the ***acetabulum*** is partly articular and partly nonarticular.
   a. The articular surface is shaped like a horse-shoe. It covers the anterior, superior and posterior walls of the acetabulum.
   b. The articular area is widest superiorly this being the area where maximum body weight is transmitted to the femur.
   c. The cartilage lining the acetabulum is thickest here.
5. The inferior part of the acetabulum is nonarticular and is called the ***acetabular fossa***.
   a. Here the rim of the acetabulum is also deficient, the gap being called the ***acetabular notch***.
   b. A part of the acetabular labrum bridges across the notch as the ***transverse ligament of the acetabulum***.
6. The ***head of the femur*** is somewhat more than half a sphere. It faces upwards, medially and slightly forwards. Near its centre it is marked by a pit called the ***fovea*** .

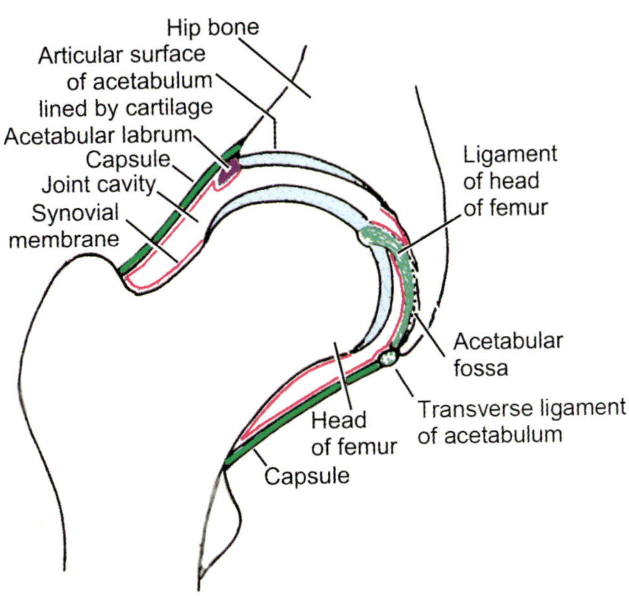


**14.2:** Schematic section across the hip joint

7. The proximal and distal articular surfaces are joined together by a capsular ligament, and directly by a ligament passing from the head of the femur to the acetabulum.
   a. This ligament is called the ***ligament of the head of the femur***.
   b. It is attached, laterally, to the fovea on the head of the femur, and medially to the two ends of the acetabular notch, and between them to the transverse ligament.
8. The ***capsular ligament*** of the hip joint is strong.
   a. Medially, it is attached to the hip bone around the margins of the acetabulum.
   b. Laterally, it covers the greater part of the neck of the femur. Anteriorly, it is attached to the trochanteric line; posteriorly to the neck of the femur a short distance medial to the trochanteric crest; above to the base of the greater trochanter; and inferiorly to the neck near the lesser trochanter (14.3, 14.4).
   c. Many of the fibres of the capsule attached to the front of the neck turn sharply to run on it towards the head: they form longitudinal bundles called ***retinacula***.
   d. The capsule itself consists of an inner layer of circular fibres (***zona orbicularis***) that form rings around the neck of the femur; and of more superficial longitudinal fibres. The capsule is strengthened by the presence of three ligaments: iliofemoral, pubofemoral and ischiofemoral.
9. The ***iliofemoral ligament*** is the strongest.
   a. It is attached above to the anterior inferior iliac spine (14.3).
   b. Inferiorly, its fibres diverge to form two bands: medial and lateral.
   c. The medial band runs vertically to be attached to the lower part of the trochanteric line.
   d. The lateral band is attached to the upper part of the same line.
   e. Because of its shape, the iliofemoral ligament is also called the Y-shaped ligament.
10. The ***pubofemoral ligament*** (14.3) is attached above and medially to the iliopectineal eminence and the superior ramus of the pubis. It passes downwards and laterally to blend with the medial band of the iliofemoral ligament and with the capsular ligament.
11. The ***ischiofemoral ligament*** (14.4) is attached medially to the ischium just beyond the acetabulum and laterally to the greater trochanter.
12. The ***synovial membrane*** of the hip joint is extensive. It lines the inside of the capsular ligament, the intracapsular part of the neck of the femur, both surfaces of the acetabular labrum, the acetabular fossa, and the ligament of the head of the femur (14.2).

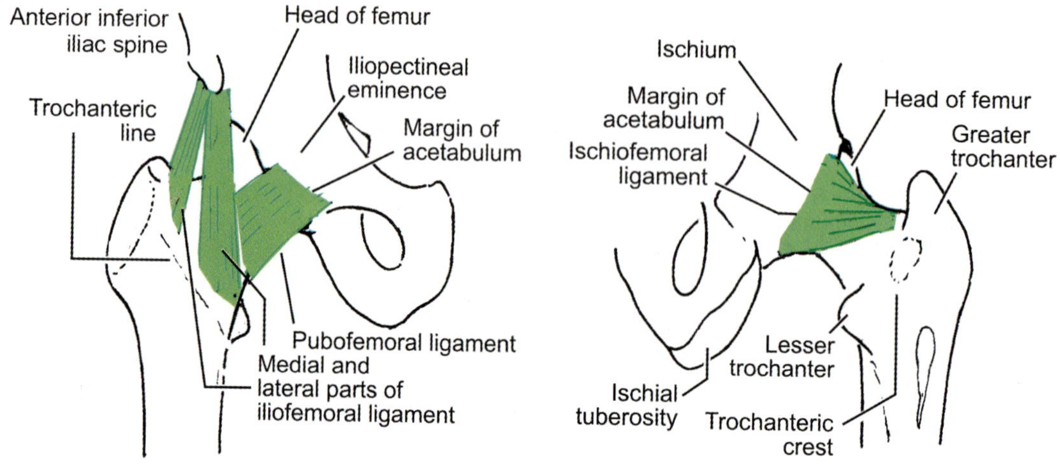


**14.3:** Hip joint: anterior aspect

**14.4:** Hip joint: posterior aspect

13. The hip joint is supplied by branches from the obturator, medial circumflex femoral, superior gluteal and inferior gluteal arteries; by the femoral, obturator and superior gluteal nerves, and by the nerve to the quadratus femoris.
14. The movements at the hip joint are flexion, extension, abduction, adduction, medial rotation and lateral rotation. The muscles responsible for them are shown in 14.5.

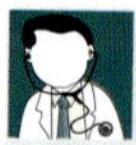

## CLINICAL CORRELATION

**Dislocations of the Hip Joint**

1. We have seen that the hip joint may be the site of congenital dislocation. The hip joint can also be dislocated as a result of injury. Dislocation can be posterior, anterior, or central.
   a. In ***posterior dislocation,*** the head of the femur passes backwards. In this process the rim of the acetabulum is usually fractured so that it is a fracture dislocation. There is serious danger of injury to the sciatic nerve which lies just behind the joint.
   b. ***Anterior dislocation*** is not common. It is caused by forced abduction and lateral rotation of the limb. After posterior dislocation the limb is medially rotated, and in anterior dislocation the limb is laterally rotated.
   c. In ***central fracture dislocation,*** the head of the femur breaks through the floor of the acetabulum to enter the pelvic cavity. There is great danger to the sciatic nerve in this dislocation.
2. As the hip joint is very stable (compared to the shoulder joint) dislocations take place only with serious injuries like car accidents, or falls from a height. Dislocation may be accompanied by fracture of the femur.

Joint Replacement

1. In old age the articular surfaces of the hip joint often undergo degeneration due to *osteoarthritis*. Movements get restricted and there is pain. The condition can be corrected by replacing the joint with one made of artificial materials.

## THE KNEE JOINT

1. The knee joint is a synovial joint of the condylar variety.
2. It is a ***compound*** joint having two distinct articular surfaces on the medial and lateral condyles of the femur, for articulation with corresponding surfaces on the medial and lateral condyles of the tibia.

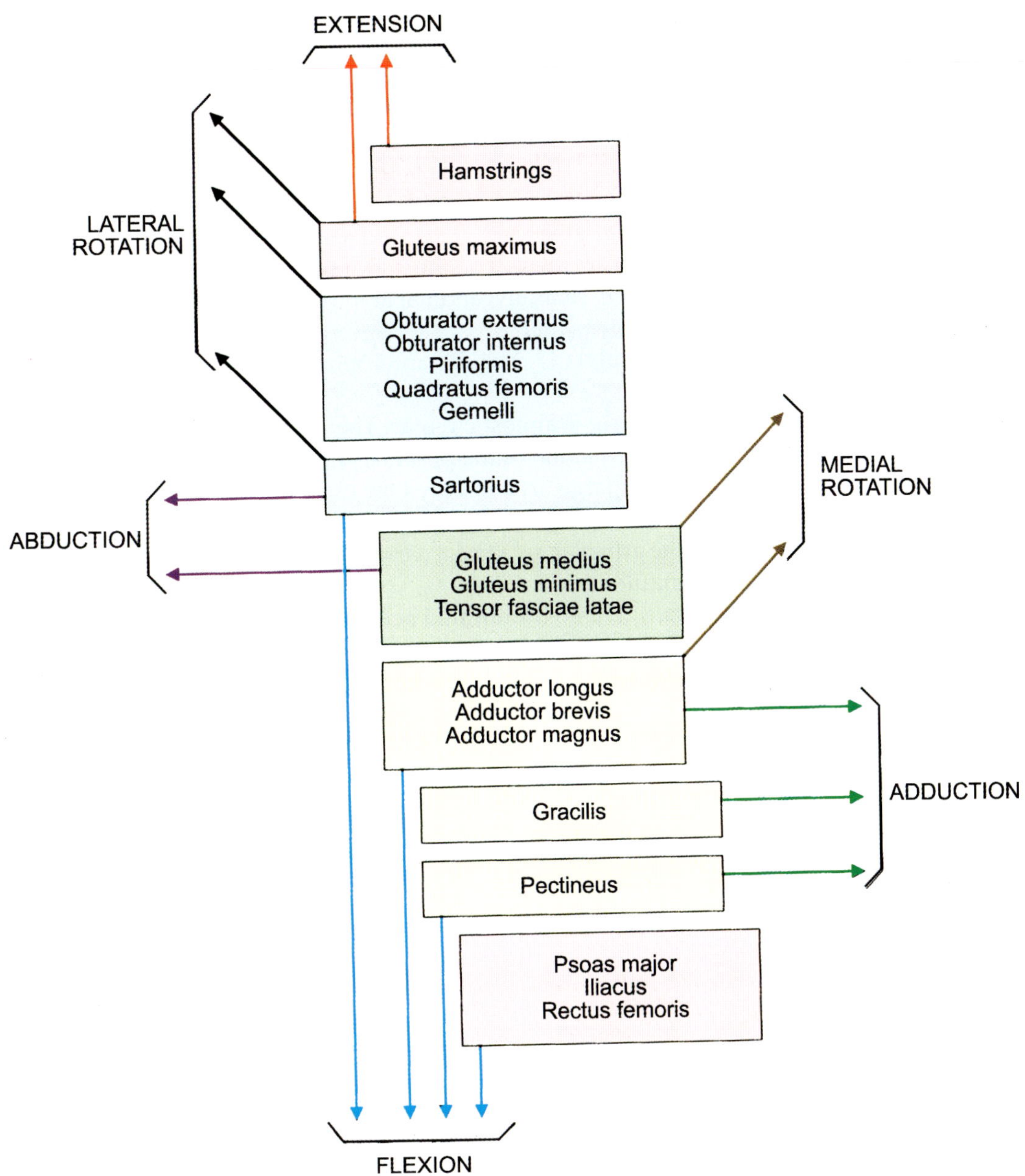


**14.5:** Scheme to show muscles responsible for movements at the hip joint

3. The anterior aspect of the lower end of the femur articulates with the posterior aspect of the patella.
4. The knee joint is a ***complex*** joint because its cavity is partially divided into upper and lower parts by plates of cartilage called the medial and lateral menisci.
5. The ***proximal articular surface*** covers the anterior, inferior and posterior aspects of the medial and lateral condyles of the femur (14.6).
   a. Anteriorly, the medial and lateral articular surfaces are continuous with each other (14.6A), but posteriorly they are separated by the intercondylar notch (6 in 14.6 B).
   b. The part of the femoral articular surface situated on the anterior aspect of its lower end articulates with the patella. It is concave from side-to-side and is subdivided by a vertical groove into a larger lateral part and a smaller medial part.

c. A small part of the inferior surface of the medial condyle, adjacent to the anterior part of the intercondylar notch comes in contact with the patella in extreme flexion of the knee. The area for the patella is marked off from the area for the tibia on each condyle by a slight groove.

d. The tibial articular surface of each femoral condyle is convex anteroposteriorly, the curvature being much more marked in the posterior part. This is most obvious when the condyle is viewed from the side. The condyles are also convex from side-to-side. The long axis of the lateral condylar articular surface is straight and is placed anteroposteriorly. The axis of the medial condylar surface shows an anteroposterior curve, the convexity of the curve being directed medially.

6. The ***distal articular surfaces*** of the knee joint are present on the upper surfaces of the medial and lateral condyles of the tibia. These surfaces are slightly concave centrally, and flat at the periphery, where they are covered by the corresponding menisci.
   a. The articular surface of the medial condyle is oval, its anteroposterior diameter being greater than the transverse diameter.
   b. The articular surface of the lateral condyle is almost circular. The posterior part of this surface is rounded and can be seen from behind (14.7B); the tendon of the popliteus muscle glides over this area.
7. The ***posterior surface of the patella*** bears a large articular area for the femur. It is convex and is divided by a ridge into a larger lateral part and a smaller medial part.
   Near the medial margin of the patella the articular area has a narrow semilunar strip that comes in contact with the medial condyle of the femur only in full flexion.
8. The attachment of the ***capsule*** of the knee joint is complicated because of the presence of the patella anteriorly, and because of the fact that anteriorly the capsule blends indistinguishably with the lower tendinous part of the quadriceps femoris muscle.

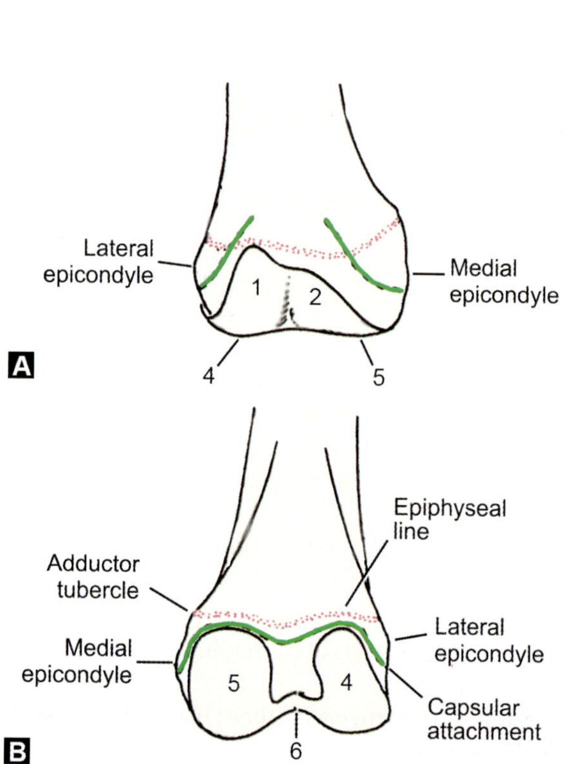


**14.6A and B:** Lower end of right femur showing attachments of the capsule of the knee joint. (A) Anterior aspect; (B) Posterior aspect

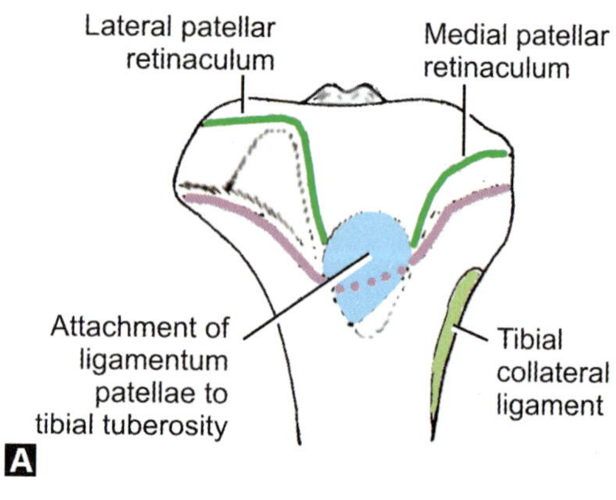


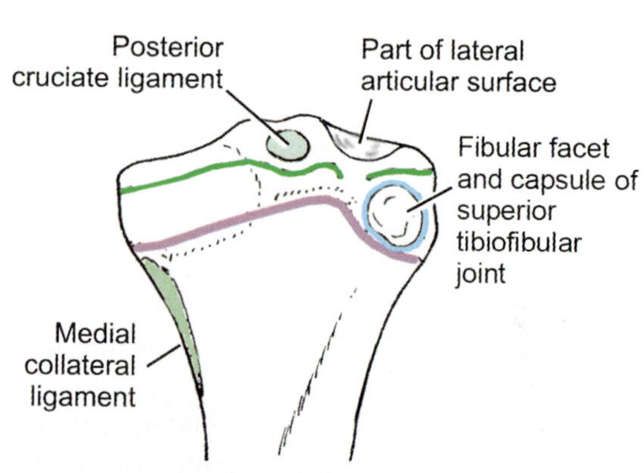


**14.7A and B:** Upper end of right tibia to show attachments of the capsule of the knee joint (green). (A) Anterior aspect; (B) Posterior aspect

## Attachment on the Femur

1. On the medial side of the femur the capsule is attached to the medial and posterior aspects of the condyle just beyond the articular surface.
2. Traced laterally, the line of attachment passes along the posterior margin of the intercondylar notch to the posterior surface of the lateral condyle (14.6B), and then to the lateral side of the condyle where it is attached above the origin of the popliteus muscle.
3. Anteriorly, the capsule merges with expansions from two muscles: The vastus medialis (medially) and the vastus lateralis (laterally). These expansions are attached to the upper, lateral and medial borders of the patella; and below the patella to the medial and lateral sides of the ligamentum patellae.

### *Inferior Attachment*

1. On the medial side (14.7) the capsule is attached to the medial margin of the medial condyle of the tibia.
2. Traced posteriorly, the line of attachment passes (in that order) onto the posterior aspect of the medial condyle (14.7B), the posterior margin of the intercondylar area, the posterior and then the lateral margin of the lateral condyle.
3. There is a gap in the capsular attachment behind the lateral condyle. The popliteus, which arises from within the knee joint, leaves it through this gap. Here the lower margin of the capsule is attached to a band of fibres called the ***arcuate popliteal ligament***. This ligament passes from the head of the fibula to the posterior margin of the intercondylar area of the tibia (14.9).
4. Anteriorly, the expansions from the vastus medialis and the vastus lateralis gain attachment to the anterior aspect of the medial and lateral condyles of the tibia: here these expansions are called the ***medial and lateral patellar retinacula*** (14.7A).
5. The capsule is strengthened in several situations by ligaments and expansions as follows:
   a. Anteriorly, below the patella the capsule is replaced by the ***ligamentum patellae***. This ligament is attached above to the nonarticular lower part of the posterior surface of the patella and below to the upper smooth part of the tibial tuberosity (14.8). Some of its fibres may extend onto the lower rough part of the tuberosity. On either side the ligament is continuous with the patellar retinacula.
   b. On the medial and lateral sides of the joint there are strong collateral ligaments.
   c. The ***tibial collateral ligament*** is attached above to the medial surface of the medial condyle of the femur just below the adductor tubercle (14.9). Inferiorly, the deeper fibres of the ligament are attached to the medial condyle of the tibia: they are adherent to the medial meniscus and blend with the capsule. The anterior and

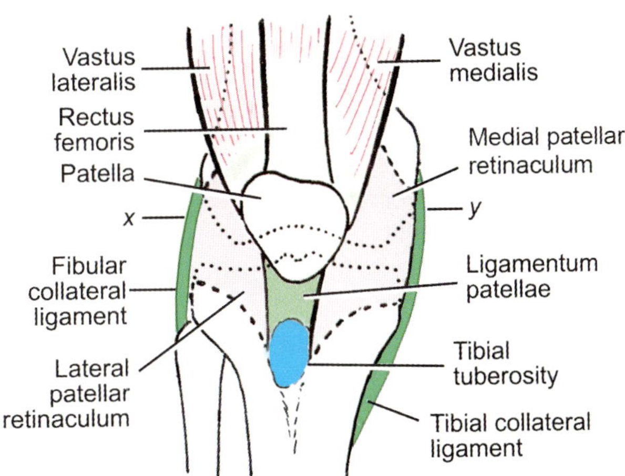


**14.8:** Schematic diagram showing structures forming the anterior wall of the knee joint

more superficial fibres of the ligament gain attachment to the upper part of the medial surface of the shaft of the tibia (14.7B, 14.9). They are separated from the capsule by an expansion from the semimembranosus, and by the medial inferior genicular vessels and nerve.

d. The ***fibular collateral ligament*** is attached above to the lateral epicondyle of the femur above the groove for the popliteus. Below it is attached to the head of the fibula. The ligament is separated from the lateral meniscus by the tendon of the popliteus and is, therefore, not adherent to the meniscus. The inferior lateral genicular vessels and nerves also lie deep to the ligament.

e. The posterior aspect of the capsule is strengthened by the ***oblique popliteal ligament***. This ligament is an expansion from the tendon of the semimembranosus (14.9). It passes upwards and laterally from the posterior aspect of the medial condyle of the tibia to be attached to the femur on the lateral part of the intercondylar line and to the lateral condyle.

The posterior aspect of the capsule is also strengthened by the origins of the medial and lateral head of the gastrocnemius.

6. Apart from the capsular ligament and its associated ligaments, the femur and tibia are united by two strong ligaments that lie within the joint. These are the anterior and posterior cruciate ligaments (so called because they cross each other).
   a. The ***anterior cruciate ligament*** is attached below to the anterior part of the intercondylar area of the tibia (14.10). It passes upwards, backwards and laterally to the medial aspect of the lateral condyle of the femur (i.e., on the lateral wall of the intercondylar notch).
   b. The ***posterior cruciate ligament*** is attached below to the posterior part of the intercondylar area of the tibia. It passes upwards, forwards and medially to attached above to the lateral surface of the medial condyle of the femur. (In respect of these ligaments, the student should associate the terms anterior and posterior with their tibial attachments).
7. The ***medial and lateral menisci*** of the knee joint are intra-articular discs made of fibrocartilage. They have a thick peripheral border and a thin inner border. They intervene between the femoral and tibial condyles (14.9).
   a. In accordance with the shape of the tibial condyles the lateral meniscus is smaller and its outline more nearly circular than that of the medial meniscus (14.10).
   b. The anterior and posterior ends of the lateral meniscus are attached to the intercondylar area of the tibia just in front of and behind the intercondylar eminence. We have noted, above, that the lateral meniscus is separated from the fibular collateral ligament by the tendon of the popliteus (14.19).

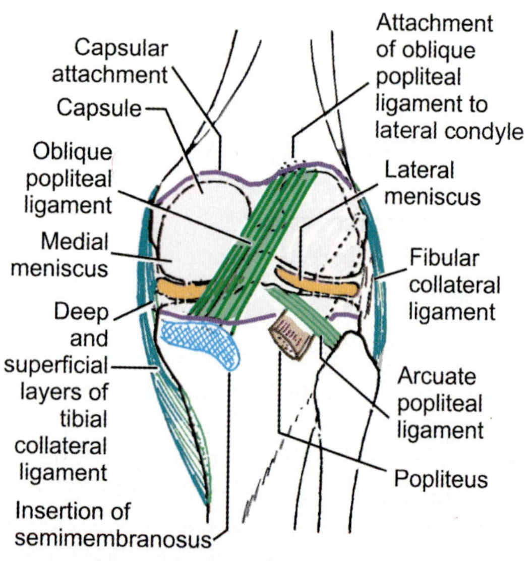


**14.9:** Schematic diagram showing some structures on the posterior aspect of the knee joint

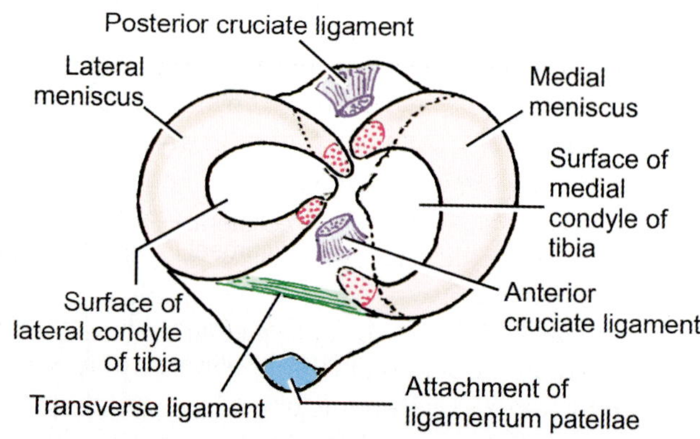


**14.10:** Menisci of the knee joint seen from above after removing the femur

c. The anterior end of the medial meniscus is attached to the most anterior part of the intercondylar area of the tibia in front of the anterior cruciate ligament. Its posterior end is attached to the posterior part of the intercondylar area in front of the attachment of the posterior cruciate ligament. We have seen that the medial meniscus blends with tibial collateral ligament.
d. When the knee is extended the anterior borders of the menisci lie against the grooves on the femur that separate the tibial and patellar articular surfaces.
e. The anterior margins of the two menisci are connected by a band of fibres called the transverse ligament (14.10).
f. The menisci provide for better adaptation of the articular surfaces of the joint. They participate in gliding movements (see below) and assist in lubrication of the joint.

8. The ***synovial membrane*** of the knee joint covers all structures within the joint except the articular surfaces and the surfaces of the menisci.
   a. It lines the inner side of the tendinous expansion of the quadriceps femoris (that replaces the capsule anteriorly) and some parts of the tibia and femur enclosed within the capsule.
   b. Just above the patella the synovial membrane forms a pouch called the ***suprapatellar bursa***: the pouch is bounded anteriorly by the quadriceps tendon, and posteriorly by the lower part of the anterior surface of the shaft of the femur.
   c. The upper edge of the synovial membrane forming the pouch is prevented from sagging downwards by a small muscle called the articularis genu.
   d. Lower down, the ligamentum patellae is separated from the synovial membrane by a large (infrapatellar) pad of fat.
   e. Folds of synovial membrane project into the joint along the medial and lateral margins of the patella: these are called the ***alar folds***.
   f. The cruciate ligaments appear to invaginate into the joint cavity from behind so that they are covered by synovial membrane on the sides and in front, but not behind.
9. The main ***movements*** at the knee joint are those of flexion and extension. However, these movements are not simple.
   a. Because of differences in the convexity of the anterior and posterior parts of the femoral condyles the axis of movement shifts forwards during extension and backwards during flexion.
   b. The tibia and menisci glide forwards relative to the femoral condyles in extension; and backwards in flexion.
   c. Further, flexion is associated with lateral rotation of the femur (or medial rotation of the tibia if the foot is off the ground); and extension is associated with medial rotation. The medial rotation of the femur is most marked during the last stages of extension.
   d. The anteroposterior diameter of the lateral femoral condyle is less than that of the medial condyle. As a result, when the lateral condylar articular surface is fully 'used up' by extension, part of the medial condylar surface remains unused.
   e. At this stage the lateral condyle serves as an axis around which the medial condyle rotates backwards (i.e., medial rotation of the femur occurs) so that the remaining medial condylar surface is also 'taken up'. This movement ***locks*** the knee joint in the position of full extension.
   f. Locking is produced by continued action of the same muscles that produce extension, namely the quadriceps femoris. When the knee is locked, the position of extension can be maintained without much muscular activity. (However, locking is not essential for stability of the extended knee, as gravity tends to cause hyperextension of the extended knee).
   g. The 'locked' knee can be flexed only after it is unlocked by a reversal of the rotation. Unlocking is brought about by the action of the popliteus muscle, which rotates the femur laterally (Rotation of the femur occurs when the feet are on the ground preventing rotation of the tibia. If the knee is flexed or extended when the foot is off the ground, it is the tibia that would rotate, in a direction opposite to that described for the femur).

10. The muscles responsible for movements of the knee joint are as follows:
    a. Flexion is produced mainly by the hamstring muscles. It is assisted by the gastrocnemius, popliteus, sartorius, gracilis and plantaris muscles.
    b. Extension is produced by the quadriceps femoris and by the tensor fasciae latae. Muscles producing locking and unlocking of the joint have been mentioned in the preceding paragraph.
11. The knee joint is supplied by branches of the descending genicular, popliteal, anterior tibial and lateral circumflex arteries; and by branches from the obturator, femoral, tibial and common peroneal nerves.
12. The knee joint is surrounded by several muscles. The posterior aspect of the joint is also related to the popliteal vessels and to the tibial nerve, and more laterally to the common peroneal nerve.
13. There are several ***bursae in the region of the knee joint***.
    a. The ***suprapatellar bursa*** has been described above. It is a part of the synovial cavity of the knee joint.
    b. The ***subcutaneous prepatellar bursa*** lies deep to the skin over the lower part of the patella.
    c. The ***deep infrapatellar bursa*** lies between the ligamentum patellae and the tibia.
    d. The ***superficial infrapatellar bursa*** lies between skin and the tibial tuberosity.
    e. Several other unnamed bursae are present in relation to tendons and ligaments around the knee.

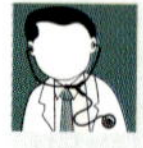

## CLINICAL CORRELATION

**Dislocation of the Knee Joint**

Dislocation at the knee joint is rare. It can result in damage to the popliteal artery, to the tibial nerve, or to the common peroneal nerve.

**Dislocation of the Patella**

1. Injury may cause lateral dislocation of the patella.
2. The dislocation may become recurrent.
3. It should be noted that the patella has a natural tendency to be displaced laterally because of the direction of pull of the quadriceps (upwards and laterally).
4. This is prevented by the patellar retinacula and is counteracted, to some extent, by the fact that the vastus medialis tends to pull the patella medially.

**Injuries in the Region of the Knee**

1. Injuries in the region can lead to effusion of a serous fluid into the joint cavity (***traumatic synovitis***).
2. If a blood vessel within the joint is injured the joint can fill with blood (***haemarthrosis***).
3. Strain or tear of the medial ligament of the knee is caused by an injury that abducts the tibia on the femur.
4. An opposite force that adducts the tibia on the femur can cause strain or tear of the lateral ligament.
5. Tears of the cruciate ligaments may occasionally occur along with those of the medial or lateral ligaments by abduction or adduction injuries. A force that drives the upper end of the tibia forwards over the tibia can rupture the anterior cruciate ligament; and a force that pushes the tibia backwards can rupture the posterior cruciate ligament.
6. A twisting force acting on a semiflexed or flexed knee can tear the medial meniscus. It is fairly common in football players. A curved tear extending through the whole length of the meniscus results in what is called a ***bucket handle tear***. As the menisci have no blood supply tears are not accompanied by bleeding into the joint cavity.
7. Torn menisci often have to be removed. The recent technique of ***arthoscopy*** allows inspection of the interior of the knee joint, without opening it. Parts of torn menisci, or parts of other loose tissue, can be removed through the same procedure.

**Housemaid's Knee**

The prepatellar bursa or the suprapatellar bursa may get inflamed (bursitis). This happens in persons who put their weight on the knee frequently e.g., housemaids.

**Knee Replacement**

1. The articular surfaces of the knee joint degenerate in many old persons due to ***osteoarthritis***.
2. In the past such patients had to depend on heavy doses of analgesics to relieve pain.
3. Now the entire joint can be replaced using artificial materials giving long-lasting relief to many.

## THE ANKLE JOINT

1. The ankle joint is a synovial joint of the hinge variety. The bones taking part are the lower end of the tibia, the lower end of the fibula, and the upper part of the talus.
2. It is, therefore, a compound joint.
3. Three distinct surfaces on the talus take part in the formation of the joint.
   a. The superior or trochlear surface (*'a'* in 14.11) is convex from front to back. It is slightly concave from side to side, so that it is like a pulley and hence the name trochlear surface. This surface is widest in its anterior part and becomes narrower posteriorly. It comes in contact with a reciprocally shaped surface on the lower end of the tibia (*'e'* in 14.12).
   b. The medial side of the talus bears a comma-shaped articular surface (*'c'* in 14.11B) that is wide anteriorly and tapers off at its posterior end. The medial surface articulates with a surface of reciprocal shape on the lateral surface of the medial malleolus of the tibia (*'f'* in 14.12).
   c. The lateral surface of the talus has a large triangular surface (*'b'* in 14.11A), the apex of the triangle being directed downwards; its base is separated from the trochlear surface by a ridge. The surface is concave from above downwards. It articulates with a surface of reciprocal shape on the medial surface of the lateral malleolus of the fibula (*'d'* in 14.12).
   d. Apart from the tibia and fibula, the upper articular surface receives a contribution from the inferior transverse tibiofibular ligament (*'g'* in 14.12). This ligament passes transversely from the malleolar fossa of the fibula to

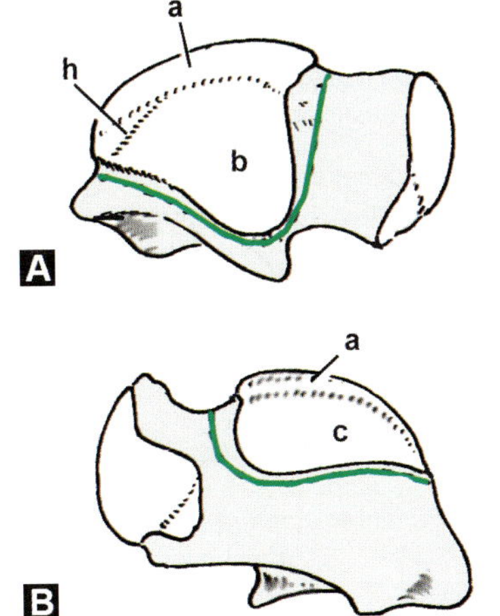


**14.11A and B:** Right talus showing attachments of the capsular ligament of the ankle joint. (A) Lateral aspect; (B) Medial aspect

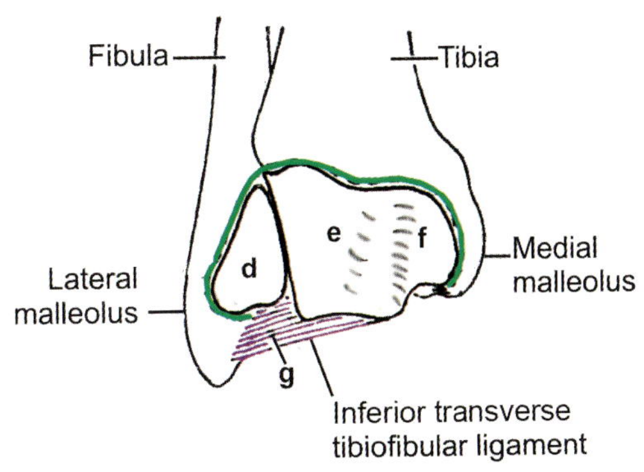


**14.12:** Superior articular surface of ankle joint seen from the anteroinferior aspect

the posterior part of the lower end of the tibia. (This is a ligament of the inferior tibiofibular joint). It comes in contact with an area between the posterior part of the trochlear and lateral articular surfaces of the talus ('h' in 14.11A).

4. The ***capsular ligament*** of the ankle joint is attached just beyond the margins of the articular surfaces. A small part of the neck of the talus is included within the joint cavity. The capsule is weak anteriorly and posteriorly, but on the medial and lateral side there are strong ligaments.
5. On the lateral side of the ankle there are three distinct bundles that constitute the ***lateral ligament*** of the joint (14.13).
   a. The ***anterior talofibular ligament*** is attached behind, to the anterior margin of the lateral malleolus. Its fibres pass forwards and medially to reach the talus anterior to its lateral articular surface.
   b. The ***posterior talofibular ligament*** is attached at its fibular end to the malleolar fossa (behind the articular surface). Its fibres pass transversely to the lateral tubercle of the posterior process of the talus.
   c. The ***calcaneofibular ligament*** is attached at its medial end to the apex of the lateral malleolus. Its fibres run downwards and backwards to the lateral surface of the calcaneus.
6. The ***medial or deltoid ligament*** is triangular (14.14). Above it is attached to the medial malleolus.
   a. Its anterior fibres pass downwards and forwards to the tuberosity of the navicular bone and constitute the ***tibionavicular ligament***.
   b. The middle fibres are attached, below, to the sustentaculum tali of the calcaneus and form the ***tibiocalcanean ligament***.
   c. Between these two bands the intervening fibres of the deltoid ligament blend with the plantar calcaneonavicular ligament.
   d. The posterior fibres pass backwards to be attached to the posterior part of the medial side of the talus. They form the ***posterior tibiotalar ligament***.
   e. Deeper fibres attached more anteriorly on the talus form the ***anterior tibiotalar ligament***.
7. The ankle joint is supplied by branches from the anterior tibial and peroneal arteries and from the deep peroneal and tibial nerves.

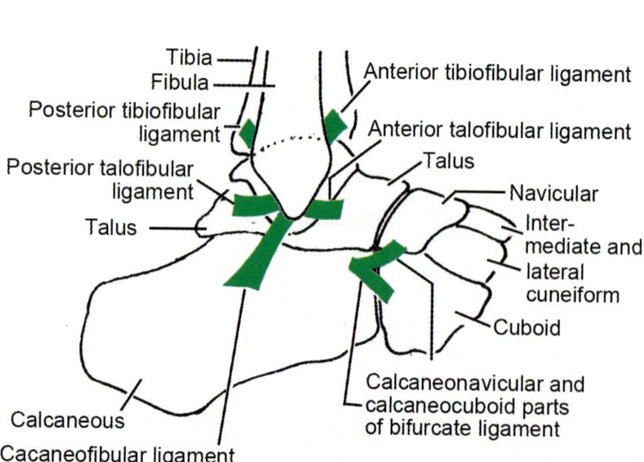


**14.13:** Ligaments on the medial aspect of the ankle joint. Some fibres of the tibiocalcaneal ligament have been cut to expose the anterior tibiotalar ligament

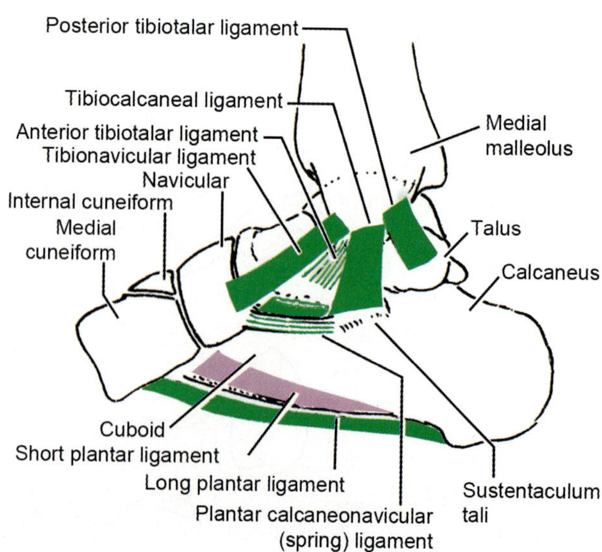


**14.14:** Ligaments on the lateral aspect of the ankle joint

8. The movements that take place at the ankle joint are those of plantar flexion and dorsiflexion. The muscles producing these movements are as follows:
   a. Dorsiflexion is produced by muscles of the anterior compartment of the leg viz., tibialis anterior, extensor digitorum longus, extensor hallucis longus and peroneus tertius.
   b. Plantar flexion is produced mainly by the gastrocnemius and soleus muscles. It is assisted by the plantaris, the tibialis posterior, the flexor hallucis longus and flexor digitorum longus.
9. Note that plantar flexion provides the propulsive force for walking, running and jumping.
   a. It is for this reason that the main muscles responsible for it (gastrocnemius and soleus) and their tendon (tendocalcaneus) are so powerful.
   b. Also note that in walking plantar flexion is accompanied by flexion at the knee joint (both movements lifting the limb off the ground); and the gastrocnemius contributes to both these movements.

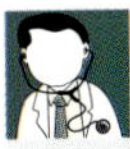

## CLINICAL CORRELATION

**Dislocations at the Ankle Joint**

As discussed above dislocations of the ankle joint may be caused by serious injuries that lead to fractures of malleoli, or separation of the lower ends of the tibia and fibula by rupture of the interosseous tibiofibular ligament.

**Injuries in the Region of the Ankle**

Injuries to ligaments in the region of the ankle have been considered under fractures of the lower end of the tibia and fibula (See above). Injuries in the region that are not enough to cause rupture result in strain of the ligaments.

## INTERTARSAL JOINTS

These will not be considered in detail, but it is important to know some facts about them. The three most important joints between the tarsal bones are:

1. The ***subtalar joint*** between the posterior facet on the inferior surface of the talus and on the superior surface of the calcaneus.
2. The ***talocalcaneonavicular*** joint in which the surfaces taking part are:
   a. The rounded head of the talus, which fits into a concavity on the posterior aspect of the navicular bone;
   b. the anterior and middle facets on the inferior aspect of the talus, and corresponding facets on the superior aspect of the calcaneus.
3. The ***calcaneocuboid*** joint in which reciprocally concavo-convex surfaces on the anterior surface of the calcaneus and the posterior aspect of the cuboid fit each other.

The talocalcaneonavicular and the calcaneocuboid joints lie along the same transverse plane and are collectively referred to as the ***transverse tarsal joint***.

Some important ligaments that connect the tarsal bones are given below:

1. The ***long plantar ligament*** is attached posteriorly to the plantar surface of the calcaneus (in front of the medial and lateral tubercles); and anteriorly to the plantar surface of the cuboid bone (distal to the groove for the peroneus longus, 14.15). It converts this groove into a tunnel. Some fibres of the ligament are prolonged into the bases of the 2nd, 3rd and 4th metatarsal bones.
2. The ***short plantar ligament*** (or ***plantar calcaneocuboid ligament***) passes from the anterior tubercle of the calcaneus to the cuboid bone proximal to the groove for the peroneus longus.
3. The ***plantar calcaneonavicular or spring ligament*** passes from the anterior margin of the sustentaculum tali of the calcaneus to the plantar surface of the navicular bone. This ligament is in contact above with the head of the talus and its upper surface forms part of the articular surface of the talocalcaneonavicular joint.

4. The ***bifurcate ligament*** (14.13) is Y-shaped. The stem of the Y is attached posteriorly to the anterior part of the upper surface of the calcaneus. Anteriorly, it splits into two bands: One passing to the dorsal aspect of the cuboid bone and another to the dorsal aspect of the navicular bone.
5. The ***interosseous talocalcaneal ligament*** lies deep between the talus and the calcaneus. It passes from the sulcus tali to the sulcus calcanei joining the talus and calcaneus in the interval between the subtalar and talocalcaneo-navicular joints.

## OTHER JOINTS OF THE LOWER LIMB

1. The tibia and fibula are joined to each other at the ***superior and inferior tibiofibular joints***. The superior joint is a synovial joint of the plane variety. The inferior tibiofibular joint is a syndesmosis.
2. Apart from the joints of the foot described above there are other ***intertarsal*** joints, ***tarsometatarsal*** and ***intermetatarsal joints*** that are plane synovial joints.
3. Their main purpose is to afford resilience to the foot.
4. The ***metatarsophalangeal joints*** and the ***interphalangeal joints*** are similar to corresponding joints in the hand, but the range of movement permitted by them is much less than in the hand.

## ARCHES OF THE FOOT

1. The bones of the foot are so arranged that they form a series of arches. There are two longitudinal arches, medial and lateral; and a number of transverse arches.
2. The ***medial longitudinal arch*** is formed (from posterior to anterior side) by:
   a. The calcaneus
   b. The talus
   c. The navicular
   d. The medial, intermediate and lateral cuneiform bones
   e. The medial three metatarsal bones.

   The arch rests posteriorly on the tubercles of the calcaneus, and anteriorly on the heads of the metatarsals. The summit of the arch is formed by the talus (14.16).

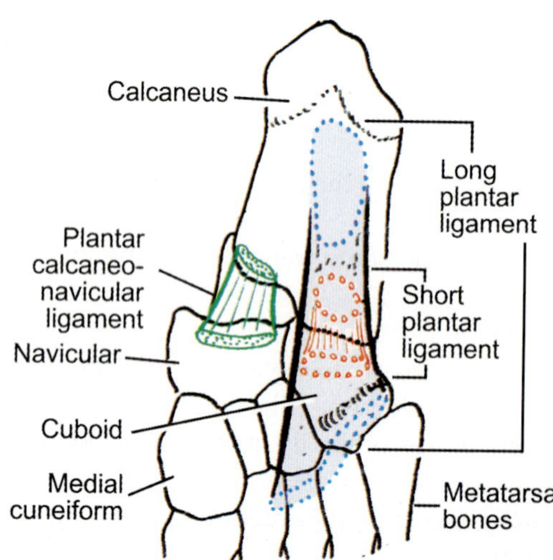


**14.15:** Posterior part of right foot (plantar aspect) to show attachments of some ligaments

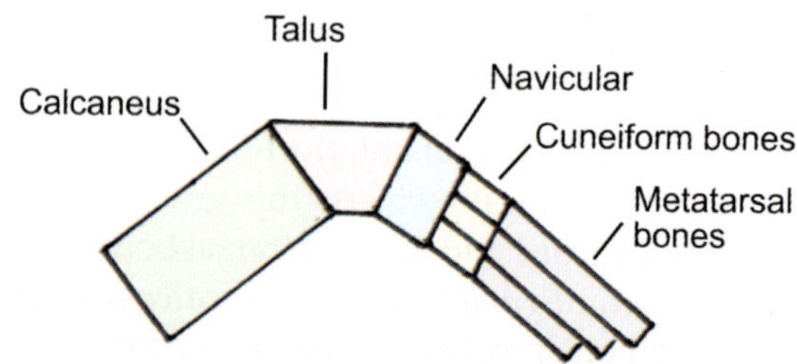


**14.16:** Scheme to show constitution of the medial longitudinal arch of the foot

3. The ***lateral longitudinal arch*** is formed by:
   a. The calcaneus
   b. The cuboid
   c. The lateral two metatarsal bones (14.17).

   The calcaneus is thus common to both arches.
4. The ***transverse arches*** are best marked in the middle of the foot i.e., in the anterior part of the tarsus, and at the bases of the metatarsal bones.
   a. As a result of the transverse arches the medial border of the foot remains off the ground in its middle part.
   b. Each foot has only half an arch the complete transverse arch being formed when the feet are placed together (14.18).
5. As a result of the presence of the arches body weight is transmitted to the ground only through the tuberosity of the calcaneus and the heads of the first and fifth metatarsal bones. The presence of the arches confers considerable resilience to the foot and makes it a more efficient lever for propulsion forwards of the body.
6. The ***factors that help to maintain the arches*** of the foot are:
   a. The configuration of the articular surfaces. The talus plays an important role in maintaining the medial longitudinal arch by acting as its keystone (14.19A and B).
   b. Flattening of the arches is prevented by ligaments, specially those that run longitudinally on the plantar aspect of the foot. These include the long and short plantar ligaments and the plantar calcaneonavicular ligament.
   c. The plantar aponeurosis plays an important role by connecting the anterior and posterior ends of the longitudinal arches like a 'tie-beam' (14.20).
   d. The muscles and tendons running longitudinally on the plantar aspect of the foot have a similar action. The tendons of the tibialis posterior and the peroneus longus together form a sling that holds the longitudinal arches up (14.20).

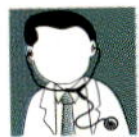

## CLINICAL CORRELATION

1. Flattening of the arches is seen in some individuals. It is called ***flat foot***, or ***pes planus.*** It causes difficulty in walking.
2. The reverse condition in which the arches are too marked is also known: it is termed ***pes cavus.***

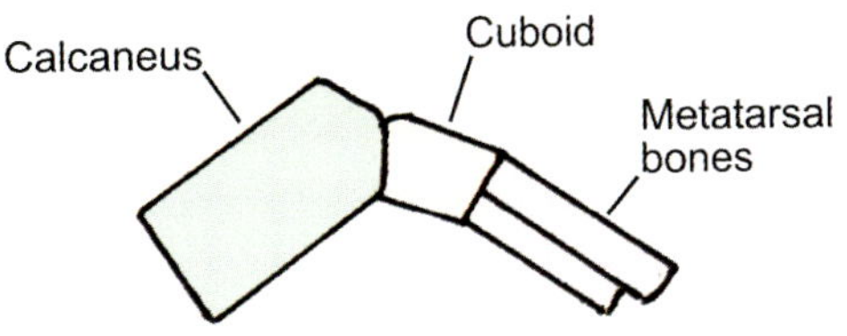


**14.17:** Scheme to show constitution of the lateral longitudinal arch of the foot

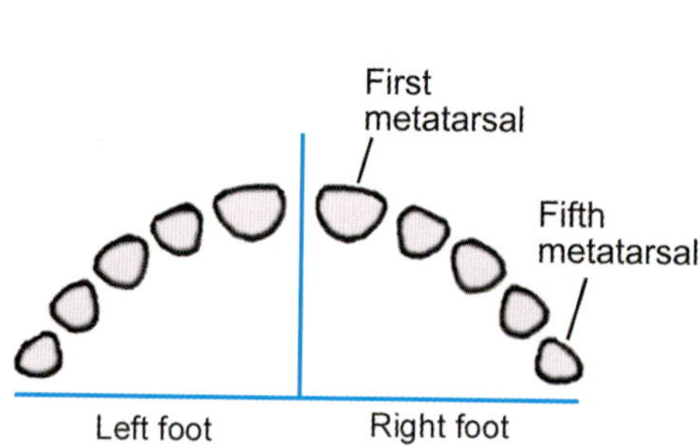


**14.18:** Scheme to show the transverse arch formed by the two feet. Note that each foot forms half of the arch

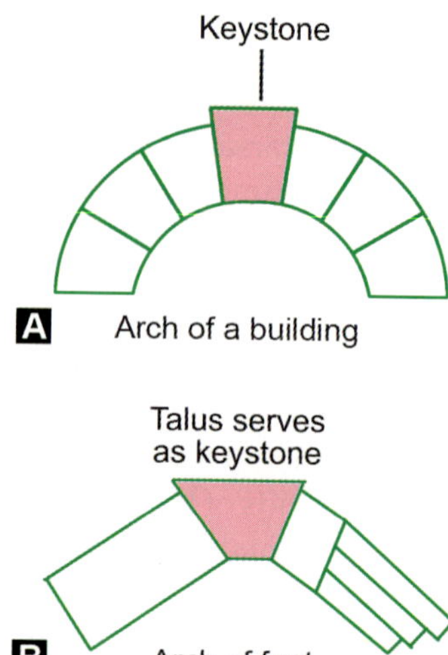


**14.19A and B:** Scheme to show how the talus serves as a keystone that helps to maintain longitudinal arches of the foot

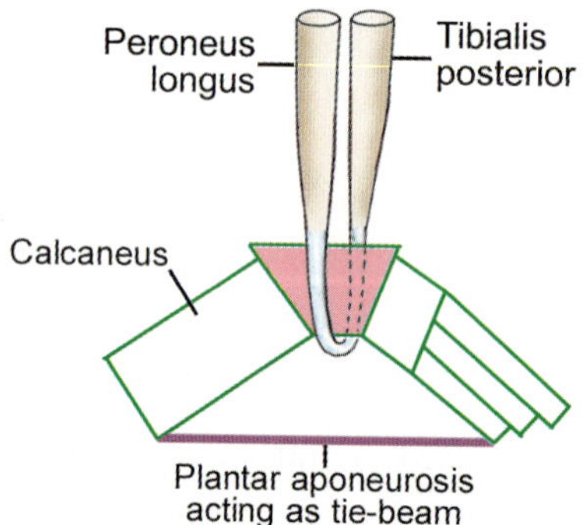


**14.20:** Scheme to show the tie-beam action of the plantar aponeurosis, and the tendinous sling, that support the archess of the foot

# 15 CHAPTER

# Surface Marking and Radiological Anatomy of Lower Limb

## SURFACE MARKING

### Femoral Artery

1. The upper end of the artery lies at the midinguinal point i.e., midway between the anterior superior iliac spine and the pubic ***symphysis***.
   (Note: Students often confuse the midinguinal point with the middle of the inguinal ligament. The two terms are not synonymous. The middle of the inguinal ligament is midway between the anterior superior iliac spine and the ***pubic tubercle***, not the symphysis).
2. The second landmark to be located for marking the artery is the ***adductor tubercle***.
   a. To locate the tubercle ask the subject to sit on a stool or chair (so that the knee is flexed approximately to a right angle).
   b. Now put your hand on the medial side of the popliteal region just above the medial condyle of the femur.
   c. Ask the subject to tighten the muscles of the thigh. You will be able to feel the cord-like tendon of the adductor magnus. The lower end of the tendon is attached to the adductor tubercle.
3. Draw a line joining the midinguinal point to the adductor tubercle. The femoral artery corresponds to the ***upper two-thirds*** of this line.
   a. The upper half of the artery lies in the femoral triangle and the lower half in the adductor canal.
   b. The lower end of the artery lies at the level of the opening in the adductor magnus. Here the femoral artery becomes continuous with the popliteal artery.

### Profunda Femoris Artery

To mark this artery, draw the same line as for the femoral artery as described above. The upper and lower ends of the profunda femoris both lie on this line.

a. The upper end is 3.5 cm below the midinguinal point.
b. The lower end is 10 cm below the midinguinal point.
c. The artery should be drawn by joining the two ends by a line that is convex laterally in its upper part.

### Popliteal Artery

This artery is marked on the posterior aspect (i.e., over the popliteal fossa).

1. The upper end of the artery (first point) lies at the junction of the middle and lower thirds of the back of the thigh, 2.5 cm medial to the midline.
2. The second point should be taken at the level of the knee joint, in the midline.
3. The third point (lower end) lies over the middle of the back of the leg at the level of the ***tibial tuberosity***. The artery is marked by joining these three points.

Note: Remember that the tibial tuberosity lies on the front of the leg, while the point you are taking is on the back. The tuberosity is to be used only as an indication of level.

## Posterior Tibial Artery

This artery is marked on the back of the leg.

1. Its upper end corresponds to the lower end of the popliteal artery. It lies over the middle of the back of the leg at the level of the tibial tuberosity (See note given on page 319).
2. Its lower end lies on the posteromedial side of the ankle midway between the medial malleolus and the tendo-calcaneus.

## Anterior Tibial Artery

This artery is marked on the front of the leg.

1. Its upper end lies about 2.5 cm medial to the head of the fibula.
2. The lower end lies in front of the ankle midway between the medial and lateral malleoli.

## Dorsalis Pedis Artery

1. This artery is the continuation of the anterior tibial artery. Hence, its upper end lies in front of the ankle midway between the malleoli.
2. It terminates at the proximal end of the space between the first and second metatarsal bones.

## Medial Plantar Artery

1. Its beginning corresponds to the termination of the posterior tibial artery on posteromedial side of ankle midway between the medial malleolus and the tendocalcaneus.
2. From here draw a line over the sole to the cleft between the great toe and second toe. (The position of the cleft can be better judged by looking at the dorsum of the foot).
3. The ***proximal half*** of this line represents the position of the medial plantar artery.

## Lateral Plantar Artery

1. Its beginning is at the same point as that for the medial plantar artery (on posteromedial side of ankle midway between the medial malleolus and the tendocalcaneus).
2. The lateral plantar artery is marked by drawing a line starting at this point and running obliquely (laterally and distally) across the sole to reach a point about 2.5 cm medial to the tuberosity of the fifth metatarsal bone.

### *Plantar Arch*

1. This is a continuation of the lateral plantar artery and ends by joining the termination of the dorsalis pedis artery. Note: While describing the marking of the dorsalis pedis artery we have seen that the lower end of this artery lies on the dorsum of the foot over the proximal end of the space between the first and second metatarsal bones. Here the artery dips ventrally to reach the sole where it joins the plantar arch. So for the purpose of marking the plantar arch the corresponding position on the sole is to be taken. This point lies 2.5 cm distal to the tuberosity of the navicular bone.
2. The plantar arch can be marked by a line drawn across the sole joining the termination of the lateral plantar artery to the point of termination of the dorsalis pedis artery (see note above). The line should be drawn with a slight distal convexity.

## Femoral Vein

1. First mark the femoral artery.
2. Now mark the vein along side the artery so that its upper end is medial to the artery, and its lower end is just lateral to the artery.
3. The vein crosses posterior to the artery.

## Popliteal Vein

1. First mark the popliteal artery.
2. Draw the vein so that its upper end is lateral to the artery and lower end medial to the artery (reverse of the relationship of the femoral artery and vein).
3. The vein gradually crosses behind the artery.

## Great Saphenous Vein

1. In a thin person it is usually possible to see the vein over the foot and leg. It begins over the medial part of the dorsum of the foot (from the medial end of the dorsal venous arch, if visible) and passes upwards in front of the medial malleolus.
2. It then ascends over the leg passing across the medial surface of the tibia, and higher up along its medial border, to reach the posteromedial aspect of the knee.
3. It then runs upwards across the medial side of the thigh to reach the saphenous opening. (Remember that the centre of the saphenous opening is 4 cm below and lateral to the pubic tubercle).

## Short Saphenous Vein

1. The vein begins over the lateral part of the dorsum of the foot (at the lateral end of the dorsal venous arch, if visible).
2. From here the vein ascends behind the lateral malleolus, and up the back of the leg, to reach the centre of the popliteal fossa.

## Femoral Nerve

1. The nerve is marked as a short vertical line (2.5 cm or 1″ long) beginning 1.2 cm (half inch) lateral to the midinguinal point.
2. The nerve ends by dividing into a number of branches.

## Sciatic Nerve

The nerve is marked over the gluteal region and back of the thigh.

1. Begin by locating:
   a. The posterior superior iliac spine
   b. The ischial tuberosity
   c. The greater trochanter.
2. Draw a line connecting the posterior superior iliac spine and the ischial tuberosity. Take a point ($x$) 2.5 cm (1″) lateral to the ***middle*** of this line. This point lies over the upper end of the nerve.
3. Next take a point ($y$) midway between the ischial tuberosity and the greater trochanter.
4. Join points $x$ and $y$ with a slight convexity to the lateral side.
5. From point $y$ carry the line downwards to the upper end of the popliteal fossa (at the level of the junction of the middle and lower-thirds of the thigh, midway between its medial and lateral margins).
6. The nerve ends here by dividing into the tibial and common peroneal nerves.

## Tibial Nerve

1. The upper end of this nerve corresponds to the lower end of the sciatic nerve (see above).
2. The nerve runs vertically to the lower angle of the popliteal fosssa (which corresponds to a point on the back of the leg, at the level of the tibial tuberosity, midway between the medial and lateral margins).
3. From here the nerve runs downwards and medially to reach the interval between the medial malleolus and the tendocalcaneus. (Here the nerve lies deep to the flexor retinaculum).

### Common Peroneal Nerve

1. The upper end of this nerve corresponds to the lower end of the sciatic nerve (see above).
2. The nerve runs downwards and laterally to reach the neck of the fibula.
3. Here the nerve turns forwards and downwards to reach the lateral side of the neck of the fibula.
4. It ends here by dividing into the deep and superficial peroneal nerves.

### Deep Peroneal Nerve

1. Its upper end corresponds to the lower end of the common peroneal nerve (lying lateral to the neck of the fibula).
2. The lower end of the nerve lies in front of the ankle midway between the medial and lateral malleoli.
3. If you wish to mark the deep peroneal nerve along with the anterior tibial artery (described above) remember that the nerve is lateral to the artery over most of its extent. It may overlap the artery over the middle one-third of the leg.

### Superficial Peroneal Nerve

1. Its upper end lies at the same point as that of the deep peroneal nerve (lateral to the neck of the fibula).
2. To find the lower end feel for the peroneal tendons just behind the lateral malleolus and pass your fingers upwards along them to recognize the peroneal muscles.
3. Take a point over these muscles at the junction of the middle and lower thirds of the leg.
   The nerve divides into branches at this level.

### Medial and Lateral Plantar Nerves

These nerves accompany the corresponding arteries and can be marked as described for the arteries.

### Retinacula

The large retinacula over the ankle are the superior and inferior extensor retinacula, and the flexor retinaculum. To mark the outlines of a retinaculum you must know (a) its position and shape, (b) its attachments, and (c) its width. Once these are known, the retinaculum can be marked easily.

## RADIOLOGICAL ANATOMY

Some aspects of the radiological anatomy of the lower limb are shown in 15.1 to 15.4.

1. Sacrum
2. Ilium
3. Ischium
4. Pubis
5. Obturator foramen
6. Head of femur
7. Greater trochanter
8. Neck of femur
9. Shaft of femur

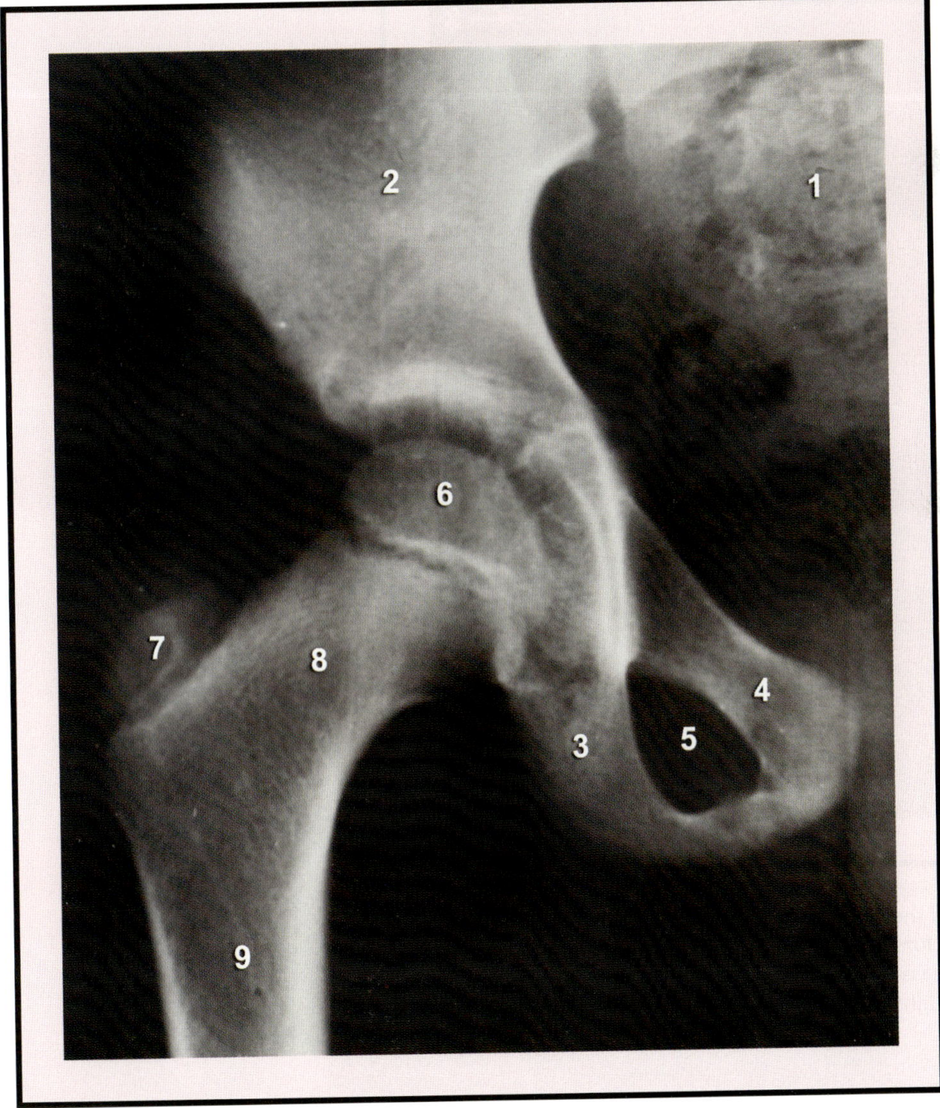


**15.1:** Radiograph of the region of the hip joint in a ten years old boy. The three parts of the hip bone (ilium, ischium and pubis) are not fused to one another, but the inferior ramus of the pubis is fused to the ischial ramus. Epiphyses for the head and greater trochanter of the femur are seen, separated from the diaphysis (which forms the shaft as well as the neck) by epiphyseal cartilages

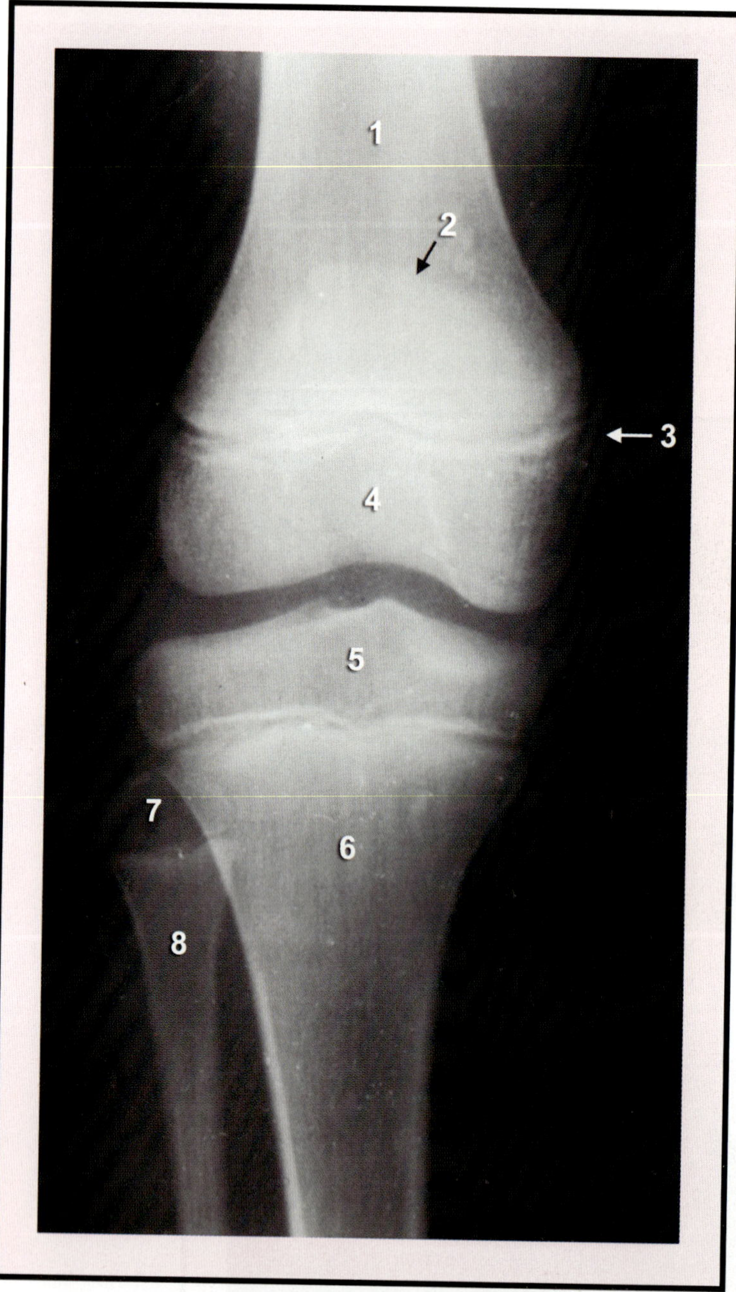


1. Shaft of femur
2. Outline of patella
3. Epiphyseal plate
4. Epiphysis of lower end of femur
5. Epiphysis of upper end of tibia
6. Shaft of tibia
7. Epiphysis of upper end of fibula
8. Shaft of fibula

**15.2:** Radiograph of the region of the knee joint in a 10 years old boy. The unfused epiphyses for the lower end of the femur, the upper end of the tibia, and the upper end of the fibula are clearly seen. The shadow of the patella is seen as a lighter area overlapping the lower end of the femur

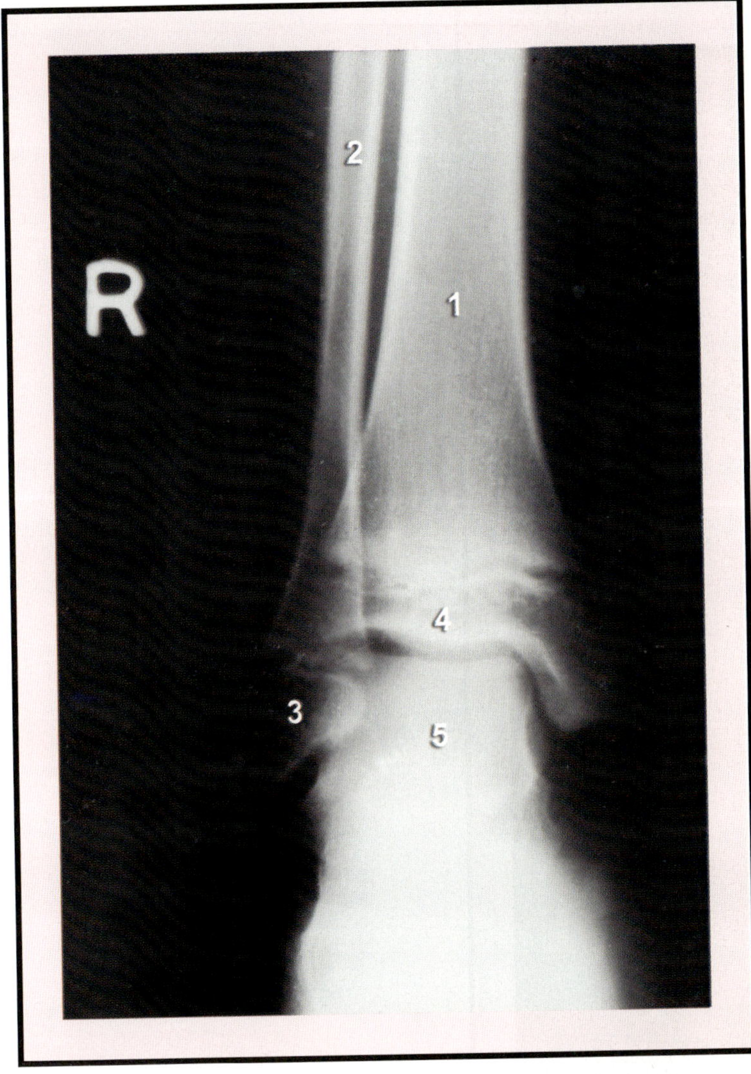


1. Shaft of tibia
2. Shaft of fibula
3. Lower fibular epiphysis
4. Lower tibial epiphysis
5. Talus

**15.3:** Radiograph of the region of the ankle in a 10 years old boy. Unfused epiphyses for the lower end of the tibia and fibula are clearly seen. The outline of the upper part of the talus is clear, but other tarsal bones cannot be demarcated because of overlap of their shadows

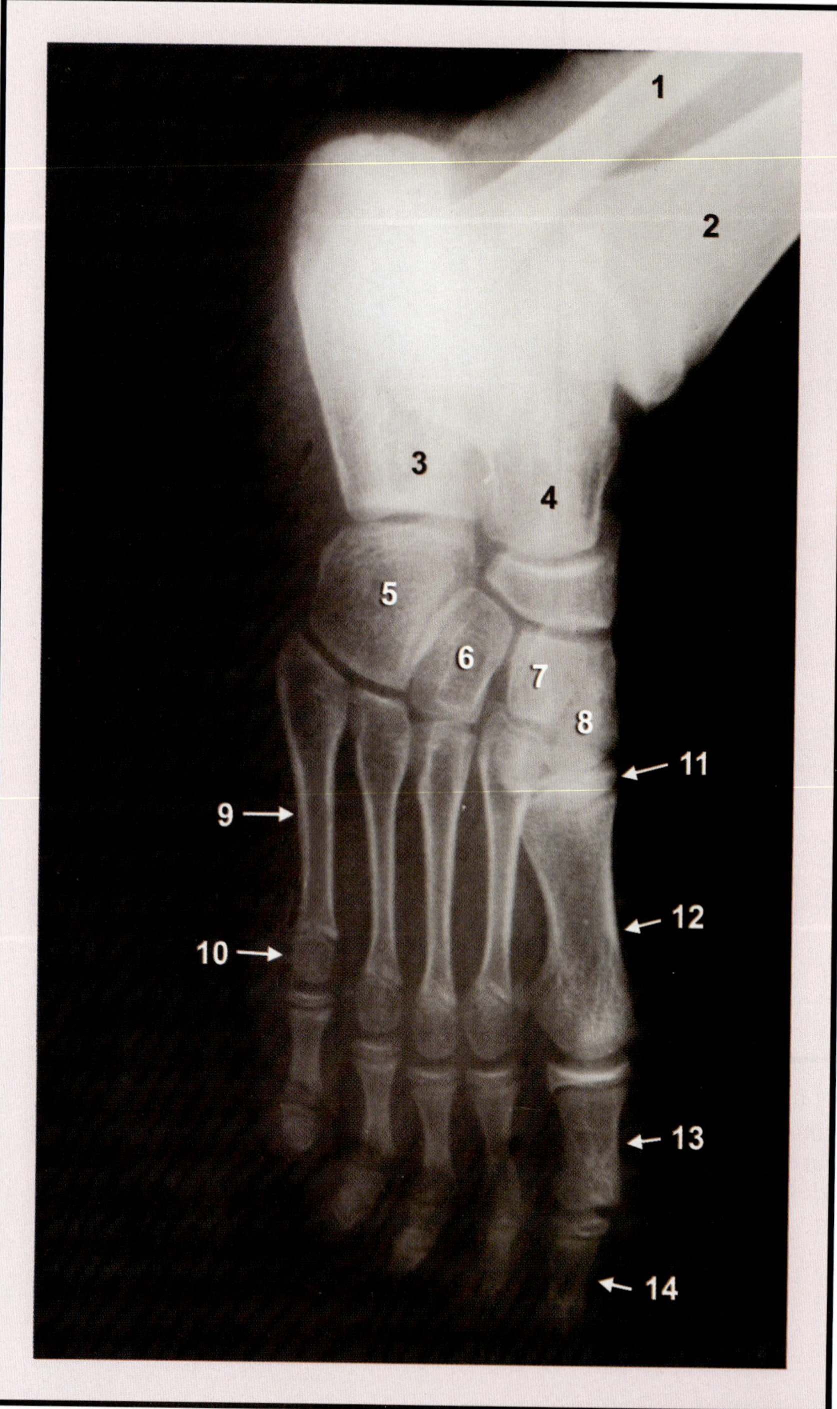


1. Lower end of fibula
2. Lower end of tibia
3. Calcaneus
4. Talus
5. Cuboid bone
6. Lateral cuneiform bone
7. Intermediate cuneiform bone
8. Medial cuneiform bone
9. Fifth metatarsal
10. Epiphysis of fifth metatarsal
11. Epiphysis of first metatarsal
12. Shaft of first metatarsal
13. Proximal phalanges with epiphyses at their proximal ends.
14. Middle phalanges with epiphyses at their proximal ends

**15.4:** Radiograph showing the skeleton of the foot in a 10 years old boy. Identify the tarsal bones, the metatarsal bones, and the phalanges. The second to fifth metatarsal bones show unfused epiphyses at their distal ends. In the first metatarsal the epiphysis is located at the proximal end. Epiphyses are also seen at the proximal ends of each of the phalanges, but the distal phalanges are not seen clearly in this skiagram

# Part 3

## Thorax

# 16 CHAPTER Bones Seen in Relation to the Thorax

## INTRODUCTION TO THE VERTEBRAL COLUMN

1. Below the skull, the central axis of the body is formed by the backbone or ***vertebral column***.
2. The vertebral column is made up of a large number of bones of irregular shape called ***vertebrae***.
   a. There are seven ***cervical vertebrae*** in the neck.
   b. Below these, there are twelve ***thoracic vertebrae*** that take part in forming the skeleton of the thorax.
   c. Still lower down, there are five ***lumbar vertebrae*** that lie in the posterior wall of the abdomen.
3. The lowest part of the vertebral column is made up of the ***sacrum***, which consists of five sacral vertebrae that are fused together; and of a small bone called the ***coccyx***. The coccyx is made up of four rudimentary vertebrae fused together.
4. There are thus thirty-three vertebrae in all. Taking the sacrum and coccyx as single bones the vertebral column has twenty-six bones.

## INTRODUCTION TO SKELETON OF THE THORAX

The skeleton of the thorax forms a bony cage that protects the heart, the lungs, and some other organs.

1. Behind, it is made up of twelve thoracic vertebrae.
2. In front, it is formed by a bone called the ***sternum***. The sternum consists of an upper part: the ***manubrium***; a middle part: the ***body***; and a lower part: the ***xiphoid process***.
3. The side walls of the thorax are formed by twelve ribs on either side.
   a. Each rib is a long curved bone that is attached posteriorly to the vertebral column.
   b. It curves round the sides of the thorax.
   c. Its anterior end is attached to a bar of cartilage (the ***costal cartilage***) through which it gains attachment to the sternum.
4. This arrangement is seen typically in the upper seven ribs (***true ribs***). The 8th, 9th and 10th costal cartilages do not reach the sternum, but end by getting attached to the next higher cartilage (***false ribs***).
5. The anterior ends of the 11th and 12th ribs are free. They are, therefore, called ***floating ribs***.
   In this chapter, we will consider the following:
   a. Vertebral column, general consideration and thoracic part.
   b. Sternum.
   c. Ribs and costal cartilages.

## STRUCTURE OF A TYPICAL VERTEBRA

1. The parts of a typical vertebra are best seen by examining a vertebra from the mid-thoracic region. Such a vertebra is seen from above in 16.1 and from behind in 16.2. A lateral view of two such vertebrae is shown in 16.3. The following parts can be distinguished:
   a. The ***body*** lies anteriorly. It is shaped like a short cylinder, being rounded from side-to-side, and having flat upper and lower surfaces that are attached to those of adjoining vertebrae through ***intervertebral discs*** (16.3).

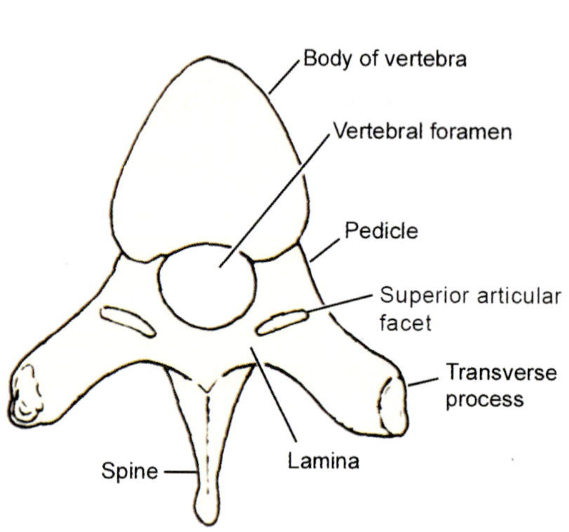


16.1: Typical vertebra seen from above

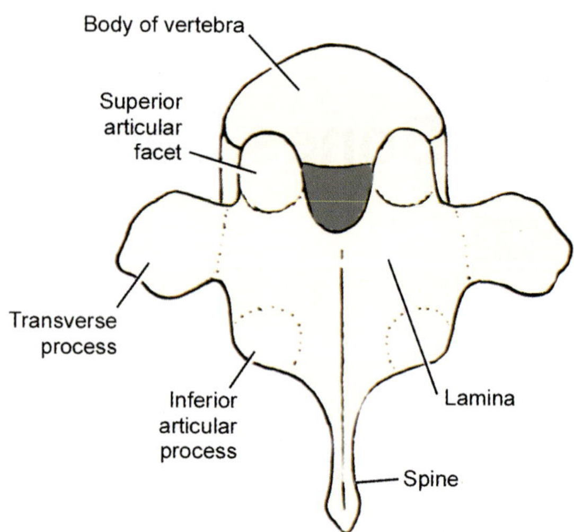


16.2: Typical vertebra seen from behind

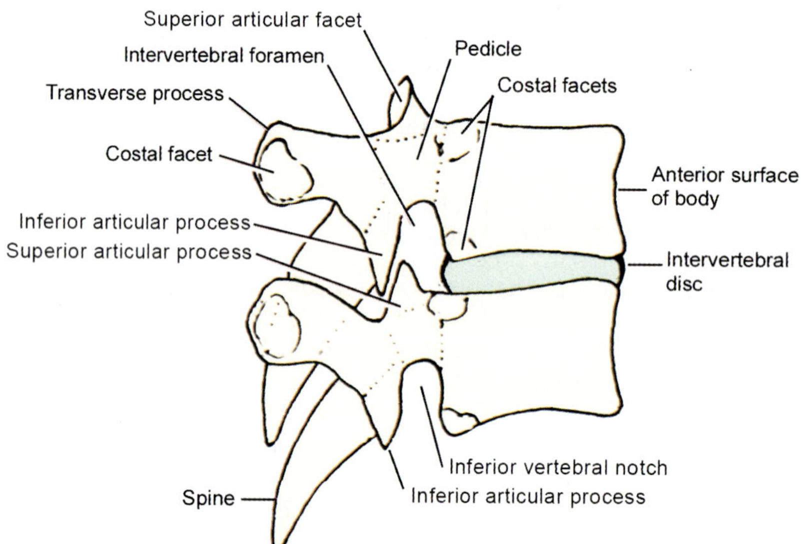


16.3: Typical vertebrae seen from the lateral side. (Costal facets, for ribs, are shown on the bodies and transverses processes. They are present only in the thoracic region)

b. The ***pedicles*** (right and left) are short rounded bars that project backwards, and somewhat laterally, from the posterior part of the body.
c. Each pedicle is continuous, posteromedially, with a vertical plate of bone called the ***lamina***. The laminae of the two sides pass backwards and medially to meet in the middle line. The pedicles and laminae together constitute the ***vertebral arch***.
d. Bounded anteriorly by the posterior aspect of the body, on the sides by the pedicles, and behind by the laminae, there is a large ***vertebral foramen***. Each vertebral foramen forms a short segment of the ***vertebral canal*** that runs through the whole length of the vertebral column and transmits the spinal cord.
e. Passing backwards (and usually downwards) from the junction of the two laminae, there is the ***spine*** (or ***spinous process***).

f. Passing laterally (and usually somewhat downwards) from the junction of each pedicle and the corresponding lamina, there is a ***transverse process***. The spinous and transverse processes serve as levers for muscles acting on the vertebral column.

2. When the vertebrae are viewed from the lateral side (16.3) we see certain additional features.
   g. Projecting upwards from the junction of the pedicle and the laminae there is, on either side, a ***superior articular process***; and projecting downwards there is an ***inferior articular process***.
      i. Each process bears a smooth articular facet. The ***superior facet*** is directed posteriorly and somewhat laterally, and the ***inferior facet*** is directed forwards and somewhat medially.
      ii. The superior facet of one vertebra articulates with the inferior facet of the vertebra above it.
      iii. Two adjoining vertebrae, therefore, articulate at three joints; two between the right and left articular processes and one between the bodies of the vertebrae (through the intervertebral disc).
   h. In 16.3, note that the pedicle is much narrower (in vertical diameter) than the body and is attached nearer to its upper border.
      i. As a result, there is a large ***inferior vertebral notch*** below the pedicle. The notch is bounded in front by the posterior surface of the body of the vertebra, and behind by the inferior articular process.
      ii. Above the pedicle, there is a much shallower ***superior vertebral notch***.
      iii. The superior and inferior notches of adjoining vertebrae join to form the ***intervertebral foramina*** which give passage to spinal nerves emerging from the spinal cord.

## Distinguishing Features of Typical Cervical, Thoracic and Lumbar Vertebrae

1. The cervical, thoracic and lumbar vertebrae can be easily distinguished from one another because of the following characteristics:
   a. The transverse process of a cervical vertebra is pierced by a foramen called the ***foramen transversarium*** (16.4).
   b. The thoracic vertebrae bear ***costal facets*** for articulation with ribs. These are present on the sides of the vertebral bodies and on the transverse processes (16.3).
   c. A lumbar vertebra (16.5) can be distinguished by the fact that it neither has foramina transversaria nor does it bear facets for ribs. It is also recognised by the large size of its body.

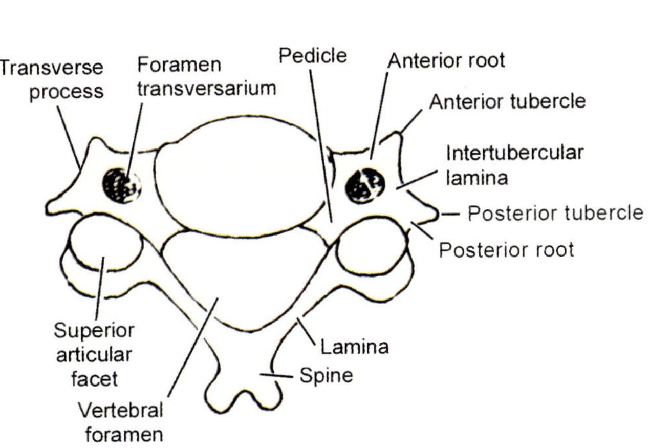


**16.4:** Typical cervical vertebra seen from above

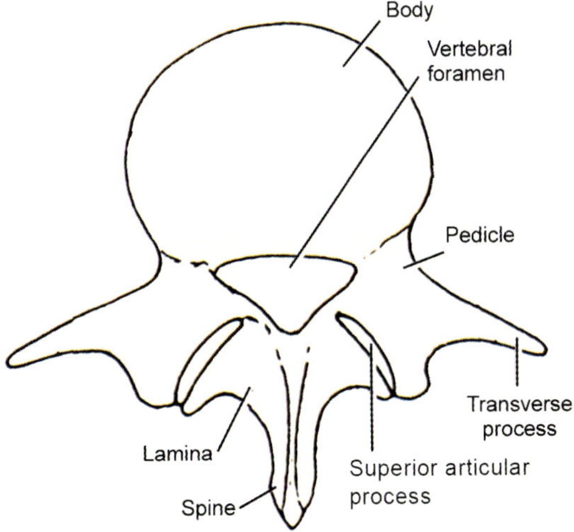


**16.5:** Typical lumbar vertebra seen from above

## WANT TO KNOW MORE?

We may now consider additional differences between cervical, thoracic and lumbar vertebrae.

1. The vertebral bodies progressively increase in size from above downwards.
   a. They are, therefore, smallest in the cervical vertebrae and largest in the lumbar vertebrae.
   b. In shape, the body is oval in the cervical and lumbar regions and triangular or heart-shaped in the thoracic region.
2. In the thoracic region, the head of a typical rib articulates with the sides of the bodies of two vertebrae (16.6).
   a. For this purpose, each side of the body of a typical thoracic vertebra bears two costal facets: upper and lower, adjoining its upper and lower borders (16.3).
   b. Each of these is really only half a facet (demifacet), the other half being on the adjoining vertebra.
   c. The upper facet is large and articulates with the numerically corresponding rib.
   d. The lower, smaller facet articulates with the next lower rib.
3. The spinous processes are short and bifid in a typical cervical vertebra (16.4).
   a. They are long and project downwards in the thoracic region (16.3).
   b. In lumbar vertebrae, they are large and quadrangular. They are more or less horizontal and have a thick posterior edge.
4. The transverse processes of typical cervical vertebrae are relatively short and, as mentioned earlier, they are pierced by foramina transversaria. When viewed from the lateral side the transverse process is seen to be grooved. The cervical nerves lie in these grooves after they pass out of the intervertebral foramina.
5. The transverse processes of a typical thoracic vertebra are large with solid blunt ends (16.1 and 16.3). They are directed backwards and laterally. Each process lies just behind the corresponding rib and bears a prominent facet for articulation with the rib.

**Attachments on Vertebrae**

1. Vertebrae give attachments to numerous muscles and ligaments. The ligaments concerned are those that hold adjoining vertebrae together.
   a. Adjoining vertebrae are connected to each other at three joints.
   b. There is one median joint between the vertebral bodies, and two joints (one right and one left) between the articular processes.

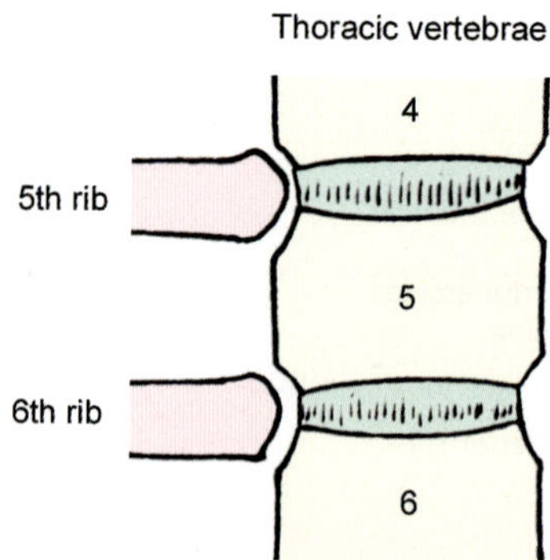


**16.6:** Scheme showing the numerical relationship of thoracic vertebrae to ribs

i. Adjoining vertebral bodies are connected to each other by ***intervertebral discs***, made up of fibrocartilage. Each disc has an outer fibrous part called the ***annulus fibrosus***, and an inner soft part called the ***nucleus pulposus***.
ii. The joints between the articular processes are synovial joints. The capsules of these joints are attached along the margins of articular facets.
iii. Apart from the intervertebral discs and the capsular ligaments, adjoining vertebrae are connected to one another by a series of ligaments that are shown schematically in 16.7.

### *Typical Thoracic Vertebrae*

1. The second to ninth thoracic vertebrae are typical and conform to the description of thoracic vertebrae given above.
2. The first, tenth, eleventh and twelfth vertebrae have some features that enable them to be distinguished.

**WANT TO KNOW MORE?**

**Some Atypical Thoracic Vertebrae**

***First Thoracic Vertebra***

This vertebra can be distinguished from a typical thoracic vertebra because of the following features (16.8 and 16.9):

a. It has a small body similar in shape to that of a cervical vertebra.
b. The posterolateral parts of the body are raised (as in cervical vertebrae) and as a result a definite superior vertebral notch can be identified.
(This is virtually absent in other thoracic vertebrae).
c. The superior costal facets (on the body) are usually complete as the first rib articulates wholly with this vertebra.
d. The spine is long and horizontal (16.9).

***Tenth, Eleventh and Twelfth Thoracic Vertebrae***

1. These vertebrae tend to resemble the lumbar vertebrae in the shape and size of their bodies, of the vertebral foramina, and of the spines (16.10).
2. They can be distinguished from typical thoracic vertebrae by the fact that they have only one costal facet on each side of the body.
3. The tenth vertebra (normally) has a costal facet on each transverse process. The transverse process is large as in typical thoracic vertebrae.
4. Facets on the transverse processes are absent in the eleventh and twelfth vertebrae that have small transverse processes.
5. The eleventh and twelfth vertebrae can be distinguished from each other by examining the inferior articular facets. These are of the thoracic type in the eleventh vertebra, but are of the lumbar type in the twelfth vertebra.
6. Further confirmation can be obtained by examining the transverse processes. Those of the twelfth vertebra show superior, inferior and lateral tubercles, which are absent or rudimentary on the eleventh vertebra.

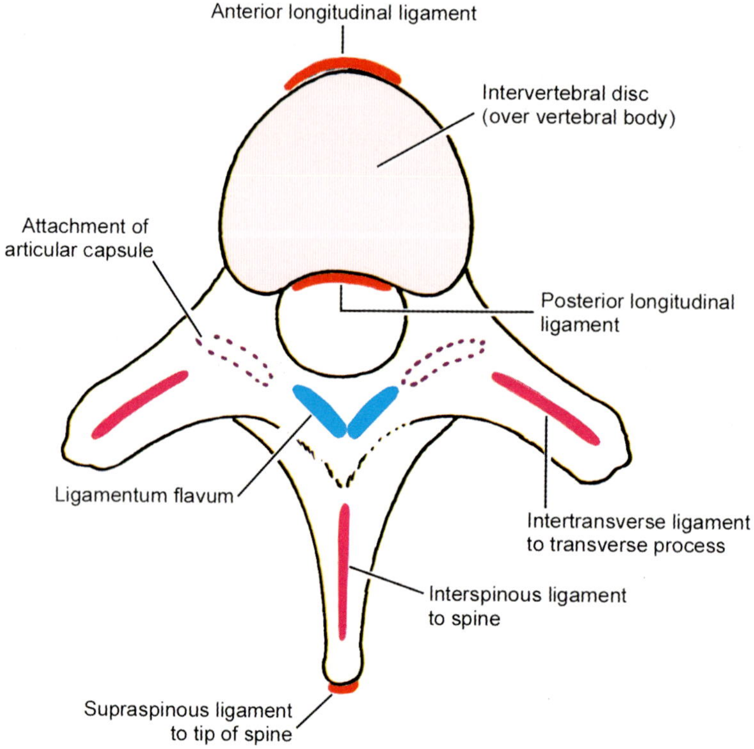


**16.7:** Scheme to show the position of various ligaments interconnecting adjoining vertebrae

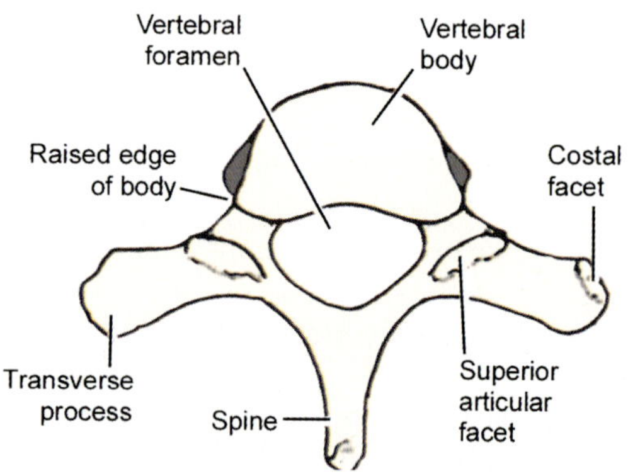


**16.8:** First thoracic vertebra seen from above

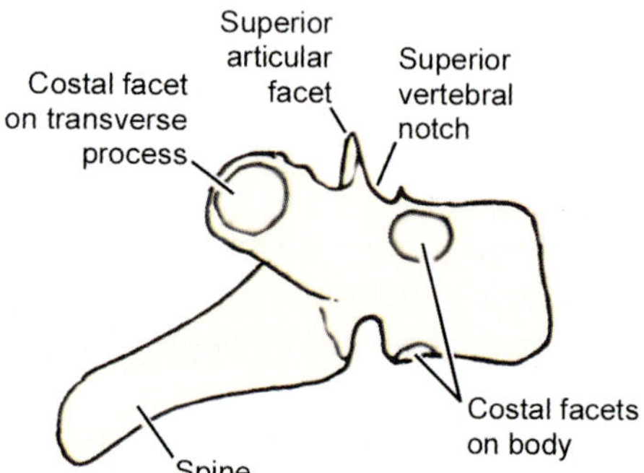


**16.9:** First thoracic vertebra seen from the lateral side

## THE STERNUM

1. The sternum lies in the anterior wall of the thorax, in the midline (16.11 to 16.13). It is elongated vertically. It is flat and has anterior and posterior surfaces.
2. Although, it is (by convention) spoken of as a single bone it consists of three separate parts. From above downwards these are the ***manubrium***, the ***body***, and the ***xiphoid process***.

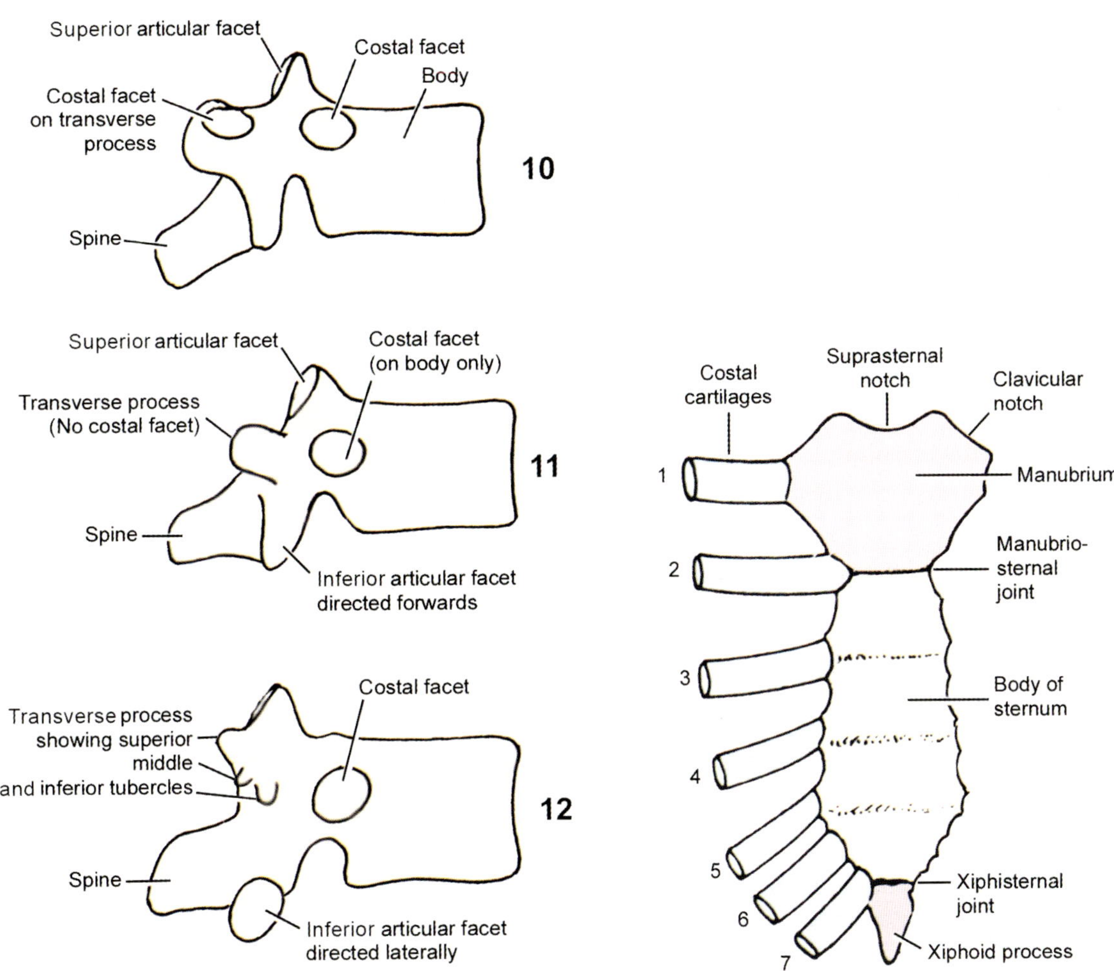


**16.10:** Tenth, eleventh and twelfth thoracic vertebrae seen from the lateral side

**16.11:** Sternum and costal cartilages seen from the front

3. The manubrium joins the body at the ***manubriosternal joint.***
4. The body joins the xiphoid process at the ***xiphisternal joint.***
5. The anterior ends of the upper seven costal cartilages are attached to the right and left margins of the sternum.
   a. The first costal cartilage is attached to the lateral margin of the manubrium.
   b. The second costal cartilage is attached partly to the manubrium, and partly to the upper end of the body.
   c. The third, fourth, fifth and sixth cartilages are attached to the lateral margin of the body.
   d. The seventh costal cartilage is attached to the lateral side of the xiphisternal joint. The area of attachment of each cartilage is marked by a notch on the lateral margin of the sternum.
6. The upper border of the manubrium articulates, on either side, with the medial end of the clavicle to form the ***sternoclavicular joint***. It bears prominent ***clavicular notches*** for this purpose.
7. Between the right and left clavicular notches, there is a median depression called the ***jugular or suprasternal notch.***
8. The manubrium and the body of the sternum lie at a slight angle to one another, and because of this fact the manubriosternal junction projects forwards. This projection forms a surface landmark and is often referred to as the ***sternal angle***. The sternal angle forms a useful guide in identifying individual costal cartilages and ribs in the living subject.

9. The body of the sternum consists of four parts or ***sternebrae*** that are united by cartilage up to the age of puberty, but fuse thereafter to form a single bone. The lines of fusion can be seen on the anterior aspect of the bone.
10. The ***manubriosternal joint*** is a symphysis.
11. The xiphoid process is cartilaginous in children, but undergoes ossification in the adult. After this happens the ***xiphisternal joint*** is said to be a symphysis. However, unlike a typical symphysis the joint disappears in old age and the xiphoid process and the body of the sternum become united by bone.
12. The junction of the first costal cartilage with the manubrium is a synchondrosis. The other sternocostal joints usually have a joint cavity (i.e., they are synovial joints).

**WANT TO KNOW MORE?**

**Attachments on the Sternum**

The muscles (and associated structures) attached to the anterior aspect of the sternum are as follows:

1. The sternal head of the ***sternocleidomastoid*** arises from the upper part of the manubrium (16.12).
2. The ***pectoralis major*** arises from the corresponding half of the manubrium and of the body of the sternum. The origin extends onto the costal cartilages.
3. The ***rectus abdominis*** is inserted into the xiphoid process. The insertion extends to the 7th, 6th and 5th costal cartilages (in that order) along a horizontal line.
4. The aponeurosis of the ***external oblique*** muscle of the abdomen, which covers the rectus abdominis, is attached just beyond the insertion of the latter(16.12).
5. The aponeuroses of the ***internal oblique*** muscle of the abdomen, and of the transversus abdominis, are attached to the sides of the xiphoid process.
6. The ***linea alba*** is attached to the apex (lower end) of the xiphoid process.

The muscles attached to the posterior surface of the sternum are as follows:

1. The ***sternohyoid*** arises from the upper part of the posterior surface of the manubrium (16.13). The area extends onto the back of the clavicle.
2. The ***sternothyroid*** arises from the posterior surface of the manubrium, below the origin of the sternohyoid. The origin extends onto the first costal cartilage.
3. The ***sternocostalis*** arises from the lower one-third of the posterior surface of the body, and of the xiphoid process (and also from the adjoining parts of the costal cartilages).
4. Sternal slips of the ***diaphragm*** arise from the back of the xiphoid process.

***Relations of the Sternum***

1. The posterior aspect of the manubrium is related to the arch of the aorta and its branches, and to the left brachiocephalic vein.
2. Its lateral part is related to lungs and pleura. The body of the sternum is also related to lungs and pleura and to pericardium.
3. The xiphoid process is related to the liver.

***Ossification of the Sternum***

1. The number of centres of ossification appearing in different segments of the sternum is variable: 1 to 3 in the manubrium, and one or two in each sternebra.
2. The centres usually appear around the 5th month of fetal life. Ossification in the xiphoid process begins around the 3rd year or later.
3. The sternebrae unite with each other between puberty and 25 years, the union starting inferiorly and proceeding upwards.

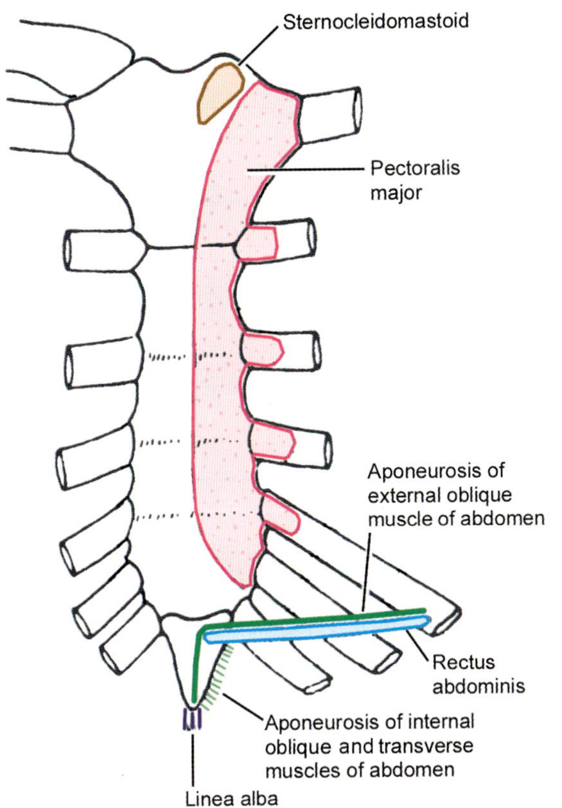


**16.12:** Attachments on the anterior aspect of the sternum

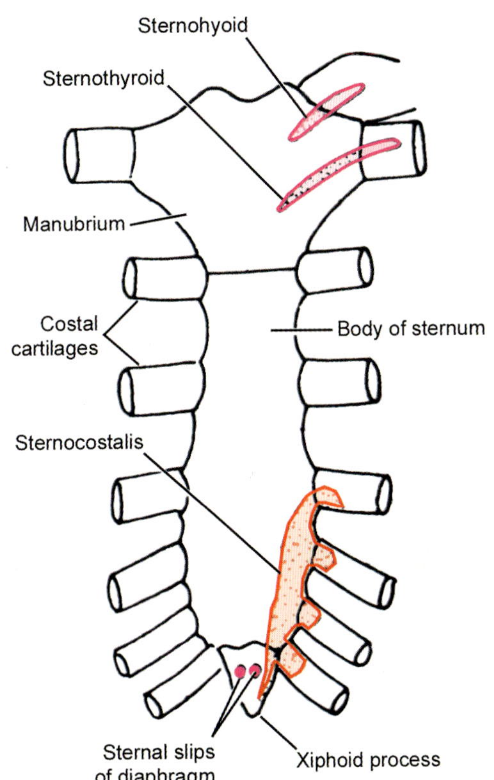


**16.13:** Attachments on the posterior aspect of the sternum

## THE RIBS

### Typical Ribs

1. The ribs are curved long bones that form the side-walls of the thorax (16.14).
2. There are twelve ribs on either side.
3. They vary considerably in length. The seventh rib is the longest, those above and below it becoming progressively shorter.
4. Adjacent ribs are separated by ***intercostal spaces***.
5. The ribs are attached behind to the thoracic vertebrae.
6. The anterior ends of the upper seven ribs are attached to bars of cartilage (***costal cartilages***) through which they gain attachment to the sternum. They are called ***true ribs***.
7. The anterior ends of the eighth, ninth and tenth ribs also end in costal cartilages. These cartilages do not reach the sternum, but end by gaining attachment to the next higher costal cartilage. They are, therefore, called ***false ribs***.
8. The anterior ends of the eleventh and twelfth ribs have small pieces of cartilage attached to their ends. These ends are free and these ribs are, therefore, called ***floating ribs***.
9. At the posterior end of a typical rib, we see a ***head***, a ***neck*** and a ***tubercle***.
   a. The head articulates partly with the superior costal facet on the body of the numerically corresponding vertebra, and partly with the inferior costal facet on the next higher vertebra. It is also attached to the intervertebral disc.

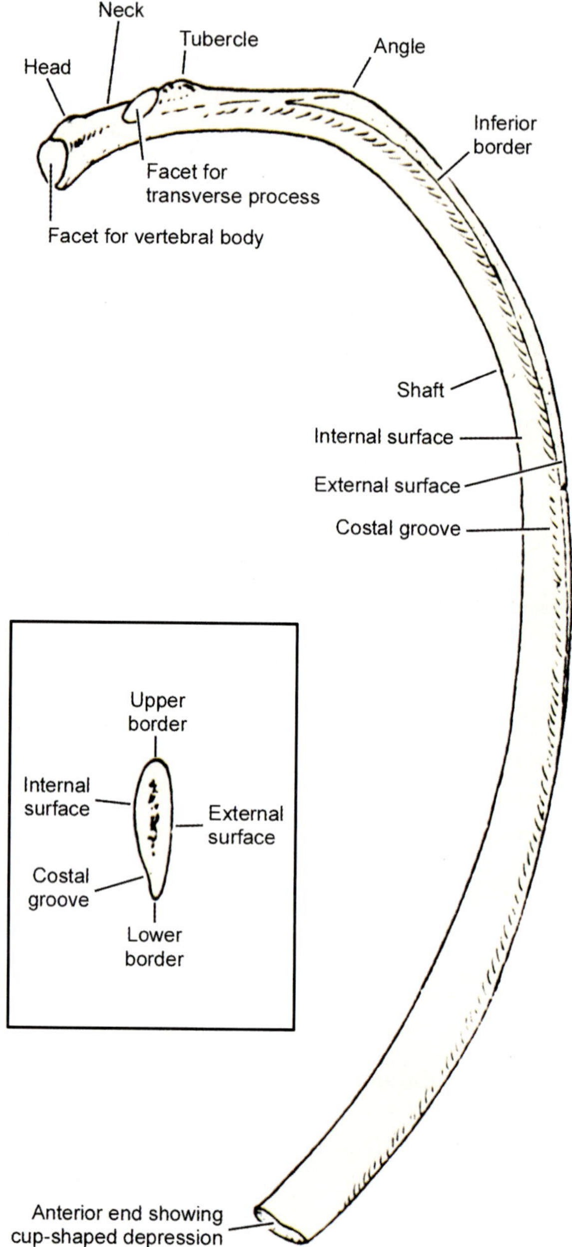


**16.14:** A typical rib seen from below

b. The part of the rib immediately lateral to the head is called the neck. It lies in front of the transverse process of the numerically corresponding vertebra. It has a sharp upper border called the ***crest*** of the neck.
c. Just lateral to the neck, the posterior aspect of the rib presents an elevation called the tubercle.
d. The tubercle has a medial articular part. It bears a facet that articulates with the costal facet on the transverse process of the corresponding vertebra.
e. The tubercle has a lateral part that is rough for attachment of ligaments.

10. The anterior end of the rib shows a cup-shaped depression for attachment of the costal cartilage concerned.
11. The part of the rib between the anterior and posterior ends is called the shaft. It is curved like the letter 'C'. The shaft is flat: it has ***inner and outer surfaces***, and ***upper and lower borders***.
12. The upper border is rounded. The lower border is sharp. The inner surface is concave.
13. Just above the lower border, the inner surface shows a ***costal groove*** running along the length of the shaft.
14. The external surface of the shaft is convex. A short distance lateral to the tubercle it is marked by a rough line. At this point the rib appears to be bent: this point is, therefore, called the ***angle***.
15. The shaft is also somewhat twisted along its long axis. As a result, the external surface faces somewhat downwards in the posterior part and somewhat upwards in its anterior part.

## WANT TO KNOW MORE?

### *Attachments and Some Relations of Typical Ribs*

1. The head of each rib gives attachment to the fibrous capsule, the radiate ligament and the intra-articular ligament of the ***costovertebral joint***.
2. The neck and tubercle give attachment to ligaments of the ***costotransverse joint***. The superior costotransverse ligament is attached to the crest of the neck; the costotransverse ligament to the posterior surface of the neck; and the lateral costotransverse ligament to the rough non-articular part of the tubercle.
3. The ***internal intercostal membrane*** is attached to the lower border and anterior surface of the neck of the rib.
4. Each ***external intercostal muscle*** is attached, superiorly, to the sharp lower border of the shaft; and inferiorly to the outer lip of the superior border (of the next lower rib).
5. The ***internal intercostal muscle*** is attached above to the floor of the costal groove; and below to the inner lip of the superior border (of the next lower rib).
6. The ***intercostalis intimus*** (***innermost intercostal***) is attached above to the upper border of the costal groove; and inferiorly to the inner lip of the superior border (of the next lower rib, along with the internal intercostal).
7. The external surfaces of typical ribs give attachment to a number of muscles, the exact attachments varying from rib to rib. The muscles include the ***serratus anterior***, the ***pectoralis minor***, the ***latissimus dorsi***, the ***external oblique*** muscle of the abdomen, the levatores costae, and the iliocostalis cervicis (part of erector spinae).
8. The ***intercostal vessels and nerve*** (of an intercostal space) lie in relation to the costal groove, but are separated from the floor of the groove by the internal intercostal muscle.
9. The sympathetic trunk descends vertically across the anterior aspect of the heads of lower ribs.
10. The internal surfaces of the ribs are covered by costal pleura.

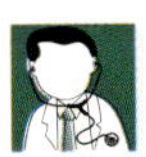

## CLINICAL CORRELATION

### Congenital Malformations of Sternum and Ribs

1. Some ribs may be underdeveloped or missing. Unilateral absence of a rib is often associated with absence of half of the corresponding vertebral body (***hemivertebra***).
   a. In the condition called ***ectopia cordis*** the sternum and the adjoining of parts of costal cartilages and ribs are missing, so that the heart can be seen from the outside.
2. Accessory ribs may be present. Such a rib may be attached to the 7th cervical vertebra (***cervical rib***) or to the first lumbar vertebra (***lumbar rib***). The clinical importance of a cervical rib is discussed in chapter 3.
3. The sternum develops in right and left halves that normally fuse in the midline. Imperfect fusion leads to partial or complete midline clefts of the sternum.
4. Various other anomalies include bifid ribs, and ribs fused to one another. The eighth costal cartilage may be directly connected to the sternum i.e., it may be an additional true rib.

*Fractures of Ribs and Sternum*

1. Ribs can be fractured by direct or indirect (crushing) injury. In a crushing injury, ribs tend to be fractured at their angles (these being the weakest points). As the upper two ribs are protected by the clavicle, injury to them is uncommon. Mobility of the last two ribs protects them from injury.
2. Injuries to ribs are rare in children as the thorax is highly elastic in them.
3. One or more ribs may be fractured by injury. Each rib may break at a single point along its length (***single rib fractures***), or may break at two or more places (***double rib fractures***). In the latter case the chest wall loses its stability as part of the wall become mobile (***flail chest***). This can result in considerable respiratory problems.
4. A special type of rib injury is commonly seen in car accidents in which the driver is violently thrown against the steering wheel. Fractures take place at the anterior ends of ribs on either side of the sternum. The sternum itself is frequently fractured near its upper end. In such injuries, again, a portion of the chest wall including the sternum becomes mobile.
5. Injuries to ribs can lead to pneumothorax, haemothorax, injury to lungs and to surgical emphysema.

*Sternal Puncture*

This is a procedure in which specimens of bone marrow can be obtained by passing a cannula into the manubrium sterni. Examination of bone marrow is useful in diagnosis of anaemias, leukaemias, and some other diseases.

*Surgical Approach*

For operations on the heart, the sternum is split into two by a cut in the midline. The two halves are retracted. After the operation the two halves are stitched together.

## WANT TO KNOW MORE?

**Atypical Ribs**

*The First Rib*

1. The first rib (16.15) can be distinguished by its small size, and by the fact that its shaft is broad and flat having upper and lower surfaces (instead of outer and inner), and inner and outer borders (instead of upper and lower).
2. The head has a single facet as this rib articulates only with the first thoracic vertebra.
3. The tubercle is prominent and coincides with the angle.
4. The upper surface of the shaft has two shallow, but wide grooves (for the subclavian artery and vein). Near the inner border of the rib these two grooves are separated by a prominence called the ***scalene tubercle***.
5. The lower surface of the rib is smooth and does not have a costal groove.

*Attachments and relations of the first rib*

1. The ***scalenus medius*** is inserted into a large rough area on the superior surface, behind the groove for the subclavian artery (16.16).
2. The ***scalenus anterior*** is inserted on the scalene tubercle, and the adjoining part of the upper surface of the rib.
3. The ***subclavius*** arises from the anterior end of the upper surface of the rib; and from the adjoining part of the first costal cartilage.
4. The first digitation of the ***serratus anterior*** arises from the outer border of the rib near the groove for the subclavian artery.
5. The outer border also gives attachment to intercostal muscles of the first space.
6. The ***costoclavicular ligament*** is attached to the rough area in front of the groove for the subclavian vein.
7. The inner border gives attachment to the ***suprapleural membrane***.

8. The inferior surface of the rib is related to pleura and lung.
9. The groove for the subclavian artery lodges this artery, and also the lower trunk of the brachial plexus. The subclavian vein lies in its own groove.
10. Three important structures lie on the anterior aspect of the neck of the first rib. From medial to lateral side these are:
    a. The sympathetic trunk (*cervicothoracic ganglion*).
    b. The superior intercostal artery (accompanied by the first posterior intercostal vein).
    c. The ventral ramus of the first thoracic nerve (which ascends across the first rib to join the brachial plexus).

### The Second Rib

1. The second rib can be distinguished from a typical rib by the fact that when placed on a flat surface the entire rib touches it. (In a typical rib, the posterior end is lifted off the surface).
2. The external surface is directed outwards and upwards (16.17) (and not directly upwards as in the first rib). Near its middle it has a prominent rough area.
3. The inner surface points medially and downwards.
4. A short costal groove is present on its posterior part.

#### *Attachments and relations*

1. The upper and lower borders of the rib give attachment to ***intercostal muscles*** (16.18).
2. The ***scalenus posterior*** is inserted into the posterior part of the outer surface.
3. The ***serratus anterior*** (first and second digitations) arises from the tubercle on the outer surface just behind the middle of the shaft.
4. A slip of the ***serratus posterior superior*** is attached just lateral to the tubercle.
5. The inner surface is related to ***lungs and pleura***.

### The Tenth, Eleventh and Twelfth Ribs

1. These ribs can be distinguished from typical ribs as each of them bears only a single articular facet on the head. This is so because each of these ribs articulates only with the corresponding vertebra.
2. In other respects, the tenth rib is similar to a typical rib.
3. The eleventh and twelfth ribs (16.19) can be distinguished from the tenth rib as they are relatively short, have no necks or tubercles, and their ends are tapering (in contrast to the broad anterior ends of typical ribs).
4. The eleventh rib can be distinguished from the twelfth as it has a slight angle, and a costal groove is discernible, but the twelfth rib has neither of these features.

#### *Attachments on the twelfth rib*

1. Near the medial end the rib gives attachment to ligaments of the costovertebral joint and (posteriorly) to the lumbocostal ligament (16.20 and 16.21).
2. The medial part of the upper border gives attachment to ***intercostal muscles***.
3. The ***diaphragm*** is attached to the lateral part of the upper border, and to the adjoining part of the anterior surface.
4. The ***quadratus lumborum*** is attached to the lower part of the medial half (or so) of the anterior surface.
5. The layers of ***thoracolumbar fascia*** are attached as follows:
    a. The anterior layer, to the anterior surface just above the attachment of the quadratus lumborum.
    b. The middle layer to the lower border just below the attachment of the quadratus lumborum.
    c. The posterior layer to the lower border, lateral to the attachment of the quadratus lumborum.
6. The ***lateral arcuate ligament*** is attached to the lower border at the lateral end of the area for attachment of the quadratus lumborum.

7. The medial part of the posterior surface of the rib gives attachment to the lowest levator costae, and to part of the erector spinae.
8. The lateral part of the posterior surface gives attachment to slips for the latissimus dorsi, the external oblique muscle of the abdomen, and the serratus posterior inferior.

*Relationship of Twelfth Rib to Pleura*

The upper part of the medial half of the anterior surface (i.e., the area above that for the quadratus lumborum) is in contact with pleura (costodiaphragmatic recess).

### *Ossification of Ribs*

1. A typical rib has a primary centre that appears in the shaft during the second month of fetal life.
2. Secondary centres appear around the age of puberty: one for the head, and one each for the articular and non-articular parts of the tubercle. The last mentioned centre is absent in the lower ribs.
3. As the eleventh and twelfth ribs have no tubercles the relevant centres are absent in them.

## THE COSTAL CARTILAGES

1. These are bars of hyaline cartilage. A typical costal cartilage has medial and lateral ends, anterior and posterior surfaces, and upper and lower borders.
2. The lateral end of each costal cartilage is attached to the anterior end of one rib.
3. The medial ends of the upper seven costal cartilages are attached to the lateral margin of the sternum.
   a. The first costal cartilage is attached to the lateral margin of the manubrium sterni.
   b. The medial end of the second cartilage is attached partly to the manubrium and partly to the first sternebra.
   c. The 3rd, 4th and 5th cartilages gain attachment to the lateral edge of the sternum at the points of junction of sternebrae; the 6th on the fourth sternebra; and the 7th at the junction of the fourth sternebra and the xiphoid process.
4. The medial ends of the 8th, 9th and 10th costal cartilages are connected to the next higher costal cartilage.
5. The cartilages of the 11th and 12th ribs are small and are attached to the tips of the ribs. Their lateral ends are free.
6. The joint between the first costal cartilage and the manubrium sterni is a synchondrosis. The 2nd to 7th costal cartilages are joined to the sternum through synovial joints. The junctions of the 8th, 9th and 10th cartilages with the next higher cartilage are also marked by the presence of synovial joints.
7. Costal cartilages make the wall of the thorax more elastic. Elasticity is lost in old people in whom the cartilages calcify.

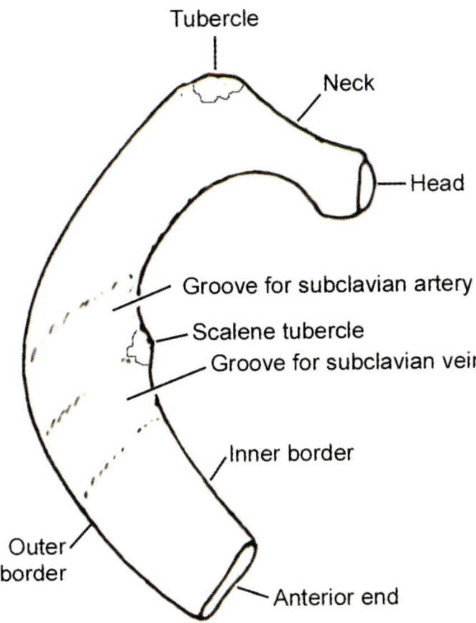


**16.15:** First rib seen from above

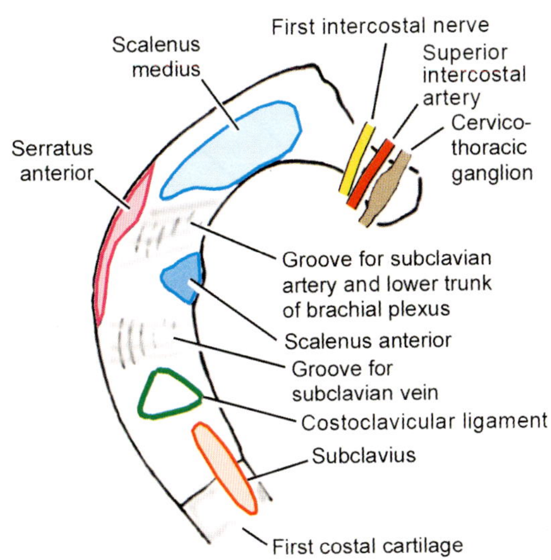


**16.16:** Attachments and relations of the first rib seen from above

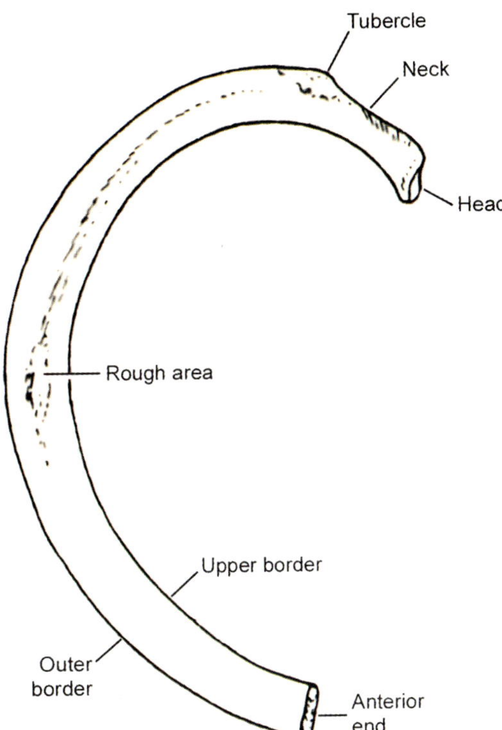


**16.17:** Second rib (right) seen from above

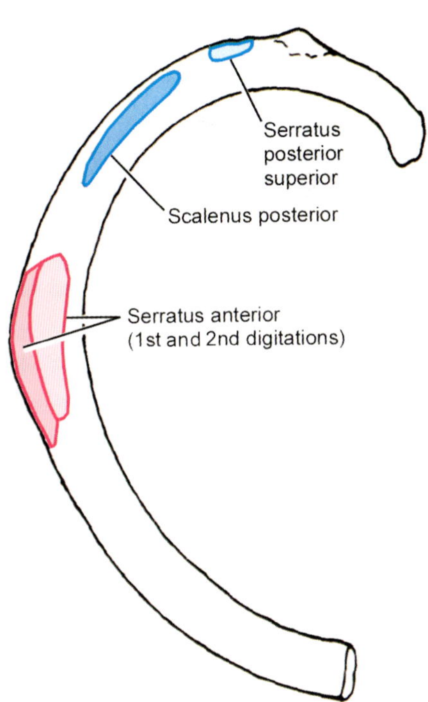


**16.18:** Attachments on the superior aspect of the second rib

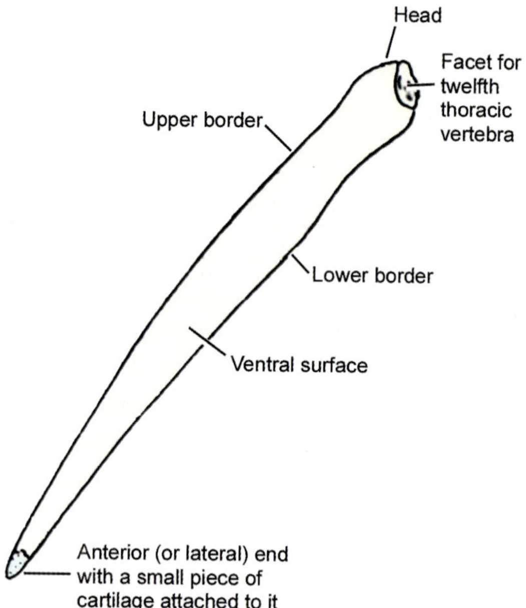


**16.19:** Twelfth rib (right) seen from the front. Note absence of neck, tubercle, angle and costal groove

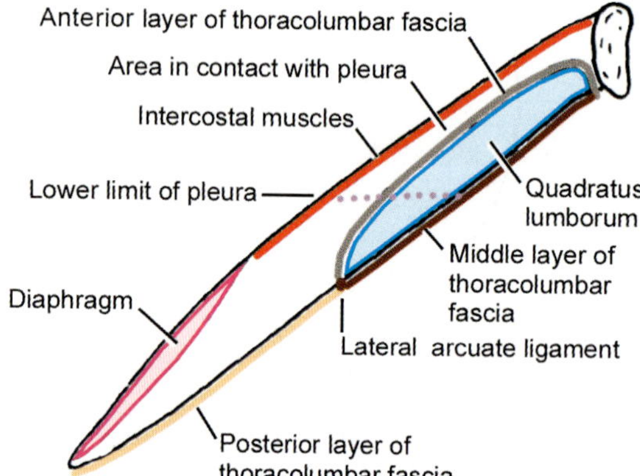


**16.20:** Attachments on the anterior aspect of the twelfth rib

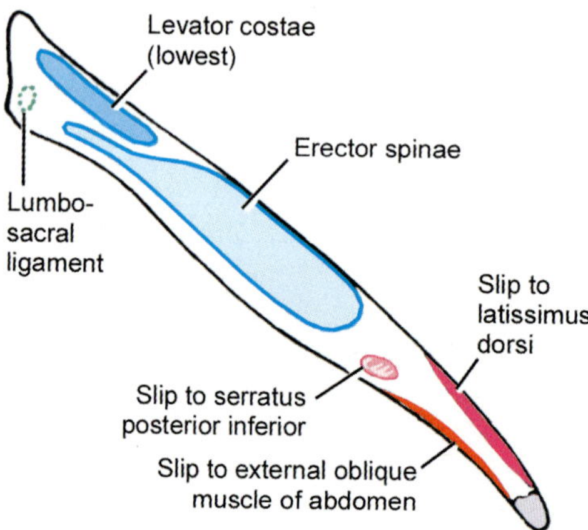


**16.21:** Attachments on the posterior aspect of the twelfth rib

# 17 CHAPTER

# Intervertebral Joints and Joints of Sternum and Ribs

In this chapter, we will consider the joints between the bones of the thorax. These are:

1. ***Intervertebral joints*** connecting adjacent thoracic vertebrae.
2. ***Sternal joints*** between different parts of the sternum.
3. ***Costovertebral joints*** between ribs and vertebrae.
4. ***Costochondral joints*** between ribs and costal cartilages.
5. ***Sternocostal joints*** or ***chondrosternal joints*** between costal cartilages and the sternum.
6. ***Interchondral joints*** amongst the lower costal cartilages.

## INTERVERTEBRAL JOINTS

Adjoining vertebrae are connected to one another through three main joints:

1. There is a median joint between the vertebral bodies.
2. There are two joints (right and left) between the articular processes.
3. The bodies, laminae, transverse processes and spinous processes of adjoining vertebrae are also united by a number of ligaments.

### Joints between Vertebral Bodies

Each vertebra has a body that is shaped roughly like a short cylinder. The body has more or less flat upper and lower surfaces.

1. The lower surface of the body of one vertebra articulates with the superior surface of the body of the next vertebra.
2. The structure of a joint between any two vertebral bodies corresponds to that of a typical symphysis.
3. The bony surfaces forming the joint are covered by thin layers of hyaline cartilage.
4. The two plates of hyaline cartilage are united to each other by a thick ***intervertebral disc*** (17.1).

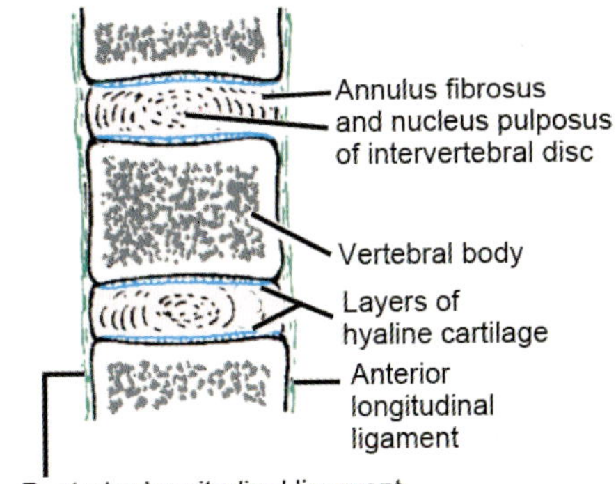


**17.1:** Schematic sagittal section across vertebral bodies and intervertebral discs

### Intervertebral Discs

1. Intervertebral discs are the chief bonds of union between adjoining vertebrae.
2. Each disc consists of an outer part called the ***annulus fibrosus***, and an inner part the ***nucleus pulposus***.
3. The superficial part of the annulus fibrosus is made up of collagen fibres. Its deeper part is of fibrocartilage.
4. In the young, the nucleus pulposus is soft and gelatinous, but this material is gradually replaced by fibrocartilage. When this happens the nucleus pulposus merges with the annulus fibrosus.
5. The intervertebral discs are very strong in the young. With advancing age, however, the annulus fibrosus becomes weak and it then becomes possible for the nucleus pulposus to burst through it. This is called ***prolapse*** of the disc (though it is really prolapse of the nucleus pulposus).

6. The thickness and shape of intervertebral discs is different in different parts of the vertebral column.
   a. The discs are thinnest in the upper thoracic region of the vertebral column (which is least mobile), and thickest in the lower lumbar region.
   b. In the cervical and lumbar regions, the discs are thicker in front than behind (and this fact is partially responsible for the forward convexity of the vertebral column in these regions).
   c. In the thoracic region, the discs are flat.
7. Intervertebral discs constitute about one fifth of the length of the vertebral column. They transmit weight, act as shock absorbers, and provide resilience to the spine. As stated above they contribute to formation of curves of the vertebral column.

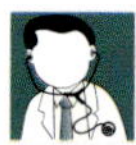

**CLINICAL CORRELATION**

**Disc Prolapse and Sciatica**

1. A prolapsed nucleus pulposus usually passes backwards and laterally and may press upon nerve roots emerging from the spinal cord at that level.
2. Prolapse results in local pain in the back.
3. When nerves are pressed upon, there is shooting pain along the course of the nerve involved. Disc prolapse occurs most frequently in the lumbosacral region and results in pain shooting down the back of the thigh and leg. This is called ***sciatica***.
4. Prolapse is also frequently seen in the cervical region.

### Joints between Vertebral Articular Processes

1. Each vertebra has four articular processes (or zygapophyses): right and left superior, and right and left inferior.
2. Each process bears an articular facet. The inferior articular facets of one vertebra articulate with the superior articular facets of the next lower vertebra forming a series of ***zygapophyseal joints***.
3. These are synovial joints having a joint cavity enclosed in a capsule. In the cervical and thoracic region, the articular facets are flat: these are, therefore, plane joints. In the lumbar region, the facets are curved from side to side.

### Ligaments Connecting Adjacent Vertebrae

Adjoining vertebrae are connected by numerous ligaments. As stated above each such union can be regarded as a fibrous joint (syndesmosis). The ligaments are as follows (17.2):

1. ***Anterior longitudinal ligament*** passing from the anterior surface of the body of one vertebra to that of another.
2. ***Posterior longitudinal ligament*** passing from the posterior surface of the body of one vertebra to that of another. This ligament lies within the vertebral canal.
3. ***Intertransverse ligaments*** interconnect adjacent transverse processes.
4. ***Interspinous ligaments*** connect adjacent spinous processes.
5. ***Supraspinous ligaments*** connect the tips of spinous processes. All the ligaments listed above are made up predominantly of collagen fibres. They limit undue movement of vertebrae on one another.
6. The ***ligamenta flava*** (= yellow ligaments) are made up of elastic tissue.
   a. They pass from the lower border of the lamina of one vertebra to the upper border of the lamina of the next lower vertebra.
   b. Medially, the right and left ligaments almost meet in the midline.
   c. Laterally, they extend up to the joints between the articular processes.
   d. They act as brakes preventing undue separation of laminae during flexion of the vertebral column.
   e. Their elasticity helps in straightening the vertebral column after flexion. By limiting movements, they probably protect intervertebral discs from undue compression and consequent injury.

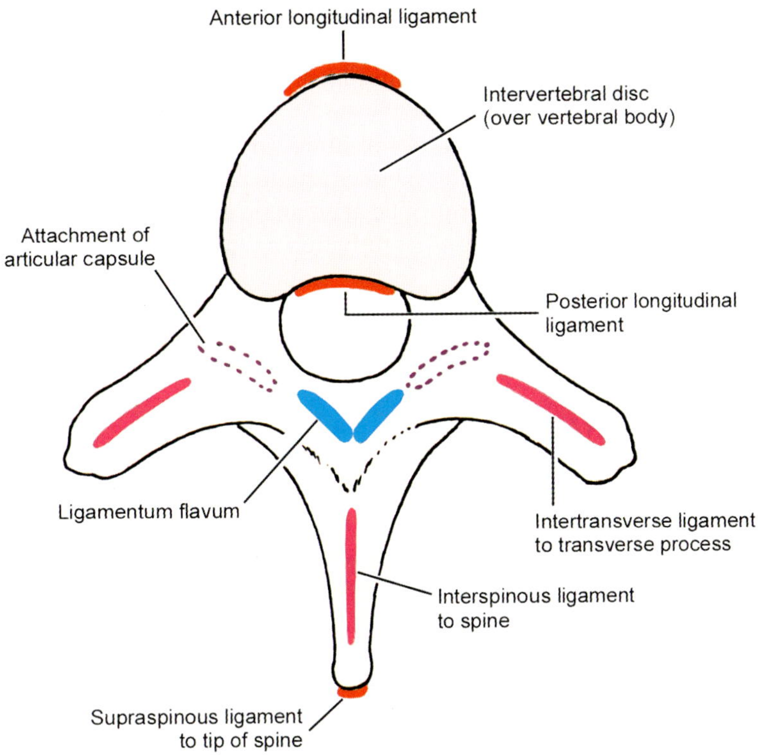


17.2: Scheme to show ligaments connecting adjacent vertebrae

In the preceding paragraphs, we have considered the basic features of typical intervertebral joints. The joint between the atlas and the axis, and the joint between the atlas vertebra and the occipital bone have special features that will be studied in the head and neck. The lumbosacral joints will be considered in the abdomen.

### Movements of the Vertebral Column

1. Movements between adjacent vertebrae take place simultaneously at the three joints connecting them.
2. The range of movement permitted between any two vertebrae is slight. However, when the movements between various vertebrae get added together, the total movement becomes considerable.
3. The vertebral column can be bent forwards (flexion), backwards (extension) and to one side (lateral flexion). Some degree of rotation is also possible (as in twisting movements of the trunk).
4. On the whole, the cervical and lumbar regions are much more flexible than the thoracic region. Stability of the thoracic region of the vertebral column facilitates respiratory movements.
5. Rotation of the spine is slight in the cervical region (and is compensated by rotation of the head). It is greater in the upper thoracic region, and greatest in the lower thoracic region. Rotation is least in the lumbar region.
6. Movements of the spine are produced by the ***erector spinae*** (which is a large muscle running along the vertebral column from the sacrum to the skull), by abdominal muscles, and by various muscles related to the vertebral column.

## JOINTS OF THE STERNUM

We have seen that the sternum consists of three parts: the manubrium, the body, and the xiphoid process. These three elements are connected by joints.

### Manubriosternal Joint

1. The lower end of the manubrium is attached to the body of the sternum at the manubriosternal joint. This joint is a symphysis. The bony surfaces are covered by thin layers of hyaline cartilage that are connected to each other by fibrocartilage.
2. As a rule, bone ends taking part in symphyses do not undergo bony union. However, the manubriosternal symphysis is atypical, bony union between the two bones taking place in many individuals after the age of 30.
3. The manubrium sterni and the body of the sternum lie at an angle of about 163° to each other (representing an angulation of 17° (17.3). The ***angulation*** increases slightly during inspiration and becomes less in expiration.

### Xiphisternal Joint

This joint is also a symphysis, but the two bones generally undergo bony union by the age of 40 years.

## JOINTS OF RIBS WITH VERTEBRAL COLUMN

### Costovertebral Joints

1. These joints (also called ***costocorporeal joints***) unite the heads of ribs to the sides of the vertebral column.
2. On the sides of the body of a typical thoracic vertebra, we see semicircular facets (demifacets) near the upper and lower margins of the body.
3. The head of a rib bears a facet that is divided into upper and lower parts by a ridge, and the two parts lie at an obtuse angle to each other (17.4).
   a. The lower part of the facet articulates with the demifacet on the superior border of the body of the numerically corresponding vertebra.
   b. The upper part of the facet articulates with the lower demifacet on the next higher vertebra.
   c. The ridge separating the facets is attached to the intervertebral disc through an ***intra-articular ligament*** that divides the joint cavity into upper and lower parts.
4. The joint is enclosed in a capsule that is strengthened in front by fibres that radiate from the head of the rib to the two vertebrae and to the intervertebral disc. These fibres constitute the ***radiate ligament*** (or triradiate ligament).
5. As the head of a rib articulates with two vertebrae the joint is classified as compound. As the joint cavity is divided into two parts, the joint can also be classified as complex.
6. Costovertebral joints of the 1st, 10th, 11th and 12th ribs are atypical in that these ribs articulate only with the corresponding vertebrae.

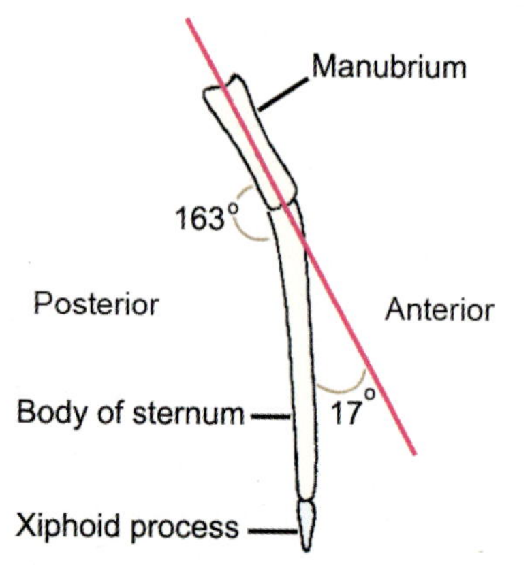


**17.3:** Scheme to show angulation at the manubriosternal junction

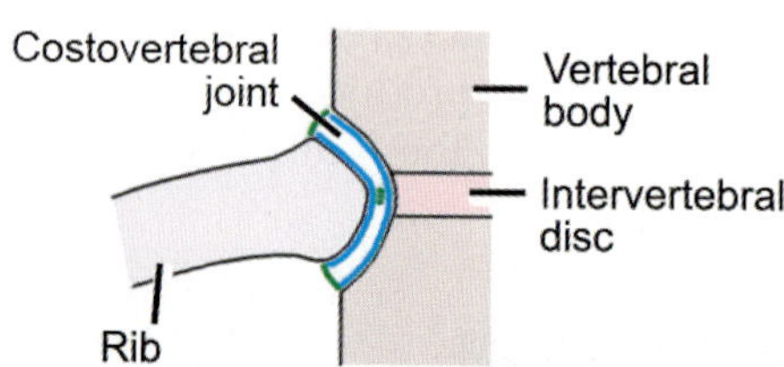


**17.4:** Schematic coronal section across a costovertebral joint

## Costotransverse Joint

1. A short distance lateral to the head, each rib bears a tubercle that is divisible into a medial articular part, and a lateral non-articular part.
   a. The medial part bears a facet that articulates with a facet on the front of the transverse process of the corresponding vertebra.
   b. The joint surfaces are enclosed in a capsule (17.5).
2. The joint is strengthened by the following ligaments (17.6 and 17.7):
   a. The ***lateral costotransverse ligament*** is attached laterally to the non-articular part of the tubercle of the rib, and medially to the tip of the transverse process.
   b. The ***superior costotransverse ligament*** passes from the upper border of the neck of a rib to the lower border of the transverse process of the ***next higher*** vertebra. The ligament has anterior and posterior laminae. Laterally, the anterior lamina blends with the internal intercostal membrane, and the posterior lamina blends with the external intercostal muscle (See chapter 18).
   c. The ***costotransverse ligament*** (or ***inferior costotransverse ligament***) passes from the posterior surface of the neck of the rib to the front of the transverse process of the ***corresponding*** vertebra(17.7).

# JOINTS BETWEEN RIBS, COSTAL CARTILAGES AND STERNUM

## Costochondral Joints

1. The anterior end of each rib bears a depression into which the rounded lateral end of a costal cartilage is fixed.
2. The two are held in position by continuity of the periosteum of the rib with the perichondrium of the cartilage. The costal cartilages are regarded as unossified extensions of the ribs.

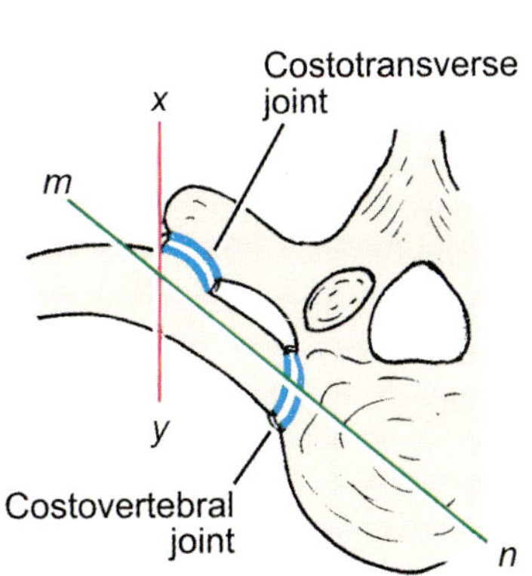


17.5: Schematic section across the posterior part of a rib to show costovertebral and costotransverse joints

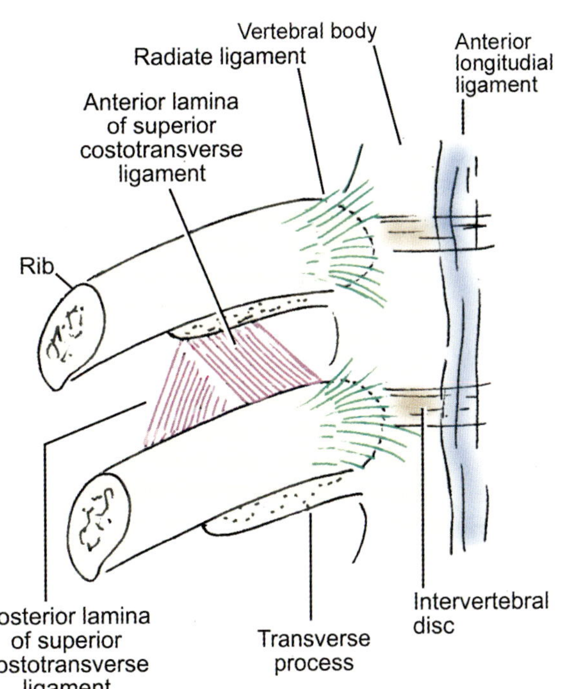


17.6: Some ligaments of costovertebral and costotransverse joints seen from the front

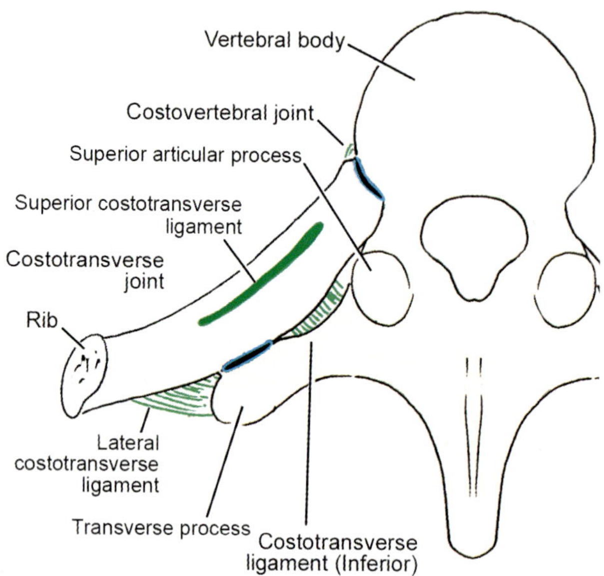


17.7: Costotransverse joint and some related ligaments. The arrow points to the attachment of the superior costotransverse ligament

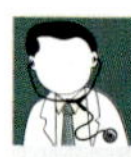

### CLINICAL CORRELATION

In ***dislocation of a costochondral joint,*** a rib separates from its costal cartilage. There is pain.

## Chondrosternal Joints

These joints are often, less accurately, referred to as sternocostal joints.

1. They are joints between the (medial ends of) 1st and 7th costal cartilages and the sternum.
2. The joint of the first costal cartilage with the manubrium sterni has been described, in the past, as a synchondrosis. However, the costal cartilage is united to the manubrium through a plate of ***fibrocartilage*** and is not a typical synchondrosis.
3. The joints between the 2nd and 7th costal cartilages and the sternum are synovial joints. They are held together by continuity of perichondrium and periosteum. They are strengthened anteriorly and posteriorly by fibres that radiate from the costal cartilage onto the sternum. The cavity of the joint between the 2nd costal cartilage and the sternum is normally divided into upper and lower parts by an intra-articular ligament.

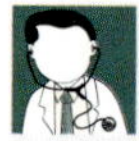

### CLINICAL CORRELATION

A costal cartilage may be displaced from the sternum. This is ***dislocation of a costosternal joint***. The condition is painful and there may be deformity.

## Interchondral Joints

The 6th to 9th costal cartilages come into contact with one another and form a number of small interchondral synovial joints.

## MOVEMENTS OF RIBS

The movements taking place at the joints of the thorax allow for rhythmic expansion and contraction of the thoracic wall during respiration.

### WANT TO KNOW MORE?

The precise nature of the movements is complex and differs in different ribs, but the two fundamental movements to be understood are as follows:

1. The anterior ends of the ribs can move up or down by rotation at the costovertebral and costotransverse joints.
   a. In expiration, the anterior ends of the ribs are lower than their posterior ends (17.8).
   b. During inspiration, the anterior end moves upwards in an arc becoming more horizontal. This increases the anteroposterior diameter of the thorax.
   c. The forward movement of the rib is made possible by an angular movement at the manubriosternal joint.
   d. Movements of the sternum have been compared to those of a ***pump handle***.
   e. Rotation of ribs on a transverse axis takes place mainly in relation to the upper six ribs. These movements are facilitated by the fact that articular surfaces on the tubercles of these ribs are convex.
2. The second movement of the ribs occurs on an axis that is roughly anteroposterior. The axis passes through the costotransverse and sternocostal joints (*xy* in 17.5).
   a. In expiration, the middle of the rib is lower than its ends.
   b. In inspiration, it is raised (like a bucket handle). This increases the transverse diameter of the thorax as shown in 17.9.
   c. These movements take place mainly in the 7th to 10th ribs. The articular surfaces on the tubercles of these ribs are flat.
3. During quiet breathing the movements of the ribs described above are produced by intercostal muscles. Elevation of ribs (during inspiration) is produced by the external intercostals, and depression (during expiration) by the internal intercostals, aided by elastic recoil of the thoracic wall. (The intercostal muscles also make the region of the intercostal spaces stiff thus resisting atmospheric pressure imposed on them because of negative intrapleural pressure).
4. In deep inspiration movements of the ribs are aided by contraction of some muscles attached to the ribs. The scaleni (present in the neck) and the sternocleidomastoid muscles elevate the first rib, while the erector spinae helps expansion of the thorax by reducing the concavity of the thoracic part of the vertebral column.
5. In forced inspiration (against resistance), the scapulae are elevated and fixed by the trapezius, the levator scapulae and the rhomboideus muscles. With the arms fixed (by holding onto a firm object) contraction of the serratus anterior and of the pectoralis major pulls upon the ribs helping expansion of the thorax. In forced expiration (as in patients with asthma), the thorax is compressed by the latissimus dorsi (but the major role is played by abdominal muscles).
6. The diaphragm plays a very important role in respiration.

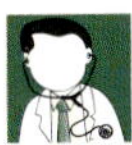

### CLINICAL CORRELATION

*Variations in Shape of the Thorax*

1. In the normal adult, the thorax is more or less oval in transverse section.
2. In infants, the thorax is more nearly circular as a result of which respiration is mostly abdominal.
3. In a condition called emphysema the lungs are dilated, and as a result the thorax can become rounded in section (***barrel chest***), making respiration much less effective.

4. Deformities seen in the thoracic cage may be congenital or may result from disease. In ***funnel chest,*** the front of the chest (in the region of the body of sternum and xiphoid process) is depressed. As a result, the costal cartilages are curved inwards near their anterior ends. (In this condition, the basic defect is that the central tendon of the diaphragm is abnormally short so that the xiphoid process is pulled inwards).
5. In ***pigeon chest,*** the thorax may project forwards in midline (as is normal in birds). These deformities can be surgically corrected.
6. Deformities may involve the thoracic spine. The spine may be bent forwards (***kyphosis***), or to one side (***scoliosis***). The two may be combined (***kyphoscoliosis***).

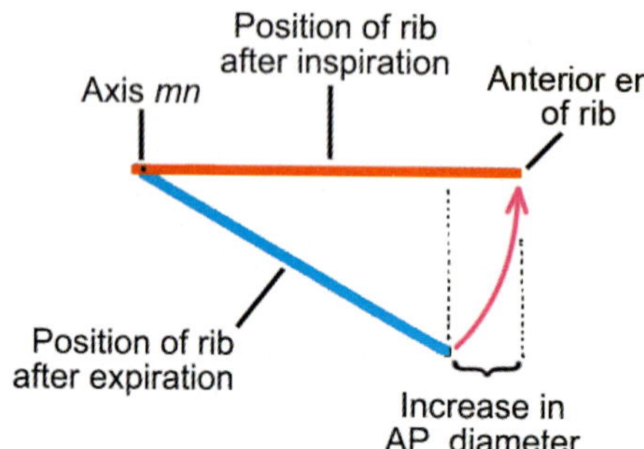


**17.8:** Scheme to show how elevation of the anterior end of a rib during inspiration increases the anteroposterior diameter of the thorax

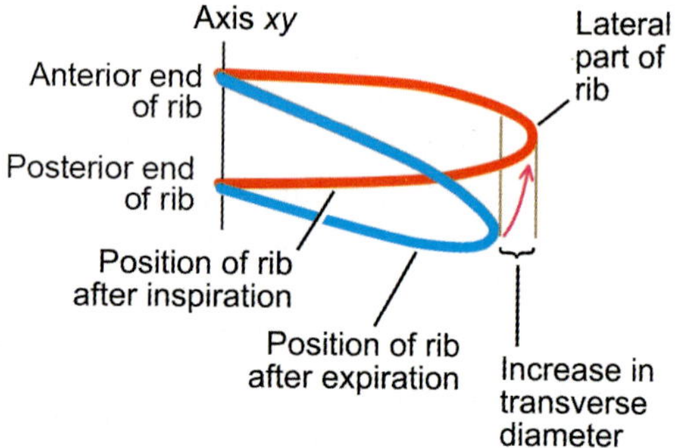


**17.9:** Scheme to show how elevation of the side of a rib increases the transverse diameter of the thorax

# 18 CHAPTER

# Walls of the Thorax

The skeletal basis of the thoracic wall has been dealt with in Chapter 16 and the joints of the thorax have been considered in Chapter 17. In this chapter, we will consider other structures to be encountered in the thoracic wall.

## MUSCLES OF THORAX

### Intercostal Muscles

1. The ***intercostal muscles*** fill the intervals between adjacent ribs. They are arranged in three layers: ***external, internal*** and ***innermost*** (18.1 to 18.3).
2. There being twelve ribs on either side, and eleven intercostal spaces between them, we have eleven sets of external and internal intercostal muscles.
3. The innermost layer is often deficient in the upper intercostal spaces.
4. Each intercostal space extends, posteriorly, up to the superior costotransverse ligaments (extending between the neck of the rib and the transverse process of the vertebra next above it). Anteriorly, the space extends to the sternum.
5. The internal intercostal muscles do not extend over the entire length of the space: anteriorly they extend right up to the sternum, but posteriorly they end at the level of the angles of the ribs beyond which they are replaced by the ***posterior intercostal membranes.***
6. The external intercostals reach the costotransverse ligaments posteriorly, but they are deficient in front. Between the costal cartilages, they are replaced by the ***anterior intercostal membranes.***

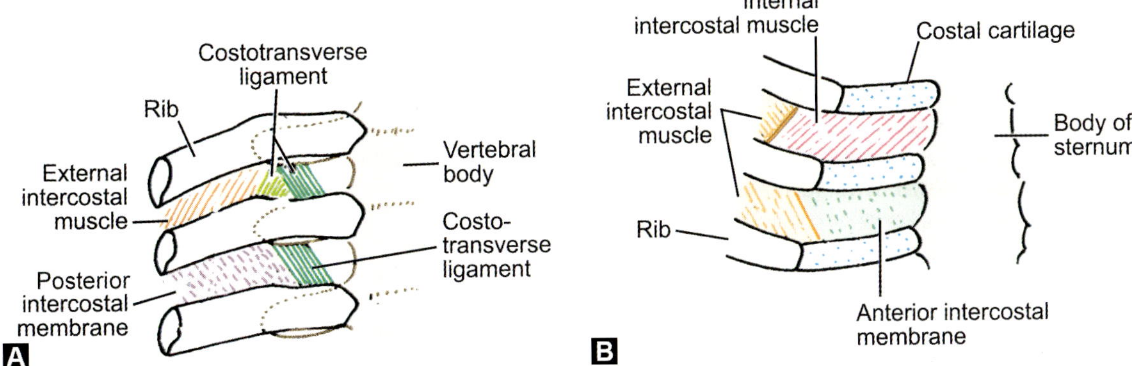


**18.1A and B:** (A) Posterior ends of two intercostal spaces viewed from within the thorax. The internal intercostal membrane has been removed in the upper space to reveal the underlying external intercostal muscle; (B) Anterior ends of two intercostal spaces viewed from the front. The external intercostal muscle and membrane have been removed in the upper space

**18.2: Intercostal muscles and sternocostalis**

| Muscle | Origin | Insertion | Direction of fibres | Action |
|---|---|---|---|---|
| External intercostal | Lower border of rib above | Upper border of rib below | Obliquely from one rib to another, the upper attachment being nearer to the vertebral end and the lower attachment being nearer to the sternal end of intercostal space | Prevent the thoracic wall from bulging inwards or outwards as a result of pressure changes during inspiration and expiration |
| Internal intercostal | Costal groove of rib above | Upper border of rib below | At right angles to external intercostal. On the front of the thorax fibres run downwards and laterally | |
| Innermost intercostal | Inner surface of adjoining rib | Inner surface of adjoining rib | | |
| Subcostales | Inner surface of rib near angle | Inner surface of rib two or three intercostal spaces below origin | | |
| Sternocostalis (18.4) | Posterior aspect of:<br>1. Lower 1/3rd of body of sternum<br>2. Xiphoid process.<br>3. Costal cartilages (adjoining parts of 4th to 7th) | 2nd, 3rd, 4th, 5th and 6th costal cartilages (lower borders and inner surfaces) | 1. Upwards and laterally from origin to insertion<br>2. Lowest fibres are transverse | Depresses costal cartilages into which it is inserted |
| Nerve Supply: All muscles described in this table are supplied by intercostal nerves of spaces concerned. | | | | |

7. The innermost layer is made up of three distinct muscles as follows:
   a. The ***intercostalis intimi*** (or ***innermost intercostal muscle***) is seen only in the middle two-fourths of the intercostal space.
   b. The ***subcostales*** are present only over the posterior part of the intercostal space (near the angles of the ribs, 18.3).
   c. In the anterior part of the thoracic wall, the innermost layer is formed by a muscle called the ***sternocostalis*** (18.4). The sternocostalis lies behind the sternum and costal cartilages.
   d. The three muscles of the inner layer lie in the same plane. Sometimes, they are collectively called the ***transversus thoracis,*** although this name is used by some authorities for the sternocostalis alone.
8. The intercostal nerves and vessels run between the muscles of the second and third layer. They supply all the muscles mentioned above. The intercostal muscles are lined on the inside by costal pleura.

#### *Attachments of Intercostal Muscles and Sternocostalis*

These are given in 18.2.

## SOME MUSCLES OF THORAX SEEN ON THE BACK

In additional to muscles seen in relation to the intercostal spaces, some small muscles are present on the back, superficial to the thoracic cage. You need to know only their names.

### Serratus Posterior Superior

This muscle is present on the back deep to the trapezius and rhomboideus muscles.

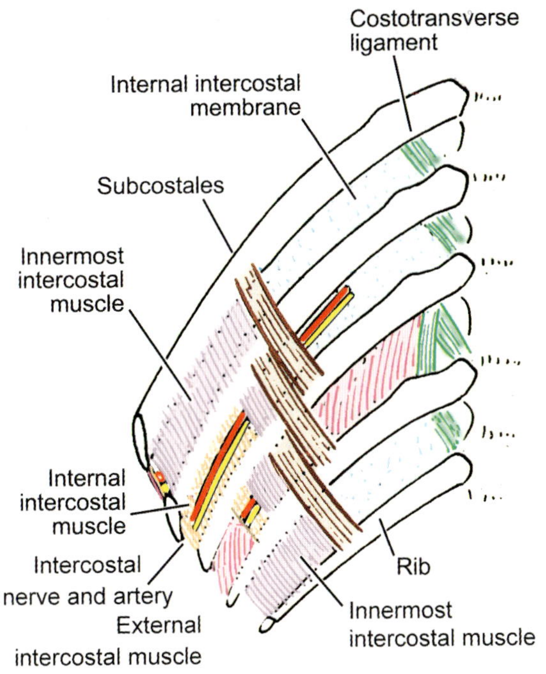


**18.3:** Diagram of the posterior ends of some intercostal spaces (internal aspect) to show the subcostales. Some layers have been removed from the 2nd and 3rd spaces drawn

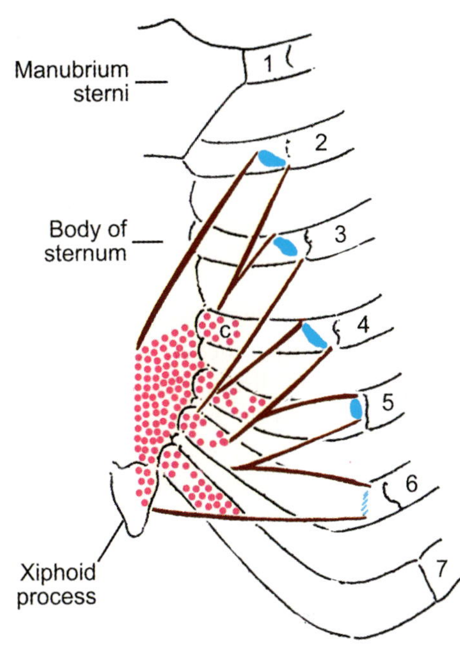


**18.4:** Scheme to show attachments of the sternocostalis

## Serratus Posterior Inferior

This muscle lies in the back deep to the latissimus dorsi, and superficial to the thoracolumbar fascia.

## Levatores Costarum

1. The levatores costarum are a series of twelve small muscles placed on either side of the back of the thorax just lateral to the vertebral column.
2. Each muscle arises from the end of a transverse process: the highest from C7 and the lowest from T11.
3. The fibres pass downwards and laterally to be inserted into rib next below.
4. Some of the lower muscles of the series have additional fasciculi that gain attachment to the second rib below the transverse process of origin. These longer fasciculi are called the ***levatores costarum longi.*** In contrast, the other fasciculi constitute the ***levatores costarum breves.***

All muscles mentioned above are supplied by the dorsal rami of thoracic spinal nerves.

These muscles can elevate the ribs to which they are attached. However, they are probably of no functional importance.

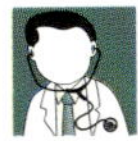

## CLINICAL CORRELATION

### Abscesses over Intercostal Spaces

*Cold Abscess*

1. Cold abscesses may be seen in relation to intercostal spaces.
2. They result from tuberculous infection of intercostal lymph nodes, or of vertebrae.

3. Pus from these sources can pass along intercostal nerves and vessels for considerable distances.
4. It generally becomes superficial at sites, where the lateral or anterior cutaneous branches emerge.

*Empyema Necessitatis*

1. An abscess over the thoracic wall can also be caused secondary to collection of pus in the pleural cavity (*empyema*).
2. The pus can perforate the chest wall (and can do so along the track of a needle used for aspiration) and present as an abscess.

**Paracentesis Thoracis**

1. Fluid in the pleural cavity can be aspirated by passing a needle into an intercostal space (usually the 6th) in the midaxillary line.
2. Remember that the neurovascular bundle of each intercostal space lies along the upper border of the space, and injury to it can be avoided by passing the needle through the lower part of the space.
3. A needle passed into one of the lower intercostal spaces, in the midaxillary line, will penetrate skin and fascia, the serratus anterior muscle, the intercostal muscles (three layers) and the parietal pleura to reach the pleural cavity.

**Thoracotomy**

1. A surgeon can enter the thoracic cavity through an opening made in the thoracic wall (thoracotomy).
2. Depending upon the region to be approached, thoracotomy can be anterior, posterior or lateral.
   a. The periosteum covering a rib is incised.
   b. A suitable length of rib is resected.
   c. An incision is made into the periosteum lying deep to the rib. This opens up the pleural cavity and organs within it can be approached.

## THE DIAPHRAGM

The diaphragm is a large muscle that forms a partition between the cavities of the thorax and the abdomen. (Its attachments are too complex to be presented in a table).

### Attachments of the Diaphragm

The diaphragm has a more or less circular origin from the thoracic outlet (18.5). The origin of the diaphragm can be divided into sternal, costal and vertebral parts.

1. The ***sternal part*** consists of two slips, right and left, that arise from the back of the xiphoid process.
2. The ***costal part*** consists of broad slips, one from the inner surface of each of the lower six ribs (i.e., 7th–12th) and their costal cartilages. These slips interdigitate with those of the transversus abdominis (a muscle of the abdominal wall).
3. The ***lumbar part*** consists of two ***crura*** (right and left) that arise from:
   a. The anterolateral aspects of the bodies of lumbar vertebrae.
   b. Fibres that arise (on either side) from two tendinous arches called the lateral and medial arcuate ligaments (See later in text) (18.5).
4. The right crus is larger than the left. It arises from the bodies of vertebrae L1, L2, L3 and from the intervening intervertebral discs.
5. The left crus arises similarly from vertebrae L1 and L2.
6. The medial margins of the two crura are joined to each other (at the level of the lower border of vertebra T12) to form the ***median arcuate ligament.*** (Do not confuse this with the ***medial*** arcuate ligament described below).
7. The descending aorta passes from thorax to abdomen under cover of this ligament.

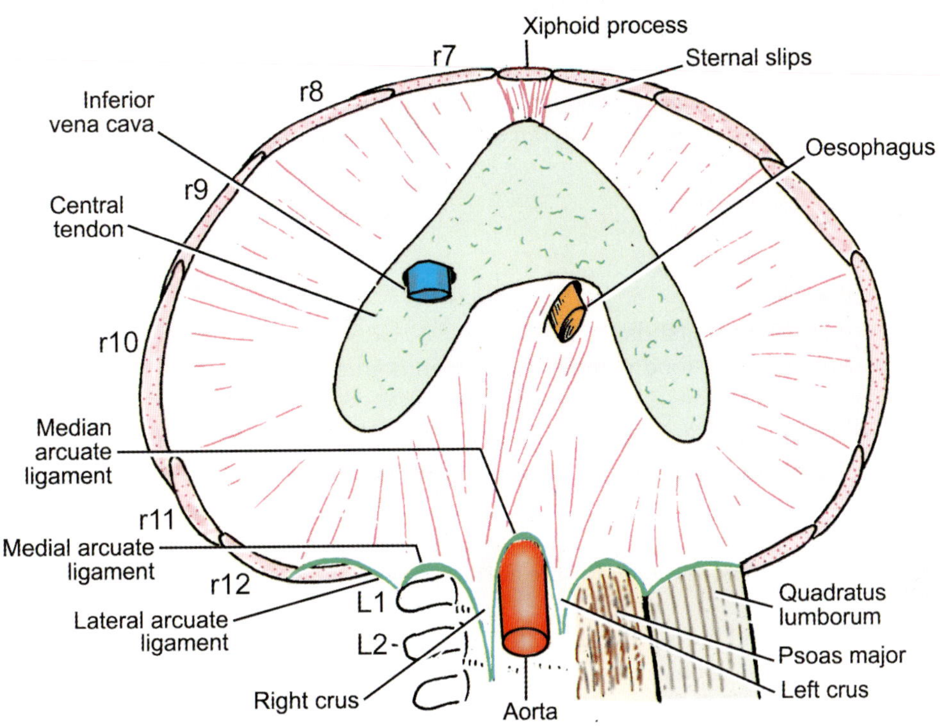


**18.5:** Scheme to show attachments of the diaphragm

8. The ***lateral arcuate ligament*** represents a thickened band of the fascia over the quadratus lumborum (a muscle in the posterior wall of the abdomen). It is attached laterally to the twelfth rib (about its middle) and medially to the transverse process of the first lumbar vertebra.
9. The ***medial arcuate ligament*** is a thickened band of the fascia covering the psoas major. It is attached laterally to the transverse process of the first lumbar vertebra. Medially, it becomes continuous with the lateral margin of the corresponding crus.
10. From its extensive origin, described above, the muscular fibres of the diaphragm run upwards and converge to be inserted on the margins of a large, flat, ***central tendon*** (18.5) that is located just below the pericardium and heart.
    a. It is usually described as being made up of three leaf-like parts (or ***folia***) that are fused together.
    b. There is an ***anterior (triangular) leaf***. Its apex is directed towards the xiphoid process and its base posteriorly, where it becomes continuous with two tongue-shaped posterior leaves. The apex of the anterior leaf receives the sternal fibres, while the sides of this leaf receive the anterior costal fibres.
    c. The posterior costal fibres reach the lateral sides of the posterior folia, while the fibres of the crura and those arising from the arcuate ligaments reach the apices and medial margins of the posterior folia.
11. The upper convex part of the diaphragm is called its ***dome***. From 18.6, it is seen that the dome bulges considerably into the bony thorax.
    a. The central part of the dome ('a' in 18.6) is formed by the central tendon and lies at the level of the xiphisternal joint. It is placed somewhat lower than the right and left muscular convexities (or ***cupolae***).
    b. The right cupola ('b' in 18.6) is slightly higher than the left ('c' in 18.6) because of the presence of the liver below it.
    c. The level of the dome rises and falls with expiration and inspiration respectively.
    d. It is also influenced by posture; being highest when the body is supine, intermediate while standing and lowest while sitting.

12. The upper surface of the diaphragm is related to thoracic contents including:
    a. The heart and pericardium in the middle.
    b. The lungs and pleura on the sides. The lungs and pleura descend in front, on the sides and behind the diaphragm (18.7) into the space between it and the thoracic wall.
13. The inferior surface of the diaphragm is related to abdominal contents including:
    a. The peritoneum
    b. The liver
    c. The stomach
    d. The spleen
    e. The right and left kidneys
    f. The right and left suprarenal glands.
    These relations will be understood when the abdomen is studied.

### *Apertures in the Diaphragm*

Many structures passing from thorax to abdomen (or ***vice versa***) pass through apertures in (or around) the diaphragm. They can be fully understood only after the study of the thorax and abdomen has been completed. However, they are listed here for completeness.

There are three large apertures, one each for the aorta, the oesophagus and the inferior vena cava, and several smaller ones (18.8A and B).

1. The ***aortic aperture*** lies behind the median arcuate ligament, and in front of the disc between vertebrae T12 and L1. The aorta, therefore, passes behind the diaphragm rather than through it.
    a. During inspiration, the pull of fibres of the muscle on the median arcuate ligament ensures that the aorta is not compressed.
    b. The aortic aperture also transmits the thoracic duct (which lies to the right side of the aorta) and sometimes the azygos and hemiazygos veins.
2. The ***aperture for the oesophagus*** is elliptical in shape. It is situated at the level of the tenth thoracic vertebra.
    a. It is formed by splitting of the fibres of the right crus a little below their attachment to the central tendon.
    b. Because the oesophagus is surrounded by muscle, it is compressed during expiration. This prevents regurgitation of the contents of the stomach.
    c. The oesophageal aperture also transmits the right and left gastric nerves that are continuations of the vagus nerves. The left nerve is placed anteriorly and the right posteriorly. Oesophageal branches of the left gastric artery also pass through the oesophageal aperture.

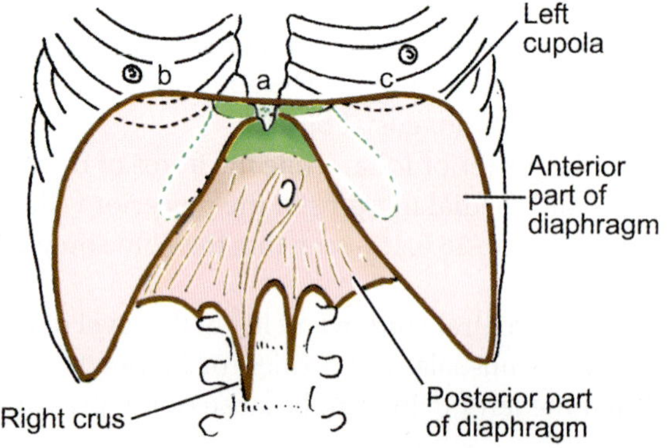


**18.6:** Diaphragm as seen from the front

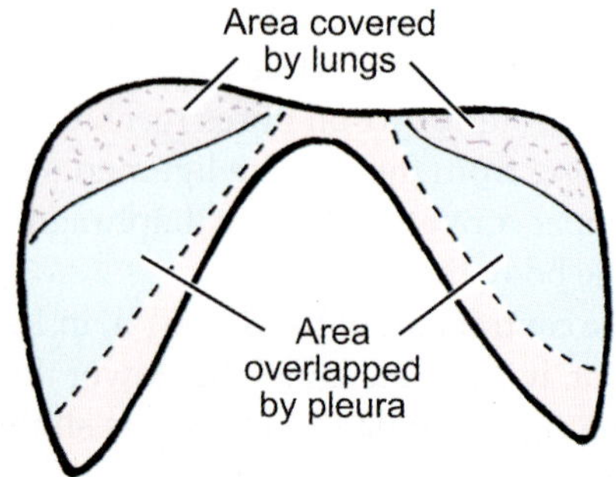


**18.7:** Structures in front of the anterior part of the diaphragm

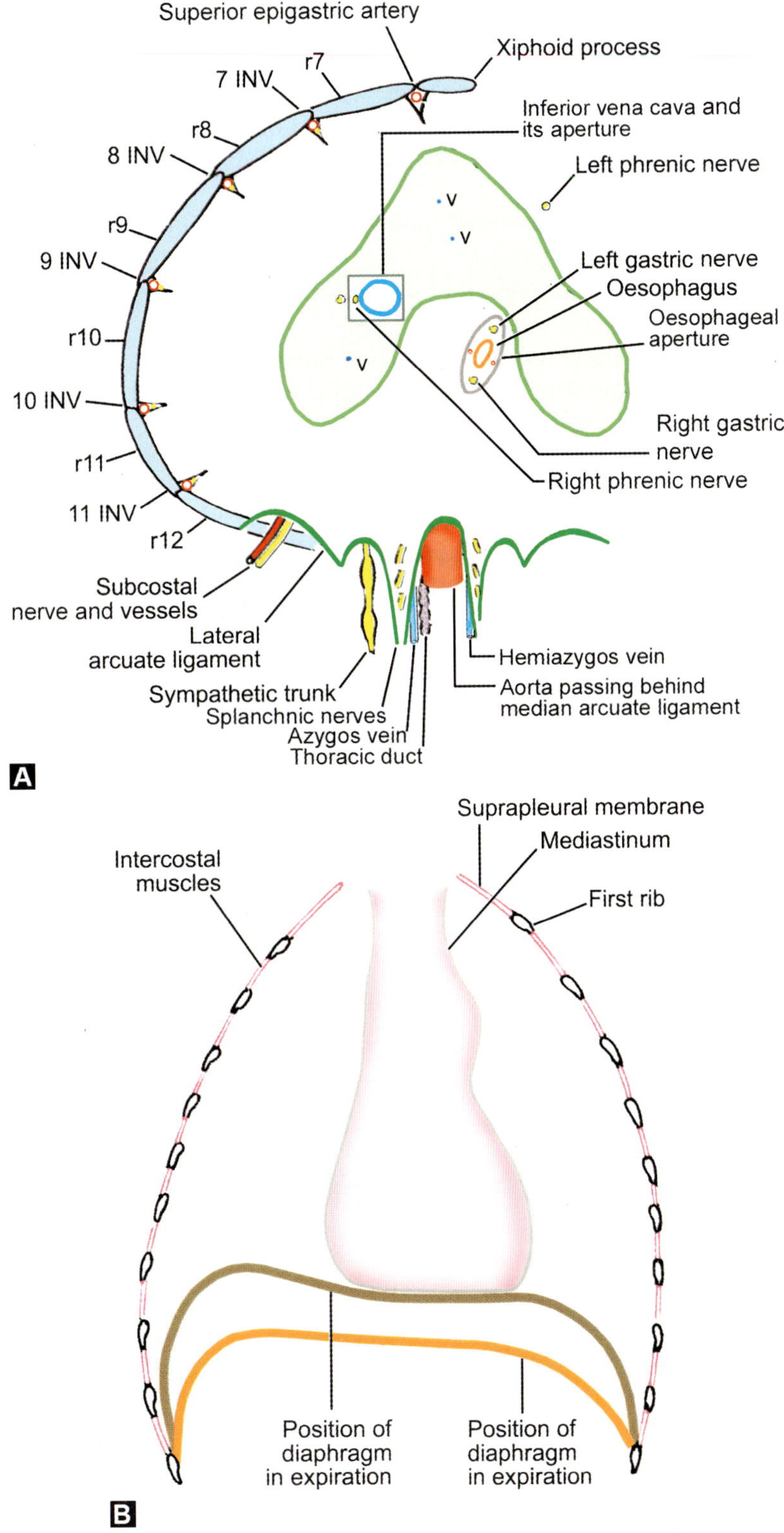


**18.8A and B:** (A) Schematic diagram to show apertures in the diaphragm. INV= Intercostal nerve and vessels; v= small vein; r7 to r12= 7th to 12th ribs; (B) Diagram to show change in level of the diaphragm during inspiration and expiration

3. The ***opening for the inferior vena cava*** lies in the central tendon at the level of the eighth thoracic vertebra (lower border). The opening is quadrilateral.
   a. The wall of the vena cava is adherent to the opening. This helps to expand the vessel during inspiration and facilitates venous return through the vessel.
   b. The vena caval opening also transmits the whole or part of the right phrenic nerve.

4.a. The left phrenic nerve passes through the muscular part of the diaphragm, to the left of the anterior folium of the central tendon.

4.b. Numerous small veins ('v') pass between the thorax and abdomen through small apertures in the central tendon.

5. There are a number of small apertures present around the periphery of the diaphragm, in gaps between various slips of origin.
   a. The ***superior epigastric artery*** (a terminal branch of the internal thoracic artery: see later in text) passes through the gap between the slip from the xiphoid process and that from the seventh rib and costal cartilage (on either side).
   b. The ***musculophrenic artery*** (another terminal branch of the internal thoracic artery) passes through the interval between slips from the 7th and 8th ribs. This interval also transmits the 7th intercostal nerve and vessels (7INV).
   c. The ***8th*** to ***11th intercostal nerves and vessels*** (labelled 8INV to 11INV in 18.8A) pass through intervals between slips from the 8th and 9th ribs, 9th and 10th ribs, 10th and 11th ribs, and 11th and 12th ribs respectively.
   d. The ***subcostal nerves and vessels*** leave the thorax by passing behind the lateral arcuate ligament.
   e. The ***sympathetic trunk*** passes behind the medial arcuate ligament.
   f. The greater, lesser and least ***splanchnic nerves*** (arising from the sympathetic trunk) enter the abdomen by piercing the corresponding crus.
   g. When the azygos vein does not pass through the aortic opening, it may pass through the right crus, or behind it. The hemiazygos vein may have a similar relationship to the left crus.

## Actions of the Diaphragm

1. The diaphragm is the chief muscle of respiration.
2. There are two phases of its action.
   a. In the first phase, it acts from its origin (the ribs being fixed by other muscles). As a result, the central tendon is pulled downwards increasing the vertical diameter of the thorax. This movement is limited by the resistance offered by the abdominal muscles and viscera.
   b. In the second phase, the central tendon is fixed as described above. The lower ribs are now drawn upwards. Through them the sternum is pushed forwards. As a result, the transverse and anteroposterior diameters of the thorax are also increased.
3. The main force for inspiration is provided by the diaphragm.
   a. When this muscle contracts, its central part (which is tendinous) is pulled downwards (pushing abdominal contents down and causing the abdominal wall to bulge).
   b. This increases the vertical diameter of the thorax (18.8).
   c. When the diaphragm relaxes, pressure of abdominal contents pushes it upwards. These up and down movements of the diaphragm (somewhat like those of a piston) provide the major force for respiration.
4. Acting along with the muscles of the anterior abdominal wall, the diaphragm helps to increase intra-abdominal pressure during acts like urination, defecation or vomiting.
5. Acts requiring forcible expulsion of air from the lungs like sneezing or laughing are preceded by a deep inspiration (diaphragm) followed by contraction of the expiratory muscles.

## Nerve Supply

1. The diaphragm receives a double nerve supply.
   a. Motor innervation is through the right and left phrenic nerves that also carry numerous sensory fibres.
   b. The diaphragm is also supplied by the lower six intercostal nerves which provide a sensory supply to the peripheral part of the muscle.
2. This innervation can be correlated with the development of the diaphragm partly from cervical myotomes and partly from the mesoderm of the body wall.

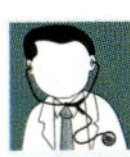

### CLINICAL CORRELATION

**Clinical Correlations of the Diaphragm**

1. The dome of the diaphragm can be seen in skiagrams of the chest.
2. It is important to remember that normally the right dome is higher than the left.
3. Movements of the diaphragm can be seen by fluoroscopy (screening) in which X-ray images are seen on a fluorescent screen.

***Congenital Diaphragmatic Herniae***

1. Parts of the diaphragm may fail to develop resulting in gaps in the muscle.
2. Abdominal contents may pass through these gaps to produce herniae.
3. Some sites at which diaphragmatic herniae may occur are as given below.

*Posterolateral hernia*

1. There is a defect in the posterolateral part of the dome of the diaphragm. (The defect is the ***foramen of Bochdalek***).
2. The hernia is more common on the left side.
3. It has no sac, there being free communication between the pleural and peritoneal cavities.
4. Herniation of abdominal contents into the thorax may produce severe respiratory distress soon after birth.
5. The condition requires immediate surgery to save the life of the infant.

*Posterior hernia*

1. This is caused by failure of development of the posterior part of the diaphragm.
2. The gap lies in front of the vertebral column. The aorta and oesophagus lie in the gap.
3. The hernia does not have a sac.

*Retrosternal hernia*

1. An abnormally large gap may exist between the sternal and costal origins of the diaphragm. (This gap is the ***foramen of Morgagni***).
2. It is more common on the right side.
3. The gap may exist without producing any symptoms.
4. When hernia occurs, it is situated anteriorly and often contains part of the transverse colon.

*Central diaphragmatic hernia*

This occurs through one dome of the diaphragm, usually the left.

*Congenital hiatus hernia*

1. A congenital hernia may occur through a wide oesophageal hiatus.
2. However, most hiatus herniae are acquired; and some authorities hold that the condition is never congenital (See later in text).

*Eventration of the diaphragm*

1. Strictly speaking this is not a diaphragmatic hernia, but it is convenient to consider it here.
2. The term is applied to a condition in which part of the diaphragm is thin and aponeurotic and bulgesabnormally upwards into the thorax.

***Acquired Hiatus Hernia***

1. This is a hernia through the oesophageal opening of the diaphragm.
2. Some authorities believe that all such herniae are acquired.
   Three varieties are described below:

*Sliding hiatus hernia*

1. In this variety, the oesophagus is short.
2. The cardio-oesophageal junction (also referred to as oesophago-gastric junction) and the adjoining part of the stomach pass through the hiatus and lie in the posterior mediastinum (18.9).
3. Factors leading to this hernia are as follows:
   a. Weakness of muscle around the oesophageal hiatus. This is often a result of degeneration with age.
   b. Increased intra-abdominal pressure from any cause.
      i. When this hernia occurs, the normal angulation between the oesophagus and the cardiac end of the stomach is lost.
      ii. Possibly as a result of this factor, the normal physiological sphincter here becomes ineffective.
      iii. Acid contents from the stomach regurgitate into the oesophagus leading to inflammation and fibrosis.
      iv. Fibrosis leads to further shortening of the oesophagus so that more of the stomach is pulled into the thorax.

*Paraoesophageal (or rolling) hiatus hernia*

1. In this variety, the oesophagus is of normal length and the cardio-oesophageal junction remains in the abdomen.
2. A part of the stomach passes through the hiatus and lies within the posterior mediastinum parallel to the oesophagus (18.10).
3. As more and more of the stomach enters the thorax, the stomach appears to 'roll' on itself, the cardiac end becoming lower than the greater part of the stomach.
4. As the cardio-oesophageal junction is normal, there is no reflux of gastric contents into the oesophagus.

*Mixed hiatus hernia*

This is a mixture of the two varieties described above (18.11).

*Treatment of hiatus hernia*

1. Some patients of hiatus hernia can obtain relief with conservative treatment.
2. Surgical procedures have been devised to bring the cardio-oesophageal junction back into the abdomen, restore its normal angulation, and prevent recurrence of the hernia by narrowing the oesophageal hiatus.

***Rupture of Diaphragm and Traumatic Hernia***

1. The diaphragm may rupture following a bullet wound or a severe crushing injury.
2. The stomach or colon may herniate through the opening into the thorax.

***Paralysis of One Half of the Diaphragm***

1. This happens if a phrenic nerve is injured.
2. Normally, both domes of the diaphragm descend during inspiration.
3. When one side is paralysed, it cannot descend. In fact pressure of abdominal viscera pushes it upwards. This can be seen by radiography.

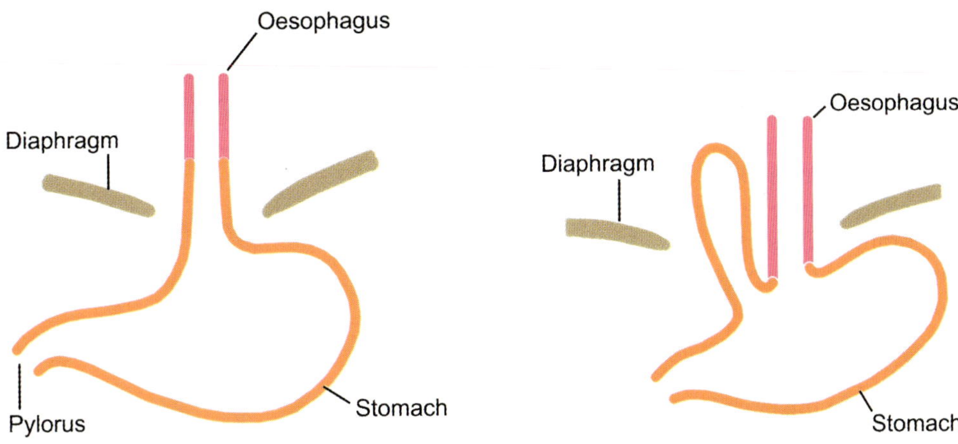


18.9: Diagram showing a sliding hiatus hernia

18.10: Diagram showing a paraoesophageal hiatus hernia

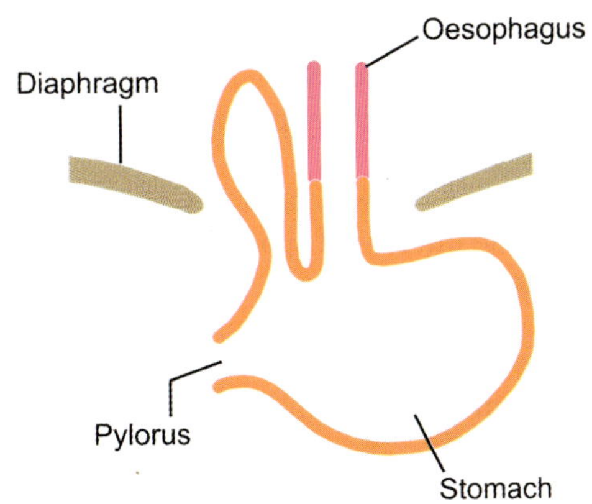


18.11: Diagram to show a mixed type of hiatus hernia

## ARTERIES OF THORACIC WALL

### Posterior Intercostal Arteries

1. The posterior intercostal arteries for the lower nine intercostal spaces arise from the back of the thoracic aorta.
2. The corresponding arteries for the first and second spaces arise from the superior intercostal artery (See later in text).
3. Each posterior intercostal artery runs backwards on the side of the body of the numerically corresponding vertebra to reach the corresponding intercostal space. Here it comes to lie in the costal groove of the rib forming the upper boundary of the intercostal space (18.12).
4. In the space, the artery lies between the internal intercostal muscle (second layer) and the innermost intercostal muscle (third layer). It is accompanied by the corresponding vein (which lies above it) and by the intercostal nerve (which lies below it).
5. Where the artery is not covered by the intercostalis intimi, it is directly in contact with the parietal pleura which separates it from the visceral pleura and lung.
6. As the descending aorta lies somewhat to the left of the median plane, the right posterior intercostal arteries (arising from it) have to cross this plane to reach the right side. They are, therefore, longer than arteries of the left side.

7. On either side, the posterior intercostal arteries pass deep to the sympathetic trunk. On the right side, they also pass deep to the azygos vein and the thoracic duct.
8. Each posterior intercostal artery gives off a number of branches that are shown in 18.9.
   a. Before entering the intercostal space the artery gives off a ***dorsal branch*** that supplies muscles and skin of the back. The dorsal branch gives off a spinal branch that supplies the spinal cord and vertebrae.
   b. The ***collateral branch*** arises near the angles of the ribs concerned.
      i. It then runs parallel to the main artery, but along the upper border of the rib below the intercostal space.
      ii. The main artery and the collateral branch reach near the anterior end of the intercostal space. Here they anastomose with two anterior intercostal arteries (see below).
   c. A number of ***muscular branches*** supply intercostal muscles, and some other muscles lying over the thoracic wall. The lower two posterior intercostal arteries continue into the abdominal wall and help to supply it.
   d. A ***lateral cutaneous branch*** arises about midway between the anterior and posterior ends of the intercostal space. It divides into anterior and posterior branches that supply skin over the thorax (and part of abdomen).
   e. The 2nd, 3rd, 4th posterior intercostal arteries give branches to the mammary gland. These are larger in the females.
   f. The right bronchial artery arises from the right third posterior intercostal artery.

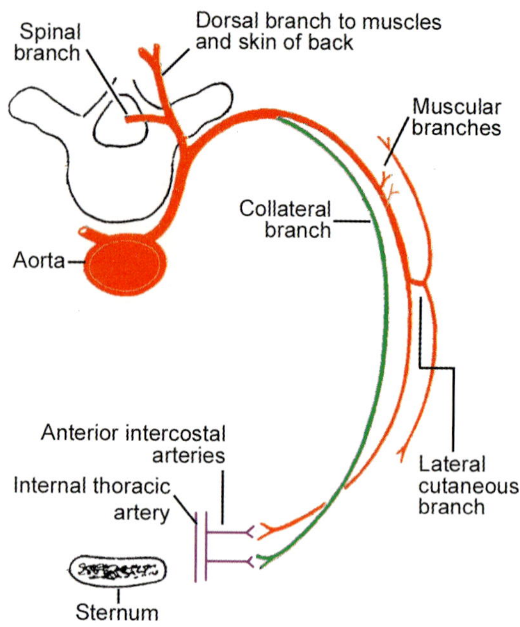


**18.12:** Scheme to show course and branches of a typical posterior intercostal artery

## Superior Intercostal Artery

The importance of this artery is that it gives off the posterior intercostal arteries for the first and second intercostal spaces.

1. The origin of this artery is shown in 18.13.
   a. Note that the subclavian artery (lying in the lower part of the neck, in front of the cervical pleura) gives off the ***costocervical trunk***.
   b. This trunk runs upwards in front of the cervical pleura, and reaching the neck of the first rib it divides into the superior intercostal and deep cervical branches.
   c. The superior intercostal artery runs downwards behind the cervical pleura. It descends across the neck of the first rib to reach the first intercostal space. Here it gives off the first posterior intercostal artery. The artery then descends across the second rib and becomes the second posterior intercostal artery.

## Subcostal Arteries

1. The subcostal arteries correspond to the posterior intercostal arteries but lie below the twelfth rib.
2. On each side, the artery runs across the lateral side of the twelfth thoracic vertebra. After a short course in the thorax the artery enters the abdomen by passing under cover of the lateral arcuate ligament. Its course in the abdomen will be studied at a later stage.
3. The subcostal artery supplies some muscles in the walls of the thorax and abdomen.
4. The artery gives off a ***dorsal branch***, the distribution of which is similar to that of the corresponding branches of the posterior intercostal arteries.

## Internal Thoracic Artery and Anterior Intercostal Arteries

1. The internal thoracic artery was earlier called the internal mammary artery. It arises (in the lower part of the neck) from the first part of the subclavian artery.
2. It descends behind the clavicle and behind the first to sixth costal cartilages (lying about 1 cm lateral to the sternal margin).
3. It terminates by dividing into the ***musculophrenic*** and ***superior epigastric*** arteries. It also gives various other branches that are as follows (18.14).
   a. Along its course, the internal thoracic artery gives off a series of ***anterior intercostal arteries***.
      i. Two arteries are given off to each of the upper six spaces.
      ii. Similar branches to the 7th, 8th and 9th spaces arise from the musculophrenic branch.
      iii. In each space, the upper of the two anterior intercostal arteries anastomoses with the main stem of the posterior intercostal artery; and the lower anterior intercostal artery anastomoses with the collateral branch.
      iv. The anterior intercostal arteries supply intercostal muscles, pectoral muscles, breast and skin.
   b. The ***pericardiophrenic branch*** is given off near the upper end of the internal thoracic artery. It runs downwards along the phrenic nerve to reach the diaphragm. It also gives branches to pleura and pericardium.

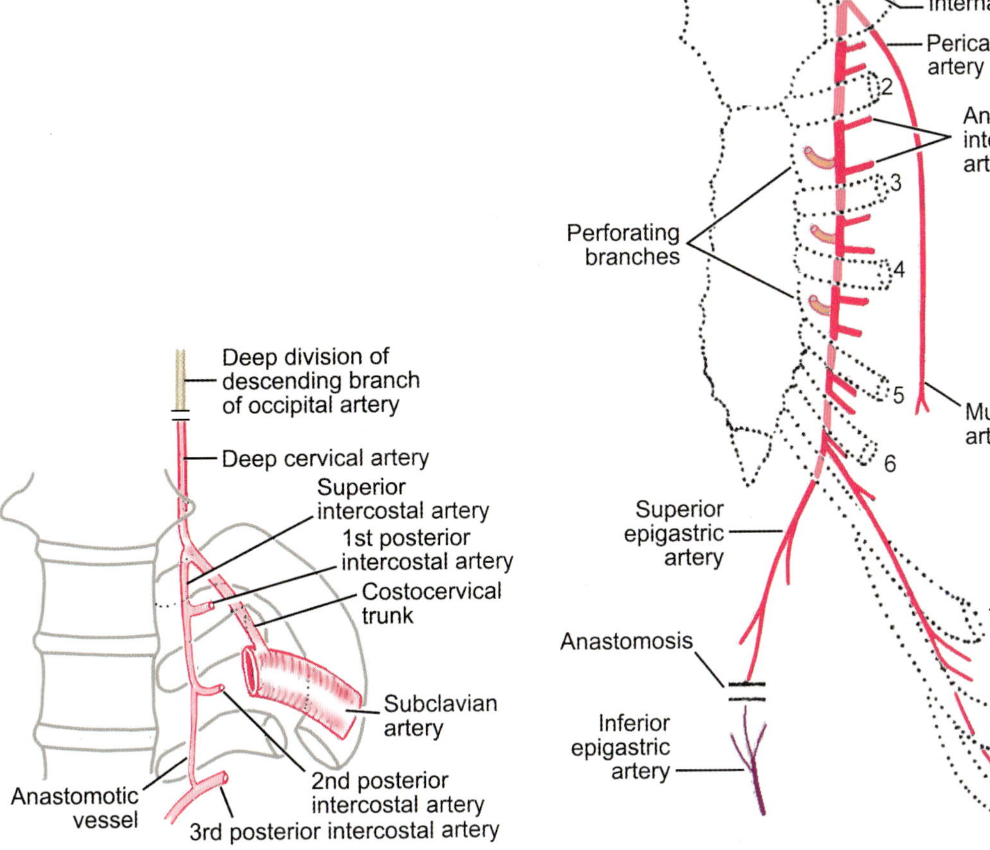


**18.13:** Scheme to show the origin of the superior intercostal artery

**18.14:** Internal thoracic artery and its branches. The skeletal elements are drawn as if transparent

c. The ***perforating branches*** pass forwards through the thickness of the upper five or six intercostal spaces to supply the pectoralis major muscle and the breast (specially arteries in the 2nd to 4th spaces). These arteries are larger in females.
d. The ***musculophrenic artery*** is the lateral terminal branch of the internal thoracic artery. It passes downwards and laterally deep to the costal margin and enters the abdominal wall by passing through an aperture in the diaphragm. We have already seen that it gives off anterior intercostal branches to the 7th, 8th and 9th intercostal spaces.
e. The ***superior epigastric artery*** is the medial terminal branch of the internal thoracic artery. Soon after its origin, it passes from the thorax into the abdomen through the interval between the costal and xiphoid origins of the diaphragm. Its course in the abdomen will be considered later. This artery gives off some branches to the anterior mediastinum (to thymus and lymph nodes), to pericardium, and to the diaphragm.

## VEINS OF THE THORACIC WALL

The thoracic wall is drained anteriorly by the internal thoracic vein and posteriorly by the azygos system of veins.

### Internal Thoracic Vein

The ***internal thoracic vein*** accompanies the corresponding artery and has tributaries corresponding to the branches of the artery (See later in text).

### Azygos System of Veins

#### *The Azygos Vein*

1. The ***azygos vein*** is present only on the right side.
2. It begins (in the abdomen) by the union of the lumbar azygos, the right subcostal and the right ascending lumbar veins (18.15).

**WANT TO KNOW MORE?**

a. The ***lumbar azygos vein*** lies to the right of the lumbar vertebrae. Its lower end communicates with the inferior vena cava.
b. The ***right subcostal vein*** accompanies the corresponding artery.
c. The ***ascending lumbar vein*** is a vertical channel connecting lumbar veins to one another.
The lumbar azygos vein is sometimes absent and in that case the azygos vein is formed only by the right subcostal and right ascending lumbar veins.

3. Thus formed, the azygos vein enters the thorax by passing behind the right crus of the diaphragm or through its aortic orifice.
4. It then ascends vertically along the right side of the vertebral column up to the level of the fourth thoracic vertebra (18.16).
5. Here, it arches forwards above the root of the right lung and ends in the superior vena cava.
6. The azygos vein is related, on its right side, to the right pleura and lung. On its left side, it is related to the aorta and to the thoracic duct.
7. Its terminal part crosses the trachea, the oesophagus and the right vagus nerve.

#### *The Hemiazygos Vein*

1. The ***hemiazygos vein*** is present only on the left side. It is formed in the same manner as the azygos vein.
2. It ascends on the left side of the bodies of the lower thoracic vertebrae.

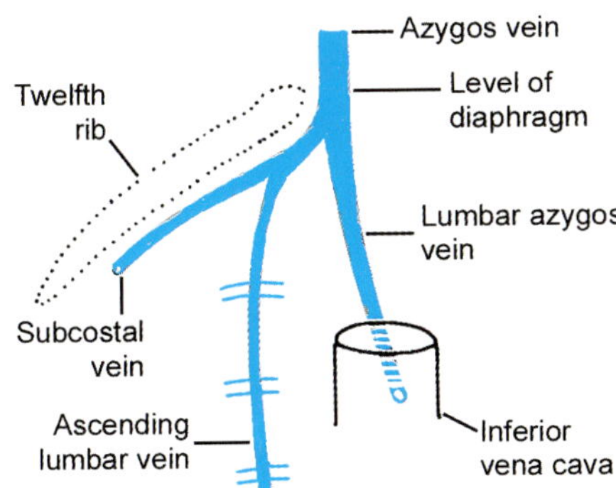


**18.15:** Azygos and hemiazygos veins. Note the manner of termination of posterior intercostal veins

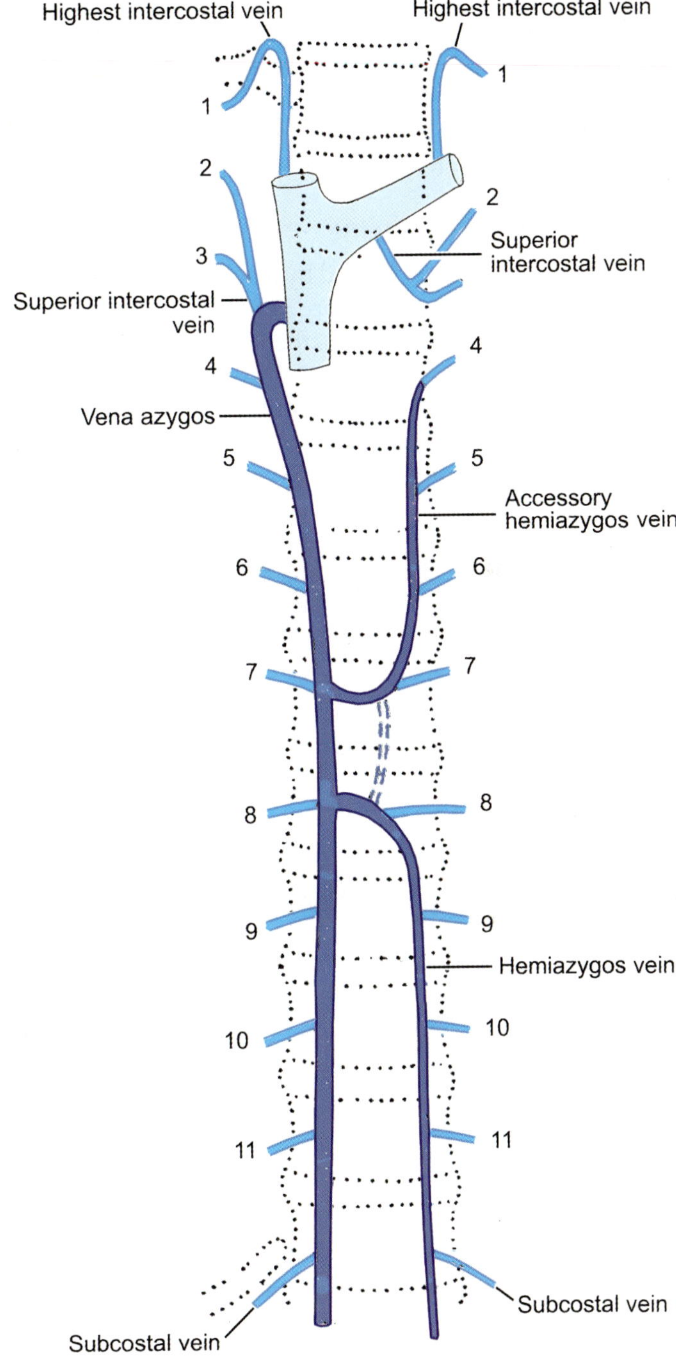


**18.16:** Scheme to show formation of azygos vein
1 to 11: Intercostal veins

3. Its upper end turns to the right in front of the body of the 8th thoracic vertebra and ends by joining the azygos vein (18.16).

### *The Accessory Hemiazygos Vein*

1. The ***accessory hemiazygos vein*** descends vertically on the left side of the bodies of upper thoracic vertebrae.
2. The lower end of the vein turns to the right across the front of the 7th thoracic vertebra and ends by joining the azygos vein.
   The terminal parts of the hemiazygos and accessory hemiazygos veins lie behind the descending thoracic aorta. They may unite to form a common channel, or may communicate with each other.

## Posterior Intercostal Veins

Each intercostal space is drained by a ***posterior intercostal vein*** that corresponds to the posterior intercostal artery. The termination of these veins are as follows (18.16):

1. On either side (right or left), the vein of the first space (called the ***highest intercostal vein***) ascends in front of the neck of the first rib, and arches over the cervical pleura to end in the corresponding brachiocephalic vein. (Compare its course with that of the superior intercostal artery).
2. The veins of the 2nd and 3rd spaces (and sometimes those of the 4th) join to form the superior intercostal veins.
   a. The ***left superior intercostal vein*** runs upwards and forwards on the left side of the arch of the aorta (18.16) and ends in the left brachiocephalic vein.
   b. The ***right superior intercostal vein*** joins the terminal part of the azygos vein (18.16).
3. On the right side, the remaining posterior intercostal veins end directly in the azygos vein.
4. On the left side of the veins from the 4th to 8th spaces end in the ***accessory hemiazygos vein.***
5. The veins of the 9th, 10th and 11th spaces (on the left side) end in the ***hemiazygos vein.***
6. The ***subcostal veins*** are in series with the posterior intercostal veins. On the right side, they end (as already mentioned) in the azygos vein. On the left side, the subcostal vein joins the corresponding ascending lumbar vein to form the hemiazygos vein.

# NERVES OF THORACIC WALL

## Ventral Rami of Thoracic Nerves

1. There are twelve pairs of thoracic nerves, each pair emerging from the vertebral canal below the corresponding vertebra.
2. Each nerve divides into a dorsal ramus and a ventral ramus.
3. The dorsal rami are smaller than the ventral rami. They pass backwards and divide into medial and lateral branches that supply muscles and skin of the back.
4. The ventral rami are considered below.

### *Typical Intercostal Nerves*

1. The ventral rami of the thoracic nerves run into the thoracic wall as the intercostal and subcostal nerves (18.17).
2. There being twelve ribs on either side, there are eleven intercostal spaces, and each space has one intercostal nerve. The intercostal nerves are numbered from above downwards.
3. The twelfth pair of nerves lie below the twelfth ribs and are called the ***subcostal nerves.***
4. The course of the third, fourth, fifth and sixth intercostal nerves can be regarded as typical. They run forwards in the intercostal spaces lying between the second and third layers of muscles (18.17).
   a. Posteriorly, each nerve lies between the pleura and the posterior intercostal membrane; next between the internal intercostal muscle on the outside, and the subcostalis and the innermost intercostal muscle on the inside.
   b. Near the anterior end of the space the nerve lies between the pleura (here posterior to it) and the internal intercostal muscle (here anterior to it).
   c. Finally, the nerve becomes superficial by piercing the internal intercostal muscle, the anterior intercostal membrane, and the pectoralis major to become the ***anterior cutaneous nerve of the thorax***. In the intercostal space, the nerve lies immediately below the intercostal artery (18.18).

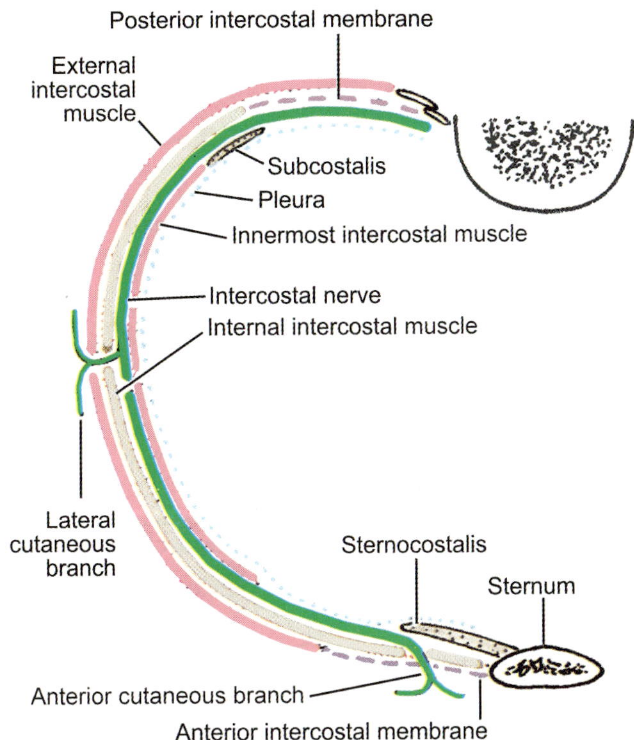


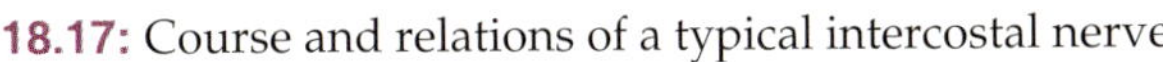

**18.17:** Course and relations of a typical intercostal nerve

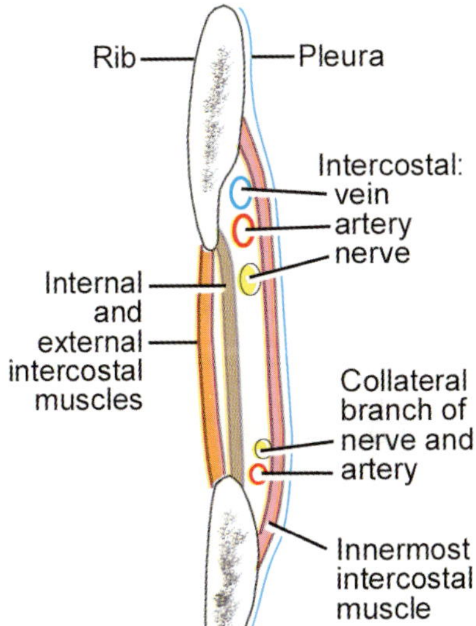


**18.18:** Vertical section through an intercostal space showing the position of nerves and vessels

5. Typical intercostal nerves are distributed to both muscles and skin through a number of branches. The main branches are the ***collateral branch*** and the ***lateral cutaneous branch*** (18.17). They are both given off near the posterior end of the intercostal space.
   a. The collateral branch runs forwards in the lower part of the intercostal space (18.18). Its relationships are similar to those of the main nerve.
   b. The lateral cutaneous branch runs along the parent nerve for some distance. It then turns laterally through the internal and external intercostal muscles (and other muscles that overlie them), and becoming subcutaneous divides into anterior and posterior branches that supply the skin over the thoracic wall.
   c. In addition to these large branches, each intercostal nerve gives several branches that supply the intercostal muscles. They also supply some other muscles as shown in 18.19.

### *Lower Intercostal Nerves*

1. The initial parts of the seventh, eighth, ninth, tenth and eleventh intercostal nerves resemble those of typical intercostal nerves described above.
2. However, on reaching the anterior end of the intercostal space concerned, each nerve passes deep to the costal margin to enter the abdominal wall.
3. The subsequent course of these nerves can be fully understood only after the abdominal wall has been studied. At this stage refer to 18.20.
   a. Note that like the thoracic wall, the abdominal wall also consists of three layers formed by the external oblique, the internal oblique and the transversus abdominis muscles.
   b. Near the midline, we see another muscle called rectus abdominis. At the lateral margin of the rectus abdominis (a muscle in the anterior wall of the abdomen), the aponeurosis of the internal oblique muscle divides into anterior and posterior layers that pass respectively in front of and behind the rectus abdominis.

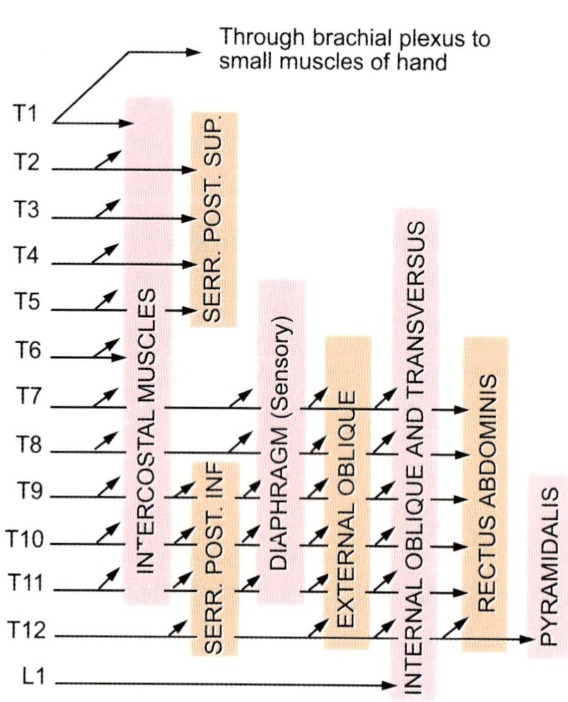


**18.19:** Scheme to show muscles supplied by ventral rami of thoracic nerves

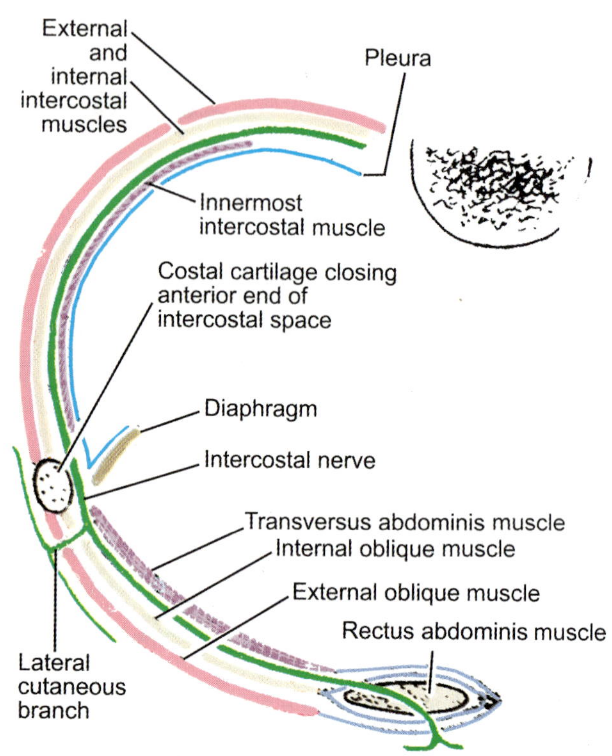


**18.20:** Scheme to show the course of one of the lower intercostal nerves. The intercostal space and the abdominal wall are cut along the course of the nerve

4. The intercostal nerves run forward in the abdominal wall lying between the second and third layers (just as in the intercostal spaces). Reaching the rectus abdominis, the intercostal nerves pierce the posterior layer of its sheath to enter the muscle.
5. The nerves pass forwards through the rectus abdominis to reach the skin and supply it (18.20).
6. The course of the seventh and eighth intercostal nerves is slightly different from that described above because the anterior ends of the corresponding spaces lie behind the rectus abdominis. These nerves, therefore, do not travel any part of their course between the internal oblique and transversus muscles, but enter the rectus sheath directly.
7. The seventh to eleventh intercostal nerves give off:
   a. ***Collateral branches*** that run parallel to the main trunks. Like the parent trunks, they enter the abdominal wall, and pierce the rectus abdominis to reach the skin over it.
   b. ***Lateral cutaneous branches*** which become superficial by piercing the internal and external intercostal muscles, or the internal and external oblique muscles of the abdomen and then divide into anterior and posterior branches that supply the skin of the trunk ('x' in 18.21).
8. From 18.21, it will be seen that the lower intercostal spaces turn upwards near the anterior ends. The seventh and eighth intercostal nerves follow this curve even after they enter the abdomen, so that they run upwards and medially in the abdominal wall. The course of the ninth nerve within the abdominal wall is horizontal. The tenth and eleventh nerves run downwards and medially.

### *First Thoracic Nerve*

1. The greater part of the ventral ramus of the first thoracic nerve ascends into the neck to join the brachial plexus (18.22) and is distributed through it to some muscles and some part of the skin of the upper limb.

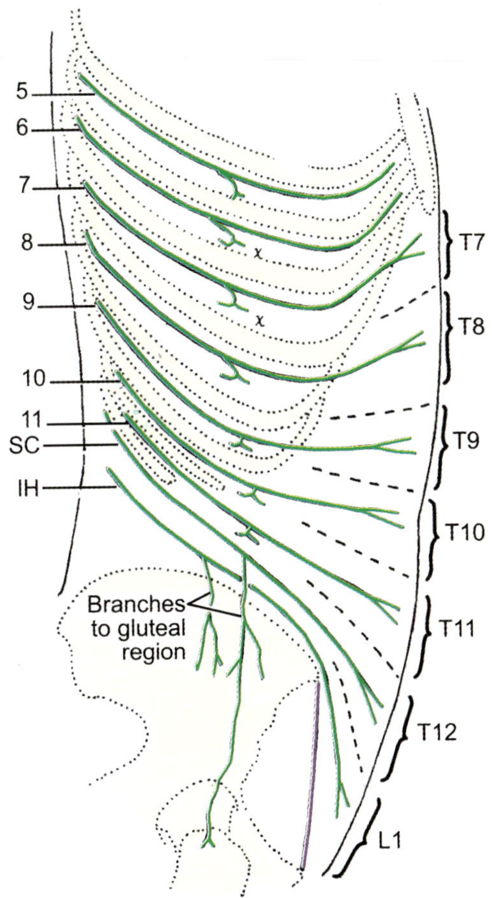


18.21: Course of intercostal nerves as seen from the lateral side.
SC: Subcostal nerve. IH: Iliohypogastric nerve

Lower trunk of brachial plexus
C8
First intercostal nerve
T1
Intercosto-brachial nerve
T2
Second intercostal nerve

18.22: Fate of ventral rami of the first and second thoracic nerves

2. The remaining part of the nerve runs forwards in the first intercostal space as the first intercostal nerve. The course and distribution of this nerve is similar to that of typical intercostal nerves considered above.

### *Second Thoracic Nerve*

1. The ventral ramus of the second thoracic nerve gives a contribution to the brachial plexus.
2. Most of it, however, forms the second intercostal nerve (18.22).
3. This nerve differs from the typical intercostal nerves described below only in that its lateral cutaneous branch forms the ***intercostobrachial nerve*** which enters the upper limb and supplies the skin on the medial side of the upper part of the arm.

### *Subcostal Nerve*

1. The subcostal nerve is the ventral ramus of the twelfth thoracic nerve. Its course is similar to that of the subcostal artery.
2. It runs along the lower border of the twelfth rib and enters the abdomen by passing behind the lateral lumbocostal arch.
3. It then passes downwards and laterally across the quadratus lumborum muscle. This part of the nerve lies behind the corresponding kidney.

4. At the lateral margin of the quadratus lumborum, the nerve enters the interval between the internal oblique and the transversus abdominis muscles. Its subsequent course is similar to that of the lower intercostal nerves (described above) (18.21).
5. The subcostal nerve gives off a collateral branch that behaves like that of an intercostal nerve.
6. It also gives off a lateral cutaneous branch that runs downwards across the iliac crest to supply the skin of the anterior part of the gluteal region.
   The distribution of the nerve is considered below along with that of the intercostal nerves.

### Distribution of Thoracic Ventral Rami

1. The muscles supplied by thoracic ventral rami are shown in 18.19.
2. Along with the subcostal and iliohypogastric nerves, the intercostal nerves supply the skin of the lateral and anterior aspects of the trunk.
   a. The areas supplied by each nerve are in the form of parallel strips.
   b. There is considerable overlap between the areas supplied by adjoining nerves so that there is hardly any area of skin supplied exclusively by one nerve.
   c. It may be remembered that the skin below the xiphoid process is supplied by the seventh intercostal nerve; that around the umbilicus by the tenth intercostal nerve and that above the pubis by the first lumbar nerve (through the iliohypogastric nerve) (18.21).

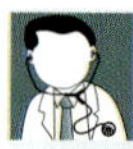

**CLINICAL CORRELATION**

**Girdle Pain**

1. When intercostal nerves are irritated (for any reason) there is pain that is felt in the front of the chest or abdomen.
2. This is known as girdle pain or root pain.

**Herpes Zoster**

1. This is characterised by the appearance of vesicles along the course of an intercostal nerve. The condition is painful.
2. It is caused by a viral infection of the dorsal nerve root ganglion concerned.

**Intercostal Nerve Block**

Sensations over the distribution of an intercostal nerve can be blocked by injecting local anaesthetic. As the territory of supply of nerves overlap more than one nerve needs to be blocked for effective anaesthesia.

### Sympathetic Trunk

1. The sympathetic trunk is a long nerve cord extending from the base of the skull to the coccyx.
2. The thoracic part lies in front of the heads of the ribs.
3. The first thoracic ganglion is fused with the inferior cervical ganglion to form the ***cervicothoracic ganglion***.
4. There are eleven thoracic ganglia (one each for nerves T2 to T12.
5. The ganglia are connected to corresponding thoracic nerves through lateral branches.
6. Medial branches supply viscera. Those arising from lower thoracic ganglia unite to form the ***greater, lesser and lowest splanchnic nerves*** that descend into the abdomen. For details see Chapter 22.

### Lymphatic Drainage of Thoracic Wall

1. The skin overlying the thorax drains mainly into the axillary lymph nodes. The vessels from the back of the thorax end in the posterior group, while those from the front end in the anterior group. The skin near the sternum is drained into the parasternal nodes (22.10).

2. The deeper tissues (including muscles covering the chest wall, and the costal pleura) drain anteriorly into the parasternal nodes and posteriorly into the intercostal nodes (22.10).
3. The ***diaphragm*** is drained by separate sets of lymph vessels on its thoracic and abdominal surfaces.
4. The ***thoracic surface*** is drained as follows (22.12).
   a. Vessels from the anterior part drain into the anterior diaphragmatic nodes, and through them to the parasternal nodes.
   b. Vessels from the middle part drain to the right and left lateral diaphragmatic nodes, and from here to the parasternal nodes and nodes around the oesophagus (part of posterior mediastinal group).
   c. Vessels from the posterior part drain into the posterior diaphragmatic nodes, and through them to nodes around the lower end of the thoracic aorta.
5. Lymphatics from the ***abdominal surface*** of the diaphragm drain into lymph nodes within the abdomen. For details see Chapter 22.

CHAPTER 19

# The Trachea, Bronchi and Lungs

## INTRODUCTION TO THE RESPIRATORY SYSTEM

The respiratory system is meant, primarily, for the oxygenation of blood. The chief organs of the system are the right and left ***lungs***. Oxygen contained in air reaches the lungs by passing through a series of respiratory passages, that also serve for removal of carbon dioxide released from the blood.

1. Air from the outside enters the body through the right and left ***anterior nares*** (or ***external nares***) that open into the right and left ***nasal cavities*** (19.1).
2. At their posterior ends, the nasal cavities have openings called the ***posterior nares*** (or ***internal nares***) through which they open into the ***pharynx.***
3. The pharynx is divisible, from above downwards, into:
   a. An upper part—the ***nasopharynx*** (into which the nasal cavities open).
   b. A middle part—the ***oropharynx*** (that is continuous with the posterior end of the oral cavity).
   c. A lower part—the ***laryngopharynx***.

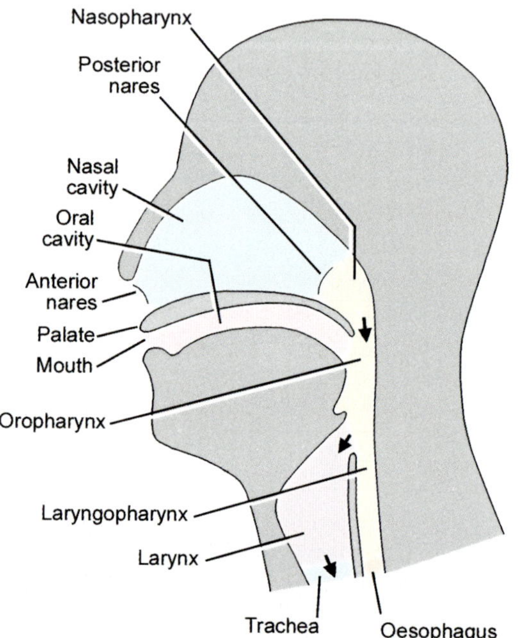


**19.1:** Simplified diagram showing intercommunications between the nasal cavities, the mouth, the pharynx, the larynx and the oesophagus

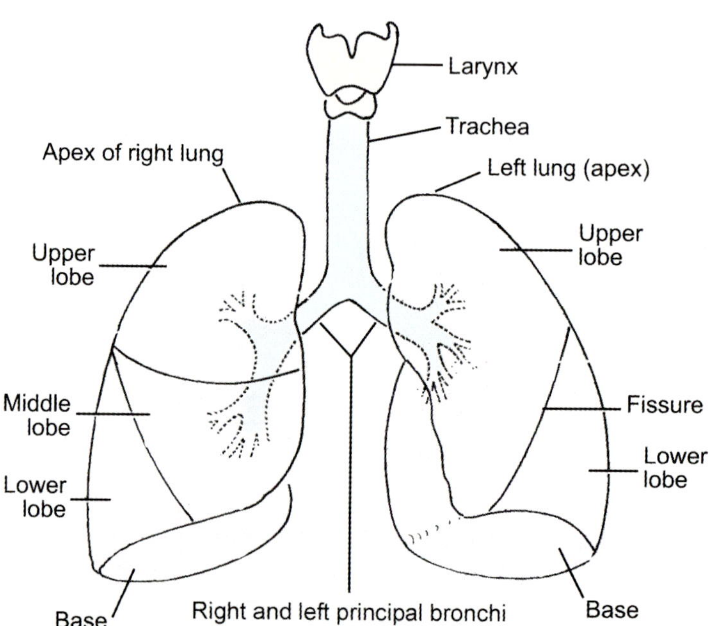


**19.2:** Larynx, trachea and lungs as seen from the front

4. Air from the nose enters the nasopharynx and passes down through the oropharynx and laryngopharynx. Air can also pass through the mouth directly into the oropharynx and from there to the laryngopharynx.
5. Air from the laryngopharynx enters a box-like structure called the ***larynx.***
   a. The larynx is placed on the front of the upper part of the neck.
   b. Apart from being a respiratory passage it is the organ where voice is produced. It is, therefore, sometimes called the voice-box.
6. Inferiorly, the larynx is continuous with a tube called the ***trachea*** that passes through the lower part of the neck into the upper part of the thorax 19.2.
7. At the level of the lower border of the manubrium sterni, the trachea bifurcates into the right and left ***principal bronchi***, that carry air to the right and left lungs.
8. Within the lung each principal bronchus divides, like the branches of a tree, into smaller and smaller ***bronchi*** that ultimately end in microscopic tubes that are called ***bronchioles.***
   a. The bronchioles open into microscopic sac-like structures called ***alveoli.***
   b. The walls of the alveoli contain a rich network of blood capillaries.
   c. Blood in these capillaries is separated from the air in the alveoli by a very thin membrane through which oxygen can pass into the blood and carbon dioxide can pass into the alveolar air.
9. Deoxygenated blood enters the lungs through pulmonary arteries; and passes into numerous pulmonary capillaries that surround alveoli.
   a. Blood in the capillaries is separated from air in alveoli only by a very thin membrane (made up mainly of flattened cells lining the alveoli, and of capillary endothelium).
   b. Gaseous exchanges take place through this membrane. The substance of the lung contains abundant elastic tissue that plays an important role in respiration.

## Respiration

1. During respiration, the lungs alternately expand (when air is drawn into them in ***inspiration***), and contract (when air is expelled in ***expiration***).
2. In these movements, the surface of the lung moves over surrounding structures.
   a. Friction during these movements is prevented because of the presence of a double layered serous membrane, the ***pleura***, around the lung.
   b. The pleura has an ***inner*** (or ***visceral) layer*** which covers the surface of the lung; and an ***outer*** (or ***parietal) layer*** which lines the inside of the cavity for the lung.
   c. The two layers of pleura are separated only by a potential space in which there is a thin film of fluid.
   d. This fluid prevents friction between the two layers of pleura.
3. During inspiration and expiration the thoracic cavity is alternately made to expand and contract. These movements are produced by muscle action.
4. When the thoracic cavity expands a negative pressure is created within the pleural cavity.
   a. This negative pressure exerts a pull on elastic tissue within the lungs causing them to expand.
   b. Expansion of the lungs draws air into them.
5. The reverse happens during expiration.
   a. Muscles that are responsible, for expansion of the thorax are now relaxed and the cavity becomes smaller expelling air to the outside.
   b. Expiration is also aided by recoil of elastic tissue within the lung.
6. The main force for inspiration is provided by the diaphragm.
   a. When this muscle contracts, its central part (which is tendinous) is pulled downwards (pushing abdominal contents down and causing the abdominal wall to bulge). This increases the vertical diameter of the thorax (18.8B).
   b. When the diaphragm relaxes, pressure of abdominal contents pushes it upwards.
   c. These up and down movements of the diaphragm (somewhat like those of a piston) provide the major force for respiration.

7. Muscles in the intercostal spaces produce movements of the ribs.
   a. As a result of these movements, and of the sternum, there is increase in the lateral and anteroposterior diameters of the thorax.
   b. Expansion of the thoracic cavity in this way is the second major factor in inspiration.
8. Respiration produced by movements of the diaphragm is called ***abdominal respiration***; and that caused by intercostal muscles is called ***thoracic respiration***.
   a. Normally, the predominant role in respiration is played by the diaphragm.
   b. In young children the thoracic cavity is almost circular in cross section and scope for anteroposterior or side-to-side expansion is limited, hence respiration is mostly abdominal.
   c. On the other hand, in a woman in an advanced stage of pregnancy descent, of the diaphragm is severely limited and respiration becomes mainly thoracic.

## Some Other Effects of Respiration

1. The fibrous pericardium is adherent to the central tendon of the diaphragm.
   a. When the diaphragm descends the heart is also pulled downwards.
   b. As a result the mediastinum becomes longer, but narrower.
   c. The reverse happens in expiration.
2. Similarly, increase in anteroposterior diameter of the thorax also stretches the mediastinum anteroposteriorly.
3. Because of the negative pressure in the pleural cavity any opening created in the thoracic wall (e.g., by injury) sucks air into the pleural cavity.
   a. Entry of air into the pleural cavity leads to collapse of the lung (with resultant loss of function).
   b. If the opening is closed, the air in the pleural cavity is gradually absorbed and the lung expands once more.
4. Entry of air (or collection of fluid in large amounts) in one pleural cavity can also exert pressure on the mediastinum (see below) and can push it the opposite side.

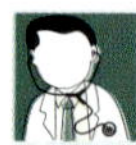

## CLINICAL CORRELATION

### Effects of Injury to Thoracic Wall on Respiratory Movements

1. It has been seen that intrapleural pressure is negative and that atmospheric pressure, therefore, tends to collapse the thoracic wall. This tendency is resisted by ribs and intercostal muscles.
2. When some ribs are fractured at two or more sites the affected part of the thoracic wall loses its integrity.
   a. The loose (or flail) segment moves inwards with inspiration and outwards during expiration.
   b. This condition is called ***flail chest***.
3. When the ribs are fractured on either side of the sternum, the sternum can also become flail.
4. If an injury to the thoracic wall creates an opening into the pleural cavity, air enters the cavity creating an ***open pneumothorax*** (see below). A broken rib may injure the underlying lung and air can then enter the pleural cavity through the lung.
5. In cases of open pneumothorax, air can also pass into subcutaneous tissues. This is called ***surgical emphysema***. This air can spread and can even enter the neck and head.

### *Paradoxical Respiration*

1. In normal respiration, pressure within the pleural cavity falls during inspiration, and this is responsible for filling of the lungs.
2. When there is an open pneumothorax the pressure in the pleural cavity ***increases*** during inspiration (because of entry of air from outside) leading to partial collapse of the lung.
3. This leads to a condition that is called ***paradoxical respiration*** because the lung expands during expiration and becomes smaller during inspiration.

*Empyema Necessitatis*

1. An abscess over the thoracic wall can also be caused secondary to collection of pus in the pleural cavity (*empyema*).
2. The pus can perforate the chest wall (and can do so along the track of a needle used for aspiration) and present as an abscess.

*Paracentesis Thoracis*

1. Fluid in the pleural cavity can be aspirated by passing a needle into an intercostal space (usually the 6th) in the midaxillary line.
2. Remember that the neurovascular bundle of each intercostal space lies along the upper border of the space, and injury to it can be avoided by passing the needle through the lower part of the space.
3. A needle passed into one of the lower intercostal spaces, in the midaxillary line, will penetrate skin and fascia, the serratus anterior muscle, the intercostal muscles (three layers) and the parietal pleura to reach the pleural cavity.

*Thoracotomy*

1. A surgeon can enter the thoracic cavity through an opening made in the thoracic wall (thoracotomy).
2. Depending upon the region to be approached thoracotomy can be anterior, posterior or lateral.

## THE THORACIC CAVITY

1. To understand the arrangement of contents of the thoracic cavity we will begin by examining a transverse section through the cavity (19.3).
2. First note the shape of the thoracic cavity. It is more or less oval, the transverse diameter being distinctly greater than the anteroposterior diameter.

3.a. Next, observe that the vertebral column projects forward into the cavity, and that on each side of it the thoracic cavity extends backwards to the level of the transverse processes of vertebrae.

3.b. The backward extensions of the thoracic cavity, on either side of the vertebral column, are called the ***paravertebral grooves***.

4. Now turn to 19.4 that is a coronal section through the thoracic cavity. Note the lateral walls formed by ribs and intercostal muscles; and the dome-shaped diaphragm closing the cavity inferiorly.
5. In 19.3 and 19.4 you will see that the thoracic cavity can be divided into three parts:
   a. To the right and left sides there are large spaces that are almost completely filled by the corresponding lungs.
   b. Separating the spaces for the right and left lungs there is a thick median partition that is called the ***mediastinum***.
   c. The most important structure in the mediastinum is the heart.
6. In 19.5, we see a sagittal section across the mediastinum. Note the following:
   a. The inlet of the thorax slopes downwards and forwards. (The level of the upper border of the manubrium sterni corresponds to the level of the intervertebral disc between T2 and T3).
   b. The diaphragm is attached anteriorly to the xiphoid process, and passes backwards to reach the vertebral column at level T12.
   c. The vertical extent of the mediastinum is greater posteriorly than anteriorly (as is true for the thoracic cavity as well).
   d. The mediastinum can be divided into upper and lower parts by a horizontal plane passing from the lower end of the manubrium sterni (sternal angle) to the intervertebral disc between vertebrae T4 and T5.
7. The part of the mediastinum lying between this plane and the inlet of the thorax is called the ***superior mediastinum***. The trachea, oesophagus, and several large vessels lie in it.

Vertebra
Thoracic duct
Right lung
Left lung
Pleura
Vena azygous
Pleura
POSTERIOR MEDIASTINUM
Descending aorta
Oesophagus
Rib
Left atrium
Right atrium
Intercostal space
MIDDLE MEDIASTINUM occupied by heart
Left ventricle
Pericardium
ANTERIOR MEDIASTINUM
Right ventricle
Manubrium sterni

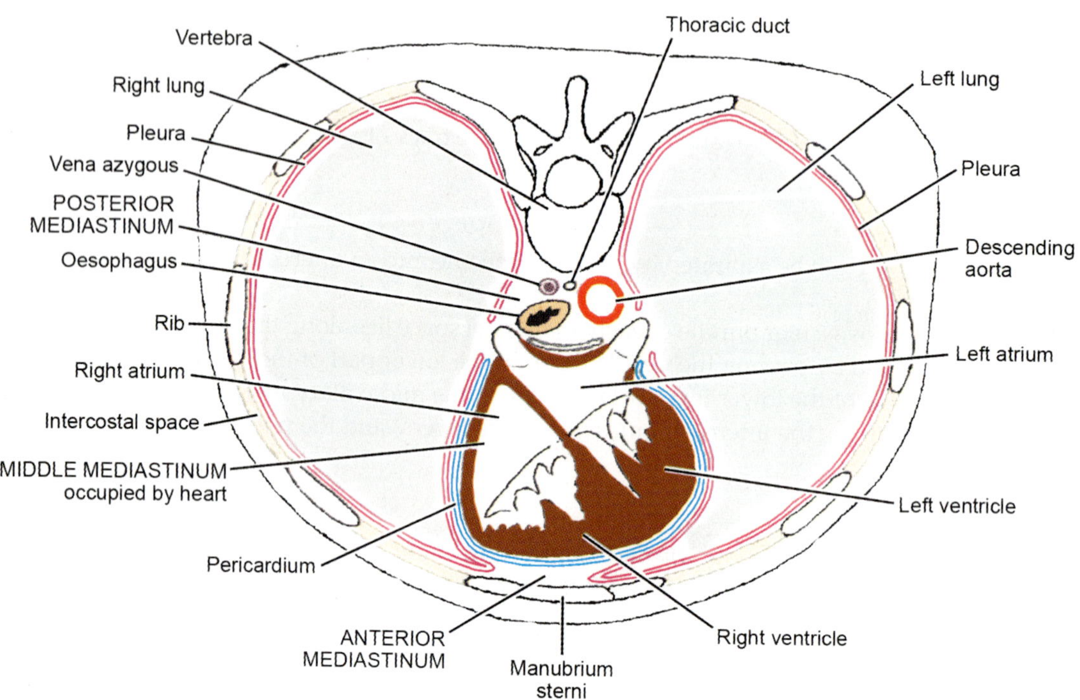

**19.3:** Transverse section through thorax showing important contents

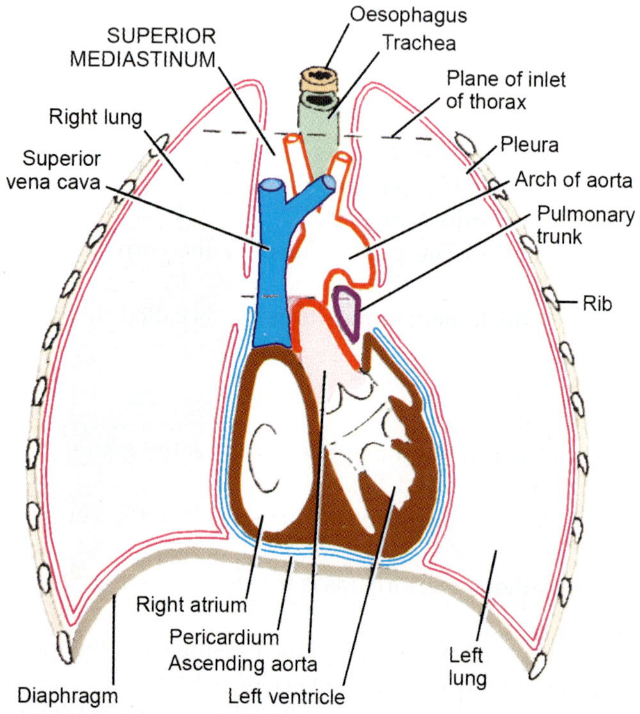

Oesophagus
SUPERIOR MEDIASTINUM
Trachea
Plane of inlet of thorax
Right lung
Superior vena cava
Pleura
Arch of aorta
Pulmonary trunk
Rib
Right atrium
Pericardium
Ascending aorta
Left lung
Diaphragm
Left ventricle

**19.4:** Schematic coronal section through thorax to show its main contents

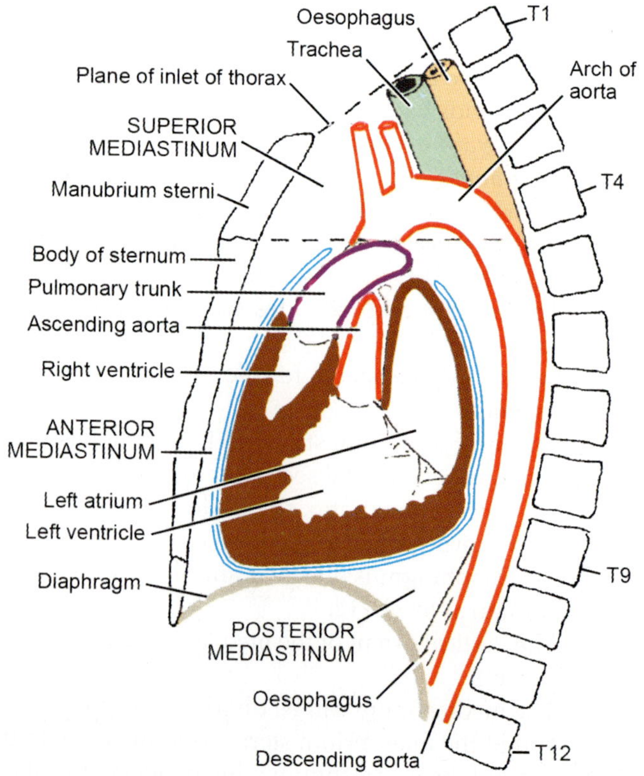

Oesophagus
T1
Trachea
Plane of inlet of thorax
Arch of aorta
SUPERIOR MEDIASTINUM
Manubrium sterni
T4
Body of sternum
Pulmonary trunk
Ascending aorta
Right ventricle
ANTERIOR MEDIASTINUM
Left atrium
Left ventricle
T9
Diaphragm
POSTERIOR MEDIASTINUM
Oesophagus
Descending aorta
T12

**19.5:** Schematic sagittal section through the thorax to show the subdivisions of the mediastinum

8. The part of the mediastinum lying below the superior mediastinum is divided into three parts as follows:
   a. The greater part of the area is occupied by the heart and by great vessels near it. This part is the ***middle mediastinum***.
   b. The part of the mediastinum in front of the heart is the anterior mediastinum. Its most important content is the ***thymus***.
   c. The part behind the heart is the ***posterior mediastinum***. Note that its main contents are the aorta and the oesophagus.

## Superior Thoracic Aperture

1. At its upper end the thoracic cage has an opening that is called the ***superior thoracic aperture***, also called the ***thoracic inlet***. (Note: Surgeons sometimes refer to this aperture as the thoracic outlet as large arteries leave the thorax through it).

2.a. This aperture is bounded posteriorly by the upper end of the body of the first thoracic vertebra, laterally, by the inner border of the first rib, and in front by the upper border of the manubrium sterni.

2.b. As the upper border of the manubrium sterni lies at the level of the lower border of vertebra T2, it follows that the superior aperture is not placed horizontally but has a slope that runs downwards and forwards.

3. The superior aperture gives passage to several structures that pass from the neck into the thorax, or ***vice versa***. These include the trachea, the oesophagus, several large blood vessels and nerves.

## Inferior Aperture of Thorax

1. At its lower end the thoracic cage has an inferior aperture that is much larger than the superior aperture. (The size of the superior aperture corresponds to the diameter of the neck; and that of the lower aperture to the diameter of the upper part of the abdomen).
2. Anteriorly, the boundary of the inferior aperture is V-shaped and is formed (in each half) by the 7th, 8th, 9th and 10th costal cartilages).
   a. This boundary passing downwards and laterally from the xiphoid process, is called the ***costal margin***.
   b. It can be easily palpated in a living person and is an important landmark.
3. Posteriorly, the inferior aperture of the thorax is bounded, in the median plane, by the lower border of the 12th thoracic vertebra, and more laterally by the 12th pair of ribs.
4. The inferior thoracic aperture is closed by the ***diaphragm***.
   a. The diaphragm is not flat, but has a marked upward convexity.
   b. The uppermost part of the abdominal cavity, therefore, lies under cover of the lower part of the thoracic cage.
   c. Structures passing from the thorax to the abdomen have to pass through apertures in the diaphragm.
   d. The largest of these are the aorta, and the oesophagus.
   e. The inferior vena cava is the largest structure entering the thorax from the abdomen.

# THE TRACHEA

1. The trachea is a wide tube lying more or less in the midline, in the lower part of the neck and in the superior mediastinum of the thorax (19.2). The trachea enters the thorax through its superior aperture. Its upper end is continuous with the lower end of the larynx. The junction lies opposite the lower part of the body of the sixth cervical vertebra.
2. At its lower end the trachea ends by dividing into the right and left principal bronchi. The level of bifurcation corresponds to the lower border of the manubrium sterni, or to the lower border of the fourth thoracic vertebra.
3. The lumen of the trachea is kept patent because of the presence of a series of cartilaginous rings in its wall. The rings are deficient posteriorly. Hence, the posterior part of the wall of the trachea is flat while the rest of it is rounded.

## Relations of the Trachea in the Thorax

The trachea is related to a large number of structures in the neck and in the thorax. The relations in the thorax are as follows:

1. Posteriorly, the trachea is related to the ***oesophagus*** that runs vertically behind it, and separates it from the bodies of the upper four thoracic vertebrae (19.7).
2. Anteriorly, the trachea is covered by skin, superficial and deep fascia, and by the ***manubrium sterni*** (19.7). The right and left sternohyoid and sternothyroid muscles (which arise from the posterior aspect of the manubrium sterni) overlap the part of the trachea near the inlet of the thorax.
3. The ***arch of the aorta*** lies in close contact with the trachea near its lower end. It is first anterior to the trachea and then on its left side (19.6).

4.a. The ***brachiocephalic trunk*** is at first in front of the trachea, but as it passes upwards it reaches the right side of the trachea.

4.b. The ***right common carotid artery*** ascends along the right side of the cervical part of the trachea (19.6 and 19.7).

5. The ***left common carotid artery*** is at first in front of the trachea. As it passes upwards it reaches the left side of the trachea.
6. The ***left subclavian artery*** arises from the part of the arch of the aorta that lies to the left of the trachea. It ascends (for some distance) along the left side of the trachea lying behind the left common carotid artery (19.7).
7. The veins related to the trachea are as follows:
   a. The ***left brachiocephalic vein*** crosses in front of the trachea just above the arch of the aorta.
   b. The ***right brachiocephalic vein***.

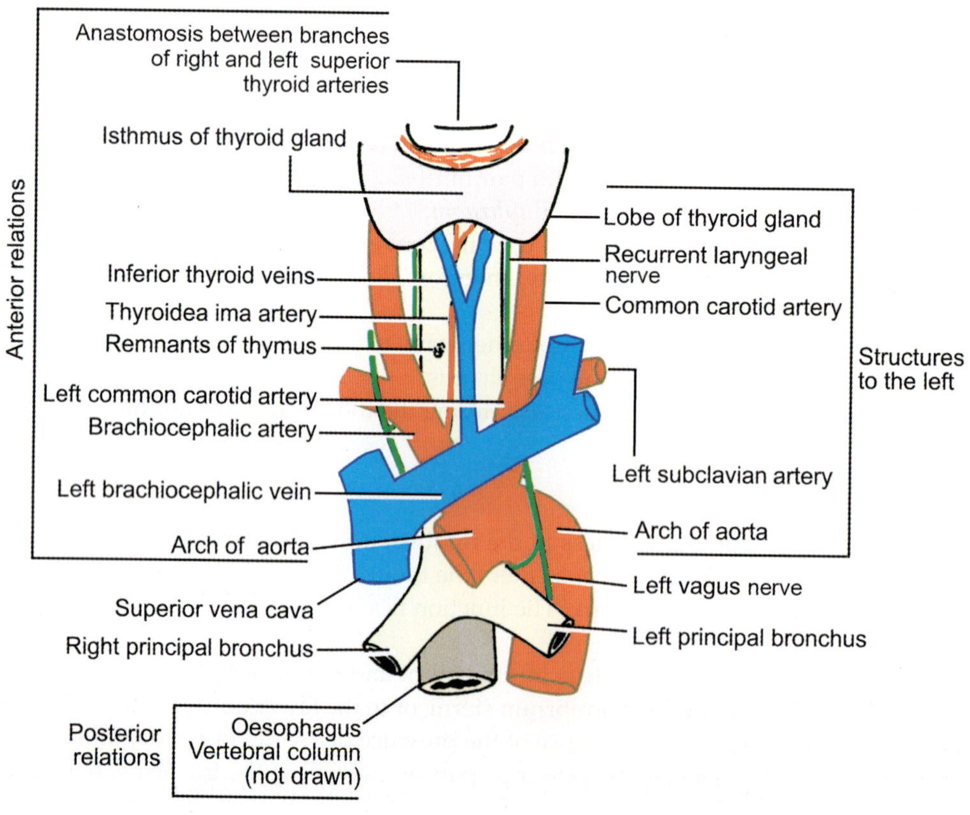


**19.6:** Some relations of the trachea as seen from the front

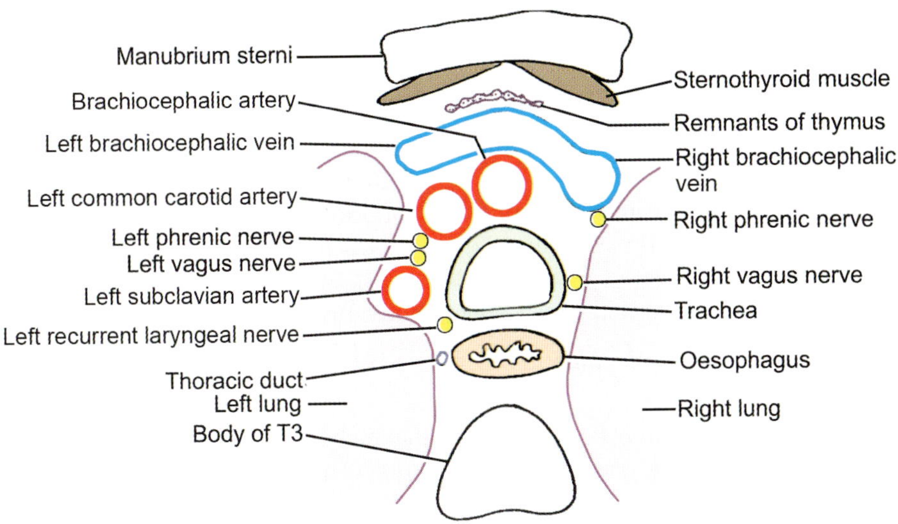


19.7: Transverse section through the superior mediastinum just above the summit of the arch of the aorta to show some relations of the trachea

c. The ***superior vena cava*** lie to the right side of the thoracic part of the trachea (19.6 and 19.7).
d. The terminal part of the ***azygous vein*** arches forwards across the right side of the trachea (near its lower end) to join the superior vena cava (19.9).

8. The left recurrent laryngeal nerve lies in the groove between the trachea and the oesophagus (19.7) (The right recurrent laryngeal nerve is related to the trachea only in the neck).
9. The right vagus nerve is closely applied to the right side of the thoracic part of the trachea (19.7).
10. On either side (right or left) the trachea is overlapped by the corresponding pleura and lung (19.7).
11. Small structures lying in front of the trachea are as follows:
    a. A small artery, the ***thyroidea ima,*** is sometimes present. It arises from the brachiocephalic trunk or from the arch of the aorta and runs upwards in front of the trachea (19.6).
    b. The deep cardiac plexus lies in front of the trachea at its bifurcation.
    c. Some lymph nodes, and some remnants of thymus also lie in front of the trachea.

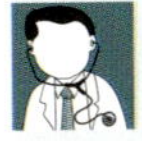

## CLINICAL CORRELATION

### The Trachea

The trachea can be palpated in the suprasternal notch. Deviation of the trachea from the midline could indicate a mediastinal shift.

#### *Tracheal Tug*

1. This is a physical sign often present in cases or aortic aneurysm.
2. To elicit the sign the examiner stands behind the patient and places his fingers just below the cricoid cartilage.
3. The patient is asked to swallow. This raises the cricoid cartilage that is retained in this position by the fingers.
4. The trachea is now stretched.
5. Pulsations of an aneurysm may then be transmitted through the trachea to the fingers of the examiner.

#### *Tracheostomy*

1. This is an operation to create an artificial opening in the trachea (in the neck).
2. It is used to provide an alternative route for supply of air to the lungs when there is obstruction in the larynx or upper end of the trachea.

3. The 2nd and 3rd (and sometimes the 4th) tracheal rings are cut and a tube inserted into the trachea through the opening.

***Stenosis of the trachea can be caused by external pressure.***

1. Such pressure can be exerted by enlargement of the thyroid gland (e.g., in carcinoma), or by enlarged lymph nodes in the region.
2. It may be pressed upon by an ***aortic aneurysm***, or by an abnormally located aortic arch.
3. Stenosis can also be produced by fibrosis of the wall of the trachea, and this may occur as an after effect of tracheostomy.
4. The lumen of the trachea can be obstructed by a foreign body, or by a tumour.

***Congenital malformations of the trachea include:***

1. Tracheo-oesophageal fistulae (19.8).
2. Diverticulae and accessory bronchi may be arising from the trachea. The accessory bronchi may be blind, may supply an accessory lobe, or may replace a normal segmental bronchus.
3. Rarely, the trachea may be absent.

## THE PRINCIPAL BRONCHI

1. At its lower end, the trachea divides into the right and left principal bronchi. Each principal bronchus begins opposite the (lower border of the body of the) fourth thoracic vertebra. It passes downwards and laterally to enter the corresponding lung (19.2).
2. There are some important differences between the right and left principal bronchi.
   a. The right bronchus is wider, shorter, and more vertical than the left bronchus (19.9).
   b. The right bronchus is about 2.5 cm (1 inch) long, while the left bronchus is approximately double this length (5 cm).
   c. The right principal bronchus enters the lung opposite the fifth thoracic vertebra, while the left principal bronchus enters the lung opposite the sixth thoracic vertebra.
   d. On reaching the hilum of the right lung, the right principal bronchus gives off a superior lobar bronchus (to the superior lobe of the lung).
      i. It then descends for a short distance before dividing into the middle and inferior lobar bronchi (which supply the middle and inferior lobes, respectively, of the right lung).
      ii. In other words, the right principal bronchus ends by dividing into three lobar bronchi.

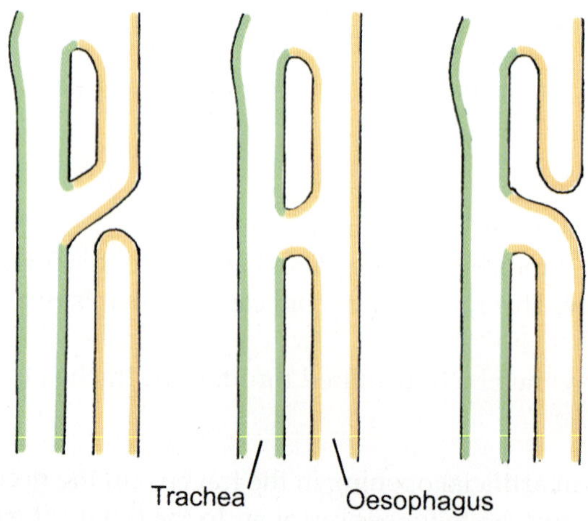


**19.8:** Three varieties of tracheo-oesophageal fistula

e. In contrast the left principal bronchus ends by dividing into two lobar bronchi, superior and inferior, corresponding to the lobes of the left lung.
   i. The length of the right principal bronchus, given above, is up to the origin of the superior lobar bronchus.
   ii. However, the part of the bronchus between the origin of the superior lobar bronchus and the origin of the middle and inferior lobar bronchi is usually described as a continuation of the principal bronchus.

3. Further subdivisions of the lobar bronchi are considered along with the lungs.

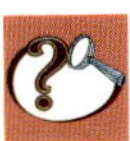

### WANT TO KNOW MORE?

*Relations of the Right Principal Bronchus*

1. The ***azygous vein*** lies just above the bronchus (near its origin) as the former arches forwards to join the inferior vena cava (19.9).
2. The ***right pulmonary artery*** is first inferior to the bronchus.
   a. It crosses in front of the bronchus, below the origin of the superior lobar bronchus.
   b. Therefore, on reaching the hilum of the lung the artery has the superior lobar bronchus above it, and the continuation of the principal bronchus below it (19.9).
3. The lower part of the right principal bronchus is also covered by the ***upper right pulmonary vein***.
   The position of the bronchus, the artery and the veins, at the hilum of the right lung is shown in 19.10.

*Relations of the Left Principal Bronchus*

1. The ***arch of the aorta*** lies above this bronchus. The ***descending aorta*** passes behind it (19.9).
2. The ***left pulmonary artery*** is first anterior to the bronchus and then superior to it.
3. The ***upper left pulmonary vein*** also crosses in front of the bronchus.
4. The position of the bronchus the artery and the veins, at the hilum of the left lung is shown in 19.10.

*Vascular and Nerve Supply of Trachea and Bronchi*

1. The trachea receives its blood supply mainly through the inferior thyroid arteries (lying in the neck). The blood is drained through the inferior thyroid veins.
2. The bronchi are supplied by bronchial arteries that also supply the lower end of the trachea.
3. The trachea and bronchi are innervated by sympathetic and parasympathetic nerves. The sympathetic nerves cause dilatation of bronchi while parasympathetic nerves cause constriction.
4. The lymph vessels of the trachea drain into the pretracheal and paratracheal lymph nodes.

## THE LUNGS

The right and left lungs lie in the corresponding halves of the thorax. They are separated from each other by structures in the mediastinum (including the heart, the great vessels, the trachea, and the oesophagus).

1. A general idea of the shape of the lungs can be had from 19.2 in which both lungs are shown as seen from the front.
2. Each lung has a relatively narrow upper end, or apex.
3. A much broader inferior surface or ***base***.
4. A rounded ***lateral*** or ***costal surface***.
5. A ***medial surface***.
6. The costal surface meets the medial surface, in front at the ***anterior border*** and behind at the ***posterior border***.
7. The costal and medial surfaces end, below, in an ***inferior border*** by which they are separated from the base.

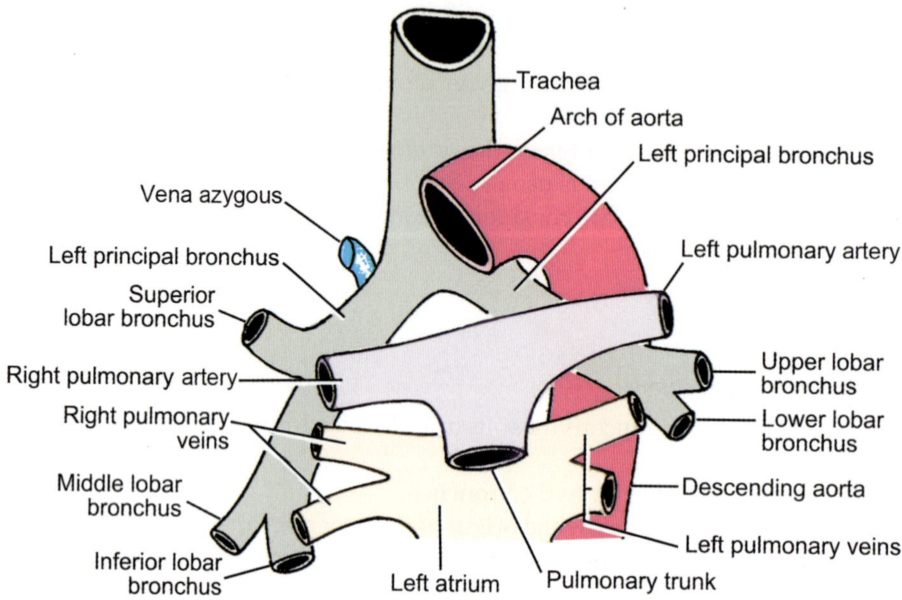


**19.9:** Diagram showing the right and left principal bronchi and their relations

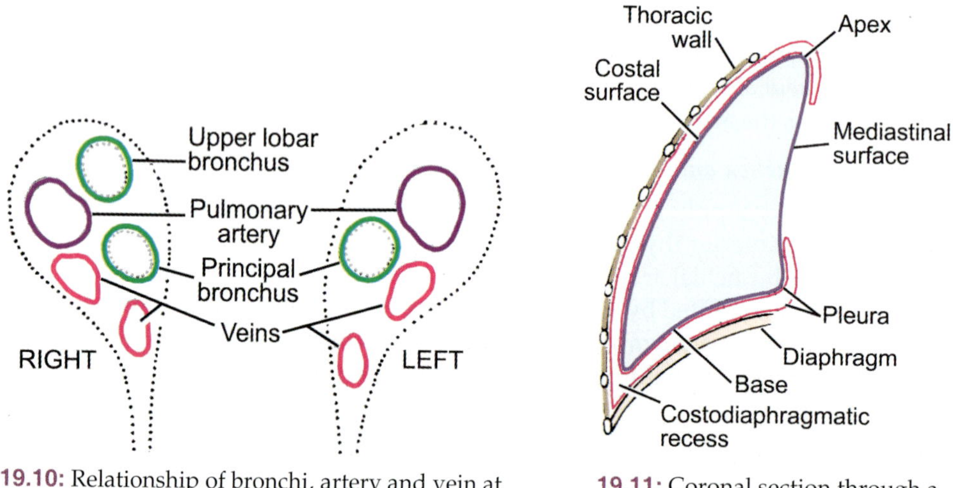


**19.10:** Relationship of bronchi, artery and vein at the hilum of right and left lungs

**19.11:** Coronal section through a lung to show its surfaces

8. The surface of the lung is free all around and is covered by pleura (visceral layer) except at an area of the medial surface called the ***hilum***. The principal bronchus and the pulmonary artery enter the lung, and the pulmonary veins leave it, at the hilum.

## Fissures and Lobes of the Lungs

1. Both the right and left lungs have a prominent ***oblique fissure***. This fissure begins at the posterior border of the lung (about 6 cm below the apex) and runs downwards and forwards through the lung substance, to emerge on the anteriormost part of the base.
2. The right lung has an additional ***horizontal fissure***. This fissure starts at the anterior border (a little below its middle) and passes backwards through the lung substance to meet the oblique fissure.

3. The part of the left lung above and in front of the oblique fissure is called the ***superior lobe.***
4. The part below and behind the oblique fissure is called the ***inferior lobe.***
5. In the right lung, the inferior lobe corresponds to that of the left lung.
6. Because of the presence of the horizontal fissure the part of the right lung in front of and above the oblique fissure is subdivided into a part above the horizontal fissure (called the ***superior lobe)*** and a part below the fissure (called the ***middle lobe).***
7. The anterior margin of the left lung has a deep cardiac notch. Because of the presence of this notch the lowest part of the superior lobe of this lung has the appearance of a tongue-like projection. This projection is called the ***lingula*** (L in 19.14A).

## Further Consideration of Surfaces and Borders of the Lungs

A transverse section across a lung is illustrated in 19.12.

1. The ***costal surface*** is rounded to conform to the shape of the ribs (and intercostal spaces). The relationship of the fissures and lobes of the lungs to this surface are shown in 19.14A.
2. The ***medial surface*** consists of an anterior (or mediastinal) part that is deeply concave, and a posterior (or vertebral) part that is convex.
   a. The concavity is meant to accommodate the heart.
   b. The convex part fits into the space between the lateral side of the vertebral bodies and the posterior parts of the ribs.
3. The medial surfaces of the right and left lungs have numerous features (and relationships) that are considered later. The relationship of the fissures and lobes to the medial surfaces of the lungs are shown in 19.14B.
4. The ***anterior border*** separates the anterior margins of the costal and medial surfaces (while the posterior border separates the posterior margins of these surfaces).
   a. The anterior border of the right lung passes straight from the apex to the base, but that of the left lung is marked by a deep cardiac notch (arrow in 19.14A).
   b. In the right lung, the anterior border is interrupted by the horizontal fissure a few centimetres from its lower end.

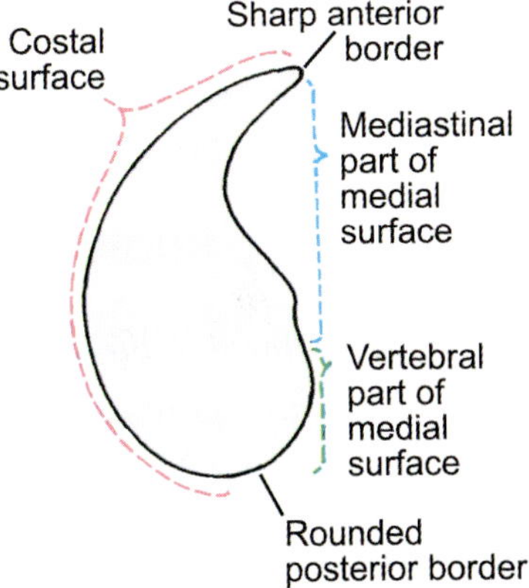


**19.12:** Transverse section through left lung to show its surfaces and borders

5. The ***base*** of the lung, is deeply concave (to fit over the corresponding cupola of the diaphragm). The part of the ***inferior border*** that separates the base from the costal surface is sharp.
   a. The part of the lung lying near this sharp border extends into the narrow costodiaphragmatic recess (between the lower ribs and intercostal spaces, on the outside, and the diaphragm, on the inside).
   b. In contrast the part of the inferior border that separates the medial surface from the base is rounded.
6. The base is formed mainly by the inferior lobe(19.14A and B). Its anteriormost part is formed by the superior lobe in the case of the left lung, and by the middle lobe in the case of the right lung.
7. The apex of the lung is rounded.
   a. When seen from the front, the apex of each lung appears to lie in the lower part of the neck.
   b. This is so because the inlet of the thorax (which represents the upper limit of the cavity of the thorax) is placed obliquely (19.13).
   c. As a result, the apex of the lung lies about one inch (2.5 cm) above the medial part of the clavicle.

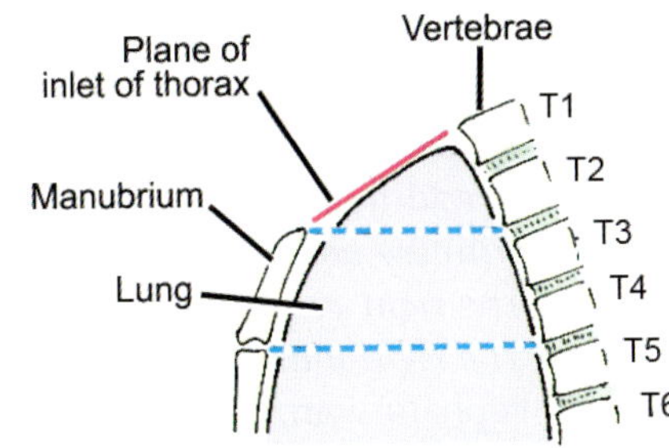


**19.13:** Scheme to show why the apical part of the lung is seen in the front of the neck

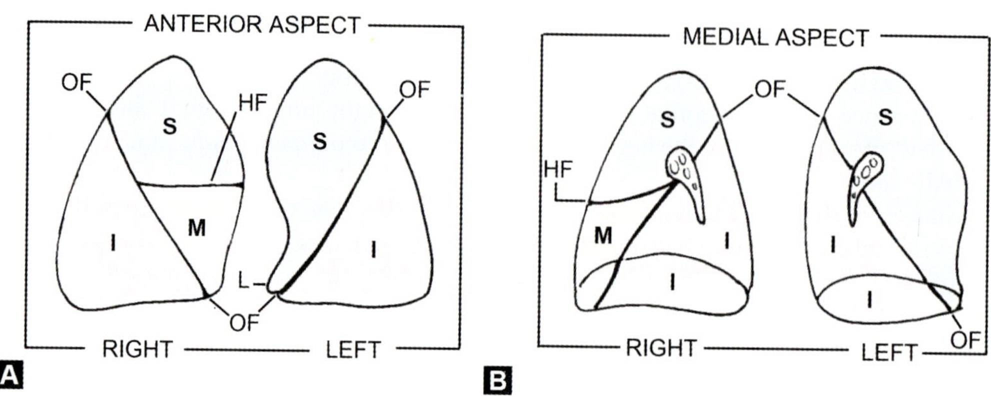


19.14A and B: Fissures and lobes of lungs. (A) Anterior aspect; (B) Medial aspect
S:Superior lobe; M:Middle lobe; I:Inferior lobe; OF:Oblique fissure; HF:Horizontal fissure; L:Lingula

## WANT TO KNOW MORE?

***Structures Related to the Medial Surface of the Right Lung***

1. The cardiac impression of the right lung is related mainly to the ***right atrium***, including its auricle. The anteriormost part of the impression comes in contact with the ***right ventricle***.
2. The posterior part of the cardiac impression is continuous below with a short but wide groove. The thoracic part of the ***inferior vena cava*** lies in this groove.
3. Continuous with the upper part of the cardiac impression there is a prominent vertical groove in which the ***superior vena cava***, and the lower end of the ***right brachiocephalic vein*** lie.
4. Continuous with the posterior margin of the groove for the superior vena cava there is a narrow, but deep groove that forms an arch above and behind the hilum. This groove is produced by the ***vena azygos***.
5. Along the posterior margin of the mediastinal area there is a wide shallow groove for the ***oesophagus***. This groove is interrupted near its middle by the groove for the vena azygos.
6. The area of the lung lying between the upper part of the groove for the oesophagus (behind) and the groove for the superior vena cava (in front) is in contact with the right side of the ***trachea***.
7. A little below the apex the anterior aspect of the lung is marked by a notch for the ***subclavian artery***.
8. Smaller structures in the mediastinum that come into contact with the right lung are as follows:
   a. In addition to the bodies of thoracic vertebrae, the vertebral part of the medial surface comes in contact with the ***posterior intercostal arteries*** and ***veins***, and with ***splanchnic nerves***.
   b. The ***right vagus*** lies between the trachea and the lung.
   c. The ***right phrenic nerve*** comes in contact (from above downwards) with the groove for the right brachiocephalic vein, the groove for the superior vena cava, the part of the cardiac impression related to the right atrium, and the groove for the inferior vena cava.

***Structures Related to the Medial Surface of the Left Lung***

In addition to the main relationships common to both lungs already described the left lung has the following important relationships:

1. The cardiac impression (which is deeper than on the right lung) is related mainly to the ***left ventricle***. The anterior part of the impression overlies the ***right ventricle***, including the ***infundibulum***.
2. Apart from the cardiac impression the most conspicuous feature to be seen is a wide groove that forms an arch above and behind the hilum, and extends below right up to the lower end of the medial surface. This groove is meant for the ***aorta***. The upper part is for the arch of the aorta, and the lower part for the descending thoracic aorta.

3. Continuous with the upper margin of the groove for the arch of the aorta there are two smaller, vertical grooves. The posterior of these lodges the ***left subclavian artery***, and the anterior one lodges the ***left common carotid artery***. As the subclavian artery passes laterally across the anterior aspect of the lung it produces a notch a little below the apex.
4. The ***oesophagus*** comes into relationship with the upper part of the left lung behind the groove for the subclavian artery. It may also be related to the lower part of the medial surface in front of the groove for the aorta.
5. Some smaller structures that are related to the medial surface of the left lung are as follows:
   a. The ***left phrenic*** and ***vagus nerves*** lie against the lung in the interval between the left subclavian and left common carotid arteries. From here both these nerves pass over the groove for the arch of the aorta. The phrenic nerve is continued downwards over the cardiac impression.
   b. The ***thoracic duct*** runs vertically between the lung and the upper part of the oesophagus.
   c. The ***left superior intercostal vein*** is related to the groove for the arch of the aorta.

The following important facts may be noted with regard to various relations of the medial surfaces of the right and left lungs.

1. The structures described as being related to the lungs are in fact separated from the lungs by:
   a. A layer of parietal pleura
   b. The pleural cavity
   c. The visceral pleura lining the surface of the lung.
2. The impressions on the medial surfaces of the right and left lungs are mirror images of the structures seen on the corresponding side of the mediastinum, and should be carefully compared with them.

*Differences Between Right and Left Lungs*

1. We have seen that the right lung normally has three ***lobes***, whereas the left lung has only two.
2. Differences in the ***bronchi*** within the lungs and in the ***bronchopulmonary segments*** are described below.
3. Differences in the arrangement of structures in the ***hila*** of the right and left lungs are shown in 19.10A and B.
4. The differences in ***impressions on the medial surfaces*** of the right and left lungs have been described before (19.15 and 19.16).
5. We have seen that the anterior border of the right lung is straight, but the anterior border of the left lung is marked by a deep ***cardiac notch*** (19.14A).
6. The right lung is more voluminous than the right lung and is, therefore, heavier.
7. The height of the right lung is less than that of the left lung (because the right cupola of the diaphragm is higher than the left).
8. The width of the right lung is greater than that of the left lung (as the heart projects more to the left side).
9. As a point of practical importance it must be remembered, however, that none of the differences described above are to be relied upon in determining the side to which a particular lung belongs. To do so identify the base, the apex, the medial and lateral surfaces, and the anterior and posterior borders; and use these features to orient the specimen correctly in the body.

## Intrapulmonary Bronchi and Bronchopulmonary Segments

1. The left lung is divided into two lobes — superior and inferior. The right lung is divided into three lobes — superior, middle and inferior.
2. Each lobe receives a lobar bronchus arising from the principal bronchus.
3. Each lobe is divisible into two or more ***bronchopulmonary segments;*** each segment is supplied by a ***segmental bronchus*** that is a branch of the lobar bronchus. The segments are summarised in 19.17.
4. The pattern of division of lobar bronchi into segmental bronchi is shown in 19.18. The extent of each bronchopulmonary segment in relation to the surfaces of the right and left lungs is shown in 19.19 A to D.

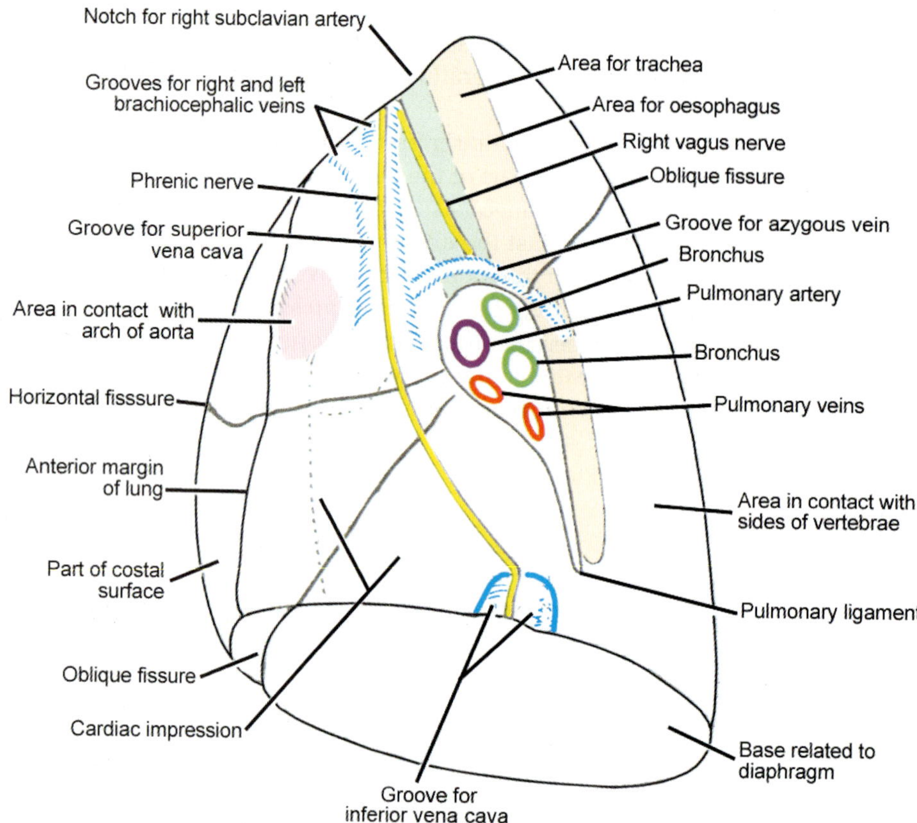


**19.15:** Right lung viewed from the medial side showing areas related to various structures

## WANT TO KNOW MORE?

***Bronchopulmonary Segments of Right Lung***

1. Near the hilum of the lung the right principal bronchus gives off the superior lobar bronchus.
2. It then descends for a short distance and divides into two lobar bronchi: one for the middle lobe and one for the inferior lobe.
3. The superior lobar bronchus divides into three segmental bronchi: ***apical, posterior*** and ***anterior.***
4. The middle lobar bronchus divides into two segmental bronchi: ***lateral*** and ***medial.***
5. The inferior lobar bronchus gives off five segmental bronchi:
   a. Superior
   b. Medial basal
   c. Anterior basal
   d. Lateral basal
   e. Posterior basal.
6. Thus, there are a total of ten bronchopulmonary segments in the right lung.

**Bronchopulmonary Segments of Left Lung**

1. The left principal bronchus divides into two lobar bronchi: ***superior*** and ***inferior***.
2. The superior lobar bronchus divides into two main branches: ***cranial*** and ***caudal***.

3. The cranial branch is the equivalent of the superior lobar bronchus of the right lung. It divides into ***apical, posterior*** and ***anterior*** segmental bronchi.
4. The caudal branch of the superior lobar bronchus is also called the ***lingular bronchus.*** It is the equivalent of the middle lobe bronchus of the right lung. It divides into ***superior*** and ***inferior lingular*** bronchi.
5. The inferior lobar bronchus gives off ***superior, medial basal, anterior basal, lateral basal,*** and ***posterior basal*** segmental branches as in the right lung.
6. Thus, the left lung also has ten bronchopulmonary segments.
   However, the following ***differences in the segmental bronchi of the right and left lungs*** are worthy of note.
   a. In the upper lobe of the left lung the apical and posterior segmental bronchi arise by a common stem. Some authorities, therefore, speak of an ***apicoposterior*** bronchopulmonary segment (combining the apical and posterior segments).
   b. In the lower lobe of the left lung, the medial basal bronchus is relatively small and appears as a branch of the anterior basal branch. Some authorities, therefore, consider the part supplied by the medial basal bronchus to be a part of the anterior basal segment.
7. Because of what has been said in points (a) and (b) above some authorities recognise only eight bronchopulmonary segments in the left lung.
8. Note that the segments of the middle lobe of the right lung are designated as medial and lateral. The corresponding segments in the left lung are designated superior and inferior.

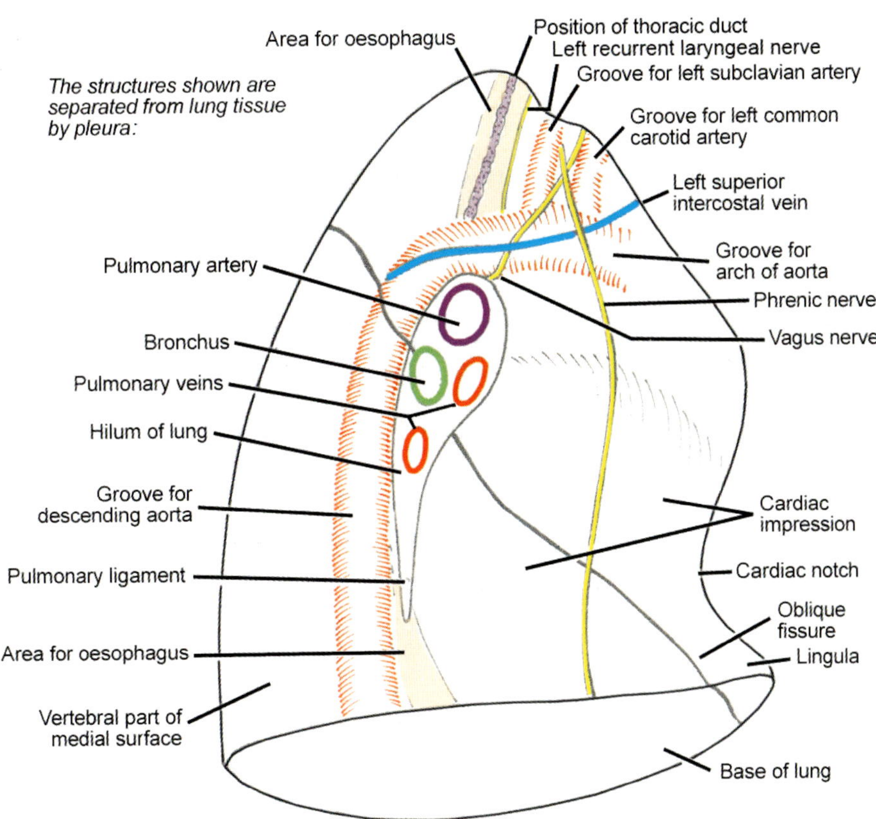


**19.16:** Left lung viewed from the medial side showing areas related to different structures

| 19.17: Bronchopulmonary segments | | | |
|---|---|---|---|
| *Right Lung* | | *Left Lung* | |
| *Lobe* | *Segments* | *Lobe* | *Segments* |
| Superior | Apical, Posterior, Anterior | Superior | Apical, Posterior, Anterior |
| Middle | Lateral, Medial | | Superior lingular, Inferior lingular |
| Inferior | Superior, Medial basal, Anterior basal, Lateral basal, Posterior basal | Inferior | Superior, Medial basal, Anterior basal, Lateral basal, Posterior |

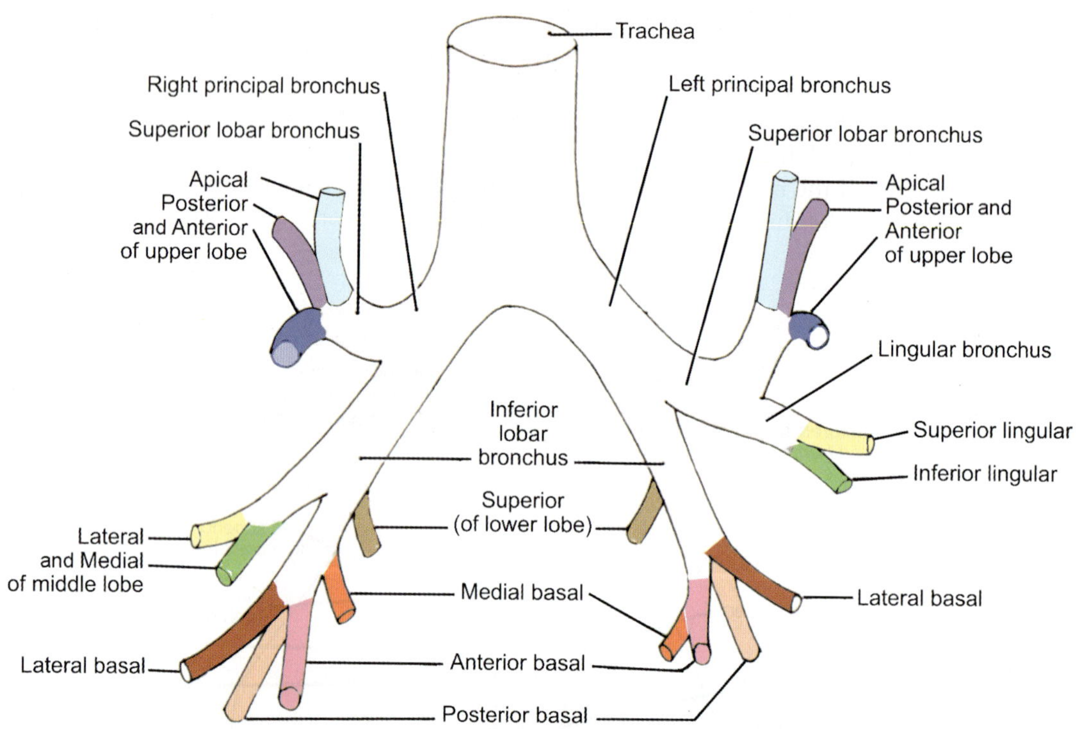


**19.18:** Scheme to show the bronchial tree as seen from the front

### Further Divisions of Bronchi

Each segmental bronchus divides into several generations of branches that ultimately end in very small tubes called ***brochioles.*** The bronchioles also undergo repeated branching and ultimately end in microscopic passages that connect them to the alveoli of the lungs (19.20).

### Blood Vessels of the Lungs

The blood supply of the lungs is peculiar in that two sets of arteries carry blood to them.

1. The pulmonary arteries convey deoxygenated blood from the right ventricle. This blood circulates through a capillary plexus intimately related to the walls of the alveoli, and receives oxygen from the alveolar air. This blood, which is now oxygenated, is returned to the heart (left atrium) through the pulmonary veins.

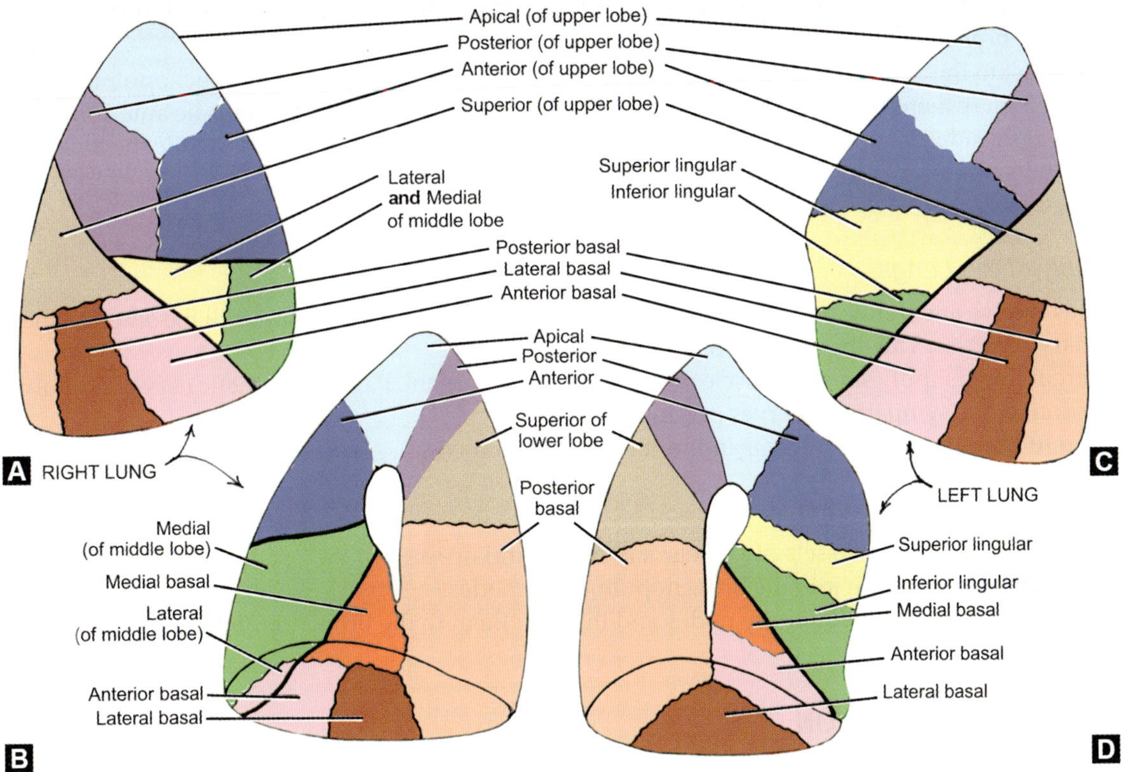


**19.19A to D:** Bronchopulmonary segments of the right and left lungs

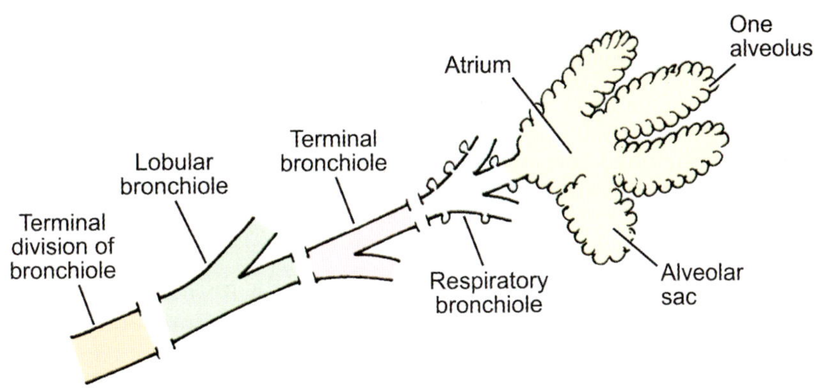


**19.20:** Scheme to show the terms used to describe the terminal ramifications of the bronchial tree

2. The lungs also receive oxygenated blood like any other tissue in the body. This is conveyed to them through the bronchial arteries. This blood supplies the walls of the bronchi and the connective tissue of the lung. Some of this blood passes into the pulmonary veins, but the rest of it is drained through bronchial veins.
   a. The extrapulmonary parts of the pulmonary arteries and veins and the bronchial arteries are described in chapter 21.
   b. Within each lung the pulmonary artery divides into branches that follow the branching pattern of the bronchi.

c. Each bronchopulmonary segment has its own artery. As a rule, the arteries lie posterolateral to the corresponding bronchi.
d. In contrast to the arteries, the pulmonary veins tend to run between adjacent bronchopulmonary segments. Each vein may therefore drain more than one segment. Near the hilum, the veins lie anterior to the bronchi.
e. On the right side, the upper pulmonary vein drains the upper and middle lobes, while the lower pulmonary vein drains the inferior lobe. On the left side, the upper and lower veins drain the superior and inferior lobes respectively.

### *Nerve Supply of the Lungs*

1. The lungs receive autonomic nerves, both sympathetic and parasympathetic through the anterior and posterior pulmonary plexuses. The fibres are both efferent and afferent.
2. The efferent fibres supply smooth muscle in the walls of the bronchi. Parasympathetic nerves produce bronchoconstriction, while sympathetic nerves produce dilatation.
3. The afferent fibres arise in the alveoli and in the bronchial mucosa.

### *Lymphatic Drainage of the Lungs*

1. The lungs are drained by two sets of vessels: superficial and deep.
2. The superficial vessels drain into the bronchopulmonary nodes.
3. Deep vessels drain first to pulmonary nodes and through them to the bronchopulmonary nodes.

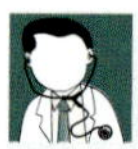

## CLINICAL CORRELATION

### The Lungs and Bronchi

**Investigating the Respiratory System**

*Clinical Examination*

1. ***Percussion and Auscultation*** of the thorax can give a great deal of information about lung diseases, and is an essential part of the physical examination of a patient suspected to have a respiratory problem.
2. A clinician examining the chest needs to know the relationship of lobes of the lungs to the thoracic wall. This is shown in 19.24 and 19.25 in which the surface projections of the borders and fissures of the lungs are shown. Details of surface projection are given after the description of pleura.

***Plain Skiagram***

1. A plain skiagram of the chest (Postero-anterior or PA view) is the most common investigation for detecting structural abnormalities within the chest. It provides useful information about the bones of the thorax, the lung fields, the heart, the diaphragm and the mediastinum. In some cases it can establish diagnosis (e.g., in pleural effusion), and in many others it may give clues that aid further investigation.
2. Right and left oblique views are also used.

***Fluoroscopy or Screening***

In this procedure, instead of recording an image on film X-ray images are seen on a fluorescent screen. Although, less detail is seen than in an X-ray film the technique allows a dynamic study. For example, movements of the domes of the diaphragm can be seen.

***Computed Tomography and Magnetic Resonance Imaging***

These are newer techniques that provide images of the chest with great detail. Sectional views can be obtained. They often help to establish diagnosis in many cases in which routine X-ray examination is inconclusive.

### *Bronchoscopy and Bronchography*

1. The interior of the trachea and bronchi can be visualised through an instrument called a ***bronchoscope***. Earlier bronchoscopes were rigid and could be passed only into larger bronchi. More recent bronchoscopes, based on fibre optics, are flexible and can be passed into smaller bronchi.
2. Apart from examining the interior of the bronchial tree, bronchoscopy can also be used to obtain bronchial secretions and tissue for examination, or to remove foreign bodies that may enter the bronchi.
3. At the bifurcation of the trachea we can see the openings into the principal bronchi. The openings are separated by a ridge called the ***carina***. The appearance of the carina alters in carcinoma and can help in diagnosis.
4. ***Bronchography*** is a procedure in which X-ray pictures of the bronchi can be obtained after instilling a radio-opaque substance into them.
5. The techniques mentioned above give information about the structural status of the respiratory system. Of equal importance are investigations of function details of which can be found in books on physiology and of medicine.

### Some Diseases of the Lungs and Bronchi

1. A foreign body can be aspirated into the trachea and bronchi. It is more likely to enter the right bronchus than the left as the right bronchus is wider, shorter and more vertical. A foreign body can become the cause of serious infection.
2. Inflammation of bronchi is called ***bronchitis***. It may be acute or chronic. In some cases there is localised or more widespread dilatation of bronchi. These dilatations can become seats of infection. This condition is called ***bronchiectasis***.
3. Inflammation in the lung is referred to as ***pneumonia*** or ***pneumonitis***. Inflammations of the lungs and bronchi can be caused by bacteria, by viruses, by allergy, or by irritant action of pollutants in the atmosphere.
4. In some cases serious lung infections cause localised necrosis of tissue leading to formation of a ***lung abscess***. ***Cavities*** can be formed within the lungs. Most lung abscesses are caused by inhalation of infective material from infected sinuses (sinusitis), tonsillitis, or dental infection.
5. Amongst bacterial infections of the lungs special mention needs to be made of ***pulmonary tuberculosis***.
   a. Until a few decades ago this was a dreaded disease usually leading to death.
   b. The disease is now treatable and preventable, but it is still prevalent especially amongst populations that live in unhygienic conditions and are poorly nourished.
   c. It is also a major killer in persons in whom immune processes are compromised (as in AIDS).
6. Sensitivity to substances of plant, animal or chemical origin in the atmosphere can also be responsible for diseases that have a predominantly allergic basis.
   a. One such condition is ***bronchial asthma*** in which spasm of bronchial muscle causes considerable difficulty in breathing. The difficulty is more pronounced during expiration.
   b. Some degree of bronchospasm may also be present in various other conditions seen in the lungs.
   c. In some cases chronic respiratory obstruction leads to considerable dilatation of alveoli. Large spaces may be formed in the lung parenchyma. This condition is called ***emphysema***. This condition may lead to a ***barrel-shaped chest***.
7. Obstruction to a bronchus from any cause can lead to collapse of the part of lung supplied by it. Collapse of part of a lung is referred to as ***atelectasis***. Partial or complete collapse of a lung can also follow pneumothorax or large accumulations of fluid in the pleural cavity,
8. Neoplasms of various kinds may be seen in the lungs. The most common of these is ***bronchogenic carcinoma***. This disease, which is a major killer, is more common in smokers than in non-smokers, and in men than in women.
9. As a result of various kinds of inflammatory and degenerative disorders the lungs can gradually undergo fibrosis. Pulmonary fibrosis can greatly reduce the efficiency of the lungs. Loss of elastic tissue makes the

lungs much less elastic. This is one reason for decreased respiratory efficiency in elderly persons, other reasons being decreased elasticity of the thoracic cage, and reduced strength of respiratory muscles.

10. Difficulty in breathing is referred to as ***dyspnoea.*** This can be a feature of any serious lung disease. Dyspnoea can also be produced by obstruction to respiratory passages; and by disturbances of the pulmonary circulation especially when they lead to pulmonary oedema which is briefly considered below.
11. In some cases, excessive accumulation of secretions in bronchi may cause respiratory embarrassment and can lead to infection. Drainage of such fluid can be facilitated by placing the patient in a posture that favours flow of such secretions by gravity (***postural drainage***). A good knowledge of bronchopulmonary segments and of the direction of each bronchus is necessary for effective use of the method.

### *Pulmonary Oedema*

This is a condition in which serous fluid seeps into lung tissue. It first invades interstitial tissue and later reaches the alveoli. It leads to great difficulty in breathing. Lack of adequate oxygenation can lead to cyanosis.

Pulmonary oedema can result from a variety of causes some of which are as follows:

1. Any ***obstruction to flow of blood*** through the left atrium and ventricle (which may be caused by left ventricular failure, mitral stenosis or mitral incompetence).
2. Excessive ***transfusion*** of fluid into the blood.
3. ***Irritation*** of lung tissue by poisonous gases, or by inflammation.
4. Sudden transportation to a ***high altitude.***

### *Pulmonary Embolism*

If a clot forming in any vein breaks loose it travels through the bloodstream into the right side of the heart and from there into pulmonary arteries. Depending upon its size such a clot gets lodged in one of the ramifications of a pulmonary artery. The clot most often originates in veins of the lower limb or pelvis. The effects of pulmonary embolism depend on the size of the vessel blocked. A very small embolism may go unnoticed, while a very large one could result in almost immediate death of the patient.

### *Lung Resection*

An entire lung or part of it can be removed by operation.

1. We have seen that each lung can be divided into a number of structural units called bronchopulmonary segments (19.12). Knowledge of these segments is essential for the clinician.
2. When disease is restricted to one bronchopulmonary segment it is possible to remove the segment without affecting the rest of the lung. This is referred to as ***segmental resection.***
3. In diseases that are more widespread an entire lobe may be removed (***lobectomy***), or even an entire lung (***pneumonectomy***).

### *Congenital Anomalies of Lungs and Bronchi*

1. Part of a lung, or even an entire lung may be missing.
2. Various abnormalities in formation of lobes and fissures of the lungs may be seen.
3. ***Accessory lobes*** may be present. They may be directly connected to the trachea, or to the oesophagus, or may have no connection.
   a. A part of the upper lobe of the right lung may lie medial to the azygos vein.
   b. This part is called the ***azygous lobe.***
   c. It is separated from the rest of the lung by a fold of pleura called the ***mesoazygos*** that contains the azygos vein at its lower end.
   d. The condition is of special interest as it can be recognised in a plain skiagram. The mezoazygos is seen as a thin line, at the lower end of which the azygos vein casts a circular shadow.
4. ***Sequestration of lung tissue***: An area of lung may not have any communication with the bronchial passages.
   a. Such tissue may form a complete lobe (***lobar sequestration***).
   b. May form a mass within a lobe (***intralobar sequestration***).
   c. Sequestration is most frequently seen in the lower lobe of the left lung.

5. Part of a lung may herniate:
   a. Through the inlet of the thorax.
   b. Through a defect in the thoracic wall.
   c. Into the mediastinum.
   d. Into the opposite pleural cavity.
6. Displaced bronchi may arise from the trachea above its bifurcation, or even from the oesophagus. They may replace a normal segmental bronchus, may supply an accessory lobe or may be blind.

## THE PLEURA

1. The right and left pleurae (singular = pleura) are thin serous membranes that are closely related to the corresponding lungs and to the corresponding half of the thoracic wall.
2. The arrangement of the pleura is best understood by thinking of it as a closed sac that is invaginated (from the medial side) by the corresponding lung. As a result of this invagination the pleura of each side comes to have:
   a. An inner or ***visceral*** layer that is closely adherent to the surface of the lung.
   b. An outer, or ***parietal*** layer that lines the wall of the thorax.
3. Apart from lining the surfaces of the lung, the visceral pleura dips into the fissures of the lungs, and lines the contiguous sides of the lobes.

4.a. The parietal and visceral layers of pleura are in contact with each other being separated only by a potential space which is called the ***pleural cavity.***

b. Under certain diseased conditions fluid or air may be present in the pleural cavity thus separating the parietal and visceral layers.

5. The parietal pleura can be subdivided into the following parts:
   a. The ***costovertebral*** pleura lines the inner aspect of the ribs and intercostal spaces, part of the inner surface of the sternum, and the sides of thoracic vertebrae (19.21).
   b. The ***diaphragmatic*** pleura lines the upper surface of the diaphragm (19.22). However, the pleura is not as extensive as the diaphragm so that some parts of the latter are not covered by pleura.
   c. The ***mediastinal*** pleura (19.22) lines structures on the corresponding side of the mediastinum.

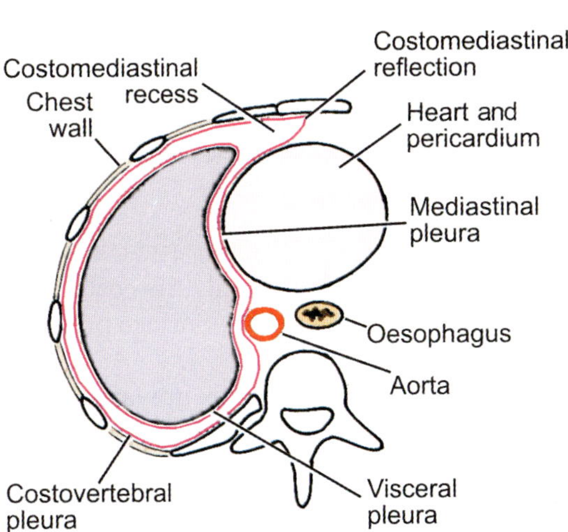


**19.21:** Schematic transverse section through the left half of the thorax to show some features of the pleura

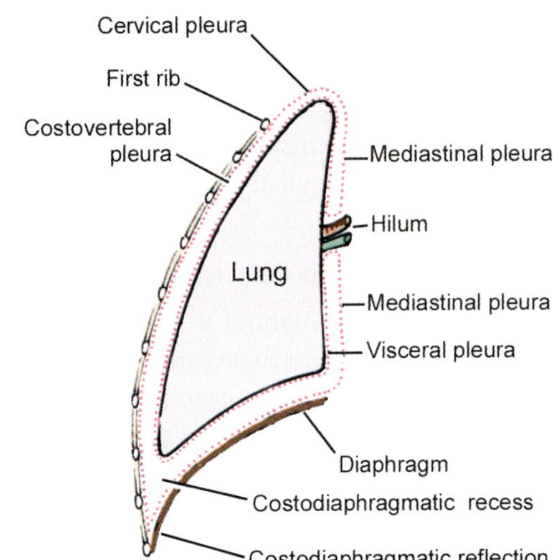


**19.22:** Schematic coronal section through one half of the thorax to show some features of the pleura

6.a. The mediastinal pleura extends as a tube over the structures passing between the mediastinum and the lung (bronchus, pulmonary artery, pulmonary veins) and becomes continuous with the visceral pleura at the hilum of the lung.

b. This pleura extends for some distance below the hilum forming a double layered fold which stretches from the mediastinum to the lung. This fold is called the ***pulmonary ligament.***

7. In 19.21 it will be seen that, when traced anteriorly, the costovertebral pleura reaches the sternum (posterior aspect) and bends sharply to become continuous with the mediastinal pleura. The line along which bending occurs is called the line of ***costomediastinal reflection*** of the pleura.

8. When traced backwards, the costovertebral pleura is reflected from the sides of the vertebral bodies onto the mediastinum.

9.a. In 19.22 it will be seen that, when the costovertebral pleura is traced downwards it bends sharply to become continuous with diaphragmatic pleura.

b. The line along which this bending takes place is called the line of ***costodiaphragmatic reflection.***

10. It is of practical importance to know the relationship of the lines of pleural reflection (described above) to the surface of the thorax.

11. In 19.22 it will be seen that, when traced upwards the costal pleura extends up to the inner margin of the first rib.
    a. Above this level, it covers the apex of the lung (that lies in the root of the neck) and is called the ***cervical pleura*** (It is also called the dome of the pleura).
    b. The cervical pleura extends upwards up to the level of the neck of the first rib (corresponding to the upper part of the first thoracic vertebra).
    c. It is covered by a sheeth of fascia called the ***suprapleural membrane*** (which stretches from the transverse process of the seventh cervical vertebra to the inner border of the first rib.

**WANT TO KNOW MORE?**

d. Both on the right and left sides the cervical pleura is related, anteriorly, to the subclavian artery and to the scalenus anterior muscle (19.23) and, posteriorly, to structures lying in front of the neck of the first rib (cervicothoracic ganglion, ventral ramus of spinal nerve T1, and superior intercostal artery).

e. The costocervical trunk runs upward in front of the cervical pleura and then arches above it to reach its posterior aspect. Here it gives off the superior intercostal artery. The superior intercostal artery descends posterior to the cervical pleura to the brachiocephalic artery and the right brachiocephalic vein.

12. The left cervical pleura is related anteromedially to the left subclavian and left common carotid arteries, and to the left brachiocephalic vein.

13. The relationship of the thoracic duct to the cervical pleura is shown in 19.23.
(The relations of the cervical pleura will be better understood after the neck has been studied).

## Surface Projection of the Pleura

1. From what has been said about the pleura and lungs it will be obvious that it is only the costal surface of the lung, and the costal pleura that come in contact with the external wall of the thorax. Surface projections, therefore, define the limits of these structures.

2.a. As seen from the front, the cervical pleura can be represented by a line that is convex upwards, and lies above the medial one-third of the clavicle.

b. The summit of the line rises 2.5 cm above the clavicle (19.24).

c. The medial end of the line lies behind the sternoclavicular joint and is continuous with the upper end of the line of costomediastinal reflection.

3. From here the line of costomediastinal runs downwards and medially to reach the midline at the level of the sternal angle, where it comes in contact with the corresponding line of the opposite side.

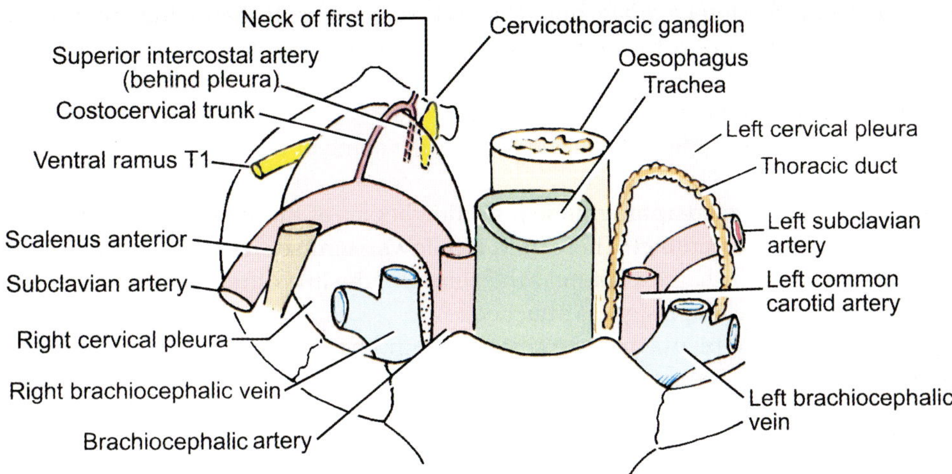


**19.23:** Some structures in the root of the neck, related to the cervical pleura. Structures on the left side are shown only in part

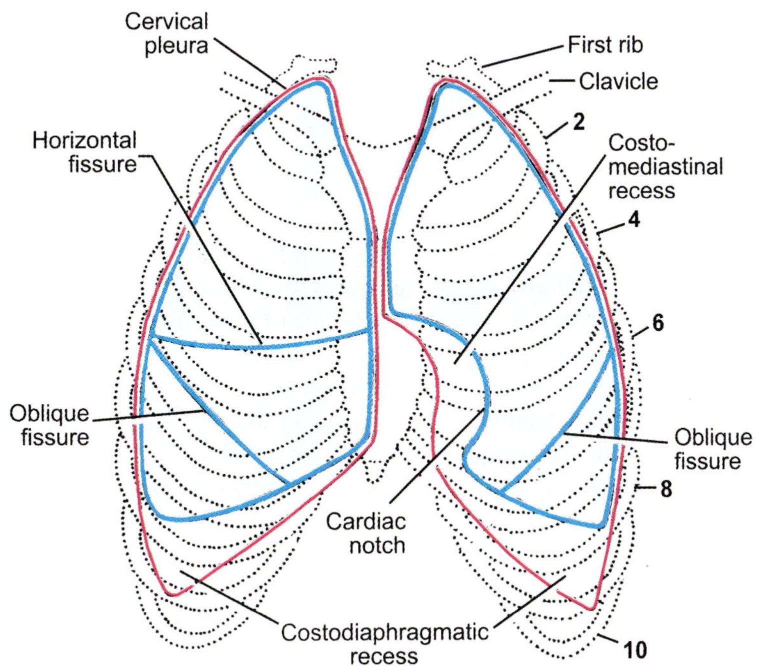


**19.24:** Scheme to show the relationship of lines of pleural reflection (red line) and of the lungs (blue line), to the skeleton of the thorax

4. On the right side the line runs downwards in the midline to reach the xiphisternal joint.

5.a. On the left side the line runs downwards in the midline up to the level of the fourth costal cartilage (the right and left pleurae being in contact with each other from the level of the sternal angle up to this level).

b. It then passes downwards and laterally to reach the lateral margin of the sternum and runs downwards a short distance lateral to this margin to reach the sixth costal cartilage about 3 cm from the midline.

6. The lower ends of the lines of costomediastinal reflection (described above) are continuous with the anterior ends of the lines of costodiaphragmatic reflection which are as follows.

7. On the right side this reflection begins behind the xiphoid process. It then winds round the anterior, lateral and posterior aspects of the thorax forming a curve convex downwards.
   a. In the midclavicular line, the line of reflection is at the level of the eighth rib.
   b. In the midaxillary line at the level of the tenth rib.
   c. At its posterior end the reflection lies at the level of the spine of the twelfth thoracic vertebra about 2 cm from the midline (19.25).
8. On the left side the line of costodiaphragmatic reflection begins at the sternal end of the sixth costal cartilage (i.e., about 2 cm lateral to the midline). Thereafter, it follows a course similar to that on the right side.

9.a. From the above it will be clear that, except near the sternum, the line of reflection of the pleura is higher than the costal margin to which the diaphragm is attached.

b. Between the lower limit of the pleura and the costal margin, the diaphragm is in direct contact with ribs and intercostal spaces.

10.a. The line along which the posterior part of the costovertebral pleura gets reflected onto the mediastinum can be represented by a vertical line about 2 cm from the middle line.

b. It extends, above up to the level of the spine of the second thoracic vertebra; and below to the level of the spine of the twelfth thoracic vertebra.

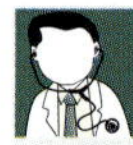

## CLINICAL CORRELATION

1. From a clinical point of view, it is important to know the relationship of the pleura to the surface of the body. This has been described above.
2. The visceral pleura is supplied by autonomic nerves (that reach it through the lung). It is relatively insensitive to pain.
3. In contrast, the parietal pleura is supplied by cerebrospinal nerves (intercostal, phrenic) and is very sensitive to pain.
   a. The lower part of the costal pleura is supplied by the lower intercostal nerves. We have seen that these nerves pass into the abdominal wall and supply skin and muscles there.
   b. Because of this fact pain arising from the lower part of the costal pleura (in pleurisy or pneumonia) can be referred to the front of the abdomen.
4. Inflammation of the pleura is referred to as ***pleurisy*** or ***pleuritis***.
   a. Pleurisy may be dry or may be accompanied by effusion of fluid into the pleural cavity.
   b. In dry pleurisy the pleura is covered by a fibrinoid exudate which makes it rough.
   c. During respiration the two layers of pleura rub against each other resulting in pain.
   d. The friction produces a sound (***pleural rub***) that can be heard through a stethoscope.
5. We have seen that normally the pleural cavity is a potential space containing a thin film of serous fluid that separates visceral and parietal pleura. Fluid or air can accumulate in the pleural cavity.
   a. Presence of air in the pleural cavity is called ***pneumothorax***.
   b. Presence of serous fluid is referred to as ***pleural effusion***.
   c. Presence of blood in the pleural cavity is called ***haemothorax***.
   d. Presence of pus is called ***empyema***.
   e. If the thoracic duct is injured, lymph may enter the pleural cavity (***chylothorax***).
6. ***Pneumothorax*** can be caused by injury to the thoracic wall resulting in entry of air from the outside (***traumatic pneumothorax***), or as a result of injury to a lung.
   a. Sometimes, there appears to be no obvious cause (***spontaneous pneumothorax***). In these cases leakage of air from lungs can result from rupture of cysts, or other lesions of various kinds.
   b. It is often associated with pulmonary tuberculosis.
   c. The presence of sufficient amount of air in the pleural cavity leads to ***pulmonary collapse***.
7. ***Haemothorax*** can follow injury or can occur after thoracic surgery. It is also seen in malignancy and any other cause leading to leakage of blood.

8. ***Pleural effusion*** (collection of fluid) can occur from various causes.
   a. In ***disturbances of osmotic*** or ***hydrostatic pressure*** the fluid is a transudate having a low protein content.
   b. In ***inflammatory lesions,*** the fluid is an exudate (and has a protein content of more than 3g/100 ml).
   c. Pleural effusions may also occur in malignancy, and in these cases the fluid is often blood stained.
   d. Pleural fluid collects in the lowest part of the pleural cavity because of gravity. Its presence can be determined by physical examination, by taking a skiagram, or by aspiration of fluid. The etiology can be established by chemical and bacteriological examination of the fluid.
9. ***Empyema,*** or collection of pus in the pleural cavity, is usually secondary to infection in the lung. It can, however, be caused by spread of infection from any site in the vicinity. Some sources of infection are:
   a. Chest wounds
   b. Postoperative infection
   c. Rupture of the oesophagus
   d. Subphrenic abscesses (collection of pus below the diaphragm).
10. Presence of fluid, blood, or pus in the pleural cavity can occur along with presence of air. These conditions are defined as ***hydropneumothorax, haemopneumothorax,*** and ***pyopneumothorax*** respectively.
11. The interior of the pleural cavity can be visualised by an instrument called a ***thoracoscope***. It is inserted through an incision in an intercostal space. The procedure is called ***thoracoscopy***. It can be diagnostic and some minor procedures can be carried out through the opening.
12. Fluid can be removed from the pleural cavity by inserting a needle through an intercostal space (***paracentesis thoracis***). The position of the needle has to be adjusted to avoid injury to blood vessels.

## Surface Projection of the Lung

1. In visualising the surface projection of the lung it may be remembered that as the lungs are surrounded by pleura, the limits of the lung must always lie within the boundaries of the pleura, already defined.
2. In some situations, the boundaries are the same as that for the pleura, but in other situations the lungs fall short of the pleura.
3. This is most evident near the costodiaphragmatic reflection of the pleura, where the costal and diaphragmatic pleura are separated by a potential space called the ***costodiaphragmatic recess*** (19.11, 19.24 and 19.25).
4. A similar space called the ***costomediastinal recess*** is present in relation to the anterior border of the left lung (19.24).
5. It may also be remembered that the limits of the lung described below represent the position in quiet respiration. In deep inspiration, the lungs extend much deeper into the costodiaphragmatic and costomediastinal recesses.
6. The outline of the apex of the lung corresponds to that of the cervical pleura.
7. The anterior border of the right lung corresponds to the costomediastinal reflection of the pleura already described.
   a. In the left lung the upper part of the anterior border (up to the fourth costal cartilage) follows the pleura, but below this level the border falls considerably short of the pleura because of the presence of the deep cardiac notch.
   b. From the midline (at the level of the fourth costal cartilage) the border passes sharply to the left and downwards so that at the level of the fifth costal cartilage it is about 3.5 cm lateral to the sternal margin (or to the line for the pleura).

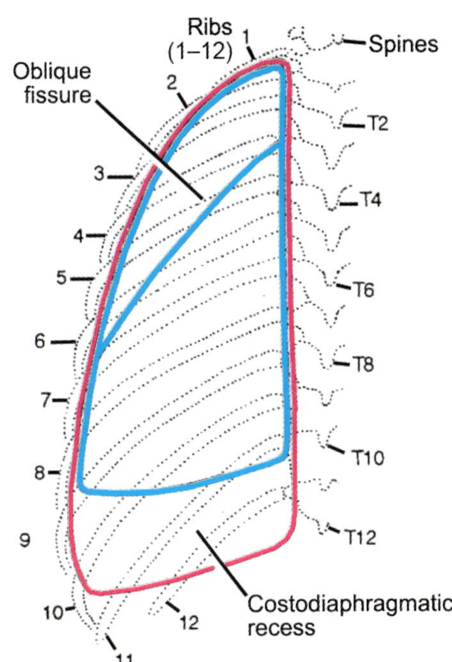


**19.25:** Projection of the pleura (red line) and lung (blue line) on the back of the thorax. The projection is similar on the right and left sides

c. It then curves downwards and medially to reach the sixth costal cartilage a short distance lateral to the line for the pleura (i.e., about 4 cm from the midline).

8. The inferior border of the lung follows a curved line lying above that for the costodiaphragmatic reflection of the pleura.
   a. On each side the line representing this border begins (anteriorly) at the lower end of the anterior border (described above).
   b. In the midaxillary line it lies over the eighth rib. Its posterior end lies at the level of the tenth thoracic spine (2 cm lateral to the midline).
   c. Note that there is a difference of two ribs in the levels of the lung and pleura over both these lines.
9. The posterior border of the lung lies 2 cm from the midline. It extends below to the level of the tenth thoracic spine and above to the level of the second thoracic spine.
10. When seen from behind the apex of the lung lies at level of the first spine about 5 cm from the midline.
11. The position of the fissures of the lungs, relative to the surface of the body are shown in 19.24 and 19.25.
12. Note that on the posterior aspect the oblique fissure corresponds to the medial border of the scapula when the arm has been fully abducted.

### *Nerve Supply of Pleura*

Note that visceral pleura is relatively insensitive to pain, but the parietal pleura is highly sensitive to pain.

### *Lymphatic Drainage of Pleura*

The parietal pleura is drained in the same way as the thoracic wall. The visceral pleura is drained by vessels that drain the lung.

The details regarding the nerve supply and lymphatic drainage of pleura have been explained in earlier chapters.

CHAPTER 20

# The Heart and Pericardium

## INTRODUCTION TO CARDIOVASCULAR SYSTEM

1. The cardiovascular system consists of the ***heart*** and ***blood vessels***. The system is responsible for the circulation of blood through the tissues of the body.
2. The heart acts as a pump and provides the force for this circulation. Blood vessels taking blood from the heart to the tissues are called ***arteries***.
3. The largest artery in the body is called the ***aorta***. Arising from the heart it divides, like the branches of a tree, into smaller and smaller branches. The smallest arteries are called ***arterioles***.
4. The arterioles end in a plexus of thin-walled vessels that permeate the tissues.
   a. These thin-walled vessels are called ***capillaries***.
   b. Oxygen, nutrition, waste products etc., can pass through the walls of capillaries from blood to tissue cells and *vice versa*.
5. In some organs, these vessels are somewhat different in structure from capillaries and are called ***sinusoids***.
6. Blood from capillaries or sinusoids is collected by another set of vessels that carry it back to the heart. These are called ***veins.***
   a. The veins adjoining the capillaries are very small and are called ***venules.***
   b. Smaller veins join together (like tributaries of a river) to form larger and larger veins.
   c. Ultimately, the blood reaches two large veins, the ***superior vena cava*** and the ***inferior vena cava***, which pour it back into the heart.
7. This blood reaching the heart through the veins has lost its oxygen.
   a. A special set of arteries and veins circulate this blood through the lungs where it is again oxygenated.
   b. This circulation through the lungs, for the purpose of oxygenation of blood, is called the ***pulmonary circulation,*** to distinguish it from the main or ***systemic circulation.***

## SOME ELEMENTARY FACTS ABOUT THE HEART

1. The heart is a muscular pump designed to ensure the circulation of blood through the tissues of the body (20.1). Both structurally and functionally, it consists of two halves namely right and left.
2. The 'right heart' circulates blood only through the lungs for the purpose of oxygenation (i.e., through the pulmonary circulation).
3. The 'left heart' circulates blood to tissues of the entire body (i.e., through the systemic circulation).
4. Each half of the heart consists of an inflow chamber called the ***atrium***, and of an outflow chamber called the ***ventricle.***
   a. The right and left atria are separated by an ***interatrial septum*** (20.2).
   b. The right and left ventricles are separated by an ***interventricular septum*** (20.2).

5.a. The right atrium opens into the right ventricle through the ***right atrioventricular orifice.*** This orifice is guarded by the ***tricuspid valve.***

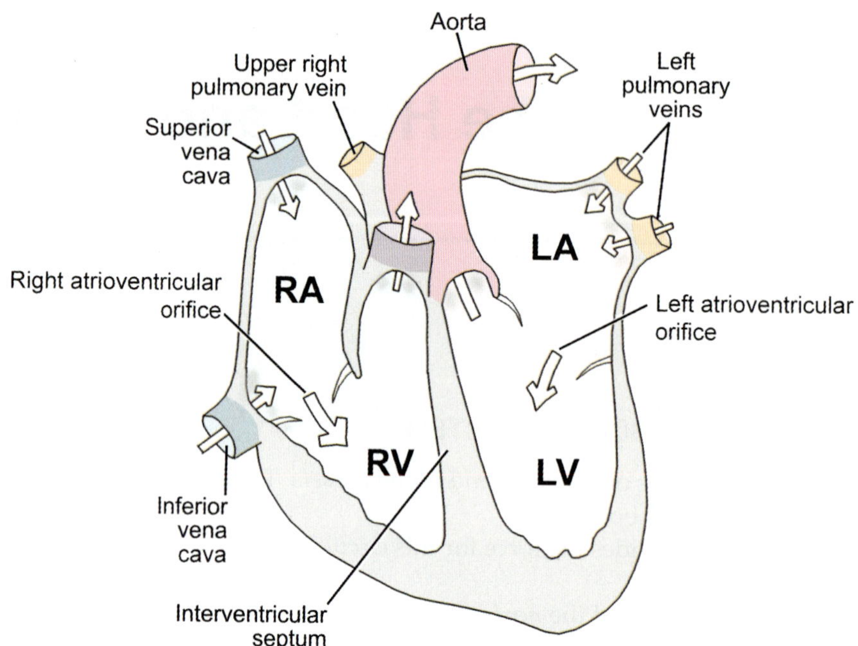


**20.1:** Schematic diagram of the heart to show its chambers and their communications

   b. The left atrium opens into the left ventricle through the ***left atrioventricular orifice.*** This orifice is guarded by the ***mitral valve.***
   c. These valves allow flow of blood from atrium to ventricle, but not in the reverse direction.
6. Each chamber of the heart is connected to one or more large blood vessels (20.1 and 20.4).
   a. The right atrium receives deoxygenated blood from tissues of the entire body through the ***superior*** and ***inferior venae cavae.***
   b. This blood passes into the right ventricle. It leaves the right ventricle through a large outflow vessel called the ***pulmonary trunk.*** This trunk divides into right and left ***pulmonary arteries*** that carry blood to the lungs.
   c. Blood oxygenated in the lungs is brought back to the heart by four ***pulmonary veins*** (two right and two left) that end in the left atrium. This blood passes into the left ventricle. The left ventricle pumps this blood into a large outflow vessel called the ***aorta***. The aorta and its branches distribute blood to tissues of the entire body.
   d. It is returned to the heart (right atrium) through the venae cavae, thus completing the circuit.

## EXTERIOR OF THE HEART

### Surfaces of the Heart

1. The heart has an anterior or sternocostal surface (20.3 and 20.4).
2. A posterior surface or base.
3. Right and left surfaces.
4. In addition to these, there is a diaphragmatic surface (20.5).
5. The ***sternocostal surface*** is shown in 20.3 and 20.4.
   a. It is made up (from right to left) by the right atrium, the right ventricle and the left ventricle. Note that the contribution of the right ventricle to this surface is much greater than that of the left ventricle.
   b. The two ventricles are separated by the ***anterior interventricular groove*** ('b' in 20.4).
   c. The right atrium and ventricle are separated by the anterior part of the ***atrioventricular groove*** ('a' in 20.4), also called the ***coronary sulcus.***

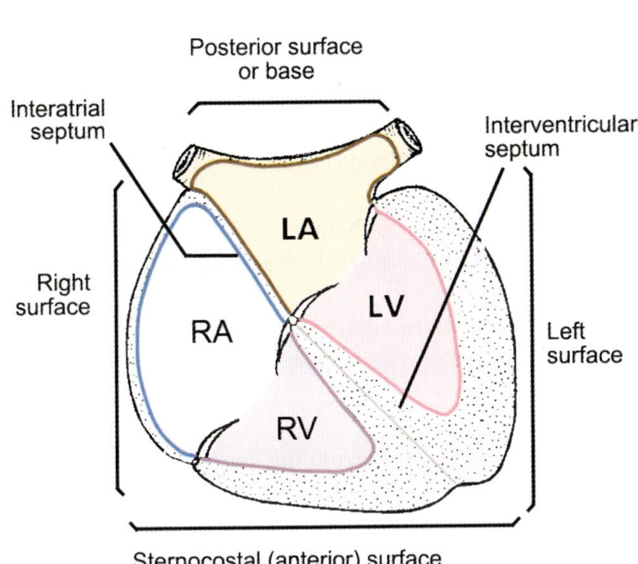


**20.2:** Schematic transverse section through the heart to show various chambers

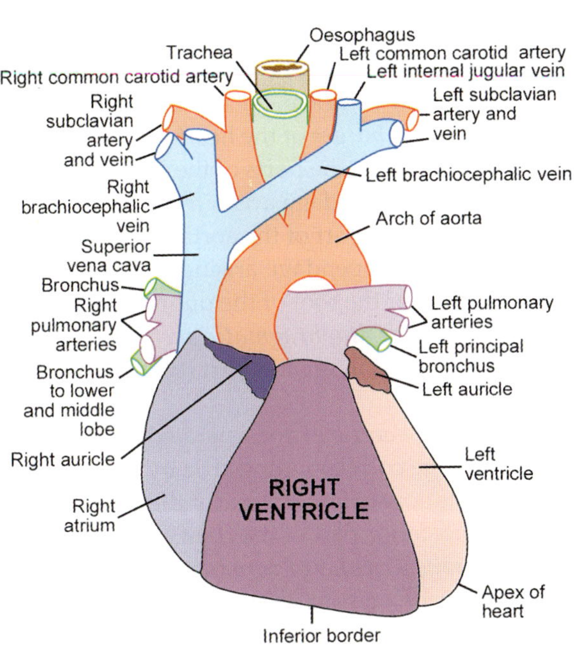


**20.3:** Heart and superior mediastinum viewed from the front

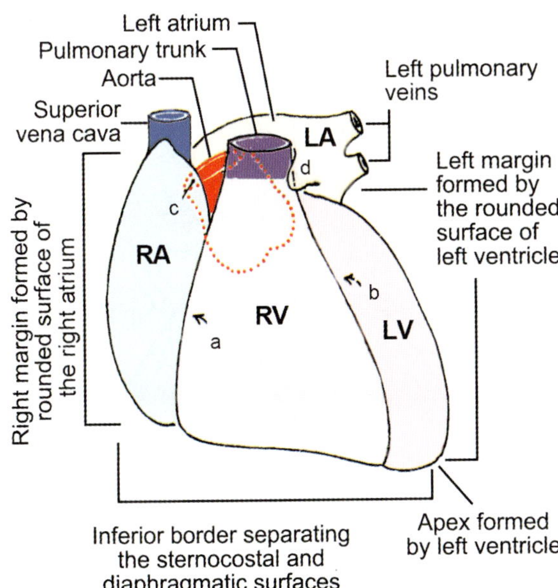


**20.4:** Sternocostal surface of the heart in which the aorta and pulmonary trunk have been cut just above their origins to show the left atrium which is hidden behind them. The outline of the root of the aorta is shown in dots

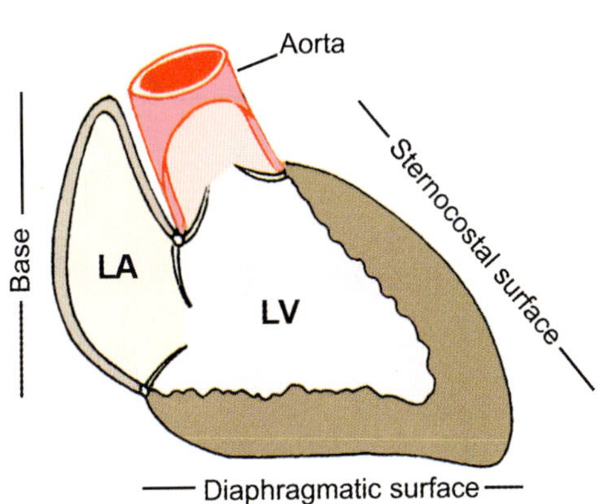


**20.5:** Schematic vertical section, in an oblique plane, passing through the left half of the heart. Note the relationship of the sternocostal and diaphragmatic surfaces to each other

   d. The sternocostal surface is bounded below by a sharp ***inferior border*** that separates it from the diaphragmatic surface.
   e. The region where the inferior border meets the left margin of the heart is called the ***apex***. The apex is formed by the left ventricle.
   f. The ***upper border*** of the heart is formed mainly by the left atrium. In the intact heart, this border is obscured from view by the parts of the aorta and the pulmonary trunk that lie in front of it.
   g. A small appendage arises from the upper and anterior part of the right atrium and overlaps the right side of the lower part of the aorta. It is called the ***auricle of the right atrium*** (20.3).
   h. A similar appendage arising from the left atrium (***auricle of the left atrium***) (20.3, 'd' in 20.4) overlaps the left side of the root of the pulmonary trunk.
6. The inferior or ***diaphragmatic surface*** is seen when the heart is viewed from below:
   a. It is formed in greater part (two-thirds) by the left ventricle, and to a lesser degree (one-third) by the right ventricle.
   b. The two ventricles are separated from each other by the ***posterior interventricular groove***. They are separated from the corresponding atria by the posterior part of the ***atrioventricular groove*** .
7. The posterior surface or base of the heart (20.6) is formed mainly by the left atrium. A small part of it is formed by the posterior part of the right atrium.
8. The ***atrioventricular*** or ***coronary sulcus***, mentioned earlier, separates the atria from the ventricles. The complete sulcus forms a circle (20.7) consisting of anterior and posterior parts.
   a. The right half of the anterior part ('a' in 20.7) is easily seen on the sternocostal surface. It runs downwards and to the right between the right atrium and the right ventricle.
   b. The part of the sulcus separating the anterior aspects of the left ventricle and atrium ('b' in 20.7) is hidden from view by the aorta and pulmonary trunk. It is shown schematically in 20.7.
   c. The posterior (or inferior) part of the sulcus lies at the junction of the diaphragmatic surface of the right ventricle with the right atrium ('c' in 20.7) and of the left ventricle with the left atrium ('d' in 20.7).
9. The ***interventricular grooves*** mark the position of attachment of the ventricular septum to the outer wall of the heart.

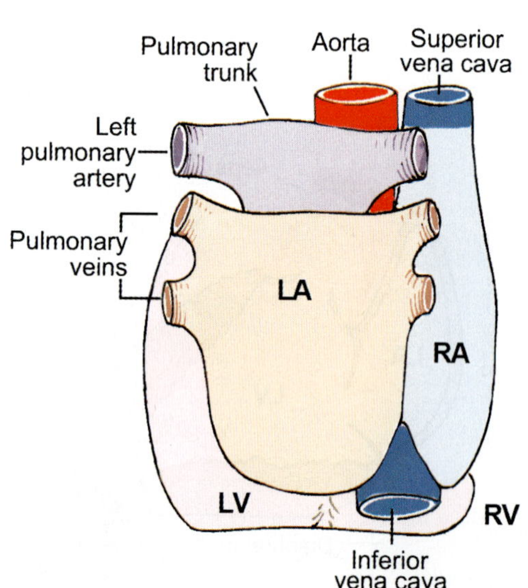


**20.6:** Heart seen from behind to show its base

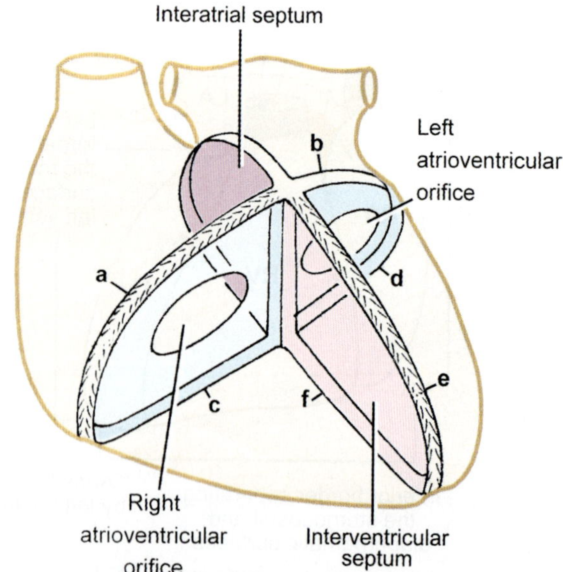


**20.7:** Schematic drawing to show the positions of the interventricular and atrioventricular junctions. The drawing is made as if the walls and septa of the heart were transparent

a. The anterior interventricular groove ('e' in 20.7) separates the right and left ventricles on the sternocostal surface.
b. The posterior (or inferior) groove ('f' in 20.7) separates the same chambers on the diaphragmatic surface.
c. As shown in 20.7, the two grooves meet each other near the apex of the heart. From here both grooves pass upwards, backwards and to the right and end by meeting the coronary sulcus.
d. Note that how the anterior and posterior parts of the coronary sulcus become continuous with each other by curving around the margins of the heart.

## INTERIOR OF THE HEART

### Interior of the Right Atrium

1. The right atrium can be divided into two main parts (20.8):
   a. The posterior part is smooth-walled and is called the ***sinus venarum***.
   b. The anterior part, or ***atrium proper*** is rough-walled.
2. In addition, the right atrium has an appendage called the ***auricle***.
   - The auricle arises from the upper and anterior part of the atrium proper, and is related to the right side of the ascending aorta (20.3 and 20.9).
3. The ***sinus venarum*** is derived, embryologically, from the sinus venosus. All the large veins entering the right atrium open into this part.
   a. The opening of the superior vena cava is situated in its upper and posterior part, and that of the inferior vena cava into its lower part, close to the interatrial septum.
   b. The opening of the inferior vena cava is bounded by a semilunar fold of endocardium called the ***valve of the inferior vena cava***.
   c. The sinus venarum presents a third opening called the coronary sinus. This opening is present just to the left of the opening of the inferior vena cava. This opening is also guarded by a valve, the ***valve of the coronary sinus***.
   d. In addition to these three major openings, there are numerous small apertures in the wall of the atrium for small veins called the ***venae cordis minimae***.

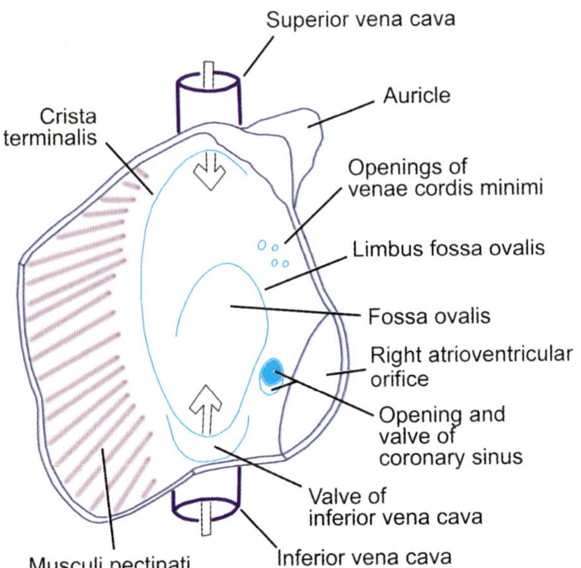


**20.8:** Right atrium viewed from the right side after cutting its wall along its upper, anterior and inferior margins, and turning the flap backwards

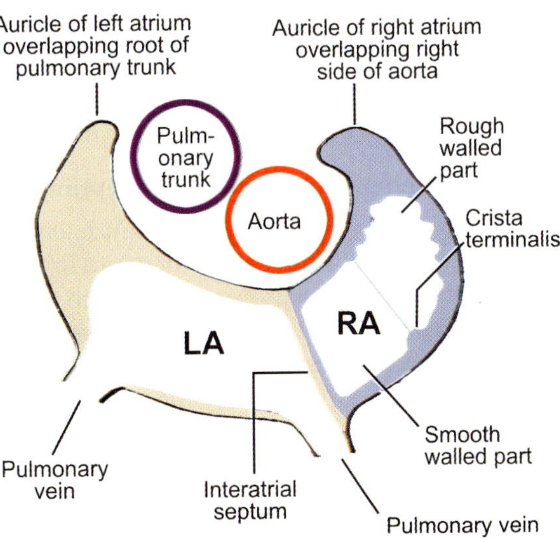


**20.9:** Transverse section through the upper parts of the atria

4. The sinus venarum and the atrium proper meet along a line that runs more or less vertically on the lateral wall of the atrium.
   a. This line is marked, on the internal surface of the atrial wall, by a muscular ridge called the ***crista terminalis***.
   b. The crista terminalis is a C-shaped ridge.
   c. It starts on the interatrial septum, passes anterior to the opening of the superior vena cava and runs along the lateral wall of the atrium to reach the opening of the inferior vena cava, where it becomes continuous with the valve of that opening.
   d. The position of the crista terminalis corresponds to a groove, the ***sulcus terminalis*** present on the external surface of the atrium.
5. The wall of the atrium proper shows the presence of a number of transversely running muscular ridges called the ***musculi pectinati***. These ridges start from the crista terminalis and run forwards. Some of them enter the auricle where they form a network.
6. The right atrium is separated from the left atrium by the interatrial septum. When viewed from within the right atrium, the septum shows some features of interest.
   a. On its lower part, there is an oval depression called the *fossa ovalis*.
   b. The upper margin of the fossa is thickened to form a curved ridge called the ***limbus fossa ovalis***.
   c. The wall of the fossa ovalis is thin and represents the embryonic ***septum primum***. The limbus fossa ovalis represents the lower curved edge of the ***septum secundum***.
7. The right atrium opens into the right ventricle through the right atrioventricular orifice which is guarded by the tricuspid valve.

### Interior of the Left Atrium

1. The left atrium is a thin walled cavity (20.9). Most of the wall is smooth. Musculi pectinati are present only in the auricle of the atrium.
2. The cavity is separated from that of the right atrium by the interatrial septum.
3. The left atrium receives four pulmonary veins, two right and two left, from the corresponding lungs. These veins open into the upper lateral part of the atrium (20.6).
4. The anteroinferior part of the atrium opens into the left ventricle through the left atrioventricular orifice which is guarded by the mitral valve.

**WANT TO KNOW MORE?**

**Summary of Development of Interatrial Septum**

1. In early embryonic life there is one atrium, one ventricle and one atrioventriclar orifice.
2. The atrioventricular orifice is divided into left and right parts by the appearance of right and left endocardial cushions that gradually grow towards each other. Their fusion forms the ***septum intermedium***.
3. The first interatrial septum to appear is the ***septum primum***. It gradually grows towards the septum intermedium. The gap between the two is the ***foramen primum***.
4. The septum primum ultimately fuses with the septum intermedium thus obliterating the foramen primum. However, before this fusion can occur the upper part of the septum primum breaks down forming the ***foramen secundum***.
5. A second septum called the ***septum secundum*** is formed to the right of the septum primum.
   a. Its growth gradually covers the foramen secundum.
   b. However an oblique passage, the foramen ovale, continues to connect the right and left atria throughout fetal life.
   c. It is obliterated after birth by fusion of the septum primum and secundum.

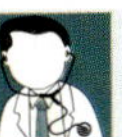

## CLINICAL CORRELATION

### Congenital Atrial Septal Defects

1. Because of the fact that the interatrial septum has a complicated developmental history, defects of the septum are common. They lead to abnormal flow of blood from the left atrium to the right atrium. (The effects are that the pulmonary circulation is overloaded and the left ventricle has to work harder and undergoes hypertrophy. If untreated, the condition can end in cardiac failure).
2. The simplest condition is one in which the septum primum and septum secundum have formed normally but have failed to fuse leading to a ***patent foremen ovale*** after birth. Such a defect may be of no functional significance and the foramen may get obliterated spontaneously.
3. In the most common variety, the lower part of the septum secundum is not properly formed leading to a central defect in the interatrial septum. This is referred to as ***septum secundum defect***.
4. In a ***septum primum defect***, the lower part of the septum primum fails to fuse with atrioventricular endocardial cushions. This defect is, therefore, seen in the lower part of the interatrial septum
5. A defect high up in the interatrial septum may be caused by defective incorporation of the sinus venosus into the atrium. These defects can be closed by open heart surgery.

## Interior of the Ventricles

The cavities of the right and left ventricles have some features in common and these will be considered first.

1. Each ventricle has an ***inflow part*** beginning just in front of the corresponding atrioventricular orifice, and running forwards and to the left i.e., towards the apex of the heart. The cavity then turns sharply upwards to form the ***outflow part***.
2. The inflow part of each ventricle has a rough inner surface because of the presence of numerous bundles of cardiac muscle called ***trabeculae carneae***. Some of these are in the form of muscular ridges while some are in the form of bundles that are free all around in the middle part and are continuous with the wall only at their ends.
3. In addition to the trabeculae carneae, the wall gives off finger-like processes attached to the ventricular wall at one end, but free at the other. These are called ***papillary muscles***. They are functionally related to the atrioventricular valves and will be considered with them.
4. In contrast to the rough walls of the inflow parts, the outflow parts of the two ventricles are smooth.
5. The outflow part of the right ventricle is called the ***infundibulum***. Its upper end becomes continuous with the pulmonary trunk, the two being separated by the pulmonary valve.
6. The inflow and outflow parts make an angle of about ninety degrees with each other. The upper part of their junction is marked by a prominent bulging of myocardium called the ***supraventricular crest***.
7. The outflow part of the left ventricle is called the ***aortic vestibule***. It becomes continuous with the ascending aorta, the two being separated by the aortic valve.
8. The aortic vestibule forms an acute angle with the inflow part, running sharply upwards and to the right to reach the aortic orifice. It crosses behind the infundibulum from left to right. This explains how the aortic orifice comes to lie to the right of the pulmonary orifice.
9. When we study a cross section across the lower parts of the two ventricles (20.10) we find that the walls of the left ventricle are much thicker than those of the right ventricle.
   a. The outline of the left ventricle is roughly circular.
   b. In contrast, the cavity of the right ventricle is crescentic in outline.
   c. This is because of the fact that the interventricular septum bulges into the right ventricle so that its right surface is convex, and its left surface is concave.

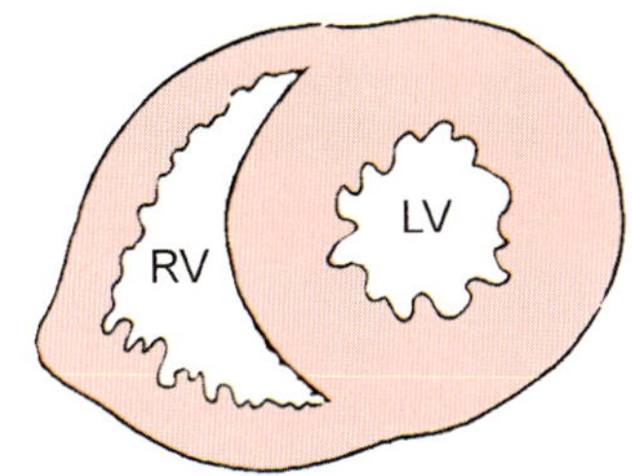


**20.10:** Transverse section across the ventricles near the apex of the heart. Note differences in thickness of wall and in shape of cavity

## Atrioventricular Orifices

1. The right and left atrioventricular orifices are oval apertures.
   a. The orientation of the apertures relative to the chambers of the heart is shown in 20.7. Note that the openings lie in a plane that is almost vertical, with a slight downward inclination. Each opening is directed forwards, to the left, and slightly downwards.
   b. Each orifice is strengthened by the presence of a variable amount of fibrous tissue around it.
   c. It is guarded by a valve which allows flow of blood from atrium to ventricle, but not in the reverse direction. The valves are made up of thin leaflets of tissue called ***cusps*** (20.11).
   d. Each cusp consists of a double fold of endocardium within which there is some fibrous tissue. It has a ventricular surface and an atrial surface. In addition, each cusp has a base which is attached to the ring of fibrous tissue around the atrioventricular orifice. It also has an apex and free margins.
   e. The margins of adjoining cusps may be fused to each other for some distance so that the cusps may in effect form a continuous membrane. The apex and margins of the cusps give attachment to delicate tendinous strands called the ***chordae tendinae***.
   f. The chordae tendinae are also attached to the ventricular surfaces of the cusps which are, therefore, rough in contrast to the atrial surfaces which are smooth. At their other end, the chordae tendinae are attached to the apices of papillary muscles.
   g. Each papillary muscle is attached (through chordae tendinae) to adjoining parts of two cusps (20.11). As a result, the adjoining margins of the two cusps are drawn together when the papillary muscle contracts.

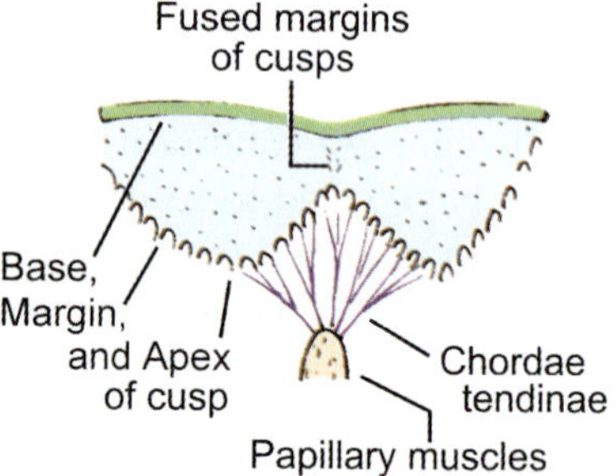


**20.11:** Schematic surface view to show the relationship of cusps to the atrioventricular ring, the chordae tendinae and a papillary muscle

2. Having considered the features common to the right and left atrioventricular orifices, we will now consider the features peculiar to each orifice.
3. The right orifice is larger than the left. The right orifice is said to be large enough to admit the tips of three fingers. In contrast, the left orifice is said to admit only two fingers.
4. Other differences between the right and left sides pertain to the arrangement of cusps and papillary muscles and these are considered below.

## The Tricuspid Valve

1. As its name implies, this valve is made up of three cusps. These cusps have traditionally been designated as ***anterior, posterior*** and ***septal*** (20.12).
2. The septal cusp is attached to the medial margin.
3. The 'anterior' cusp is attached to the superolateral part of the margin.
4. The 'posterior' cusp is attached to the inferolateral part of the margin. The anterior cusp separates the inflow part of the right ventricle from the infundibulum.
5. The chordae tendinae attached to these cusps arise from:
   a. A large anterior papillary muscle.
   b. A large posterior papillary muscle.
   c. Directly from the interventricular septum or from small papillary muscles attached to the septum (20.12 and 20.13).
6. The chordae tendinae arising from the anterior papillary muscle are attached to the anterior and posterior cusps; those from the posterior muscle to the posterior and septal cusps; and those from the septal muscles to the anterior and septal cusps (20.12).
7. The base of the anterior muscle is attached to the sternocostal wall of the right ventricle.

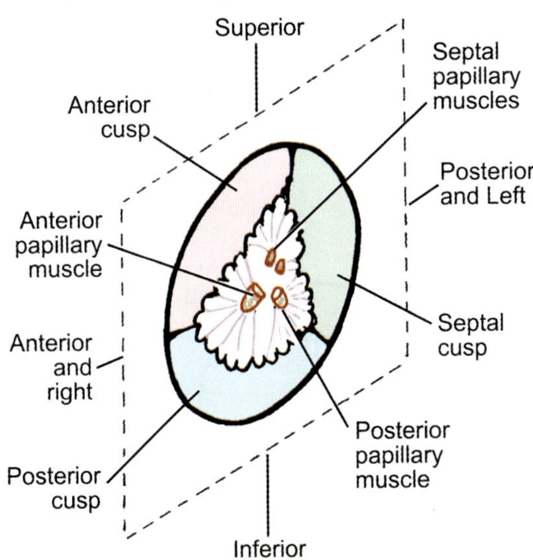


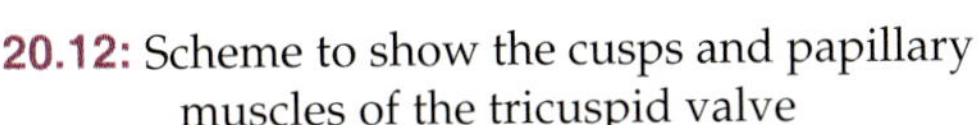
**20.12:** Scheme to show the cusps and papillary muscles of the tricuspid valve

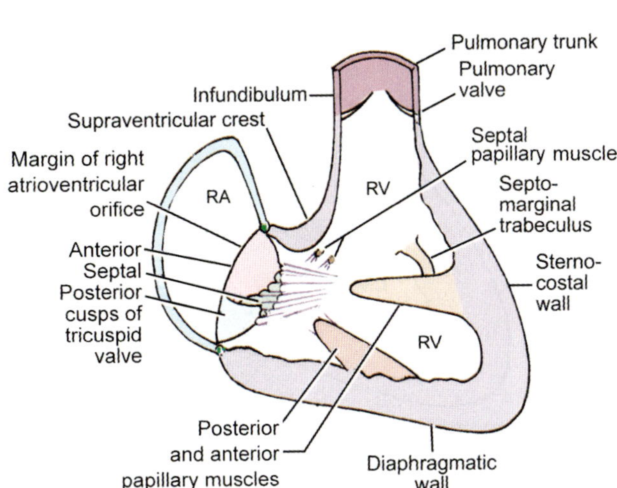


**20.13:** Schematic diagram to show the main features in the interior of the right ventricle

8. The base of the posterior muscle is attached near the angle between the diaphragmatic wall and the interventricular septum.
9. We have already seen that the septal papillary muscles are attached to the interventricular septum.
10. The base of the anterior papillary muscle is connected to the interventricular septum by a special band of cardiac muscle called the ***septomarginal trabecula*** (also called the ***moderator band***).

## The Mitral Valve

1. The mitral valve has the same basic features as those of the tricuspid valve.
2. It has two cusps namely ***anterior*** and ***posterior*** (20.15).
   a. The 'anterior' cusp (which is larger than the posterior cusp) is attached on the upper-right part of the margin of the left AV orifice.
   b. The 'posterior' cusp is attached to the lower-left part.
3. The anterior cusp intervenes between the mitral and aortic orifices (20.14).
   a. As a result, there is forceful blood flow along both surfaces (atrial and ventricular) of this cusp.
   b. In keeping with this fact both surfaces of this cusp are smooth, nearly all the chordae tendinae being attached at or near the margin of the cusp (and not on the ventricular surface as in the posterior cusp, or in the cusps of the tricuspid valve).
4. The papillary muscles connected to the cusps of the mitral valve are also termed anterior and posterior ('a' and 'p' respectively in 20.15).
   a. The anterior muscle arises from the sternocostal wall of the ventricle near its lower end (20.14).
   b. The posterior muscle arises from the diaphragmatic wall near its anterior end.
5. The origins of the two papillary muscles are close together.
   a. The two muscles run backwards almost parallel to each other and the 'anterior' muscle being placed to the left of and slightly above the 'posterior' muscle.
   b. The chordae tendinae arising from each papillary muscle pass to adjoining parts of the two cusps of the mitral valve.
   c. Those of the anterior muscle pass to the left half of each cusp and those of the posterior muscle to the right half.

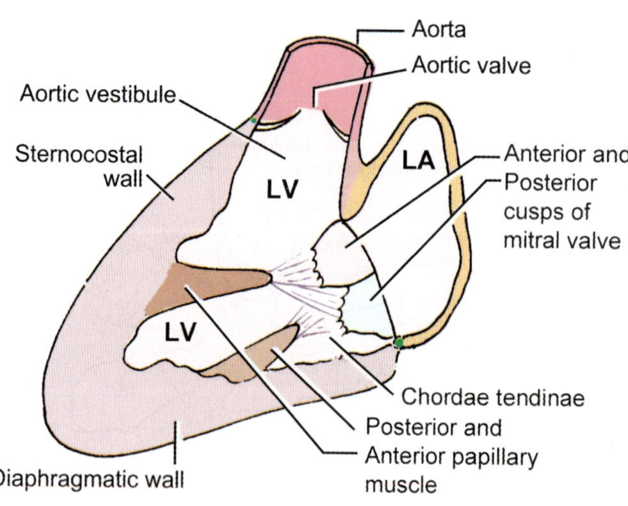


**20.14:** Schematic diagram to show the main features in the interior of the left ventricle

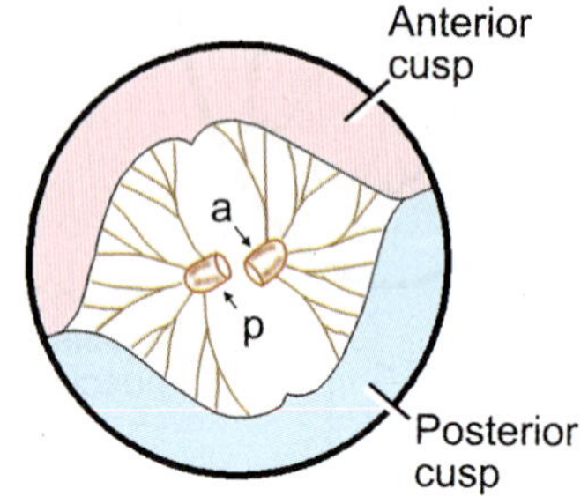


**20.15:** Scheme to show the cusps and papillary muscles of the mitral valve

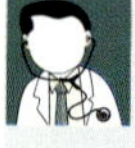

## CLINICAL CORRELATION

### Endocarditis

1. Inflammation of the endocardium is referred to as ***endocarditis***, and that of the myocardium as ***myocarditis***.
2. Bacterial endocarditis often follows rheumatic infection in childhood and can damage cusps of valves. Most frequently it affects the mitral and aortic valves.

### Mitral Valve Disease

1. As a result of infection, and of subsequent fibrosis, the cusps become thickened with reduced mobility, and often fuse with each other.
2. This leads to a narrowed mitral orifice (***mitral stenosis***).
   a. Blood flow from left atrium to left ventricle is reduced and requires greater force.
   b. Mitral stenosis is often combined with regurgitation (some blood flowing back from ventricle to atrium).
   c. All this adds greatly to load on the left atrium leading to its dilatation.
   d. Back pressure leads to pulmonary hypertension.
   e. In an effort to push blood through the pulmonary circulation, the right side of the heart has to work harder and eventually there is right heart failure.
3. Surgical correction of mitral stenosis is one of the most common operations on the heart.
   a. Initially most of the cases underwent closed mitral valvulotomy, but at present open surgery is favoured as it allows scope for repair of the valve.
   b. In some cases, the diseased valve may be replaced by an artificial one.

## Aortic and Pulmonary Orifices

1. These orifices are located at the upper ends of the outflow parts of the left and right ventricles respectively. Each orifice is circular.
2. The pulmonary orifice is somewhat larger than the aortic orifice, the diameters of the orifices being about 3 cm and 2.5 cm respectively.

3. The aortic orifice is placed in front and to the right of the mitral orifice.
4. The pulmonary orifice is placed above and to the left of the tricuspid orifice, the aortic orifice intervening between them.
5. The aortic orifice is guarded by the ***aortic valve***, and the pulmonary orifice by the ***pulmonary valve***.
6. Each valve consists of three semilunar cusps.
   a. Each cusp is roughly triangular.
   b. It has a convex edge that is attached to a part of the margin of the orifice.
   c. It also has two free margins that meet at the apex of the cusp.
   d. Each cusp consists of a double fold of endocardium with some fibrous tissue enclosed in it.
   e. The region of the apex is thickened to form a ***nodule***, while crescentic parts near the free edges, called the ***lunules***, contain very little connective tissue.
7. It is important to note the position of the three cusps of the pulmonary and aortic valves.
   a. In the fetus (20.16A), the pulmonary valve lies directly in front of the aortic valve.
   b. It has one anterior cusp ('a' in 20.16), and two posterior cusps ('b' and 'c' in 20.16).
   c. The aortic valve has two anterior cusps ('d' and 'e' in 20.16) and one posterior cusp ('f' in 20.16).
   d. Subsequently, the aorta and pulmonary trunk undergo a rotation so that the pulmonary orifice comes to lie somewhat to the left of the aortic orifice (20.16B).
   e. The rotation affects the position of the cusps.
   f. The pulmonary valve now has one posterior cusp ('b' in 20.16) and two anterior cusps ('a' and 'c' in 20.16) whereas the aortic valve has one anterior cusp ('e' in 20.16) and two posterior cusps ('d' and 'f' in 20.16).
   g. As an aid to memory, it may be noted that the Aorta has one Anterior cusp and that the Pulmonary trunk has one Posterior cusp.

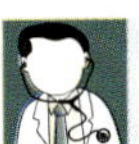

## CLINICAL CORRELATION

### Aortic and Pulmonary Valves

1. These orifices may be too narrow (stenosis) or may show regurgitation.
2. The conditions can be corrected by open heart surgery. Recently such cases have also been treated by a technique in which a cardiac catheter with a balloon is passed into the region and the valve is dilated (***percutaneous balloon valvulotomy***).

***Acquired Aortic Valve Disease***

1. As a consequence of endocarditis, the aortic valve may undergo stenosis, or may show regurgitation.
2. In either case, load on the left ventricle is greatly increased and in untreated cases, this can lead to left heart failure.
3. At present, the favoured surgical treatment is valve replacement.

## The Interventricular Septum

1. This septum separates the right and left ventricles. Its position, relative to the surfaces of the heart, corresponds to the anterior and inferior interventricular grooves (20.7).
2. From 20.10, it is seen that its right side is convex and bulges into the right ventricle.
3. From 20.7, it is seen that the right side of the septum faces forwards and to the right and that its left surface faces backwards and to the left.
4. The septum has a posterosuperior border that separates the right and left AV orifices, and is continuous with the interatrial septum (20.7).
5. The greater part of the septum is thick and muscular, but a small area near the posterior margin is membranous (20.17).

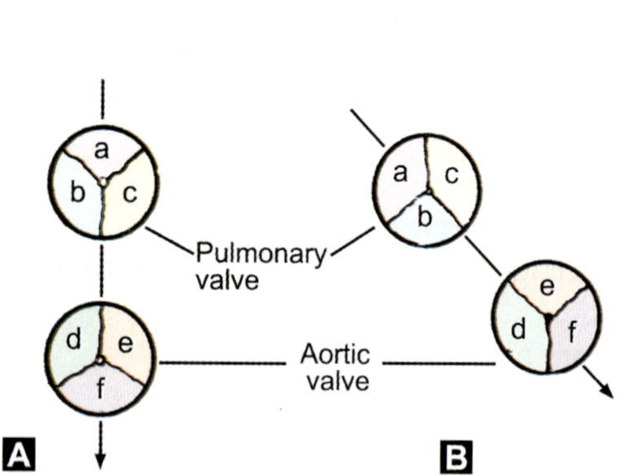


**20.16A and B:** Position of cusps of pulmonary and aortic valves A. Before rotation; B. After rotation

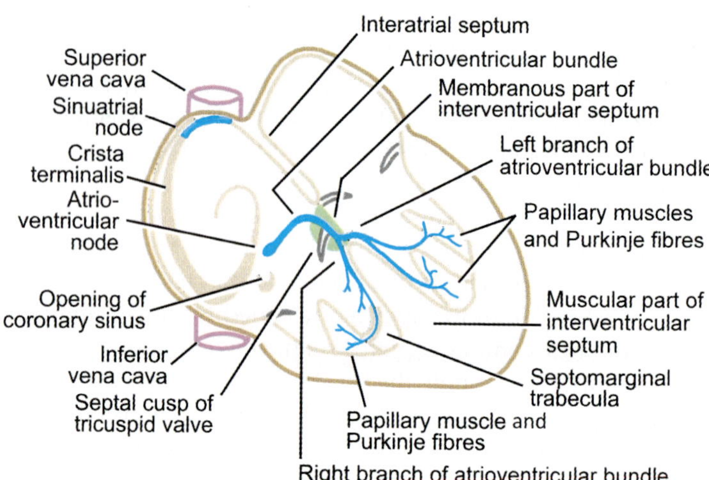


**20.17:** Schematic view of the interior of the heart to show the parts of the conducting system

6. The septal cusp of the tricuspid valve is attached vertically on this part of the septum and divides it into:
   a. An anterior part that separates the right and left ventricles.
   b. A posterior part that separates the left ventricle from the right atrium.
7. The latter part is, therefore, referred to as the ***atrioventricular septum***.

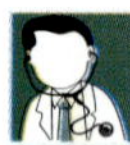

## CLINICAL CORRELATION

### Congenital Ventricular Septal Defect

1. An isolated defect of the ventricular septum is a common cardiac anomaly seen at birth. In many cases, the defects disappear by about one year of age, and some even later.
2. Most of the defects involve the membranous part of the septum which is close to the aortic and pulmonary valves. As a result, ventricular septal defects are often found in association with abnormalities of these orifices.
3. The physiological effects are those of a left-right shunt leading to excessive pressure in the pulmonary circulation (***pulmonary hypertension***), and excessive load on the left ventricle eventually leading to cardiac failure.
4. The defect can be corrected by open heart surgery.

### Fallot's Tetralogy

1. This is a congenital anomaly. The four features that make up this tetralogy are as follows:
   a. There is an interventricular septal defect.
   b. There is pulmonary stenosis.
   c. The aortic opening over-rides the free upper edge of the ventricular septum. In other words, the aorta communicates with both the right and left ventricles.
   d. There is hypertrophy of the wall of the right ventricle.
2. Surgical treatment of Fallot's tetralogy aims ideally at complete correction of all defects.
3. Shortage of this blood flow into the lungs can be increased by anastomosing the aorta or one of its branches to the pulmonary artery.
4. One common operation is that described by Blalock, in which the left subclavian artery is anastomosed with the left pulmonary artery.

## CONDUCTING SYSTEM OF THE HEART

1. For proper working of the heart, it is essential that the chambers contract in a definite sequence.
2. The rate at which the heart contracts is determined by a small area of specialised tissue called the ***sinuatrial node*** (commonly abbreviated as SA node).
3. It is located in the right atrium along the anterior margin of the opening of the superior vena cava (20.17). The greater part of the node lies in the sinus venarum part of the atrium, but anteriorly it extends into the crista terminalis.
4. Impulses originating here spread out into the atrial musculature.
5. Some of these impulses reach another node of specialised tissue called the ***atrioventricular node*** (or AV node). This node lies in the wall of the right atrium formed by the interatrial septum, just above the opening of the coronary sinus.
6. Arising from this node, there is the ***atrioventricular bundle***.
   a. This bundle passes forwards in the interatrial septum to reach the membranous part of the interventricular septum.
   b. It passes between the right side of this septum and the septal cusp of the tricuspid valve to enter the right ventricle.
   c. The bundle now divides into right and left branches.
7. The right branch runs forwards on the right side of the muscular part of the interventricular septum, towards the apex of the heart.
   a. It passes through the septomarginal trabecula to reach the base of the anterior papillary muscle.
   b. The bundle now breaks up into a plexus of the fine ***Purkinje fibres*** which spread out deep to the endocardium to reach all parts of the right ventricle.
8. The left branch of the AV bundle enters the left ventricle by piercing the interventricular part of the membranous interventricular septum.
   a. It then runs deep to the endocardium and divides into branches that reach the bases of the papillary muscles.
   b. Here, the branches end in Purkinje fibres that are distributed to the entire musculature of the left ventricle.
9. The SA node, the AV node, the atrioventricular bundle and its branches, and the Purkinje fibres, are all made up of specialised tissue that has a partial resemblance to the structure of cardiac muscle. This tissue conducts impulses faster than cardiac muscle, but slower than nerve fibres.

10.a. Impulses arising in the SA node and spreading into the atrial musculature cause the atria to contract.

10.b. These impulses reach the AV node, pass through the AV bundle and its branches to reach the ventricular muscle.

11. This conduction takes time. As a result, the contraction of the ventricles is not simultaneous with that of the atria, but follows after a definite interval.
12. Within the ventricles themselves, the papillary muscles are the first to contract (as the branches of the AV bundle reach here first). This ensures closure of the mitral and tricuspid valves before the ventricles contract.

### Blood Suppy of the Heart

This is a very important topic. It is considered in detail in Chapter 21.

### Lymphatic Drainage of the Heart

Lymphatics from the heart drain into the brachiocephalic and inferior tracheobronchial nodes. See Chapter 22.

## THE PERICARDIUM

1. The heart is surrounded by a sac called the pericardium. The pericardium has an outer fibrous layer called the ***fibrous pericardium***. Some parts of the great vessels attached to the heart are also encosed by the sac.

2. The fibrous pericardium surrounds the heart like a bag (20.18).
   a. Its upper end is continuous with the fibrous tissue covering the aorta and the pulmonary trunk.
   b. Inferiorly, it is partially fused to the central tendon of the diaphragm.
3. The inner surface of the fibrous pericardium is lined by a ***thin serous membrane***, the ***parietal serous pericardium***. A similar membrane lines the outside of the heart. This is the ***visceral serous pericardium***.
4. The aorta and pulmonary trunk are enclosed in a common tube of pericardium. They lie in front of the atria from which they are separated by a tubular recess of the pericardial cavity called the ***transverse sinus***.
5. At the venous end, the veins are arranged as shown in 20.19. As a result a pouch of the pericardial cavity comes to lie behind the heart.
6. This pouch which lies behind the left atrium is called the ***oblique sinus***. Its boundaries are formed as follows:
   a. Anteriorly by the visceral serous pericardium lining the left atrium.
   b. Posteriorly by the parietal serous pericardium lining the fibrous pericardium.
   c. Above by continuity of the parietal and visceral layers along the upper margin of the left atrium.
   d. To the left by continuity of the parietal and visceral layers along the upper and lower left pulmonary veins.
   e. To the right by continuity of these layers along the superior vena cava, the upper and lower right pulmonary veins and the inferior vena cava.
7. Note that the oblique sinus opens into the rest of the pericardial cavity below and to the left.
8. The reflections of pericardium as seen in a transverse section are shown in 20.20.

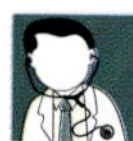

## CLINICAL CORRELATION

### Pericarditis

1. Inflammation of the pericardium is called ***pericarditis***. It may be acute or chronic. In some case, a ***pericardial rub*** may be heard on auscultation.
2. The pericardial cavity may be filled by fluid (***pericardial effusion***).
3. When the quantity of fluid is large its pressure may interfere with the filling of the heart during diastole. This is called ***cardiac tamponade***.
4. Pericardial fluid can be drained by passing a needle immediately to the left of the xiphoid process (i.e., in the angle between the xiphoid process and left costal margin). The needle is passed upwards and backwards at an angle of 45 degrees. Note that in this position the needle does not injure the pleura.
5. In ***chronic pericarditis***, which is usually due to tuberculosis, the pericardium may become very thick and may restrict movements of the heart. Surgical removal of the pericardium then becomes necessary.

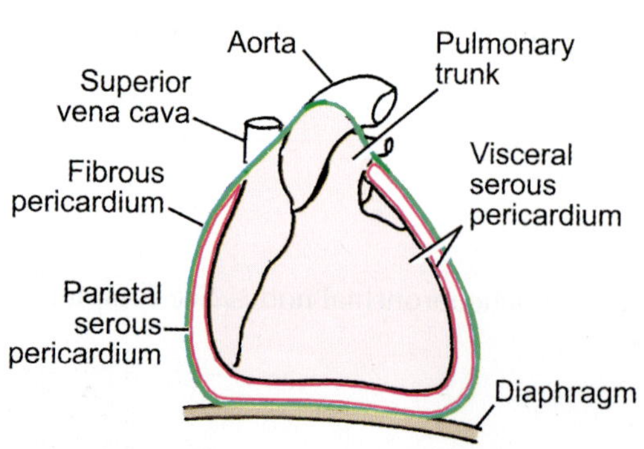


**20.18:** Diagram to show layers of pericardium

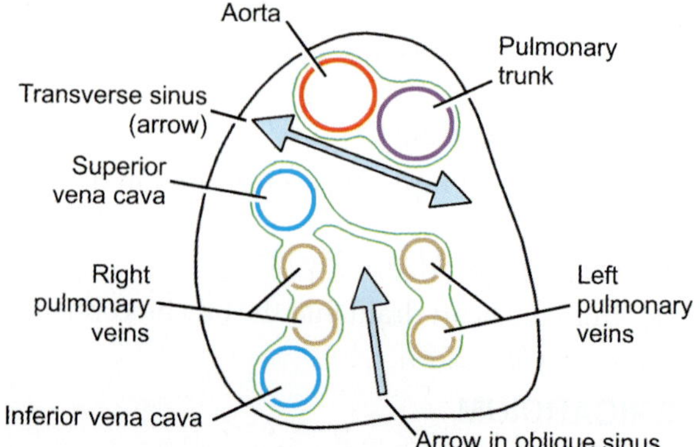


**20.19:** Schematic drawing to show the relationship of the developing heart to the pericardial sac

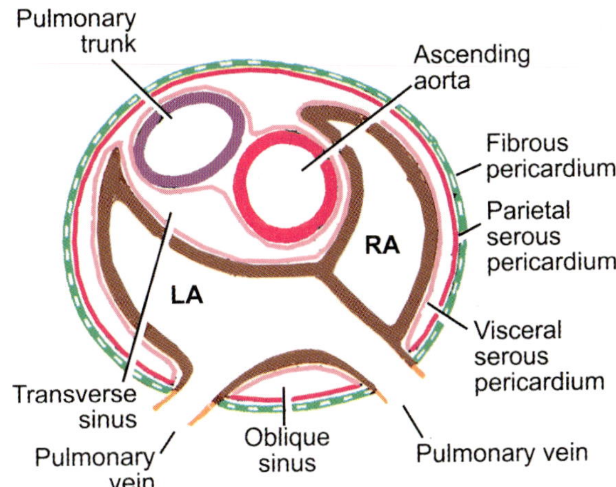


**20.20:** Schematic transverse sections through the upper part of the heart and pericardium

## SURFACE PROJECTION OF THE HEART

1. The borders of the heart can be projected on to the surface of the body by using the points A, B, C and D, shown in 20.21, as landmarks.
2. The ***right border*** can be drawn by joining points A and B by a line convex to the right, the convexity being greatest in the fourth space.
3. The ***left border*** can be drawn by joining points C and D by a line that is convex to the left.
4. The ***upper border*** can be drawn by joining points A and C.
5. The ***lower border*** is formed by joining points B and D. The line is slightly convex downwards at its right and left end, and concave downwards in the middle part. It passes through the xiphisternal joint.
6. The ***valves of the heart*** lie along a line that joins points B and C.
    a. The ***pulmonary valve*** ('p' in 20.21) is about 2.5 cm broad and lies partly behind the left third costal cartilage, and partly behind the sternum.
    b. The ***aortic valve*** ('a' in 20.21) is about 2.5 cm broad. It is placed obliquely behind the left half of the sternum at the level of the third intercostal space.

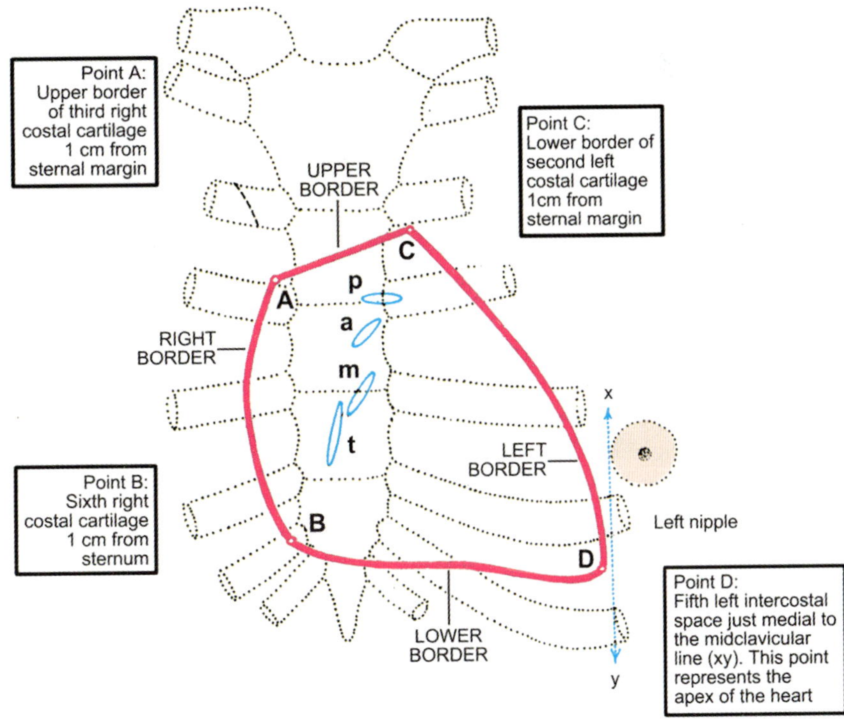


**20.21:** Surface projection of the heart

c. The ***mitral valve*** ('m' in 20.21) is about 3 cm wide. It is placed obliquely deep to the left half of the sternum at the level of the fourth costal cartilage.
d. The ***tricuspid valve*** ('t' in 20.21) is about 4 cm broad. It is placed almost vertically behind the sternum. Its upper end lies in the midline at the level of the fourth costal cartilage. Its lower part inclines slightly to the right and reaches the level of the fifth costal cartilage.

The blood vessels supplying the heart are described in Chapter 21. The nerve supply of the heart is considered in Chapter 22.

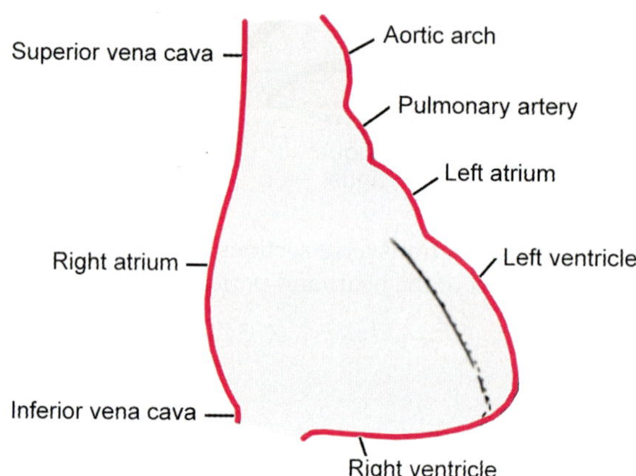


**20.22:** Outline tracing of heart shadow in a PA skiagram to show bulgings produced by some structures

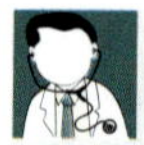

## CLINICAL CORRELATION

### The Heart and Pericardium

**Some Investigative Procedures**

1. Plain X-rays of the chest can give useful information about some parts of the heart or great vessels. In a plain skiagram of the chest, the heart and other structures produce a shadow in which several individual prominences can be recognized (20.22).
2. Along the left border of the shadow, we can see (from above downwards) prominences produced by:
   a. The aortic arch
   b. The pulmonary artery
   c. The left auricle
   d. The left ventricle
3. Along the right border of the shadow, there are (from above downwards):
   a. The superior vena cava
   b. The right atrium
4. The inferior border of the shadow is formed mainly by the right ventricle.
5. Enlargement of any of these structures can produce alterations in the appropriate part of the heart shadow.

***Cardiac Catheterisation and Angiography***

1. A fine catheter introduced into the brachial or femoral artery can be made to pass into the left side of the heart.
2. Similarly, a catheter introduced into the femoral vein can reach the right side of the heart. The procedure is done under X-ray control.

3. Cardiac catheterization is used to collect samples of blood from individual chambers for analysis.
   a. Pressures within the chambers can also be recorded.
   b. Dyes can be injected into specific parts to obtain angiograms.
   c. The coronary vessels and their branches can also be visualised (***coronary angiography***) and sites of narrowing can be determined.
4. With increasing sophistications of technique of cardiac catheterisation, some operative procedures are being done through them.

*Echocardiography*

1. Echocardiography is a technique in which the structure of the heart and its functioning can be seen on a screen using ultrasound waves.
2. By use of the Doppler principle blood flow, velocities can be measured.

**Other Investigations**

More sophisticated recent innovations in investigation of the heart include the use of magnetic resonance imaging and radioactive materials.

1. The various techniques mentioned above refer mainly to visualisation of structural defects in the heart.
2. Various other tests that cannot be considered here are used to assess cardiac function.
3. Diagnosis of disease, and planning of its treatment is dependent on overall assessment of the patient using all these methods.

**Ischaemic Heart Disease**

1. With increasing age all arteries of the body undergo atherosclerosis. As a result of this, their lumen becomes narrower. This process also takes place in the coronary arteries reducing oxygen supply to the myocardium.
2. Narrowing of coronary arteries produces no symptoms as long as enough oxygen is available to meet the requirements of the person.
3. At a later stage, the oxygen supply becomes insufficient at certain levels of activity (like exercise, or climbing stairs) and insufficient oxygen supply then leads to severe pain and a sense of constriction in the chest (***angina pectoris***).
   a. The pain is predominantly in the region of the sternum.
   b. It can radiate to the left shoulder and arm, into the neck and jaw, or to the back. It can also radiate in other directions.
4. In addition to physical narrowing of coronary arteries, angina pectoris can be produced by spasm of muscle in the walls of coronary arteries. Such spasm can be relieved by appropriate drugs that can, therefore, relieve and prevent the occurrence of angina.
5. Complete blockage of a branch of a coronary artery leads to death of the part of the myocardium supplied by that branch (***myocardial infarction***). Myocardial infarction (or heart attack in layman's language) can result in death.
6. The state of the coronary arteries can be determined by ***coronary angiography***. Sites of narrowing, or occlusion, of the arteries can be determined.
7. In suitable cases, coronary bypass surgery can enable a person with ischaemic heart disease to lead a much more normal life. Two main types of bypass are as follows:
8. In ***aortocoronary bypass***, an isolated segment of the long saphenous vein (of the patient) is used as a graft.
   a. At one end, it is connected to the ascending aorta, and the other end to a coronary artery beyond the site of obstruction.
   b. When more than one vessel is obstructed multiple grafts are used, or multiple anastomoses are made with one graft.
9. Another technique is to use the internal thoracic (internal mammary) artery.
   a. The origin of the artery from the subclavian artery is left intact.
   b. The artery itself is mobilized and its distal end anastomosed to a coronary artery (the right or left internal thoracic artery being used as appropriate).

10. In a recent technique called ***percutaneous transluminal coronary angioplasty,*** blockage in coronary arteries can be removed through cardiac catherization in suitable cases.
    a. A flexible guide wire is passed into a coronary artery and taken through the site of obstruction.
    b. A catheter with a miniature balloon is passed along the guide wire into the area of narrowing.
    c. Repeated inflation of the balloon can correct the stenosis.

**Cardiac Arrest**

1. This term is used to describe stoppage of the beating of the heart. Cardiac arrest may result from a wide range of causes.
2. A patient with cardiac arrest can be saved if immediate resuscitative measures are taken.
3. Mouth to mouth breathing, and external cardiac massage are relatively simple procedures that can be learnt even by a lay person and they can save the life of a person in cardiac arrest if used immediately.
4. In some cases in whom closed chest cardiac massage does not succeed in restarting the heart an ***open cardiac massage*** can be done by opening the thorax.

**Cardiac Transplantation**

1. In 1967, it was shown for the first time (by the surgeon Christian Barnard) that the heart of one person could be transplanted into another person.
2. In the years that have passed cardiac transplants have been done with success in many centres in the world.
3. The procedure is attempted only on persons who are likely to die in the absence of an implant (because of advanced disease that cannot be treated by other means).
4. The main problem of all transplantation surgery is that tissues of the body tend to reject any tissues that are foreign to it. The risks of rejection can be minimised by careful matching of the donor and recipient and by the use of immunosuppressive drugs.
5. From the point of view of the student of anatomy, it is easy to understand the complexity of this kind of procedure. Each of the vessels entering or leaving the heart has to be anastomosed. These include the aorta, the pulmonary trunk, the superior and inferior venae cavae, and the four pulmonary veins.

# CHAPTER 21

# Blood Vessels of the Thorax

## THE PULMONARY TRUNK AND ARTERIES

### The Pulmonary Trunk

1. The pulmonary trunk arises from the right ventricle, the junction between the two being guarded by the pulmonary valve.
2. The trunk runs upwards and backwards and ends by dividing into the right and left pulmonary arteries (21.1).
3. The lower end of the trunk lies opposite the sternal end of the left third costal cartilage.
4. Its upper end (bifurcation) lies in front of the fifth thoracic vertebra.
5. The lower part of the trunk lies in front of, and to the left of, the ascending aorta; and higher up on its left side (21.2). The two vessels are enclosed in a common sheath of serous pericardium. They are separated from the left atrium by the transverse sinus of pericardium.
6. The bifurcation of the pulmonary trunk lies below the arch of the aorta (21.1).
7. Anteriorly, the pulmonary trunk is overlapped by the left lung (21.2). Near its lower end, it is overlapped on the left side by the auricle of the left atrium.

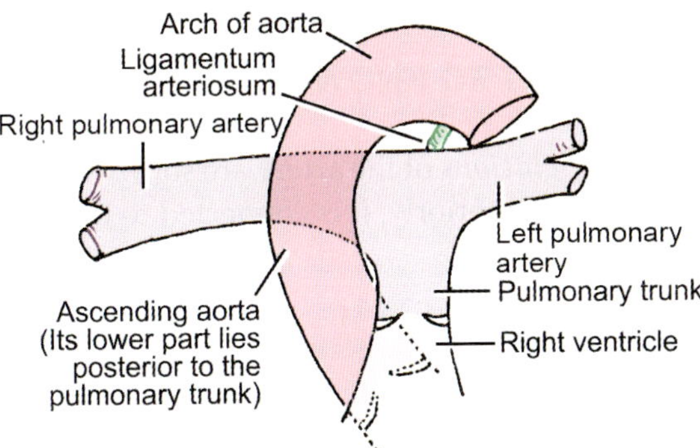


**21.1:** Diagram to show the pulmonary trunk and pulmonary arteries, and their relationship to the aorta

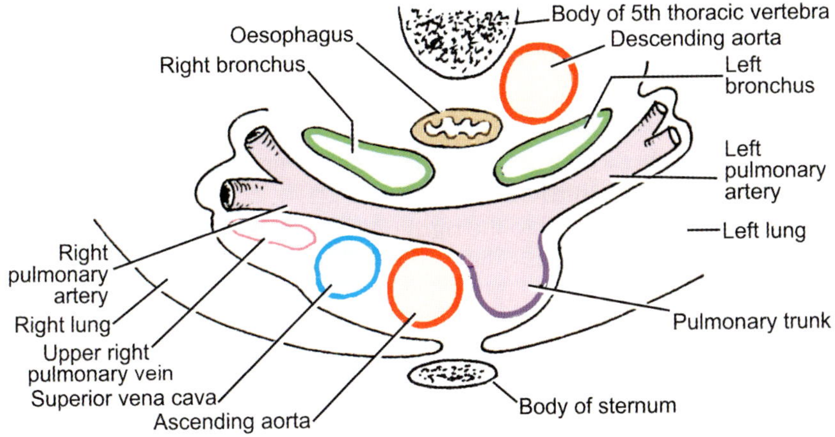


**21.2:** Diagram to show the relations of the uppermost part of the pulmonary trunk, and of the pulmonary arteries. (TS at level of vertebra T5)

### The Right Pulmonary Artery

1. The right pulmonary artery arises from the upper end of the pulmonary trunk (21.1) and runs to the right to reach the hilum of the right lung.
2. Here, it divides into two main branches. The upper branch supplies the upper lobe of the lung and the lower branch supplies the lower lobe.
3. Each of these branches subdivides to accompany the branches of the corresponding bronchi.

**WANT TO KNOW MORE?**

4. The ***relations*** of the artery are shown in 21.2. Anterior to it, there are the ascending aorta, the superior vena cava and the upper right pulmonary vein. Behind it, there are the oesophagus and the right bronchus.

### The Left Pulmonary Artery

1. The left pulmonary artery arises from the upper end of the pulmonary trunk (21.1) and runs to the left to reach the hilum of the left lung.
2. Here, it divides into two main branches that are distributed to the two lobes of the left lung.

**WANT TO KNOW MORE?**

3. The ***relations*** of the artery are shown in 21.2. It is related posteriorly to the left bronchus and to the descending aorta. Superiorly, it is connected to the arch of the aorta by the ligamentum arteriosum (21.1).

## THE AORTA

1. The heart distributes blood to the entire body through an elaborate arterial tree. The 'main stem' of this tree is called the ***aorta.***
2. The aorta arises from the left ventricle of the heart, the junction between the two being guarded by the aortic valve.
3. The aorta is the largest artery in the body. At its origin, it is about 3 cm in diameter.
4. For convenience of description, it is divided into the ***ascending aorta,*** the ***arch of the aorta*** and the ***descending aorta***.
5. The descending aorta is divisible into the ***descending thoracic aorta*** and the ***abdominal aorta*** (21.3).

### The Ascending Aorta

1. The junction of the ascending aorta ('a' in 21.3, 21.4) with the left ventricle is situated behind the left half of the body of the sternum at the level of the third intercostal space (21.4).
2. From here it passes upwards, forwards and to the right up to the junction of the body of the sternum with the manubrium sterni. The ascending aorta, thus, lies within the middle mediastinum. It is surrounded by the pericardium.
3. The following additional points may be noted:
   a. Just above the aortic valve, the wall of the ascending aorta is marked by three dilatations called the ***aortic sinuses*:** one anterior, and right and left posterior (21.9).
   b. At the junction of the ascending aorta with the arch the right wall of the vessel bulges outwards to form the ***bulb of the aorta***.
   c. The only branches of the ascending aorta are the right and left coronary arteries that supply the heart.

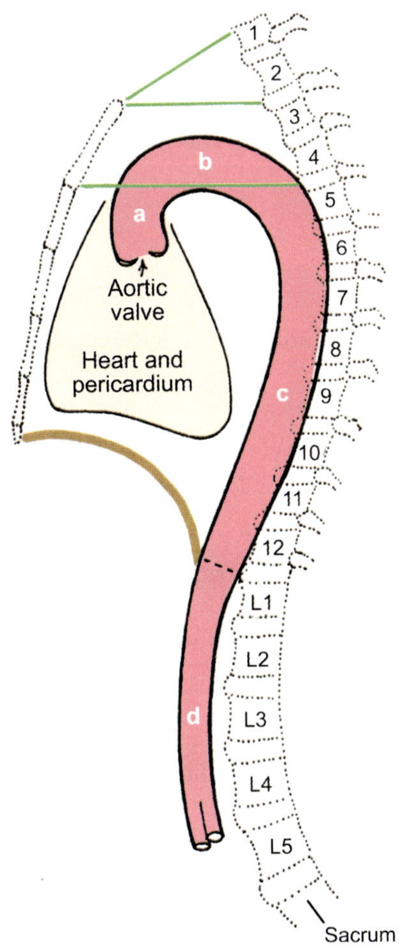


**21.3:** Scheme to show the parts of the aorta as seen from the left side

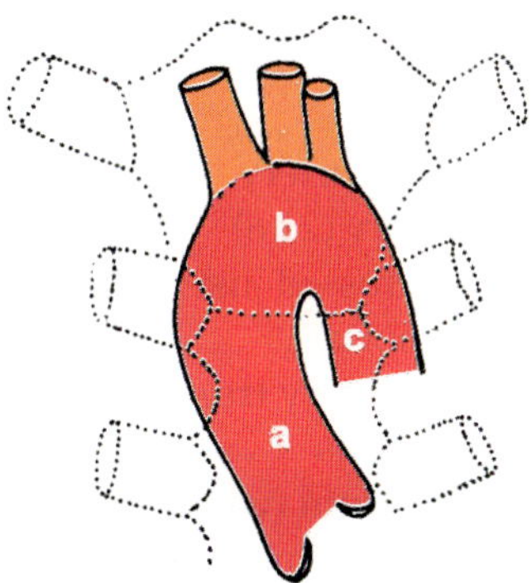


**21.4:** Relationship of ascending aorta and arch of aorta to the sternum as viewed from the front

### WANT TO KNOW MORE?

4. The relations of the ascending aorta are as follows:
   a. ***Anteriorly***, the ascending aorta is related, in its upper part to the right lung and pleura. Its middle part is related to the pulmonary trunk. The lowest part is related to the auricle of the right atrium and part of the atrium proper, and to the infundibulum of the right ventricle.
   b. ***Posteriorly***, the ascending aorta is related (in its upper part) to the right pulmonary artery and the right principal bronchus and lower down to the left atrium.
   c. ***To the right*** of the ascending aorta there is the superior vena cava, and lower down there is the right atrium.
   d. ***To the left side***, there is the pulmonary trunk and (lower down) there is part of the left atrium.

## The Arch of the Aorta

1. The arch of the aorta ('b' in 21.4) passes ***backwards and to the left*** forming a convexity directed upwards.
2. The summit of the arch reaches the level of the middle of the manubrium.
3. Its posterior end lies on the left side of the lower border of the fourth thoracic vertebra.

### WANT TO KNOW MORE?

**Relations of Arch of Aorta**

The structures related to the arch of the aorta can be divided into those that lie anteriorly and to the left, or posteriorly and to the right (21.5) and into those that are above and below it (21.6).

1. ***Anteriorly and to the Left***
   a. Left lung and pleura
   b. Left vagus and left phrenic nerves
   c. Left superior intercostal vein
   d. Smaller nerves present are the superior cervical cardiac branch of the left sympathetic trunk, and the inferior cervical cardiac branch of the left vagus nerve.
2. ***Posteriorly and to the Right*** (from behind forwards)
   a. Vertebral column
   b. Oesophagus
   c. Trachea
   d. Superior vena cava
   e. Small structures present are the thoracic duct, the left recurrent laryngeal nerve, and the deep cardiac plexus (21.5).
3. ***Above the arch*** of the aorta, there are branches arising from the arch itself which are as follows:
   a. Brachiocephalic artery
   b. Left common carotid artery
   c. Left subclavian artery (21.6)
   d. These arteries are crossed just above the arch by the left brachiocephalic vein.
4. ***Below the arch*** of the aorta
   a. Bifurcation of pulmonary trunk
   b. Left principal bronchus
   c. Ligamentum arteriosum (which connects the left pulmonary artery to the arch)
   d. Left recurrent laryngeal nerve that winds round the ligamentum arteriosum and then below the arch of the aorta to reach its right side.

## The Descending Aorta

1. The descending thoracic aorta ('c' in 21.3 and 21.4) is continuous with the lower end of the arch. It descends in front of the thoracic verterbrae gradually passing from the left side towards the median plane.
2. At the level of the lower border of the twelfth thoracic vertebra it passes through the aortic orifice of the diaphragm to enter the abdomen.
3. The descending thoracic aorta becomes continuous with the ***abdominal aorta*** ('d' in 21.3) that descends in front of the lumbar vertebrae.
4. It terminates in front of the fourth lumbar vertebra by dividing into two terminal branches called the ***common iliac arteries***.
5. The abdominal aorta will be studied in detail, when we consider the abdomen.

### WANT TO KNOW MORE?

**Relations of Descending Thoracic Aorta**

***Relationship to Vertebral Column***

1. The upper end of the descending thoracic aorta lies at the upper border of the fifth thoracic vertebra (21.7). Here, the aorta lies to the left of the vertebral column.

2. It descends gradually passing to the front of the vertebrae. Its lower end lies in front of the lower border of the twelfth thoracic vertebra.
3. The hemiazygous veins pass from left to right between the aorta and the vertebral column.

### *Relationship to the Oesophagus*

1. After passing deep to the arch of the aorta the oesophagus lies to the right of the upper end of the descending aorta.
2. The oesophagus gradually passes to the front of the aorta. Its lower end lies in front, and to the left, of the aorta (21.7).

### *Relationship to Root of Lung*

The structures comprising the root of the left lung cross in front of the upper part of the descending aorta (21.6).

### Anterior Relations

The ***anterior relations*** of the descending thoracic aorta are given below (21.8) (from above downwards).

1. The root of the left lung consisting of the left pulmonary artery (LPA), the left principal bronchus (LPB) and the left pulmonary veins (LPV).
2. The left atrium of the heart separated by the fibrous pericardium and the oblique sinus.
3. The oesophagus.
4. The diaphragm.

### *Structures to the Right Side*

1. Oesophagus (in the upper part) (21.7)
2. Vena azygous
3. Thoracic duct
4. The upper part of the aorta is separated from the right lung and pleura by the oesophagus, but its lower part is in contact with them.

### *Structures to the Left Side*

Left lung and pleura.

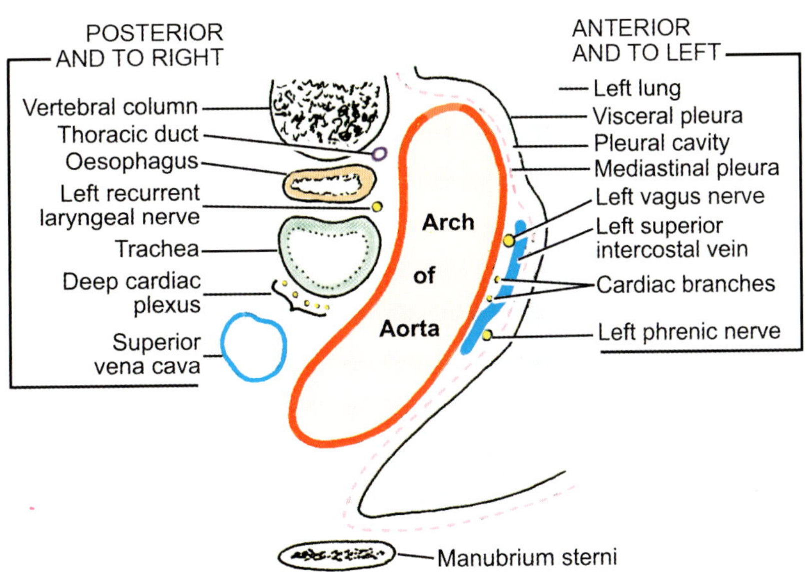


**21.5:** Transverse section through the arch of the aorta and surrounding structures

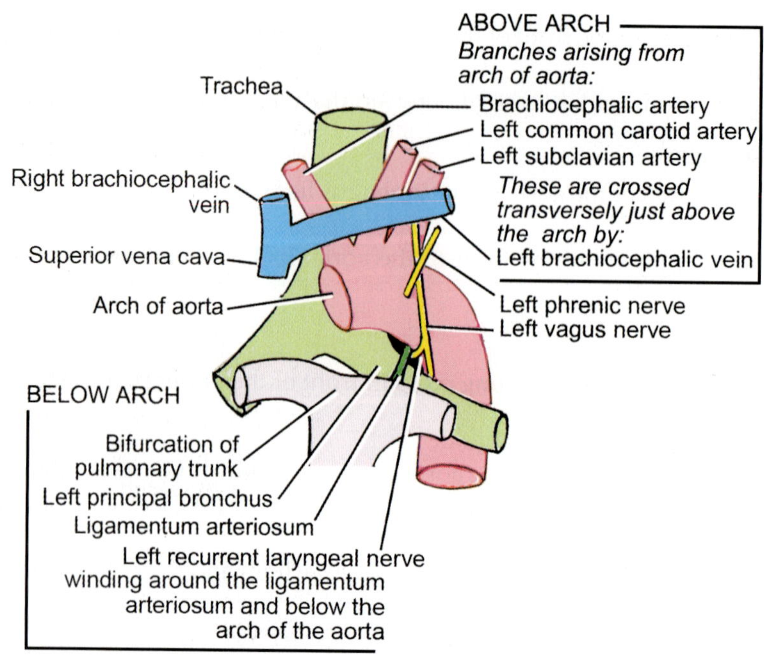


**21.6:** Diagram to show the structures above and below the arch of the aorta

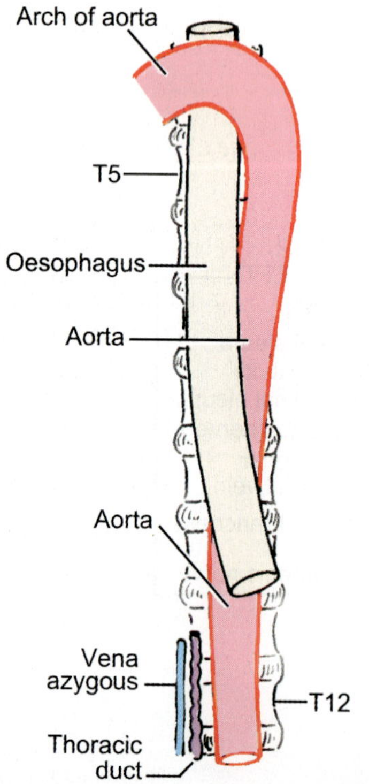


**21.7:** Diagram to show relationship of the aorta to the vertebral column and to the oesophagus

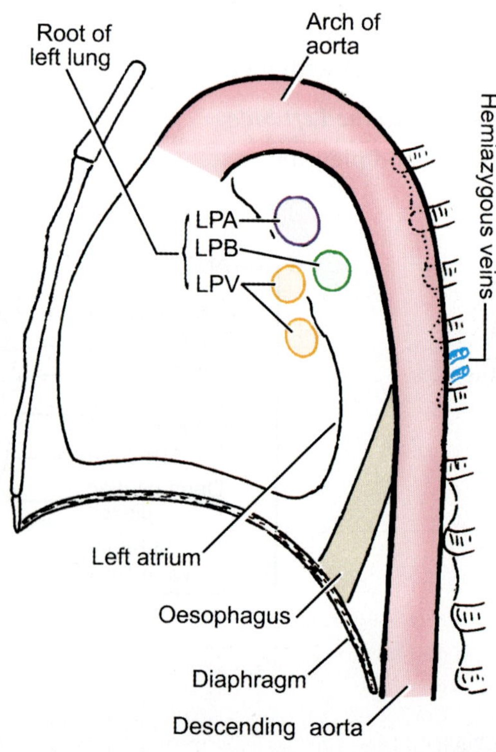


**21.8:** Schematic diagram to show some relations of the descending thoracic aorta

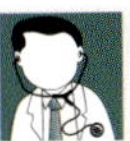

## CLINICAL CORRELATION

**Patent Ductus Arteriosus**

1. In the fetus, the ductus arteriosus connects the left pulmonary artery to the arch of the aorta just distal to the origin of the left subclavian artery.
2. Normally, the ductus is obliterated very soon after birth.
3. If the ductus remains patent after birth, blood from the aorta enters the pulmonary arteries. The effects are that:
   a. The pulmonary circulation is overloaded
   b. The left ventricle has to work harder and undergoes hypertrophy.
4. If untreated, the condition can end in cardiac failure.
5. The patent ductus can be closed surgically.

**Coarctation of the Aorta**

1. This term refers to a condition in which the aorta is abnormally narrow near the attachment of the ligamentum arteriosum.
2. Coarctation may be of two types:
   a. The ***preductal*** type is common in infants.
      i. The narrowing is proximal to the attachment of the ductus arteriosus that usually remains patent and feeds blood to the part of the aorta distal to the coarctation.
      ii. As this blood is unoxygenated the lower part of the body shows cyanosis.
   b. In the ***postductal*** variety, seen in adults, the ductus arteriosus is usually not patent.
      i. Blood reaches the distal part of the body through an elaborate collateral circulation.
      ii. Part of this collateral circulation is through the intercostal arteries. Blood enters them through the internal thoracic artery and flows backwards in them to reach the thoracic aorta.
      iii. These arteries enlarge and produce characteristic notching on ribs that can be seen in a skiagram.
3. a. When coarctation is present there is hypertension in the part of the body supplied by branches arising above the level of constriction, and hypotension in parts supplied by branches arising below the level of constriction.
   b. Hence, blood pressure recorded from the upper limbs is much higher than that recorded from the lower limbs.
4. At present, coarctation can be surgically corrected by removing the narrow segment and anastomosing the two cut ends of the aorta.

**Aortic Aneurysms**

1. A dilatation of a segment of the aorta is referred to as ***aneurysm***.
   a. The dilatation may be fusiform or may take the form of a sac attached to the main vessel.
   b. In some cases an aneurysm splits the wall of the aorta into two layers (***dissecting aneurysm***).
2. Surgical repair of aortic aneurysms is now possible. Some pressure effects of an aneurysm have been described above.
3. A physical sign called ***tracheal tug*** may sometimes be elicited when an aneurysm of the aorta is present (See Chapter19).

## BRANCHES OF AORTA

The aorta gives off a large number of branches in the thorax. These are shown in 21.9. Some of the branches are large and have a wide distribution, while others are small. They will be considered one by one in the pages that follow.

## The Coronary Arteries

1. The coronary arteries supply the blood to heart. There are two of them: right and left.
2. The importance of a knowledge of their course and branches has increased considerably in recent years as these arteries are often visualised in the living ***(coronary angiography)*** for diagnosis of possible obstruction to them (21.13).
3. The pattern of branching of the coronary arteries shows considerable variation. The description given below refers only to the most common pattern.

### *Course of Right Coronary Artery*

The ***right coronary artery*** arises from the ascending aorta, from its anterior sinus (21.9). For convenience of description, the artery may be divided into three parts.

1. The first part passes forwards for a short distance between the pulmonary trunk (to its left) and the auricle of the right atrium (to its right).
2. The second part runs downwards on the sternocostal surface of the heart between the right atrium and right ventricle (i.e., in the anterior part of the atrioventricular groove seen in 21.10).

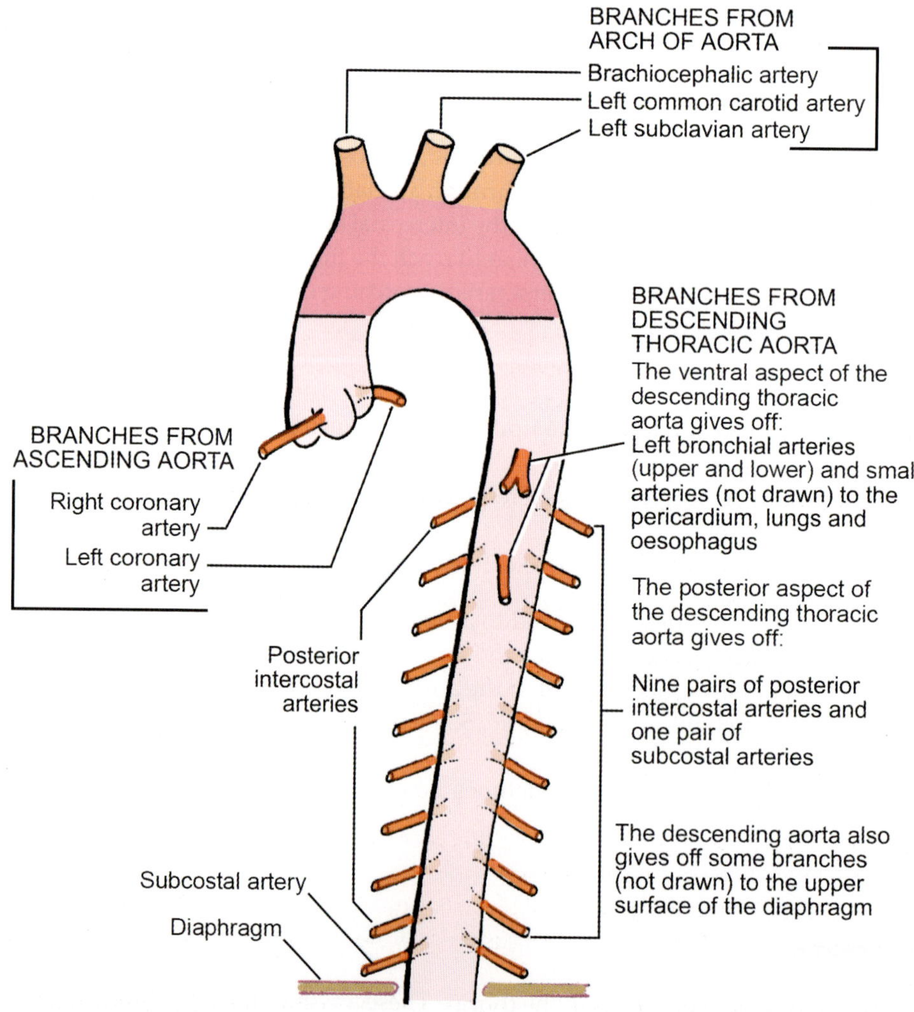


**21.9:** Scheme to show branches arising from the aorta in the thorax

3. Reaching the inferior (or acute) margin of the heart the artery curves round it to become the third part, which lies in the posterior part of the atrioventricular groove (between the right atrium and ventricle). It runs upwards and to the left and ends by anastomosing with the circumflex branch of the left coronary artery (see below).
4. Just before its termination, it gives off the ***posterior interventricular*** branch that runs downwards, forwards and to the left in the posterior interventricular groove (21.10).
5. The branches of the right coronary artery are considered here.

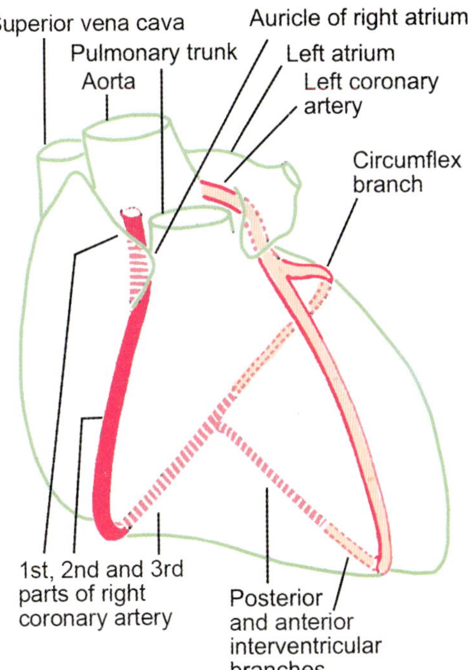


**21.10:** Schematic diagram to show the coronary arteries and their interventricular branches

### *Course of Left Coronary Artery*

1. The ***left coronary artery*** arises from the left posterior sinus of the ascending aorta (21.9).
2. It passes to the left between the pulmonary trunk and the left atrium and appears on the sternocostal surface of the heart after passing deep to the auricle of the left atrium (21.10).
3. Here, the artery divides into two main branches that are more or less equal in diameter. These are the ***circumflex*** and ***anterior interventricular*** arteries.
   a. The circumflex branch runs to the left in the anterior part of the atrioventricular groove (between the left atrium and the left ventricle, 21.10).
   b. It then curves round the left border of the heart and runs downwards and to the right in the posterior part of the same groove. It ends by anastomosing with the terminal part of the right coronary artery.
4. a. Note that the right coronary artery, and the left coronary artery along with its circumflex branch, form an arterial ring lying in the atrioventricular groove.
   b. This ring is responsible for the name 'coronary' (meaning crown).
   c. It will be obvious that the circumflex branch represents the main continuation of the left coronary artery.
5. a. The anterior interventricular branch runs downwards and to the left in the anterior interventricular groove (i.e., between the right and left ventricles).
   b. Near the apex of the heart it curves round the lower border and runs for a short distance in the posterior interventricular groove where it ends by anastomosing with the posterior interventricular branch of the right coronary artery (21.10).
6. From the foregoing description and from 21.10, the basic configuration of the coronary arteries should be clear. We can now proceed to consider the further distribution of each artery.

### *Branches of the Right Coronary Artery*

1. The first part of the artery gives off the following branches:
   a. The ***right conus artery*** is small and ramifies over the lower part of the pulmonary trunk and the upper part of the infundibulum (21.11).
   b. The ***artery of the sinoatrial node*** passes backwards between the aorta and the auricle of the right atrium to reach the superior vena cava. It gives branches that form a ring round the vena cava and descend to supply the right atrium including the sinoatrial node.
2. The second part of the artery gives off a series of branches to the right atrium (21.11), and to the anterior wall of the right ventricle. The largest of these branches runs along the lower border of the heart and is called the ***right marginal branch.***
3. The third part of the artery also gives off atrial and ventricular branches to the right atrium and to the diaphragmatic wall of the right ventricle. One of the atrial branches supplies a part of the wall of the left atrium.

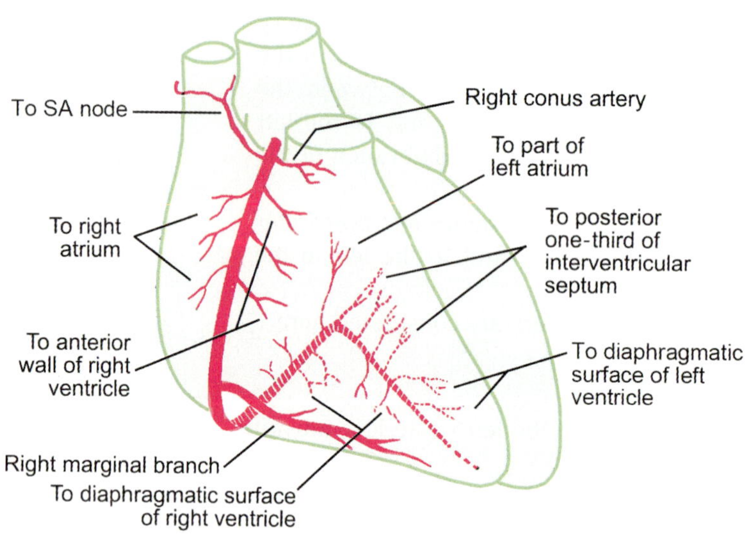


**21.11:** Scheme to show the distribution of the right coronary artery

4. The posterior interventricular branch of the right coronary artery gives off branches to the diaphragmatic wall of the right ventricle; and some to the left ventricle. Some branches run upwards and forwards into the posterior one-third of the interventricular septum.

### *Branches of the Left Coronary Artery*

1. The ***anterior interventricular branch*** gives off several large branches to the anterior wall of the left ventricle (21.12).
2. One of these is specially prominent and runs downwards and to the left between the anterior interventricular and circumflex arteries. It is called the ***diagonal*** branch. Sometimes the diagonal branch arises directly from the trunk of the left coronary artery.
3. The anterior interventricular branch also gives off a few small branches to the right ventricle. One of these ramifies on the infundibulum and is called the ***left conus artery.*** It anastomoses with the right conus artery.
4. The anterior interventricular branch also sends several branches downwards into the interventricular septum. They supply the anterior two-thirds of the septum. Some branches to the septum arise from the terminal part of the artery after it has entered the posterior interventricular groove.
5. The ***circumflex branch*** gives off several branches to the wall of the left ventricle. One of these branches is specially prominent. It is called the ***left marginal artery.*** It runs down along the rounded left margin of the heart and supplies it.
6. The circumflex artery also gives some branches to the diaphragmatic surface of the left ventricle.
7. a. Almost the whole of the left atrium is supplied by branches of the circumflex artery.
   b. One of these branches sometimes passes across the back of the left atrium to reach the SA node. When present, it replaces the branch to the node from the right coronary artery.
8. Instead of ending in the atrioventricular groove, the circumflex branch may continue into the posterior interventricular groove replacing the posterior interventricular branch of the right coronary (21.13).
9. From the foregoing descriptions of the distribution of the right and left coronary arteries, it is seen that the right atrium and ventricle are supplied mainly by the right coronary artery, and the left atrium and ventricle by the left coronary artery. However, small parts of each ventricle, and of the left atrium are supplied by the artery of the opposite side.
10. The anterior two-thirds of the interventricular septum is supplied by the left coronary artery, and its posterior one-third by the right coronary artery. The SA node, the AV node, the AV bundle and the proximal parts of its

right and left branches are supplied by the right coronary artery. The distal parts of the bundle branches are supplied by the left coronary artery.

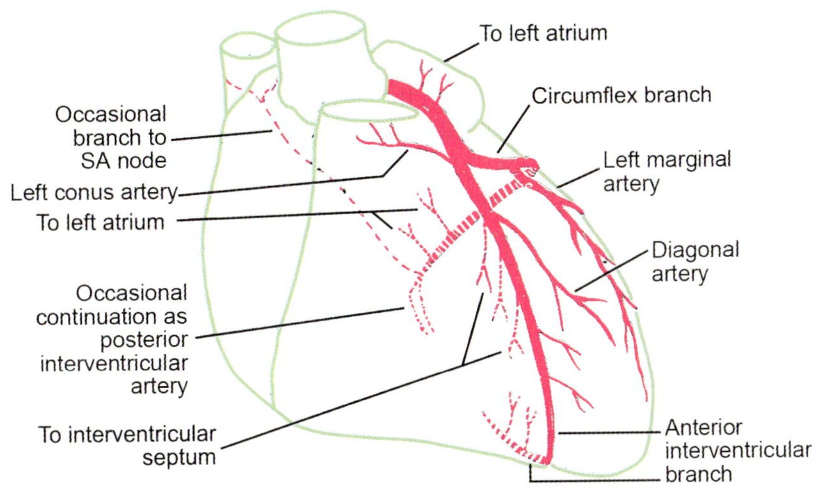


**21.12:** Scheme to show the distribution of the left coronary artery. Some small branches given by the anterior interventricular branch to the right atrium are not drawn for sake of clarity

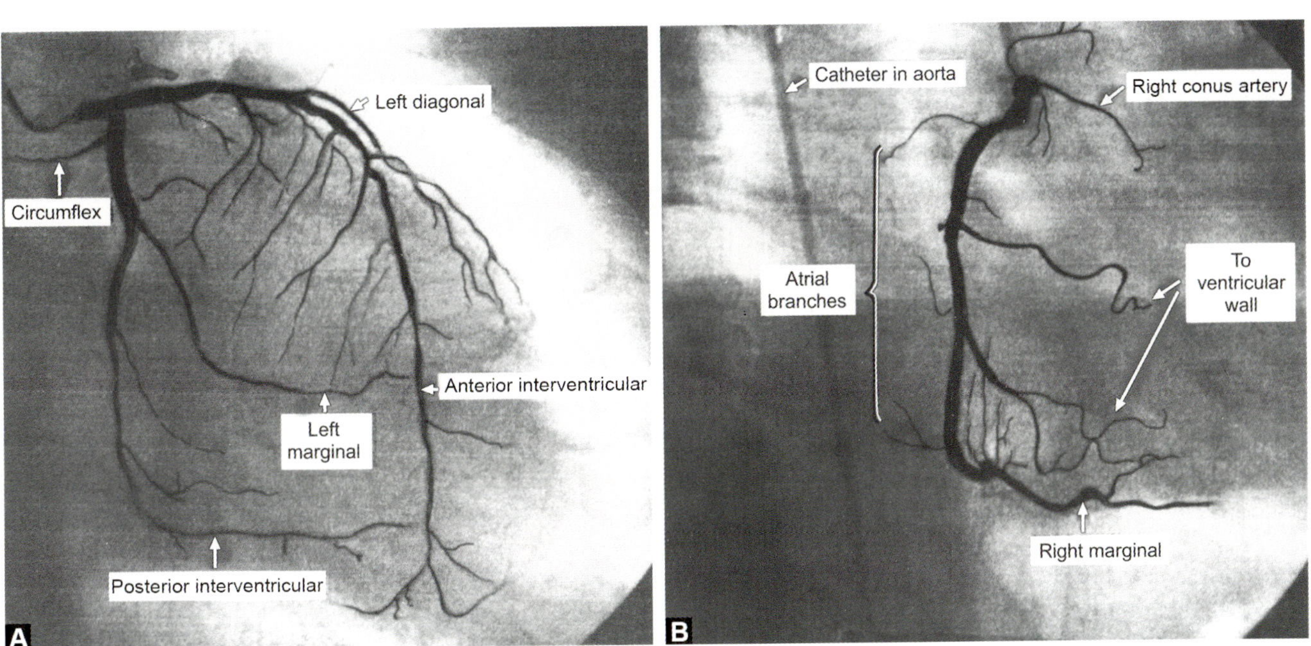


**21.13A and B:** Coronary angiography. Oblique views. A catheter is passed into the femoral artery, and upwards to reach the aorta. Its tip is then made to enter one coronary artery and a contrast medium injected. The left coronary artery and its branches are seen in A, and the right coronary artery in B. Both figures are from the same person. In this case the posterior interventricular branch is derived from the left coronary artery (instead of the more common derivation from the right coronary). Such a condition is referred to as left dominance

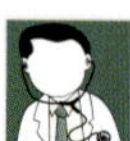

## CLINICAL CORRELATION

### Coronary Angiography

1. The coronary arteries and their branches can be visualised by coronary angiography and sites of narrowing determined (21.13).
2. In this connection, it is necessary for the student to know that the nomenclature used in clinical texts for some branches of the coronary arteries are different from those in textbooks of anatomy as follows:
   a. The anterior interventricular branch of the left coronary artery is described as the ***anterior descending branch.***
   b. The posterior interventricular branch of the right coronary artery is described as the ***posterior descending branch.***
   c. The right marginal branch of the right coronary artery is named the ***acute marginal branch.***
   d. The left marginal branch of the left coronary artery (which may be multiple) is referred to as the ***obtuse marginal branch.***

## BRANCHES OF THE ARCH OF THE AORTA

1. These are the brachiocephalic, left common carotid and left subclavian arteries. The branches of the arch of the aorta are shown in 21.14.
2. They are meant for distribution of blood to the head and neck and to the upper limbs.
3. They reach the head and neck by passing through the superior mediastinum of the thorax. Their course and relations here are important and are considered below.
4. All these arteries arise from the summit of the arch of the aorta that lies at the level of the middle of the manubrium sterni (or the disc between the third and fourth thoracic vertebrae).

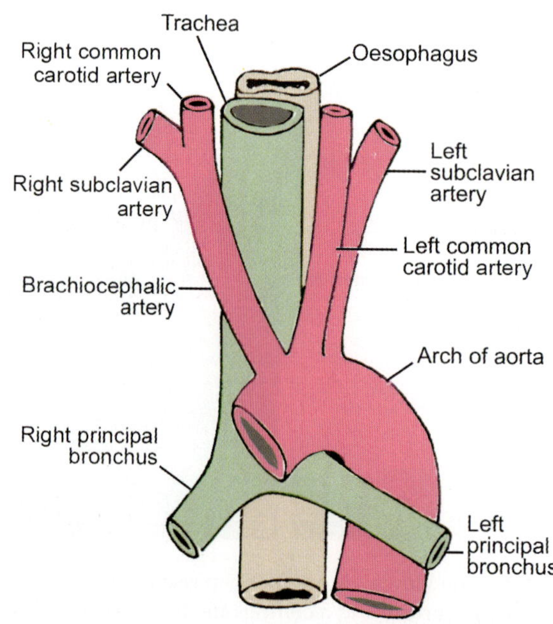


**21.14:** Diagram to show the branches of the arch of the aorta

## Brachiocephalic Artery

1. This is the first branch of the arch of the aorta. Its origin lies more or less in the median plane, in front of the trachea.
2. From here, it runs upwards and backwards and as it does so it winds round the trachea to reach its right side.
3. It ends behind the right sternoclavicular joint by dividing into the right common carotid and right subclavian arteries.

### WANT TO KNOW MORE?

**Relations**

*Anteriorly* to:

1. The manubrium sterni
2. The sternoclavicular joint of the right side
3. The right sternohyoid and sternothyroid muscles
4. The remnants of the thymus
5. The left brachiocephalic vein.

*Posteriorly* to:

1. The trachea
2. Right pleura and lung
3. The right vagus nerve.

*On its right side* to:

1. The right brachiocephalic vein
2. The upper part of the superior vena cava
3. The right lung and pleura.

*On its left side* to:

1. The remnants of the thymus
2. The inferior thyroid veins
3. The left common carotid artery
4. The trachea.

## Left Common Carotid Artery

1. The left common carotid artery arises from the arch a little to the left of the brachiocephalic artery. Its origin also lies in front of the trachea.
2. From here, it passes upwards winding around the trachea to reach its left side. It enters the neck by passing deep to the left sternoclavicular joint.

### WANT TO KNOW MORE?

**Relations of Thoracic Part**

*Anteriorly* to:

1. The manubrium sterni
2. The left sternohyoid and sternothyroid muscles
3. The remnants of the thymus
4. The left brachiocephalic vein.

*Posteriorly* to:
1. The trachea
2. The left subclavian artery
3. The left vagus and left phrenic nerves.

*On its right side* to:
1. The brachiocephalic artery
2. Trachea.

*On its left side* to:
1. The left lung and pleura
2. The left vagus and phrenic nerves.

### Left Subclavian Artery

1. The left subclavian artery arises from the arch of the aorta a little to the left of and behind the left common carotid artery, the origin lying to the left of the trachea.
2. The artery runs almost vertically along the left side of the trachea to enter the neck at the level of the left sternoclavicular joint, where it lies behind the common carotid artery.

### WANT TO KNOW MORE?

**Relations of Thoracic Part**

*Anteriorly* to:
1. The left common carotid artery
2. The left brachiocephalic vein
3. The left vagus and phrenic nerves.

*Posteriorly* to:
1. The left lung and pleura
2. The left edge of the oesophagus
3. The left recurrent laryngeal nerve
4. The thoracic duct.

*On the right side* to:
1. The trachea
2. The left recurrent laryngeal nerve
3. The oesophagus.

*On its left side* to:
1. The left lung and pleura.

## BRANCHES OF DESCENDING THORACIC AORTA

1. The branches of the descending thoracic aorta are shown in 21.9.
2. Apart from several small branches to the oesophagus, the pericardium, the diaphragm (phrenic branches) and to lymph nodes in the posterior mediastinum (mediastinal branches) it gives off the bronchial, posterior intercostal and subcostal arteries.
3. The posterior intercostal and subcostal arteries have already been described (Chapter 18). The bronchial arteries are described below.

### The Bronchial Arteries

1. These arteries supply the bronchi, the connective tissue of the lung and related lymph nodes. (Note that in contrast the blood reaching the lungs through the pulmonary arteries passes through capillaries related to the alveoli where oxygenation takes place).
2. Generally, there are two left bronchial arteries: upper and lower. They arise from the front of the thoracic aorta.
3. Usually, there is one right bronchial artery. It may arise from the upper left bronchial artery or from the third right posterior intercostal artery.
4. The number and origin of bronchial arteries is subject to considerable variation.

### Other Arteries in the Thorax

The ***internal thoracic artery***, and the ***superior intercostal artery*** arise in the neck and descend into the thoracic wall.

## VEINS OF THE THORAX

The veins of the thorax are as follows:

### Veins That Drain the Wall of the Thorax

These include the intercostal and subcostal veins, the azygos and hemiazygos veins, and the internal thoracic vein. These have been described in Chapter 18.

### Veins that Drain the Heart

These are the coronary sinus and its tributaries; and some small veins.

### Large Veins Present in the Mediastinum

These are the superior vena cava, the right and left brachiocephalic veins, the inferior vena cava, and the pulmonary veins.

## VEINS OF THE HEART

In order to understand the disposition of the veins of the heart, it is desirable to be familiar with the position of the atrioventricular and interventricular grooves and the course of the coronary arteries (described earlier in this chapter).

### The Coronary Sinus

1. Most of the veins draining the heart wall end in a wide vein, about two centimeters long, called the coronary sinus (21.15 and 21.16).
2. This sinus lies in the posterior and left part of the atrioventricular groove i.e., along the posterior edge of the diaphragmatic surface of the left ventricle. Its right end opens into the right atrium.
   The coronary sinus receives the following veins:
   a. The great cardiac vein
   b. The small cardiac vein
   c. The middle cardiac vein
   d. The posterior vein of the left ventricle
   e. The oblique vein of the left atrium (21.15 and 21.16).

### The Great Cardiac Vein

1. The great cardiac vein is seen mainly on the sternocostal aspect of the heart (21.15). It ascends in the anterior interventricular groove (parallel to the anterior interventricular branch of the left coronary artery).

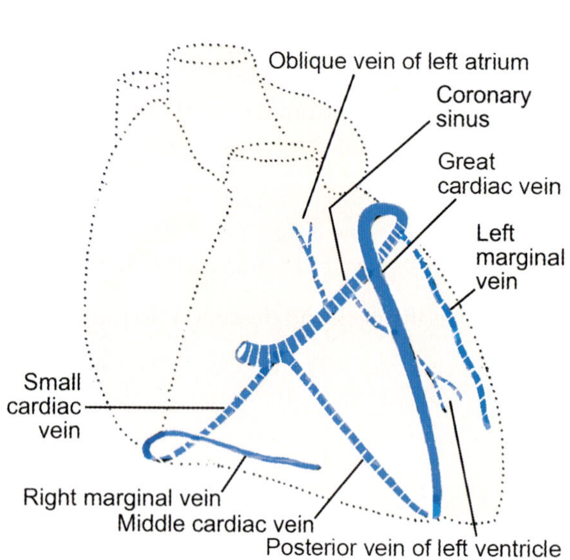


**21.15:** Scheme to show veins of the heart as seen from the front. Veins not normally seen from the front are drawn as if the walls of the chambers of the heart were transparent

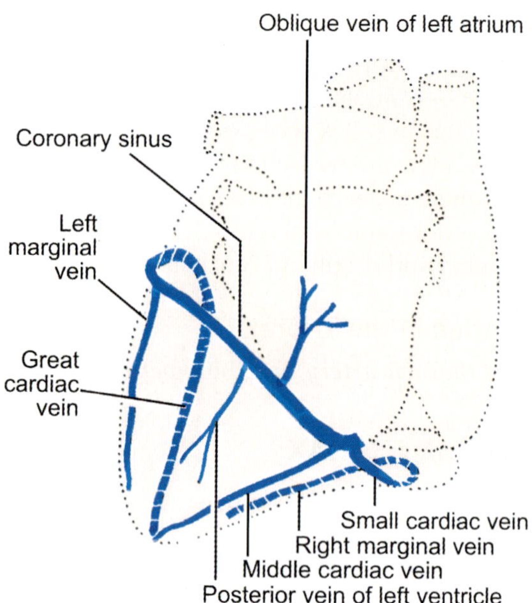


**21.16:** Veins of the heart as seen from behind. Veins not normally seen from the back are drawn as if the walls were transparent

2. At the upper end of the groove the vein turns to the left in the coronary sulcus (alongside the circumflex branch of the left coronary artery), winds round the left margin of the heart and ends in the left extremity of the coronary sinus.
3. It receives a large left marginal vein which corresponds to the left marginal branch of the left coronary artery.

## The Small Cardiac Vein

1. The small cardiac vein is situated at the junction of the base of the heart and its diaphragmatic surface (21.15 and 21.16). It lies in the posterior and right part of the coronary sulcus.
2. It thus runs along side the terminal part of the right coronary artery.
3. The small cardiac vein ends by joining the coronary sinus near its termination.
4. The small cardiac vein receives the ***right marginal vein*** which is seen on the sternocostal surface just above the inferior border of the heart. Its position thus corresponds to that of the right marginal branch of the right coronary artery.

## The Middle Cardiac Vein

1. The middle cardiac vein begins near the apex of the heart and runs backwards on the diaphragmatic surface (21.15 and 21.16).
2. It lies in the posterior interventricular groove i.e., it accompanies the posterior interventricular branch of the right coronary artery.
3. The vein ends in the coronary sinus near its termination.

## Other Veins of the Heart

1. The ***posterior vein of the left ventricle*** runs backwards on the diaphragmatic surface of the ventricle and ends in the coronary sinus.

2. The ***oblique vein of the left atrium*** lies behind this chamber i.e., on the base of the heart. (Its importance is that it represents a remnant of the left common cardinal vein).
3. In addition to the above some ***anterior cardiac veins*** lying on the right ventricle open into the right atrium. A number of small ***venae cordis minimae*** drain directly into the chambers of the heart.

## THE PULMONARY VEINS

1. There are four pulmonary veins, two each (superior and inferior), on the right and left sides.
2. Each of them is formed by union of smaller veins draining the alveoli of the lungs.
3. On the left side the superior and inferior veins drain the upper and lower lobes of the lung, respectively. The veins of the left side pass anterior to the descending aorta.
4. On the right side the upper and middle lobes drain through the superior vein and the lower lobe through the inferior vein. The superior vein crosses behind the superior vena cava; and the inferior vein crosses behind the right atrium.

## THE SUPERIOR VENA CAVA

1. The superior vena cava is formed by the union of the right and left brachiocephalic veins. Large veins draining into the superior vena cava are illustrated in 21.17.
2. Its upper end is situated at the lower border of the first right costal cartilage.
3. It descends behind the first intercostal space, the second costal cartilage and the second intercostal space to end at the level of the third right costal cartilage by opening into the right atrium.
4. The vessel is about 7 cm long. The lower half of the vessel is enclosed within the fibrous pericardium.
5. Apart from the brachiocephalic veins the superior vena cava receives the azygos vein which joins it on the right side about its middle.

### WANT TO KNOW MORE?

**Relations**

***To the right side*** the superior vena cava is related to:
1. The right lung and pleura
2. The right phrenic nerve descends in contact with the right side of the vena cava.

***Anteromedially***, the vena cava is related to:
1. The ascending aorta.

***Posteromedially***, it is related to:
1. The trachea
2. The right vagus nerve.

***Anteriorly***, the superior vena cava is related to:
1. The internal thoracic artery
2. The 1st and 2nd costal cartilages
3. The anterior margin of the right lung.

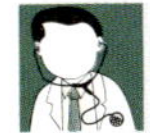

### CLINICAL CORRELATION

**Obstruction of Superior Vena Cava**

1. In obstruction to the superior vena cava, the azygous vein becomes an important channel for maintaining venous return from the upper part of the body.

2. In this context, it is very important to remember that at its lower end the azygous vein usually communicates with the inferior vena cava; and at its upper end it opens into the superior vena cava at about its middle.
3. When the superior vena cava is obstructed above the entry of the azygous vein, blood from the upper half of the body reaches intercostal veins through anastomoses between these veins and other veins of the region (including the internal thoracic vein). Through the intercostal veins this blood passes into the azygous vein and into the superior vena cava.
4. When the superior vena cava is obstructed below the entry of the azygous vein, blood in the vena cava can pass through the azygos vein into the inferior vena cava and hence to the heart.
5. Blood also passes through superficial veins that connect the lateral thoracic vein (a tributary of the axillary vein) with the superficial epigastric tributary of the femoral vein. This connecting vein is the ***thoracoepigastric vein***.
6. The vertebral venous plexuses are also important channels of communication between the superior vena caval and inferior vena caval systems.

## Right Brachiocephalic Vein

1. This vein is formed by union of the right internal jugular and subclavian veins.
2. It ends by joining the left brachiocephalic vein to form the superior vena cava.
3. The vein is about 2.5 cm long. Its upper end (beginning) lies behind the sternal end of the right clavicle; while its lower end (termination) lies at the level of the lower border of the first right costal cartilage.

### WANT TO KNOW MORE?

The ***relations*** of the vein are as follows:

***To its right side*** the right brachiocephalic vein is related to:

1. The right lung and pleura
2. The right phrenic nerve.

***Posteromedially,*** the vein is related to:

1. The brachiocephalic artery
2. The right vagus nerve.

***Anteriorly,*** the vein is related to

1. The first costal cartilage
2. The sternal end of the clavicle.

The ***tributaries*** of the right brachiocephalic vein are:

1. Right vertebral vein
2. Right internal thoracic vein
3. An inferior thyroid vein
4. Right first intercostal vein.

## Left Brachiocephalic Vein

1. This vein is formed by union of the left internal jugular and subclavian veins.
2. The vein begins behind the sternal end of the left clavicle.
3. This vein is about twice as long as the right brachiocephalic vein as it has to run obliquely behind the manubrium to reach its termination at the lower border of the first right costal cartilage.
4. Here, it joins the right brachiocephalic vein to form the superior vena cava.

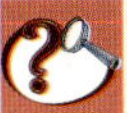

## WANT TO KNOW MORE?

The ***relations*** of the vein are as follows (21.18):

*Anteriorly*

1. Manubrium sterni
2. Sternohyoid and sternothyroid muscles
3. Remnants of the thymus.

*Posteriorly*

1. Arteries arising from the arch of the aorta i.e., the brachiocephalic, left common carotid and left subclavian arteries.
2. Trachea.
3. Left vagus and left phrenic nerves.

The ***tributaries*** of the left brachiocephalic vein are:

1. The left vertebral vein
2. The left first intercostal vein
3. The left superior intercostal vein
4. An inferior thyroid vein.

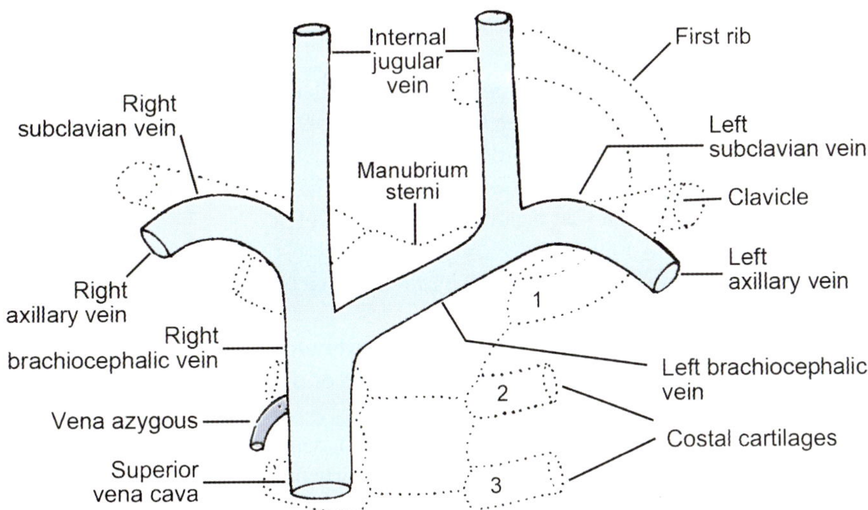


**21.17:** Large veins draining into the superior vena cava

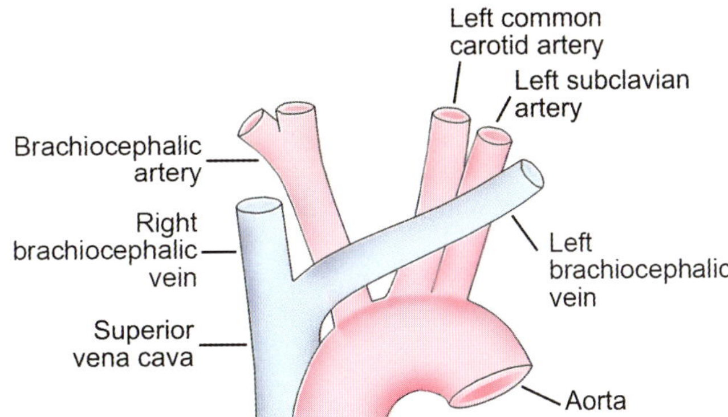


**21.18:** Drawing to show the relationship of the left brachiocephalic vein to the arch of the aorta

22

CHAPTER

# The Oesophagus, The Thymus, Lymphatics and Nerves of the Thorax

## THE OESOPHAGUS

1. The oesophagus (22.1) is a tubular structure which starts (in the neck) at the lower end of the oropharynx (i.e., in front of the sixth cervical vertebra). It descends through the lower part of the neck, and enters the thorax through its inlet (22.17).
2. Within the thorax, the oesophagus descends first through the superior mediastinum, and then through the posterior mediastinum.
3. It leaves the thorax by passing through an aperture in the diaphragm: this aperture lies at the level of the tenth thoracic vertebra.
4. After a very short course in the abdomen, the oesophagus ends by joining the stomach. The junction with the stomach lies at the level of the eleventh thoracic vertebra.
5. The upper end of the oesophagus lies in the midline (22.1).
   a. As the oesophagus descends in the neck, it deviates slightly to the left side so that at the root of the neck, it is somewhat to the left of the midline.
   b. As it passes through the superior mediastinum it again approaches the midline that it reaches at level T5.
   c. It is approximately in the midline from levels T5 to T7, but below this level it again deviates to the left so that its lower end is distinctly to the left of the midline.
   d. Here its position corresponds to that of the left seventh costal cartilage 2.5 cm from the junction of the latter with the sternum.
6. a. The transverse diameter of the oesophagus is about 2.5 cm (one inch). Its total length is about 25 cm (10 inches).
   b. It is sometimes necessary to introduce instruments into the oesophagus and for this purpose it is useful to know that the upper end lies 15 cm from the incisor teeth, and its lower end lies 40 cm from them.
7. The oesophagus has numerous relations, in the neck, in the thorax, and in the abdomen. The relations in the thorax are described below. (Relations in the neck and in the abdomen will be described in the relevant sections).

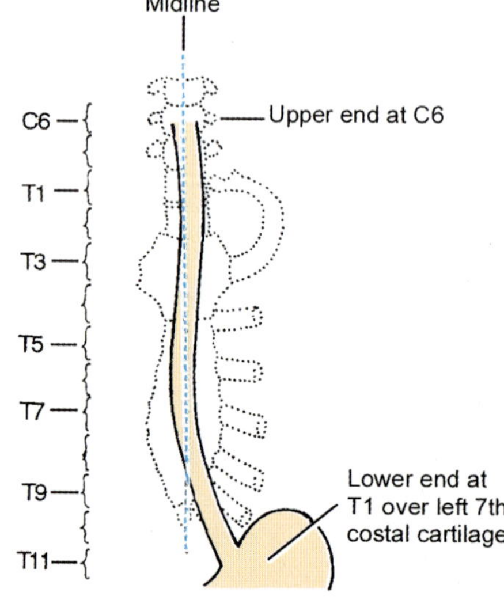


**22.1:** Lateral curvatures of the oesophagus and the levels of its upper and lower ends

### Relations in the Thorax

#### *Main Relations*

1. The oesophagus first lies in the superior mediastinum and then in the posterior mediastinum.
2. a. In the superior mediastinum, the oesophagus lies in front of the vertebral column and behind the trachea (21.5).

b. On either side, it is related to the corresponding pleura and lung.

c. As the oesophagus enters the lower part of the superior mediastinum, it passes behind and to the right of the arch of the aorta.

3. a. Descending into the posterior mediastinum the oesophagus first lies to the right of the descending thoracic aorta (and in front of the vertebral column), but lower down it gradually passes anterior to the aorta.

b. As the oesophagus and aorta descend through the posterior mediastinum, they both lie first behind the heart, and then behind the posterior part of the diaphragm.

c. In the upper part of the posterior mediastinum, the oesophagus is in contact with the right lung, but is separated from the left lung by the aorta.

d. In the lower part of the mediastinum, the oesophagus crosses to the left (in front of the aorta) and it, therefore, comes into contact with the left lung.

 **WANT TO KNOW MORE?**

**Other Structures Related to the Oesophagus**

1. The left subclavian artery, and the left recurrent laryngeal nerve, lie anterior and to the left of the oesophagus.
2. Just below the arch of the aorta, the oesophagus is crossed by the right pulmonary artery and the left principal bronchus (22.2).
3. The thoracic duct lies behind the oesophagus in the posterior mediastinum (22.3) and along its left side in the superior mediastinum (22.3).
4. The vena azygos ascends behind the oesophagus in the posterior mediastinum (22.3). Above the root of the right lung, the vein crosses the right side of the oesophagus to reach the superior vena cava.
5. Apart from the thoracic duct and the vena azygos other structures intervening between the oesophagus and the vertebral column are (22.3):
   a. The hemiazygos and accessory hemiazygos veins (as they cross from left to right).
   b. The right posterior intercostal arteries (which arise from the aorta and cross behind the oesophagus to reach the right side).
   c. The prevertebral muscles and ligaments.
6. Below the roots of the lungs the right and left vagus nerves form a plexus around the oesophagus. Branches of the left nerve tend to lie in front of the oesophagus, and those of the right vagus nerve behind it.

**Blood Supply**

1. The cervical part of the oesophagus receives branches from the inferior thyroid artery.
2. The thoracic part receives small branches from the aorta and from the bronchial arteries.
3. The abdominal part receives branches from the left gastric artery and from the left inferior phrenic branch of the abdominal aorta.
4. Veins from the cervical part join the inferior thyroid veins.
5. Those from the thoracic part drain into the azygos, hemiazygos and accessory hemiazygos veins.
6. Veins from the abdominal part of the oesophagus drain into the left gastric vein and into the azygos vein. The lymphatic drainage of the oesophagus is described later in this Chapter (page 450).

**Nerve Supply**

1. The oesophagus is supplied by autonomic nerves, both sympathetic and parasympathetic.
2. Sympathetic nerves reach it through splanchnic branches of the sympathetic trunk.
3. Parasympathetic branches are received from the vagal plexus around the oesophagus.

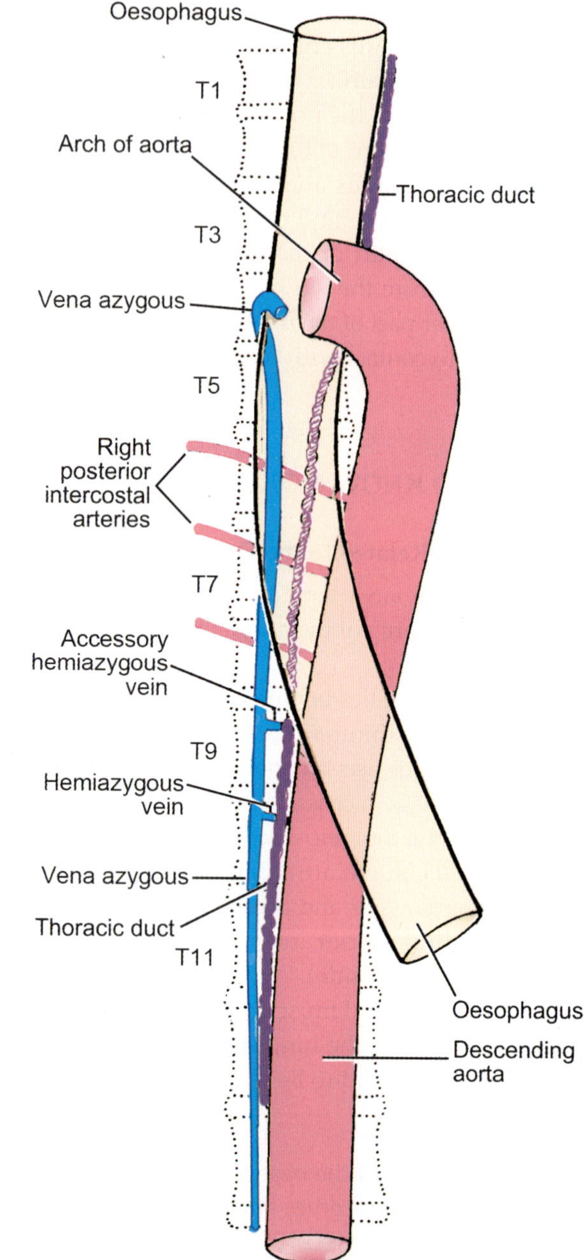


**22.2:** Scheme to show that the oesophagus is crossed by the left principal bronchus and the right pulmonary artery

**22.3:** Scheme to show posterior relations of the oesophagus (which is drawn as if transparent)

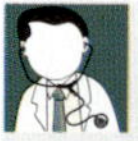

## CLINICAL CORRELATION

### The Oesophagus

#### Congenital Malformations

The oesophagus may show congenital stenosis (narrowing) or atresia (non-development of a segment). Atresia is often accompanied by abnormal communications (fistulae) between the oesophagus and the trachea (19.11).

**Constrictions**

1. The lumen of the oesophagus normally shows constrictions at the following sites:
   a. At its upper end.
   b. Where it is crossed by the arch of the aorta.
   c. Where it is crossed by the left principal bronchus.
   d. Where it pierces the diaphragm.
2. For the purpose of passing a tube through the oesophagus, it is important to know that these constrictions lie 6″, 9″, 11″, and 15″ from the incisor teeth.

**Cardio-oesophageal Junction**

1. a. The junction of the lower end of the oesophagus and the stomach (cardio-oesophageal junction) is guarded by a sphincteric mechanism, the structure of which is uncertain.
   b. This 'sphincter' prevents regurgitation of stomach contents into the oesophagus.

***Cardiospasm***

1. a. Neuromuscular incoordination at the lower end of the oesophagus may cause difficulty in passage of food from oesophagus to stomach (***achalasia cardia*** or ***cardiospasm***).
   b. When severe, the condition may lead to accumulation of food in the oesophagus and its dilatation.

***Oesophageal Varices***

1. Veins from the abdominal part of the oesophagus drain partly into the left gastric vein and partly into the azygous vein.
2. Note that the azygous vein is a systemic vein, whereas the left gastric vein is a tributary of the portal vein.
3. When venous flow through the liver is obstructed (in liver disease) blood may flow from the left gastric vein into the azygous vein through anastomoses between the two at the lower end of the oesophagus.
4. The anastomoses then enlarge and are called ***oesophageal varices***. They can be a source of bleeding into the stomach and can lead to haematemesis (vomiting of blood).

**Barium Swallow**

1. The lumen of the oesophagus can be visualised in the living subject by taking a skiagram immediately after the subject swallows a meal containing a suitable barium salt. The procedure is referred to as ***barium swallow***.
2. Apart from diseases of the oesophagus itself, this procedure can be used to detect enlargement of the left atrium of the heart. An enlarged left atrium presses on the oesophagus and produces an indentation in its outline (23.3).

**Dysphagia**

1. The oesophagus may be compressed by a mass in the mediastinum (see below).
2. Compression causes difficulty in swallowing (***dysphagia***).

**Hiatus Hernia**

For the relationship of the oesophagus to hiatus hernia see chapter 18.

**Carcinoma of Oesophagus**

1. Carcinoma of oesophagus can form a mass in the mediastinum and can press on neighbouring structures (see below).
2. It should be remembered that lymphatics from the lower one-third of the oesophagus pass into coeliac lymph nodes located in the abdomen.
3. For excision of the tumour, the affected part of the oesophagus has to be resected and lymph nodes also have to be removed.
4. The cut end of the oesophagus is then anastomosed to the jejunum (***oesophagojejunostomy***) to restore continuity of the gut. It will be obvious that the operation requires opening of both the thorax and the abdomen.

## THE THYMUS

1. The thymus is one of those organs the importance of which has been recognized only in recent years.
2. a. On superficial examination, it appears to be just a collection of lymphoid tissue.
   b. Recent studies have shown, however, that the thymus plays a vital role in making lymphocytes competent to react to the invasion of the body by foreign proteins.
   c. The thymus is, therefore, now regarded as the 'central organ' of the lymphoid system.
3. The thymus is difficult to recognise as a distinct organ in the usual dissection hall cadaver because of rapid degeneration after death.
4. The organ is easy to see up to the age of puberty (22.4).
5. a. It consists of two pear shaped lobes, right and left, that may be joined to each other by connective tissue.
   b. These lobes are placed in the anterior part of the superior mediastinum (i.e., just behind the manubrium sterni) and in the anterior mediastinum (i.e., behind the upper part of the body of the sternum and the upper four costal cartilages).
   c. A cord like prolongation from each lobe may extend into the neck, reaching the lower border of the thyroid gland.
6. a. At birth, the total weight of the thymus is about 10 g.
   b. It increases in size till the age of puberty when it may weigh as much as 30 g.
   c. Thereafter, it retrogresses in size and the lymphoid tissue in it is gradually replaced with fat.
7. We have seen that the thymus (or its remnants) are related anteriorly to the manubrium and body of the sternum. Posteriorly they rest on pericardium, the arch of the aorta and its branches, the left brachiocephalic vein and the trachea.
8. Each lobe of the thymus has a connective tissue capsule. Connective tissue septa passing inwards from the capsule incompletely subdivide the lobe into a large number of lobules.

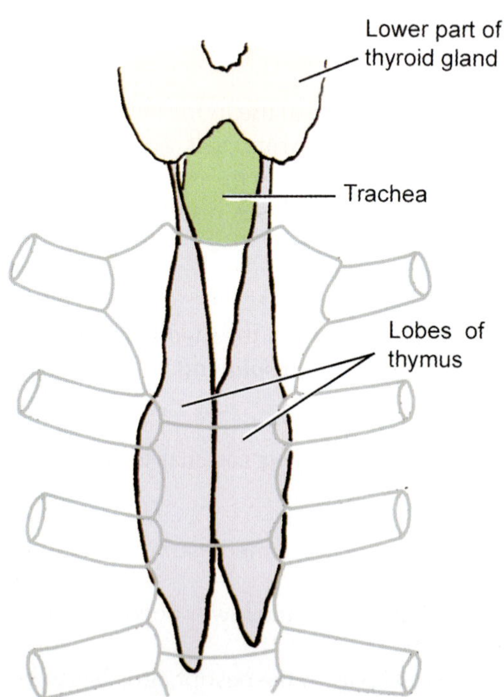


**22.4:** Diagram to show location of the thymus in a person at puberty

9. Each lobule is about 2 mm in diameter. It has an outer cortex and an inner medulla.
   a. Both the cortex and medulla contain cells of two distinct lineages.
   b. These are epithelial cells derived from the endodermal lining of the third pharyngeal pouch and lymphocytes (***thymocytes***) which are derived from stem cells in bone marrow.
   c. The lymphocytes undergo a process of maturation in the thymus where they become immunologically competent T-lymphocytes.
   d. These enter the circulation and reach lymph nodes, spleen and other collections of lymphocytes. Because of this fact, the thymus is regarded as the *primary lymphoid organ*.
10. It is now known that the thymus produces a number of hormones and is, therefore, to be regarded as an *endocrine gland*.
11. The thymus is supplied by branches from the internal thoracic and inferior thyroid arteries. Veins from the thymus drain into corresponding veins or into the left brachiocephalic vein.

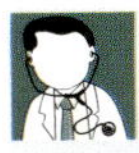

## CLINICAL CORRELATION

1. Enlargement of the thymus (or the presence of a tumour in it) is often associated with a disease called ***myasthenia gravis***.
2. In this condition, there is great weakness of skeletal muscle. Removal of the thymus may result in considerable improvement in the condition.
3. Myasthenia gravis is now considered to be an autoimmune disease. Proteins that normally bind acetylcholine to motor end plates are destroyed by antibodies present in patients having this disease.

### SOME CLINICAL CORRELATIONS OF THE MEDIASTINUM AS A WHOLE

#### Mediastinal Shift

1. The mediastinum may be displaced to the opposite side if there is a large collection of air or of fluid in a pleural cavity.
2. In open pneumothorax, the mediastinum can move from side to side with each respiration.
3. Extensive fibrosis in a lung, or collapse of a lung may shift the mediastinum to the affected side.
4. Clinically, the presence of mediastinal displacement may be indicated by displacement of the trachea away from the midline, and also by displacement of the apex beat.

#### Mediastinitis

1. Inflammation in the mediastinum is called mediastinitis. It may be acute or chronic.
2. The most common cause of acute mediastinitis is perforation of the oesophagus.
3. It may also follow surgical procedures involving splitting of the sternum (median sternotomy).
4. Chronic infection may be caused by spread from infected lymph nodes in the region and such infection can be tubercular.
5. The superior mediastinum is continuous with tissues in the neck. Infections from the neck can, therefore, pass into the superior mediastinum and from there into the posterior mediastinum.

#### Pneumomediastinum

Air may sometimes be present in the mediastinum. It may be caused by rupture of the trachea, a bronchus, or oesophagus. Air can also enter the mediastinum from the neck.

#### Mediastinal Masses

1. A mediastinal mass may be a tumour, an aneurysm, a cyst, or a mass of enlarged lymph nodes.
2. An enlarged thyroid may extend into the mediastinum (***retrosternal goitre***).

3. A mass in the mediastinum can press upon various structures. Such pressure may also be exerted by an aneurysm of the aorta.
   a. Pressure on the left recurrent laryngeal nerve causes hoarseness of voice.
   b. Pressure on the phrenic nerve can cause paralysis of the diaphragm on that side.
   c. Pressure on intercostal nerves can produce pain in their region of supply (***intercostal neuralgia***).
   d. Pressure on the trachea or on a bronchus obstructs breathing and can cause dyspnoea and cough.
   e. Compression of the oesophagus results in dysphagia.
   f. If the superior vena cava is pressed upon venous return from the head and neck and upper limbs is reduced, and there is engorgement of veins in the head and neck and upper limbs (see below). Abnormal fullness of the face is seen.
   g. Pressure on the sympathetic chain results in Horner's syndrome (small pupil, ptosis and absence of sweating on the affected side of the face).
   h. A mass in the mediastinum may cause erosion of vertebral bodies.
4. Symptoms resulting from pressure effects on structures in the mediastinum are described as the ***mediastinal syndrome***.

**Aortic Aneurysms**

An aortic aneurysm can behave like a mediastinal mass. See chapter 21.

## LYMPHATICS OF THE THORAX

### Thoracic Duct

1. The thoracic duct is the largest lymph vessel in the body. It looks like a vein. It is about 40 cm long.
2. It begins in the abdomen as the upward continuation of a sac called the ***cisterna chyli*** (22.5).
3. It enters the thorax by passing through the aortic opening of the diaphragm within the opening it lies to the right of the aorta. The vena azygous lies to the right of the thoracic duct.
4. Having entered the thorax, the thoracic, duct ascends between the aorta and the vena azygous up to the fifth thoracic vertebra. It then continues upwards, but inclines towards the left side and passes deep to the arch of the aorta.
5. The thoracic duct now comes to lie along the left margin of the oesophagus. In this position, it runs upwards through the superior mediastinum and into the lower part of the neck.
6. At the level of the transverse process of the seventh cervical vertebra, the thoracic duct arches laterally behind the carotid sheath (containing the common carotid artery, the internal jugular vein and the vagus nerve).
7. The terminal part of the duct descends in front of the first part of the subclavian artery and ends by opening into the junction of the left subclavian vein and the internal jugular vein (22.5).

#### *Other Important Relations*

1. In the lower part of the posterior mediastinum, the duct lies behind the diaphragm. Higher up it lies behind the oesophagus and gradually courses behind it to reach its left side. This position is maintained in the superior mediastinum.
2. As the duct passes laterally behind the carotid sheath it passes in front of the vertebral artery and vein, the sympathetic trunk, the thyrocervical trunk (or its branches), the phrenic nerve and the medial margin of the scalenus anterior. These structures are seen in the neck.

#### *Area of Drainage*

1. As a generalisation, it may be said that the thoracic duct carries lymph from both sides of the body below the diaphragm and from the left side above the diaphragm.

2. In other words, it carries lymph from both lower limbs, the pelvis, the abdomen, the left half of the thorax, the left half of the head and neck and the left upper limb (22.6).

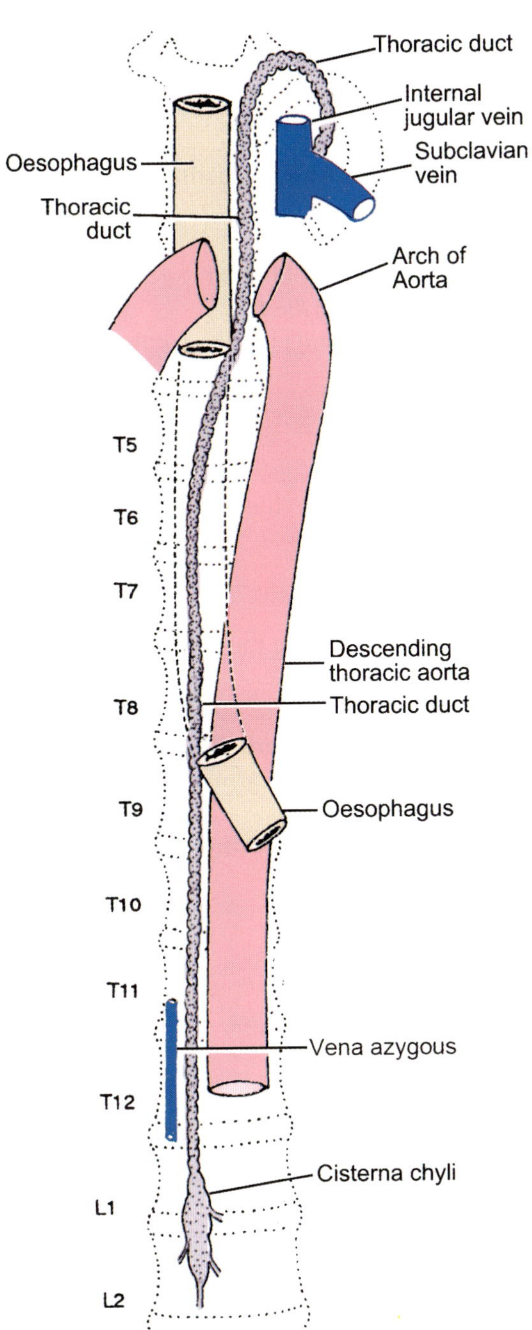


**22.5:** Course and relations of the thoracic duct as seen from the front

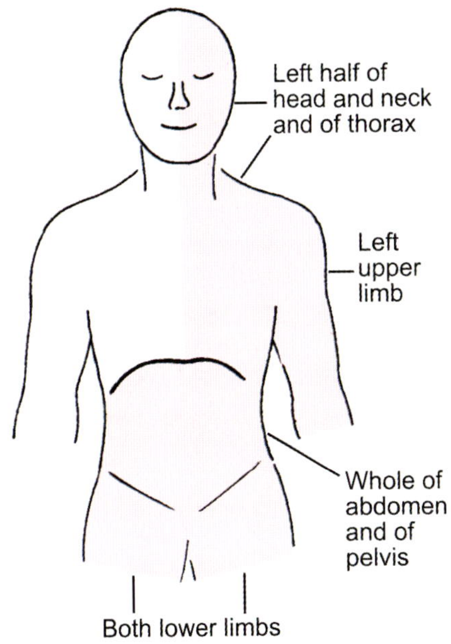


**22.6:** Scheme to show the area of the body draining through the thoracic duct

### *Tributaries of Thoracic Duct*

1. Most of the lymph from the abdomen reaches the thoracic duct through the cisterna chyli, but the thoracic duct also receives some vessels directly from the upper lumbar lymph nodes (lying in the abdomen).
2. Within the thorax, the duct receives vessels from lymph nodes of the region.
3. Near its termination the thoracic duct receives the ***left subclavian trunk*** from the left upper limb and a ***left jugular trunk*** from the left half of the head and neck.
4. It may also receive the ***left bronchomediastinal trunk*** from the upper part of the thorax, but this trunk usually enters the subclavian vein independently (22.7).

## Right Bronchomediastinal Trunk

1. Lymph from the right half of the thorax is drained by the right bronchomediastinal lymph trunk (22.7 and 22.11).
2. This trunk also drains lymph from the convex upper surface of the liver.
3. It ascends into the neck where it joins the ***right jugular trunk*** from the right half of the head and neck, the ***right subclavian trunk*** from the right upper limb, to form the ***right lymphatic duct.***
4. The position, course and relations of the right lymphatic duct corresponds to those of the terminal part of the thoracic duct (on the left side).

# LYMPH NODES OF THE THORAX

The lymph nodes of the thorax may be divided into those present in relation to the thoracic wall and those present in relation to the contents of the thorax (22.8).

## Nodes Present in Relation to Thoracic Wall

1. The ***parasternal*** nodes lie at the anterior ends of the intercostal spaces, along the course of the internal thoracic artery.
2. The ***intercostal*** lymph nodes lie at the posterior ends of the intercostal spaces.
3. The ***diaphragmatic*** lymph nodes lie on the thoracic surface of the diaphragm. They consist of the following subgroups:
   a. The ***anterior group*** lies behind the xiphoid process.
   b. The right and left ***lateral groups*** lie near the points where the corresponding phrenic nerves pierce the diaphragm.
   c. The ***posterior group*** lies behind the crura of the diaphragm.

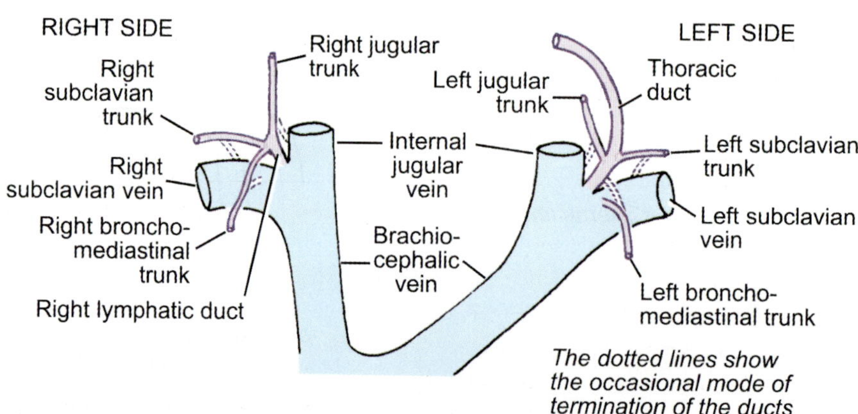


**22.7:** Scheme to show the main lymphatic ducts

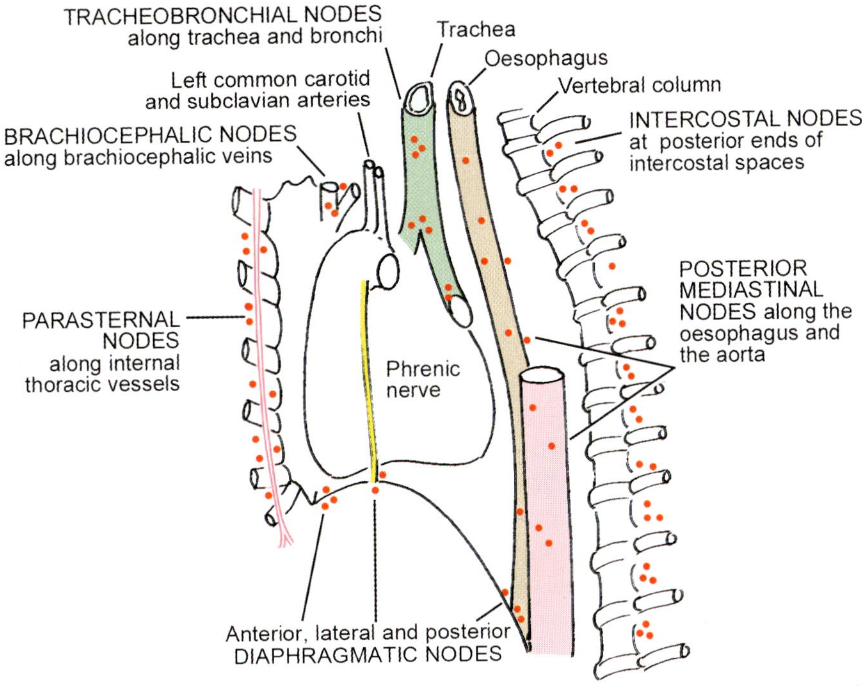


**22.8:** Scheme to show the lymph nodes of the thorax

## Nodes Present in Relation to Contents of the Thorax

1. The ***brachiocephalic*** lymph nodes lie in the superior mediastinum, in front of the brachiocephalic veins (22.8).
2. The ***posterior mediastinal*** lymph nodes are present in relation to the oesophagus and the descending thoracic aorta.
3. The ***tracheobronchial*** lymph nodes lie along the trachea and bronchi (22.9). They consist of the following subgroups:
   a. The ***paratracheal nodes*** lie on either side of the trachea.
   b. The ***superior tracheobronchial*** nodes lie in the angle between the trachea and the principal bronchus (right or left).
   c. The ***inferior tracheobronchial*** nodes lie below the bifurcation of the trachea.
   d. The ***bronchopulmonary*** nodes are situated at the hilum of the right and left lungs.
   e. The ***pulmonary*** nodes lie along the bronchi within the substance of the lungs.

## Lymphatic Drainage of the Thoracic Wall

1. The skin overlying the thorax drains mainly into the axillary lymph nodes. The vessels from the back of the thorax end in the posterior group, while those from the front end in the anterior group. The skin near the sternum is drained into the parasternal nodes (22.10).
2. The deeper tissues (including muscles covering the chest wall, and the costal pleura) drain anteriorly into the parasternal nodes and posteriorly into the intercostal nodes (22.10).
   a. Efferents from the parasternal nodes (along with those from the tracheobronchial and brachiocephalic nodes) form the bronchomediastinal lymph trunk.
   b. On the left side, this trunk may join the thoracic duct, but it usually opens into the subclavian vein independently. On the right side, the bronchomediastinal trunk joins the right lymphatic duct.

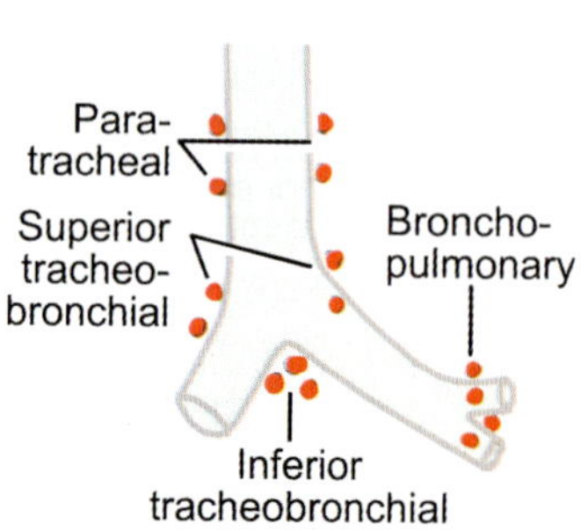


**22.9:** Tracheobronchial lymph nodes

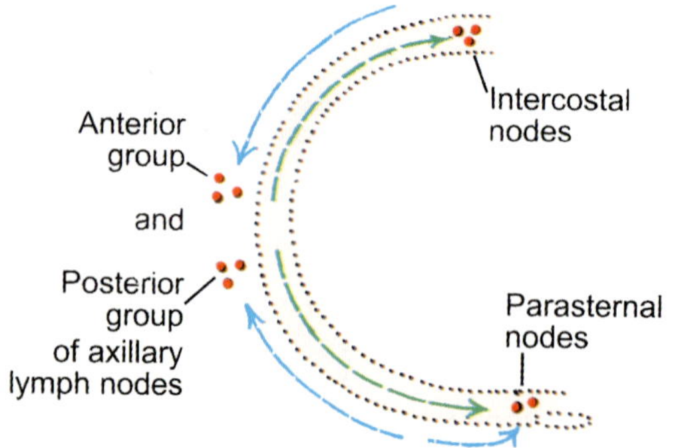


**22.10:** Scheme to show lymphatic drainage of skin and deeper tissues of thoracic wall

   c. Efferents from the intercostal nodes of the left side end in the thoracic duct (22.11). Those from the lower nodes of the right side also end in the thoracic duct, but efferents of the upper nodes reach the right bronchomediastinal trunk.

3. The ***diaphragm*** is drained by separate sets of lymph vessels on its thoracic and abdominal surfaces.
4. The ***thoracic surface*** is drained as follows (22.12):
   a. Vessels from the anterior part drain into the anterior diaphragmatic nodes, and through them to the parasternal nodes.
   b. Vessels from the middle part drain to the right and left lateral diaphragmatic nodes, and from here to the parasternal nodes and nodes around the oesophagus (part of posterior mediastinal group).
   c. Vessels from the posterior part drain into the posterior diaphragmatic nodes, and through them to nodes around the lower end of the thoracic aorta.
5. Lymphatics from the ***abdominal surface*** of the diaphragm drain into lymph nodes within the abdomen. The right and left halves of the diaphragm are drained by separate sets of vessels.
   a. On the right side, the vessels end in ***nodes lying along the inferior phrenic artery***, and in the right ***lateral aortic nodes*** (on right side of abdominal aorta).
   b. On the left side, the lymph vessels end in the ***preaortic nodes*** (in front of the aorta) and in nodes around the lower end of the oesophagus.

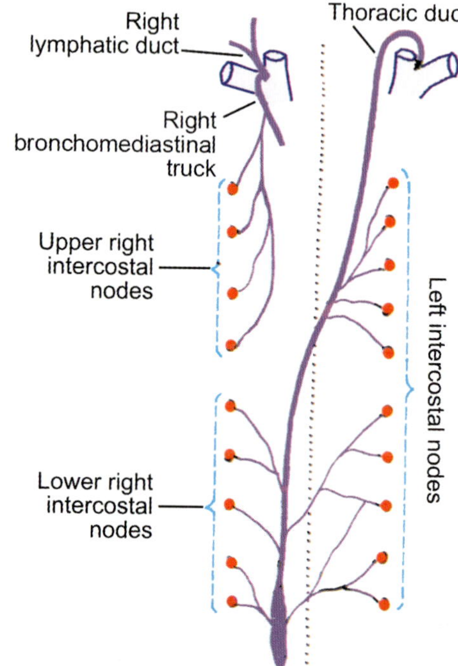


**22.11:** Scheme to show efferent vessels arising from intercostal lymph nodes

## Lymphatic Drainage of Thoracic Organs

### *Lymphatic Drainage of the Lungs*

1. The ***lungs*** are drained by two sets of vessels, superficial and deep (22.13).
2. The superficial vessels lie near the surface of the lung. Curving around its surfaces, borders and fissures they converge onto the bronchopulmonary nodes (lying near the hilum of the lung).
3. The deep vessels follow the bronchi. They drain first into the ***pulmonary nodes*** (in the substance of the lung) and then into the bronchopulmonary nodes.
4. The superficial and deep pathways are usually distinct. When the deep vessels are obstructed by disease lymph from the deeper parts of the lung may drain through superficial vessels.
5. Vessels arising from the bronchopulmonary nodes pass to the tracheo-bronchial nodes and from there into the bronchomediastinal trunk (22.14).

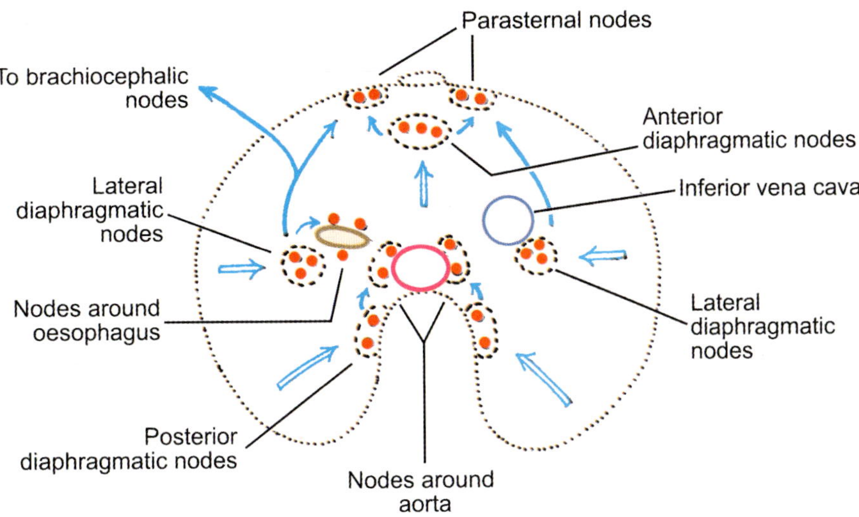


**22.12:** Scheme to show lymphatic drainage of thoracic surface of diaphragm

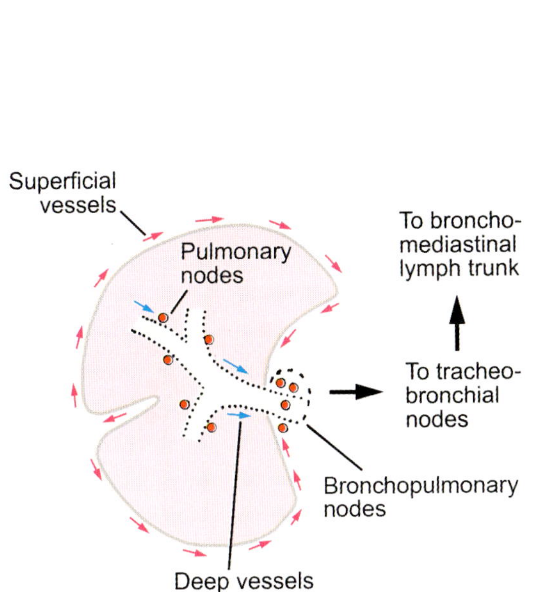


**22.13:** Lymphatic drainage of the lungs

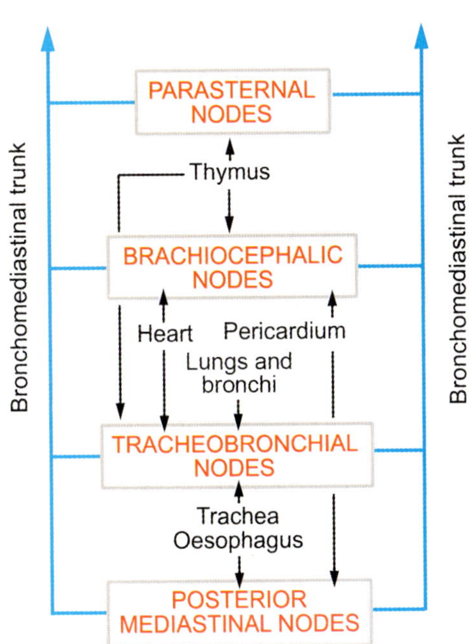


**22.14:** Scheme to show interconnections of major lymph nodes draining the thoracic viscera

### *Lymphatic Drainage of the Heart*

1. The heart is drained through vessels that travel mainly in the interventricular and atrioventricular grooves (22.15).
2. One set runs in the anterior part of the atrioventricular groove. The vessels of this set cross the aorta to reach the brachiocephalic nodes.
3. Another set of vessels runs along the anterior interventricular groove and ends in the inferior tracheobronchial nodes.

### Lymphatic Drainage of Thymus

The thymus drains into the parasternal, brachiocephalic and tracheobronchial nodes.

### Lymphatic Drainage of Trachea

1. The ***cervical part*** of the trachea drains into the ***deep cervical nodes*** directly and also through the ***pretracheal*** and ***paratracheal*** nodes (22.16).
2. The ***thoracic part*** of the trachea drains into the right and left superior tracheobronchial nodes and into the inferior tracheobronchial nodes.

### Lymphatic Drainage of Oesophagus

1. The ***cervical part*** of the oesophagus drains into the deep cervical nodes. Some of these lymph vessels pass through the paratracheal nodes (22.17).
2. The ***thoracic part*** of the oesophagus drains into the posterior mediastinal lymph nodes.
3. The ***abdominal part*** of the oesophagus drains into nodes present in relation to the left gastric artery.

## NERVES OF THE THORAX

### Introductory Remarks

The nerves of the thorax belong to two distinct functional categories.

1. Branches of spinal nerves (including the intercostal nerves) supply mainly skeletal muscle and skin.
   a. Most of the nerves of the body that we have studied so far are of this type. (These are sometimes referred to as ***cerebrospinal nerves*** in contrast to the ***autonomic nerves*** mentioned in this chapter).

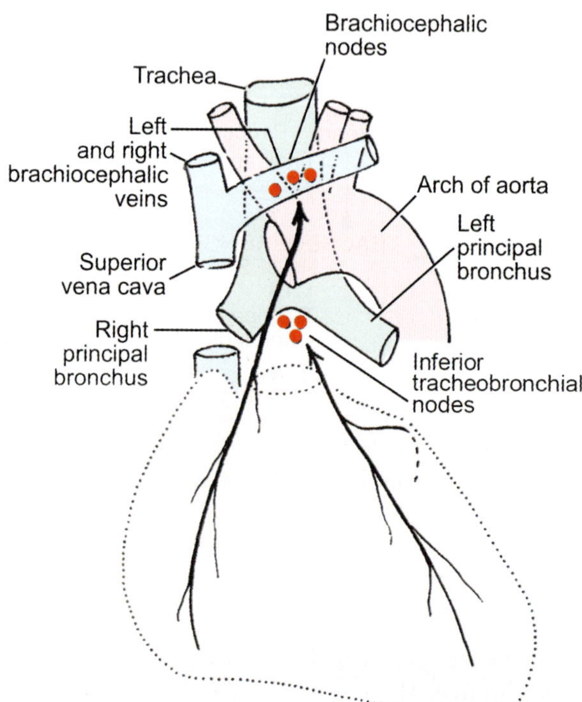


**22.15:** Scheme to show the lymphatic drainage of the heart

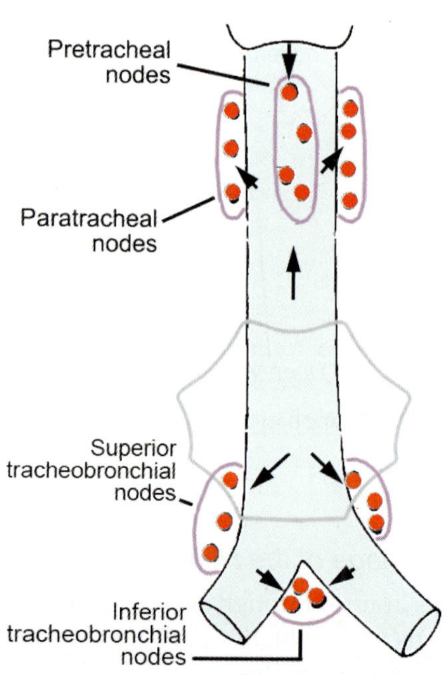


**22.16:** Lymphatic drainage of trachea

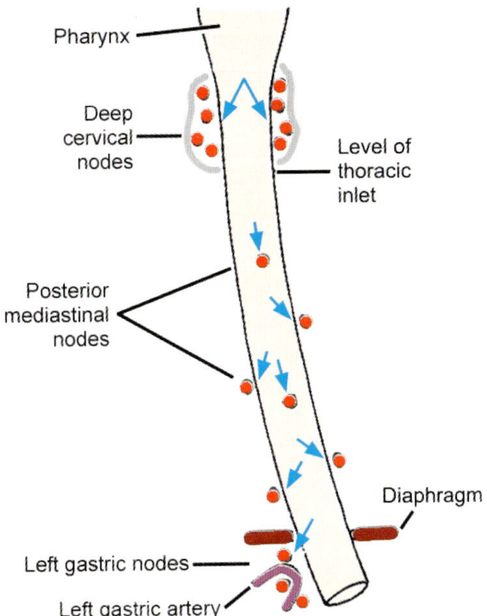


22.17: Lymphatic drainage of oesophagus

   b. In the thorax, the nerves belonging to this category are the intercostal, subcostal and phrenic nerves.
   c. The intercostal and subcostal nerves have been described in chapter 18. The phrenic nerve is described below.
2. The viscera, including smooth muscle in the walls of blood vessels and glands are supplied by ***autonomic nerves***. Before the arrangement of autonomic nerves can be properly understood some general principles about them need to be known. These are described below.
3. Both cerebrospinal and autonomic nerves carry motor (or efferent) and sensory (afferent) fibres.

## THE PHRENIC NERVES

1. The phrenic nerves are amongst the most important nerves in the body as they are the only motor supply to the diaphragm.
2. Each nerve (right or left) arises from the (anterior primary rami of) spinal nerves C3, C4 and C5. The contribution from C4 is the greatest.
3. The nerve descends vertically through the lower part of the neck and then through the thorax to reach the diaphragm. Some terminal branches enter the abdomen.
4. a. In the neck, the phrenic nerve descends vertically across the scalenus anterior muscle (22.20).
   b. Crossing the medial (or lower) border of the muscle, it crosses in front of the first part of the subclavian artery.
   c. On the right side, however, the nerve is usually separated from the artery by a part of the scalenus anterior.
5. Throughout its course in the neck the nerve lies deep to the sternocleidomastoid muscle. Other relationships of the nerve in the neck will be considered when we study the head and neck.
6 a. The ***relations in the thorax*** are as follows:
   b. On entering the thorax, the nerve passes medially crossing in front of the internal thoracic artery and comes into relationship with structures in the mediastinum. Subsequent relations are different on the right and left sides.

7. The ***relations of the left phrenic nerve*** are as follows:
    a. Above the arch of the aorta the nerve lies in the interval between the left common carotid and left subclavian arteries.
        i. It, at first lies posterior and lateral to the vagus nerve, but crosses the latter superficially and comes to lie in front and medial to it.
        ii. Just above the arch of the aorta, the left brachiocephalic vein crosses these structures.
    b. The nerve then crosses the aortic arch lying on its anterolateral side. Here, the nerve crosses superficial to the left superior intercostal vein.
    c. Below the arch of the aorta, the phrenic nerve crosses in front of the structures comprising the root of the left lung and then descends across the heart (left ventricle) lying between the parietal pericardium and the mediastinal pleura.
8. The ***relations of the right phrenic nerve*** are as follows:
    a. After crossing the internal thoracic artery, the nerve reaches the right brachiocephalic vein. It runs downwards lateral to this vein and at its lower end the nerve passes onto the lateral side of the superior vena cava.
    b. Leaving the vena cava the nerve descends over the right side of the heart (right atrium) lying between the parietal pericardium and the mediastinal pleura.
    c. Just above the diaphragm, the nerve lies lateral to the inferior vena cava.
9. The ***relationship of the phrenic nerves to the diaphragm*** is as follows:
    a. The nerves pierce the diaphragm and divide into branches that ramify within its substance, or on its ***inferior*** surface.
    b. The right phrenic nerve passes through the opening for the inferior vena cava, or pierces the central tendon just lateral to this opening.
    c. The left phrenic nerve pierces the muscular part of the diaphragm in front of the central tendon.

**WANT TO KNOW MORE?**

10. Apart from motor fibres to the diaphragm, each phrenic nerve carries a number of afferent fibres as follows:
    a. It carries proprioceptive fibres from the diaphragm.
    b. In the thorax, it gives off sensory branches to the pericardium and the parietal pleura.
    c. The nerve also carries sensations from some organs within the abdomen including the suprarenal glands, the inferior vena cava and the gallbladder.

*Accessory Phrenic Nerve*

1. The root of the phrenic nerve from C5 may sometimes follow a complicated course.
2. Instead of arising from C5 itself, it may arise from the nerve to the subclavius.
3. From here, the root descends through the neck lateral to the main phrenic nerve and joins it in the upper part of the thorax.
4. Such a root from C5 constitutes the accessory phrenic nerve.

## PRELIMINARY REMARKS ON THE AUTONOMIC NERVOUS SYSTEM

1. The autonomic nervous system is responsible for the nerve supply of viscera and blood vessels. It is subdivided into two main parts.
    a. These are the ***sympathetic*** and ***parasympathetic*** nervous systems. Both these divisions contain efferent as well as afferent fibres.

2. The efferent fibres supply smooth muscle throughout the body. The influence of these nerves may be either to cause contraction or relaxation.
   a. In a given situation, the sympathetic and parasympathetic nerves generally produce opposite effects.
   b. For example, sympathetic stimulation causes dilatation of the pupil, whereas parasympathetic stimulation causes constriction.
3. In addition to the supply of smooth muscle autonomic nerves supply glands. Such nerves are described as ***secretomotor***. The secretomotor nerves to almost all glands are parasympathetic. The only exceptions are the sweat glands which have a sympathetic supply.
4. In the thorax, the parasympathetic nervous system is represented by the vagus nerve and the sympathetic nervous system by the right and left sympathetic trunks and their branches.

## Basic Arrangement of Efferent Autonomic Pathways

1. A pathway for supply of smooth muscle or gland always consists of two neurons that synapse in a ganglion.
2. The cell body of the first, or ***preganglionic*** neuron is located within the brain or spinal cord. Its axon enters a peripheral nerve and after a variable course it ends in a ganglion.
3. The cell body of the second, or ***postganglionic***, neuron is located in the ganglion. Its axon reaches the smooth muscle or gland and supplies it (22.18).
   These remarks apply to both sympathetic and parasympathetic pathways.

## Autonomic Plexuses

1. Autonomic fibres, both sympathetic and parasympathetic, reach the thoracic and abdominal viscera through a number of plexuses.
2. Although they are called plexuses, they contain numerous neurons and are in fact equivalent to ganglia.
3. Most of the sympathetic fibres passing through them are postganglionic (having relayed in ganglia on the sympathetic trunk). Some are preganglionic and relay in the plexuses.
4. Parasympathetic fibres reaching the plexuses (through the vagus) are entirely preganglionic. The neurons in the plexuses are mostly parasympathetic postganglionic neurons.
5. The autonomic plexuses to be seen in the thorax are as follows:
   a. Cardiac plexuses
      i. Superficial cardiac plexus
      ii. Deep cardiac plexus.

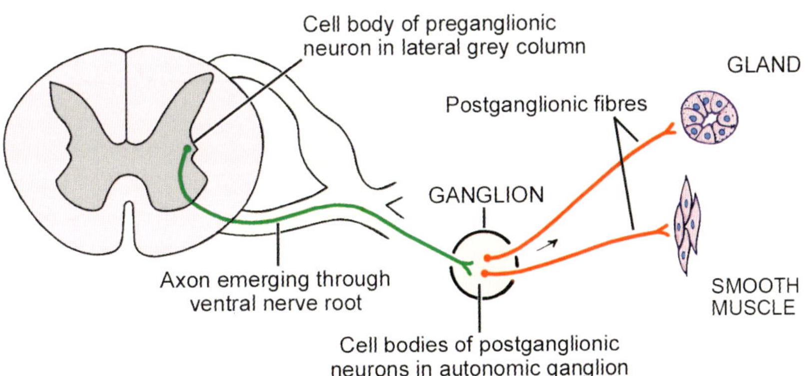


**22.18:** Scheme to show arrangement of nerve pathways supplying smooth muscle or gland

b. Pulmonary plexuses
   i. Anterior pulmonary plexus
   ii. Posterior pulmonary plexus.
c. Oesophageal plexuses
   i. Anterior oesophageal plexus
   ii. posterior oesophageal plexus.

## Basic Arrangement of Parasympathetic Pathways

The parasympathetic nervous system consists of a cranial part and a sacral part (22.19).

1. ***Preganglionic neurons*** of the ***cranial part*** are located in the brainstem (general visceral efferent nuclei of the cranial nerves). Details of these will be considered in the section on the head and neck.
   a. The preganglionic fibres arising from them pass through the third, seventh, ninth and tenth cranial nerves. They collectively constitute the ***cranial parasympathetic outflow***.
   b. The only fibres of this outflow relevant to the thorax and abdomen are those that travel through the vagus nerve.
2. ***Postganglionic neurons*** of the cranial part of the parasympathetic nervous system are located in a number of ganglia present in association with branches of the cranial nerves concerned.
   a. They will be studied in the head and neck.
   b. Postganglionic neurons related to the vagus nerve are scattered in the autonomic plexuses mentioned above.
3. Preganglionic neurons of the ***sacral part*** of the parasympathetic nervous system are located in the sacral segments of the spinal cord (intermediolateral grey column in spinal segments S2, S3 and S4).
   a. Their axons constitute the ***sacral parasympathetic outflow*** (22.19).
   b. They are concerned with the innervation of some viscera in the abdomen and pelvis and will be dealt with later.

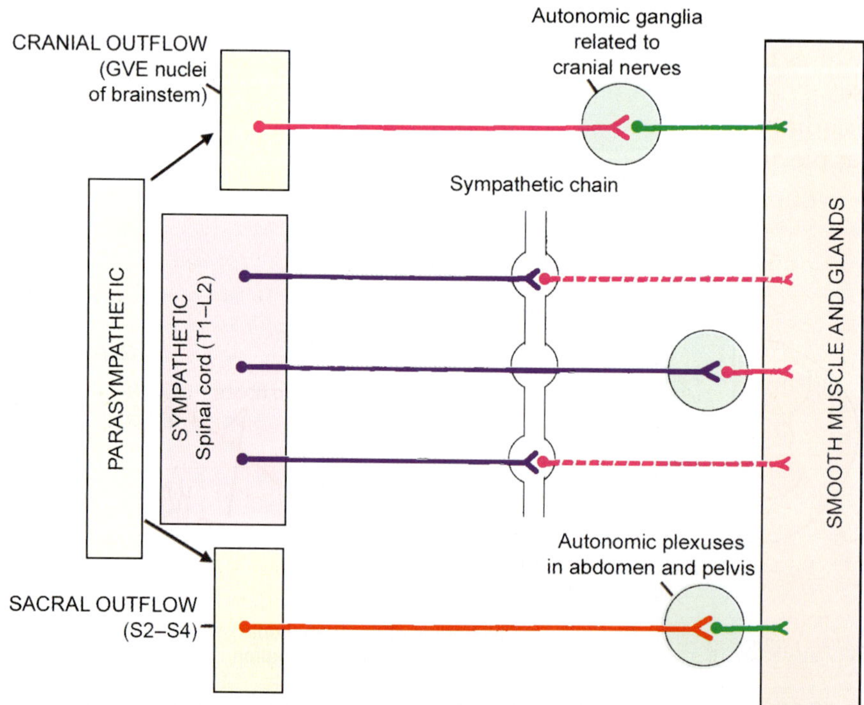


**22.19:** Basic plan of the sympathetic and parasympathetic nervous systems

## THE VAGUS NERVE

1. The vagus nerve arises from the brain (medulla oblongata).
2. It descends vertically in the neck in close relationship to the internal or common carotid artery and the internal jugular vein.
3. In the lower part of the neck, the nerve crosses anterior to the first part of the subclavian artery (22.20) and enters the thorax.

### Course and Relations of Vagus Nerve in the Thorax

1. a. In the superior mediastinum, ***the right vagus nerve*** lies on the right side of the trachea.
   b. Here it is posteromedial first, to the right brachiocephalic vein and then to the superior vena cava.
   c. The nerve passes deep to the vena azygos to reach the posterior side of the root of the right lung.
2. a. In the superior mediastinum, ***the left vagus nerve*** descends between the left common carotid and left subclavian arteries.
   b. It passes behind the left brachiocephalic vein and then crosses the left side of the arch of the aorta to reach the posterior aspect of the root of the left lung.
   c. The nerve is related laterally to the left lung and pleura. Above the arch of the aorta the vagus is crossed by the left phrenic nerve. Over the arch of the aorta, it is crossed by the left superior intercostal vein (21.5 and 21.6).
3. Having reached the root of the lung each vagus nerve (right or left) divides into a number of branches. At this level, the vagi cease to exist as distinct trunks.
4. The distribution of the vagus nerves in the thorax is as follows. (Branches given off to structures in the neck, or in the abdomen will be considered in appropriate sections).

### Branches of the Vagus Nerve to Structures in the Thorax

Note at the outset that some branches arising from the vagi, in the neck, descend into the thorax. These will also be considered here.

#### *Recurrent Laryngeal Nerve*

1. The course of the recurrent laryngeal nerve is different on the right and left sides (22.21).
2. ***On the right side,*** the nerve is confined to the neck and does not enter the thorax.
   a. It arises from the vagus as the latter passes in front of the subclavian artery.
   b. It passes backwards below the artery and then upwards behind the artery forming a loop.
   c. The nerve then runs upwards and medially to reach the side of the trachea.
3. ***On the left side,*** the recurrent laryngeal nerve arises from the vagus in the thorax, as the latter crosses lateral to the arch of the aorta (21.6).
   a. The nerve winds below the arch, immediately behind the ligamentum arteriosum and then passes upwards and medially (deep to the arch of the aorta) to reach the side of the trachea (22.21).
   b. Having reached the trachea, the nerve ascends in the groove between it and the oesophagus, and passes into the neck.
4. The recurrent laryngeal nerves provide the motor supply to most of the intrinsic muscles of the larynx. The nerves also provide the sensory supply to the mucous membrane of the lower half of the larynx. Details of the supply to the larynx will be considered in the section on the neck.

**WANT TO KNOW MORE?**

5. The recurrent laryngeal nerves also give sensory branches to the trachea and the oesophagus. Some branches are given off to the deep cardiac plexus (see below).

### Cardiac Branches and Cardiac Plexuses

1. While descending through the neck each vagus nerve gives off one (or more) superior cervical cardiac branch and an inferior cervical cardiac branch.
   a. These branches descend into the thorax and take part in forming the cardiac plexuses described below.
   b. Additional cardiac branches arise from the nerve in the superior mediastinum and also from the recurrent laryngeal branches.
2. a. The ***superficial cardiac plexus*** is located just below the arch of the aorta, close to the ligamentum arteriosum (22.21).
   b. It is formed by the inferior cervical cardiac branch of the left vagus nerve and the superior cervical cardiac branch of the left sympathetic trunk.
3. The deep cardiac plexus is situated in front of the bifurcation of the trachea.
4. It receives several branches from the right and left vagus nerves as follows:
   a. Right superior and inferior cervical cardiac branches.
   b. Left superior cervical cardiac branch.
   c. Branches from right and left vagi arising in the thorax.
   d. Branches from the right and left recurrent laryngeal nerves.
5. The plexus also receives numerous cardiac branches from the right and left sympathetic trunks.
6. Branches from the superficial and deep cardiac plexuses supply the heart.

### Pulmonary Branches

1. On reaching the root of the lung each vagus divides into a number of branches that form the posterior pulmonary plexus (right or left).
2. Each plexus also receives several branches from the sympathetic trunk.
3. Some branches of the vagus reach the front of the root of the lung and forms a less prominent anterior pulmonary plexus. Branches from these plexuses accompany the bronchi and supply the smooth muscle in their wall.

### Oesophageal Branches

1. Fibres of the right and left vagus nerves emerge from the posterior pulmonary plexuses and descend on the oesophagus forming an anterior and a posterior oesophageal plexus.
2. Although both plexuses receive fibres from the nerves of both sides, the anterior plexus is formed mainly by fibres from the left vagus and the posterior plexus mainly by fibres from the right vagus.
3. Branches from these plexuses supply the oesophagus and the posterior part of the pericardium.
4. Fibres emerging from the lower end of the anterior oesophageal plexus collect to form the anterior vagal trunk which is made up mainly of fibres from the left vagus.
5. Similarly fibres arising from the posterior oesophageal plexus (mainly right vagus) collect to form the posterior vagal trunk.
6. The anterior and posterior vagal trunks enter the abdomen through the oesophageal opening in the diaphragm. Their distribution will be taken up in the section on the abdomen.

## Basic Arrangement of Sympathetic Pathways

1. The ganglia related to the sympathetic nerves are located mainly in the sympathetic trunk (right or left).
2. Each trunk is a long nerve cord placed on either side of the vertebral column and extending from the base of the skull above, to the coccyx below. The sympathetic ganglia are seen as enlargements along the length of the trunk.

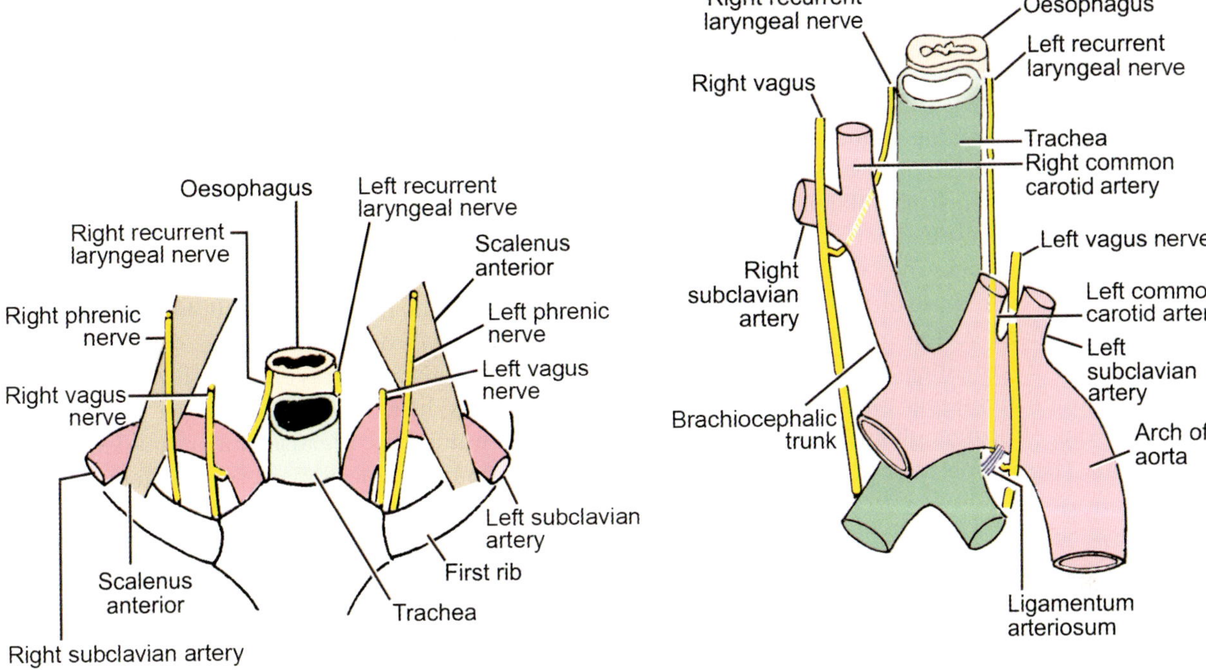


**22.20:** Relationship of subclavian artery to the vagus nerve. The phrenic nerve is also shown

**22.21:** Course of recurrent laryngeal nerves on the right and left sides

3. Basically, there is one ganglion corresponding to each spinal nerve, but in many situations the ganglia of adjoining segments fuse so that they appear to be fewer in number than the spinal nerves.
4. The ventral primary ramus of each spinal nerve receives fibres from a sympathetic ganglion through a delicate communication called the ***grey ramus communicans***.
5. In the case of spinal nerves T1 to L2 (or L3) there is, in addition to the grey ramus, a ***white ramus communicans*** through which fibres pass from the spinal nerve to the ganglion (22.22).
6. The cell bodies of sympathetic preganglionic neurons are located in the ***intermediolateral grey column*** of the spinal cord in spinal segments T1 to L2 (or L3) (22.22). Their axons leave the spinal cord through the anterior nerve root to enter the corresponding spinal nerve.
7. After a very short course through the ventral primary rami these fibres pass into the white rami communicantes and reach the sympathetic ganglia.
8. These preganglionic fibres leaving the spinal cord through spinal nerves T1 to L2 (or L3) collectively form the ***thoracolumbar outflow*** (22.19).
9. On reaching the sympathetic trunk, the preganglionic fibres may behave in one of the following ways (22.23).

## WANT TO KNOW MORE?

a. They may terminate in relationship to cells of the sympathetic ganglion concerned.
b. They may travel up or down the sympathetic trunk to terminate in ganglia at higher or lower levels in the trunk.
c. They may leave the sympathetic trunk through one of its branches to terminate in relation to neurons located in a peripheral autonomic plexus.

10. Sympathetic postganglionic neurons are located primarily in ganglia located on the sympathetic trunks (22.22 and 22.23). Some are located in peripheral autonomic plexuses. Axons arising from them behave in one of the following ways (22.24):
    a. The axons may pass through a grey ramus communicans to reach a spinal nerve. They then pass through the spinal nerve and its branches to innervate sweat glands and arrectores pilorum muscles of the skin in the region to which the nerve is distributed.
    b. The axons may reach a cranial nerve through a communicating branch and may be distributed through it as in the case of a spinal nerve.
    c. The axons may pass into vascular branches which form plexuses over the vessels and their branches. Some fibres from these plexuses may pass to other structures in the neighbourhood of the vessels. Fibres meant for blood vessels may also reach them through spinal nerves or their branches.
    d. The axons of postganglionic neurons located in sympathetic ganglia may travel through visceral branches and through autonomic plexuses to reach some viscera (e.g., the heart).
    e. The axons of postganglionic neurons located in peripheral autonomic plexuses innervate neighbouring viscera. These fibres often travel along blood vessels. Confirm the connections described above in 22.19.

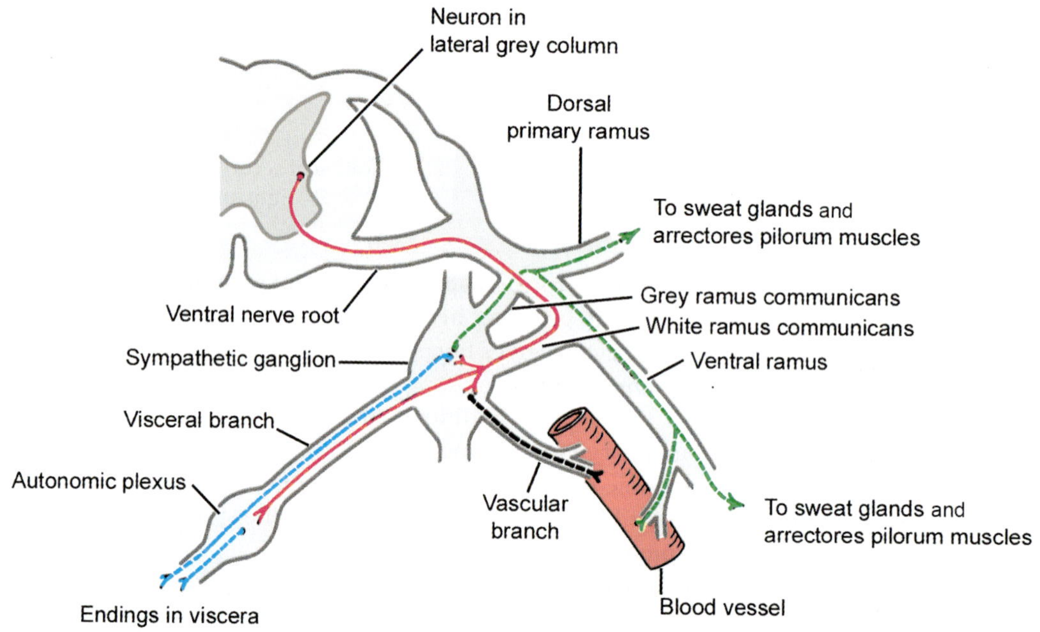


**22.22:** Grey and white rami connecting a spinal nerve to the sympathetic trunk, and the fibres passing through them. Preganglionic fibres are shown in red line and postganglionic fibres in blue or green

## THE SYMPATHETIC TRUNK

1. We have seen that the sympathetic trunk (right or left) is a long nerve cord extending from the base of the skull to the coccyx, and that it bears a number of ganglia along its length.
2. In the neck the trunk lies posterior to the carotid sheath, anterior to the transverse processes of the cervical vertebrae.
3. In the thorax the trunk descends in front of the heads of the ribs, and in the abdomen it is anterolateral to the lumbar vertebrae.
4. Lower down, the trunk descends anterior to the sacrum. Passing medially as they descend the right and left sympathetic trunks join each other in front of the coccyx.

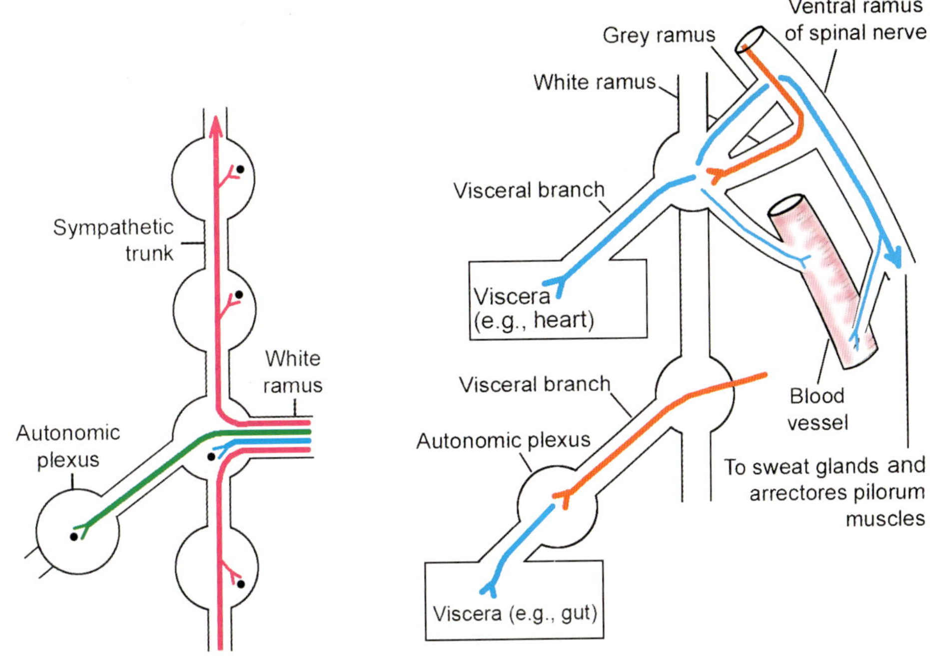


**22.23:** Mode of termination of sympathetic preganglionic neurons

**22.24:** Course and termination of sympathetic post-ganglionic neurons

5. We have also seen that basically the sympathetic trunk bears one ganglion for each spinal nerve, but the number is reduced by fusion of some of the ganglia.
   a. In the cervical region, there are usually three ganglia; superior, middle and inferior.
   b. The first thoracic ganglion is usually fused to the inferior cervical ganglion the two forming the ***cervicothoracic ganglion***.
   c. There are usually eleven ganglia in the thorax, four in the lumbar region, and four or five in the sacral region.
   d. The lower fused ends of the right and left sympathetic trunks are thickened by the presence of a midline ganglion called the ***ganglion impar***.
6. Details of the thoracic part of the sympathetic trunk are considered below. Some cardiac branches arising from the cervical part of the sympathetic chain descend into the thorax. They will also be considered here.

## WANT TO KNOW MORE?

### Cardiac Branches of Cervical Part of Sympathetic Trunk

1. We have seen that the cervical part of each sympathetic trunk bears three ganglia: superior, middle and inferior.
2. Each ganglion gives off a cardiac branch, so that there are a total of six cardiac branches (three right and three left).
3. The left superior cervical cardiac branch descends into the thorax along the common carotid artery. It runs across the lateral side of the arch of the aorta and ends in the superficial cardiac plexus.
4. All other cervical sympathetic cardiac branches (left middle and inferior; right superior, middle and inferior) end in the deep cardiac plexus.

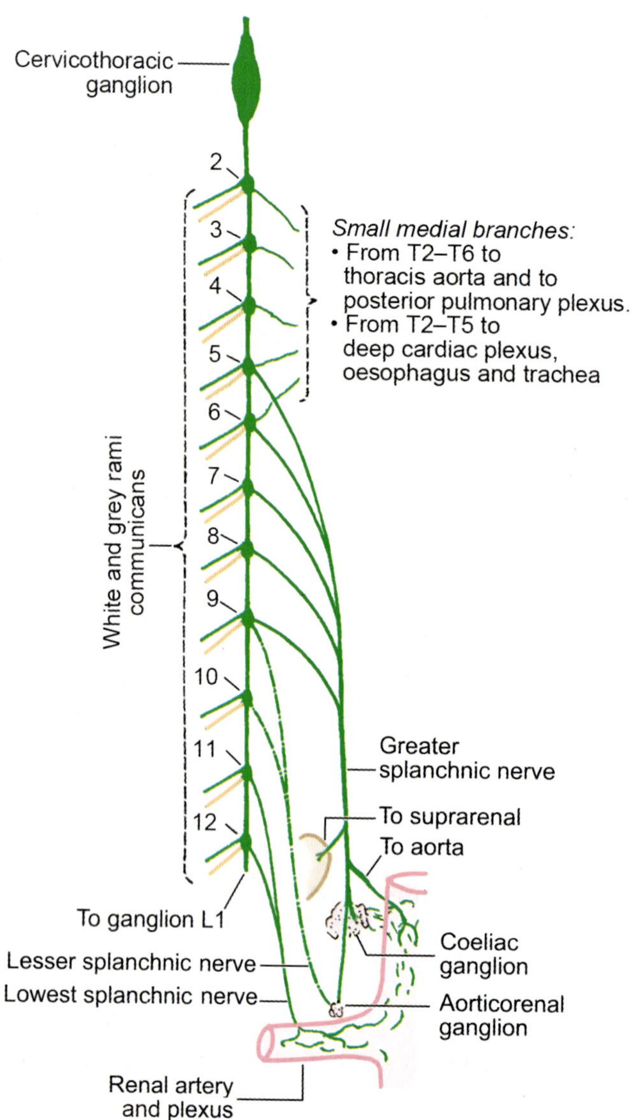


**22.25:** Branches of the thoracic part of the sympathetic trunk

## Thoracic Part of Sympathetic Trunk

1. The first thoracic ganglion is fused with the inferior cervical ganglion to form the ***cervicothoracic ganglion*** (22.25).
2. There are usually eleven thoracic ganglia, there being one each for nerves T2 to T12. These ganglia give off medial and lateral branches.
   a. Lateral branches arising from each ganglion connect it to the corresponding spinal nerve by white and grey rami communicans as already described (22.22).
   b. The medial branches arising from the ganglia supply viscera.
      i. Those arising from the upper thoracic ganglia are small. They supply the thoracic aorta (T2 to T6); join the posterior pulmonary plexus (T2 to T6), or join the deep cardiac plexus (T2 to T5).
      ii. Some of them supply the trachea and the oesophagus.

3. The lower thoracic ganglia give origin to prominent medial branches called the ***greater, lesser and lowest splanchnic nerves*** (22.25). Their origin is highly variable.

**WANT TO KNOW MORE?**

   a. The ***greater splanchnic nerve*** is usually formed by branches from ganglia T5 to T9.
   b. The ***lesser splanchnic nerve*** by branches from ganglia T9 to T10.
   c. The ***lowest splanchnic nerve*** from ganglion T11.
4. All these nerves pass through the diaphragm and enter the abdomen.
   a. The greater splanchnic nerve ends mainly in the ***coeliac ganglion.***
   b. The lesser splanchnic nerve ends in the ***aorticorenal ganglion.***
   c. The lowest splanchnic nerve ends in the ***renal plexus.***

   Details of these will be studied in the abdomen.
5. Afferent fibres accompany almost all efferent sympathetic fibres. These afferent fibres are peripheral processes of unipolar neurons located in dorsal nerve root ganglia of spinal nerves T1 to L2 or L3. For some details see Figure 22.26.

   In this chapter, we have so far concentrated our attention on the arrangement of sympathetic nerves, and of parasympathetic nerves as represented by the vagus nerves. We will conclude by summarising the nerve supply of the heart and lungs and pleura. The nerve supply of the trachea and that of the oesophagus is considered with these organs.

**Nerve Supply of the Heart**

1. The heart is supplied by nerves passing through the superficial and deep cardiac plexuses. The nerves contributing to these plexuses have been mentioned above.
2. ***Parasympathetic preganglionic neurons*** for the heart are located in the medulla oblongata of the brain (dorsal nucleus of the vagus). They reach the heart through cardiac branches of the vagus.
3. ***Parasympathetic postganglionic neurons*** are located within the superficial and deep cardiac plexuses and also in the walls of the atria.
4. ***Preganglionic sympathetic neurons*** are located in segments T1 to T5 of the cord.
5. On reaching, the sympathetic trunk their axons synapse with ***postganglionic neurons*** in the upper thoracic ganglia. Some of them run upwards in the sympathetic trunk to end in cervical ganglia. Postganglionic fibres leave these ganglia through their cardiac branches and join the vagal fibres in forming the cardiac plexuses.
6. Contraction of cardiac muscle is not dependent on nerve supply. It can occur spontaneously. The nerves supplying the heart, however, influence heart rate. Sympathetic stimulation increases heart rate and parasympathetic stimulation slows it.
7. Sympathetic nerves supplying the coronary arteries cause vasodilatation increasing blood flow through them.
8. Afferent fibres from the heart travel through both sympathetic and parasympathetic pathways.
   a. Impulses of pain arising in the heart travel along sympathetic pathways.
   b. They are carried mainly by the cardiac branches of the middle and inferior cervical ganglia. Some fibres also pass through cardiac branches of thoracic ganglia.
   c. These fibres pass through the sympathetic trunks and enter the spinal cord through spinal nerves T1 to T5.
   d. The cell bodies of the neurons concerned are located in the dorsal nerve root ganglia on these nerves. These pathways convey impulses of pain produced as a result of anoxia of heart muscle (angina).
9. Afferent fibres running along the vagus are concerned with reflexes controlling the activity of the heart.

**Nerve Supply of Lungs and Bronchi**

1. ***Parasympathetic*** preganglionic neurons that supply the bronchi are located in the dorsal nucleus of the vagus. The fibres travel through the vagus and its branches, to reach the anterior and posterior pulmonary plexuses.

2. Postganglionic neurons are located near the roots of the lungs. Their axons run along the bronchi and supply them.
3. The ***sympathetic*** preganglionic neurons concerned are located in spinal segments T2 to T5. Their axons terminate in the corresponding sympathetic ganglia.
4. Postganglionic fibres arising in these ganglia reach the bronchi through branches from the sympathetic trunks to the pulmonary plexuses.
5. Parasympathetic stimulation causes bronchoconstriction, while sympathetic stimulation causes bronchodilatation. Parasympathetic stimulation also produces vasodilatation and has a secretomotor effect on mucous glands in the bronchi. Sympathetic stimulation produces vasoconstriction.
6. Afferent fibres arise in alveoli and bronchial mucosa. They are important in respiratory reflexes.

**Nerve Supply of Pleura**

1. The parietal pleura receives its nerve supply through nerves supplying the thoracic wall, while the visceral pleura receives branches from nerves that supply the lungs.
2. Thus, the parietal pleura is supplied by branches from intercostal and phrenic nerves.
3. The visceral pleura is innervated by sympathetic and parasympathetic nerves that supply the lungs.
4. An important result of this difference in nerve supply is that the parietal pleura is much more sensitive to pain than the visceral pleura.

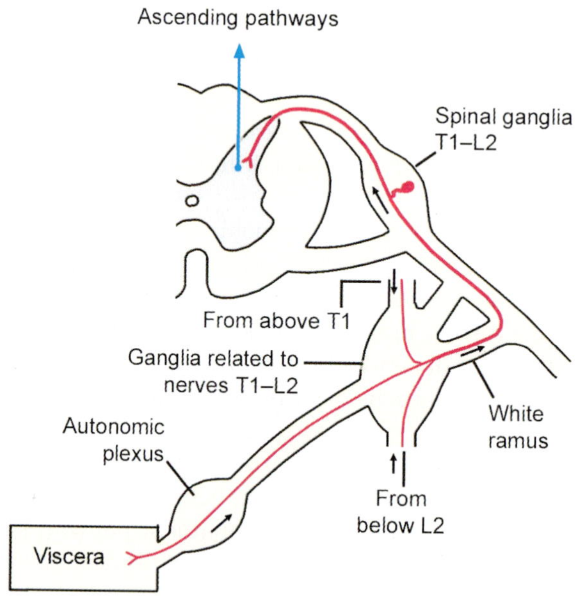


**22.26:** Afferent autonomic pathway involving the sympathetic nerves

# 23 CHAPTER

# Surface Marking and Radiological Anatomy of the Thorax

## SURFACE MARKING

1. The thorax is a region of considerable clinical importance. Having a clear idea of the relationship of internal organs within it to the surface of the body is, therefore, very useful.
2. The most important organs within the thorax are the heart and lungs. The surface projection of the pleura and lungs has already been described on pages 397 and 399 (19.24 and 19.25).
3. The surface projection of the borders and valves of the heart has been described on page 418 (20.21). The projections of some other structures are described below.

### Some Landmarks on the Thorax

1. Before going on to understand the surface markings of structures in the thorax, it is necessary that the students have a clear idea of the formation of the thoracic cage. The clavicle, the sternum, the costal cartilages and the ribs serve as important landmarks that help us to mark projections of individual structures on the surface of the body.
2. Beginners often have difficulty in correctly identifying individual costal cartilages and ribs. The anterior part of the first rib is overlapped by the clavicle and because of this it cannot be felt. Identify some landmarks on the front of the thorax as follows.
3. Begin by placing your fingers over the clavicle.
   a. Trace the clavicle to its expanded medial end that forms a marked projection.
   b. Now put one finger in the interval between the medial ends of the right and left clavicles and feel for the upper border of the manubrium sterni.
   c. Notice that this border is concave and lies at a distinctly lower level than the medial ends of the clavicles.
4. Pass one finger downwards over the manubrium sterni (in the midline) till you come to a ridge-like prominence.
   a. This prominence is the manubriosternal junction or ***sternal angle***.
   b. At this level pass the fingers laterally and you will be able to feel the ***second*** costal cartilage. (Remember that the second costal cartilage meets the sternum at the junction of the manubrium and the body of the sternum).
5. Passing further laterally along the second costal cartilage you can feel the second rib.
   a. Other ribs and costal cartilages can be felt by counting downwards from the second.
   b. Trace each rib laterally up to the midaxillary line. Remember that the lowest rib here is the tenth.
6. The ribs can be traced beyond the midaxillary line onto the back of the thorax.
7. The spines of thoracic vertebrae can be identified as follows:
   a. Put your fingers on the back of the neck, in the midline, and feel for the ligamentum nuchae.
   b. When the fingers are run down the midline they reach the spine of the 7th cervical vertebra.
   c. Thoracic vertebral spines can be identified by counting downwards from here.

## Surface Marking of the Trachea

1. Place a finger just above the upper border of the manubrium sterni and pass it upwards for about one inch.
   a. You will feel the firm prominence of the cricoid cartilage.
   b. Just below this level, you can feel the softer cartilages of the trachea.
2. a. To mark the trachea, draw two vertical lines parallel to each other, and about 2 cm apart, starting just below the cricoid cartilage and ending at the level of the sternal angle.
   b. Near its lower end, the trachea inclines slightly to the right side.
   c. The trachea ends at this level by dividing into the right and left principal bronchi.

## Surface Marking of Right Principal Bronchus

1. The upper end of the right principal bronchus lies, more or less in the midline, at the level of the sternal angle.
2. Its lower end lies over the sternal end of the right third costal cartilage.
3. The bronchus is marked by drawing two lines 1 cm apart, running downwards and to the right, joining these two levels.
4. The bronchus is about 2.5 cm long.

## Surface Marking of Left Principal Bronchus

1. Before trying to mark this bronchus remember that, as compared to the right bronchus, it is twice as long (5 cm), and is placed more transversely.
2. Like the right bronchus its upper end lies at the level of the sternal angle.
3. Its lower end lies over the left third costal cartilage, 4 cm from the median plane.
4. The bronchus is marked by two lines, 1 cm apart joining these two levels.

## Surface Marking of Oesophagus

1. The upper end of the oesophagus lies at the lower border of the cricoid cartilage that can be located as described for the trachea.
2. a. From here draw two lines, 2.5 cm apart, descending to the upper border of the manubrium sterni.
   b. Continue the two lines downwards till they reach the sternal angle.
3. a. These lines should be drawn so that at the level of the cricoid cartilage and at the level of the sternal angle, the oesophagus is seen to be in the middle line.
   b. However, at the level of the thoracic inlet (i.e., the upper border of the manubrium sterni) the lines should deviate slightly to the left side.
4. a. To mark the part of the oesophagus that lies in the posterior mediastinum continue the same lines downwards, but with a distinct inclination to the left side.
   b. The lines should end at the level of the left 7th costal cartilage.
   c. Here the centre of the oesophagus should be 2.5 cm to the left of the midline.
5. The lowest half inch of the oesophagus marked as described above outlines the abdominal part.

## Internal Thoracic Artery

1. The upper end of this artery lies in the neck, 1 cm above the sternal end of the clavicle, 3.5 cm from the median plane.
2. The lower end of the artery lies in the sixth intercostal space 1.2 cm from the lateral border of the sternum.
3. The line joining these two points runs downwards behind the upper six costal cartilages and lies about 1.2 cm lateral to the sternum.

## Pulmonary Trunk

1. a. Note that the pulmonary valve is about 2.5 cm broad. It lies transversely, partly behind the left third costal cartilage and partly behind the sternum.
   b. This gives us the lower end (beginning) of the pulmonary trunk.

2. a. From here draw two vertical parallel lines upwards to the level of the left second intercostal cartilage.
   b. This gives us the level at which the pulmonary trunk divides into the right and left pulmonary arteries.

## Ascending Aorta

1. The first point to remember is that this vessel lies entirely in the middle mediastinum.
2. a. Its lower end corresponds to the position of the aortic valve.
   b. This valve is placed obliquely behind the left half of the body of the sternum at the level of the third intercostal space.
   c. It is about 2.5 cm broad.
3. Mark the valve as described above.
4. From the ends of the line representing the valve draw two parallel lines passing upwards and to the right to reach the sternal angle (right half).

## Arch of the Aorta

The projection of the arch onto the anterior wall of the thorax is shown in 21.4 (page 421). Note the following points:

1. The lower end of the arch of the aorta corresponds to the upper end of the ascending aorta described above. In other words, the anterior end of the arch lies behind the right half of the sternal angle.
2. The posterior end of the arch also lies at the level of the sternal angle.
   a. It lies partly behind the left half of the sternal angle and partly behind the second left costal cartilage.
   b. Do not forget that the posterior end really lies against the posterior wall of the thorax, at the level of the lower border of the fourth thoracic vertebra.
3. The summit of the arch reaches up to the level of the middle of the manubrium sterni.
4. When viewed from the front the arch looks much smaller than it actually is because of foreshortening.
5. a. To mark the convex upper border of the arch begin, the line at the right end of the sternal angle and carry it upwards and to the left with a curve that reaches the middle of the manubrium sterni.
   b. From there, continue the convexity downwards and to the left to end over the second left costal cartilage near the sternal margin.
   c. You can draw the lower border in the form of a sharply convex short line as shown in 21.4.

## Descending Thoracic Aorta

1. a. The upper end of the descending thoracic aorta corresponds to the lower end of the arch of the aorta.
   b. It lies at the level of the lower border of the fourth thoracic vertebra.
2. Its projection onto the anterior wall of the thorax lies over the left part of the sternal angle and the adjoining part of the second left costal cartilage. In other words, the upper end of the descending aorta lies to the left of the midline.
3. a. The lower end has to be marked at the level of the lower border of the twelfth vertebra. This level lies over the anterior abdominal wall.
   b. To mark it you have to first mark the ***transpyloric plane.*** (This is an imaginary transverse line drawn on the anterior abdominal wall midway between the upper end of the sternum and the upper border of the pubic symphysis. It lies roughly at a hand's breadth below the xiphoid process).
4. Take a point 2.5 cm above this plane, in the midline. Remember that the lower end of the thoracic aorta is about 2.5 cm broad and lies in the median plane.
5. The aorta can now be marked merely by drawing two parallel lines, 2.5 cm apart joining the upper and lower ends. As the vessel descends it gradually passes from the left side to a median position.

## Branches of Arch of Aorta

1. These are the brachiocephalic artery, the left common carotid artery and the left subclavian artery.
2. They all arise from the summit of the arch of the aorta.
3. Therefore, to mark any of these arteries first mark the upper border of the arch of the aorta as described above.

### Brachiocephalic Artery

1. Its lower end lies over the centre of the manubrium sterni.
2. Its upper end lies behind the right sternoclavicular joint.
3. Join these two levels by two parallel lines about one-fourth inch (8 mm) apart.

### Left Common Carotid Artery in Thorax

1. Its origin from the arch of the aorta lies just to the left of the centre of the manubrium (i.e., just to the left of the origin of the brachiocephalic artery).
2. From here it passes upwards and to the left to reach the left sternoclavicular joint. (At this level, the artery enters the neck).
3. To mark the artery join the two levels by two parallel line about one-fourth inch (8 mm) apart. The lines pass upwards and somewhat to the left.

### Left Subclavian Artery in Thorax

1. The origin of this artery from the arch of the aorta is to the left of that of the left common carotid i.e., it is near the left border of the manubrium sterni.
2. The artery is marked by two parallel, vertical, lines that extend to the left sternoclavicular joint. The lines should be about one-fourth inch (8 mm) apart.

## Superior Vena Cava

1. This vessel lies partly in the superior mediastinum and partly in the middle mediastinum. Its surface projection is, therefore, partly above the level of the sternal angle and partly below this level.
2. The surface projection of the superior vena cava is shown in 21.17 (page 437). Note that the vessel lies along the right side of the sternum.
3. The vena cava can be represented by two parallel and vertical lines 2 cm apart.
   a. Its upper end (beginning) lies over the lower border of the first right costal cartilage.
   b. Its lower end (termination) is at the level of the upper border of the third right costal cartilage.

### Right Brachiocephalic Vein

1. The upper end of the vein lies behind the medial end of the clavicle.
2. The lower end (termination) of this vein corresponds to the upper end of the superior vena cava (and lies over the lower border of the first right costal cartilage).
3. The lines representing the vein should be vertical and 1.5 cm apart.

### Left Brachiocephalic Vein

1. The upper end of the vein lies deep to the medial end of the left clavicle.
2. The lower end of this vein (termination) corresponds to the upper end of the superior vena cava (and lies over the lower border of the first right costal cartilage).
3. The vein is represented by two lines 1.5 cm apart joining these two levels.
4. Note that the vein runs obliquely and crosses behind the left sternoclavicular joint and the manubrium sterni.

## RADIOLOGICAL ANATOMY OF THE THORAX

The radiological anatomy of the thorax is shown in 23.1 to 23.4.

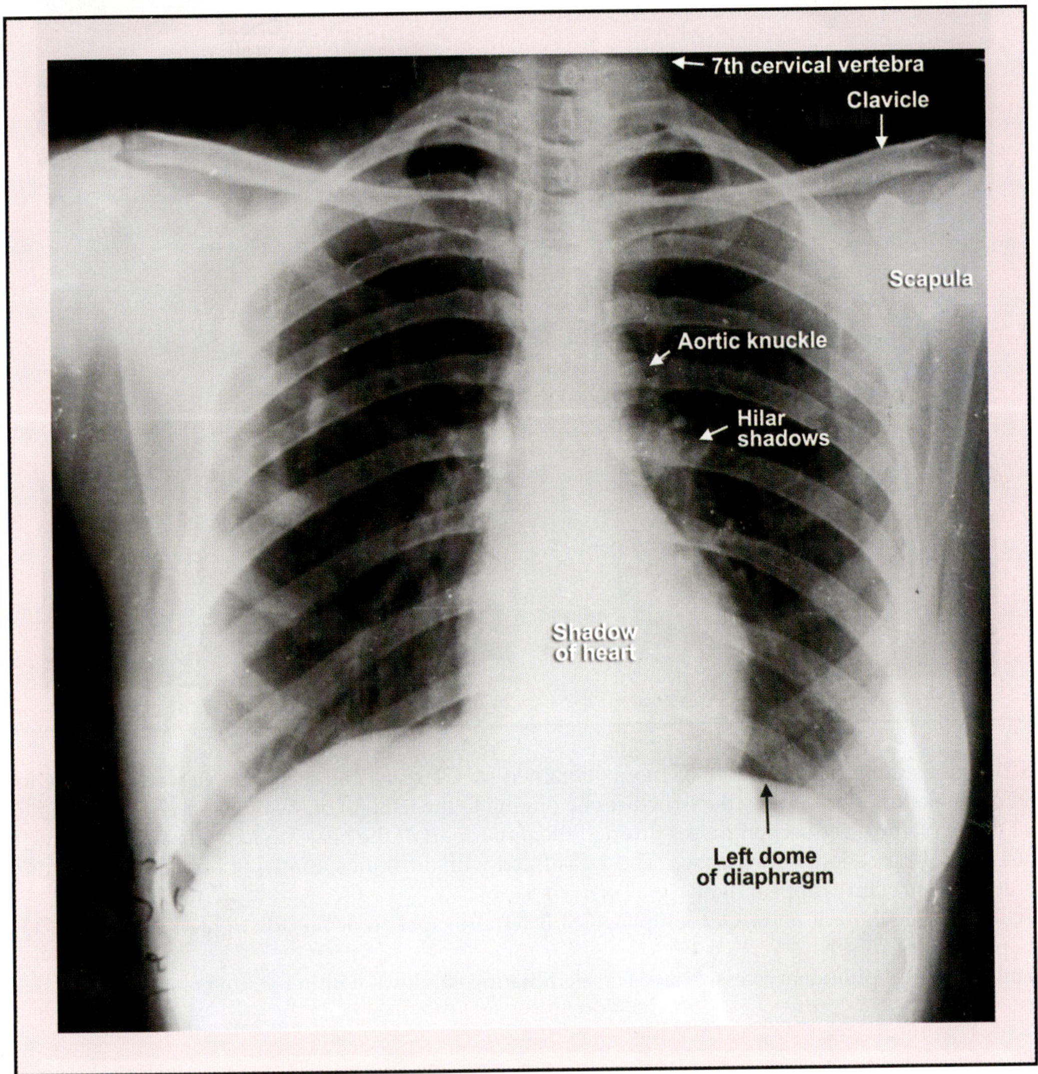


**23.1:** Plain radiograph of the chest. Posteroanterior view, in a female adult.

Observe the following in 23.1:

1. *Skeletal elements*: The posterior parts of the ribs form a series of shadows running laterally and downwards. The anterior parts of ribs are seen (in the lateral part) as less prominent shadows curving downwards and medially. (The costal cartilages do not case any shadows). The vertebrae can be made out in the upper part of the radiograph. Lower down, the vertebrae and the sternum cannot be made out as they are overlapped by the shadow of the heart, and of structures in the mediastinum. The clavicle and scapula are seen, on each side, in the upper lateral part of the radiograph.
2. The *heart* casts a shadow as it is full of blood. The right and left borders of the heart can be made out. When traced upwards, the left border becomes continuous with a shadow convex to the left. This shadow is produced by the arch of the aorta and is referred to as the aortic knuckle. Just below the aortic knuckle, the border of the heart shadow represents the pulmonary trunk. When this is enlarged it may be seen as a projection called the pulmonary conus. The right border of the heart merges, above and below, with the corresponding vena cava.
3. The *areas occupied by the lungs* are seen as dark areas (as they are full of air). However, just lateral to the cardiac shadow irregular shadows are produced by structures in the hilum of each lung.
4. Finally, note the *shadow cast by the diaphragm* (and structures below it). Note the domes of the diaphragm. The right dome is higher than the left.

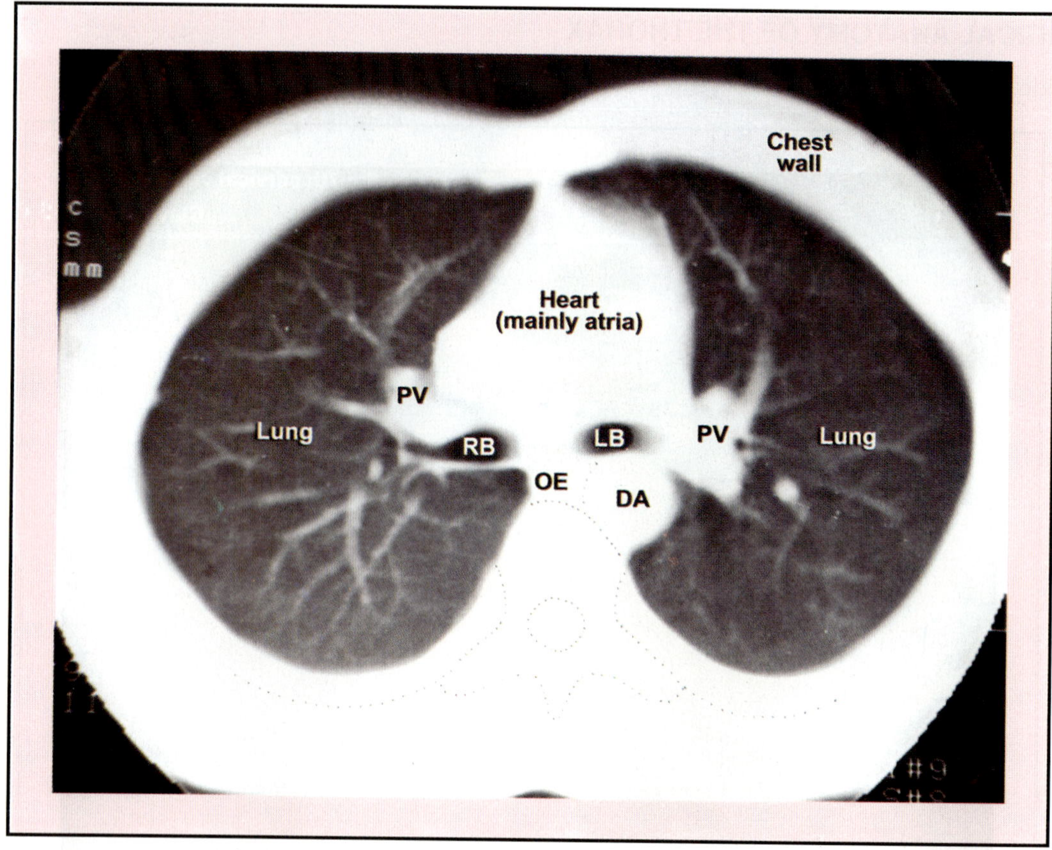


**23.2:** Cross-section (axial section) of thorax obtained by CT scan. The section is viewed from the foot end of the patient. That is why the structures belonging to the left half of the thorax are seen in the right half of the picture. The section passes through the upper part of the heart (mainly atria), just below the level of the bifurcation of the trachea. The areas filled with air (lungs, lumen of bronchi) appear dark, while other structures appear light.

DA: descending thoracic aorta; OE: oesophagus; LB: left principal bronchus; RB: right principal bronchus; PV: pulmonary vessels.

Ramifications of pulmonary vessels are seen as radiating shadows within the lungs.

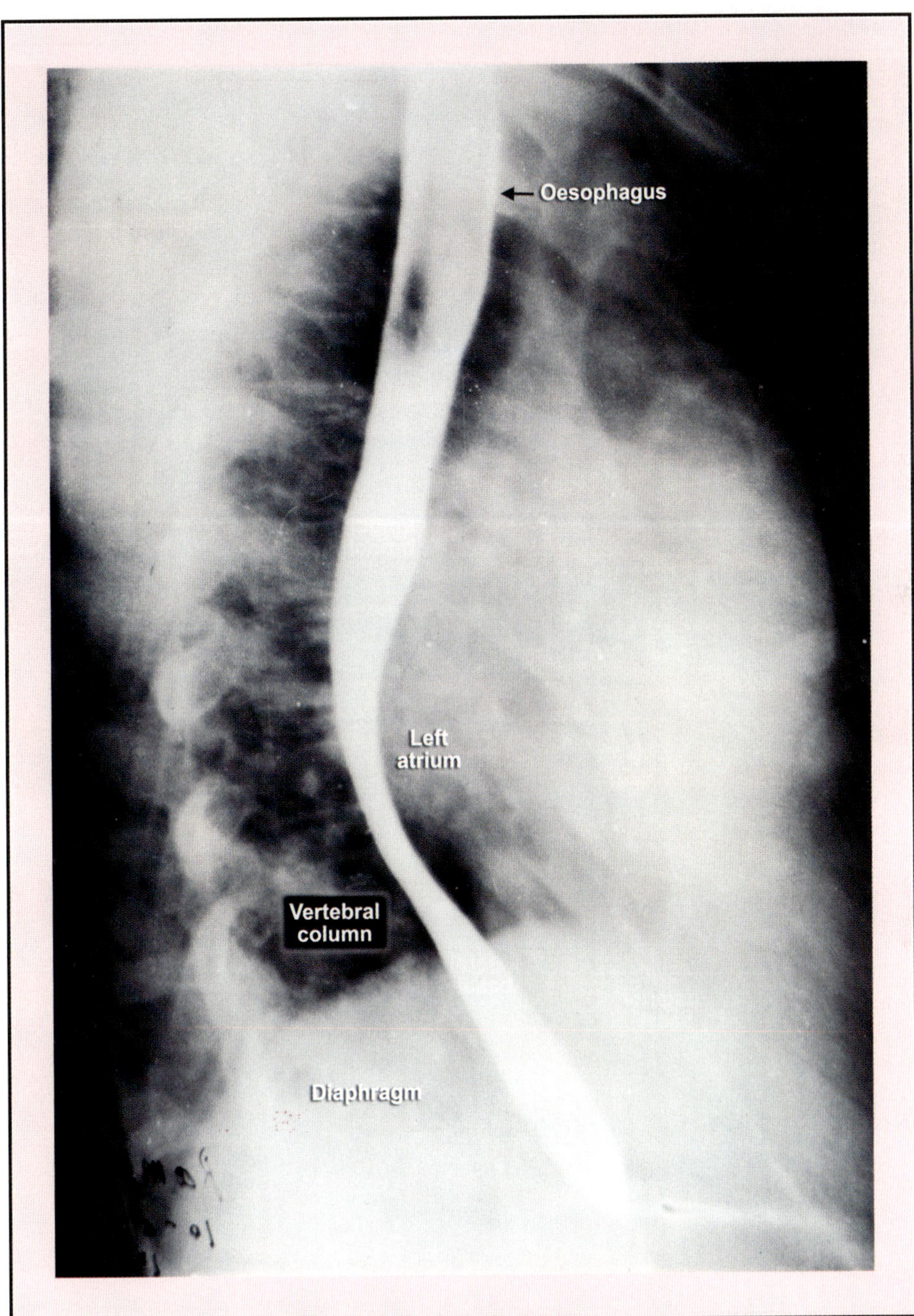


23.3: Radiograph taken immediately after the patient had swallowed a suspension of barium sulphate (which is opaque to X-rays). The oesophagus is clearly outlined. Any defects in the lumen produced by disease can be made out. An enlarged left atrium (abnormal) produces an indentation on the shadow of the oesophagus

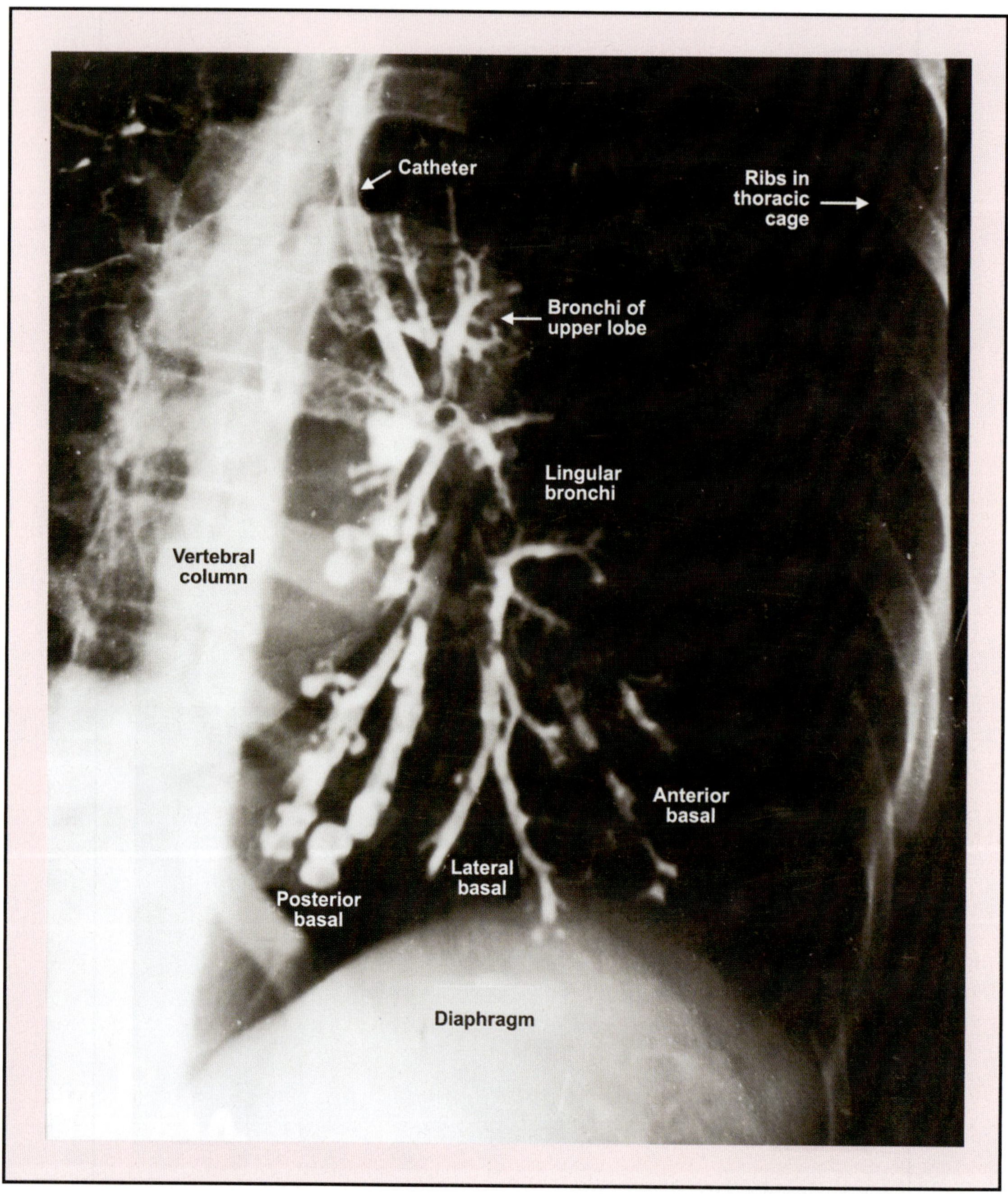


**23.4:** Bronchogram showing bronchi of the left lung (oblique view). A catheter was passed into the trachea, and then into the left principal bronchus, and a contrast medium was injected to outline the bronchi. See 21.13 (page 429) (Coronary angiography)

# PART 4

# Abdomen and Pelvis

# 24 CHAPTER Bones and Joints of the Abdomen

## BONES OF THE ABDOMEN

The bones that belong exclusively to the abdomen are:

1. Lumbar vertebrae
2. Sacrum
3. Coccyx

### Other Bones Related to Structures in the Abdomen

1. The inner surfaces of the hip-bones are closely related to structures in the abdomen and pelvis. They have been described in Chapter 9. This chapter also describes the pelvis as a whole.
2. The lower ribs and costal cartilages give attachment to, and are related to, many structures in the abdomen. They have been described in Chapter 16.

## LUMBAR VERTEBRAE

### Distinguishing Features of Typical Cervical, Thoracic and Lumbar Vertebrae

The structure of a typical vertebra has been described in Chapter 16. The cervical, thoracic and lumbar vertebrae can be easily distinguished from one another because of the following characteristics:

1. The transverse process of a cervical vertebra is pierced by a foramen called the ***foramen transversarium***.
2. The thoracic vertebrae bear ***costal facets*** for articulation with ribs. These are present on the sides of the vertebral bodies and on the transverse processes.
3. A lumbar vertebra (24.1) can be distinguished from thoracic and cervical vertebrae by the fact that it neither has foramina transversaria nor does it bear facets for ribs. It is also recognised by the large size of its body.

#### *Some Features of Typical Lumbar Vertebrae*

1. The vertebral bodies progressively increase in size from above downwards. They are, therefore, largest in the lumbar vertebrae. The body of a lumbar vertebra is oval in shape.
2. The vertebral foramen is triangular (24.1).
3. The pedicles are thick and short in the lumbar region and are directed backwards and somewhat laterally (24.1).
4. The laminae of lumbar vertebrae are short and broad, but do not overlap each other.
5. The spinous processes of lumbar vertebrae are large and quadrangular. They are more or less horizontal and have a thick posterior edge (24.2).
6. The articular facets of lumbar vertebrae are vertical. They are curved from side-to-side.
   a. The superior facets are slightly concave (24.1) and are directed equally backwards and medially.
   b. The inferior facets are slightly convex, and are directed equally forwards and laterally (24.2).
   c. Each superior articular process of a lumbar vertebra bears a rough projection called the mamillary process, on its posterior border.

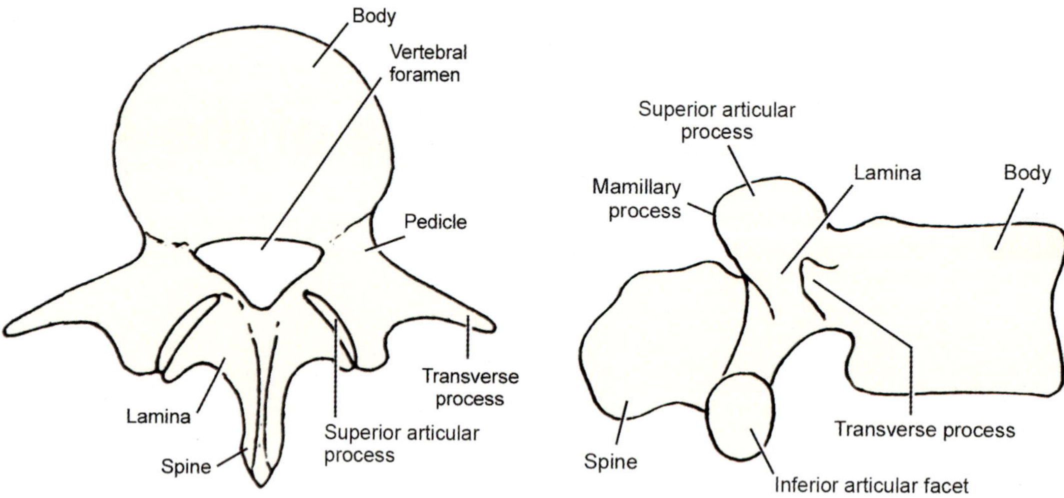


**24.1:** Typical lumbar vertebra seen from above

**24.2:** Typical lumbar vertebra seen from the lateral side

The first to fourth lumbar vertebrae are typical and show the features described above. The fifth lumbar vertebra is atypical.

## Fifth Lumbar Vertebra

1. The fifth lumbar vertebra is the largest of lumbar vertebrae.
2. In contrast to the small and tapering transverse processes of typical lumbar vertebrae the transverse processes of the fifth lumbar vertebra are very large. They form a distinguishing characteristic of this vertebra (24.3).

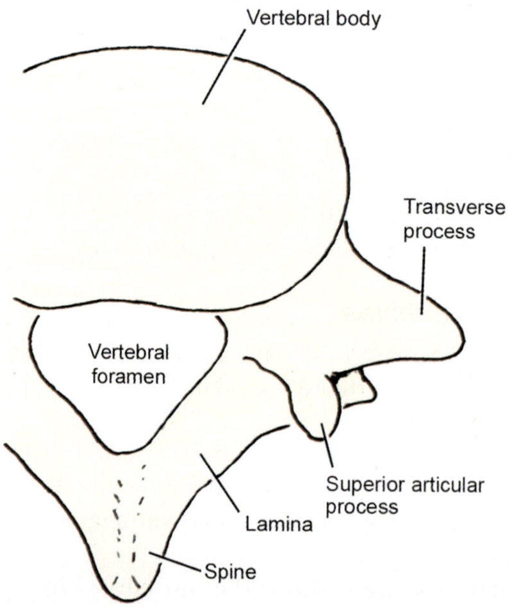


**24.3:** Fifth lumbar vertebra seen from above

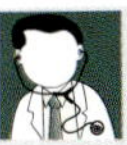

## CLINICAL CORRELATION

### Congenital Malformations

Vertebrae have a complex developmental history, and abnormalities resulting from maldevelopment are frequently seen.

1. The two halves of the neural arch may fail to fuse in the midline. This condition is called ***spina bifida***.
   a. If the gap between the neural arches is small, no obvious deformity may be apparent on the surface (***spina bifida occulta:*** occult = hidden).
   b. When the gap is large, meninges and nerves may bulge out through the gap forming a visible swelling.
   c. When the swelling contains only meninges and CSF it is called a ***meningocoele***.
   d. When neural elements are also present in the swelling the condition is called ***meningomyelocoele***.
2. Two or more vertebrae that are normally separate may be fused to one another. The fifth lumbar vertebra may be partially, or completely fused to the sacrum (***sacralisation of 5th lumbar vertebra***).
3. Alternatively, the first piece of the sacrum may form a separate vertebra (***lumbarisation of first sacral vertebra***).
4. Abnormality in ossification of a vertebra may result in a condition in which the spine, laminae and inferior articular processes are not fused to the rest of the vertebra.
   a. Normally, vertebral bodies do not slip forwards over one another because of the restraining influence of the inferior articular processes.
   b. However, when the abnormality described above is present, body weight can cause the body of the 5th lumbar vertebra to slip forward over the sacrum.
   c. This condition is called ***spondylolisthesis***.
5. Sometimes, a similar condition may affect the 4th lumbar vertebra that may then slip forwards over the 5th lumbar vertebra. Spondylolisthesis can be a cause of persistent low back pain.

### Fractures of Lumbar Vertebrae

1. Like other vertebrae those in the lumbar region can be fractured by direct injury.
   a. Such injury usually results in fracture of the spinous process, transverse process or lamina.
   b. If the lumbar spine is forcibly flexed (as in a fall from a height) the body of a vertebra can be compressed.
   c. In a compression injury, the vertebral arch and the ligaments around the body can remain intact and can prevent the spinal cord from being injured.
2. In more severe injuries, compression of the body of a lumbar vertebra may be combined with fracture of the articular processes (***fracture dislocation***). The vertebrae involved become unstable and injury to structures within the spinal canal can result.
3. Such injury in the lumbar region leads to the ***cauda equina syndrome***.
   a. The patient has a flaccid paraplegia.
   b. Sensations are lost over the perineum and upper medial area of thighs (the area corresponding to that which comes in contact with a saddle).
   c. There is incontinence of urine and of faeces.

### Lumbar Puncture

1. The term lumbar puncture is applied to a procedure in which a long needle is passed into the subarachnoid space through the interval between the 3rd and 4th lumbar vertebrae, or sometimes through the interval between the 4th and 5th vertebrae.
2. a. In this connection, it is important to note that the lower end of the spinal cord lies at the level of the lower border of the first lumbar vertebra.
   b. The subarachnoid space (containing cerebrospinal fluid) extends down to the level of the lower border of the second sacral vertebra.
   c. Hence, a needle passed into the lower lumbar part of the vertebral canal does not injure the spinal cord.

3. a. Remember, however, that here the subarachnoid space contains nerve roots forming the cauda equina.
   b. They are not injured as they are mobile.
4. Lumbar puncture has several uses as follows:
   a. Samples of cerebrospinal fluid (CSF) can be obtained for examination. Important points to note about CSF are its colour, its cellular content, and its chemical composition (specially the protein and sugar content).
   b. The pressure of CSF can be estimated.
   c. Air or radio-opaque dyes can be introduced into the subarachnoid space for certain investigative procedures. A skiagram taken after injecting iodinized oil into the subarachnoid space outlines the space.
   d. Anaesthetic agents injected into the subarachnoid space act on the lower spinal nerve roots and render the lower part of the body insensitive to pain. This procedure, called ***spinal anaesthesia***, is frequently used for operations on the lower abdomen and on the lower extremities.

**Prolapse of Intervertebral Disc**

1. a. The intervertebral discs are very strong in the young.
   b. With advancing age, however, the annulus fibrosus becomes weak and it then becomes possible for the nucleus pulposus to burst through it.
   c. This is called prolapse of the intervertebral disc (though it is really prolapse of the nucleus pulposus).
2. A prolapsed nucleus pulposus usually passes backwards and laterally and may press upon nerve roots attached to the spinal cord at that level.
3. Prolapse results in local pain in the back.
4. a. When nerves are pressed upon there is shooting pain along the course of the nerve involved.
   b. Disc prolapse occurs most frequently in the lumbosacral region and results in pain shooting down the back of the leg and thigh. This is called *sciata*.

**Psoas Abscess**

1. Tubercular infection of thoracic or lumbar vertebrae (commonly seen a few decades ago) can lead to formation of pus.
2. As the bodies of lumbar vertebrae are closely related to the psoas major this pus passes into the potential space deep to the fascia enclosing the muscle.
3. It then descends along the fascia to reach the femoral triangle where it forms a swelling.
4. Such a swelling may sometimes be confused with a femoral hernia.
5. A tubercular abscess is referred to as a cold abscess because the usual signs of inflammation are missing.

## THE SACRUM AND COCCYX

### The Sacrum

1. The sacrum lies below the fifth lumbar vertebra.
2. It is made up of five sacral vertebrae that are fused together (24.4 and 24.5).
3. It is wedged between the two hip-bones and takes part in forming the pelvis.
4. As a whole the bone is triangular.
   a. It has an upper end or ***base*** which articulates with the fifth lumbar vertebra.
   b. A lower end or ***apex*** which articulates with the coccyx.
   c. A concave ***anterior (or pelvic) surface***.
   d. A convex ***posterior or (dorsal) surface*** (24.5).
   e. Right and left lateral surfaces that articulate with the ilium of the corresponding side.
5. When viewed from the front (24.4) the pelvic surface of the sacrum shows the presence of four pairs of ***anterior sacral foramina***. The first foramen is the largest and the fourth the smallest.

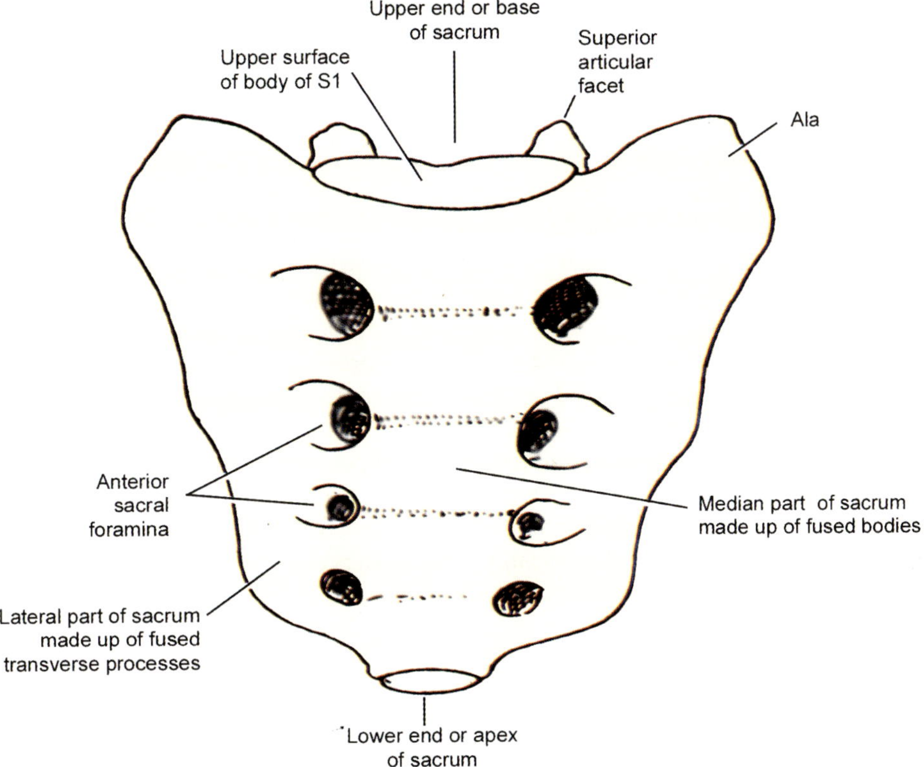


**24.4:** Sacrum seen from the front

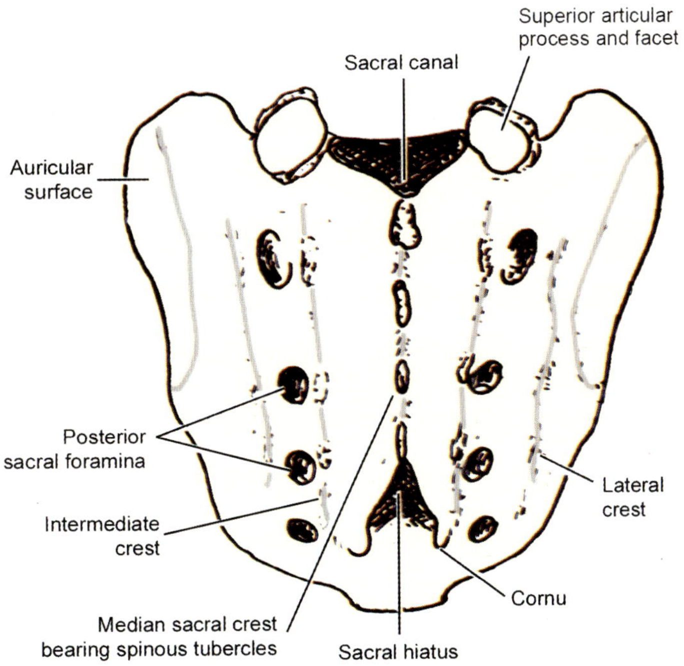


**24.5:** Sacrum seen from behind

6. The foramina separate the ***medial part*** of the bone from the ***lateral part***.
   a. The medial part is formed by the fused bodies of the sacral vertebrae.
   b. The lateral part represents the fused transverse processes, including the costal elements.
7. The anterior sacral foramina, seen on the pelvic surface, are continued into the substance of the bone and become continuous posteriorly with the ***posterior sacral foramina*** that open onto the dorsal surface.
8. The canals connecting the anterior and posterior foramina open medially into the ***sacral canal*** that is a downward continuation of the vertebral canal.
9. When viewed from above, we see the base of the sacrum. It is seen formed by the first sacral vertebra.
   a. It has a large oval body that articulates with the body of the fifth lumbar vertebra.
   b. The body has a projecting anterior margin called the ***sacral promontory***.
10. Behind the body of the sacrum, there is a triangular vertebral (or sacral) canal bounded by thick pedicles and laminae. Where the laminae meet there is a small tubercle representing the spine.
11. Arising from the junction of the pedicles and laminae there are the superior articular facets that articulate with the inferior articular facets of the fifth lumbar vertebra.
12. Lateral to the body, we see the superior surface of the lateral part, which is also called the ala.
13. When the sacrum is viewed from behind (24.5) we see the dorsal surface.
   a. We can again distinguish medial and lateral parts separated by four pairs of posterior sacral foramina.
   b. These foramina give passage to the dorsal rami of sacral nerves.
   c. The medial part of the dorsum of the sacrum is formed by the fused laminae of sacral vertebrae.
14. The laminae of the fifth sacral vertebra (sometimes also of the fourth) are deficient leaving an inverted U-shaped or V-shaped gap called the ***sacral hiatus***.
15. The midline is marked by a ridge called the ***median sacral crest*** on which four ***spinous tubercles*** (representing the spines) can be recognised.
16. Just medial to the dorsal sacral foramina, we see four small tubercles that represent fused articular processes. They collectively form the ***intermediate crest***.
17. Lateral to the foramina, we see a prominent lateral sacral crest formed by the fused transverse processes. The crest is marked by tubercles that represent the tips of transverse processes.
18. The lower end of the bone (apex) bears an oval facet for articulation with the coccyx.
19. At the sides of the sacral hiatus, we see two small downward projections called the ***sacral cornua***. They represent the inferior articular processes of the fifth sacral vertebra. They are connected to the coccyx by ligaments.
20. When the sacrum is viewed from the side, we see that the pelvic aspect of the bone is concave forwards, while the dorsal aspect is convex backwards.
21. The lateral surface bears a large L-shaped ***auricular area*** (or facet) for articulation with the ilium. (It is so called because its shape resembles that of the auricle or pinna).
   a. It consists of a cranial limb present on the first sacral vertebra.
   b. A caudal limb that lies on the second and third sacral vertebrae.
22. The area behind the auricular surface is rough and gives attachment to strong ligaments that connect the sacrum to the ilium.

**WANT TO KNOW MORE?**

**Sex Differences in the Sacrum**

1. The female sacrum is wider and shorter than in the male. This is to be correlated with the fact that the female pelvis is also shorter and broader than the male pelvis.
2. The forward concavity is more pronounced in the female.
3. The auricular surface is shorter in the female.
4. However, for practical purposes the sex of a given sacrum is most easily found out by examining the base.
   a. In the female, the transverse diameter of the body is approximately equal to the width of the ala.
   b. But in the male, the diameter of the body is distinctly larger than that of the ala.

The attachments on the sacrum, and its ossification, are described below along with those of the coccyx.

## THE COCCYX

1. The coccyx consists of four rudimentary vertebrae fused together (24.6). It has pelvic and dorsal surfaces.
2. The base or upper end has an oval facet for articulation with the apex of the sacrum.
3. Lateral to the facet, there are two cornua that project upwards and are connected to the cornua of the sacrum by ligaments.
4. The first coccygeal vertebra has rudimentary transverse processes. The remaining vertebrae are represented by nodules of bone.

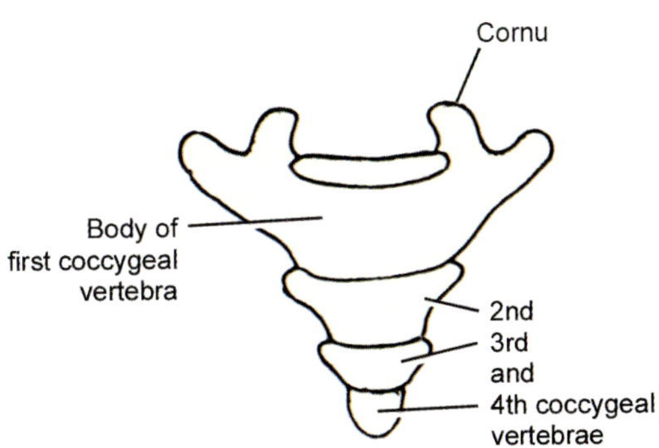


**24.6:** Coccyx seen from the front

### WANT TO KNOW MORE?

**Attachments on the Sacrum and Coccyx**

The following muscles are attached (24.7 and 24.8):

1. The ***iliacus*** arises from the anterolateral part of the upper surface of the ala (or lateral part).
2. The ***piriformis*** arises from the pelvic surface. The medial part of the origin is in the form of three digitations that arise from the areas between the sacral foramina.
3. The ***coccygeus*** is inserted into the lateral side of the pelvic aspect of the last piece of the sacrum and to the coccyx.
4. The ***levator ani*** is inserted into the sides of the lower two segments of the coccyx.
5. The ***gluteus maximus*** arises from the lateral margin of the lowest part of the sacrum, and that of the coccyx.
6. The ***erector spinae*** has a linear U-shaped origin from the dorsal aspect of the sacrum. The medial limb of the 'U' is attached to the spinous tubercles, and the lateral limb to the transverse tubercles.
7. The ***multifidus*** arises from a large area within the U-shaped origin of the erector spinae.

The following ligaments are attached:

1. Ligaments of the joints between the fifth lumbar vertebra and the sacrum correspond to those of other intervertebral joints.
2. The area around the auricular surface gives attachment to the ***ventral, dorsal*** and ***interosseus ligaments*** of the sacroiliac joint.
3. The ***iliolumbar ligament*** is attached to the lateral part of the ala.
4. The ***sacrotuberous ligament*** is attached to the lower lateral part of the dorsal surface of the sacrum.
5. The ***sacrospinous ligament*** is attached to the lower part of the lateral margin of the sacrum and to the adjoining lateral margin of the coccyx.

**Important Relations of the Sacrum**

1. The rectum is in contact with the ventral surface of the 3rd, 4th and 5th pieces of the sacrum.
2. The ventral surfaces of the first three pieces of the sacrum are covered by peritoneum and give attachment to the sigmoid mesocolon.
3. Deep to the peritoneum and rectum, the ventral surface is crossed by the right and left sympathetic trunks, the median sacral vessels, the right and left lateral sacral vessels, and the superior rectal vessels.
4. The ala is covered by the psoas major muscle and is crossed by the lumbosacral trunk.
5. The sacral canal contains the cauda equina, the spinal meninges and the filum terminale. The subarachnoid and subdural spaces end at the level of the middle of the sacrum.
6. The ventral and dorsal sacral foramina give passage to the corresponding rami of sacral nerves.

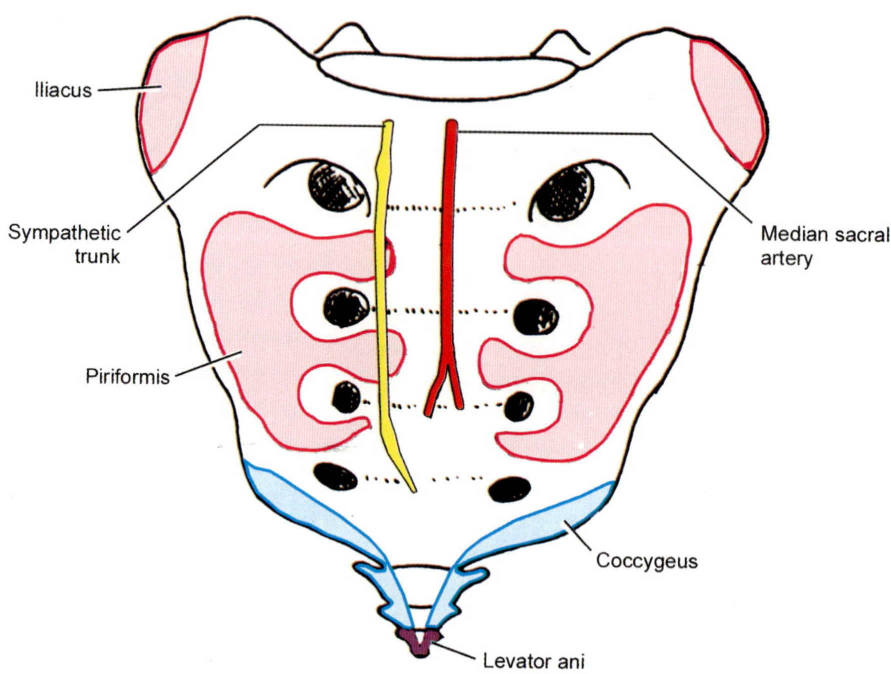


**24.7:** Attachments on the pelvic aspect of the sacrum and coccyx. Some related structures are also shown

## JOINTS OF THE ABDOMEN

### Intervertebral Joints

The joints between the lumbar vertebrae are similar to typical intervertebral joints. These have been described in Chapter 17.

### Lumbosacral Joint

1. This joint is similar to an intervertebral joint. Because of the large size of the vertebral bodies the intervertebral disc is thick and large. It is deepest anteriorly.
2. The fifth lumbar vertebra and the pelvis are connected by two additional ligaments.
   a. The ***iliolumbar ligament*** connects the tip of the transverse process of the fifth lumbar vertebra to the posterior part of the iliac crest.
   b. The ***lumbosacral ligament*** is attached above to the inferior margin and anterior aspect of the transverse process. Below it is attached to the sacrum near the anterior sacroiliac ligament.

### Pubic Symphysis

1. The two pubic bones are united in front at the ***pubic symphysis***.
2. This is a ***secondary cartilaginous joint***. Such cartilaginous joints are permanent structures that do not disappear with age. They are also called ***symphyses***.
3. The bone ends forming the joint are covered by a thin layer of hyaline cartilage. The two layers of hyaline cartilage are united by an intervening layer of fibrocartilage.

### Sacroiliac Joints

1. The sacrum articulates on each side with the corresponding ilium forming the right and left sacroiliac joints. These are synovial joints.

2. a. The iliac and sacral surfaces are both shaped like the auricle (pinna) and are, therefore, called ***auricular surfaces***.
   b. The surfaces are covered by cartilage, but because of the presence of a number of raised and depressed areas the joint allows little movement.
3. The capsule of the joint is attached around the margins of the articular surfaces.
4. It is thickened in its anterior part to form the ***ventral sacroiliac ligament***.
5. The main bond of union between the sacrum and ilium is, however, the ***interosseous sacroiliac ligament*** that is attached to rough areas above and behind the auricular surfaces of the two bones.
6. The posterior aspects of the sacrum and ilium are connected by a strong ***dorsal sacroiliac ligament*** that covers the interosseous ligament from behind.
7. The stability of the sacroiliac joints is important as body weight is transmitted from the sacrum to the lower limbs through them.

Two other ligaments that connect the sacrum to the hip-bone are the sacrotuberous and the sacrospinous ligaments that are seen in the gluteal region (24.9).

## Sacrotuberous Ligament

1. The sacrotuberous ligament is large and strong. It has a broad upper medial end and a narrower lower lateral end.
2. The upper end is attached (from above downwards) to:
   a. The posterior superior and posterior inferior iliac spines.
   b. The lower part of the posterior surface of the sacrum (transverse tubercles).
   c. The lateral margin of the lower part of the sacrum and the upper part of the coccyx.
3. Its lower end is attached to:
   a. The medial margin of the ischial tuberosity.
   b. Some fibres that are continued onto the ramus of the ischium constitute the ***falciform process***.

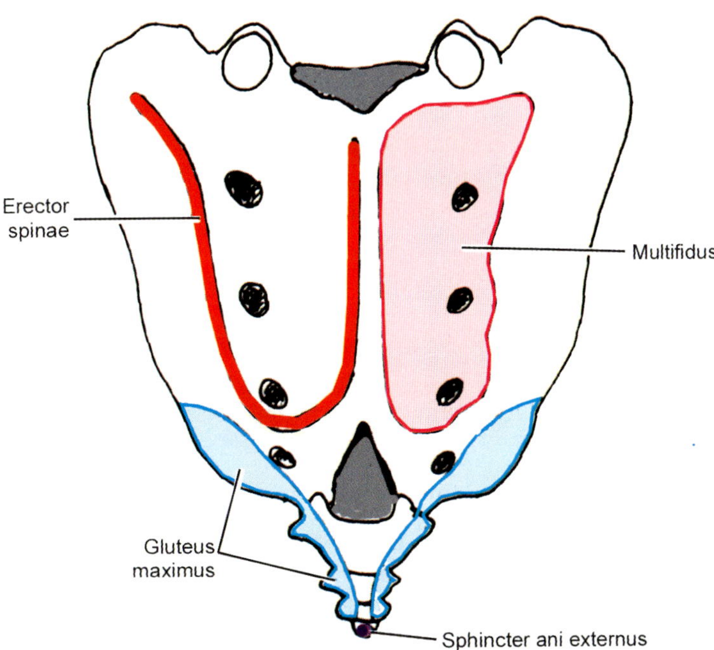


**24.8:** Attachments of muscles on the posterior aspect of the sacrum and coccyx

## Sacrospinous Ligament

The sacrospinous ligament is attached medially to the sacrum and coccyx and laterally to the ischial spine.

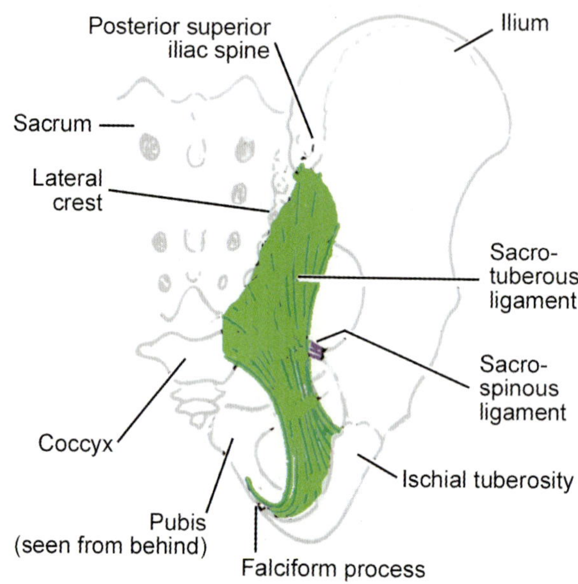


**24.9:** Sacrotuberous and sacrospinous ligaments

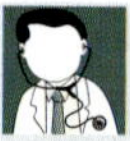

### CLINICAL CORRELATION

**Joints of Pelvis**

1. During pregnancy, the ligaments of joints of the pelvis are softened by the action of hormones (oestrogen, progesterone, relaxin) produced by the ovaries and the placenta. (Other soft tissues of the pelvic wall are also similarly influenced).
2. Softening of ligaments increases the range of movement permitted at the sacroiliac joint and this facilitates the passage of the head of the fetus through the pelvis.
3. However, softened ligaments render the sacroiliac joint more liable to strain and the effects of such stain may persist even after the end of pregnancy.
4. As ligaments tighten after pregnancy the joint may sometimes get locked in an abnormal position. This is called ***subluxation*** of the joint.
5. Strain in the sacroiliac joint leads to pain over the region of the joint. The pain may also radiate into the upper part of the thigh.
6. The sacroiliac joint may also undergo inflammation (arthritis) that may sometimes be tubercular. Symptoms are similar to those of strain.

**Dimensions of the Female Pelvis and their Importance in Obstetrics**

1. During childbirth, the fetus has to pass through the true pelvis. The largest part of the fetus is the head and for smooth passage of the fetus the dimensions of the true pelvis have to be large enough for the fetal head to be able to pass through it.
2. In cases where the passage is not large enough serious difficulties can arise during childbirth, and in the absence of adequate medical facilities this can be a cause of death of both the mother and the fetus.

3. Because of these facts, one of the important aspects of antenatal care is to examine the expectant mother to make sure that the pelvis is of normal size. Various methods have been used for this purpose as follows:

*External Pelvimetry*

1. In this procedure, an attempt is made to judge to size of the birth canal by making measurements between bony landmarks of the pelvis that can be felt on the surface of the body.
2. They include:
   a. The distance between the two anterior iliac spines (***interspinous diameter***).
   b. The distance between the outermost points on the right and left iliac crest (***intercristal diameter***).
   c. The anteroposterior distance between the lowest sacral spine and the pubic symphysis (***external conjugate***).

   However, experience has shown that information provided by such measurements is of little value and the procedure is of historical importance only.

*Internal Pelvimetry*

1. A better estimate of pelvic dimensions can be made by trying to palpate some features of the pelvis by fingers introduced into the vagina (vaginal examination).
   a. Such examination can be done most usefully in the later weeks of pregnancy as, by this time, the actions of hormones make the tissues of the pelvis much softer than normal.
   b. Ligaments are also affected and joints are less rigid. However, the procedure requires considerable experience.
2. During vaginal examination, the obstetrician tries to estimate the side to side dimension of the pelvis by feeling for the width and shape of the pubic arch, and the distance between the right and left ischial tuberosities.
3. To get an estimate of the anteroposterior diameter, a finger is placed against the sacral promontory and the distance of this point from the pubic symphysis is estimated. This measurement that is referred to as the ***diagonal conjugate*** is normally at least 11.5 cm.
4. The actual anteroposterior diameter at the inlet of the pelvis (***true conjugate***) can be estimated from the diagonal conjugate as it is 1.5 to 2 cm less than the diagonal conjugate.
5. Apart from the above, the obstetrician tries to palpate the lateral and posterior walls of the bony pelvis to find out if the curvatures are normal.

*X-ray Pelvimetry*

1. The most reliable estimates of pelvic dimensions can be made by taking skiagrams of the pelvis. An added advantage is that the dimension of the fetal head can also be determined at the same time.
2. However, exposure of a fetus to X-rays is far from desirable (as it can lead to abnormalities in the fetus) and the procedure has to be reserved for specially difficult cases only.

**Abnormalities in Shape of the Pelvis**

1. The shape of the pelvis can be congenitally abnormal, but most abnormal pelves result from lack of adequate nutrition. The shape of the pelvis can also become abnormal after injury.
2. In the typical female pelvis, the pelvic inlet is oval and the transverse diameter is slightly larger than the anteroposterior diameter. This is referred to the ***gynaecoid*** type of pelvis (or as the ***mesatipellic*** pelvis).
3. We have seen that in contrast to the female pelvis, the inlet of the male pelvis tends to be triangular so that the greatest transverse diameter is placed more posteriorly than in the female. When a female pelvis resembles the male pelvis it is described as ***android*** (or ***brachypellic***).
4. In anthropoid apes, the anteroposterior diameter of the pelvis is clearly greater than the transverse diameter. Such a condition is sometimes seen in the female pelvis that is then referred to as being of the ***anthropoid*** type. An anthropoid pelvis tends to be long and narrow.
5. In some pelves, the transverse diameter of the inlet is normal but the anteroposterior diameter is small (so that the pelvis appears to be flattened from front to back). This is referred to as the ***platypelloid*** type of pelvis.

6. It is important to note that the different types of pelvis described above are to be regarded as variants of the normal female pelvis and are compatible with normal childbirth ***provided*** the dimensions are adequate. According to one survey the pelvis is gynaecoid only in about 41% of women, android in about 33%, and anthropoid in about 24%. The platypelloid type is a rarity.
7. Absolute dimensions are more important than relative proportions of various dimensions. In some cases, the pelvis may have a normal shape but its dimensions may be small. Such a ***contracted pelvis*** is not compatible with normal labour. Many other terms are used to described different types of pelves but reference to them is not relevant here.

   The diameters of the pelvic inlet and outlet as measured on the bony pelvis have been given in Chapter 9.

**Fractures of the Pelvis**

1. These are not common. They may occur through the superior or inferior ischiopubic ramus, near the junction of the pubis and ischium (when they may involve the acetabulum), or the lateral part of the ilium.
2. Isolated fractures of one part of the pelvis are usually not serious as long as the ring formed by the two hip bones and sacrum is not disrupted.
3. Disruption of the ring occurs when it is broken (or dislocated) at two points (e.g., fracture of both ischiopubic rami combined with dislocation at the sacroiliac joint).
4. When disruption occurs, there can be injury to the urinary bladder, the urethra, the rectum, or the vagina.
5. Injury to a large artery in the pelvic wall can cause severe bleeding.
6. In serious disruption of the pelvis, there may be permanent damage to nerves of the lumbosacral plexus.
7. When a fracture of the pelvis involves the acetabulum, it can eventually lead to osteoarthritis at the hip joint.
8. Extremely strong contraction of muscles (in competitive sports) can tear off a tendon from its attachment along with a small piece of bone. The anterior superior and anterior inferior iliac spines can be torn off. These are called ***avulsion fractures***.

# 25 CHAPTER

# Introduction to the Abdomen and the Anterior Abdominal Wall

## INTRODUCTION TO THE ABDOMEN

### Extent of the Abdominal Cavity

1. The cavity within the abdomen can be divided into a large upper part, the ***abdominal cavity proper***; and a lower part, the ***pelvic cavity***, which lies within the true pelvis (25.1 and 25.2). The pelvic cavity is the part that lies below and behind the pelvic brim.
2. Superiorly, the abdominal cavity is bounded by the diaphragm, which separates it from the cavity of the thorax. We have seen that the domes of the diaphragm reach much above the level of the costal margin. As a result of this fact, a considerable part of the abdominal cavity lies deep to the thoracic cage.
3. The abdominal organs lying in this part of the cavity are separated from pleurae and lungs only by the diaphragm.

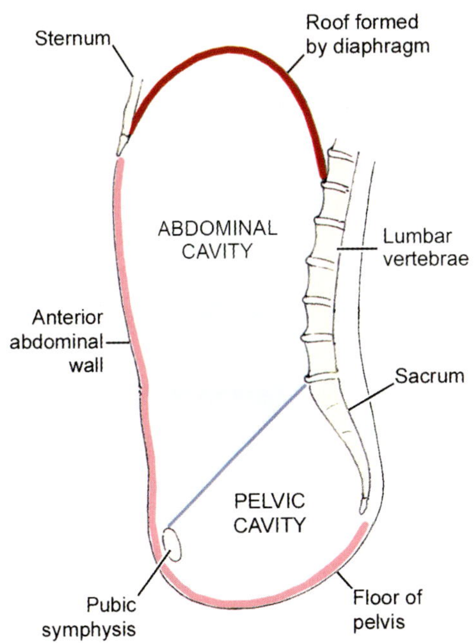


**25.1:** Schematic sagittal section to show extent and walls of the abdominal cavity

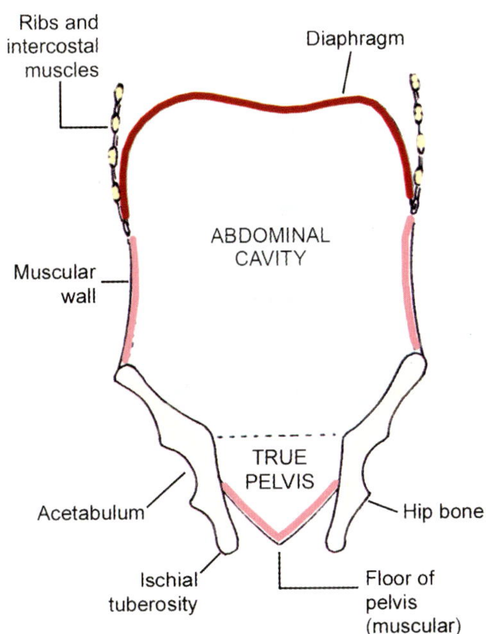


**25.2:** Schematic coronal section through abdominal cavity to show its extent and its walls

4. Inferiorly, the abdominal cavity extends into the false pelvis (i.e., the part of the pelvis above the pelvic brim). It is directly continuous with the cavity of the true pelvis.
5. Note that the gluteal region lies behind the lower part of the abdominal cavity, and the pelvic cavity.

## Preliminary Review of Walls of the Abdomen

1. The constitution of the anterior and posterior walls of the abdomen can be understood by examining a transverse section through the wall (25.3).
2. The ***posterior abdominal wall*** is made up:
   a. In the median plane, by the lumbar vertebrae.
   b. Lying along each side of the vertebral bodies there is the ***psoas major*** muscle.
   c. Still more laterally, the posterior wall is formed by a muscle called the ***quadratus lumborum***.
3. The part of the abdominal wall extending all the way from the midline (in front) to the lateral edge of the quadratus lumborum is referred to as the ***anterior abdominal wall***. However, note that it is not confined to the anterior aspect of the abdomen, but covers it from the lateral side as well.
4. Next to the midline, the wall is formed by the ***rectus abdominis muscle*** that runs vertically. This muscle is seen in transverse section in 25.3.

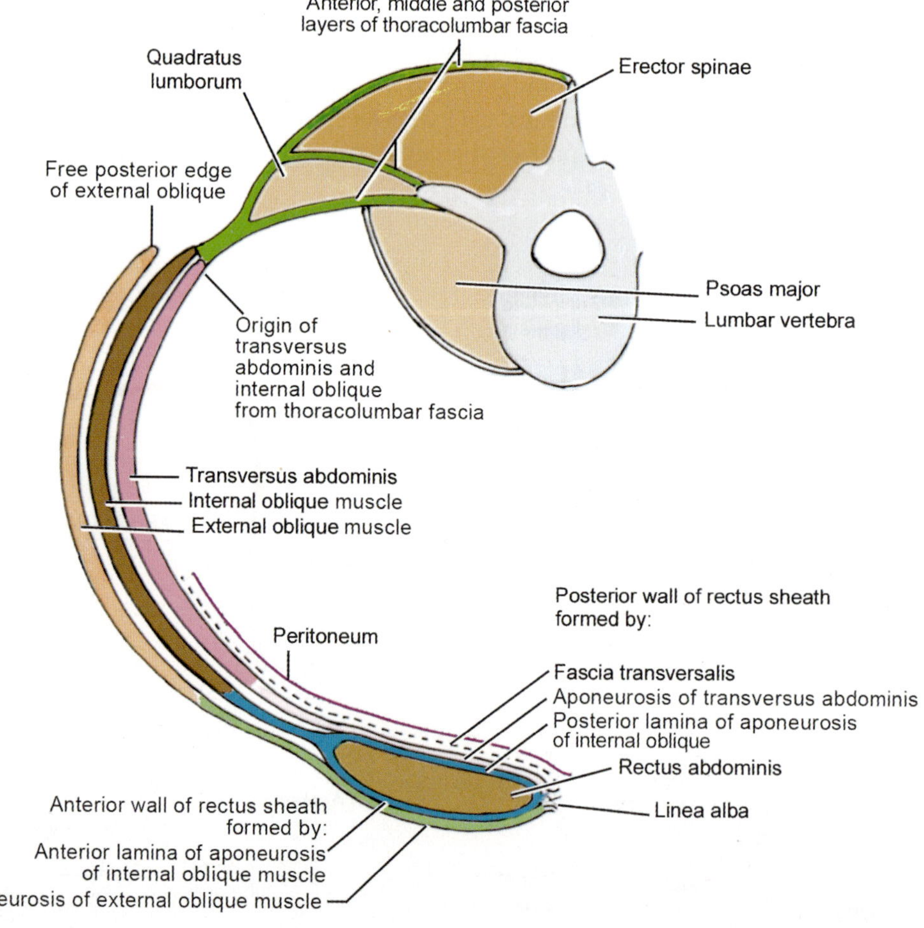


**25.3:** Schematic transverse section through abdominl wall to show its layers

5. Between the lateral edge of the rectus abdominis and the lateral edge of the quadratus lumborum the anterolateral wall is made up of three layers of muscle. From outside to inside, these layers are formed by the ***external oblique, internal oblique*** and ***transverse muscles of the abdomen***. These three are collectively referred to as the anterolateral muscles of the abdominal wall.
6. The innermost layer of muscle is lined by a fascia called the ***fascia transversalis***.
7. The fascia transversalis is covered on the inside by ***parietal peritoneum***, the two being separated by a layer of ***extraperitoneal fat***.
8. At the costal margin, the anterior abdominal wall becomes continuous with the thoracic wall. An intercostal nerve can pass from an intercostal space into the abdominal wall. Both the thoracic and abdominal walls have three layers of muscle:
   a. The external oblique muscle of the abdomen corresponds in position, and in the direction of its fibres, to the external intercostal muscle.
   b. The same is also true about the internal oblique muscle of the abdomen and the internal intercostal muscle.
   c. In the abdomen, the third layer is formed by the transversus abdominis muscle that is so called because its fibres run transversely. It corresponds to the transversus thoracis (even though the fibres of its constituent parts do not run transversely).
   d. Finally, note that both in the thorax and in the abdomen the nerves (and vessels) lie between the second and third layers of muscles.

## Superficial Fascia of Abdomen

1. The abdominal cavity is required to expand and contract with each respiration.
2. It expands when the stomach is full of ingested food. It is capable of expanding enormously in pregnancy; as a result of accumulation of fluid; or because of the presence of a large tumour within it.
3. It follows that unlike the limbs the abdomen cannot be enclosed in a tight sleeve of deep fascia. In fact deep fascia is not present over the front and sides of the abdomen.
4. The superficial fascia over the abdomen shows some special features. Over the lower part of the anterior abdominal wall (and over the perineum), the superficial fascia consists of two layers. There is a superficial ***fatty layer*** (also called the ***fascia of Camper***), and a deeper ***membranous layer***. (The membranous layer is also called the ***fascia of Scarpa***. In the perineum, it is called the ***fascia of Colles***). The fatty layer corresponds to superficial fascia elsewhere in the body.

### WANT TO KNOW MORE?

5. When traced upwards the membranous layer ends by merging with the fatty layer.
6. When traced downwards (near the midline) it passes across the pubic symphysis, over the penis and into the scrotum.
7. However, when traced laterally it is seen to be firmly adherent to underlying bone or underlying deep fascia (of the thigh) as follows:
   a. The membranous layer passes into the upper part of the thigh across the inguinal ligament. However, the layer ends a short distance below the ligament by fusing with deep fascia along a horizontal line extending laterally from the pubic tubercle. (The line of fusion is ***Holden's line***) (25.4).
   b. Near the midline, the membranous layer passes downwards over the pubic symphysis, but a little lateral to the midline it is fused to the body of the pubis.
   c. In the anterior part of the perineum, the membranous layer is attached to the pubic arch.
   d. The posterior edge of the fascia reaches the posterior border of the perineal membrane and fuses with it.

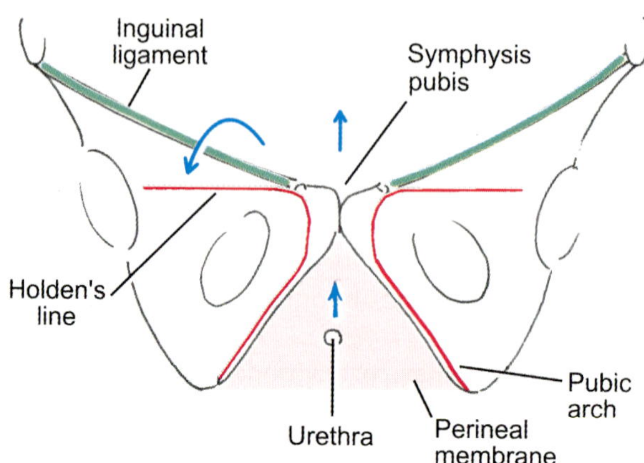


**25.4:** Diagram to show lines along which the membranous layer of superficial fascia is firmly united to underlying structures. Anterior view. Arrows indicate the path that can be taken by extravasated urine if the urethra is ruptured.

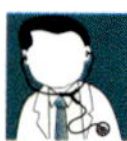

### CLINICAL CORRELATION

8. These attachments acquire significance in case of rupture of the urethra in the perineum. In such cases, urine leaking out of the urethra passes into the space between the membranous layer and deeper structures.
   a. It cannot pass backwards beyond the perineal membrane because the membranous layer of fascia is fused to the posterior border of the perineal membrane.
   b. However, it can pass forwards over the scrotum, over the penis, and upwards over the pubic symphysis into the lower part of the anterior abdominal wall.
   c. It cannot spread laterally into the thigh because of the attachment of the membranous layer to the ischiopubic rami.
   d. However, it can pass laterally over the lower part of the abdominal wall and can then pass downwards across the inguinal ligament into the thigh (25.4).
   e. However, its descent into the thigh is limited by the fusion of the membranous layer of superficial fascia to the deep fascia of the thigh along Holden's line.

## REGIONS OF THE ABDOMEN

1. The relationship of the abdominal viscera to the surface of the body is of considerable importance.
2. As the anterior and lateral walls of the abdomen are devoid of skeletal landmarks (except at their upper and lower ends), reference has to be made to some imaginary planes.
3. The abdomen can be divided into nine regions by using two transverse and two vertical planes which are as follows (25.5):
   a. The upper transverse plane is called the ***transpyloric plane***.
      i. This lies midway between the upper border of the manubrium sterni (suprasternal notch) and the upper border of the symphysis pubis.
      ii. The plane is roughly midway between the lower end of the body of the sternum (not of xiphoid process) and the umbilicus; or a hand's breadth below the lower end of the body of the sternum.
      iii. The transpyloric plane passes through the lower part of vertebra L1 (body). It cuts the costal margin at the tip of the ninth costal cartilage.

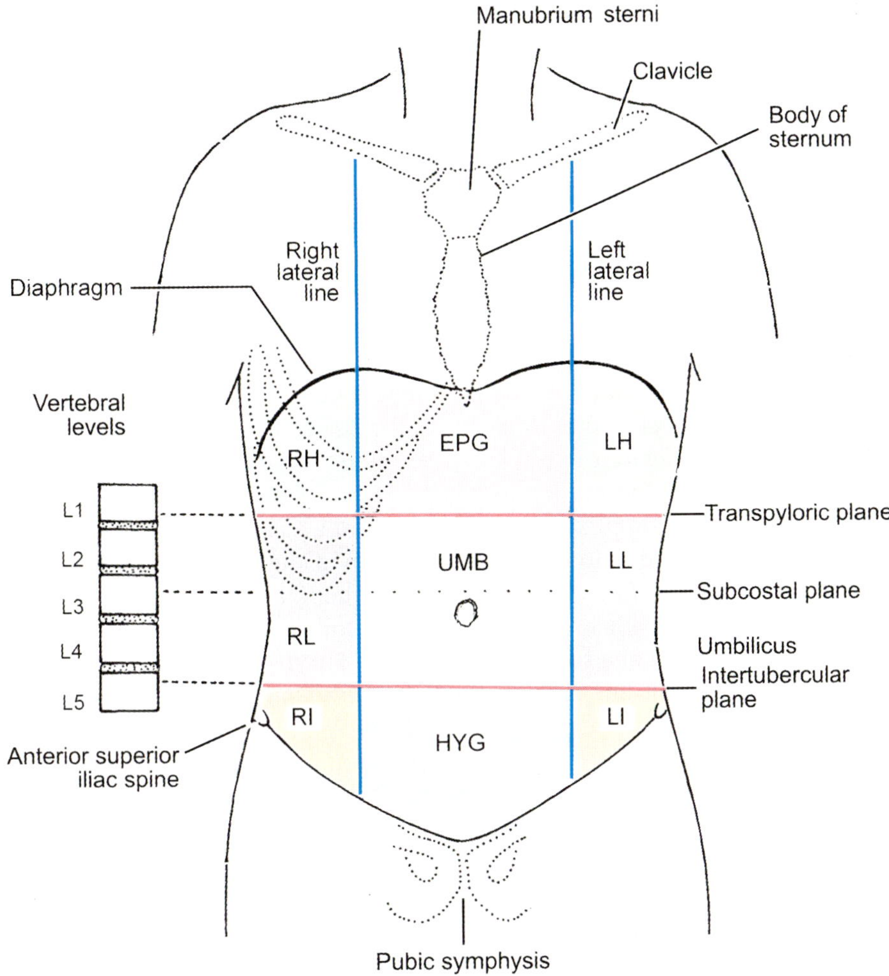


**25.5:** Regions of the abdomen and the lines demarcating them

b. The lower transverse plane is called the ***transtubercular plane***.
   i. It lies at the level of the tubercles of the iliac crests. (These are prominences on the outer lip of each iliac crest about 5 cm behind the anterior superior iliac spines).
   ii. The transtubercular plane passes through the upper part of vertebra L5 (body).
c. The vertical planes used for subdividing the abdomen into regions are the ***right*** and ***left lateral planes***. On the anterior aspect of the body, they are represented by the right and left lateral lines.
   i. The upper end of each line is at the midpoint between the medial and lateral ends of the clavicle.
   ii. Its lower end is midway between the anterior superior iliac spine and the pubic symphysis.
   iii. The right and left lateral lines are commonly referred to as the ***midclavicular lines***.
d. We have seen that the upper limit of the abdomen is demarcated by the diaphragm. Roughly, it can be said to lie at the level of the lower end of the body of the sternum. The lower limits of the abdominal cavity (excluding the true pelvis) are marked by the right and left inguinal ligaments.
e. Keeping in mind the planes and limits defined above, the abdomen can be divided into the following nine regions (25.5):
   i. In the midline from above downwards there are:
      - The ***epigastrium*** (EPG)

- The ***umbilical region*** (UMB)
- The ***hypogastrium*** (HYG) which is also called the ***pubic region***.

ii. Lateral to the epigastrium there are:
- The ***right hypochondrium*** (RH)
- The ***left hypochondrium*** (LH).

iii. Lateral to the umbilical region there are:
- The ***right lumbar region*** (RL)
- The ***left lumbar region*** (LL). The lumbar regions are also called ***lateral regions.***

iv. Lateral to the hypogastrium there are:
- The ***right inguinal region*** (RI), also called the ***right iliac fossa***.
- The ***left inguinal region*** (LI), also called the ***left iliac fossa***.

f. Two additional planes sometimes referred to are as follows:
   i. The ***subcostal plane*** is at the level of the lowest part of the costal margin (formed by the tenth costal cartilage). It lies at the level of the upper part of vertebra L3 (body). Some authorities use this plane (instead of the transpyloric) for dividing the abdomen into the regions mentioned above.
   ii. The ***supracristal plane*** is at the level of the highest points of the iliac crests. When drawn on the posterior surface of the body this plane cuts the spine of vertebra L4, and is used as a guide to locate this spine.

g. The midline of the anterior abdominal wall is marked by a slight groove. When skin over the midline is removed a white line is seen in this situation. It is called the ***linea alba***.

h. When the rectus abdominis is made to contract (e.g., by asking a lying person to sit up) we can see the lateral edge of this muscle in the form of a curved line extending from the pubic tubercle (below) to the tip of the 9th costal cartilage (above). This line is called the ***linea semilunaris***. Its junction with the costal margin (9th costal cartilage) lies at the level of the transpyloric plane.

i. The ***umbilicus*** is a prominent feature on the anterior abdominal wall, but is not a useful landmark because of variability in its position. In the healthy young adult it usually lies at the level of the intervertebral disc between L3 and L4. The umbilicus marks the point at which the umbilical cord is attached during fetal life.

## SOME INTRODUCTORY REMARKS ABOUT THE PERITONEUM

1. The abdominal cavity and most of the viscera within it are lined by a serous membrane called the ***peritoneum***.
2. Like the pleura, the peritoneum is a closed sac that is invaginated by viscera.
3. It, therefore, comes to have a ***parietal*** layer lining the abdominal wall; and a ***visceral*** layer that is in intimate relationship to the viscera.

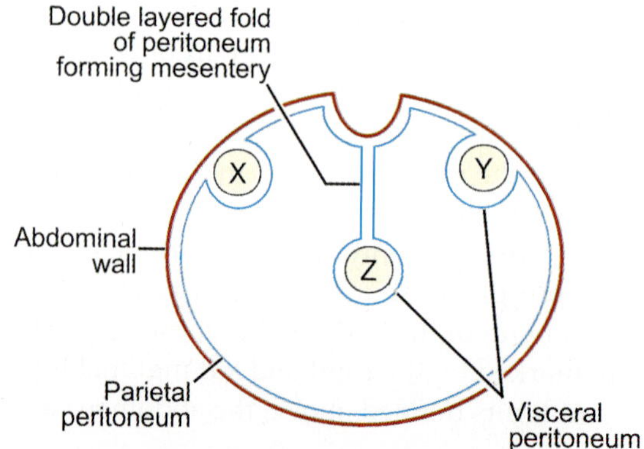


**25.6:** Scheme to show two basic types of relationship between viscera and peritoneum

4. The parietal and visceral layers of peritoneum are separated only by a potential space called the ***peritoneal cavity***. This space contains a thin film of fluid that allows free movement of the viscera against the abdominal wall and against each other.
5. Notice carefully the distinction between the terms 'abdominal cavity' and 'peritoneal cavity'. The abdominal cavity contains all the contents of the abdomen, while the peritoneal cavity is only a potential space.
6. The basic arrangement of the peritoneum relative to the viscera is shown in 25.6. Viscus 'X' and 'Y' project only partially into the peritoneal cavity. As a result, they are in contact with the posterior abdominal wall, and are only partly lined by peritoneum. Such viscera (and other structures) are described as being ***retroperitoneal***. It will be obvious that such a viscus will have very limited mobility. Examples of retroperitoneal viscera are the duodenum, the ascending colon, the descending colon and the kidneys.
7. In contrast to such viscera others ('Z' in figure) are suspended from the abdominal wall by double layered 'folds' of peritoneum passing from the abdominal wall to the viscera.
8. The best example of such a viscus is the small intestine. The fold of peritoneum by which it is attached to the posterior abdominal wall is called the ***mesentery***.
9. Some other similar folds are ***meso-gastrium, meso-colon,*** and ***mesovarium***.
10. Blood vessels and nerves reach the viscera concerned through these folds.

# THE ANTERIOR ABDOMINAL WALL

## ANTEROLATERAL MUSCLES OF ABDOMINAL WALL

These are:

1. Obliquus Abdominis Externus (External Oblique of Abdomen).
2. Obliquus Abdominis Internus (Internal Oblique of Abdomen).
3. Transversus Abdominis (Transverse, of Abdomen).
   In addition to these anterolateral muscles, the anterior abdominal wall has a vertically running muscle, the rectus femoris, which is considered separately.

The attachments of the three anterolateral muscles are given in 25.7. They are shown in 25.8 to 25.10.

### Notes about the External Oblique Muscle

1. The external oblique is the most superficial of the anterolateral muscles of the abdomen (25.8).
2. The upper slips of the muscle interdigitate with those of the serratus anterior; and the lower ones with those of the latissimus dorsi.
3. The uppermost slip (from the 5th rib) arises a little behind the junction of the rib with its costal cartilage.
4. Succeeding slips arise further back on the ribs so that the line of origin is, on the whole, oblique passing downwards and backwards to reach the 12th rib.
5. The ***inguinal ligament*** is the lower edge of the aponeurosis of the muscle folded on itself.

### Notes about the Internal Oblique Muscle

1. The fibres arising from the middle one-third of the inguinal ligament are closely related to the inguinal canal.
2. They first pass upwards and medially in front of the lateral part of the canal (forming its anterior wall); then turn backwards and medially above the canal (forming its roof) and finally dip downwards and medially behind it. Here the fibres become tendinous and join those of the transversus abdominis to form the conjoint tendon through which they are attached to the pubic crest and the pecten pubis.
3. The conjoint tendon forms the medial part of the posterior wall of the inguinal canal.

### Notes about the Transversus Abdominis

The aponeurosis of the transversus abdominis muscle takes part in forming the sheath for the rectus abdominis muscle along with those of the external and internal oblique muscles.

**25.7: Anterolateral muscles of abdomen**

| | *Obliquus Externus Abdominis* | *Obliquus Internus Abdominis* | *Transversus Abdominis* |
|---|---|---|---|
| Direction of fibres | The fibres run downwards and forwards | The fibres run forwards and upwards (at right angles to externus) | The fibres run forwards |
| Origin | Fifth to twelfth ribs (external surfaces and lower borders) | 1. Uppermost fibres from thoracolumbar fascia (at lateral border of the quadratus lumborum muscle)<br>2. Middle fibres from iliac crest (anterior two-thirds of ventral segment, intermed, zone)<br>3. Lowest fibres from inguinal ligament (lateral 2/3 of deep aspect) (grooved upper surface) | 1. Upper fibres from inner aspect of lower 6 costal cartilages<br>2. Middle fibres from thoracolumbar fascia (at lateral border of quadratus lumborum)<br>3. Lower fibres from ventral segment of iliac crest (anterior 2/3 of inner lip)<br>4. Lowest fibres from lateral 1/3 of inguinal ligament (upper grooved surface) |
| Insertion | 1. All fibres except those arising from the 11th and 12th ribs end in an extensive aponeurosis. The aponeurosis is attached to:<br>a. Xiphoid process<br>b. Linea alba (entire length)<br>c. Pubic crest and pubic tubercle<br>d. Lateral to the pubic tubercle the aponeurosis has a free lower border that forms the inguinal ligament. This ligament is attached laterally to the ant. sup. iliac spine<br>2. The fibres that arise from the 11th and 12th ribs are inserted into the iliac crest (anterior half of outer lip) | 1. Fibres arising from lumbar fascia and the posterior part of iliac crest are inserted into lower three ribs (lower border)<br>2. Fibres from anterior part of iliac crest and lateral part of inguinal ligament end in an aponeurosis. Its upper part is attached to the costal margin. Its lower part is attached to entire length of linea alba<br>3. Fibres from middle 1/3 of inguinal ligament are related to the inguinal canal. They first lie in front of the canal, then in its roof, and then behind the canal. Here the fibres join those of the transversus to form the conjoint tendon. This tendon is inserted into the pubic crest and pecten pubis | 1. Fibres end in aponeurosis inserted chiefly into linea alba<br>2. Lowest part of aponeurosis joins that of internal oblique to form conjoint tendon (inserted into pecten pubis and pubic crest) |
| Nerve supply | For all muscles: Lower six thoracic nerves. | | |
| Action | 1. Support abdominal viscera.<br>2. Increase intra-abdominal pressure that helps to expel contents of viscera (as in defecation, micturition, vomitting and child birth) | | |

## Some Structures Closely Related to Anterolateral Muscles

### *The Linea Alba*

1. This is a tendinous raphe present in the midline of the anterior abdominal wall.
2. It is attached above to the xiphoid process and below to the symphysis pubis.
3. It is formed by the interlacing of the fibres of the aponeuroses of the external oblique, the internal oblique and the transversus abdominis muscles.
4. It separates the two rectus abdominis muscles from each other.

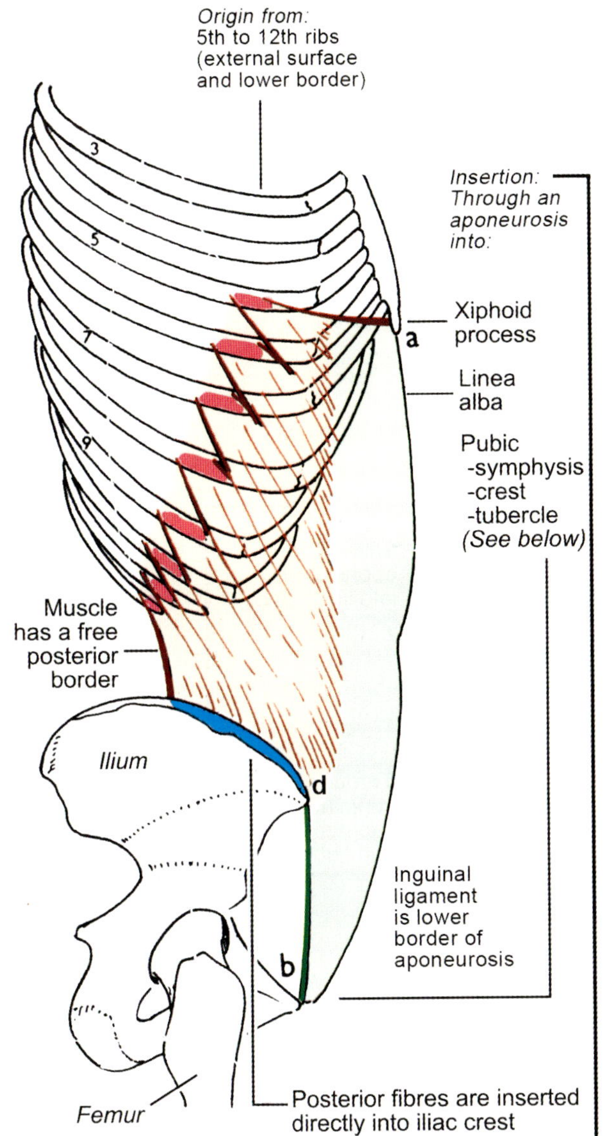


**25.8:** Lateral view of the trunk to show the attachments of the external oblique muscle of the abdomen

Origin from:
Thoraco-
lumbar
fascia
Iliac crest
Inguinal
ligament
(lateral 2/3)
a
b
c
Insertion:
(a) 9th, 10th
11th, 12th ribs.
(b) Costal
margin.
(c) Linea alba
(d) Through
conjoint
tendon to
pecten pubis
and pubic crest

**25.9:** Lateral view of the trunk to show attachments of the internal oblique muscle of the abdomen

### The Inguinal Ligament

1. This is a thick curved band of fibres that lies at the junction of the abdomen and the front of the thigh.
2. It is attached medially to the pubic tubercle and laterally to the anterior superior iliac spine (25.11).
3. It represents the lower border of the aponeurosis of the external oblique muscle, which is folded on itself.
4. As a result, the ligament comes to have a grooved upper surface that can be seen if the ligament is viewed from its deep aspect.

### The Lacunar Ligament

1. This is also called the ***pectineal part of the inguinal ligament.***
2. It is a triangular membrane placed horizontally, behind the medial most part of the inguinal ligament.
3. Its base, directed laterally, is free: it forms the medial boundary of the femoral ring.

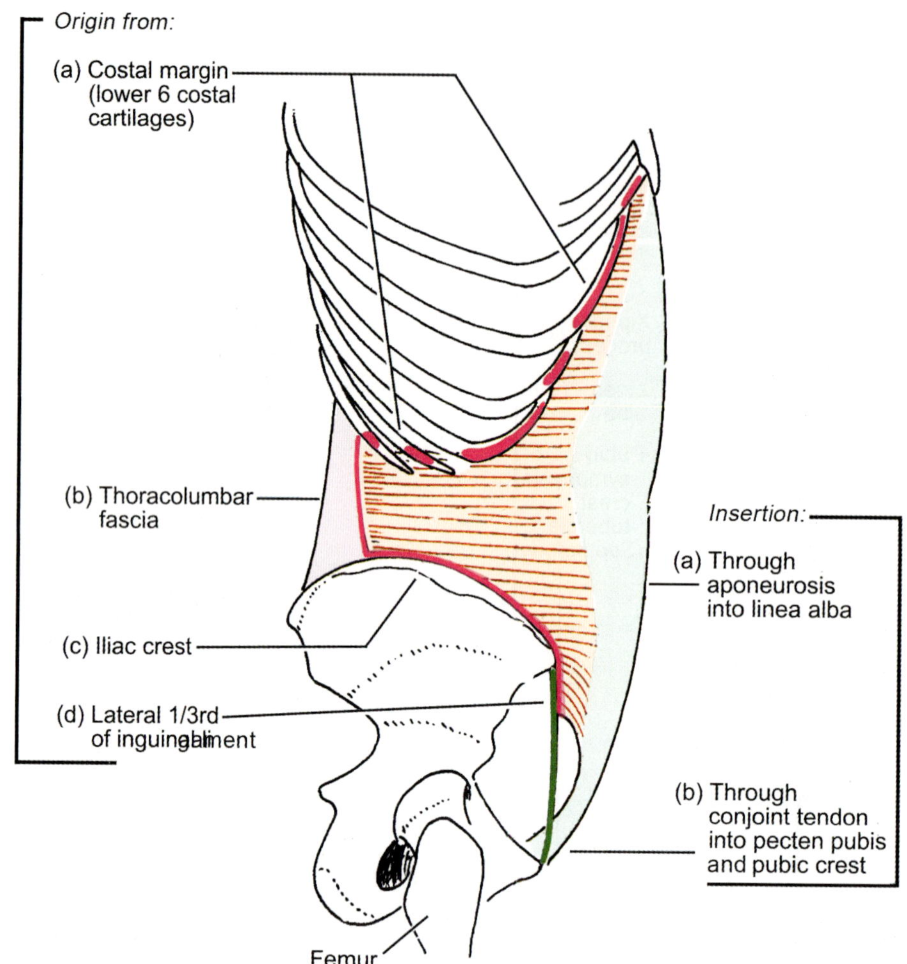


**25.10:** Lateral view of the trunk to show the attachments of the transversus abdominis muscle

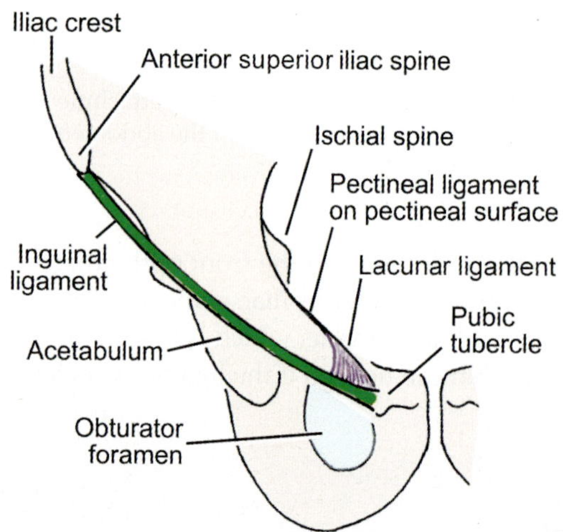


**25.11:** Diagram to show the inguinal ligament and some related structures

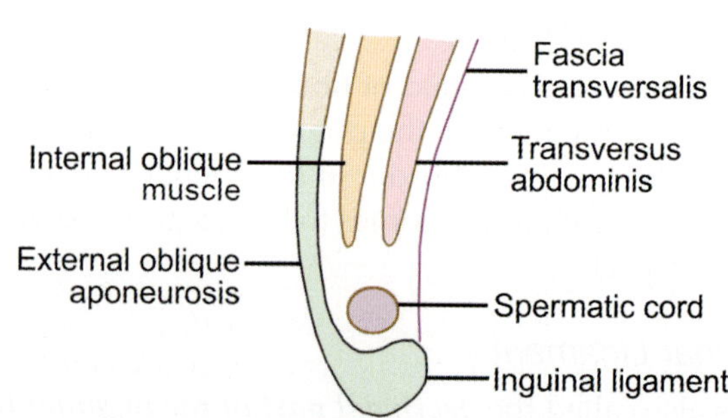


**25.12:** Diagram to show the position of the inguinal canal

### *Pectineal Ligament*

1. Some fibres (continuous with the lacunar ligament) extend laterally along the pecten pubis beyond the base of the lacunar ligament.
2. They constitute the pectineal ligament, the fibres of which are firmly adherent to the pecten pubis.

### *Superficial Inguinal Ring*

1. Just above the medial part of the inguinal ligament, there is an aperture in the aponeurosis of the external oblique muscle called the superficial inguinal ring (25.12).
2. The so called ring is really an obtuse angled triangle. The base of the triangle is formed by the pubic crest.
3. The two sides of the triangle form the lateral (or lower) and the medial (or upper) margins of the opening: these are referred to as crura.
4. The lateral crus is nothing but the medial part of the inguinal ligament: We have seen that it is attached to the pubic tubercle and has a grooved upper surface.
5. The medial crus is attached to the front of the symphysis pubis.
6. The superficial inguinal ring is the external opening of the inguinal canal.

### *Reflected Part of the Inguinal Ligament*

1. This is made up of fibres that pass upwards and medially from the lateral crus of the superficial inguinal ring and disappear under its medial crus (25.14).
2. The fibres of the ligaments of the two sides decussate in the linea alba.

### *The Conjoint Tendon (or Falx Inguinalis)*

1. This is made up of some fibres of the aponeuroses of the internal oblique and transversus abdominis muscles that join together and descend to be inserted into the pubic crest and the medial part of the pecten pubis.
2. The conjoint tendon lies behind the superficial inguinal ring.
3. Traced medially the fibres of the tendon become continuous with the rectus sheath.
4. The aponeuroses of the internal oblique and transversus muscles fuse lateral to the rectus abdominis in the lower part of the abdominal wall. The more lateral fibres run downwards forming the conjoint tendon, while the more medial ones form the anterior sheath of the rectus abdominis.

## The Inguinal Canal

1. This is an oblique passage through the anterior abdominal wall placed a little above the medial part of the inguinal ligament (25.12 and 25.15).

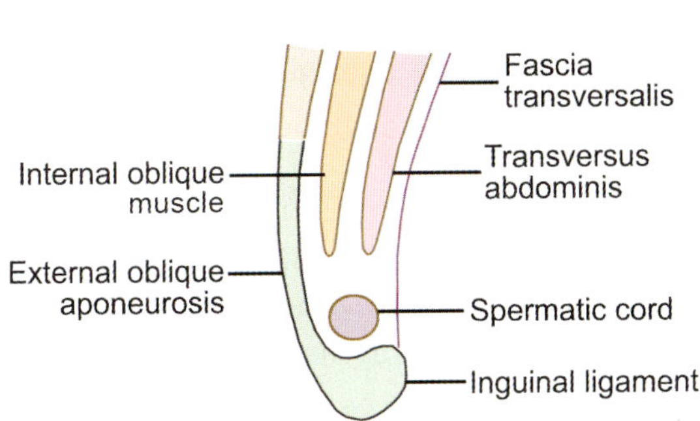


**25.13:** Sagittal section through inguinal canal

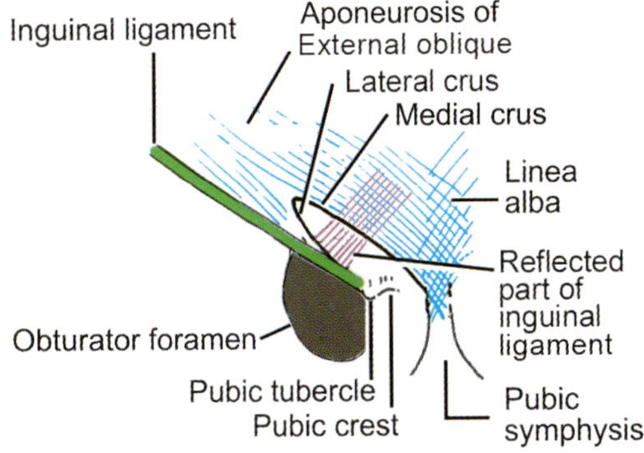


**25.14:** Diagram to show the structure of the superficial inguinal ring

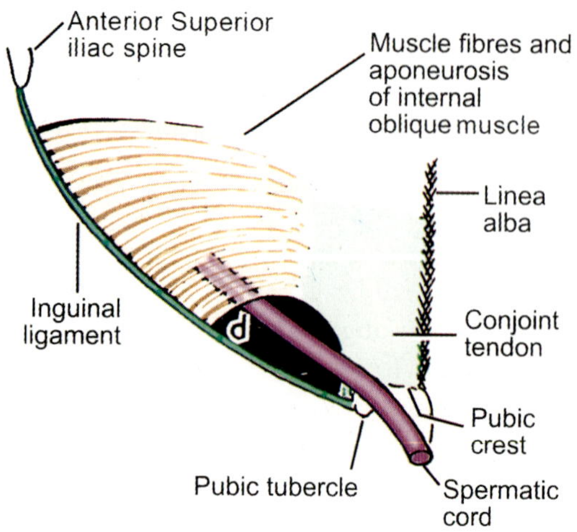


**25.15:** Diagram to show relationship of the internal oblique muscle to the inguinal canal

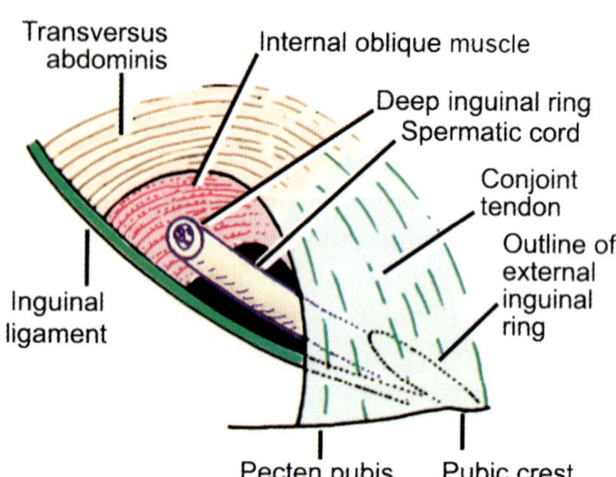


**25.16:** Inguinal canal seen from behind

2. It begins at the deep inguinal ring. This ring is situated in the trasversalis fascia midway between the anterior superior iliac spine and the pubic symphysis, half an inch above the inguinal ligament.
3. The inguinal canal passes downwards and medially to reach the superficial inguinal ring. It gives passage to the spermatic cord in the male, and the round ligament of the uterus in the female.
4. The canal has an anterior wall, a posterior wall, a roof and floor.
5. The ***floor*** is formed by the grooved upper surface of the inguinal ligament, and more medially by the lacunar ligament (25.13). The fascia transversalis is adherent to the back of the inguinal ligament and helps to close the canal below.
6. The ***roof*** of the canal is formed by the fibres of the internal oblique (25.16). The fibres of the transversus abdominis may or may not take part in forming the roof depending on the level to which they descend.
7. The ***anterior wall*** of the inguinal canal is formed by:
   a. Fleshy fibres of internal oblique (over lateral one-third of canal).
   b. Aponeurosis of external oblique (over entire length of canal).
   c. Skin and superficial fascia.
8. The ***posterior wall*** of the canal is formed by:
   a. The fascia transversalis (over entire extent of canal). The fascia transversalis is separated from peritoneum by extraperitoneal fat.
   b. Conjoint tendon (over medial half of canal).
   c. Reflected part of inguinal ligament (over medial one-third of canal).
9. Note that the anterior wall is strong where the posterior wall is weakened by the deep inguinal ring; and that the posterior wall is strong where the anterior wall is weakened by the presence of the superficial ring.
10. The importance of the inguinal canal is that an inguinal hernia frequently takes place through it.

### *Spermatic Cord and its Coverings*

We have seen that the inguinal canal gives passage to the spermatic cord in the male. The structures that constitute the spermatic cord are as follows:

1. The ***ductus deferens*** is a thick walled tube that carries spermatozoa formed in the testis to the male excretory passages.
2. Arteries present in the spermatic cord are:
   a. The testicular artery to the testis.

b. An artery to the ductus deferens.
c. Another artery to the cremaster muscle descends along the cord.

3. The veins draining the testis and epididymis form a plexus around the ductus deferens. This is called the ***pampiniform*** plexus. Near the superficial inguinal ring, the plexus ends in three or four longitudinal veins that pass through the inguinal canal.
4. The genital branch of the genitofemoral nerve enters the spermatic cord at the deep inguinal ring. It supplies the cremaster muscle and gives some branches to the skin of the scrotum.
5. A plexus of sympathetic nerves runs along the testicular artery.
6. The lymphatic vessels from the testis also pass through the spermatic cord.

### Coverings of the Cord

1. In early embryonic life the testes lie within the abdomen, but in later months of pregnancy they descend through the inguinal canal into the scrotum.
2. As each testis passes through the abdominal wall it carries extensions from its layers.
3. These extensions which form the coverings of the testis, and of the cord, are as follows (within outwards) (25.17).
   a. ***The internal spermatic fascia*** is a prolongation of transversalis fascia from the margins of the deep inguinal ring.
   b. The ***cremasteric fascia*** is an extension from the internal oblique muscle. The fascia contains several muscle bundles that constitute the cremaster muscle (see below).
   c. The ***external spermatic fascia*** is an extension from the margins of the superficial ring (i.e., from the aponeurosis of the external oblique). It surrounds the cord below the level of the superficial inguinal ring.

## Rectus Abdominis

The attachments of this muscle are given in 25.18A. They are shown in 25.18B.

### Pyramidalis

1. The pyramidalis is a small muscle placed in front of the rectus abdominis, within its sheath (25.18).
2. It is triangular. Its base (or origin) is attached to the front of the pubis and of the symphysis pubis. Its apex is inserted into the linea alba.
3. It is supplied by the subcostal nerve.

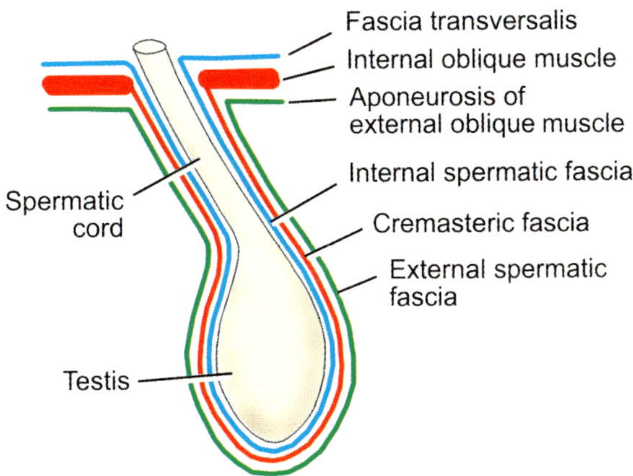


**25.17:** Schematic diagram to show coverings of the spermatic cord and of the testis.

| 25.18A: Rectus abdominis | |
|---|---|
| Origin | The muscle has two tendons of origin:<br>1. The medial tendon is attached to the front of the symphysis pubis.<br>2. The lateral tendon is attached to the pubic crest. |
| Insertion | 5th, 6th, and 7th costal cartilages along horizontal line. |
| Nerve supply | Lower 6 or 7 thoracic nerves. |
| Action | 1. Bends the trunk forwards.<br>2. Supports abdominal viscera.<br>3. Increases intra-abdominal pressure. |
| Notes | 1. The lower end is the origin, the upper end the insertion.<br>2. The origin is narrow, the insertion is broad.<br>3. The muscles of the two sides are separated by the linea alba.<br>4. The medial tendon of origin is superficial, the lateral deep.<br>5. A number of tendinous intersections (usually three) run transversely across the muscle. |

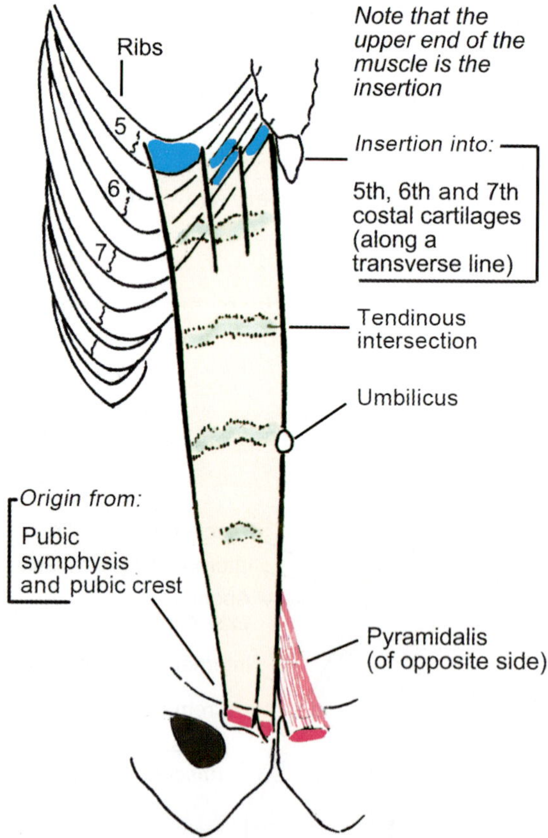


**25.18B:** Scheme to show the attachments of the rectus abdominis

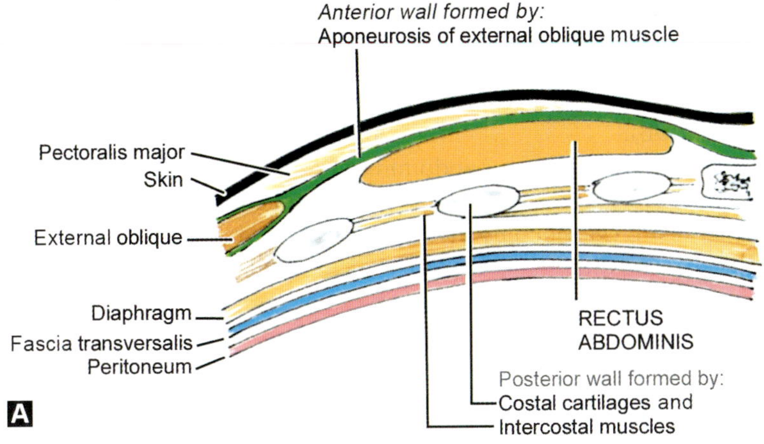


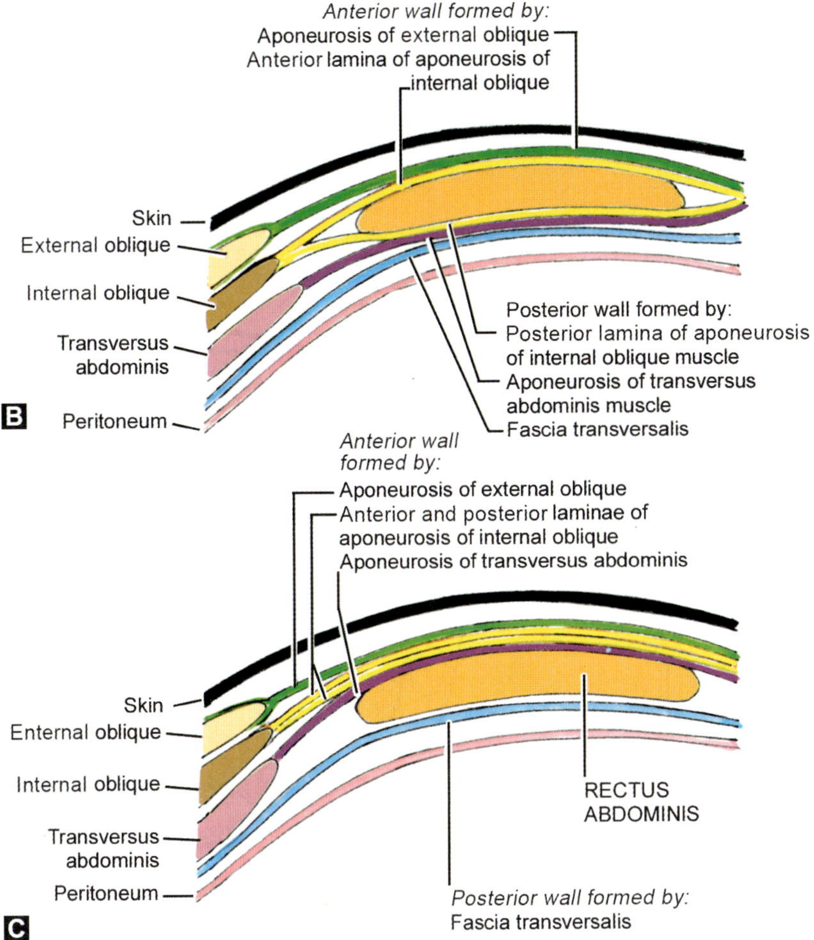


**25.19A to C:** Schematic transverse sections through the rectus abdominis muscle and its sheath at upper, middle and lower layers

## The Rectus Sheath

The rectus abdominis is enclosed in a sheath formed by the aponeuroses of the oblique and transverse muscles. The manner in which the sheath is formed is shown in 25.19A to C.

1. The typical arrangement is seen from the level of the costal margin above to that midway between the umbilicus and the pubic symphysis (25.19B).
   a. On reaching the lateral margin of the rectus abdominis, the aponeurosis of the internal oblique muscle splits into anterior and posterior laminae.
   b. The anterior wall of the sheath is formed by the external oblique aponeurosis, and the anterior lamina of the aponeurosis of the internal oblique.
   c. The posterior wall is formed by the posterior lamina of the aponeurosis of the internal oblique, and the aponeurosis of the transversus abdominis.
2. Below this level the arrangement is as follows:
   a. The lower part of the rectus abdominis rests directly on transversalis fascia, the posterior part of the sheath being deficient.
   b. The aponeurosis of the transversus abdominis, and both laminae of the internal oblique join the external oblique aponeurosis in forming the anterior wall of the sheath.
   c. The posterior part of the sheath has a lower free margin, called the ***arcuate line*** (25.20) lying on the transversalis fascia.

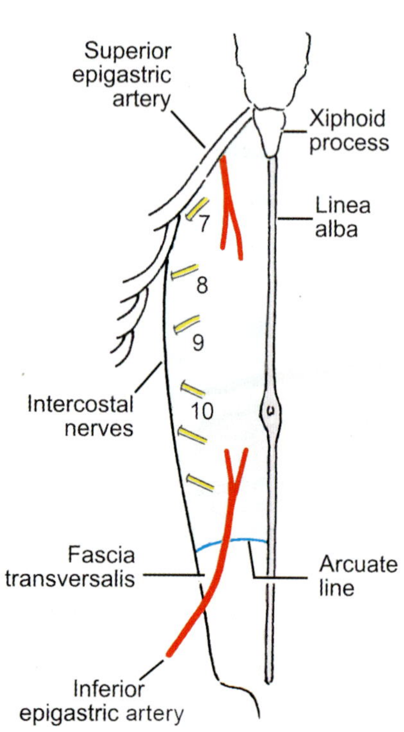


**25.20:** Diagram showing contents of the rectus sheath

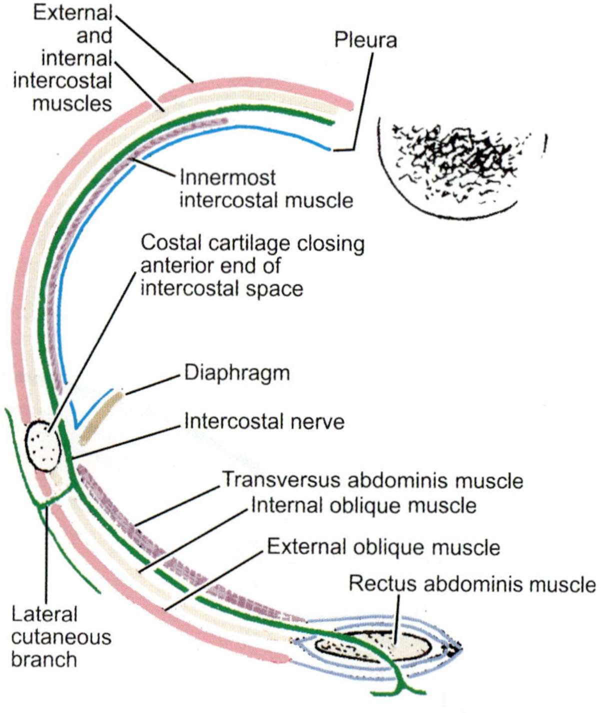


**25.21:** Scheme to show the course of one of the lower intercostal nerves

3. When traced upwards the aponeurosis of the transversus abdominis and the posterior lamina of the internal oblique end by gaining attachment to the costal margin.
   a. Just below the costal margin, the posterior wall of the sheath contains some fleshy fibres of the transversus abdominis.
   b. Above the level of the costal margin, the rectus abdominis lies directly on the costal cartilages and intercostal muscles that separate it from the diaphragm.
4. The ***contents of the rectus sheath*** are shown in 25.20 in which the posterior wall of the sheath has been shown after the muscle has been removed.
   a. The superior epigastric artery enters the sheath at its upper end by piercing the posterior wall.
   b. The inferior epigastric artery runs upwards over the transversalis fascia and enters the sheath by passing anterior to the arcuate line.
   c. The lower intercostal nerves run forwards between the internal oblique and the transversus abdominis muscles. They enter the sheath by piercing the posterior lamina of the internal oblique in its lateral part( 25.21).

### *Nerve Supply of Muscles of Anterior Abdominal Wall*

The muscles of the anterior abdominal wall are supplied by:
1. Branches from the lower six intercostal nerves (T6 to T11)
2. The subcostal nerve (T12)
3. The iliohypogastric and ilioinguinal nerves (both L1).
   a. The intercostal nerves and the subcostal nerve give branches to the external and internal oblique muscles, the transversus abdominis and the rectus abdominis.
   b. The iliohypogastric nerve gives branches only to the internal oblique and transversus muscles.
   c. The ilioinguinal nerve gives branches only to the internal oblique.
   d. The subcostal nerve also supplies the pyramidalis (25.25).

## Nerves of Anterior Abdominal Wall

The various nerves to be seen in relation to each half of the anterior abdominal wall are (25.23):
1. Anterior parts of the lower five pairs of intercostal nerves
2. The subcostal nerve
3. The iliohypogastric nerve
4. The ilio-inguinal nerve (25.23)
5. The genitofemoral nerve (25.24).

### *Cutaneous Innervation of Anterior Abdominal Wall*

The cutaneous innervation of the anterior abdominal wall is through the lower five intercostal nerves, the subcostal nerve and the iliohypogastric nerves. Some points of interest are as follows:
1. Each intercostal nerve gives off a lateral cutaneous branch that divides further into anterior and posterior branches. Anteriorly, the intercostal nerve terminates by becoming superficial as the anterior cutaneous branch.
2. The lowest two lateral cutaneous branches (from T10 and T11) become superficial by piercing the external oblique muscle.
3. Apart from the lower five intercostal nerves (T7, T8, T9, T10, T11), anterior cutaneous branches arise from the subcostal nerve (T12), and from the iliohypogastric nerve (L1).
5. Apart from intercostal nerves lateral cutaneous branches are given off by the subcostal and iliohypogastric nerves also (25.22), but these descend into the gluteal region.
6. Finally observe the direction taken by intercostal nerves after they enter the abdominal wall. The 10th nerve runs horizontally towards the umbilicus, but those above it run medially and upwards with increasing degree of obliquity.

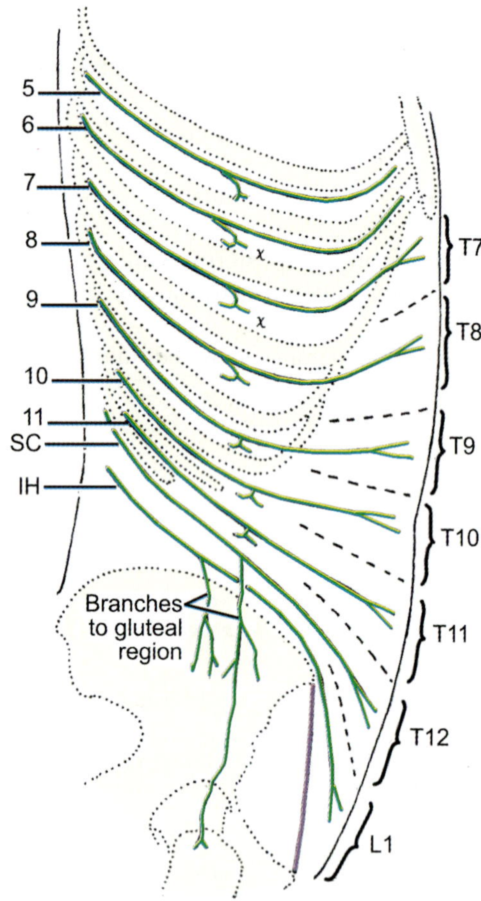


25.22: Course of intercostal nerve as seen from the lateral side. SC=subcostal nerve. IH=Iliohypogastric nerve

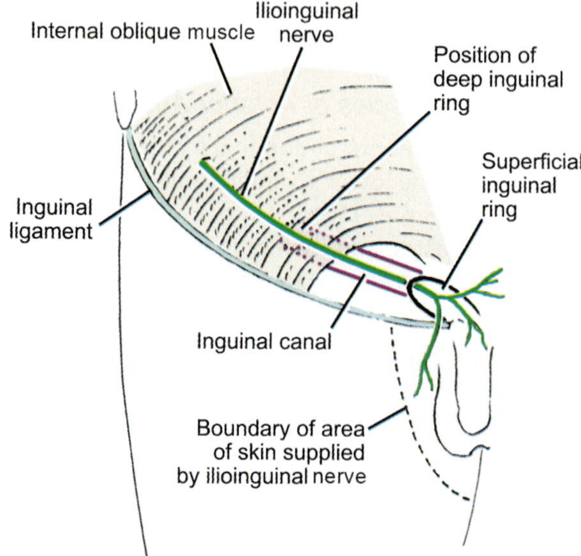


25.23: Scheme to show the course of the anterior part of the ilioinguinal nerve

### *Blood Vessels of Anterior Abdominal Wall*

The various arteries that supply the abdominal wall are as follows:

1. Lower two (10th and 11th) posterior intercostal arteries (branches of descending thoracic aorta).
2. Subcostal artery (branch of descending thoracic aorta).
3. Musculophrenic and superior epigastric arteries (which are terminal branches of the internal thoracic artery).
4. Inferior epigastric and deep circumflex iliac branches of external iliac artery (25.27).
5. Three superficial branches arising from the upper part of the femoral artery are:
   a. The superficial epigastric
   b. Superficial circumflex iliac
   c. Superficial external pudendal arteries (see below).
6. Terminal parts of lumbar arteries (lying in the posterior abdominal wall) also supply the anterolateral abdominal wall.

## Inferior Epigastric Artery

1. The inferior epigastric artery arises from the external iliac artery just above the inguinal ligament (25.26).
2. Its initial part is intimately related to the deep inguinal ring. It first runs medially inferior to the ring and then runs upwards medial to the ring.

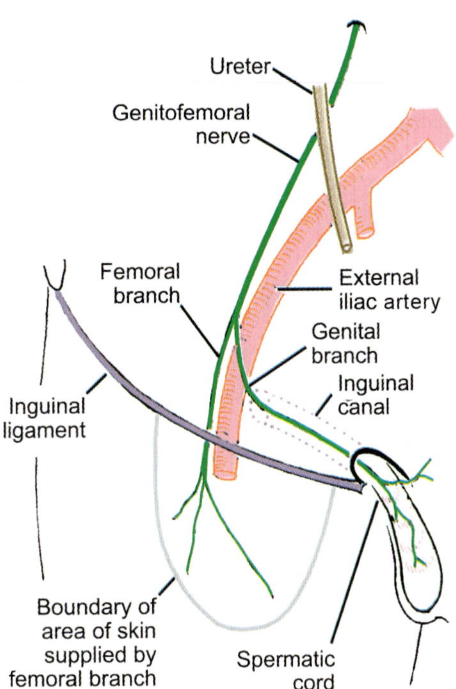


25.24: Scheme to show the course of the genitofemoral nerve

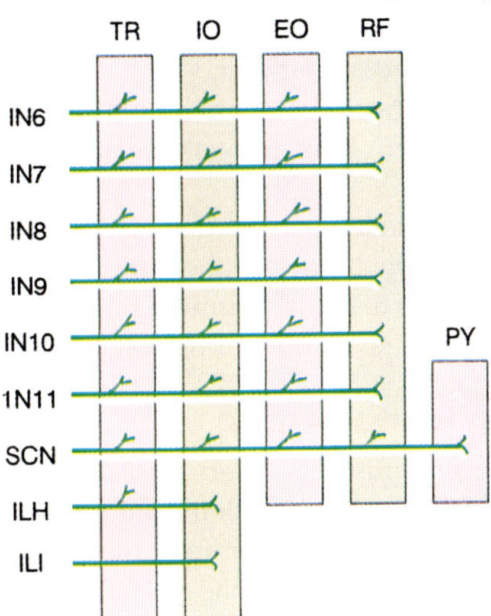


25.25: Scheme to show innervation of muscles of the anterior abdominal wall. IN6 to IN11 = 6th to 11th intercostal nerves; SCN= Subcostal nerve;
ILH= Iliohypogastric nerve; ILI= Ilioinguinal nerve; TR= Transversus abdominis;
IO= Internal oblique; EO= External oblique;
RF= Rectus femoris; PY= Pyramidalis.

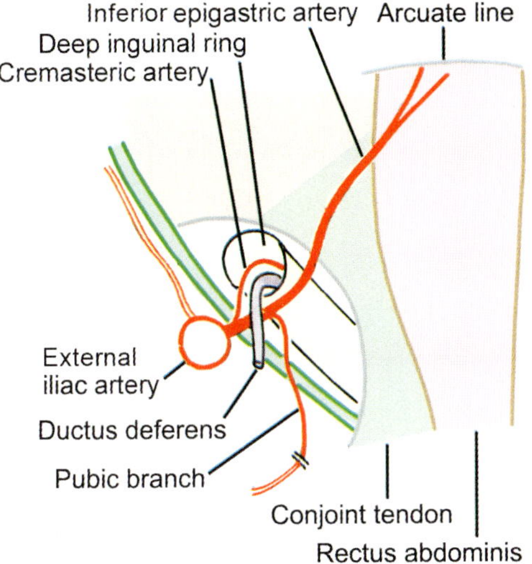


25.26: Scheme to show the course of the inferior epigastric artery. The inguinal region and the lower part of the anterior abdominal wall are viewed from behind

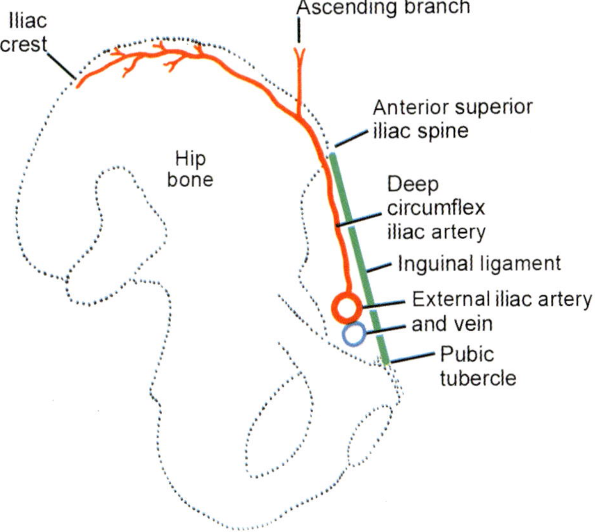


25.27: Scheme to show course of the deep circumflex iliac artery

3. The artery continues upwards and medially on the posterior aspect of the anterior abdominal wall and enters the rectus sheath by passing in front of the arcuate line (25.20). Within the sheath it anastomoses with the superior epigastric artery.
4. Apart from its relationship to the deep inguinal ring, mentioned above, the artery is related to the ductus deferens (in the male) or to the round ligament of the uterus (in the female). These wind round its lateral side to enter the deep inguinal ring (25.26). The artery raises a fold of peritoneum called the ***lateral umbilical ligament*** on the back of the anterior abdominal wall.
5. The inferior epigastric artery gives off the following branches:
   a. The ***cremasteric*** branch enters the deep inguinal ring along with the spermatic cord. It supplies the cremaster muscle.
   b. The ***pubic*** branch passes medially and downwards in close relation to the femoral ring. It anastomoses with the pubic branch of the obturator artery. Occasionally, this branch is large and the obturator artery then appears to be its continuation.
   c. Branches are given off to muscles of the anterior abdominal wall and to the skin overlying them.

## Deep Circumflex Iliac Artery

1. The deep circumflex iliac artery arises from the lateral side of the external iliac artery. It runs laterally behind the inguinal ligament to reach the anterior superior iliac spine.
2. It then passes along the inner lip of the iliac crest, deep to the transversus abdominis muscle.
3. At about the middle of the iliac crest, it pierces the muscle and continues to run backwards between it and the internal oblique. It gives branches to the muscles of the anterior abdominal wall.

### *Superficial Branches of Femoral Artery that Supply the Abdominal Wall*

1. These branches arise from the femoral artery just below the inguinal ligament. They become superficial by piercing the femoral sheath and the cribriform fascia. They contribute to the supply of the lower part of the abdominal wall.
2. The ***superficial circumflex iliac artery*** runs laterally towards the anterior superior iliac spine.
3. The ***superficial epigastric artery*** ascends across the inguinal ligament and runs towards the umbilicus.
4. The ***superficial external pudendal artery*** runs medially to supply skin over the external genitalia and over the lower part of the abdomen.
5. Branches from the various arteries described above supply muscles in the abdominal wall.

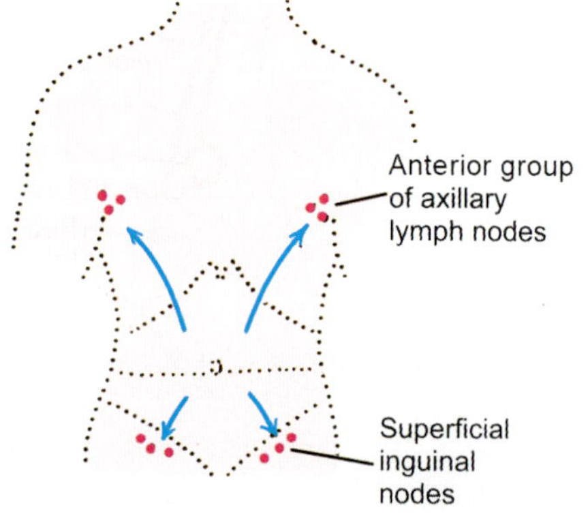


**25.28:** Lymphatic drainage of anterior aspect of trunk

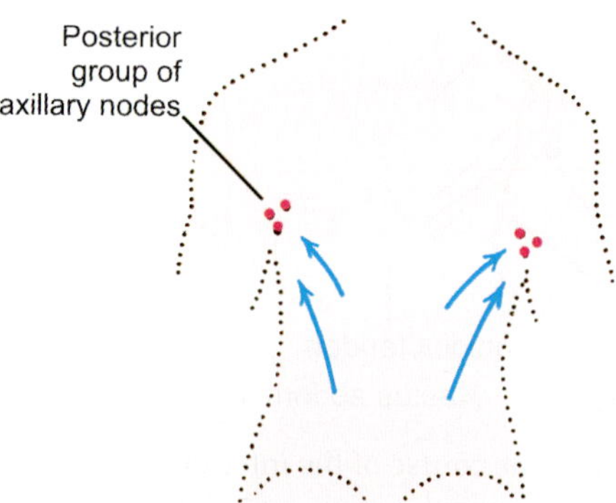


**25.29:** Posterior aspect of trunk to show its lymphatic drainage.

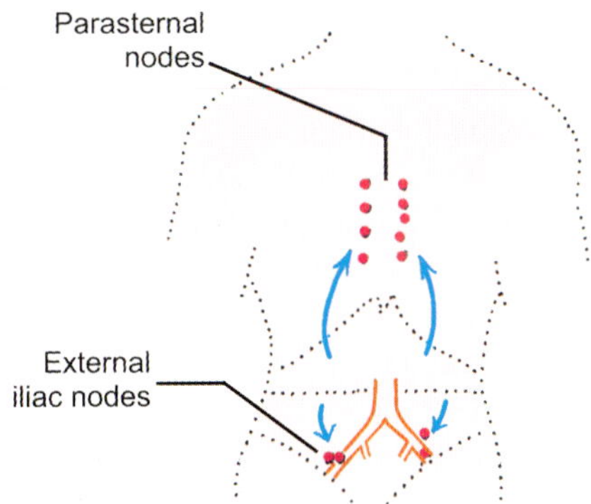


**25.30:** Lymphatic drainage of deeper tissues of anterior abdominal wall

## Cutaneous Arteries

1. The skin of the abdomen is supplied by lateral cutaneous branches arising from intercostal and subcostal arteries;
2. By anterior cutaneous arteries arising from the superior and inferior epigastric arteries.
3. And by superficial branches of the femoral artery.

## Veins of Anterior Abdominal Wall

The veins of the anterior abdominal wall correspond to the arteries described above. The veins that accompany the superficial branches of the femoral artery drain into the long saphenous vein (not into the femoral vein).

## Lymphatic Drainage of the Anterior Abdominal Wall

### *Lymphatic Drainage of the Skin*

1. The skin above the level of the umbilicus (in front) and above the iliac crest (at the back) drains into the axillary lymph nodes (25.28 and 25.29).
2. The skin of the anterior abdominal wall below the umbilicus drains into the superficial inguinal lymph nodes.

### *Lymphatic Drainage of Deeper Tissues*

1. The vessels from the upper part of the abdominal wall travel along the superior epigastric vessels to reach parasternal lymph nodes.
2. The vessels from the lower part of the anterolateral abdominal wall travel along the inferior epigastric and circumflex iliac vessels. Passing through nodes placed along these vessels they reach the external iliac nodes (25.30) lying along the external iliac artery.

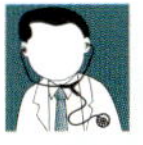

## CLINICAL CORRELATION OF ABDOMINAL WALL

### Lymphatic Drainage

The lymphatic drainage of the abdominal wall described above is important. Infections or malignancy in relation to the abdominal wall can drain into widely separated lymph nodes.

#### *Superficial Veins*

The superficial veins over the anterior abdominal wall are normally inconspicuous. In some conditions they become prominent.

1. a. The umbilicus is one of the sites at which tributaries of the portal vein communicate with systemic veins.

   b. In case of obstruction to the portal vein, these communications become very prominent and are seen as veins that radiate from the umbilicus.
   c. This appearance is given the name ***caput medusae***.
2. Superficial veins running more or less vertically over the lateral part of the anterior abdominal wall connect tributaries of the lateral thoracic vein with tributaries of the superficial epigastric vein. The main channel of communication is called the ***thoraco-epigastric vein***.
3. We have seen that the lateral thoracic vein drains into the axillary vein. The superficial epigastric vein joins the great saphenous vein that, in turn, joins the femoral vein. The superficial veins referred to above, therefore, provide channels of communication between the axillary and femoral veins.
4. In case of obstruction to either the superior or inferior vena cava these superficial veins enlarge considerably and serve as alternative channels through which blood can flow one vena cava to the other and thus reach the heart. The direction of blood flow in superficial veins gives a clue to the identity of the blocked vena cava.

**Umbilicus**

1. See remarks on lymphatic drainage and superficial veins in the preceding section.
2. Typically, the umbilicus lies at the level of the intervertebral disc between vertebral bodies L3 and L4. However, it is not a reliable guide to structures within the abdomen due to variability in its position.
3. The cutaneous nerve supply of the skin at the level of the umbilicus is derived from the tenth intercostal nerve.
4. Early in fetal life the region of the future umbilicus is marked by a large gap in the future abdominal wall. Several structures pass through the gap as follows:
   a. The ***vitello-intestinal duct*** connects the embryonic gut to the yolk sac.
      i. In the normal course of development, this duct disappears.
      ii. If the duct remains patent, there is a channel through which intestinal contents flow out at the umbilicus (***fecal fistula***).
      iii. Sometimes, the vitellointestinal duct may not communicate with the exterior but part of it may remain patent as a diverticulum communicating with the gut. This is called ***Meckel's diverticulum***.
      iv. Remnants of the vitellointestinal duct may also give rise to tumours at the umbilicus.
   b. The ***allantoic diverticulum*** is a tube like structure that is connected, at one end, to the distal part of the embryonic gut (the part called the cloaca).
      i. In later development, the cloaca is partitioned into a part that forms the rectum and another part that forms the urinary bladder, and after this partition is established the allantoic diverticulum comes to communicate with the urinary bladder.
      ii. The other end of the allantoic diverticulum is blind. This end passes through the umbilical opening.
      iii. Normally, the allantoic diverticulum is occluded and forms a fibrous band called the ***urachus***. This band connects the apex of the urinary bladder to the umbilicus.
      iv. Occasionally, however the urachus remains patent resulting in a communication between the urinary bladder and the umbilicus (***urinary fistula***).
   c. In the early embryo, the abdominal cavity is small. Meanwhile the gut undergoes rapid growth and the abdomen is unable to accommodate it.
      i. As a result, some coils of intestine pass out of the abdomen through the umbilical opening (This is referred to as ***physiological hernia***).
      ii. Later, as the abdomen becomes larger in size, the coils return into the abdominal cavity.
      iii. In some cases, the coils of gut fail to return, and the infant is born with coils of gut protruding out of the abdomen in the region of the umbilicus.
      iv. This is referred to as ***congenital umbilical hernia*** or ***exomphalos***.
   d. The original umbilical opening is obliterated by growth of tissue into it from all sides.
      i. In some cases, growth of the wall below the future umbilicus is deficient resulting in a gap in the abdominal wall.
      ii. Simultaneously, the anterior wall of the urinary bladder is also absent.

iii. Hence, we have a condition in which the posterior wall of the urinary bladder can be seen on the surface of the body. The condition is called ***ectopia vesicae.***

**Surgical Incisions in Anterior Abdominal Wall**

1. The abdomen is a region that is frequently operated upon. To reach any of the viscera the abdominal wall has to be incised (cut across) to enter the peritoneal cavity. This is called ***laparotomy***.
2. Incisions in the abdominal wall are not made at random, but are based on certain principles.
3. The primary objective of an incision is to provide good exposure of the region to the operated upon.
4. At the same time, the surgeon is equally concerned about the integrity of the abdominal wall and plans his incisions in such a way that after healing the abdominal wall returns to as near a condition as it was before the operation.
5. Some of the factors that influence the placing of incisions are the direction of muscle fibres, and the position of nerves.
6. Some commonly used incisions are as follows:
   a. ***Midline incisions*** are made through the linea alba. No muscles are cut across.
      i. In this connection note that the rectus abdominis muscles are closer together in the lower part than they are at higher levels, and that the linea alba is broader in its upper part.
      ii. For this reason median incisions are easier above the umbilicus, but the resulting scar may sometimes be weak and an ***epigastric hernia*** (see below) may take place in the region.
      iii. Midline incisions below the umbilicus are less likely to lead to hernia as this region is protected by the recti which are close to each other.
   b. ***Paramedian incisions*** are made about one inch lateral to the midline.
      i. They may be supraumbilical or infraumbilical.
      ii. The anterior wall of the rectus sheath is incised and the rectus muscle retracted laterally. (Remember that nerves to the rectus abdominis enter it from the lateral side and are safe when the muscle is pulled laterally).
      iii. The posterior wall of the sheath, the underlying fascia and the peritoneum are then incised to gain access to the peritoneal cavity.
   c. ***Pararectal incisions*** are explained as follows:
      i. A vertical cut is made along the lateral margin of the rectus abdominis, and the muscle is retracted medially.
      ii. As this is done, the nerves passing into the muscle from the lateral side come into view and have to be carefully preserved by retracting them up and down.
      iii. The posterior wall of the sheath is now incised.
      iv. The incision is not favoured as access provided is small, and the incision cannot be enlarged without cutting one or more nerves.
   d. ***Vertical incision through the rectus abdominis (transrectal incision).***
      i. In this incision, the rectus abdominis muscle and its sheath are cut vertically.
      ii. Such an incision is not to be favoured as nerve supply to part of the rectus abdominis medial to the incision is destroyed and this part of the muscle degenerates.
   e. ***Transverse incisions*** may be made through the abdominal wall, and the incision can include the rectus abdominis.
      i. Injury to nerves can be prevented by placing the cut parallel to the course of the nerves.
      ii. In any case, injury to more than one nerve is unlikely.
   f. From the point of view of retaining integrity of the abdominal wall the best incisions are those that split each layer of muscle along the length of its fibres. As the fibres of different layers run in different directions the area of exposure is small. The best known muscle splitting incision is the ***grid-iron*** (or ***McBurney's***) incision used for operations on the appendix.
      i. A line is drawn joining the umbilicus to the right anterior superior iliac spine. A point on this line at the junction of the medial two-thirds and lateral one-third is called ***McBurney's point***.

ii. The grid iron incision is made through this point at right angles to the line drawn. The length of the line depends on the degree of exposure desired. As each layer of muscle is exposed its fibres are split along the line of the fibres and retracted till the fascia transversalis and peritoneum are exposed.

g. In addition to the incisions described above various others are used for special purposes. An abdominothoracic incision is used when it is necessary to enter both the abdominal and thoracic cavities.

**Herniae through Abdominal Wall**

1. The term hernia is applied to a condition in which the contents of a cavity protrude out of it through a weak area in its wall. Most hernias are seen in relation to the abdomen. Before going onto consider individual types of hernia some terms need to be defined.
2. Abdominal viscera exert pressure on the abdominal wall, and this pressure is increased considerably during acts like coughing or defecation.
   a. If there is a gap (or weakened area) in the abdominal wall repeated pressure against it can cause a process of peritoneum to pass out through the gap into subcutaneous tissues.
   b. Further pressure gradually increases the size of the peritoneal process that gradually becomes sac like.
3. As the sac enlarges coils of intestine (or other abdominal contents) may enter it.
   a. Such a ***hernial sac*** can become very large, but the site of the original protrusion remains narrow and is referred to as the ***neck of the hernial sac***.
   b. Skin and other tissues that cover the sac are called ***coverings of the hernia***.
   c. Abdominal contents that enter the sac are the ***contents of the hernia***.
4. Usually pressure over a hernia can push its contents back into the abdominal cavity. Such a hernia is said to be ***reducible***.
5. a. Sometimes sudden increase in intra-abdominal pressure may push contents into the hernia, but thereafter they may be unable to return.
   b. Pressure exerted by the margins of the narrow neck of the hernia may cut off vascular supply of the contents.
   c. This is then called a ***strangulated hernia*** (which is an emergency requiring urgent surgery).

**Inguinal Hernia**

*Preliminary Remarks*

1. The inguinal canal is a passage through the entire thickness of the abdominal wall. It represents a site of weakness through which hernia may occur. However, structures in the wall of the canal are so arranged that they resist the tendency to herniation to a great extent. Some of the factors that do this are as follows:
   a. Because of the fact that the inguinal canal passes through the abdominal wall obliquely, the deep inguinal ring and the superficial ring do not lie opposite each other.
   b. Further, the weakness produced in the posterior wall of the canal (in its lateral part) because of the presence of the deep inguinal ring, is compensated by the thickening of the anterior wall by fibres of the internal oblique muscle.
   c. The weakness produced in the anterior wall (in its medial part), because of the presence of the superficial inguinal ring is compensated for by the presence of the conjoint tendon and the reflected part of the inguinal ligament in the posterior wall.
   d. When intra-abdominal pressure increases the anterior and posterior walls of the canal get pressed together closing the canal. This is sometimes referred to as the ***flap valve mechanism***.
   e. The internal oblique muscle reinforces the inguinal canal from the front (laterally), from above, and from behind (medially). Contraction of this muscle effectively obliterates the canal, the action being reinforced by contraction of the transversus abdominis.
   f. Contraction of the external oblique muscle tends to plug the superficial inguinal ring. Simultaneous contraction of the cremaster pulls the spermatic cord upwards and makes it thicker thus helping to plug the superficial ring.

2. In spite of the presence of all these mechanisms, the inguinal region is a fairly common site of hernia. The reasons for this are as follows:
   a. In fetal life, the inguinal canal serves as a passage through which the testis passes through the abdominal wall to descend into the scrotum.
   b. A tubular process of peritoneum called the ***processus vaginalis*** passes through the canal and facilitates the descent of the testis.
   c. Normally, the greater part of the processus vaginalis is obliterated, but the part around the testis becomes the tunica vaginalis.
   d. Sometimes, the processus vaginalis (or parts of it) may persist as a patent channel into which herniation of abdominal contents may occur.
   e. In such a hernia, the contents pass through the deep inguinal ring, the inguinal canal, and the superficial ring and can pass into the scrotum. This type of hernia is called an ***indirect inguinal hernia***.
   f. In some cases, the processus vaginalis gets obliterated, but weakness remains in the region of the inguinal canal leading to formation of hernia.
   g. Another reason for occurrence of inguinal hernia can be weakening of muscles with age. This results in a ***direct inguinal hernia*** described below.

*Indirect Inguinal Hernia*

1. This type of hernia is seen in young individuals.
2. It is seen more commonly on the right side (probably because the right testis descends into the scrotum later than the left testis).
3. Indirect inguinal hernias are much more common in the male than in the female (the inguinal canal being much narrower in the female as the ovary does not pass through it).
4. The herniae are frequently bilateral.
5. An indirect inguinal may be of various types as follows:
   a. When the processus vaginalis remains fully patent the contents of the hernia reach right up to the scrotum. This is a ***congenital vaginal hernia*** or ***complete hernia***.
   b. In some cases, the processus vaginalis remains patent but has no communication with the tunica vaginalis. Hernial contents do not enter the scrotum, but are present in relation to the spermatic cord. This is a ***congenital funicular hernia***.
   c. The processus vaginalis may persist only in the region of the inguinal canal (i.e., it does not persist beyond the superficial inguinal ring). In such cases the hernial swelling is small (***bubonocele***).
6. The neck of the sac of an indirect inguinal hernia lies at the deep inguinal ring, and is ***lateral*** to the inferior epigastric vessels.
7. The coverings of an indirect inguinal hernia are the same as the coverings of the testis. From deep to superficial these are:
   a. Extraperitoneal tissue
   b. Internal spermatic fascia
   c. Cremasteric fascia
   d. External spermatic fascia
   e. Skin.

*Direct Inguinal Hernia*

1. In this type of hernia, the sac does not pass through the deep inguinal ring, but enters the inguinal canal by pushing through the posterior wall of the canal.
2. Because of this the neck of the sac lies ***medial*** to the inferior epigastric vessels.
3. The region of the anterior abdominal wall through which a direct inguinal hernia takes place is seen from behind in 25.26. The area is triangular. It is bounded:
   a. Laterally by the inferior epigastric artery.
   b. Medially by the lateral border of the rectus abdominis.
   c. Inferiorly by the inguinal ligament. This is ***Hesselbach's triangle***.

4. The triangle is divided into medial and lateral parts by the obliterated umbilical artery.
   a. The importance of these details is that a direct inguinal hernia can occur through either the lateral or medial part of Hesselbach's triangle.
   b. These are named ***lateral direct inguinal hernia*** and ***medial direct inguinal hernia*** respectively.
5. In 25.26 note the relationship of the inferior epigastric artery to the deep inguinal ring. From this figure it will be clear that the sac of a direct inguinal hernia will always lie ***medial*** to the artery, while the sac of an indirect hernia will always be ***lateral*** to the artery.
6. Sometimes, a small inguinal hernia may be confused with a femoral hernia. The two can be distinguished by the fact that:
   a. A femoral hernia takes place into the femoral canal which is ***lateral to the pubic tubercle.***
   b. In contrast, an inguinal hernia passes through the superficial inguinal ring that lies ***medial to the pubic tubercle.***
7. The coverings of a direct inguinal hernia are as follows:
   a. In a lateral direct hernia they are (from deep to superficial) are:
      i. Extraperitoneal tissue
      ii. Fascia transversalis
      iii. Cremasteric fascia
      iv. External spermatic fascia
      v. Skin.
   b. In a medial direct hernia the coverings are the same as given above except that the cremasteric fascia is replaced by the conjoint tendon (which lies in the posterior wall of the medial part of the inguinal canal).

**Umbilical Hernia**

1. At an early stage in embryonic life some coils of intestine project out of the abdominal cavity, constituting a ***physiological umbilical hernia***. After some time these coils return to the abdominal cavity, and the gap at the umbilicus is gradually closed.
2. In some cases, a child may be born with coils of intestine projecting out of the umbilicus.
   a. This is caused by failure of the physiological hernia to get reduced.
   b. The coils are not covered by peritoneum. They are covered by amnion to which the umbilical cord is attached.
   c. This condition is called ***congenital umbilical hernia, exomphalos***, or ***omphalocoele***.
3. Even in later life the umbilicus represents an area of weakness.
   a. In some infants, a small protrusion of peritoneum may take place in the region resulting in a small swelling.
   b. This is called ***acquired infantile umbilical hernia***.
4. An ***acquired umbilical hernia*** may also be seen in old people (specially in women) in whom the abdominal muscles have become weak. Such hernias are really paraumbilical and lie to one side of the umbilicus.

***Other Midline Herniae***

1. The linea alba is widest in its upper part. A midline protrusion through the linea alba anywhere above the umbilicus is called an ***epigastric hernia***.
2. Below the level of the umbilicus, the region of the linea alba is narrow and is strengthened by close approximation of the right and left rectus muscles.
   a. However, in women whose abdominal muscles have become very weak as a result of repeated pregnancies a hernia may take place in the midline.
   b. As it increases in size, it pushes the rectus muscles apart creating a condition called ***divarication of recti***.

**Some other Herniae**

1. Abdominal contents may pass into the upper part of the thigh through the femoral canal constituting a ***femoral hernia***.
2. Various types of diaphragmatic hernias may occur and have been described in chapter 18. They may be congenital or acquired.
3. Other rare sites where herniation may occur are the lumbar region (inferior lumbar triangle), perineal (through the pelvic floor), obturator (through the obturator canal), gluteal (through the greater sciatic foramen) and sciatic (through the lesser sciatic foramen). Ischiorectal hernia is described in an earlier chapter.
4. Hernia can also take place in the region of an operative incision (***incisional hernia***). This is more likely to occur in persons who are obese, who have abdominal distension, and in whom there is postoperative infection.

# 26 CHAPTER

# The Perineum and Related Genital Organs

## INTRODUCTION TO THE PERINEUM

1. As seen on the surface of the body, the perineum is the region where the external genitalia and the anus are located.
2. In relation to the skeleton, the boundaries of the perineum correspond to those of the pelvic outlet (26.1).
3. This outlet is rhomboid in shape, and can be divided into anterior and posterior triangular areas. These are the ***uro-genital triangle*** placed anteriorly, and the ***anal triangle*** placed posteriorly.
4. a. The apex of the ***urogenital triangle*** lies anteriorly and is formed by the pubic symphysis.
   b. On either side the triangle is bounded by the corresponding ischiopubic ramus.
   c. Posteriorly, the base of the triangle is formed by an imaginary line joining the two ischial tuberosities.
   d. Some genital organs are located in this region.
   e. In the male, these are the scrotum (containing the right and left testis and epididymis), and the penis.
   f. In the female, we see the external genitalia which are present around the external openings of the urethra and the vagina.

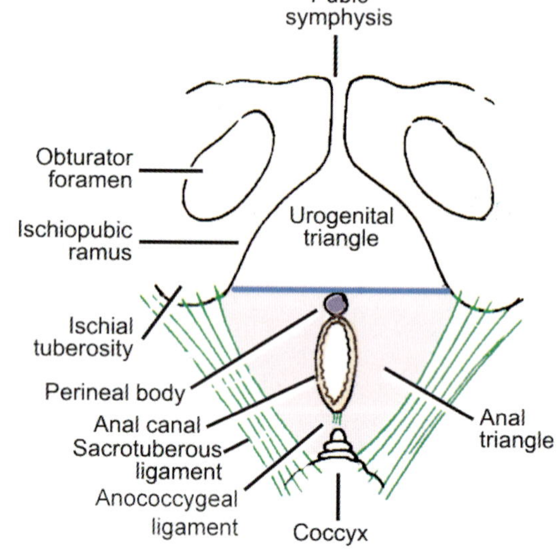


**26.1:** Boundaries of the perineum

5. a. The apex of the ***anal triangle*** is placed posteriorly, and is formed by the coccyx.
   b. Laterally, the triangle is bounded by the sacrotuberous ligaments (passing from the sacrum to the ischial tuberosity). (More superficially, the boundary is formed by the inferior margin of the gluteus maximus muscle).
   c. The base of the anal triangle is the imaginary line joining the right and left ischial tuberosities. The anal canal passes through this triangle to open to the exterior at the anus.

### The Scrotum

1. a. The scrotum is a sac that is lined on the outside by skin.
   b. Closely united to the skin there is a layer of smooth muscle that constitutes the ***dartos muscle***.
   c. Contraction of the muscle produces corrugations on the skin and makes it tight.
2. a. The scrotum consists of two halves, right and left that are separated from each other by a septum.
   b. The dartos muscle extends into this septum.
   c. Deep to the dartos muscle each half of the scrotum is lined by the coverings of the testis shown in 26.6.
3. Each half of the scrotum contains the corresponding testis, epididymis, and the initial part of the ductus deferens. These are described below. The coverings of the testis are described as additional 'layers' of the scrotum.

4. a. The scrotum is supplied by:
   i. The scrotal branches of the internal pudendal artery and by.
   ii. The superficial and deep external pudendal branches of the femoral artery.
   iii. The cremasteric artery (a branch of the inferior epigastric) also reaches the scrotum.
   b. The veins follow the corresponding arteries.
5. The nerves supplying the scrotum are:
   a. The ilioinguinal
   b. The genital branch of the genitofemoral
   c. The posterior scrotal branches of the perineal nerve
   d. The perineal branch of the posterior cutaneous nerve of the thigh.
6. Lymph vessels from the scrotum end in the superficial inguinal lymph nodes.

## THE TESTIS AND EPIDIDYMIS

1. a. Each testis (right or left) is an oval shaped structure about 4 cm in its longest (vertical) diameter.
   b. It is about 2.5 cm broad and about 3 cm in anteroposterior diameter.
2. a. The two testes lie in the scrotum (26.2 and 26.3).
   b. They are placed obliquely the upper pole being slightly anterior and lateral to the lower pole.
   c. The left testis is usually somewhat lower than the right.
3. a. For descriptive convenience, the surface of the testis is divided into medial and lateral surfaces that are separated by anterior and posterior borders.
   b. The anterior border is rounded there being no definite demarcation between the medial and lateral surfaces.
   c. The posterior border can be identified because the epididymis is attached to it.
4. a. The epididymis is a mass formed by tortuous tubules.
   b. Its upper end lies near the upper pole of the testis. It is enlarged and is called the ***head***.
   c. The middle part of the epididymis is of medium size and called the ***body***.
   d. Its lower part is thin and is called the ***tail*** (26.3).
5. a. On each side, the testis and epididymis lie in a closed sac which is called the ***tunica vaginalis*** (26.4).
   b. The wall of the sac is formed by a thin membrane similar in structure to peritoneum.
   c. It has a visceral layer lining the testis and a parietal layer. The two layers are separated by a potential space.
6. The visceral layer covers the entire surface of the testis except along its posterior aspect. On reaching the posterior end of the medial surface the visceral layer becomes continuous with the parietal layer.
7. a. At the posterior end of the lateral surface of the testis, the visceral layer is reflected on to the medial aspect of the body of epididymis.
   b. Here, it lines a recess which separates the two surfaces. This recess is called the ***sinus of the epididymis*** (26.4).

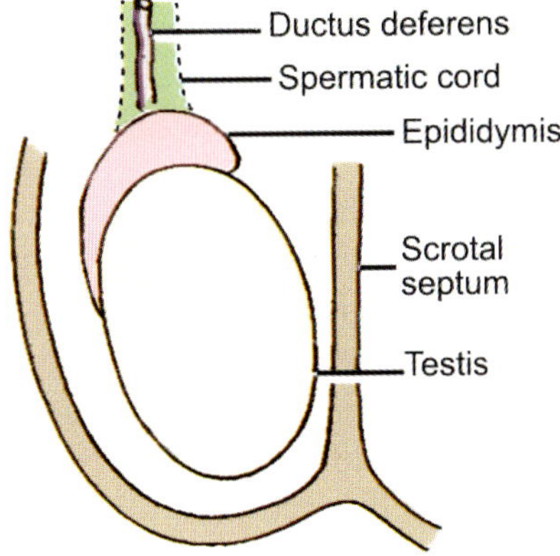


**26.2:** Right testis seen from the front

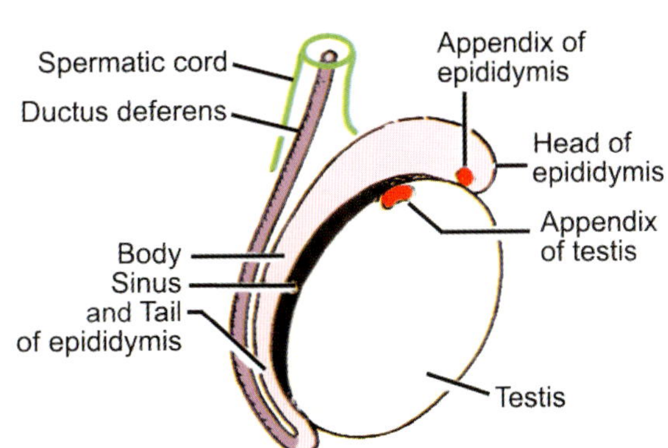


**26.3:** Right testis seen from the lateral side

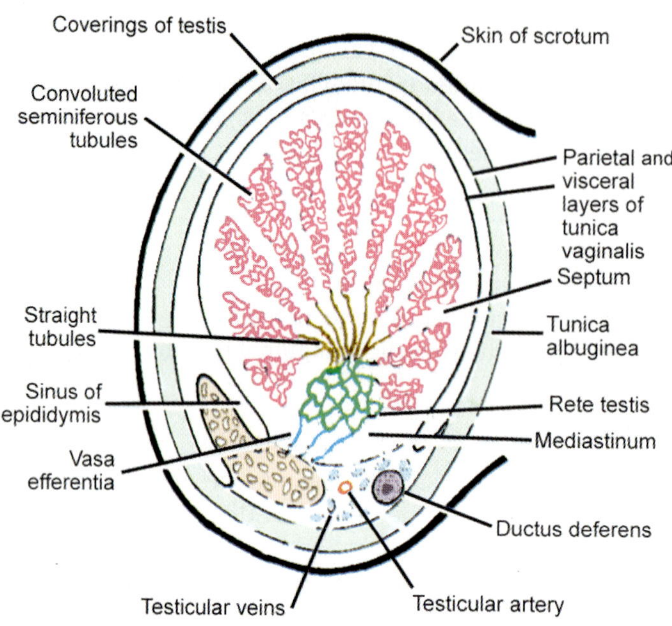


**26.4:** Schematic transverse section through testis

8. a. In an isolated specimen, the presence of the sinus enables the lateral aspect of the testis to be distinguished from the medial aspect; while the upper pole can be identified because the head of the epididymis is attached to it.
   b. These features enable the right and left testes to be distinguished from each other.
9. a. In 26.4 note that the posterior 'border' is broad.
   b. The epididymis is attached on the lateral part of the 'border'.
   c. While the ductus deferens ascends along its medial part.
   d. The posterior aspect is also related to the testicular artery and a plexus of veins.
10. a. In 26.4 also note that deep to the visceral layer of the tunica vaginalis, the outermost layer of the testis is formed by a dense fibrous membrane called the ***tunica albuginea***.
    b. In the posterior part of the testis, the connective tissue forming the tunica albuginea is thicker than elsewhere and projects into the substance of the testis. This projection is called the ***mediastinum testis***.
11. a. Numerous septa pass from the mediastinum testis to the tunica albuginea, and divide the substance of the testis into a large number of lobules.
    b. Each lobule contains one or more highly convoluted ***seminiferous tubules***.
12. a. These tubules are lined by an epithelium the cells of which are concerned with the production of spermatozoa.
    b. It has been estimated that each testis has about 200 lobules, and that each lobule has one to three seminiferous tubules. The total number of tubules is between 400 and 600.
13. a. From 26.4, it will be seen that each lobule is roughly conical, the apex of the cone being directed towards the mediastinum testis.
    b. Near the apex of the lobule, the seminiferous tubules lose their convolutions and join one another to form about twenty to thirty larger ***straight tubules***.
    c. These enter the fibrous tissue of the mediastinum testis and unite to form a network called the ***rete testis***.
14. a. At its upper end, the rete testis gives off 12 to 20 ***efferent ductules*** (an old name for which is vasa efferentia).
    b. These ductules pass from the upper part of the testis into the head of the epididymis. Within the head, these tubules become highly convoluted.
    c. The head of the epididymis is in fact nothing but a mass of these convoluted tubules.

15. a. At the lower end of the head of the epididymis, these tubules end in a single tube called the ***duct of the epididymis***.
    b. The body and tail of the epididymis are formed by convolutions of this duct.
    c. At the lower end of the tail, the duct of the epididymis becomes continuous with the ductus deferens.
16. a. Deep to the tunica albuginea, there is a layer of vascular tissue called the ***tunica vasculosa***, which also lines the septa bounding the lobules of the testis.
    b. The visceral layer of the tunica vaginalis, the tunica albugina and the tunica vasculosa collectively form the ***capsule*** of the testis.
    c. Apart from this capsule the testis is covered by a number of 'coverings' that form part of the wall of the scrotum.

### Blood Vessels, Lymphatics and Nerves of the Testis

1. a. The testis is supplied by the testicular artery, a direct branch of the abdominal aorta.
   b. Each artery (right or left) runs down over the posterior abdominal wall to reach the external iliac artery. It runs along this vessel to reach the deep inguinal ring.
   c. The testicular artery then passes through the inguinal canal (as part of the spermatic cord) to reach the testis and supply it.
2. a. The testis is drained through the testicular vein.
   b. The 'vein' travels through the spermatic cord in the form of a plexus (pampiniform plexus).
   c. At the deep inguinal ring the plexus drains into one, or more, channels that run along the testicular artery.
   d. Ultimately, one vein is formed.
   e. Note that the right testicular vein ends in the inferior vena cava, but the left vein ends by joining the left renal vein.
3. Lymph vessels from the testis pass along the testicular vessels directly to the lateral aortic lymph nodes (lying along the sides of the abdominal aorta).
4. a. The nerves to the testis are sympathetic.
   b. They are derived from the 10th and 11th thoracic segments of the spinal cord.
   c. They pass through the aortic plexus and then along the testicular vessels to reach the testis.

### Descent of the Testis and Processus Vaginalis

1. Each testis develops in relation to the posterior abdominal wall, but in later fetal life it descends towards the scrotum reaching it at about the time of birth.
2. a. This process of descent is facilitated by the formation of a pouch like extension of the peritoneum called the ***processus vaginalis***.
   b. The processus vaginalis passes through the abdominal wall into the region of the future scrotum.
   c. The passage through the abdominal wall becomes the inguinal canal.
   d. The testis descends along the posterior margin of the processus vaginalis (not within it) and gradually invaginates it from behind.
   e. The distal part of the processus vaginalis (which is invaginated by the testis) becomes the tunica vaginalis. The remaining part of the processus is obliterated.
   f. As the processus passes through the inguinal canal it carries with it a number of coverings that surround it and the spermatic cord. These are described below.

## THE DUCTUS DEFERENS

1. The ductus deferens begins in the scrotum (as a continuation of the epididymis). It passes through the inguinal canal to enter the abdomen.
2. It then runs backwards (over the lateral wall of the pelvis) and finally turns medially to reach the posterior aspect of urinary bladder.

3. Here, the ductus deferens terminates by joining the duct of the seminal vesicle to form the ejaculatory duct.
4. From 26.4, it is seen that the initial part of the ductus deferens passes upwards along the posterior aspect of the testis. This part lies medial to the epididymis.
5. a. The part of the ductus deferens that lies in the inguinal canal forms part of the spermatic cord.
   b. This cord extends from the upper pole of the testis up to the deep inguinal ring.
   c. At the deep inguinal ring, the ductus deferens enters the abdomen.
   d. Here it hooks around the lateral side of the inferior epigastric artery (26.5).
6. a. The ductus then runs backwards (and somewhat downwards).
   b. Crossing medial to the external iliac vessels the ductus deferens comes to lie in the lateral wall of the true pelvis.



**26.5:** Scheme to show relationship of ductus deferens to inferior epigastric artery. Also note relationship of the artery to the deep inguinal ring.

7. The further course of the ductus deferens will be studied in the pelvis (chapter 33). For the time being just note that the ductus terminates by joining the duct of the seminal vesicle to form the ejaculatory duct.
8. a. The ductus deferens has a very narrow lumen, but has a thick wall.
   b. When palpated it feels like a cord. Its initial part (lying behind the testis) is highly convoluted, but the rest of it is straight.
   c. Near the seminal vesicle the ductus bears a dilatation called the ***ampulla;*** but the terminal part of the ductus again narrows down before joining the duct of the seminal vesicle.

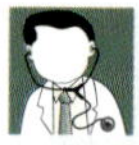

## CLINICAL CORRELATION

**Vasectomy**

1. a. This operation is very frequently performed in India as a family limiting measure.
   b. The operation can be done using local anaesthesia.
   c. The right and left ductus deferens are approached through small incisions in the upper part of the scrotal wall, and are cut. The cut ends are ligated.
   d. The operation is called vasectomy as an old name for the ductus deferens is vas deferens.
2. a. Following the operation spermatozoa do not reach the exterior.
   b. Normal ejaculation takes place, the ejaculate consisting of prostatic and other secretions.
   c. In case of need the two ends of the ductus deferens can be re-anatomosed in many cases. This is easier if a segment of the ductus deferens has not been removed during vasectomy.

## THE SPERMATIC CORD

1. The spermatic cord extends from the upper pole of the testis, through the inguinal canal, to the deep inguinal ring.
2. Apart from the ductus deferens (described above) it contains:
   a. The testicular artery.
   b. The testicular veins which are in the form of the pampiniform plexus.
   c. The cremasteric artery (a branch of the inferior epigastric artery).
   d. The artery to the ductus deferens (a branch of the superior vesical artery).
   e. The genital branch of the genitofemoral nerve.
   f. Lymph vessels and a plexus of sympathetic nerves are also present.
3. The spermatic cord has a number of coverings that are described as follows:

## Coverings of Spermatic Cord and of Testis

1. When the testis descends through the inguinal canal during development, it carries with it prolongations from various layers of the abdominal wall.
2. These provide a series of coverings for the testis and for the spermatic cord (26.6). These are as follows:
   a. The innermost covering is derived from the fascia transversalis and is called the ***internal spermatic fascia.*** It starts at the deep inguinal ring.
   b. The next covering is derived from the internal oblique muscle of the abdomen. This layer is partly muscular and partly fibrous. It is called the ***cremasteric fascia***. The muscle fibres constitute the ***cremaster muscle***.
   c. The outermost layer is a prolongation of the aponeurosis of the external oblique muscle of the abdomen. It is called the ***external spermatic fascia.*** This fascia surrounds the spermatic cord below the level of the superficial inguinal ring.
   d. In addition to the above, the testis is surrounded by the wall of the scrotum.

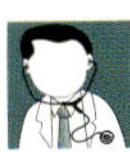

## CLINICAL CORRELATION

### Clinical Correlation of Scrotum and Testes

*Understanding Terminology*

1. Scrotum is the Latin word for a bag.
2. The Latin word for testis is ***orchis***.
3. Some words derived from orchis are ***orchitis*** (inflammation of testis from any cause), ***orchidectomy*** or ***orchiectomy*** (surgical removal of testis) and ***orchidopexy*** (surgical fixation of testis).

*Some Facts About the Scrotum*

1. a. The condition of the skin of the scrotum shows variations.
   b. In young persons, and in cold weather, the scrotal wall contracts (by action of the dartos muscle) making the scrotum small and firm.
   c. In old persons and in warm weather the scrotum tends to hang loosely.
2. a. The skin of the scrotum and groin are often sites of infection specially if personal hygiene is not good.
   b. Fungal or other infections may occur.
   c. Because of the presence of hair and sebaceous glands, sebaceous cysts are not uncommon.
   d. Sometimes infection of the scrotum can lead to gangrene. This is a very serious condition.
3. In filarial infection (in which lymph vessels get choked) stasis of substances normally drained through lymphatics can lead to enormous enlargement of the scrotum.
4. Two common causes of scrotal swelling are inguinal hernia (discussed above) and hydrocele (see below).

*Hydrocele*

1. In the section on inguinal hernia, we have seen that the processus vaginalis is a prolongation of peritoneum that passes through the inguinal canal into the scrotum. Its distal part forms the tunica vaginalis that surrounds the testis, while the proximal part normally disappears. We have also seen that abnormally various parts of the processus vaginalis may persist.
2. The tunica vaginalis, or any persisting part of the processus vaginalis, may become filled with a collection of fluid. This condition is called ***hydrocele*** that can be of various types.
   a. Most commonly fluid is confined to the tunica vaginalis. This condition is termed ***vaginal hydrocele***.
   b. Sometimes the entire processus vaginalis remains patent and the hydrocele fluid can pass into the peritoneal cavity. This is called ***congenital hydrocele***.
   c. In ***infantile hydrocele*** fluid extends upwards from the tunica vaginalis around the spermatic cord right up to the deep inguinal ring.
   d. Sometimes there is no fluid in the tunica vaginalis, but there is a collection of fluid in a patent segment of processus vaginalis present in relation to the spermatic cord (***encysted hydrocele of the cord***).

3. Fluid of a typical vaginal hydrocele can be removed by passing a needle of suitable bore into it. The needle has to pass through the various coverings of the testis (skin, membranous layer of superficial fascia containing fibres of dartos muscle, external spermatic fascia, internal spermatic fascia and the outer layer of tunica vaginalis (26.6).

*Varicocele*

1. The pampiniform plexus of veins drains the testis. When these veins become tortuous and dilated (varicose) and form a palpable mass (that feels like a mass of worms) the condition is called ***varicocele***.
2. The condition may be harmless and may cause no symptoms, but in some patients there is discomfort and a dragging sensation.
3. The condition is much more common on the left side. This is often said to be due to the fact that the left testicular vein ends in the left renal vein, in which the pressure is higher than in the inferior vena cava (into which the right testicular vein opens).
4. Any factor that tends to obstruct flow in the testicular veins can predispose to the formation of varicocele. e.g.,
   a. Pressure by the colon
   b. By growth of cells of a hypernephroma into the veins.
5. 1. Veins of the pampiniform plexus communicate with cremasteric veins that drain into the inferior epigastric vein.
   2. This provides an alternative path for drainage of blood.
   3. In some cases of varicocele the enlarged veins are cremasteric veins.
6. Surgical treatment is necessary if varicocele causes discomfort.
7. Varicocele can also interfere with spermatogenesis by raising the temperature within the scrotum and this is another indication for treatment.
8. Treatment consists of ligation of the testicular artery above the inguinal ligament, accompanied if necessary by removal of the enlarged veins of the pampiniform plexus.

**Congenital Anomalies of Testis and Epididymis**

*Descent of the Testes*

1. The testes develop in relation to the lumbar region of the posterior abdominal wall.
   a. During fetal life they gradually descend to the scrotum, reaching the iliac fossa in the third month.
   b. They lie at the deep inguinal ring up to the seventh month of intrauterine life, and pass through the inguinal canal during the seventh month.
   c. Normally, the testes reach the scrotum by the end of the eighth month.
2. Descent of the testis may fail to occur or may be incomplete (***cryptorchidism***, literally hidden testis). The organ may lie anywhere along the path of descent.
3. It is important to note that an undescended testis may complete its descent normally after birth. Failure of a testis to descend to the scrotum can lead to several complications.
   a. Spermatogenesis may fail to occur (as it appears to depend on the lower temperature provided in the scrotum).
   b. Malignancy is more common in an undescended testis.
   c. A testis lodged in the inguinal canal may be subject to repeated trauma that can lead to orchitis.
   d. The condition of undescended testis is very commonly accompanied by the presence of an indirect inguinal hernia.
   e. In suitable cases, the testis can be brought into the scrotum and fixed there by surgery (***orchiopexy*** or ***orchidopexy***).
4. Instead of descending into the scrotum, the testis may get lodged at an abnormal site (***ectopic testis***). It may come to lie:
   a. Under the skin of the front of the abdomen
   b. Under the skin of the thigh

   c. In the femoral canal
   d. Under the skin of the penis
   e. In the the perineum behind scrotum.
5. The position of the testis within the scrotum may be abnormal.
   a. In ***anterior inversion,*** the relative position of the testis and the epididymis is reversed so that the epididymis lies in front of the testis.
   b. In polar inversion the vertical position of the testis is reversed and the head of the epididymis (globus major) can be felt below the testis.
6. A number of small vestigial elements are present in relation to the testis and epididymis and can lead to formation of cysts. The vestigial structures include:
   a. The appendix of the testis (or hydatid or Morgagni).
   b. The appendix of the epididymis.
   c. The superior or inferior aberrant ductules.
   d. The paradidymis.

**Some Other Clinical Correlations of the Testis and Epididymis**

1. Infections of the epididymis (***epididymitis***), or of the testis (***orchitis***) may occur alone but are usually combined (***epididymo-orchitis***).
2. The infection usually reaches the region from the urethra or prostate through the ductus deferens. The infection may be acute or chronic.
3. The testis may be a site of malignancy and many varieties of tumours are encountered.
   a. Malignancy can spread through lymphatics to the para-aortic nodes and spread can be bilateral.
   b. If the scrotum is invaded by the growth the inguinal lymph nodes can be involved.

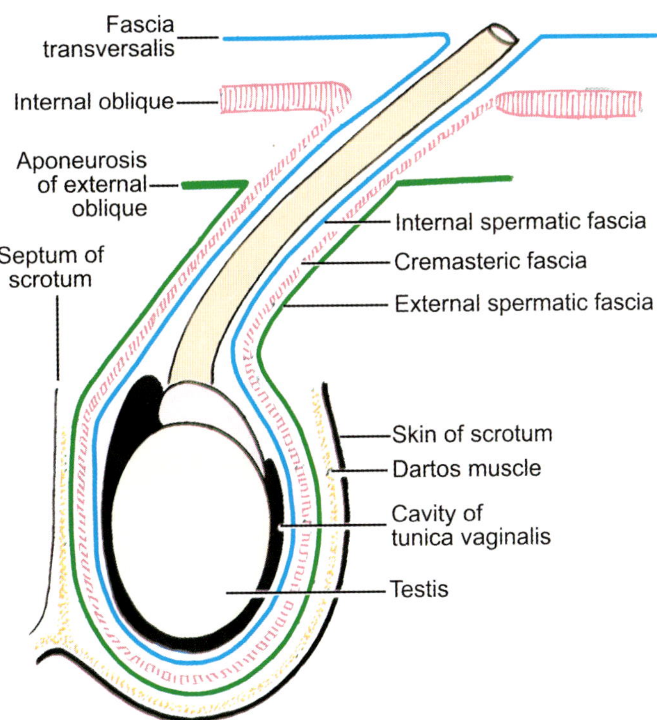


**26.6:** Scheme to show the coverings of the spermatic cord and testis

## THE PENIS

1. The penis consists of a ***root*** that is fixed to the perineum, and of a free part that is called the ***corpus*** (or body). The free part is lined all round by skin.
2. a. The apical part of the penis is enlarged and conical. This part is called the ***glans penis*** (26.8).
   b. The glans penis has a projecting posterior margin that is termed the ***corona glandis***. Immediately proximal to the corona the penis shows a slight constriction that is referred to as the ***neck of the penis***.
3. a. The skin covering the penis is loosely attached except over the glans. Here, it is firmly attached to underlying tissues.
   b. The glans is also covered by a fold of skin that extends from the neck of the penis towards the tip. This fold is called the ***prepuce*** (26.8).
4. The posteroinferior part of the prepuce is attached to the adjoining part of the glans by a fold called the ***frenulum***.
5. a. The prepuce normally covers the greater part of the glans, but can be retracted to expose the latter.
   b. The space between the surface of the glans and the prepuce is called the ***preputial sac***.
6. a. For descriptive purposes, the surface of the penis that is continuous with the anterior abdominal wall is called the ***dorsum***.
   b. The surface towards the scrotum is the ventral surface.
7. A transverse section through the free part of the penis is shown in 26.7. The substance of the penis is made up of three masses of spongy tissue, two dorsal and one ventral.
8. The dorsal masses are the right and left ***corpora cavernosa*** (singular = corpus cavernosum). They lie side by side and are separated only by a median fibrous septum. The septum is part of a fibrous sheath that surrounds each corpus cavernosum.
9. a. The ***corpus spongiosum*** is placed in the midline ventral to the corpora cavernosa.
   b. It is tranversed by the penile part of the urethra.
   c. The corpus spongiosum is surrounded by a fibrous sheath.
   d. In addition, there is an outer sheath that is common to the corpora cavernosa and the corpus spongiosum. This sheath is covered on the outside by superficial fascia and skin.
10. a. The substance of the corpora cavernosa and of the corpus spongiosum contains numerous small spaces separated by delicate partitions. These spaces are in communication with blood vessels.
    b. Most of them are normally empty, but during erection of the penis the spaces become filled with blood leading to enlargement and rigidity of the penis.

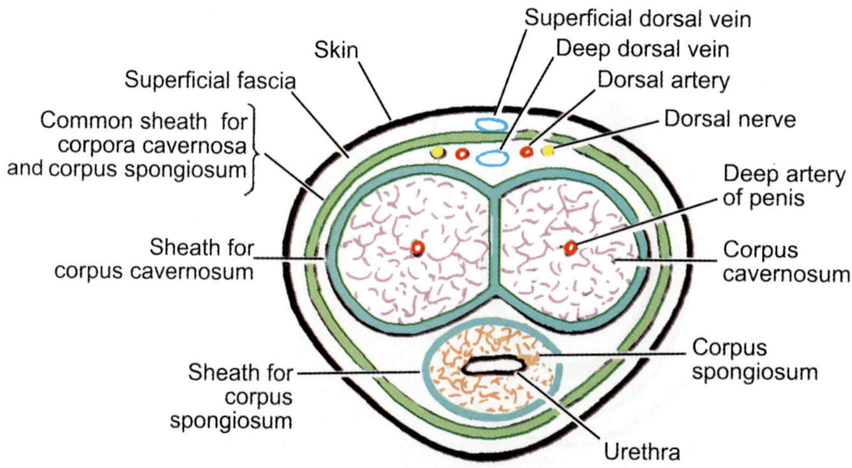


**26.7:** Schematic cross section through the free part of the penis

11. a. A longitudinal section through the penis, a little to one side of the midline is shown in 26.8. From this figure, it is seen that the distal part of the corpus spongiosum is greatly enlarged to form the substance of the glans penis.
    b. The distal ends of the corpora cavernosa fit into a hollow on the proximal aspect of the glans.
12. a. When traced into the perineum (i.e., into the root of the penis) the right and left corpora cavernosa separate to form the right and left ***crura*** (singular = crus) of the penis.
    b. The crura lie in the superficial perineal space, on the inferior aspect of the perineal membrane (26.9).
    c. Each crus is firmly attached to the corresponding margin of the pubic arch i.e., to the inferior ramus of the pubis and the ramus of the ischium.
    d. Note that this ramus has a prominent everted edge for attachment of the crus.
13. a. The corpus spongiosum also extends into the superficial perineal space where it is firmly attached to the inferior aspect of the perineal membrane, in the midline.
    b. Its proximal end is enlarged to form the ***bulb*** of the penis.
    c. The urethra enters the bulb after piercing the perineal membrane.
14. The right and left crura of the penis are covered by the corresponding ischiocavernosus muscle; while the bulb is covered by the bulbospongiosus muscle (see later in text).

## Vessels and Nerves of Penis

1. The arteries supplying the penis are the deep and dorsal arteries of the penis. These are branches of the internal pudendal artery (26.18).
2. The right and left dorsal arteries lie along the dorsum of the penis on either side of the deep dorsal vein (26.7).
3. The right and left deep arteries enter the corresponding crus penis in the perineum and run forward in the centre of the corpus cavernosum.
4. The main veins draining the penis are the superficial and deep dorsal veins.
    a. The superficial vein lies deep to the skin.
    b. While the deep vein is deep to the common fibrous sheath surrounding, the corpora cavernosa and the corpus spongiosum.
    c. Both veins are unpaired and lie in the midline.
5. a. At the posterior end of the penis, the superficial vein ends by joining the right or left external pudendal vein (which drains into the great saphenous vein).
    b. The deep dorsal vein ends by joining the prostatic plexus of veins through which it drains into the internal iliac veins.

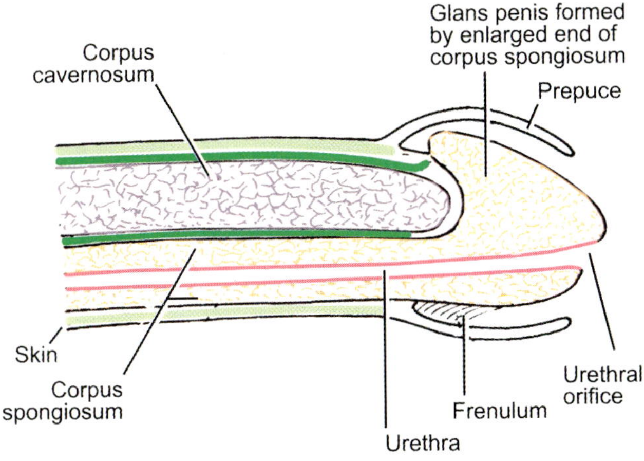


**26.8:** Schematic parasagittal section through the penis

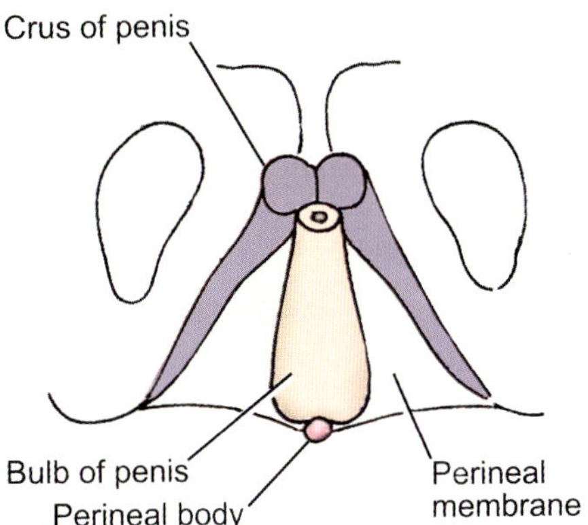


**26.9:** Parts of the root of the penis lying on the perineal membrane

6. a. The lymphatics from the penis drain into the superficial inguinal nodes (upper medial group).
   b. Those from the glans penis drain into the deep inguinal nodes.
7. The main nerve to the penis is the dorsal nerve of the penis. It is a branch of the pudendal nerve and lies lateral to the dorsal artery of the corresponding side (26.7).

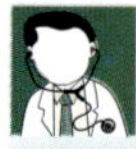

## CLINICAL CORRELATION

### Congenital Malformations of External Genitalia

A. Both male and female external genitalia are derived from the same primordia.
B. The female external genitalia represent the more primitive state of development, and when the development of male external genitalia is deficient the appearances tend to resemble the female condition.

#### *Anomalies of the Penis*

1. Clinically, the most common abnormality of the penis is ***phimosis***, in which the prepuce is too narrow to be retracted.
   a. Accumulation of secretions under the prepuce can lead to infection, and in the long term it can also a predisposing factor in development of malignancy.
   b. A narrow phimosis can be a cause of urinary retention.
   c. Phimosis is corrected surgically by removing part of the prepuce (***circumcision***).
2. Circumcision (removal of prepuce) is practised as a religious ritual in Muslims and Jews.
3. Rare anomalies of the penis include:
   a. Partial or complete absence
   b. A double or bifid penis
   c. A penis placed behind the scrotum.
4. The penile urethra may open at an abnormal site.
   a. If the opening is located on the undersurface of the penis the condition is called ***hypospadias***.
   b. When (much more rarely) it is on the dorsal surface the condition is called ***epispadias***.

### Congenital Malformations of Scrotum

1. The scrotum is formed by fusion of right and left genital swellings.
2. In the female, the two genital swellings remain separate and form the labia majora.
3. Sometimes the genital swellings may fail to fuse in a male, and the scrotum is in two halves and the external genitalia resemble those of the female.
4. Rarely, the scrotum may lie in front of the penis.

## THE PERINEUM

1. The perineum is divisible into an anterior urogenital triangle, and a posterior anal triangle.
2. Boundaries of these triangles have been noted. We will now take up detailed consideration of these regions.

### Urogenital Triangle

1. The ***urogenital triangle*** is placed between the two ischiopubic rami.
2. Stretching transversely across the rami, there are three membranes between which are enclosed two spaces as shown in 26.10. From above downwards, the membranes are as follows:
   a. Part of the pelvic fascia, that is continuous laterally with the fascia on the obturator internus, constitutes the ***superior fascia of the urogenital diaphragm.***
   b. The second membrane is the ***inferior fascia of the urogenital diaphragm.*** It is thick and is also called the ***perineal membrane.***
   c. The most superficial membrane is the membranous layer of superficial fascia.

3. a. Between the upper and middle membranes, there is the ***deep perineal space*** (or pouch).
   b. Between the middle and lower membranes, there is the ***superficial perineal space (or pouch).***
4. Posteriorly, all the three membranes are attached to the perineal body and to each other thus closing the superficial and deep perineal spaces behind (26.11).
5. Anteriorly, the superior and inferior fasciae of the urogenital diaphragm (i.e., the upper and middle membranes) fuse a little behind the pubic symphysis and form the ***transverse ligament of the pubis.***
6. The interval between this ligament and (the arcuate pubic ligament of) the pubic symphysis gives passage to the dorsal vein of the penis.
7. Traced anteriorly, the membranous layer of superficial fascia is continued cranially into the anterior abdominal wall.

## Contents of Deep Perineal Space

1. The ***deep perineal space*** contains two muscles (26.12 and 26.13).
   a. The ***sphincter urethrae*** stretches between the two ischiopubic rami. It is pierced by the urethra.
   b. Parallel to the posterior edge of the sphincter urethrae, there are the ***deep transverse perinei*** muscles of the two sides. They are attached laterally to the ramus of the ischium, and medially to the perineal body.

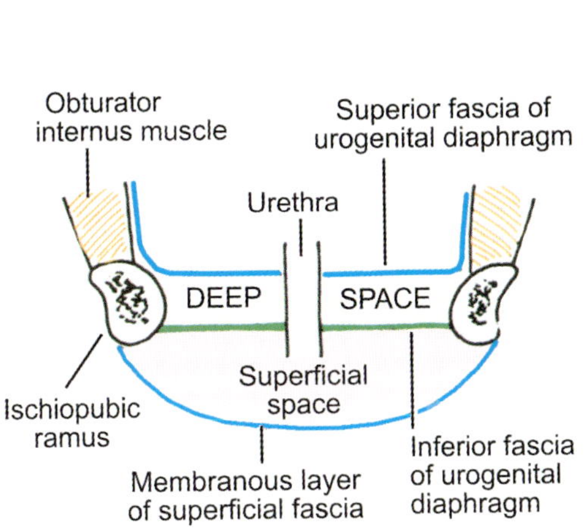


**26.10:** Schematic coronal section through urogenital triangle to show formation of superficial and deep perineal spaces

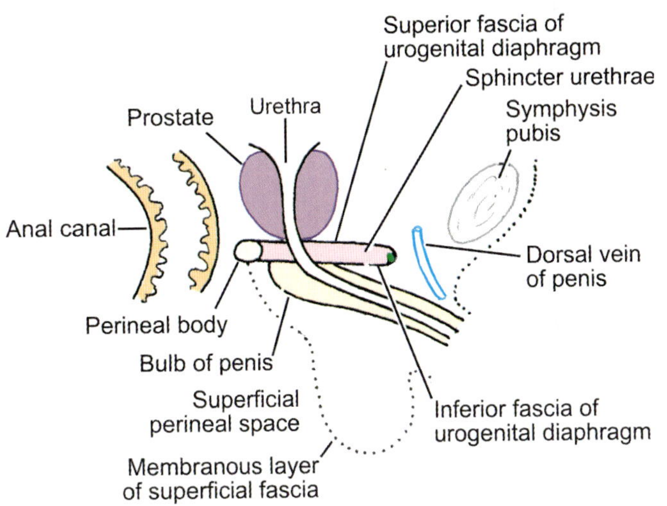


**26.11:** Sagittal section through the male urogenital triangle

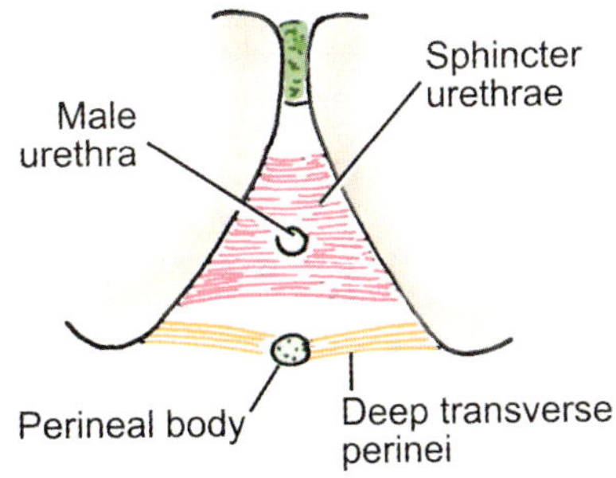


**26.12:** Muscles present in deep perineal space (as seen in the male)

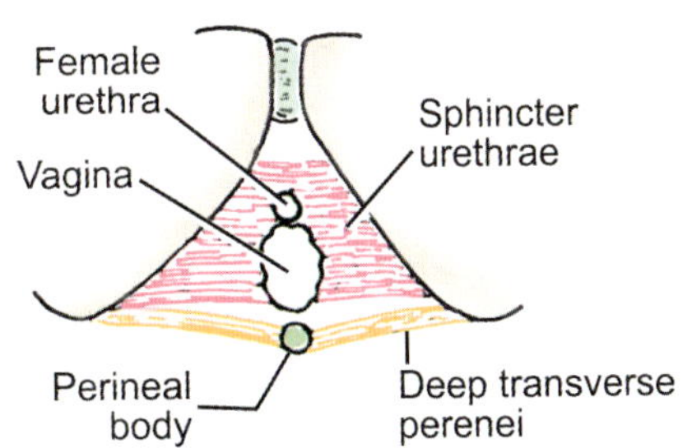


**26.13:** Muscles present in deep perineal space (as seen in the female)

2. The sphincter urethrae and the deep transverse perinei muscles, along with the two layers of fascia enclosing them constitute the ***urogenital diaphragm.***
3. The urogenital diaphragm is pierced by the membranous part of the urethra in the male.
4. a. In the female (26.13, the diaphragm is pierced by the urethra and vagina.
   b. As a result of the presence of a wide vaginal opening, the muscles and membranes of the urogenital diaphragm are much less developed in the female.
   c. The posterior fibres of the sphincter urethrae are attached to the vaginal wall.
5. Other contents of the deep perineal space are as follows:
   a. The ***bulbourethral glands*** (of Cowper) lie on each side of the membranous urethra in the male. Their ducts pierce the perineal membrane to enter the superficial perineal space where they open into the urethra.
   b. Several nerves and vessels pass through the deep perineal space.

## Superficial Perineal Space in the Male

1. The superficial perineal space contains parts of the external genitalia, and the muscles associated with them.
2. In the male, it contains the ***root of the penis*** that is made up of
   a. The ***bulb of the penis*** lying in the median plane.
   b. Right and left ***crura*** attached to the ischiopubic rami (26.9).
3. The bulb becomes continuous, anteriorly, with the ***corpus spongiosum*** of the penis, while each crus becomes continuous with the corresponding ***corpus cavernosum.***
4. After piercing the urogenital diaphragm, the urethra enters the bulb and passes forwards in it into the corpus spongiosum.

### *The Following Muscles are Present*

1. The ***bulbospongiosus*** overlies the bulb of the penis.
   a. Its fibres arise from a median raphe lying on the inferior aspect of the bulb (26.14A). The raphe is continuous posteriorly with the perineal body that also gives origin to some fibres of the muscle.
   b. The fibres pass round the sides of the bulb.
   c. The posteriormost fibres are inserted into the perineal membrane (26.14D).
   d. The middle fibres go right round the bulb, and the posterior part of the corpus spongiosum and end in another raphe on the dorsal aspect (26.14C).
   e. The anterior fibres of the muscles of the two sides pass forwards round the anterior parts of the crura (Fig. 40.15A) to meet in an aponeurosis on the dorsal aspect of the penis (26.14B).
2. The ***ischiocavernosus muscle*** covers the crus of the penis. It is attached to the ischiopubic rami around the attachment of the crus. It runs forwards and is inserted into the anterior part of the crus.
3. The ***superficial transverse perinei*** muscle is a narrow slip that runs transversely along the posterior margin of the superficial perineal space. It is attached laterally to the ischial tuberosity; and medially to the perineal body.

### *Nerve Supply*

All muscles of the urogenital triangle are innervated by the perineal branch of the pudendal nerve (S2, S3, S4).

### *Actions*

1. The bulbospongiosus helps in emptying the urethra in the terminal phases of micturition, and in ejaculation.
2. The anterior fibres that pass right round the penis assist in its erection by compressing the deep dorsal vein.
3. The ischiocavernosus may play a part in erection by compressing the crus.
4. The transverse perinei appear to act like ligaments keeping the perineal body in place.

## Superficial Perineal Space in the Female

The superficial perineal space in the female contains the female external genitalia and the muscles associated with them.

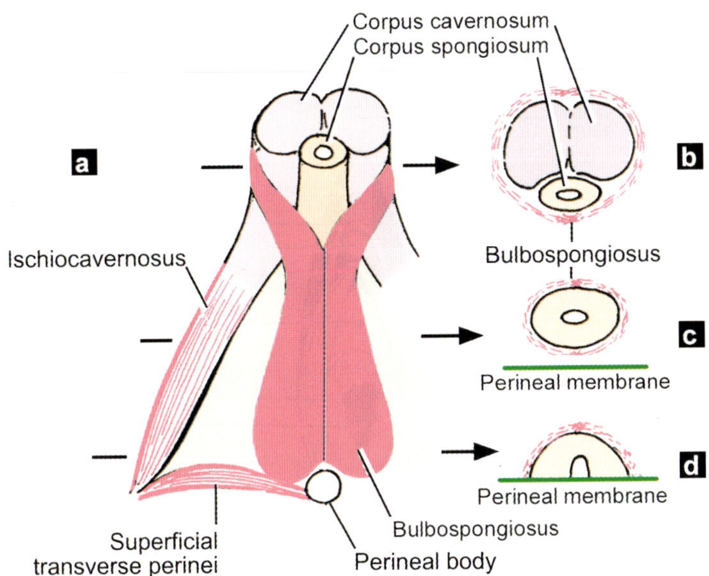


26.14: (a) Diagram to show muscles related to the root of the penis; (b to d) are transverse sections at levels indicated in 'a'

### Female External Genitalia

1. The region of the female external genitalia is referred to as the ***vulva*** or the ***pudendum.*** It is seen in surface view in 26.15.
2. When viewed from the surface, we see a midline ***pudendal cleft.*** The vagina and the urethra open to the exterior through this cleft.
3. The cleft is bounded on either side by an elevation called the ***labium majus.***
   a. The labia majora are folds of skin. The space between the anterior and posterior layers of skin is filled by connective tissue and fat.
   b. The labia majora are developmentally equivalent to the scrotum. This explains the termination of the round ligaments of the uterus in them. Like the scrotum the superficial fascia in the labia majora has some smooth muscle in it.
   c. The right and left labia majora are joined anteriorly by a fold called the ***anterior labial commissure*** and posteriorly by the ***posterior labial commissure.***
4. When the labia majora are separated, we see two smaller and thinner folds of skin deep to them. These are the ***labia minora*** placed on either side of the vaginal orifice (26.15).
   a. Posteriorly, the two labia minora are joined together by a fold called the ***frenulum***. This fold is conspicuous only in a virgin.
   b. Anteriorly, the labia minora join each other near the clitoris (see below).
   c. The space between the right and left labia minora is called the ***vestibule.***
5. The ***clitoris*** is a small median rod-like structure placed between the anterior parts of the labia majora.
   a. In structure, it resembles a miniature penis with the exception that the urethra does not pass through it.
   b. Like the penis, it has a ***glans***, a ***body*** and a ***root.***
   c. The body is made up of ***corpora cavernosa*** that extend into the perineum as the crura of the clitoris.
   d. The bulb and corpus spongiosum (of the penis) are represented in the female by two masses of erectile tissue placed on either side of the vaginal orifice. These are called the ***bulbs of the vestibule.*** Anteriorly, the two bulbs become very thin and meet at the glans of the clitoris.

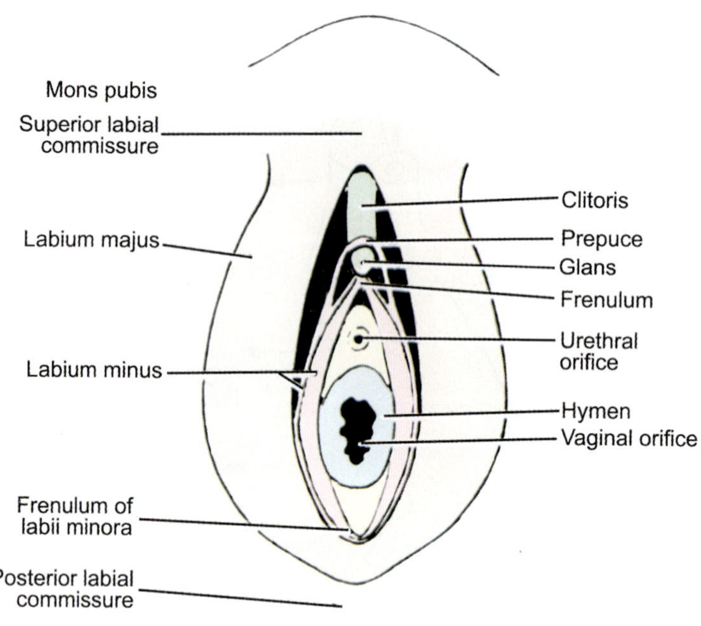


**26.15:** Female external genitalia

   e. On reaching the clitoris each labium minus divides into one part that passes dorsal to the clitoris and one part that is ventral to it. The dorsal parts of the two sides fuse to form a membrane called the ***prepuce*** of the clitoris. The ventral parts fuse to form the ***frenulum*** of the clitoris.
   f. The crura of the clitoris and the bulbs of the vestibule are placed in the superficial perineal space (26.16).
6. Deep to the labia minora the vaginal orifice is partially closed by a circular fold of mucous membrane called the ***hymen.***
   a. It is well defined only in the virgin.
   b. In married womenm, its position is marked by rounded elevations called the ***carunculae hymenales.***
7. The external orifice of the female urethra is located a short distance in front of the vaginal opening.
8. Near the posterior end of each bulb of the vestibule, there is one ***greater vestibular gland*** (which corresponds to the bulbourethral glands of the male). A duct arises from each gland and opens into the vestibule in the space between the labium minus and the hymen.
9. The ***mons pubis*** is a surface elevation overlying the pubic symphysis. It is produced by a mass of fat present just under the skin. The mons pubis is included in the female external genitalia.
10. a. The female external genitalia are supplied by the superficial and deep external pudendal branches of the femoral artery, and by the labial branches of the internal pudendal artery.
   b. The veins accompany the arteries.
   c. Lymph vessels end in the superficial inguinal lymph nodes.
11. The nerves supplying the region are the ilioinguinal nerve, the genital branch of the genitofemoral nerve, and the perineal branch of the posterior cutaneous nerve of the thigh.

### *Muscles Associated with Female External Genitalia*

These are similar to those in the male (26.17).

1. The ***bulbospongiosus*** covers each bulb of the vestibule.
   a. Posteriorly, its fibres merge with the perineal body.
   b. Anteriorly, they are attached to the body of the clitoris.
   c. Some of its fibres wind round the sides of the clitoris to reach its dorsal aspect (just as in the male).

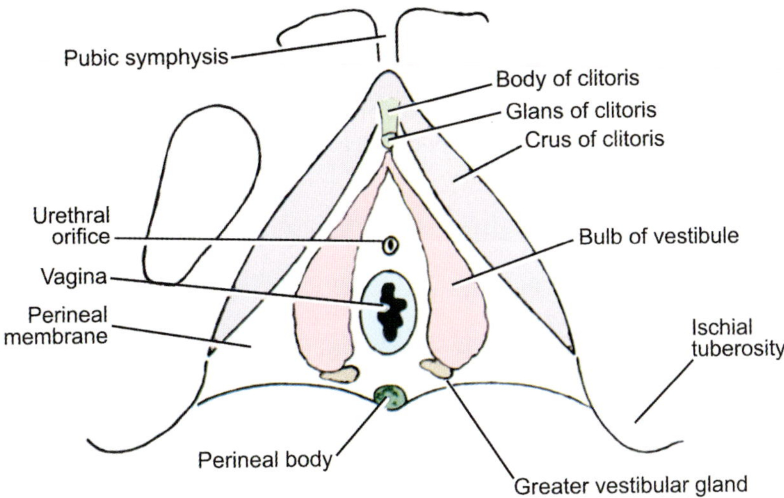


**26.16:** Some deeper structures in the female perineum

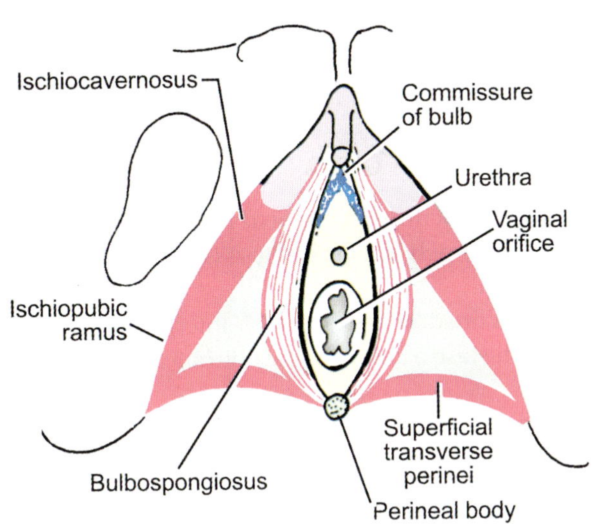


**26.17:** Muscles present in the superficial perineal space in the female

2. The ***ischiocavernosus*** muscle of each side covers the crus of the clitoris and has similar attachments as in the male.
3. The ***superficial transverse perinei*** are similar to those in the male. Medially, some of their fibres are attached to the vagina.

### *Nerve Supply*

As in the male all muscles of the urogenital triangle are supplied by the perineal branch of the pudendal nerve (S2, S3, S4).

*Actions*

1. In the female, the bulbospongiosus may serve as a sphincter for the vaginal orifice and may assist in erection of the clitoris.
2. The ischiocavernosus may also play a part in erection of the clitoris by compressing the crus.
3. The transverse perinei muscles help to keep the perineal body in place.

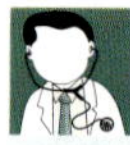

### CLINICAL CORRELATION

**Anomalies of Female External Genitalia**

1. The clitoris may be absent, double or bifid. It is enlarged in hermaphroditism (see below).
2. The labia minora may show partial fusion.
3. Instead of opening into the vestibule, the female urethra may open on the anterior wall of the vagina (this being the female equivalent of hypospadias in the male).

**Hermaphroditism**

1. Abnormal development of gonads and genitalia gives rise to various types of hermaphroditism, in which there is a mixture of male and female characters.
2. A person in whom both testis and ovary are present is a ***true hermaphrodite***.
3. In contrast a ***pseudohermaphrodite*** is one in whom the external genitalia resemble those of one sex, whereas the gonad is of the opposite sex.

## ANAL TRIANGLE AND ISCHIORECTAL FOSSA

1. To understand the arrangement of structures in the anal triangle, it is essential to have a clear picture of two muscles present in relation to the true pelvis. One of these is the ***obturator internus*** studied in the lower limb. The second muscle is the ***levator ani***.
2. The lateral wall of the true pelvis is lined by the obturator internus muscle (40.21).
3. The levator ani takes origin from the fascia covering the obturator internus, and runs downwards and medially towards the midline.
4. The levator ani muscles of the right and left sides meet in the midline and form the ***pelvic diaphragm***.
5. This diaphragm cuts off the cavity of the true pelvis from the exterior.
6. The perineum is the region lying inferior to the pelvic diaphragm.
7. The part of the obturator internus lying inferior to the origin of the levator ani comes into direct relationship with some structures in the perineum.
8. The obturator internus is lined by a thick ***obturator fascia***.
9. The inferior surface of the levator ani is lined by fascia that is a part of the pelvic fascia.

### Anal Triangle

1. The anal canal passes through the anal triangle to reach the exterior.
2. The anal canal is surrounded by a number of sphincters. When the anal triangle is dissected, we see that the anal canal is surrounded by prominent muscle fibres of the external anal sphincter (***sphincter ani externus***).
3. Immediately anterior to the anal canal, there is the perineal body (see below). Posteriorly, the anal canal is connected to the coccyx by the ***anococcygeal ligament***.
4. On either side of the anal canal, there is a triangular space called the ***ischiorectal fossa*** described as follows.

### Ischiorectal Fossa

1. The ischiorectal fossa is a space between the obturator internus and the levator ani (26.19).
2. The ischiorectal fossa is a wedge shaped space. Its ***base*** (situated inferiorly) is formed by skin overlying the fossa.
3. Its ***medial wall*** is formed, in its upper part, by fascia lining the inferior surface of the levator ani (inferior fascia of the pelvic diaphragm). Lower down the medial wall is formed by the sphincter ani externus.
4. The ***lateral wall*** of the fossa is formed by the ischial tuberosity and by the fascia covering the obturator internus below the level of the origin of the levator ani. The apex of the fossa lies where the levator ani and the obturator internus meet.
5. The ***posterior boundary*** of the fossa is formed by the gluteus maximus muscle (superficially) and by the sacrotuberous ligament (more deeply).
6. ***Anteriorly***, the space is bounded by the posterior edge of the urogenital diaphragm.
7. In addition to the inferior fascia of the pelvic diaphragm and the obturator fascia the walls of the ischiorectal fossa are lined by another fascia called the ***lunate fascia.*** The lunate fascia is really the deep fascia of the region that is pushed into the fossa by the thick pad of fat that fills the fossa.
8. The ischiorectal fossa is often the site of infection.

### Pudendal Canal

1. On the lateral wall of the ischiorecatal fossa, we see the pudendal canal (26.19).
2. The canal is bounded laterally by obturator fascia, and medially by the lunate fascia.
   a. The canal begins posteriorly, near the lesser sciatic foramen.
   b. It ends anteriorly, near the posterior margin of the urogenital diaphragm (26.18).
   c. Inferiorly the canal comes into relationship with the falciform process of the sacrotuberous ligament.
3. The contents of the canal are as follows:
   a. The internal pudendal artery (see below).
   b. The pudendal nerve runs forwards in the canal and divides within it into the dorsal nerve of the penis and the perineal nerve.

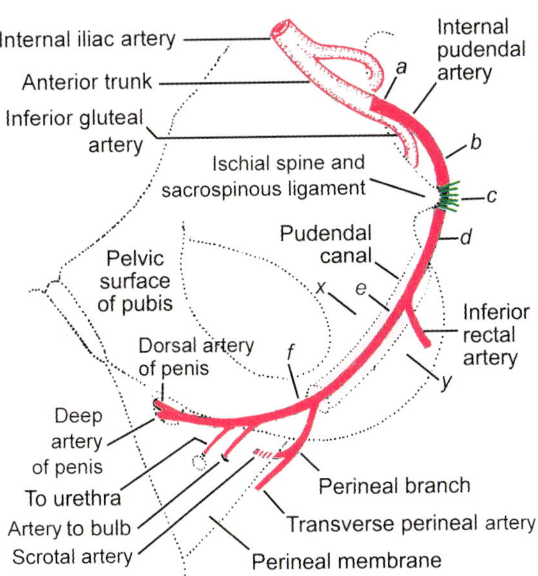


**26.18:** Scheme to show course and branches of the internal pudendal artery

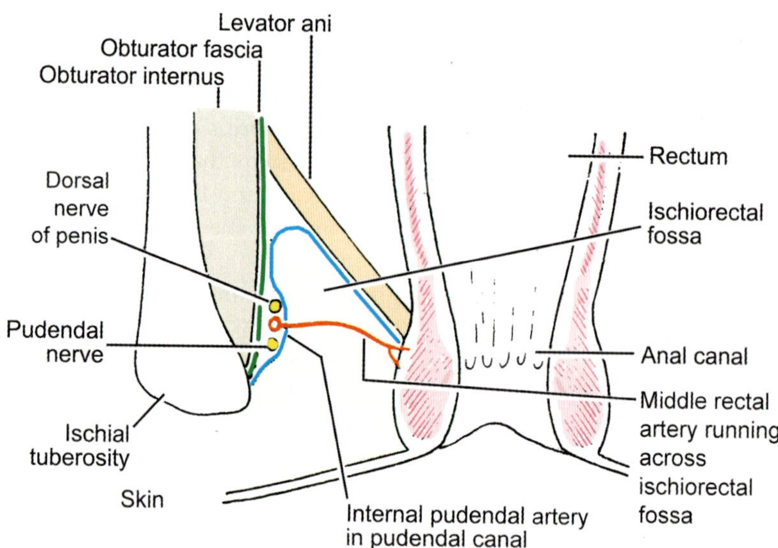


**26.19:** Section through the ischiorectal fossa and the pudendal canal in plane xy shown in 26.18

c. The main trunk of the pudendal nerve and the dorsal nerve of the penis lie above the internal pudendal artery. The perineal branch lies belows the artery.
d. The medial wall of the pudendal canal is pierced by the inferior rectal artery and nerve that run medially through the ischiorectal fossa.

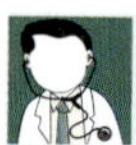

## CLINICAL CORRELATION

**Ischiorectal Fossa**

The boundaries of the ischiorectal fossa have been described above.

1. The fossa can be the site of an abscess.
2. The region is particularly vulnerable to infection because of the presence of poorly vascularised fat in the fossa.
3. Infections can reach the fossa from the anal canal.
4. They can also reach it from overlying skin of the perineum and, occasionally, by downward rupture of a pelvirectal abscess (through the levator ani).
5. The right and left ischiorectal fossae communicate with each other posterior to the anal canal, and infection can pass from one fossa to the other.
6. Bursting of an ischiorectal abscess on to the perineal skin results in a sinus. If the abscess also bursts into the anal canal an anal fistula (ischiorectal type) is produced.

***Hiatus of Schwalbe and Ischiorectal Hernia***

1. The ***hiatus of Schwalbe*** is a gap that may exist between the obturator fascia and the origin of the levator ani from it (i.e., in relation to the upper end of the ischiorectal fossa).
2. Herniation of some pelvic contents can take place through the gap constituting an ***ischiorectal hernia***.

### *The Perineal Body*

1. The perineal body (or central tendon of the perineum) is a fibromuscular body placed in the median plane at the junction of the anal and urogenital triangles.

2. Through the muscles attached to it can help to maintain the rectum and vagina in position.
3. Damage to it during child-birth can weaken the perineum and may lead to prolapse of pelvic organs.

## VESSELS OF THE PERINEUM

The arteries to be seen in the perineum are the superficial and deep external pudendal branches of the femoral artery and various branches from the internal pudendal artery that is described below.

### Internal Pudendal Artery

1. The internal pudendal artery supplies the external genitalia. It follows a complicated course.
2. Starting within the pelvic cavity ('a' in 26.18) the artery passes out of it through the greater sciatic foramen to enter the gluteal region ('b').
3. Here, it lies inferior to the piriformis muscle. It descends across the back of the ischial spine ('c') and leaves the gluteal region through the lesser sciatic foramen ('d').
4. It now comes to lie in the lateral wall of the ischiorectal fossa ('e'), within the pudendal canal. At the anterior end of this canal it reaches the posterior end of the deep perineal space ('f').
5. It runs forwards in the deep perineal space lying above the inferior fascia of the urogenital diaphragm (or perineal membrane).
6. Its terminal part pierces this fascia to enter the superficial perineal space.

#### *The Branches of the Artery are as Follows*

1. The ***inferior rectal*** artery is given off while the internal pudendal artery is in the pudendal canal. This branch runs medially through the ischiorectal fossa to supply the anal canal (26.18 and 26.19).
2. The ***perineal*** branch arises near the anterior end of the pudendal canal (26.18 and 26.19). It runs forwards into the superficial perineal space (i.e., below the inferior fascia of the urogenital diaphragm).
   a. It gives off ***scrotal*** branches to the scrotum (or labial branches in the female).
   b. A ***transverse perineal*** branch that runs medially along the superficial transverse perinei muscle.
3. The remaining branches are given off by the internal pudendal artery as it lies in the deep perineal space (26.20).
   a. It gives a branch to the bulb of the penis (26.18 and 26.19).
   b. Another to the urethra.
   c. Finally, it divides into the deep and dorsal arteries of the penis that pass through the inferior layer of the urogenital diaphragm to enter the superficial perineal space.

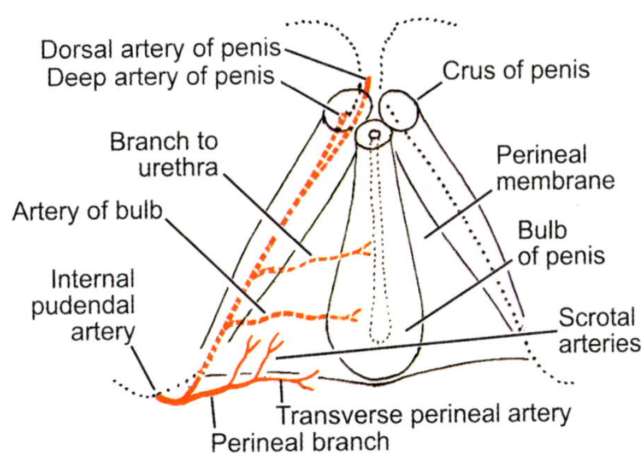


**26.20:** Terminal part of internal pudendal artery as seen in the male perineum (viewed from below). Compare with 26.18

4. The deep artery of the penis enters the corresponding crus of the penis, and runs forwards in the centre of the crus.
5. The dorsal artery reaches the dorsum of the penis, and runs forwards in this situation up to the glans penis.

## NERVES OF THE PERINEUM

The nerves seen in the perineum that have already been described are:

1. The ilioinguinal nerve (page 162, 182).
2. The genitofemoral nerve (page 163, 182).
3. The perineal branch of the posterior cutaneous nerve of the thigh (page 163, 195).
4. The main nerve of the region is the pudendal nerve that is described below.

### The Pudendal Nerve

1. The pudendal nerve arises from the sacral plexus and derives its fibres from spinal nerves S2, S3 and S4.
2. The nerve passes from the pelvis to the gluteal region through the greater sciatic foramen. Within the foramen the nerve lies below the piriformis muscle.
3. The nerve has a short course through the gluteal region.
   a. Emerging at the lower border of the piriformis it crosses the sacrospinous ligament and disappears into the lesser sciatic foramen.
   b. Here the nerve lies medial to the internal pudendal vessels.
4. The nerve now enters the pudendal canal (26.21) in the lateral wall of the ischiorectal fossa (26.19).
5. It ends within the canal by dividing into:
   a. The perineal nerve
   b. The dorsal nerve of the penis (or of the clitoris).
6. The branches and distribution of the pudendal nerve are as follows:

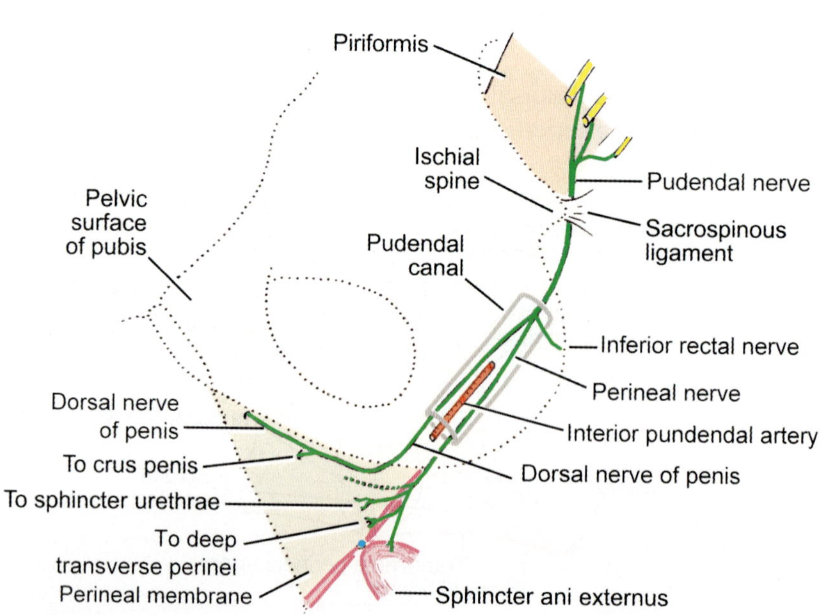


**26.21:** Scheme to show the course and distribution of the pudendal nerve

### Sensory Branches

1. The ***inferior rectal nerve*** arises from the pudendal nerve before the latter divides into its terminal branches.
   a. This branch passes medially through the ischiorectal fossa (accompanied by the inferior rectal artery (26.19).
   b. It supplies the skin lining the lower part of the anal canal and that around the anus.
2. The ***perineal nerve*** is a terminal branch of the pudendal nerve.
   a. In the pudendal canal it lies below the internal pudendal vessels.
   b. At the anterior end of the canal, it divides into posterior scrotal (or posterior labial) branches and into muscular branches (see below).
   c. The posterior scrotal branches are distributed to the skin of the scrotum. In the female, the scrotal branches are replaced by the posterior labial branches that supply the labium majus (and possibly the lower part of the vagina).
   d. Some fibres of the perineal nerve reach the mucous membrane of the urethra through the nerve to the bulbospongiosus (see below).
3. The ***dorsal nerve of the penis*** is the other terminal branch of the pudendal nerve.
   a. It passes forwards through the pudendal canal lying above the internal pudendal vessels.
   b. At the anterior end of the canal, the nerve enters the deep perineal space. Here, it gives off a branch to the crus penis (26.21).
   c. After passing through the deep perineal space the nerve reaches the dorsum of the penis, and ends by supplying the glans penis.
   d. In the female, the nerve is replaced by the much smaller dorsal nerve of the clitoris.

### Muscular Branches

1. The inferior rectal branch supplies the sphincter ani externus.
2. The muscular branches arising from the perineal nerve supply:
   a. The anterior part of the superficial transverse perinei ('a' in 26.22)
   b. The deep transverse perinei (26.21)
   c. The bulbospongiosus
   d. The ischiocavernosus
   e. The sphincter urethrae (26.21)
   f. They also supply the anterior parts of the sphincter ani externus ('b' in 26.22)
   g. The levator ani.

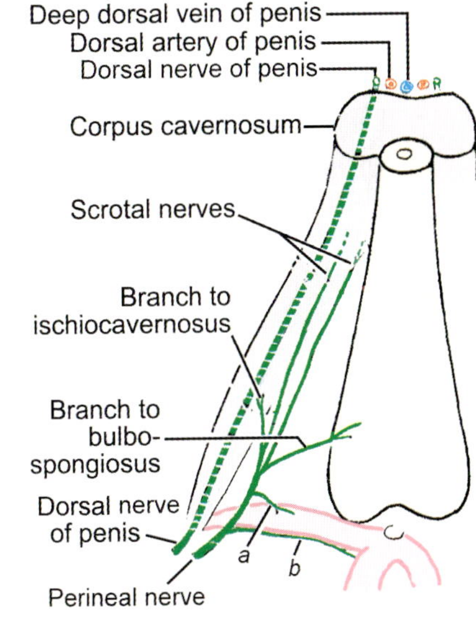


**26.22:** Branches of the perineal nerve as seen in the male perineum

## Perineal Membrane

In the preceding sections numerous references have been made to the perineal membrane, also called the inferior fascia of the urogenital diaphragm. Some facts about it may be summarised here.

1. It is a triangular membrane. Its apex is directed anteriorly and base posteriorly.
2. On each side it is attached to the corresponding ischiopubic ramus.
3. Its posterior edge is attached, in the midline to the perineal body.
   a. The border is fused to the superior fascia of the urogenital diaphragm.
   b. It is also fused to the membranous layer of superficial fascia.
4. Its anterior end or apex lies a short distance behind the pubic symphysis.
   a. Here again, the membrane is fused to the superior fascia of the urogenital diaphragm to form a thickened band called the ***transverse perineal ligament***.
   b. A small gap is present between this ligament and the ***arcuate pubic ligament*** that covers the inferior aspect of the pubic symphysis.

5. a. Posteriorly, near its lateral ends, the deep perineal space is confluent with the anterior end of the pudendal canal.
   b. The internal pudendal artery, the dorsal nerve of the penis and the perineal nerve therefore pass directly into the deep perineal space.
   c. However, their branches meant for the superficial perineal space have to pierce the perineal membrane to reach that space.
6. There are numerous apertures in the perineal membrane as follows.

### *Apertures in the Perineal Membrane*

1. The central part of the membrane is pierced by
   a. The urethra
   b. In the female, the vagina pierces the membrane posterior to the aperture for the urethra
   c. In the male, the bulbourethral glands lie in the deep perineal space. Their ducts pierce the perineal membrane lateral to the aperture for the urethra.
2. Along its posterior margin the membrane is pierced by scrotal (or labial) nerves and vessels.
3. In 26.23 note that the internal pudendal artery runs forwards along the lateral margin of the membrane, on its deep aspect. Note the apertures for the following branches of this artery:
   a. Artery to the bulb
   b. Artery to the ureter
   c. Deep artery of the penis
   d. The dorsal artery of the penis.
4. The apertures for branches of nerves are as follows:
   a. The perineal nerve and its scrotal branches enter the superficial perineal space by piercing the perineal membrane near its posterior edge.
   b. The dorsal nerve of the penis runs along the lateral edge of the membrane and gives off branches for the bulb, and a branch for the crus of the penis.
   c. The dorsal nerve of the penis itself reaches the dorsum of the penis by passing through the space between the transverse perineal ligament and the arcuate pubic ligament.
5. The deep dorsal vein of the penis also passes through this gap.

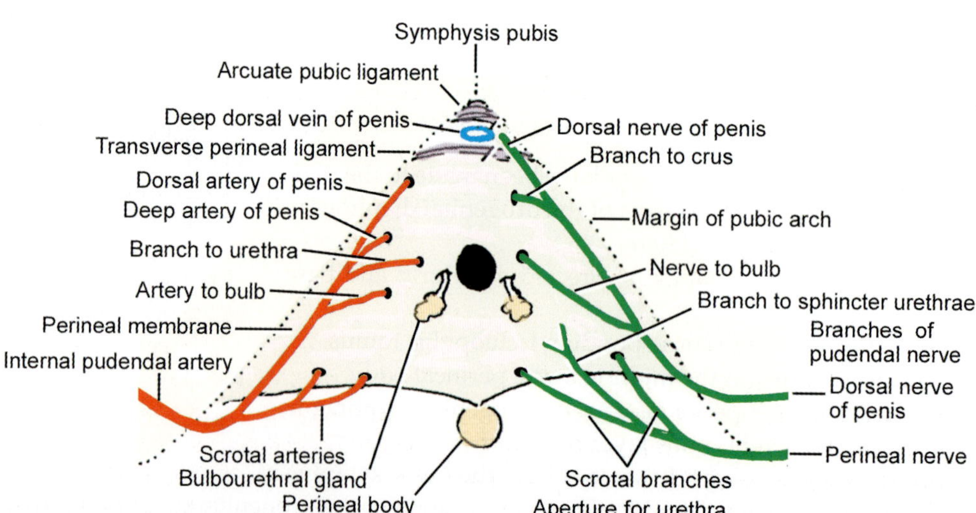


**26.23:** Perineal membrane viewed from behind and above to show apertures in it. The left half of the drawing shows related arteries; and the right half shows related nerves, and apertures for them

27

CHAPTER

# Oesophagus, Stomach and Intestines

## ABDOMINAL PART OF OESOPHAGUS

1. The orifice in the diaphragm through which the oesophagus enters the abdomen is located at the level of the $10^{th}$ thoracic vertebra, slightly to the left of the median plane.
2. The orifice has muscular walls formed by fibres of the right crus of the diaphragm.
3. From the orifice, the oesophagus passes downwards and to the left to end (at the level of the eleventh thoracic vertebra) by joining the cardiac end of the stomach.
4. Some relations of the abdominal part of the oesophagus are shown in 27.1. The relations will be better understood after the liver and the peritoneum have been studied.

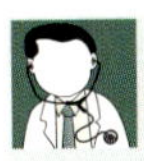

### CLINICAL CORRELATION

#### Abdominal Part of Oesophagus

1.a. Histological studies of the oesophago-cardiac junction have failed to reveal the presence of an anatomical sphincter.

b. However, the musculature here acts as a physiological sphincter that normally keeps the cardiac orifice closed, but relaxes to allow passage of swallowed food.

c. In some persons failure of the sphincter to relax leads to dysphagia (difficulty in passage of food leading to discomfort). The defect is believed to be a functional one and is referred to as ***achalasia cardia*** (achalasia = failure to relax).

2.a. Normally, acid in the stomach does not regurgitate into the oesophagus.

b. However, in some cases such regurgitation occurs and results in inflammation of the oesophagus (***oesophagitis***), and formation of ulcers.

c. This could be a factor explaining the frequent occurrence of cancer at the lower end of the oesophagus.

3. See hiatus hernia (Chapter 18).

4. See oesophageal varices (Chapter 22).

## THE STOMACH

1. The stomach is a sac-like structure that serves as a reservoir of swallowed food, and plays an important part in digesting it. It has a capacity of about one litre. It is the most dilated part of the alimentary canal.
2. Its shape varies considerably depending upon whether it is full or empty; and is also influenced by posture. However, for purposes of description we can presume it to have the form shown in 27.2.
3. The cranial end of the stomach is continuous with the oesophagus. As this end lies close to the heart it is named the ***cardiac end***.
4. The caudal end of the stomach is continuous with the duodenum. This end is called the ***pyloric end***, or simply the ***pylorus***. (The word pylorus is derived from a Greek word meaning 'gate keeper').

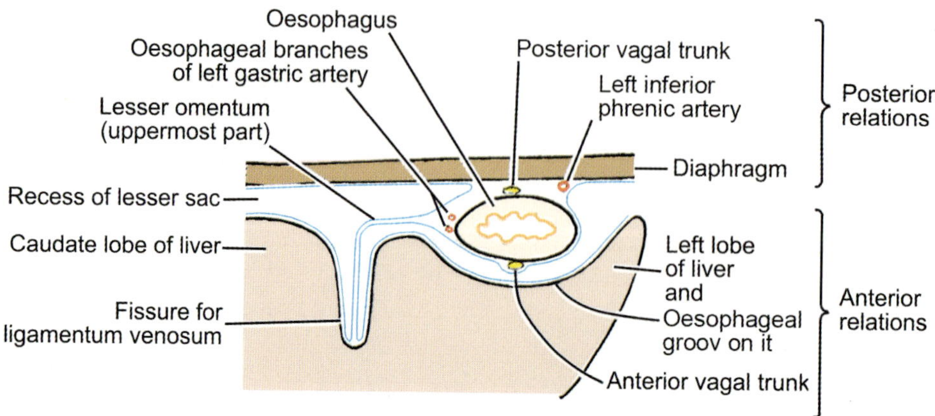


**27.1:** Schematic transverse section through the abdominal part of the oesophagus to show some related structures

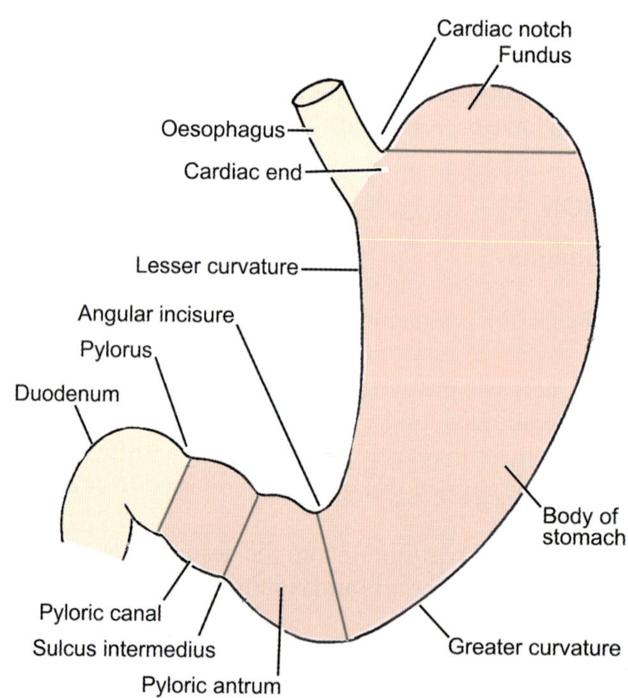


**27.2:** Subdivisions of the stomach

5. The stomach has two surfaces, anterior and posterior (or more strictly anterosuperior and posteroinferior). These surfaces meet at a concave upper border, and at a lower border that is convex.
6. The concave upper border is called the ***lesser curvature***, and the convex lower border is called the ***greater curvature***. In 27.2 note that the lesser curvature faces to the right in its upper part, and upwards in its lower part.
7. Proceeding from the cardiac end to the pyloric end the convexity of the greater curvature has a part facing upwards, then a part facing the left side, and finally a part facing downwards.
8. The stomach is lined by peritoneum on both its surfaces. At the lesser curvature, the layers of peritoneum lining the anterior and posterior surfaces meet and become continuous with the ***lesser omentum*** (33.29). At the greater

curvature the anterior and posterior layers of peritoneum become continuous with the ***gastrosplenic ligament*** (33.29), and with the ***greater omentum*** (33.31).

9. The stomach is divided into a number of parts as follows (27.2):
   a. At the junction of the left margin of the oesophagus with the greater curvature of the stomach, there is a deep ***cardiac notch***. Because of the upward convexity of the adjoining part of the greater curvature a part of the stomach lies above the level of the cardio-oesophageal junction. This part of the stomach is called the ***fundus***.
   b. We have seen that the upper part of the lesser curvature faces to the right, while its lower part faces upwards. The junction of these parts of the curvature is often marked by a notch called the ***angular incisure***. The part of the stomach to the left of the incisure is more or less rounded and is called the body (excluding the part already defined as the fundus).
   c. The part of the stomach to the right of the angular incisure is the ***pyloric part***. It consists of a relatively dilated left part (continuous with the body) called the ***pyloric antrum;*** and a narrower right part called the ***pyloric canal***. The greater curvature may show slight bulgings corresponding to the pyloric antrum and canal. These bulgings may be separated by a notch called the ***sulcus intermedius.*** The position of the pylorus (or pyloric orifice) is indicated on the surface by a groove that marks the junction of the stomach with the duodenum.
10. The position of the stomach relative to the surface of the body is shown in 27.3.
   a. The cardiac end (or orifice) is situated to the left of the median plane, behind the left seventh costal cartilage, 2.5 cm (one inch) from the midline. This point lies at the level of the eleventh thoracic vertebra.
   b. The pylorus (or pyloric orifice) lies about 1 cm (half inch) to the right of the midline, at the level of the transpyloric plane. (This explains the name transpyloric given to this plane). We have seen that this plane lies at the level of the lower part of the first lumbar vertebra.
   c. However, when the stomach is full the pylorus may move downwards to the level of the second lumbar vertebra, or even the third vertebra.
   d. The highest part of the stomach is the fundus. It reaches the left fifth intercostal space, just below the nipple.
   e. The greater curvature cuts the costal margin at the level of the tenth costal cartilage.
   f. The lowest part of the stomach is formed by the pyloric antrum. In the full stomach, it may lie below the level of the umbilicus.
   g. From 27.3 note that parts of the stomach extend into the epigastrium, the umbilical region, the left hypochondrium and the left lumbar region.

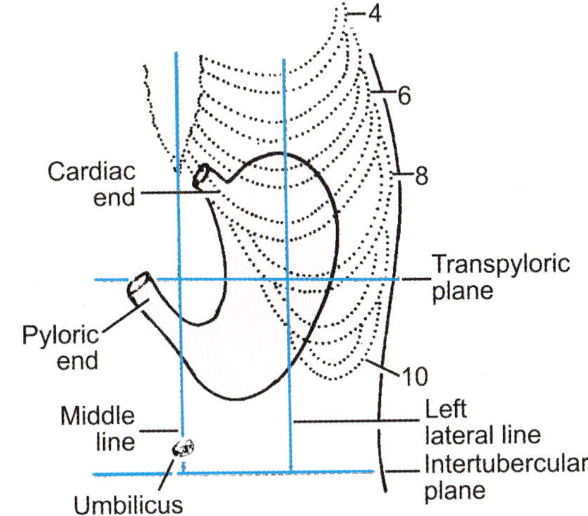


**27.3:** Surface projection of the stomach

11. The shape of the stomach can be studied in the living by taking skiagrams after giving a meal containing barium sulphate (***barium meal***).
   a. Commonly, the stomach is J-shaped having a long vertical part (above and to the left) and a shorter horizontal part (below and to the right) (27.4B).
   b. Sometimes, the stomach may be orientated almost transversely. This is described as a ***steer-horn*** type of stomach (27.4A).
   c. Various forms intermediate between these two types may be seen (27.2).

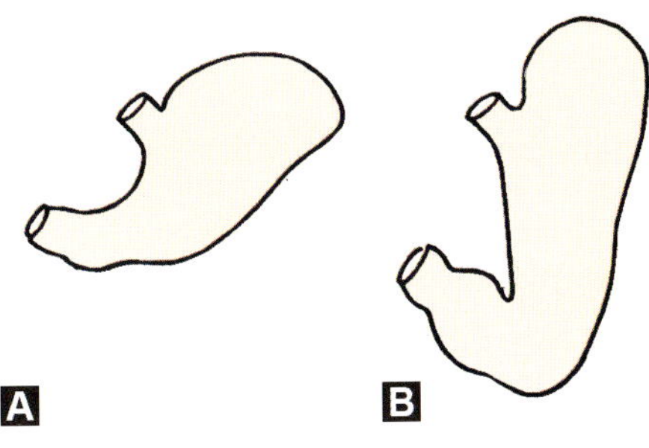


**27.4A and B:** (A) Steer-horn stomach; (B) J-shaped stomach

## WANT TO KNOW MORE?

### Relations of the Stomach

*Anterior Surface*

1. From 27.5 it will be seen that a considerable part of the stomach lies above the costal margin (Also see 27.3). Most of this part of the anterior surface is in contact with the diaphragm that separates the stomach from the left pleura and lung.
2. Part of the anterior surface of the stomach is in contact with the liver, and part of it with the anterior abdominal wall.
3. The extreme left part of what is called the anterior surface really faces backwards and to the left. This part comes into contact with the spleen.

*Posterior Surface*

1. The posterior surface of the stomach is separated by the cavity of the lesser sac from several structures lying on the posterior abdominal wall. These structures are described collectively as forming the ***stomach bed***.
2. They include:
   a. The posterior part of the diaphragm
   b. The left kidney
   c. The left suprarenal gland
   d. The pancreas
   e. The left colic flexure and the transverse mesocolon (27.6)
   f. The spleen (which we have seen is related to the anterior surface) is often included amongst the structures forming the surface bed.

### Vessels and Nerves Supplying the Stomach

All the arteries supplying the stomach are derived from the coeliac trunk or one of its branches (29.3).

1. Along the lesser curvature (within the 2 layers of the lesser omentum), there are the right and left gastric arteries. The left gastric artery is a direct branch of the coeliac trunk. The right gastric artery is a branch of the gastroduodenal artery.
2. Along the greater curvature (between the 2 layers of the greater omentum), there are the right and left gastroepiploic arteries. The right gastroepiploic artery arises from the common hepatic artery, while the left gastroepiploic artery is a branch of the splenic artery.
3. The stomach also receives short gastric arteries which are branches of the splenic artery.
4. The veins from the stomach drain into the splenic and superior mesenteric veins. This blood passes through the portal vein to the liver. In other words, the veins of the stomach form part of the portal venous system.
5. Lymph vessels from different parts of the stomach drain in different directions and reach the following nodes:
   a. Pancreaticosplenic nodes lying along splenic artery.
   b. Left gastric notes lying along left gastric artery.
   c. Right gastroepiploic nodes along artery of same name.
   d. Pyloric nodes in angle between first and second parts of duodenum.
   e. Hepatic nodes along hepatic artery.

   Lymph from all these nodes ultimately reaches the coeliac nodes (around coeliac trunk). For details see Chapter 34.
6. The nerves supplying the stomach are sympathetic and parasympathetic. The sympathetic nerves are derived from the coeliac plexus and run along the arteries. Some direct splanchnic branches also reach the stomach from the sympathetic trunk. The parasympathetic nerves are derived from the vagus nerves. For details of nerve supply see Chapter 34.

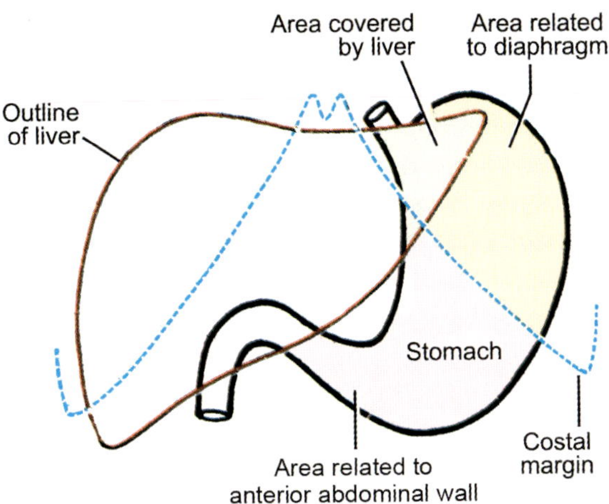


**27.5:** Scheme to show the chief structures in contact with the anterior surface of the stomach

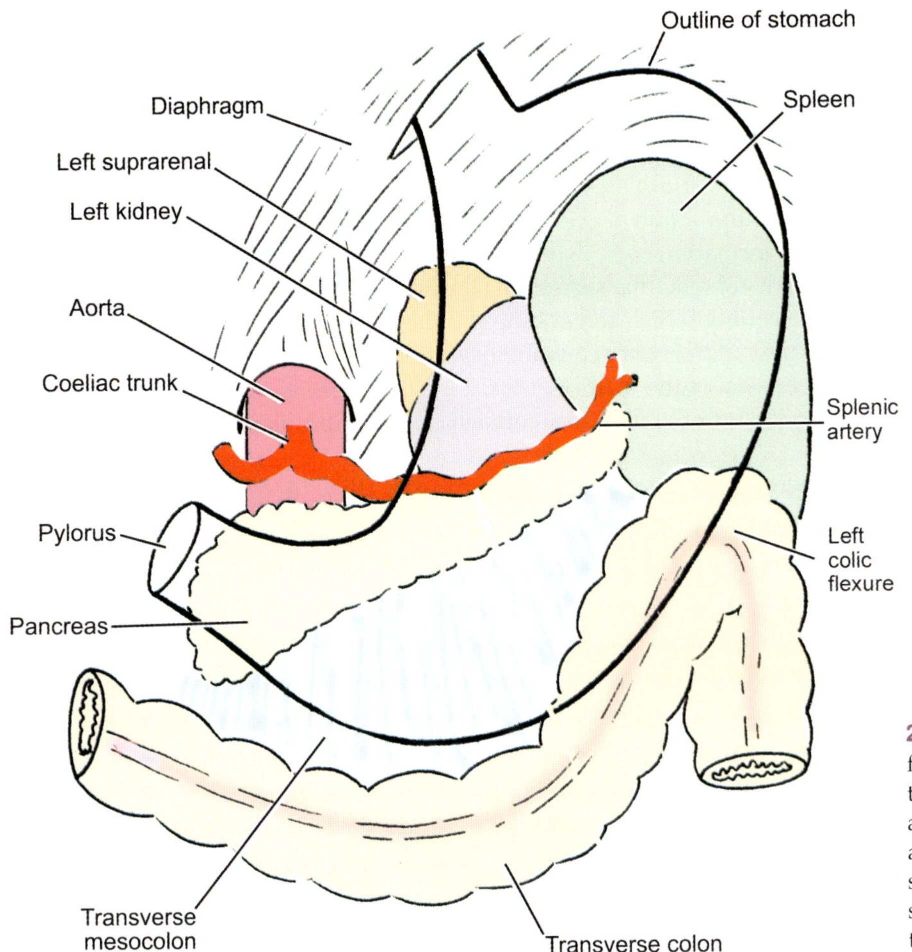


**27.6:** Scheme to show the structures forming the stomach bed. Note that the spleen is separated from the stomach by the gastrosplenic ligament, and is really related to the 'anterior' surface. The remaining structures are separated from the posterior surface of the stomach by the lesser sac

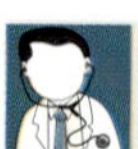

## CLINICAL CORRELATION

### Stomach

1. The Greek word for stomach is *gaster*. From this, we have the adjectives gastric and gastroa that are used in relation to the stomach. Inflammation of the stomach is ***gastritis***. An instrument that is used to visualise the interior of the stomach is a ***gastroscope***, and the procedure is called ***gastroscopy***.
2. Gastric pain is referred to the epigastrium. It is produced by spasm of muscle, or by overdistension of the organ. Irritation of gastric mucosa in gastritis can cause abdominal discomfort, nausea and vomiting.

*Sphincters of Stomach*

1. See ***achylasia cardia*** under oesophagus.
2. The condition called ***congenital pyloric stenosis*** is a developmental anomaly.
   a. There is great thickening of muscle at the pyloric end of the stomach.
   b. The thickening of muscle extends into the pyloric antrum as well.
   c. The condition appears to be genetically determined and is much more common in male infants.
   d. It can be successfully treated by surgically incising the thickened mass of muscle longitudinally. The incision is carried into the entire thickness of the muscle without damaging the mucosa.

*Gastric Ulcer*

1. The term peptic ulcer is applied to ulcers in the stomach, in the duodenum, and in unusual sites like Meckel's diverticulum. To avoid confusion, it is better to refer to ulcers in the stomach as gastric ulcers.
2. a. From a functional point of view the mucosa of the stomach can be divided into an acid secreting proximal part (consisting of the fundus and greater part of the body); and a distal area (pyloric antrum and pyloric canal) the secretions of which are rich in mucous and are mildly alkaline.
   b. The distal region also secretes gastrin which stimulates acid secretion by the proximal part.
3. a. The normal gastric mucosa is resistant to the action of acid present in the stomach. However, in some cases, the mucosa gets eroded leading to the formation of a gastric ulcer.
   b. Such ulcers are usually formed in the distal (alkaline secretion producing) area, near the lesser curvature.
4. An ulcer can be a source of pain, and of bleeding which can at times be serious.
5. As the ulcer erodes further into the thickness of the stomach wall, it can result in adhesion of the stomach wall to surrounding structures, or to perforation of the wall.
6. a. Perforation of an ulcer located on the posterior wall of the stomach can lead to leakage of contents into the lesser sac.
   b. It can also lead to erosion of the pancreas, and even of the splenic artery (the latter leading to fatal haemorrhage).
7. a. Perforation of an ulcer on the anterior wall of the stomach can lead to escape of gastric contents into the greater sac.
   b. Such an ulcer can adhere to and involve the liver substance. Patients of gastric ulcer are treated by drugs that block acid secretion. In some cases, a ***partial gastrectomy*** (removing the distal gastrin producing part) can cure an ulcer.

*Gastric Carcinoma*

1. The stomach is a frequent site of carcinoma.
   a. The cancer cells can spread through lymphatics.
   b. Surgical treatment involves removal of the entire stomach (***total gastrectomy***).
   c. The lower end of the oesophagus and the first part of the duodenum are also removed.
2. a. In an effort to remove the lymph nodes involved the surgeon may also remove:
   i. The spleen (along with the gastrosplenic and lienorenal ligaments).
   ii. The greater omentum.

iii. Part of the pancreas.
iv. The splenic vessels.

2. b. Continuity of the gut is established by anastomosing the oesophagus with the jejunum.
3. In cases of suspected gastric ulcer or carcinoma, the interior of the stomach can be viewed through a gastroscope. Biopsies can also be taken through the instrument.
4. Radiologically, the gastric mucosa can be studied by taking skiagrams after a barium meal.

## THE SMALL INTESTINE

The small intestine is a tube about five metres long. It is divided into three parts. These are (in cranio-caudal sequence): the ***duodenum,*** the ***jejunum*** and the ***ileum.***

### The Duodenum

1. The duodenum forms the first 25 cm (10 inches) of the small intestine. It is in the form of a roughly C-shaped loop which is retroperitoneal and, therefore, fixed to the posterior abdominal wall.
2. It is continuous at its cranial end with the stomach. The junction between the two is called the ***pyloroduodenal junction***. At its caudal end, the duodenum becomes continuous with the jejunum at the ***duodenojejunal flexure***.
3. The duodenum is subdivided into four parts as follows (27.7):
   a. The ***first or superior part*** begins at the pylorus and passes backwards, upwards and to the right. It is about 5 cm long.
   b. The ***second or descending part*** is about 8 cm long. It passes downwards (with a slight convexity to the right).
   c. The ***third or horizontal part*** is about 10 cm long. It passes from right to left (with a slight downward convexity) and crosses the midline at the level of the third lumbar vertebra.
   d. The ***fourth or ascending part*** is about 2 cm long. It runs upwards and to the left and ends by joining the jejunum at the duodenojejunal flexure.
4. The junction of the superior and descending parts of the duodenum is called the ***superior duodenal flexure***; while that between the descending and horizontal part is called the ***inferior duodenal flexure***.

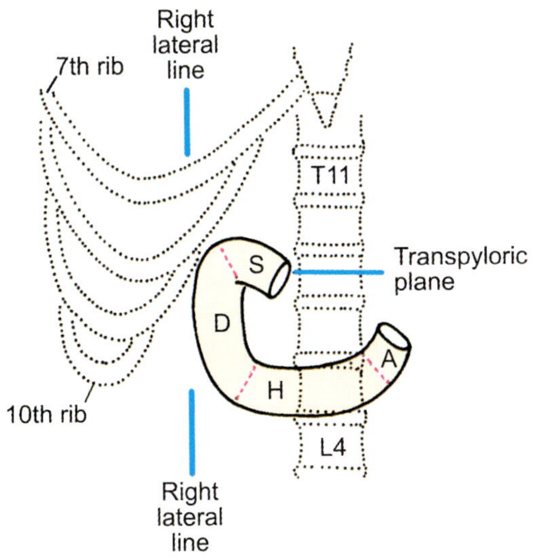


27.7: Parts of the duodenum and their surface projection.
S: Superior part; D: Descending part;
H: Horizontal part; A: Ascending part

## WANT TO KNOW MORE?

**Relations of the Duodenum**

***Superior (First) Part***

*Anteriorly*

1. Liver (quadrate lobe)
2. Gall bladder.

*Posteriorly*

1. Inferior vena cava, separated by a part of the lesser sac.
2. The bile duct, the portal vein and the gastroduodenal artery.

*Superiorly*

- Aditus to the lesser sac.

*Inferiorly*

- Pancreas (head and neck).

***Descending (Second) Part***

*Anteriorly*

1. Crossed by transverse colon and transverse mesocolon
2. Part above colon is overlapped by the liver
3. Part below the colon is overlapped by coils of jejunum.

*Posteriorly*

1. Medial margin of right kidney and right renal vessels.
2. Right edge of inferior vena cava
3. Right psoas major.

*Medially (or left)*

1. Pancreas
2. Bile duct
3. Pancreatic ducts.

*Laterally (or right)*

- Right colic flexure.

***Horizontal (Third) Part***

*Anteriorly*

1. Crossed by mesentery and superior mesenteric vessels.
2. Covered by transverse mesocolon, and sometimes by transverse colon, and/or loops of jejunum.

*Posteriorly*

1. Right psoas major
2. Inferior vena cava
3. Aorta
4. Right ureter
5. Right testicular or ovarian vessels
6. Inferior vena cava and aorta separate it from vertebra L3.

ABOVE: Pancreas.

BELOW: Coils of jejunum.

*Ascending (Fourth) Part*

*Anteriorly*

a. Transverse mesocolon
b. Transverse colon.

*Posteriorly*

Left psoas major separated by:
a. Left sympathetic trunk
b. Left renal and testicular vessels
c. Inferior mesenteric artery.

ABOVE: Pancreas
BELOW: Jejunum
RIGHT: Aorta
LEFT: Left kidney and ureter.

***Peritoneal Relations of Duodenum***

1. Most of the duodenum is retroperitoneal and is covered by peritoneum only on its anterior aspect.
2. The proximal portion of the superior part of the duodenum is however lined on both its anterior and posterior aspects by peritoneum (continuous with that on the anterior and posterior surfaces of the stomach).
3. The two layers lining the proximal part of the duodenum meet above to form the extreme right part of the lesser omentum. This part of the lesser omentum passes to the liver as the right free margin.
4. Immediately posterior to the right free margin of the lesser omentum we see the aditus to the lesser sac.
5. Peritoneum lining the posterior surface (of the proximal half) of the superior part of the duodenum is reflected onto the front of the pancreas. This reflection forms the right margin of the lesser sac in this position.

### *Features on Interior of Duodenum*

1. Like the rest of the small intestine the mucous membrane of the duodenum is marked by transverse folds.
2. In the posterolateral portion of the descending part, the mucous membrane also shows a prominent vertical fold. The lower part of this fold is marked by a projection called the ***major duodenal papilla***.
3. The papilla bears an opening of a common channel, the hepatopancreatic ampulla, into which the bile duct and the main pancreatic duct open.
4. A short distance cranial to, and in front of, the major duodenal papilla, there is a smaller projection called the ***minor duodenal papilla***. The minor papilla has an opening for the accessory pancreatic duct.

## WANT TO KNOW MORE?

**Vessels and Nerves of Duodenum**

1. In keeping with their development from the foregut, the superior part of the duodenum, and the upper portion of the descending part (cranial to the major duodenal papilla) are supplied by branches derived from the coeliac trunk (hepatic, right gastric, supraduodenal, right gastroepiploic and superior pancreaticoduodenal arteries).
2. The remaining part of the duodenum (caudal to the major duodenal papilla) is derived from the midgut. This part is supplied by the inferior pancreaticoduodenal branch of the superior mesenteric artery.
3. The veins of the duodenum end in the splenic and superior mesenteric veins. Some veins end directly in the portal vein.
4. The lymphatic drainage of the duodenum is into the ancreaticoduodenal nodes. From here lymph passes to the hepatic, coeliac and superior mesenteric nodes. For details see Chapter 34.
5. Like other parts of the gut, the duodenum receives sympathetic and parasympathetic nerve fibres.

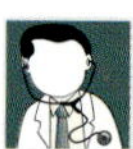

**CLINICAL CORRELATION**

**Duodenum**

*Duodenal Ulcers*

1. These frequently occur in the first part of the duodenum this being the part most exposed to acid entering from the stomach. (Note that both in the stomach and duodenum ulcers occur in alkaline secreting mucosa).
2. Perforation of an ulcer located on the anterior wall of the duodenum lead to leakage of intestinal contents into the greater sac of peritoneum.
3. The leaked fluid tends to gravitate to the right iliac fossa and can give rise to symptoms resembling those of acute appendicitis.
4. Ulcers on the posterior wall of the first part of the duodenum sometimes erode the gastroduodenal artery resulting in serious haemorrhage.

Note the following points as well:

1. a. The relations of the duodenum have been described above. These are very important for a surgeon operating on the region.
   b. Because of the close relationship of the gall bladder to the duodenum, gall stones sometimes erode right through the walls of these organs to enter the duodenum.
2. Internal hernias may take place into one of the peritoneal recesses related to the duodenum.
3. See congenital malformations described under intestines.

## THE JEJUNUM AND ILEUM

1. The jejunum and ileum are in the form of a long coiled tube suspended from the posterior abdominal wall by *the* mesentery.
2. The jejunum is proximal to the ileum. It is about two metres long, whereas the ileum is about three meters long. There is no hard and fast point of demarcation between the jejunum and ileum.
3. The jejunum and ileum are distinguished mainly on the basis of the structure of their walls.
   a. The mucous membrane of the jejunum is marked by the presence of numerous, large, transverse, folds. These are few or absent in the ileum.
   b. The submucosa of the ileum contains large aggregations of lymphoid tissue that can be seen with the naked eye and are called the ***aggregated lymphatic follicles*** or ***Peyer's patches***. There are no such patches in the proximal jejunum. The distal jejunum has some patches, but these are smaller and fewer than those in the ileum.
4. Because of the mobility of the jejunum and ileum, their relations are highly variable.
   a. The coils occupy the central and lower part of the abdominal cavity, in the interval between the ascending colon (on the right) and the descending colon (on the left).
   b. They are covered anteriorly by the greater omentum, the transverse colon and transverse mesocolon.
   c. On the whole the coils of jejunum lie above those of the ileum.
   d. The first coil of the jejunum lies in front of the left kidney, behind the transverse mesocolon.
   e. The terminal part of the ileum lies in the true pelvis. It passes to the right across the right psoas major to join the caecum.

### The Mesentery

1. The fold of peritoneum through which coils of jejunum and ileum are suspended from the posterior abdominal wall is called *the* mesentery.
2. The attachment of the mesentery to the posterior abdominal wall is referred to as the ***root*** of the mesentery (27.8). The root is about 15 cm long.

3. When traced towards the gut the mesentery increases very greatly in length so that it can give attachment to the entire length of the jejunum and ileum (which is about 5 m). This is why the mesentery is often described as fan-shaped.
4. a. The upper end of the root of the mesentery corresponds in position to that of the duodenojejunal flexure. It lies a little to the left of the median plane at the level of the second lumber vertebra.
   b. In relation to the anterior abdominal wall the upper end lies about 3 cm below and medial to the tip of the left ninth costal cartilage.
5. a. The attachment of the mesentery runs downwards and to the right, its lower end lying to the right of the median plane in front of the right sacroiliac joint.
   b. This point corresponds to the junction of the right lateral and intertubercular planes (27.8).

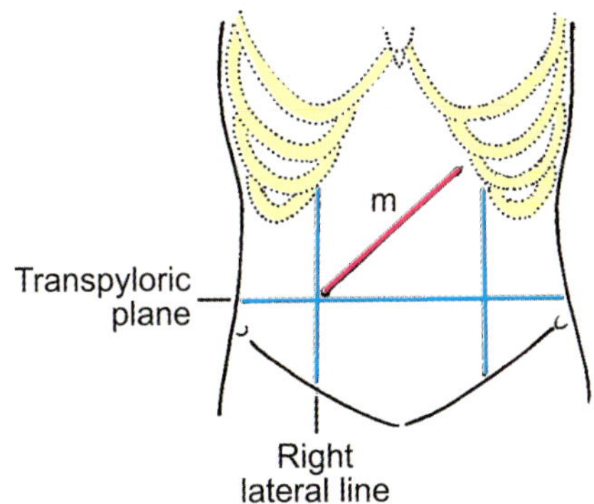

27.8: Attachment of root of mesentery (M) to posterior abdominal wall

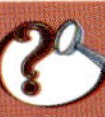

**WANT TO KNOW MORE?**

6. The attachment of the root of the mesentery crosses several structures on the posterior abdominal wall. These are:
   a. The horizontal part of the duodenum
   b. The abdominal aorta
   c. The inferior vena cava
   d. The psoas major
   e. The right ureter and the testicular (or ovarian) vessels cross behind the root as they descend over the psoas major.

*Vessels and Nerves of Jejunum and Ileum*

1. The jejunum and ileum are supplied by several branches arising from the superior mesenteric artery (Chapter 29). These branches travel to the gut through the mesentery.
2. As they do so they divide into smaller branches that anastomose with each other to form a series of ***arcades*** (27.9 A and B). The arcades are fewer (1 – 3) in the jejunum than in the ileum (5 – 6).
3. ***Straight arteries*** arising from the arcades reach the gut and supply it. The straight arteries are long in the case of the jejunum and short in the case of the ileum.
4. The intervals between the vessels (in the mesentery) are filled with fat. The layer of fat extends right up to the gut in the case of the ileum; but in the case of the jejunum empty spaces (often called windows) can be seen when the mesentery is held up against a source of light.
5. The veins from the jejunum and ileum end in the superior mesenteric vein (Chapter 29).
6. The lymphatic drainage of the jejunum and ileum is through nodes present in the mesentery along branches of the superior mesenteric artery and the ileocolic artery. Ultimate drainage is into superior mesenteric nodes.
7. See innervation of gut later in the text.

## THE LARGE INTESTINE

### Introductory Remarks about the Large Intestine

1. The large intestine is about one and a half metres long. The main subdivisions of the large intestine are shown in 27.11. These are the ***caecum***, the ***ascending colon***, the ***transverse colon***, the ***descending colon***, the ***sigmoid*** (***or pelvic***) ***colon***, the ***rectum*** and the ***anal canal***.

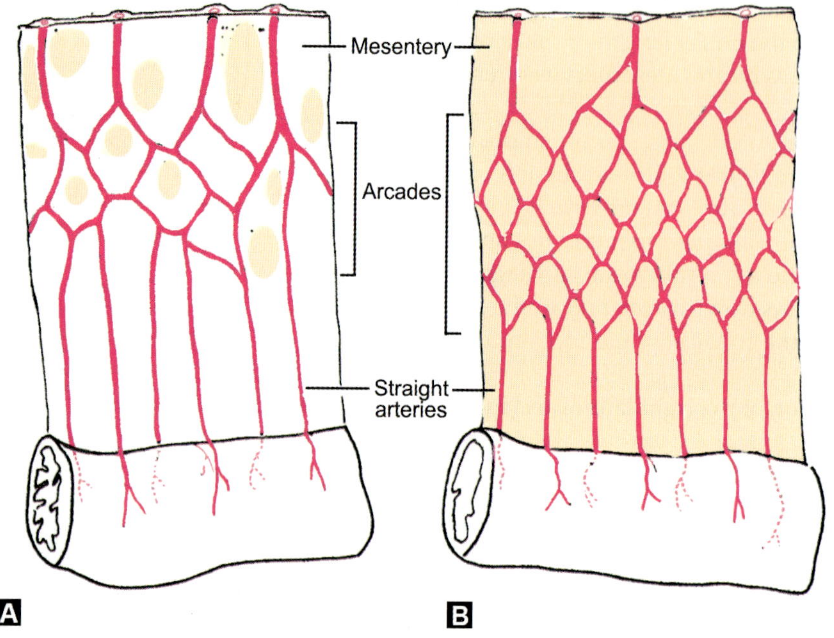


**27.9A and B:** Comparison of the pattern of the arteries supplying the jejunum (27.12A) and the ileum (27.12B). Note that the arcades are fewer, and the straight arteries longer, in the jejunum. Fat (yellow) is much more abundant in the mesentery of the ileum

Appendices epiploicae
*Taenia coli*
Sacculation

**27.10:** A segment of the colon

2. The large intestine forms a curve within which the small intestine lies. The terminal part of the ileum becomes continuous with the large intestine at the ***ileocaecal junction***.
3. Near this junction the caecum is also joined by a short, narrow, blind tube called the ***vermiform appendix***.
4. The ascending colon meets the transverse colon at the ***right colic flexure***. The junction of the transverse colon with the descending colon is called the ***left colic flexure***.
5. ***Peritoneal relations***
   a. The ascending colon, and the descending colon are retroperitoneal; they are covered by peritoneum on the front and sides, but posteriorly they are in direct contact with the abdominal wall.
   b. The transverse colon is suspended from the posterior abdominal wall by the transverse mesocolon; and the sigmoid colon by the sigmoid mesocolon.
   c. The caecum is usually surrounded all round by peritoneum and, therefore, has considerable mobility.
   d. Its posterior aspect of the caecum is separated from the posterior abdominal wall by a recess of the peritoneal cavity called the ***retrocaecal recess***. The vermiform appendix often lies in this recess.
   e. The rectum is partially covered by peritoneum, while the anal canal does not come in contact with peritoneum at all.
6. ***Differences between small and large intestine***

   The following differences enable a segment of the colon to be easily distinguished from a segment of small intestine.
   a. The colon is much wider than the small intestine. That is why it is called the 'large' intestine.
   b. The outer diameter of a segment of small intestine is more or less uniform. In contrast a segment of the colon shows a series of ***sacculations*** (also called ***haustrations***).
   c. In the case of the small intestine, the layer of longitudinal muscle is of uniform thickness all round its circumference.
      i. In the caecum and colon, however, the longitudinal muscle layer shows thickenings at three places on the circumference.

ii. These thickenings of muscle form three prominent bands that run along the length of the colon, approximately equidistant from each other.

iii. These bands are called the ***taenia coli***.

d. The taenia coli appear to be shorter than the rest of the wall of the colon. This may be one reason for presence of sacculations in the wall of the colon.

e. Attached to the outer wall of the colon there are numerous irregular projections called the ***appendices epiploicae***. Each of these consists of a small mass of fat enclosed by a covering of peritoneum.

## The Caecum

1. The terminal ileum joins the large intestine in the right iliac fossa. The part of the large intestine lying (here) below the level of the ileocaecal junction is called the caecum.
2. It is so called as its lower end is blind (caecum = blind recess).
3. Superiorly, the caecum is in open communication with the ascending colon.
4. The caecum is about 6 cm in height, and about 7.5 cm in width. (The width is greater than the length).
5. In relation to the anterior abdominal wall the caecum lies in a triangle bounded as follows:
   a. Above by the transtubercular plane.
   b. Medially by the right lateral line.
   c. Below (and laterally) by the inguinal ligament (27.11).
6. The ileocaecal junction lies at the intersection of the right lateral and transtubercular planes.
7. The vermiform appendix opens into the caecum about 2 cm below this point.

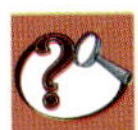

### WANT TO KNOW MORE?

***Relations of the Caecum***

The caecum is surrounded all round by peritoneum which separates it from the following structures.

1. In front of it there is the anterior abdominal wall.
2. Posteriorly, the vermiform appendix frequently lies in the retrocaecal recess.
   a. Behind this recess the caecum rests on the iliacus and the psoas major muscles.
   b. The lateral cutaneous nerve of the thigh intervenes between the iliacus and the caecum.

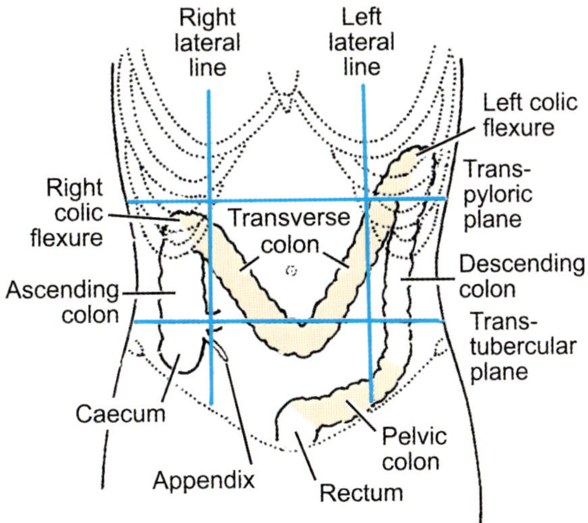


**27.11:** Surface projection of the large intestine. Note that the position of the transverse colon, and of the pelvic (sigmoid) colon is highly variable

### *Lymphatic Drainage of Caecum*

Lymph passes through ileocolic nodes to superior mesenteric nodes.

## The Ileocaecal Junction

Some features to be seen at the junction of the ileum and the large intestine are as follows:

1. Firstly, note that the ileum enters the posteromedial aspect of the large intestine. The junction marks the plane of demarcation between the caecum and the ascending colon.
2. A valvular or sphincteric function is often ascribed to the junction, although this is not supported by physiological evidence.

**WANT TO KNOW MORE?**

3. a. When viewed after opening the caecum (27.13) the junction presents a transverse slit bounded by upper and lower 'lips'.
   b. At the edges of the slit the lips fuse with each other and become continuous with folds of mucous membrane called the ***frenula.***
4. The wall of the ileum projects for some distance into the cavity of the large intestine. It is this projection that is responsible for the formation of prominent upper and lower 'lips' of the ileocaecal orifice.

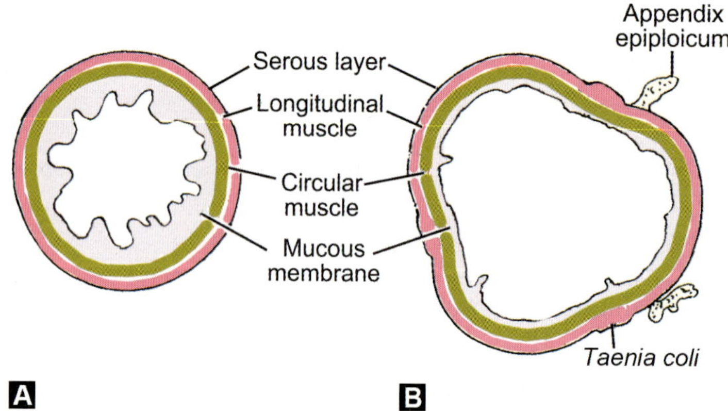


**27.12A and B:** Transverse sections through the (A) small intestine and (B) large intestine to show differences in basic structure

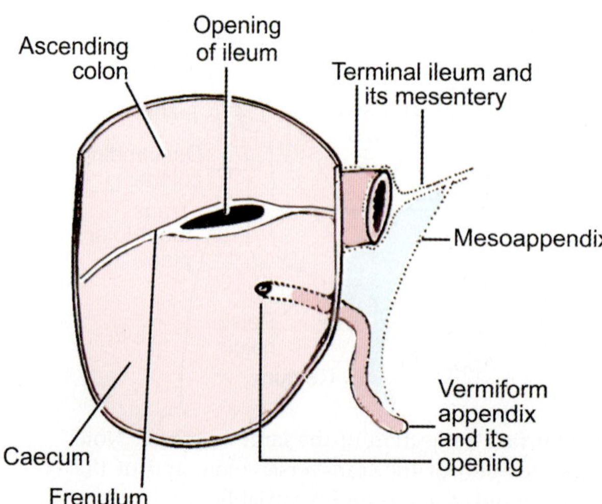


**27.13:** Some features in the interior of the caecum seen after opening it

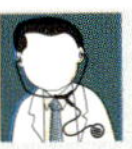

## CLINICAL CORRELATION

### Intestines

This section on clinical correlations of the gut applies to most parts of the gut. Additional correlations are given along with descriptions of some parts of the gut.

***Identification of Coils of Intestine Seen at Operation***

1. It is of vital importance for a surgeon to be able to correctly identify coils of intestine seen at operation. For this purpose, it is essential to know differences between the jejunum and ileum (page 544), and those between the small and large intestines (page 546).
2. It is also essential to be able to identify the proximal and distal ends of a loop of intestine. This can be done by tracing the mesentery to its attachment to the posterior abdominal wall to make sure that the mesentery is not twisted on itself. If there is no such twist the upper end of the loop is the proximal end.

**Congenital Malformations of the Gut**

Congenital malformations follow a common pattern throughout the length of the gut. Malformations of all parts of the gut are described here.

***Congenital Obstruction***

1. ***Atresia*** (non-continuity of lumen) or ***stenosis*** (narrowing of lumen) may occur anywhere along the length of the gut. Stenosis or atresia in the region of the rectum and anal canal gives rise to various kinds of ***imperforate anus***.
2. Obstruction can be caused by hypertrophy of muscle (as in ***congenital pyloric stenosis***).
3. Obstruction can also be caused by non-development of nerve plexuses over a length of the gut wall leading to interference with peristalsis and to passage of contents through the affected part.
   a. This has been observed most typically in the distal part of the colon.
   b. The part of the colon proximal to the defect becomes dilated with intestinal contents and becomes large.
   c. The condition is called ***megacolon*** or ***Hirschsprung's disease***.
   d. Surgical treatment of the condition involves resection of the aganglionic segment.
4. Obstruction to the gut can also be caused by external pressure from abnormal peritoneal bands, or blood vessels.
5. The duodenum can be obstructed by:
   a. The ***cystocolic band*** passing from the gall bladder to the transverse colon.
   b. By pressure of the superior mesenteric vessels.
   c. By an ***annular pancreas*** (which completely surrounds the duodenum).

***Fistulae***

1. Abnormal communications may be seen between the gut and other cavities near them.
2. They are most common in regions where the gut normally undergoes a process of septation.
3. Defects in the process of separation of the trachea from the oesophagus lead to various varieties of ***tracheo-oesophageal fistulae***.
4. Defects in septation of the cloaca lead to fistulae between:
   a. The rectum and urinary bladder (***rectovesical fistula***).
   b. The rectum and vagina (***rectovaginal fistula***).
5. Such fistulae can also be produced in later life by trauma caused during childbirth.

***Duplication***

A part of the gut may be duplicated. The duplicated part may form only a small cyst or may be of considerable length.

*Diverticulae*

These tend to arise most commonly in the duodenum near the major duodenal papilla. This region has a normal tendency to formation of outgrowths. The liver and biliary apparatus, and the pancreas are derived from buds arising in this region.

*Meckel's Diverticulum*

1. The embryonic gut is connected to the yolk sac through the vitello intestinal duct. This duct passes through the embryonic umbilical opening.
2. Later in fetal life, this duct undergoes complete obliteration and disappearance. However, in some persons its proximal part (near the gut) persists and forms a diverticulum arising from the terminal part of the ileum. This is ***diverticulum ilei*** or ***Meckel's diverticulum***.
3. The diverticulum is of surgical importance as it may undergo inflammation resulting in symptoms similar to those of appendicitis.
4. The mucosa in the diverticulum can show abnormalities and may have patches of gastric mucosa that can even be the site of a peptic ulcer.
5. Some facts of interest about the diverticulum are as follows:
   a. It is attached to the ileum about two feet proximal to the ileocaecal junction.
   b. It length is variable and is usually two inches.
   c. It is seen in about two percent of the population.
6. Persistence of remnants of the vitello-intestinal duct can also result in other anomalies as follows:
   a. If the entire duct remains patent there is a fecal fistula at the umbilicus.
   b. The part of the duct between Meckel's diverticulum and the umbilicus may become a fibrous band. Pressure from such a band may cause intestinal obstruction. It can also cause volvulus (see below).
   c. Sometimes the part of the vitello-intestinal duct near its junction with the gut disappears but part of the duct persists near the umbilicus. Such remnants may form:
      i. An umbilical sinus.
      ii. A cyst attached to or embedded in the anterior abdominal wall, or a malignant growth at the umbilicus.

*Errors of Rotation and Fixation*

The normal placing of various parts of the gut within the abdomen depends on orderly rotation of the gut during development. Abnormalities in rotation can lead to various anomalies.

1. The small intestine (which normally occupies mainly the lower left part of the abdominal cavity) may lie on the right side, and the entire large intestine may lie towards the left.
2. Normally, the transverse colon lies in front of the superior mesenteric vessels, while the duodenum lies behind them. The arrangement may be reversed.
3. The caecum and appendix may lie just below the liver (***subhepatic caecum***), or may descend only to the lumbar region.
4. All organs in the abdomen may show side to side reversal (***situs inversus***).
5. A part of the gut that normally has a mesentery (and is mobile) may be fixed; and conversely a part that is normally fixed may become mobile.
6. Abnormal mobility may result in twisting of the intestine leading to obstruction to blood supply. The condition is called ***volvulus***.

**Acquired Clinical Conditions**

***Pain of Intestinal Origin***

1. Pain arising in relation to parts derived from the midgut (middle of second part of duodenum to left two-thirds of transverse colon) is referred to the area around the umbilicus.
2. Pain arising from derivatives of the hindgut is referred to the hypogastrium.
3. When parietal peritoneum is inflamed pain is felt over the area of inflammation.

*Trauma to the Intestines*

1. The intestines can be involved in injuries by sharp weapons or gunshots. Rupture of the small intestines can also take place as a result of blunt injuries.
2. A blow is most likely to cause rupture of the intestine if it is over a bony projection like the promontory of the sacrum.
3. Rupture of the colon is relatively rare, but can be produced by blast injuries.
4. Rupture of the intestines is always serious as it leads to peritonitis.

*Infections in the Intestines*

1. Numerous infections can affect the intestine as they can enter them through ingested food.
2. Infection of the small intestine (***enteritis***) or of the colon (***colitis***) can be acute or chronic.
3. It can be produced by bacteria, by viruses, and by parasites like entamoeba histolytica (***amoebiasis***).
4. A bacterial infection can be tubercular. Another serious bacterial infection is ***typhoid*** that is accompanied by typhoid fever (or enteric fever). In such infection ulcers form and these can lead to intestinal perforation.

*Diverticulosis*

We have seen that diverticuli can occur in any part of the gut as a congenital anomaly and that these are most common in the duodenum.

1. Diverticuli can also be acquired. In congenital diverticuli, all three coats of the gut wall are present, but in acquired diverticuli only the mucosa is present as it herniates out through gaps in the muscle coat.
2. Such herniation is almost always on the mesenteric side of the gut and may be present in relation to points of entry of blood vessels.
3. Acquired diverticuli in the duodenum may be a result of weakening of the wall produced by an ulcer.
4. Jejunal diverticuli are usually single, while in the colon rows of diverticuli are sometimes seen.
5. Diverticuli can be sites of infection, and, occasionally, of perforation.

*Neoplasms of the intestines*

1. Neoplasms may be benign or malignant.
2. They are seen much more commonly in the colon than in the small intestine. Within the small intestine, carcinoma is more frequent in the jejunum than in the ileum.
3. Cancers of the colon are usually slow growing, and if recognised in time they can be removed completely.
4. Histologically, the neoplasms can be of various types. A relatively uncommon type is a ***carcinoid tumour*** arising from argentaffin cells. Such tumours secrete large amounts of 5-hydroxytryptamine.
5. In surgery for removal of a carcinoma of the colon, it has to be remembered that lymphatic drainage takes place alongside blood vessels. Hence, it may be necessary to ligate and remove a large artery to the region. The entire area of gut supplied by that artery has to be removed.
6. For example in carcinoma of the caecum the operation involves removal of the terminal part of the ileum, the caecum and ascending colon, and part of the transverse colon (***right hemicolectomy***). It has to be ensured that the parts of gut left behind have an adequate blood supply.

*Intestinal Obstruction*

1. Intestinal obstruction may be acute or chronic.
2. Acute intestinal obstruction is a surgical emergency for which many cases need operation.
3. Congenital causes of intestinal obstruction have been considered earlier. Some other causes are given below.

*Strangulation in hernias*

Coils of intestine can be constricted at the neck of the sac of a hernia and can undergo obstruction and strangulation. An internal hernia can also be a cause for obstruction. Internal hernias can occur into:

1. The aditus to the lesser sac
2. A defect in the mesentery

3. A defect in the transverse mesocolon
4. A defect in the broad ligament
5. One of the peritoneal recesses around the duodenum or the caecum.

*Intussusception*

This term is used for a condition in which one part of gut invaginates into another part leading to obstruction.

*Volvulus*

This condition results if a loop of gut rotates on itself. Such rotation may take place around a fibrous band. Volvulus may occur in the ileum, the caecum, or the pelvic colon.

*Bands and adhesions*

Pressure from peritoneal adhesions, or fibrous bands can lead to intestinal obstruction. The bands may be congenital or may be formed following peritonitis.

*Strictures*

Strictures of the small intestine can follow ulceration e.g., in tuberculosis. They can lead to intestinal obstruction.

*Paralytic ileus*

In this condition, there is no physical cause of obstruction. The condition is due to a failure of the neuromuscular mechanism governing peristalsis. The condition may occur after an abdominal operation, or after peritonitis.

*Embolism and thrombosis in blood vessels*

Embolism in an artery, or thrombosis in a vein supplying a part of a gut leads to loss of blood supply. There is infarction of tissue that leads to swelling and obstruction.

***Investigation of the gut***

1. Any radiological procedure in the abdomen should be preceded by careful preparation of the patient.
2. The objective of preparation is remove gas and fecal matter from the intestines as they cast shadows that may obscure significant findings.
3. This is achieved by restricting feeding for some hours, and by the use of laxatives and substances that absorb gas (e.g., charcoal tablets).

***Plain skiagram***

1. A plain skiagram shows shadows of bones in the region.
2. Some soft tissues also cast faint shadows.
   a. The domes of the diaphragm can be made out.
   b. The psoas major muscle, the kidneys the liver and the spleen may cast light shadows.
   c. Swallowed air present in the fundus of the stomach is usually seen under the left dome of the diaphragm.

***Barium meal***

Skiagrams taken after administering a barium meal (barium sulphate suspension) can reveal many details about the mucosa of the stomach, the duodenum and the small intestine.

1. The pattern of mucosal folds in the stomach can be seen.
2. Barium filling the first part of the duodenum casts a characteristic shadow that is referred to as the ***duodenal cap***.
3. Mucosal folds in the distal part of the duodenum and in the jejunum produce a feathery appearance.
4. The large intestine shows characteristic haustrations.

***Barium enema***

A barium sulphate suspension can be introduced into the large intestine through the anus. The large intestine is much better visualised than with a barium meal.

**Newer Imaging Techniques**

Investigation of the abdomen (and other parts of the body) has been revolutionised in recent years by the introduction of several new techniques. The following are now in common use.

***Ultrasonography***

The principle of the method is that ultrasound waves applied to any part of the body are reflected back by various structures. The reflected waves can be picked up and visualised on a screen. Images of internal organs can be obtained in this way.

***Computed Tomography***

1. The term tomography has been applied to radiological methods in which tissues lying in a particular plane are visualised.
2. In recent years, a technique has been developed in which images at a series of levels are analysed using computers. Such analysis provides images giving a remarkable degree of detail.

***Magnetic Resonance Imaging***

1. This is a complex technique in which, strong magnetic fields, and radio pulses are used to create images of outstanding clarity.
2. The images are distinctly superior to those of CT scans.
3. Using MRI, sectional appearances in sagittal, coronal and transverse planes can be obtained. The ability to image structures in multiple planes makes spatial localisation and differentiation of lesions more accurate.
4. In additional to sectional images in different planes three dimensional pictures can also be produced (by combining information from a series of sectional views).
5. The main advantages of MRI are high contrast, good soft tissue discrimination, absence of bone and metal artefacts, and the use of non-ionizing radiation.
6. However, like all other techniques, MRI has its limitations.
   a. These are high cost, long time required for collecting data.
   b. The fact that the patient being investigated has to be confined within a tube for a prolonged period (during which there can be difficulty in monitoring a critically ill patient).
   c. The machine is very noisy.
   d. Very fat persons or those with metallic implants or pacemakers cannot be subjected to this technique.

***Endoscopic Examination***

The interior of many part of the gut can be viewed directly through endoscopic instruments. The range has been greatly extended by the development of flexible instruments. These inlude oesophagoscopy, gastroscopy, sigmoidoscopy and colonoscopy.

## THE VERMIFORM APPENDIX

1. The vermiform appendix looks very much like a round worm: hence the name vermiform. It is a tube only a few millimetres wide, and about 9 cm in length. The length is, however, highly variable being anything between 2 to 20 cm.
2. At one end, the ***apex***, the appendix is blind and at the other end, the ***base***, it opens into the (posteromedial part of the) caecum.
3. The opening into the caecum lies about 2 cm below the opening of the ileum.
4. The appendix has a short mesentery called the ***mesoappendix***. Unlike other mesenteries, the mesoappendix is not attached to the posterior abdominal wall, but to the mesentery of the terminal part of the ileum (27.13).

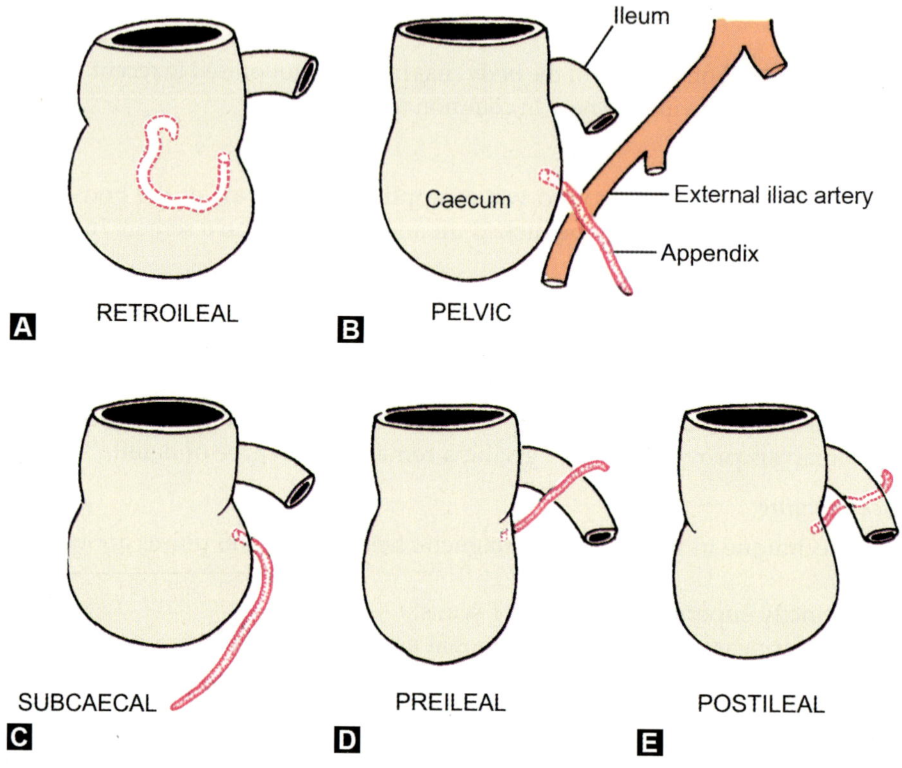


**27.14A to E:** Various positions of the vermiform appendix

5. The appendix is mobile and highly variable in position.
   a. In about 60 percent of individuals it lies behind the caecum, in the retrocaecal recess of the peritoneal cavity. (Part of it may lie behind the lower end of the ascending colon).
   b. In about 30 percent of individuals the appendix extends downwards and medially into the true pelvis. In this case, the appendix crosses the right external iliac artery. In the female, it may lie close to the right ovary and uterine tube.
   c. The appendix may be subcaecal — inferior to the caecum.
   d. It may be preileal: in front of the terminal ileum.
   e. It may be postileal: behind the terminal ileum.
6. In relation to the abdominal wall the position of the base of the appendix is found as follows:
   a. Draw a line joining the anterior superior iliac spine to the umbilicus and divide it into three equal parts.
   b. The base lies at the junction of the lateral and middle thirds of this line.
   c. This is referred to as ***Mc Burney's point***. In operations for removal of the appendix the usual incision passes through this point, at right angle to the line mentioned above (***Mc Burney's incision***).
7 Some other facts of importance about the appendix are as follows:
   a. The three taenia of the caecum converge towards the point at which the appendix is attached. They become continuous with the longitudinal muscle coat of the appendix which is uniformly thick all round. The taenia in front of the caecum is, therefore, a useful guide in locating the appendix.
   b. The appendix is supplied by a branch of the ileocolic artery.
      i. This artery runs in the mesoappendix.
      ii. However, over the distal part of the appendix the mesoappendix becomes very short and the artery may come into direct contact with the wall of the appendix.

iii. The basic structure of the appendix is similar to that of the large intestine (27.12B). The submucosa contains large amounts of lymphoid tissue that pushes the mucosa towards the lumen and narrows the latter. With age, or as a result of infection, the lumen may be partially or completely obstructed.

iv. The human vermiform appendix is often regarded as a vestigeal organ of no functional importance. However, some authorities feel that its rich blood supply, and the abundant lymphoid tissue present in it are not consistent with such a view.

8. Lymph from the appendix drains through the ileocolic node to superior mesenteric nodes.

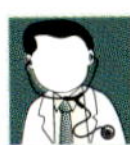

## CLINICAL CORRELATION

Some clinical correlations about the appendix have already been presented above. Some additional facts may be noted as follows.

1. Inflammation of the appendix is ***appendicitis***.
   a. Pain of appendicitis is first felt around the umbilicus. This is referred pain. It is vaguely localised, and of relatively low intensity.
   b. When inflammation reaches the parietal peritoneum pain shifts to the right iliac fossa. Here, the pain is precisely localised and severe.
2. Variations in position of the appendix have been mentioned above. The position can influence symptoms observed in appendicitis.
   a. If the appendix is retrocaecal (as it very often is) tenderness may be difficult to elicit over the right iliac fossa, specially if the caecum is distended with gas.
   b. Such an appendix comes into contact with the psoas major muscle. Because of this, pain may be felt on extending the right hip joint (the muscle being stretched in this position). So, the patient tends to keep the right thigh flexed.
   c. When the appendix is in the pelvic position tenderness may be present in the hypogastrium instead of the right iliac fossa.
      i. Tenderness may also be elicited by rectal or vaginal examination.
      ii. A pelvic appendix may irritate the obturator internus muscle, and the patient may find relief in keeping the hip laterally rotated.
      iii. Flexion and internal rotation of the right hip joint (which causes the obturator internus to be stretched) may produce pain in the hypogastrium.
   d. In situs inversus, the appendix may be located on the left side.
   e. In incomplete descent of the caecum the appendix may be subhepatic and appendicitis may be confused with cholecystitis.
3. The greater omentum plays an important role in trying to localise the infection in appendicitis.
4. We have seen above that the ileocolic artery may be closely related to the distal part of the appendix.
   a. The importance of this fact is that when the appendix is inflamed (***appendicitis***) infection may spread to the artery resulting in thrombosis.
   b. If this happens the distal part of the appendix undergoes necrosis, with danger of its bursting.
5. Bursting of the appendix is a very serious complication of appendicitis as infection then spreads to the peritoneum (***peritonitis***).
6. Apart from appendicitis other conditions that may affect the appendix are
   a. Malignant growths, the appendix being the most common site for a carcinoid tumour.
   b. Diverticulosis.
   c. Intussusception.

## The Ascending Colon

1. The ascending colon lies vertically in the right lateral region of the abdomen. It is about 15 cm long.
2. Its lower end is continuous with the caecum at the level of the intertubercular plane.
3. Its upper end meets the transverse colon at the right colic flexure. This flexure lies about an inch below the transpyloric plane (to the right of the right lateral line).
4. The ascending colon is covered by peritoneum in front and on either side, but posteriorly it is in direct contact with structures on the posterior abdominal wall.
   a. Its lowermost part may be separated from this wall by an upward extension of the retrocaecal recess.
   b. Rarely, the ascending colon may have a short mesocolon. It is then covered all round by peritoneum.

### WANT TO KNOW MORE?

5. The posterior relations of the ascending colon are as follows:
   a. Its lower part rests on the iliacus muscle.
   b. Just above this muscle it rests on the iliac crest.
   c. Above the iliac crest, it lies on the quadratus lumborum (medially) and the transversus abdominis (laterally).
   d. The lateral cutaneous nerve of the thigh, and the iliac branch of the iliolumbar artery intervene between the colon and the iliacus.
   e. The quadratus lumborum and transversus abdominis are partly separated from the colon by the lower part of the right kidney, and by the iliohypogastric and ilioinguinal nerves.
6. Anteriorly, the ascending colon is in contact with anterior abdominal wall.
7. Its upper end (right colic flexure) lies deep to the liver, and just to the right of the duodenum and gall bladder.

## The Transverse Colon

1. The transverse colon is the longest subdivision of the large intestine. It begins at the right colic flexure (which lies in the right lateral region a short distance below the transpyloric plane). It ends at the left colic flexure.
2. The left colic flexure is distinctly higher than the right flexure, and extends above the transpyloric plane into the left hypochondrium (27.11).
3. Between the right and left colic flexures, the transverse colon forms a downward loop of varying size. Its lowest part frequently descends to a level below the umbilicus and may even descend into the pelvis. Its total length is about 50 cm (27.15).

### WANT TO KNOW MORE?

4. Anteriorly, the transverse colon is overlapped by the greater omentum which separates it from the anterior abdominal wall.
5. Posteriorly, its right end crosses in front of the descending part of the duodenum and the pancreas. The rest of it lies in front of coils of jejunum and ileum.
6. Along its upper margin, the transverse colon lies close to (or in contact with) the liver, the gall bladder, stomach and spleen.
7. At its left extremity (i.e., the left colic flexure), it lies just below the spleen and the tail of the pancreas. The left kidney lies immediately medial to the left colic flexure.

*The Transverse Mesocolon*

1. The transverse colon is attached to the posterior abdominal wall through the transverse mesocolon.
2. The attachment of this mesocolon to the posterior abdominal wall is transverse.
   a. It is attached to the anterior aspect of the head of the pancreas. and to
   b. The anterior border of the body of the pancreas.
3. The greater omentum and transverse mesocolon are attached to the posterior abdominal wall parallel to each other, the attachment of the greater omentum being superior.
4. On reaching the posterior abdominal wall the posterior layer of the greater omentum is immediately reflected off again to form the anterior layer of the transverse mesocolon.
   a. These two layers of peritoneum are often adherent with each other.
   b. It may, therefore, appear that the greater omentum is attached to the transverse colon.
   c. However, the two can be easily separated from each other.

## The Descending Colon

1. The descending colon begins at the left colic flexure. Its upper end, therefore, lies in the left hypochondrium a little above the transpyloric plane.
2. From here the descending colon descends through the left lateral region, and the left inguinal region to reach the left side of the brim of the true pelvis (just above the inguinal ligament).
3. It ends here by becoming continuous with the sigmoid colon.
4. The descending colon is retroperitoneal and, therefore, has very limited mobility. It is covered by peritoneum on the front and sides, but posteriorly it rests directly on the abdominal wall. Rarely, however, it may have a short mesocolon.
5. The upper end of the descending colon (i.e., the left colic flexure) is anchored to the diaphragm by a fold of peritoneum called the ***phrenicocolic ligament***.

### WANT TO KNOW MORE?

6. The descending colon is about 25 cm in length.
7. The posterior relations of the descending colon are as follows:
   a. The left kidney (lower lateral part)
   b. The left transversus abdominis
   c. The left quadratus lumborum
   d. The left iliacus
   e. Psoas major muscles.
8. Smaller structures deep to the descending colon are similar to those related to the ascending colon and caecum on the right side. They include:
   a. The iliohypogastric
   b. Ilioinguinal nerves
   c. The lateral cutaneous nerve of the thigh
   d. The iliac branch of the iliolumbar artery.
9. Just above the inguinal ligament, the descending colon lies over the external iliac artery, the femoral nerve, the genitofemoral nerve and the testicular vessels (in the male).
10. Anteriorly, the descending colon is related to the anterior abdominal wall, but in its upper part coils of jejunum may intervene between it and this wall.

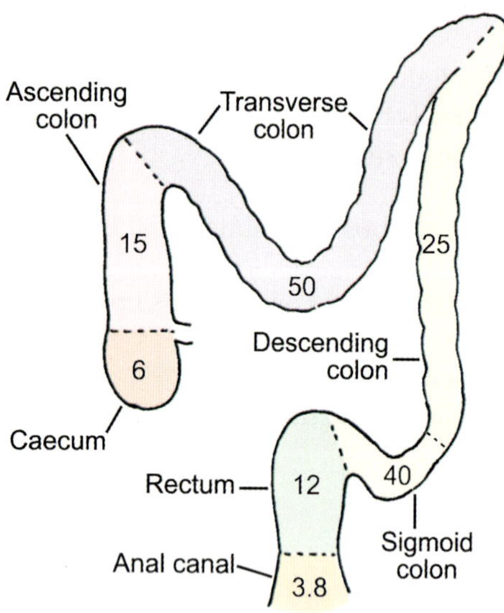


27.15: Scheme to show the lengths (cm) of the various subdivisions of the large intestine. The coils of sigmoid colon are not drawn

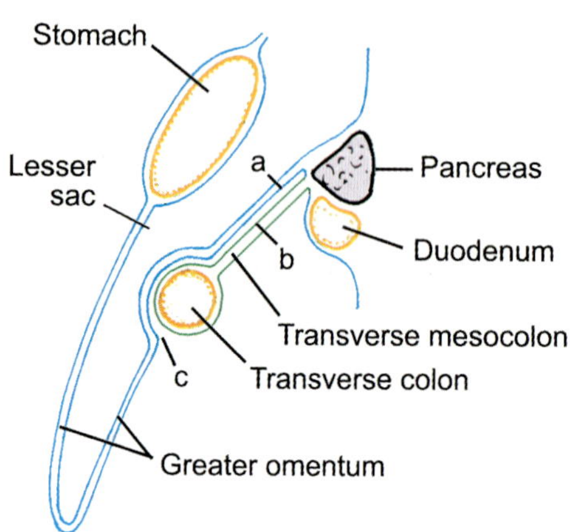


27.16: Scheme to show the relationship of the transverse mesocolon to the greater omentum

## THE SIGMOID COLON

1. The sigmoid, or pelvic, colon is highly variable in length, but is usually about 40 cm long.
2. It is continuous at one end with the lower end of the descending colon, and at the other end with the rectum. The junction with the descending colon lies over the pelvic brim (left half). The junction with the rectum is more or less in the median plane.
3. Between these ends, the sigmoid colon forms a convoluted loop that is enclosed all round by peritoneum and is attached to the posterior abdominal wall by the sigmoid mesocolon (see below).
4. Being located in the true pelvis the sigmoid colon is related to structures on its wall (particularly on the left side) as well as to viscera.
5. The structures on the pelvic wall include:
   a. The internal and external iliac vessels.
   b. The obturator nerve, the ductus deferens (in the male).
   c. The ovary (in the female).
6. A part of the sigmoid colon frequently lies between the rectum and the urinary bladder in the male and between the rectum and the uterus in the female.

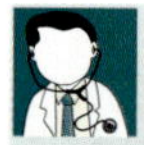

### CLINICAL CORRELATION

***Sigmoidoscopy***

The interior of the sigmoid colon can be viewed directly through a ***sigmoidoscope***. Recently, flexible sigmoidoscopes have been introduced. These allow more complete examination of the sigmoid colon.

 **WANT TO KNOW MORE?**

*The Sigmoid Mesocolon*

1. The line of the attachment of the sigmoid colon to the posterior abdominal and pelvic walls is shaped like an inverted 'V'.
2. The apex of the 'V' overlies the bifurcation of the left common iliac artery.
3. The left ureter crosses the artery just deep to the apex of the mesocolon.
4. The left limb of the 'V' runs downwards along the external iliac artery, on the medial side of the psoas major, to reach the junction of the sigmoid colon with the descending colon.
5. The right limb of the 'V' runs downwards and medially over the pelvic wall to reach the junction of the sigmoid colon with the rectum, in the median plane.

*Blood Vessels, Lymphatics and Nerves of the Colon*

1. The caecum, ascending colon and the right two-thirds of the transverse colon are supplied by the branches of the superior mesenteric artery. These are:
   a. The ileocolic branch (to the appendix, caecum, and lower one-third of the ascending colon).
   b. The right colic branch (to the upper two-thirds of ascending colon).
   c. The middle colic branch (to the transverse colon) (Chapter 29).
2. The left one-third of the transverse colon, the descending colon and the sigmoid colon are supplied by branches of the inferior mesenteric artery (left colic and sigmoid branches).
3. The veins from the colon drain through the superior and inferior mesenteric veins. This blood ultimately reaches the portal vein through which it reaches the liver (Chapter 29).
4. The lymphatic drainage of the region is as follows. The ascending colon and the transverse colon drain into the superior mesenteric nodes. The descending colon and sigmoid colon drain into the inferior mesenteric nodes. For details see Chapter 34.
5. See innervation of the gut described below.

### *Rectum and Anal Canal*

The rectum and anal canal will be considered along with other pelvic viscera in Chapter 33.

## INNERVATION OF THE GUT

1. The gut is innervated by sympathetic and parasympathetic (vagal) nerve fibres.
2. The distribution of the vagus nerve in the abdomen is described below.
3. The abdominal part of the sympathetic trunk is described in Chapter 34.

### Vagus Nerve in the Abdomen

1. The fibres of the right and left vagus nerves emerge from the posterior pulmonary plexuses (within the thorax) and descend on the oesophagus forming an ***anterior*** and a ***posterior oesophageal plexus.***
2. Although both plexuses receive fibres from the nerves of both sides the anterior plexus is formed mainly by fibres from the left vagus and the posterior plexus mainly by fibres from the right vagus.
3. Fibres emerging from the lower end of the anterior oesophageal plexus collect to form the ***anterior vagal trunk*** which is made up mainly of fibres from the left vagus.
4. Similarly, fibres arising from the posterior oesophageal plexus (mainly right vagus) collect to form the ***posterior vagal trunk.*** The anterior and posterior vagal trunks enter the abdomen through the oesophageal opening in the diaphragm and are distributed as follows:

**WANT TO KNOW MORE?**

5. The ***anterior vagal trunk*** supplies:
    a. The anterosuperior surface of the stomach.
    b. The superior and descending parts of the duodenum.
    c. The head of the pancreas and the liver.
6. The ***posterior vagal trunk*** supplies:
    a. The posteroinferior surface of the stomach.
    b. The posterior vagal trunk gives a large ***coeliac branch*** which ends in the ***coeliac plexus***. This plexus surrounds the coeliac trunk and stretches between the right and left ***coeliac ganglia*** (which lie on the corresponding crus of the diaphragm).
    c. Fibres from the coeliac plexus pass into several secondary plexuses that surround branches of the abdominal aorta. These are the splenic, hepatic, renal, suprarenal and superior mesenteric plexuses.
7. Fibres passing through these plexuses provide parasympathetic innervation to the whole of the small intestine, the large intestine up to the junction of the right two thirds and left one third of the transverse colon, the liver, the kidneys, and the spleen.
8. It may be noted that all these plexuses also receive numerous sympathetic fibres and that many fibres in them are afferent.

## Autonomic Innervation of the Gut

1. As a rule, parasympathetic nerves stimulate intestinal movement and inhibit the sphincters. They are also secretomotor to the glands in the mucosa. Sympathetic fibres are distributed chiefly to blood vessels.
2. The parasympathetic nerve supply to the greater part of the gastrointestinal tract (from pharynx to the right two-thirds of the transverse colon) is through the vagus.
3. The left one-third of the transverse colon, the descending colon, the sigmoid colon, the rectum and the upper part of the anal canal are supplied by the sacral part of the parasympathetic system.

**WANT TO KNOW MORE?**

   a. The preganglionic neurons concerned are located in segments S2, S3 and S4 of the spinal cord. They emerge through the ventral nerve roots of the corresponding nerves, and pass into their ***pelvic splanchnic branches***.
   b. The fibres to the rectum and the upper part of the anal canal pass through the ***inferior hypogastric plexus***.
   c. The remaining fibres pass through the ***superior hypogastric plexus*** and are distributed along the inferior mesenteric artery.
4. The postganglionic parasympathetic neurons are located in the myenteric and submucosal plexuses in the region to be supplied.
5. Preganglionic sympathetic neurons for the gut are located in the thoracolumbar region of the spinal cord.
6. Their axons pass through the sympathetic trunk without relay. They travel through the splanchnic nerves to terminate in plexuses (or ganglia) related to the coeliac trunk, the superior mesenteric artery, the inferior mesenteric artery and the aorta itself.
7. Postganglionic neurons are located in these plexuses. They travel along the branches of the arteries mentioned above to reach the gut.
8. Afferent fibres from the gut travel along both sympathetic and parasympathetic pathways.
9. Those from the rectum and lower part of the pelvic colon are carried by the pelvic splanchnic nerves.

# 28 CHAPTER The Liver, Pancreas and Spleen

## THE LIVER

1. The liver is one of the largest organs in the body weighing about 1.5 kg. It is by far the largest gland.
2. It is included amongst the accessory organs of the alimentary system because it produces a secretion, the bile, which is poured into the duodenum (through the bile duct) and assists in the digestive process.
3. All the blood circulating through the capillary bed of the abdominal part of the alimentary canal (excepting the lower part of the anal canal) reaches the liver through the portal vein and its tributaries.
   a. In this way, all substances absorbed into the blood from the stomach and intestines are filtered through the liver, where some of them are stored and some toxic substances may be destroyed.
   b. Numerous other functions essential to the well being of the individual are performed in the liver that is, therefore, regarded as one of the vital organs.
4. The liver lies in the upper, right part of the abdominal cavity (28.1). It lies mainly in the right hypochondrium and in the epigastrium, but part of it extends into the left hypochondrium and part of it into the right lateral region.
5. When seen from the front (28.1) the liver is roughly triangular and appears to have upper, lower and right borders.
6. a. In the midline, the upper border lies at the level of the xiphisternal joint.
   b. To the right of the midline, the upper border follows the upward convexity of the right dome of the diaphragm reaching to a level just below the right nipple.
   c. To the left of the midline, the upper border follows the curve of the medial part of the left dome of the diaphragm, and ends a little below and medial to the left nipple.
7. The right border runs vertically, with an outward convexity and ends at the level of the tip of the tenth costal cartilage.
8. a. The lower border runs obliquely upwards and to the left.
   b. It crosses the midline at the level of the transpyloric plane.
   c. From 28.1 note that most of the liver is placed deep to the costal margin and comes into contact with the anterior abdominal wall in the epigastrium.
   d. A liver extending below the level of the lateral part of the right costal margin is considered to be enlarged.
9. a. The liver has basically two surfaces (28.2).
   b. Above it has a convex ***diaphragmatic surface***, and below it has an inferior or ***visceral surface***.
      i. The diaphragmatic surface is extensive. Part of it faces forwards, part of it upwards, and part of it backwards. These parts are sometimes referred to as anterior, superior and posterior surfaces but there are no features that demarcate them from one another.
      ii. The diaphragmatic and visceral surfaces meet in front at a sharp ***inferior border***.
      iii. Posteriorly, the junction of the two surfaces is rounded and not sharply defined.

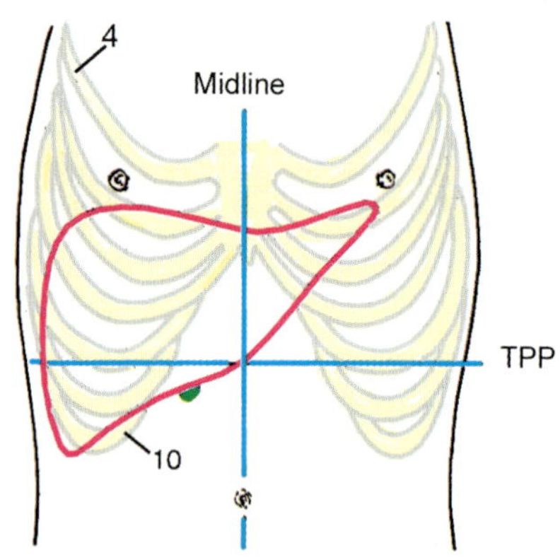


28.1: Surface projection of the liver as seen from the front

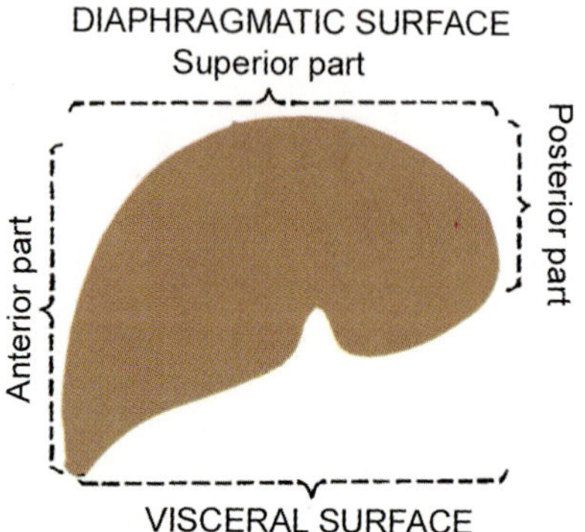


28.2: Schematic sagittal section through the liver to show its surfaces

10. Before proceeding to study the features to be seen on individual surfaces of the liver, it is necessary to briefly consider the basic peritoneal relationships of the organ.
    a. At an early stage in development, the stomach has a ventral mesogastrium that passes from its ventral border (future lesser curvature) to the developing diaphragm and anterior abdominal wall (28.3 and 28.4). The liver develops in intimate relation to this mesogastrium.
    b. After the formation of the liver the peritoneum of the ventral mesogastrium passes from the stomach to the liver, covers the greater part of the liver, and is then reflected from the liver to the diaphragm and anterior abdominal wall (28.5).
    c. The part of the ventral mesogastrium between the stomach and the liver becomes the lesser omentum.
    d. The lesser omentum gains attachment (partly) to an area on the visceral surface of the liver called the porta hepatis (28.6). Here, the two layers of the peritoneum forming it separate to cover the greater part of the liver surface.
    e. The peritoneum from the surface of the liver is reflected on to the diaphragm (and anterior abdominal wall) in the form of a number of ligaments that are identified in the paragraphs that follow.
11. a. The liver is shown as seen from the front in 28.7 and as seen from above in 28.8. In both these figures, we see the anterior and superior parts of the diaphragmatic surface.
    b. The anterior part of the diaphragmatic surface is lined by peritoneum except along a line near the median plane.
    c. Along this line, the peritoneum is reflected off from the liver to the diaphragm, and to the upper part of the anterior abdominal wall as the ***falciform ligament***.
12. a. The line of attachment of the falciform ligament has traditionally been used to divide the liver into a larger right lobe and a much smaller left lobe.
    b. However, most authorities agree that the division of the liver into right and left lobes should be based on the areas drained by the right and left hepatic ducts. This plane of division is shown in 28.7 in red line.
13. Apart from the falciform ligament, peritoneum from the superior part of the diaphragmatic surface is reflected on to the diaphragm in the form of:
    a. The left triangular ligament.
    b. The superior layer of the coronary ligament.
    c. The right triangular ligament (28.8 and 28.9).
14. a. The posterior aspect of the liver is marked by a deep notch for the vertebral column (28.8).
    b. To the right of this notch, there is a deep groove for the inferior vena cava.

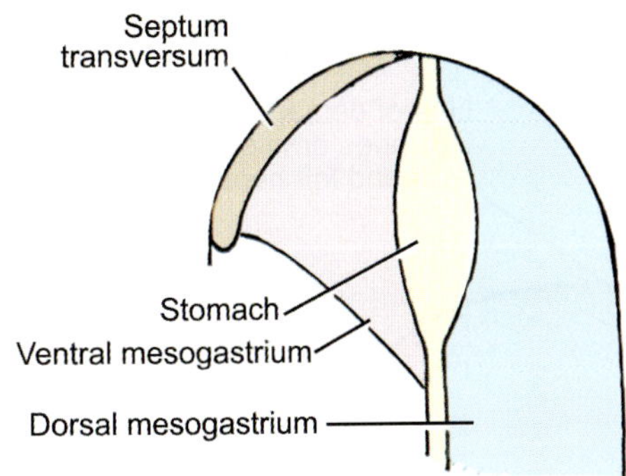


**28.3:** Ventral and dorsal mesogastrium as seen from the left side

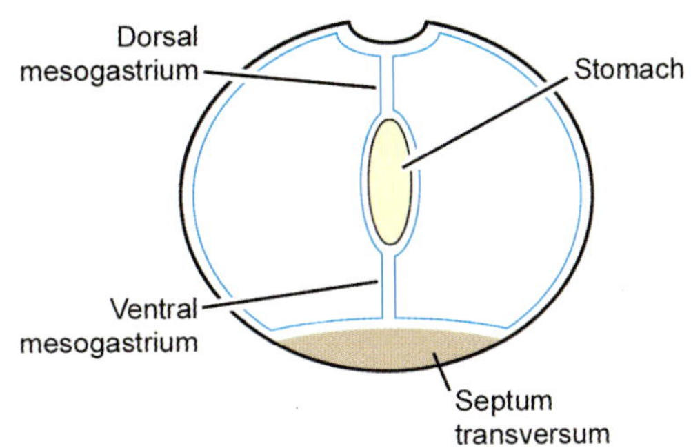


**28.4:** Ventral and dorsal mesogastrium as seen in transverse section

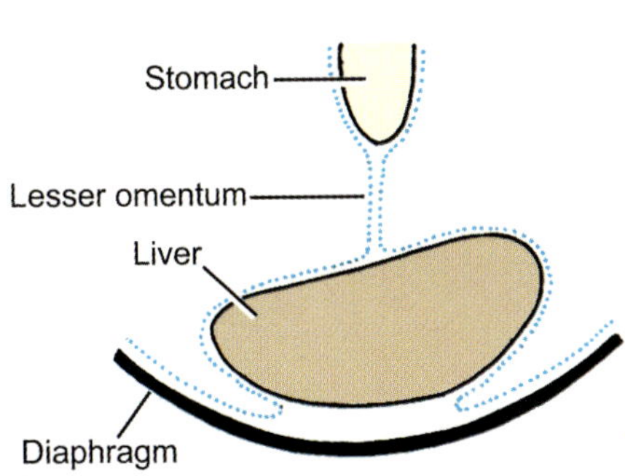


**28.5:** Transverse section at a later stage than in 28.4 to show the fate of the ventral mesogastrium

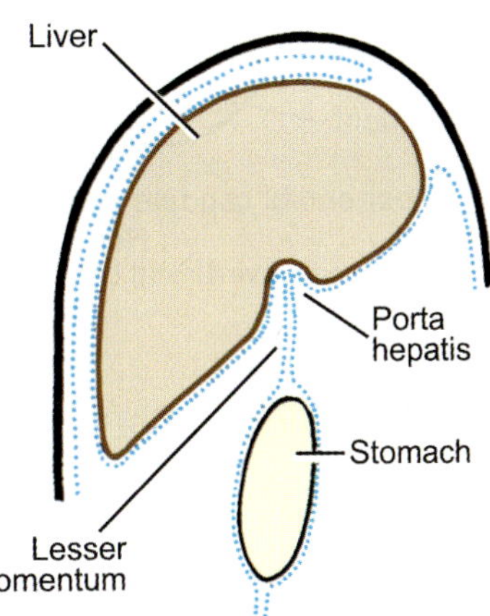


**28.6:** Schematic parasagittal section through the liver to show its basic peritoneal relations

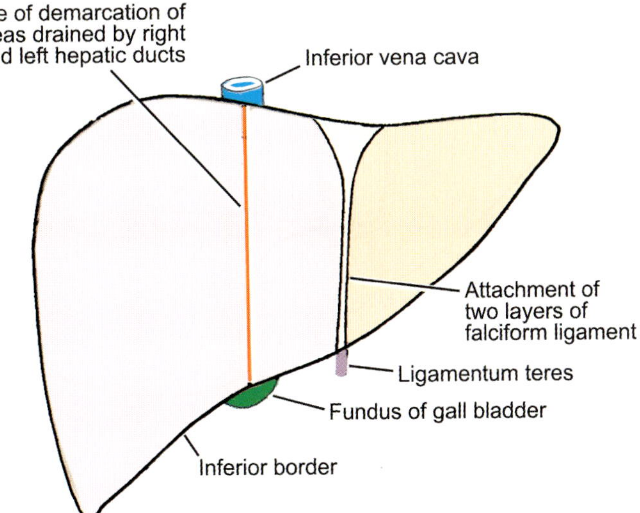


**28.7:** Liver viewed from the front

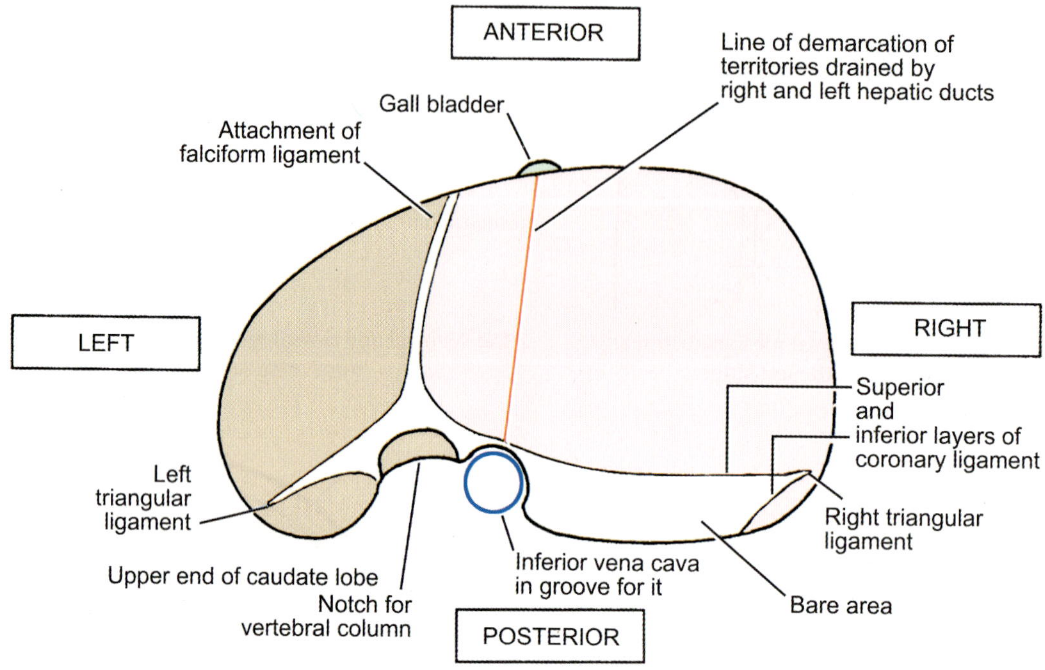


28.8: Liver viewed from above

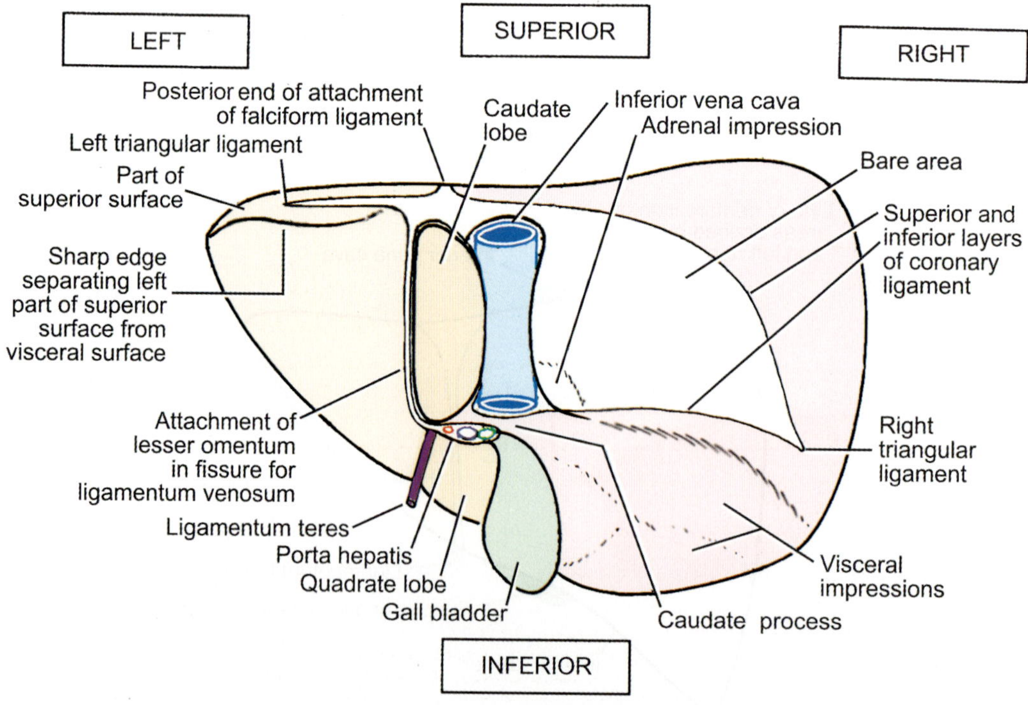


28.9: Liver viewed from behind

15. The liver is shown as seen from behind in 28.9. The upper part of this figure shows the posterior part (and adjoining superior part) of the diaphragmatic surface. The lower part of the figure shows the visceral surface (better seen in 28.10).
    a. In 28.9 identify some features already noticed in 28.8. These are the attachments of the left triangular ligament, the upper layer of the coronary ligament, the right triangular ligament, and the groove for the inferior vena cava.
    b. A considerable area on the posterior part of the diaphragmatic surface of the liver is not covered by peritoneum and is, therefore, called the ***bare area***.
        i. It includes the groove for the inferior vena cava and a large triangular area on the right of it.
        ii. The triangle is bounded above by the attachment of the superior layer of the coronary ligament and below by the attachment of the inferior layer of the same ligament.
        iii. These two layers meet towards the right side to form the right triangular ligament.
    c. To the left of the groove for the inferior vena cava there is a circumscribed part of the posterior surface that is called the ***caudate lobe***.
    d. The caudate lobe is bounded on its left side by a deep groove called the ***fissure for the ligamentum venosum***.
    e. Inferiorly, the caudate lobe is separated from the visceral surface by the ***porta hepatis*** (which is in the form of a transverse groove).
    f. The porta hepatis is the 'hilum' of the liver. The hepatic artery and portal vein enter the liver here, while the right and left hepatic ducts leave it.
16. a. The porta hepatis and the fissure for the ligamentum venosum give attachment to the two layers of the lesser omentum.
    b. The attachment is L-shaped when seen from behind, and in the form of an inverted 'L' when visualised from the front.

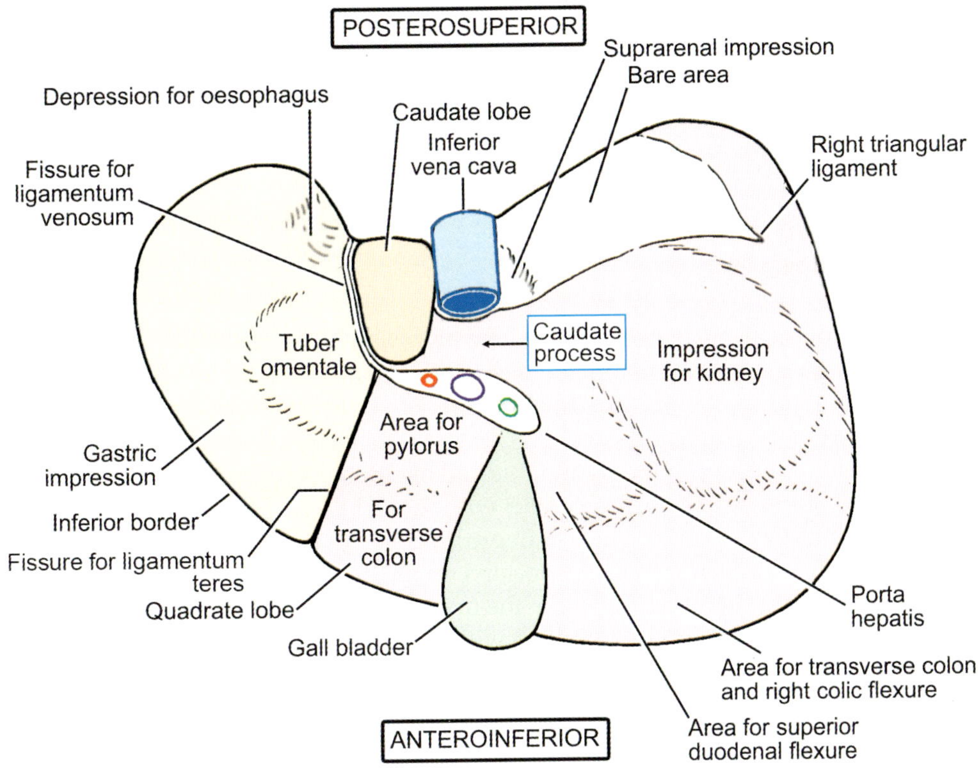


**28.10:** Ventral surface of the liver seen from behind and below

17. a. The structures entering or leaving the liver at the porta hepatis (portal vein, hepatic artery, bile duct) are enclosed between the two layers of peritoneum forming the lesser omentum.
    b The two layers become continuous with each other at the right end of the porta hepatis. This represents the upper end of the right free margin of the lesser omentum.
18. a. A narrow strip of liver tissue intervenes between the posterior aspect of the porta hepatis and the groove for the inferior vena cava.
    b. This strip projects downwards and is called the ***caudate process***.
    c. It connects the caudate lobe (on the left) to the visceral surface of the right lobe (on the right).
    d. The caudate process forms the upper boundary of the aditus to the lesser sac (41.10).
19. The most conspicuous feature on the visceral surface of the liver is the gall bladder.
    a. It lies in a depression on the liver surface called the ***fossa for the gall bladder***. This fossa is not usually exposed to view as the gall gladder is fixed to the liver by peritoneum as shown in 28.11.
    b. Starting near the right end of the porta hepatis the gall bladder runs downwards and forwards across the visceral surface of the liver.
20. a. Another conspicuous feature to be seen on the visceral surface is the ***fissure for the ligamentum teres***.
    b. This fissure runs from the left end of the porta hepatis to the inferior margin of the liver. It lodges the ligamentum teres.
21. a. The part of the visceral surface between the fissure for the ligamentum teres and the fossa for the gall bladder is called the ***quadrate lobe*** (because of its quadrangular shape).
    b. It is bounded posteriorly and above by the porta hepatis, and anteriorly and below by the inferior margin of the liver.

Liver tissue
Gall bladder
Peritoneum

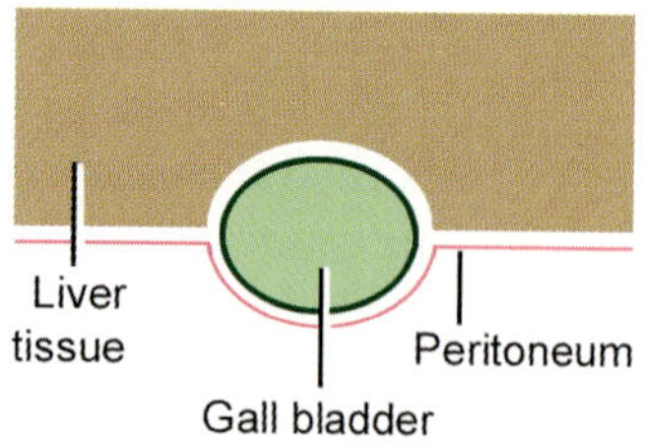

**28.11:** Section through the fossa for the gall bladder

22. a. In relation to the diaphragmatic surface, it has been mentioned that the attachment of the falciform ligament is used to divide the liver into right and left lobes.
    b. On the visceral surface, the line of division runs along the fissure for the ligamentum venosum and the fissure for the ligamentum teres.
    c. However, in terms of the territory of drainage of the right and left hepatic ducts the caudate and quadrate lobes are to be regarded as parts of the 'left' lobe.

## WANT TO KNOW MORE?

23. The visceral surface of the liver comes into contact with several viscera that are as follows (28.9 and 28.10).
    a. A strip along the inferior margin of the liver comes in contact with the transverse colon. It includes:
       i. The lower (anterior) part of the quadrate lobe.
       ii. The lower part of the gall bladder.
       iii. The lower part of the area to the right of the gall bladder.
       iv. The right end of this strip comes in contact with the right colic flexure.
    b. The oesophagus comes in contact with a depression to the left of the upper end of the fissure for the ligamentum venosum. The depression is located on the posterosuperior margin of the visceral surface.
    c. The part of the visceral surface to the left of the fissure for the ligamentum venosum and the ligamentum teres comes in contact with the stomach, and with the lesser omentum.
       i. The area for the stomach is in the form of a shallow depression called the ***gastric impression***.
       ii. The area in contact with the lesser omentum is raised. The elevation is called the ***tuber omentale***.
    d. The pylorus comes in contact with the posterosuperior part of the quadrate lobe.
    e. The first part of the duodenum crosses the upper part of the gall bladder, while the superior duodenal flexure comes into contact with an area immediately to the right of the upper part of the gall bladder.

f. To the right of the area for the superior duodenal flexure, and above the area for the transverse colon, the visceral surface bears a large impression for the right kidney.
g. The liver comes in contact with the right suprarenal gland above and medial to the impression for the kidney. The suprarenal produces a depression on the bare area immediately to the right of the lower part of the inferior vena cava.

**Lobes and Segments of the Liver**

1. a. The liver has been traditionally divided into right and left lobes using certain surface features.
   b. On the anterior and superior parts of the diaphragmatic surface, the line of demarcation is the attachment of the falciform ligament.
   c. On the posterior part of the diaphragmatic surface, the line of demarcation is the fissure for the ligamentum venosum.
   d. On the visceral surface, the demarcation is by the fissure for the ligamentum teres.
   e. According to this plan of division, the caudate and quadrate lobes form part of the right lobe.
2. The liver is drained by two ***hepatic ducts***, right and left which join to form the ***common hepatic duct***. It is rational to regard the territory drained by the right hepatic duct as the true right lobe and that drained by the left hepatic duct as the true left lobe.
3. The lines of demarcation between the two territories are as follows:
   a. On the visceral surface, the line of demarcation between these territories lies roughly along the fossa for the gall bladder.
   b. On the posterior part of the liver, the line lies along the groove for the inferior vena cava.
   c. On the anterosuperior part of the diaphragmatic surface, the line is not marked by any surface feature. It can be represented roughly by a line joining the fundus of the gall bladder and the upper end of the inferior vena cava (red lines in 28.7 and 28.8).
   d. Note that the caudate and quadrate lobes lie in the territory drained by the left hepatic duct.
4. Each lobe, thus defined is divisible into a number of segments based on the branching pattern of the hepatic ducts within the liver. A simplified scheme of these segments is shown in 28.12.
5. The 'left' lobe is divided into medial and lateral parts.
   a. The lateral part corresponds to the traditional left lobe.
   b. The medial part lies to the right of the attachment of the falciform ligament. On the visceral surface it corresponds to the quadrate lobe, and the caudate lobe.
   c. The medial and lateral parts of the left lobe are each divided into superior and inferior segments.
   d. The caudate lobe is described as an independent segment .
6. The 'right' lobe is divided into the anterior and posterior parts each of which is subdivided into the superior and inferior segments. There are thus a total of nine segments.
7. It is important to remember, however, that there are no surface features to outline the segments, and that there is considerable individual variation in the size and relationship of individual segments to the surface of the liver. The subdivision is, therefore, not very useful to a surgeon wanting to remove a part of the liver.

## Further Consideration of Peritoneal Folds Attached to the Liver

### *The Lesser Omentum*

1. The lesser omentum consists of two layers of peritoneum that are continuous with the peritoneum lining the anterior and posterior surfaces of the stomach (28.13).
2. It is attached by its lower edge to the lesser curvature of the stomach and to the proximal portion of the first part of the duodenum.
3. Its upper edge has an inverted 'L' shaped attachment to the liver. This attachment is to the fissure for the ligamentum venosum and to the lips of the porta hepatis (28.10).

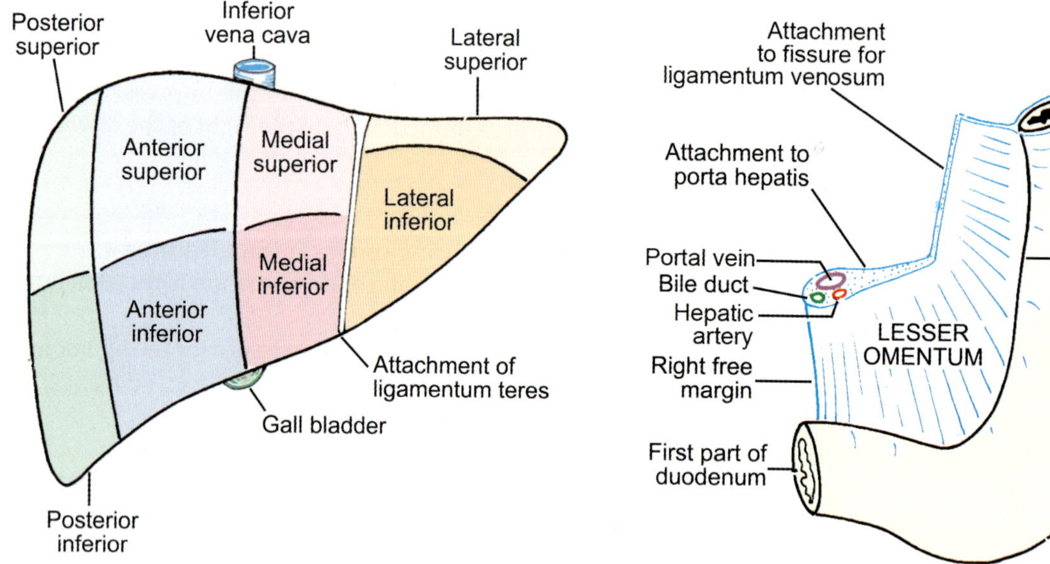


**28.12:** Scheme to show the segments of the liver

**28.13:** Scheme to show the arrangement of the lesser omentum

4. a. Extending between the duodenum and the right extremity of the porta hepatis the lesser omentum has a free edge formed by continuity of the anterior and posterior layers.
   b. The structures that lie between the two layers of the omentum near its free edge are:
      i. The portal vein
      ii. The bile duct
      iii. The hepatic artery.
5. Along the lesser curvature of the stomach, the right and left gastric arteries and veins lie within the omentum. Some lymph nodes are also present.

## WANT TO KNOW MORE?

6. a. The lesser omentum forms part of the anterior wall of the lesser sac.
   b. The right margin of the omentum forms the anterior boundary of the aditus to the lesser sac.
7. The anterior layer of peritoneum forming the omentum can be traced down to the front of the pylorus and the commencement of the duodenum.

### *Relationship of Peritoneum to the Caudate Lobe*

1. The caudate lobe is bounded on the left side by the fissure for the ligamentum venosum. The lesser omentum is attached to this fissure (28.10).
2. The lesser omentum extends to the bottom of the fissure where its layers are reflected on to the walls of the fissure.
3. At the right margin of the posterior surface of the caudate lobe (i.e., near the inferior vena cava) the peritoneum is reflected from the caudate lobe to the diaphragm.
4. a. In this way, a narrow recess of the cavity of the lesser sac comes to lie behind the caudate lobe.
   b. This is called the ***superior recess of the lesser sac.***
   c. The peritoneum lining the posterior surface of the caudate lobe is reflected on to the diaphragm along the upper border of the lobe thus forming the upper limit of the superior recess of the lesser sac.

### The Falciform Ligament

1. The falciform ligament is attached on the anterior and superior parts of the diaphragmatic surface of the liver.
2. a. The ligament is shaped like a sickle (falciform = sickle shaped).
   b. Its lower part is attached anteriorly to the anterior abdominal wall, the attachment extending up to the level of the umbilicus and posteriorly it has a free edge formed by continuity of the two layers of peritoneum (right and left) that form it.
3. The upper part of the ligament is a short fold passing from the diaphragm to the liver.
4. a. The ligamentum teres is enclosed within the falciform ligament (near its free edge).
   b. It passes from the umbilicus to the inferior border of the liver within the ligament.

### The Coronary Ligament

1. This 'ligament' is made up of two layers (superior and inferior) of peritoneum that pass from the diaphragm to the posterior part of the diaphragmatic surface of the liver (28.8 and 28.9).
2. The superior and inferior layers form the upper and lower boundaries of the bare area of the liver.
3. Towards the right side the superior and inferior layers meet at an acute angle to form the right triangular ligament.
4. When traced to the left side the superior layer of the coronary ligament becomes continuous with the right layer of the falciform ligament.
5. When traced to the left the inferior layer passes in front of the groove for the inferior vena cava, along the posterior edge of the caudate process and becomes continuous with the line of reflection of peritoneum along the right margin of the caudate lobe (28.9).

## Peritoneal Spaces around the Liver

1. Surrounding the liver there are a number of regions where the peritoneum covering the surface of the liver is separated from the peritoneum lining the diaphragm, or adjoining viscera, only by a potential space.
2. The spaces lying between the diaphragm and the liver are referred to as ***subphrenic spaces***.
3. Spaces inferior to the liver are called ***subhepatic spaces.***
4. The importance of the subphrenic and subhepatic spaces is that they are sites where abnormal fluids (like pus) can collect.
5. Normally, all parts of the peritoneal cavity are in communication with each other, but in the presence of infection abnormal adhesions may form and pockets may become isolated. From this point of view it is of importance to define the regions where this may happen.

### WANT TO KNOW MORE?

1. a. The ***right subphrenic space*** is bounded, on the left side by the falciform ligament, and behind by the superior layer of the coronary ligament.
   b. Anteriorly and to the right it becomes continuous with the rest of the peritoneal cavity at the lower border of the liver.
2. a. The ***left subphrenic space*** is bound on the right side by the falciform ligament, and behind by the left triangular ligament.
   b. Anteriorly and to the left it is in communication with the part of the peritoneal cavity intervening between the stomach and spleen (below) and the diaphragm (above).
3. a. The ***right subhepatic space*** is also called the ***hepatorenal*** or ***Morrison's pouch***.
   b. It lies below the right half of the visceral surface of the liver.
   c. The gall bladder also lies anterior to the pouch.
   d. Posteriorly (and below) the pouch is related to the right kidney the transverse colon and the descending part of the duodenum.
   e. Inferiorly, the space is continuous with the rest of the peritoneal cavity.

4. The *left subhepatic space* is merely another name for the lesser sac (omental bursa). We have noted the intimate relationship of the superior recess of this sac to the caudate lobe (28.14).

## Blood Vessels of the Liver

1. The liver receives oxygenated blood through the hepatic artery. This artery is a branch of the coeliac trunk, and is described in Chapter 29. Entering the liver at the porta hepatis it divides into two main branches that are distributed to the 'true' right and left lobes.
2. The branching pattern of the artery corresponds to that of the hepatic ducts. Each hepatic segment (28.12) receives one major branch.
3. The terminal branches of the hepatic artery are functional end arteries, the anastomoses between them being insignificant.
4. The liver receives blood from the gastrointestinal tract through the portal vein. This vein is described in Chapter 29.
5. At the porta hepatis, the portal vein divides into right and left branches that accompany branches of the hepatic artery.
6. Blood from the liver is drained by a number of hepatic veins that open directly into the inferior vena cava (Chapter 31).

### *Significance of Ligamentum Teres and Ligamentum Venosum*

1. In fetal life oxygenation of blood takes places not in the lungs, but in the placenta.
2. Blood from the placenta is brought to the fetus initially through right and left ***umbilical veins***.
3. a. The right vein is transitory and soon disappears so that all blood now comes to the fetus through the left umbilical vein.
   b. The left umbilical vein ends initially in the left horn of the sinus venosus, but later in fetal life it ends by joining the left branch of the portal vein.

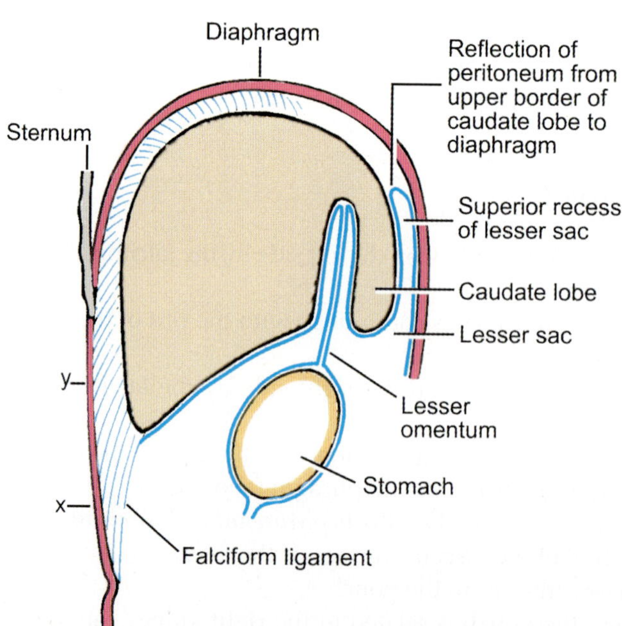


**28.14:** Sagittal section through the caudate lobe of the liver showing its peritoneal relations

4. For some time during fetal life all blood coming from the placenta has to filter through the liver before reaching the heart.
5. a. However, at a later stage a new channel, the ***ductus venosus***, short circuits a large part of this blood to the inferior vena cava.
   b. The ductus venosus is connected at one end to the left branch of the portal vein, and at the other end to the inferior vena cava.
6. After birth, the left umbilical vein and the ductus venosus are no longer functional. They retrogress into fibrous structures.
7. The left umbilical vein becomes the ligamentum teres, and the ductus venosus becomes the ligamentum venosum (28.15).
8. The ligamentum teres, therefore, begins at the umbilicus and ends by joining the left branch of the portal vein, while the connections of the ligamentum venosum are those of the ductus venosus.

## WANT TO KNOW MORE?

**Lymphatic Drainage and Nerve Supply of the Liver**

1. The lymphatic drainage of the liver is into the following nodes:
   a. Nodes around upper end of inferior vena cava
   b. Nodes in porta hepatis
   c. Coeliac nodes.
   For details see Chapter 34.
2. The nerve supply is through autonomic nerves that travel along the hepatic artery.

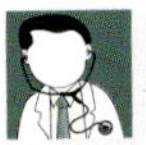

## CLINICAL CORRELATION

### The Liver

*Palpation of the liver*

1. The surface projection of the liver is shown in 28.1. Note that part of the anterior surface of the liver comes into contact with the anterior abdominal wall in the epigastrium.
2. However, the liver cannot be palpated here because it is covered by the rectus abdominis muscles.
3. Dullness in the area can, however, be elicited on percussion.
4. The lower border of an enlarged liver extends beyond the right costal margin and can be palpated, especially after a deep breath.

**Congenital Anomalies**

These are rare and mostly involve abnormalities in formation of fissures and lobes. Part of the liver may be missing. Ectopic liver tissue may be present in the falciform ligament.

**Liver biopsy**

1. A small piece of liver tissue can be obtained for examination by introducing a needle into the organ.
2. The needle is usually introduced through the right 8th or 9th intercostal space and pierces through the diaphragm.
3. Biopsy can also be obtained through the epigastrium.

**Injury**

Injury to the liver can occur by fracture of the lower ribs. Injury to the organ is common in automobile accidents. Laceration of the liver leads to considerable haemorrhage.

*Liver Infections and Damage*

1. Liver tissue can be damaged by infections and by toxic substances reaching it through the bloodstream.
2. Inflammation of the liver is called ***hepatitis*** (hepar = liver). Hepatitis is often viral. The infection can reach the liver through contaminated drinking water. Hepatitis can also be spread through needles used for injection.
3. Severe viral infections can lead to serious liver damage. They can also predispose to cancer.
4. a. Infection with amoeba histolytica leads to ***amoebic hepatitis***.
   b. This is usually secondary to intestinal infection. Amoebic hepatitis can lead to the formation of an ***amoebic abscess***.
   c. Various other infections may occur.
5. a. All substances absorbed into the bloodstream from the gut pass, through the portal vein, into the liver.
   b. Apart from nutrients these include alcohol and drugs. The liver tries to detoxify harmful substances before they are passed into the systemic circulation, but in the process liver tissue can itself undergo damage.
   c. In persons who consume excessive amounts of alcohol over long periods, the liver tissue undergoes fibrosis (***cirrhosis of liver***).
6. a. The liver tissue has considerable reserve and continues to carry out its normal functions even after large amounts of it are damaged.
   b. However, as damage progresses liver failure can set in.
   c. Coma occurring as a result of liver failure is called ***hepatic coma***.

*Tumours of the Liver*

1. Tumours of the liver may arise either from liver cells or from cells lining bile capillaries.
   a. They may be benign (hepatoadenoma, cholangioadenoma).
   b. Malignant (hepatocarcinoma, cholangiocarcinoma).
2. The liver is also a common site for secondary growths (metastases) caused by malignancy elsewhere in the body.

*Surgery on the liver*

1. In cases of injury, the main aim of surgery is to control bleeding.
2. For excision of tumours, parts of the liver may require surgical removal. The surgeon tries to remove as little liver tissue as possible. For this purpose knowledge of the segments of the liver is essential.
3. Sometimes the entire right lobe may have to be removed (***right hemihepatectomy***).

Other topics of clinical importance discussed in the book:

1. Peritoneal spaces around the liver (subphrenic spaces).
2. Portal hypertension.

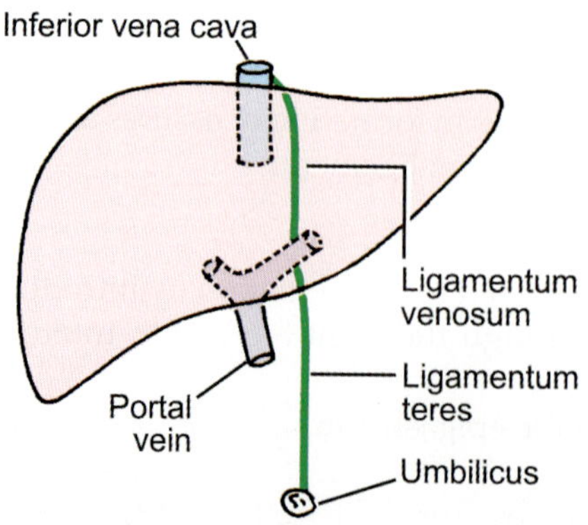


**28.15:** Scheme to show the ligamentum teres and the ligamentum venosum

## EXTRAHEPATIC BILIARY APPARATUS

The passages through which bile, produced in the liver, passes before entering the duodenum are seen in 28.16.

1. The ***right*** and ***left, hepatic ducts*** emerge at the porta hepatis and join to form the ***common hepatic duct***.
2. At its lower end, the common hepatic duct is joined by the ***cystic duct*** from the ***gall bladder*** to form the ***bile duct***. The bile duct opens into the duodenum.
3. The gall bladder and bile duct are considered in detail below.

### The Gall Bladder

1. The gall bladder is a small sac attached to the visceral surface of the liver (28.10). It is held in place by peritoneum that covers its inferior (or posterior) surface (28.11).
2. Its superior (or anterior) aspect is in direct contact with liver tissue.
3. The lowest part of the gall bladder, which is called the ***fundus***, projects beyond the inferior border of the liver (28.7) and is surrounded all round by peritoneum.
4. The central part of the gall bladder is called the ***body***.
5. The narrow part succeeding the body is called the ***neck***.
6. The neck is connected to the ***cystic duct*** through which the gall bladder drains into the bile duct.

### WANT TO KNOW MORE?

***Relations of the Gall Bladder***

1. Anteriorly, the body and neck of the gall bladder are in contact with the liver.
2. a. The fundus comes in contact with the anterior abdominal wall just below the ninth costal cartilage.
   b. The area of contact corresponds to the point where the lateral margin of the right rectus abdominis muscle crosses the costal margin.
3. The posterior (or inferior) relations of the gall bladder are:
   a. The transverse colon (near its right end).
   b. The duodenum (first part and beginning of second part).
4. The mucous membrane lining the neck of the gall bladder is folded in a spiral manner forming the so-called ***spiral valve***. This 'valve' extends into the cystic duct also.
5. The gall bladder is supplied by the cystic artery (branch of the hepatic artery). It is drained by the cystic veins. Some of these enter liver tissue directly, while others join veins draining the bile duct and ultimately drain into the portal vein.
6. The gall bladder has a capacity of about 40 ml.

### The Bile Duct

1. The bile duct extends from just below the porta hepatis to the middle of the descending part of the duodenum. It is about 7 cm long. From above downwards it lies:
   a. In the right margin of the lesser omentum (28.13).
   b. Behind the first part of the duodenum.
   c. Behind the head of the pancreas.
2. a. Within the lesser omentum, the duct lies to the right of the hepatic artery and in front of the portal vein (28.13).
   b. All these structures lie anterior to the aditus to the lesser sac by which they are separated from the inferior vena cava.
3. Behind the duodenum, the gastroduodenal artery lies to the left of the bile duct.
4. Behind the pancreas, the duct lies in front of the inferior vena cava. This part of the duct may be embedded in pancreatic tissue.

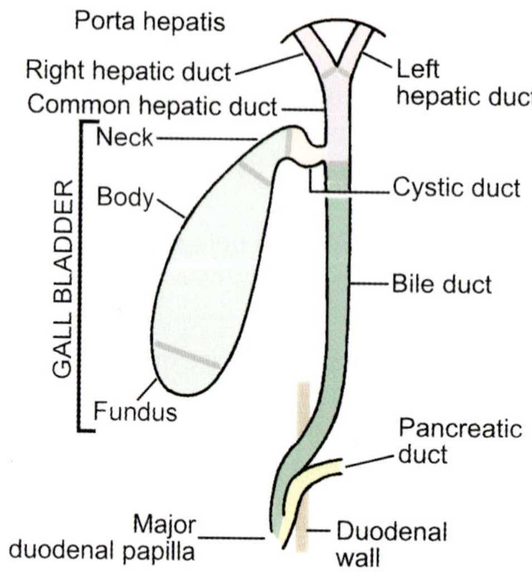


**28.16:** Scheme to show the parts of the extrahepatic biliary apparatus

5. a. Just outside the duodenal wall the bile duct is joined by the pancreatic duct.
   b. The two ducts pierce the muscular wall of the duodenum obliquely (28.17) and then descend in the submucosa.
   c. The bile and pancreatic ducts may open separately on the major duodenal papilla, or may join (at a variable distance above the papilla) to form a common passage called the ***hepatopancreatic ampulla***.

## WANT TO KNOW MORE?

6. The bile duct is supplied by branches from the hepatic, cystic and superior pancreaticoduodenal arteries (Chapter 29). The veins join those from the gall bladder and ultimately end in the portal vein.
7. Lymphatics from the gall bladder and bile duct drain to hepatic nodes (including cystic node) and coeliac nodes.

## Sphincters Related to the Bile and Pancreatic Ducts

1. a. The terminal part of the bile duct is surrounded (just above its junction with the pancreatic duct) by a ring of smooth muscle that forms the ***sphincter choledochus*** (choledochus = bile duct) (28.18). This sphincter is always present.
   b. It normally keeps the lower end of the bile duct closed. As a result, bile formed in the liver keeps accumulating in the gall bladder (and also undergoes considerable concentration).
2. a. When food enters the duodenum (especially a fatty meal) the sphincter opens and bile stored in the gall bladder is poured into the duodenum.
   b. The sphincter choledochus is, therefore, essential for filling of the gall bladder.
3. Another less developed sphincter is usually (but not always) present around the terminal part of the pancreatic duct. This is the ***sphincter pancreaticus***.
4. A third sphincter surrounds the hepatopancreatic ampulla and is called the ***sphincter ampullae***. The sphincter ampullae may extend upwards to enclose the lower parts of the bile and pancreatic ducts.

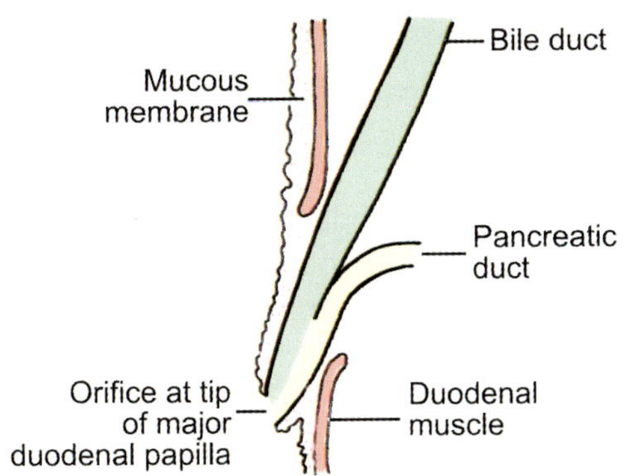


**28.17:** Terminal parts of the bile and pancreatic ducts

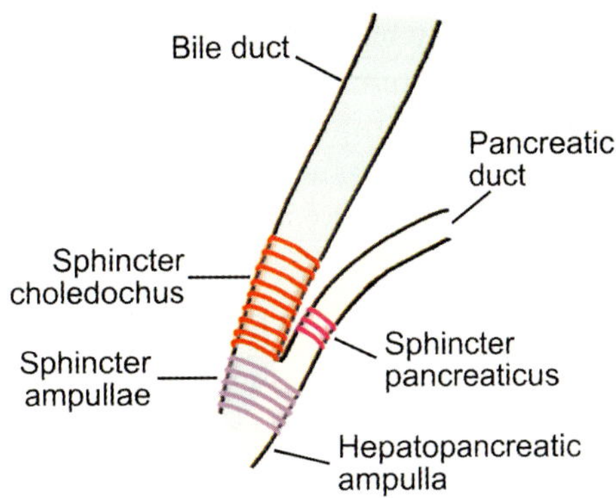


**28.18:** Sphincters around the terminal parts of the bile and pancreatic ducts

5. The sphincters named above are often referred to collectively as the ***sphincter of Oddi*** (although this term strictly applies only to the sphincter ampullae).

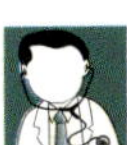

## CLINICAL CORRELATION

### Clinical Correlation of Gall Bladder and Biliary Ducts

#### *Oral Cholecystography*

1. This is a method to visualise the gall bladder.
2. A suitable radio-opaque dye is given by mouth. It is absorbed by the gut and reaches the liver through the portal circulation.
3. It is then secreted into bile that is concentrated in the gall bladder making it visible in a skiagram.

#### *Intravenous Cholangiography*

1. A suitable radio-opaque dye is injected intravenously.
2. It reaches the liver and is secreted into bile.
3. It permits visualisation of the bile ducts.

### CONGENITAL MALFORMATIONS

The extrahepatic biliary apparatus shows many variations in its anatomy. A surgeon operating on the region has to be familiar with them.

#### Gall Bladder

1. The fundus of the gall bladder may be folded on itself to form a cap like structure called the ***phrygian cap***.
2. The wall of the infundibulum may project downwards as a pouch (***Hartmann's pouch***) that may be adherent to the cystic duct or even to the bile duct.
3. In the condition called ***floating gall bladder,*** the gall bladder is lined by peritoneum on all sides. Such a gall bladder can undergo torsion.
4. Alternatively, the gall bladder may be embedded in liver substance.
5. Instead of lying in its normal position the gall bladder may lie transversely under the right lobe, or may lie under the left lobe of the liver.
6. The gall bladder may open directly into the bile duct (***sessile bladder***), the cystic duct being missing.
7. Agenesis, atresia, or duplication may affect the gall bladder or one of the ducts.

#### Duct System

1. Any of the ducts may show abnormalities of length, atresia, or duplication.

2. The cystic duct may have an abnormal termination.
   a. It may join the common hepatic duct on its left side (instead of the normal right side).
   b. It may end in the right hepatic duct.
   c. May even open into the stomach.
3. Sometimes, the cystic duct is very long and descends anterior to the duodenum before joining the common hepatic duct.

***Some Other Correlations of Gall Bladder and Biliary Ducts***

1. Inflammation of the gall bladder is called ***cholecystitis***.
2. Chronic cholecystitis is often associated with the formation of stones in the gall bladder (***cholelithiasis***).
3. Surgical removal of the gall bladder is called ***cholecystectomy***.
4. a. Pain arising in the gall bladder is felt over the right hypochondrium.
   b. The pain may radiate to the right scapula or right shoulder especially if the subdiaphragmatic parietal peritoneum is involved.
5. To test for gall bladder inflammation, the physician places a finger over the site where the right costal margin meets the linea semilunaris (or at the tip of the 9th costal cartilage) and asks the patient to take a deep breath. The presence of sharp pain is referred to as ***Murphy's sign***.
6. When a gall stone tries to pass through the bile duct it causes severe pain called ***biliary colic*** which is felt in the epigastrium.
7. Obstruction to the biliary duct system from any cause leads to the development of jaundice. Such obstruction is often associated with a tumour of the pancreas.
8. a. In many cases, the bile and pancreatic ducts retain separate lumens right up to the tip of the major duodenal papilla.
   b. In some cases, they open into a common hepatopancreatic duct (or ampulla of Vater) that is highly variable in length.
   c. When this common duct is long, obstruction near the orifice (by a calculus, or by spasm of muscle) can lead to regurgitation of bile into the pancreatic duct.
   d. This can lead to pancreatitis.
9. a. The wall of the gall bladder may become adherent to that of the duodenum and erosion here may lead to the formation of a fistula between the two.
   b. Gall stones can thus pass into the duodenum.
10. Following operations on the biliary tract an ***external biliary fistula*** may form.
11. A radiological technique for investigation of the gall bladder (cholecystography) is described above.

## THE PANCREAS

1. The pancreas is a large gland present in close relationship to the duodenum and stomach (28.19).
2. It lies obliquely on the posterior abdominal wall, partly to the right of the median plane and partly to the left.
3. Its right end is enlarged and is called the ***head***.
4. Next to the head there is a short, somewhat constricted part called the ***neck***.
5. The neck is continuous with the main part of the gland that is called the ***body***.
6. The left extremity of the pancreas is thin and is called the ***tail.***
7. The head lies in the C-shaped space bounded by the duodenum. The neck is placed behind the pylorus and the body of the pancreas lies behind the body of the stomach.
8. The neck and body are separated from the stomach by the lesser sac.
9. The tail lies in the lienorenal ligament and its tip comes in contact with the spleen.
10. A projection arising from the lower left part of the head is called the ***uncinate process*** of the pancreas (28.19).

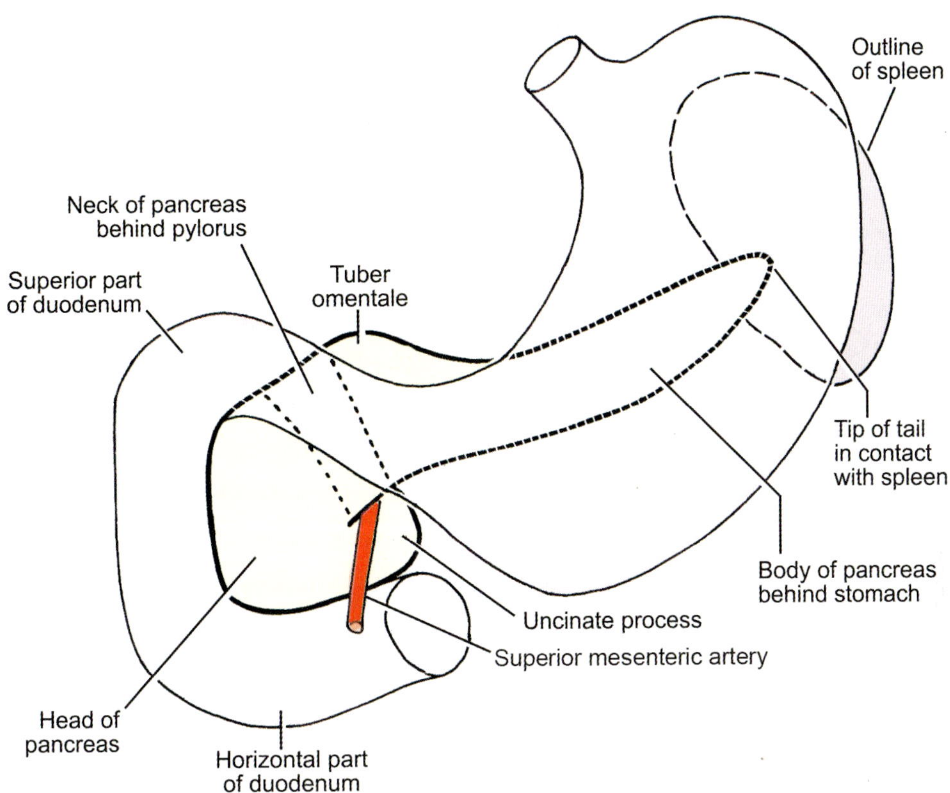


**28.19:** Parts of the pancreas and their relationship to the stomach, the duodenum and the spleen

11. a. The head and neck of the pancreas have anterior and posterior surfaces.
    b. The body of the pancreas has three surfaces (28.20).
       i. The anterior surface faces anteriorly and upwards.
       ii. The inferior surface faces downwards and somewhat forwards.
       iii. The posterior surface faces backwards.
       iv. The anterior and inferior surfaces meet at the anterior border. The anterior and posterior surfaces at the superior border and the inferior and posterior surfaces meet at the inferior border.
12. A part of the body of the pancreas projects upwards beyond the lesser curvature of the stomach and comes in contact with the lesser omentum. This projection is called the ***tuber omentale*** (28.19).
13. With this preliminary orientation, we can now proceed to consider the other relationships of the pancreas that are as follows.
14. The pancreas is placed in front of the inferior vena cava, the abdominal aorta, and the left kidney.
    a. The head of the pancreas is placed in front of the inferior vena cava.
    b. The aorta is related to the right end of the body of the pancreas.
    c. Between the abdominal aorta and the left kidney the body of the pancreas lies on the left crus of the diaphragm, the left suprarenal gland, and the left renal vessels.
15. The superior mesenteric artery arises from the aorta deep to the pancreas. Lower down the artery lies in front of the uncinate process that intervenes between the superior mesenteric artery and the abdominal aorta (28.19).
16. In 28.21 shows the relationship of the pancreas to the superior mesenteric and splenic veins as they join to form the portal vein.
    a. The portal vein lies behind the neck of the pancreas, intervening between it and the inferior vena cava.
    b. The splenic vein lies behind the body of the pancreas, partially separating it from the other structures behind it.

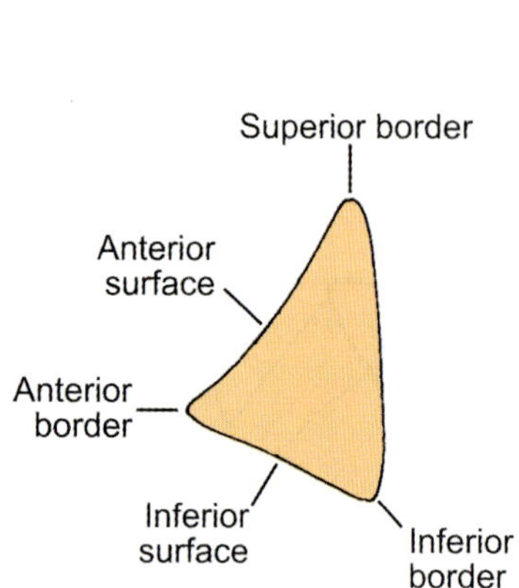


**28.20:** Sagittal section through the body of the pancreas to show its surfaces and borders

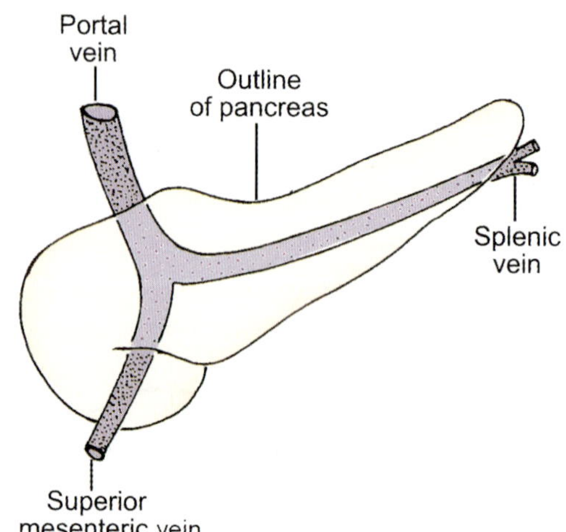


**28.21:** Relationship of portal vein, superior mesenteric vein and splenic vein to the pancreas

17. The posterior edge of the greater omentum and the upper end of the transverse mesocolon are attached to the anterior aspect of the pancreas.
    a. On the body of the pancreas, the attachment is along the anterior border.
    b. The anterior surface of the body of the pancreas is covered by peritoneum continuous with the anterior of the two layers forming the greater omentum, and lies in the posterior wall of the lesser sac.
    c. The body of the pancreas (anterior surface) is related anteriorly to the stomach from which it is separated by the lesser sac.
18. The inferior surface of the body of the pancreas is lined by peritoneum continuous with the posterior layer of the transverse mesocolon. It is related to the greater sac.
19. The head of the pancreas is related anteriorly to the transverse colon.
20. The neck of the pancreas is related anteriorly to the pylorus.
    a. The peritoneum lining the posterior aspect of the pylorus is reflected on to the anterior aspect of the neck of the pancreas.
    b. This is how the right boundary of the lesser sac of peritoneum is formed at this level.
21. The gastroduodenal artery descends over the pancreas immediately in front of the neck.
22. Superiorly, the head of the pancreas is related to the superior part of the duodenum.
23. The body of the pancreas is related superiorly to the coeliac trunk (which lies just above the tuber omentale), the hepatic artery and the splenic artery.
24. Inferiorly, the head of the pancreas is related to the horizontal part of the duodenum.
25. The inferior surface of the body of the pancreas is in the contact with the duodenojejunal flexure, the left colic flexure, and coils of jejunum.

## Ducts of the Pancreas

Secretions of the pancreas are poured into the duodenum through two ducts (28.22).

1. The ***main pancreatic duct*** begins in the tail of the pancreas, and passes to the right through the body.
    a. At the neck of the pancreas, it turns downwards and backwards and ends by joining the bile duct just outside the duodenal wall.
    b. The walls of the bile and the main pancreatic ducts join each other here, but their lumina remain separate as the ducts descend through the muscle wall and submucosa of the duodenum (28.17).

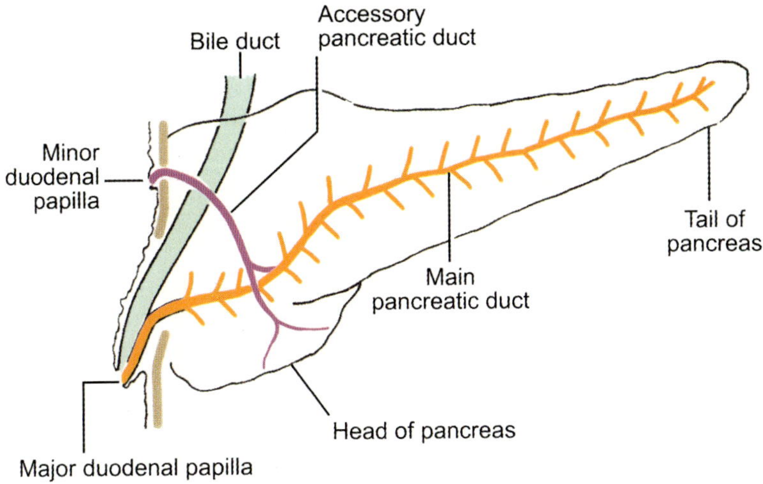


28.22: Schematic diagram of the ducts of the pancreas

c. Usually, the two ducts unite a short distance above the major duodenal papilla to form the hepatopancreatic ampulla. They may, however, have separate openings on the papilla.
d. The terminal part of the main pancreatic duct is surrounded by the sphincter pancreaticus.

2. The ***accessory pancreatic duct*** begins in the lower part of the head of the pancreas.
   a. It runs upwards crossing in front of the main duct and opens into the duodenum at the minor duodenal papilla (which lies a short distance above and in front of the major papilla).
   b. The main and accessory pancreatic ducts usually anastomose with each other. Occasionally, the duodenal end of the accessory duct may be blind. In that case the duct drains into the duodenum through the anastomosis with the main duct. The accessory duct may be surrounded near its termination by a sphincter.

## WANT TO KNOW MORE?

### Blood Supply, Lymphatic Drainage and Nerve Supply of Pancreas

1. The pancreas is supplied by branches from the splenic artery and from the superior and inferior pancreaticoduodenal arteries (Chapter 29).
2. The veins drain into the splenic, superior mesenteric and portal veins. We have seen (28.21) that these veins are closely related to the pancreas.
3. Lymphatics of the pancreas drain to pancreaticosplenic nodes along the splenic artery; and to pancreatico-duodenal and coeliac nodes. Some vessels reach the superior mesenteric nodes. For details see Chapter 34.
4. The pancreas is innervated by autonomic nerves, both sympathetic and parasympathetic that travel to it through the plexus around the splenic artery.

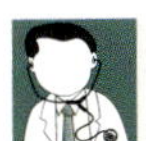

## CLINICAL CORRELATION

### Clinical Correlation of Pancreas

#### *Congenital Malformations*

1. The pancreas is derived from ventral and dorsal buds that later fuse. Most of the organ is derived from the dorsal bud. The parts derived from the two buds may remain separate resulting in a ***divided pancreas***.

2. The parts of the pancreas arising from dorsal and ventral buds have independent ducts.
   a. The duct draining the part of the pancreas derived from the dorsal bud at first opens into the duodenum at the minor duodenal papilla.
   b. The duct of the ventral bud opens at the major duodenal papilla (along with the bile duct).
   c. When the dorsal and ventral parts of the pancreas fuse their ducts anastomose.
   d. The main pancreatic duct is formed as follows. Its distal part is derived from the (distal part of the) duct of the dorsal bud while its proximal part is derived from the duct of the ventral bud.
   e. The proximal part of the duct of the dorsal bud remains narrow and forms the accessory pancreatic duct.
   f. In some cases, the duct of the dorsal bud retains its embryonic form and in that case the main drainage of the pancreas is at the minor duodenal papilla. This condition is referred as ***inversion of pancreatic ducts***.
3. Pancreatic tissue may develop all round the duodenum (***annular pancreas***) and can be a cause of obstruction to the duodenum.
4. ***Accessory pancreatic tissue*** may be present in the walls of the stomach, the duodenum, the jejunum, or the gall bladder. It can also be present in the spleen, and in the wall of a Meckel's diverticulum.
5. ***Cystic fibrosis*** is a congenital anomaly affecting the secretory elements of the pancreas. Pancreatic insufficiency leads to malabsorption.
6. ***Congenital cysts*** may be present in the pancreas.

*Other Correlations*

1. The beta cells of pancreatic islets produce insulin, deficiency of which causes ***diabetes mellitus***.
2. Inflammation of the pancreas is called ***pancreatitis***. It is often associated with collection of fluid in the lesser sac (***pseudopancreatic cyst***). A stricture may develop in the transverse colon where it overlies the pancreas.
3. *Tumours*:
   a. Carcinoma of the pancreas is relatively common. It can lead to biliary obstruction and jaundice. It can also cause obstruction at the pylorus or duodenum, and ascites by pressure on the portal vein.
   b. In some cases of carcinoma of the head of the pancreas, the organ is removed along with the duodenum (***pancreatico-duodenectomy***).
   c. Tumours arising from beta cells of pancreatic islets (***beta cell tumours*** or ***insulinoma***) can produce features of hyperinsulinism.
   d. A gastrin producing cell tumour can be responsible for repeated formation of peptic ulcers (***Zollinger Ellison syndrome***).
4. The pancreas may be eroded by an ulcer on the posterior wall of the stomach.

## THE SPLEEN

1. The spleen is a solid organ, irregularly oval in shape.
   a. It is about 12 cm long and 7 cm broad.
   b. It lies in the left hypochondrium, behind the stomach.
2. Posteriorly, the spleen rests on the diaphragm opposite the ninth, tenth and eleventh ribs (28.23). Its long axis corresponds to that of the tenth rib.
3. The spleen has a ***medial end*** that is directed medially, upwards and backwards. A ***lateral end*** that is directed laterally, forwards and downwards.
4. The medial end lies about 4 cm from the midline at the level of the spine of the tenth thoracic vertebra. The lateral end reaches up to the midaxillary line.
5. The medial and lateral ends are joined by ***upper*** and ***lower borders***. The upper border is sharp, while the lower is blunt. One or more notches are present on the upper (or anterior) border.
6. The spleen has a ***diaphragmatic surface*** and a ***visceral surface*** that are separated from each other by the upper and lower borders.

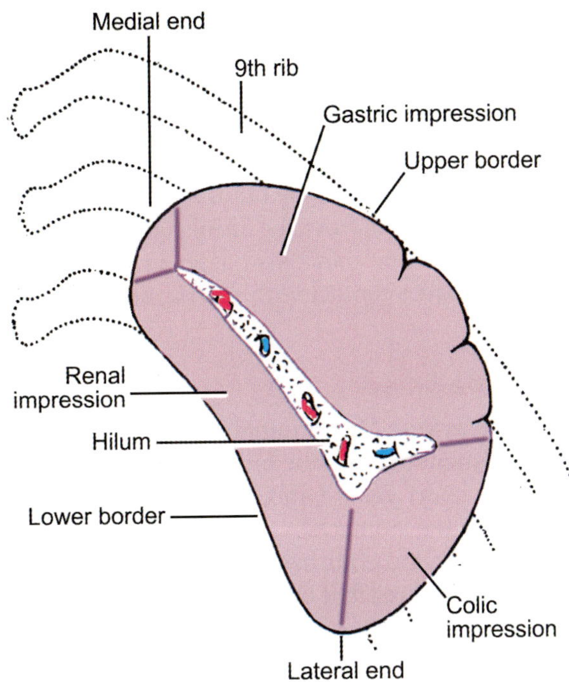


**28.23:** Spleen as seen from the front

7. The diaphragmatic surface is convex and is separated from the diaphragm only by peritoneum. The diaphragm separates this surface from the lower parts of the left lung and pleura. The lung is related only to the upper part of the spleen, but the pleura extends to its lower margin.
8. The visceral surface of the spleen is shown in 28.23. It is divided into three roughly triangular areas:
   a. The largest of these areas, placed anterosuperiorly, comes into contact with the stomach and is called the ***gastric impression***.
   b. The posteromedial part of the visceral surface comes into contact with the left kidney. This part is therefore, called the ***renal impression***.
   c. Anteroinferiorly the spleen has a ***colic impression*** that comes in contact with the left colic flexure.
9. The region lying along the junction of these three impressions of the visceral surface is the ***hilum***. The spleen is penetrated here by branches of the splenic artery and vein.
10. The tail of the pancreas comes in contact with the hilum of the spleen, near the colic impression.
    Further details of the relations of the spleen are as follows.

## WANT TO KNOW MORE?

*Peritoneal Relations*

1. The spleen develops in the upper part of the dorsal mesogastrium.
   a. In later life this part of the mesogastrium is represented by the ***gastrosplenic ligament*** that passes from the greater curvature of the stomach to the hilum of the spleen.
   b. It is also represented by the ***lienorenal*** (or ***splenorenal) ligament*** that passes from the hilum to the front of the left kidney.
2. When the peritoneum lining the posterior surface of the stomach is traced to the greater curvature, it becomes continuous with the anterior (or right) layer of the gastrosplenic ligament. At the hilum of the spleen this layer becomes directly continuous with the right layer of the lienorenal ligament.

3. When the peritoneum lining the anterior surface of the stomach is traced to the greater curvature it becomes continuous with the posterior (or left) layer of the gastrosplenic ligament.
   a. At the hilum of the spleen, this layer passes on to the surfaces of the spleen lining (in that order) its gastric impression, the diaphragmatic surface and the renal impression, and thus returns to the hilum.
   b. Here, it becomes continuous with the left layer of the lienorenal ligament. In this way, the spleen comes to be lined all round by peritoneum except at the hilum.
4. The spleen is separated from the diaphragm, from the kidney and from the stomach, by a part of the greater sac of peritoneum. However, the tail of the pancreas passes in the interval between the two layers of the lienorenal ligament and comes into direct contact with splenic tissue.

## Blood Supply and Innervation of the Spleen

1. The spleen is supplied by the splenic artery. The terminal part of the artery divides into a number of branches that pass through the lienorenal ligament to enter the hilum of the spleen.
2. The splenic artery also gives off the short gastric and left gastroepiploic branches. These branches enter the gastrosplenic ligament and thus reach the stomach.
3. The splenic vein accompanies the artery and ends in the portal vein.
4. The spleen receives autonomic nerves that reach it by running along the plexus surrounding the splenic artery.

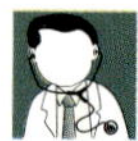

## CLINICAL CORRELATION

### Spleen

*Congenital Malformations*

1. The spleen may show lobulation.
2. Accessory spleens (***splenuneuli***) may be present in structures near the organ including the gastrosplenic and lienorenal ligaments, the hilum of the spleen itself, the pancreas, and along the splenic artery.
3. Rarely, the spleen may be absent.
4. Congenital cysts may be present in the spleen.

*Other Correlations*

1. Enlargement of the spleen (***splenomegaly***) occurs in many diseases.
   a. In India, the most common cause of enlargement is malaria.
   b. Enlargement also takes place in portal hypertension.
   c. A normal spleen does not extend anteriorly beyond the midaxillary line. When enlarged considerably (to almost twice its normal size) the spleen projects from under the costal margin and can be felt on palpation of the abdomen.
2. Surgical removal of the spleen is called ***splenectomy***. Because of the close relationship of the tail of the pancreas to the hilum of the spleen the former can be injured during splenectomy.
3. The spleen can be ruptured as a result of trauma (specially when enlarged). This can lead to death from internal haemorrhage. Immediate splenectomy may save the patient.
4. Radio-opaque dyes can be introduced into the portal venous system through a needle introduced into the spleen (***splenovenography*** or ***splenoportography***). The technique has now been largely replaced by coeliac angiography during the venous filling phase.

29

CHAPTER

# Blood Vessels of Stomach, Intestines, Liver, Pancreas and Spleen

## INTRODUCTION

1. The arteries that supply the stomach, the intestines, the liver, the pancreas and the spleen are the ***ventral branches*** of the abdominal aorta. These are:
   a. The ***coeliac trunk***
   b. The ***superior mesenteric artery***
   c. The ***inferior mesenteric artery***.
2. The veins draining these organs do not drain directly into the systemic circulation.
   a. Blood in them first drains into the portal vein through which it reaches the liver.
   b. After passing through the sinusoids of the liver the blood reaches the inferior vena cava through hepatic veins.

## THE COELIAC TRUNK AND ITS BRANCHES

1.a. The coeliac trunk arises from the front of the uppermost part of the abdominal aorta just below the aortic opening in the diaphragm.

b. The trunk is only about one centimeter long. It passes forwards and terminates by dividing into three branches: These are:
   i. The left gastric artery
   ii. The hepatic artery
   iii. The splenic arteries.

### WANT TO KNOW MORE?

2. The coeliac trunk is covered in front by the peritoneum lining the posterior wall of the lesser sac.
   a. It is related above to the diaphragm.
   b. The caudate process of the liver lies above and to its right.
   c. The stomach lies below and to its left.
   d. The pancreas and splenic vein lie below it.
   e. On either side, the coeliac trunk is related to the corresponding crus of the diaphragm and to the coeliac ganglion.
   f. The coeliac trunk is surrounded by branches of the ***coeliac plexus*** of nerves.

### The Left Gastric Artery

1. This artery arises from the coeliac trunk and passes upwards and to the left ('a' in 29.1) on the posterior abdominal wall (formed here by the diaphragm).

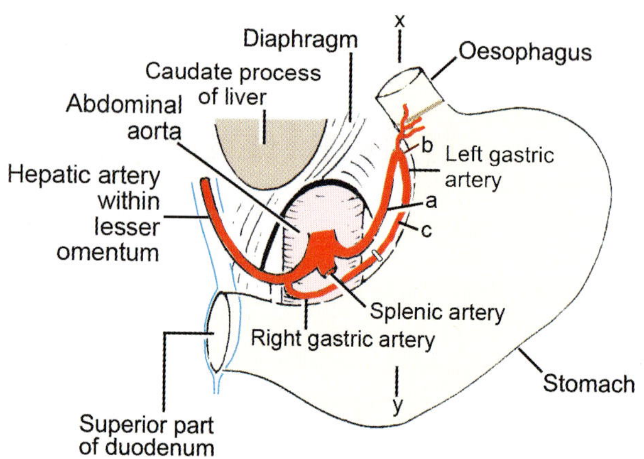


**29.1:** Scheme to show course of the left and right gastric arteries

2. Reaching near the cardiac end of the stomach the artery turns forwards and passes from the diaphragm to the lesser curvature of the stomach ('b' in 29.1).
3. The artery then runs to the right along the lesser curvature of the stomach ('c' in 29.1) between the two layers of the lesser omentum.
4. It ends by anastomosing with the right gastric artery.
5. The left gastric artery gives branches to:
   a. The oesophagus
   b. Both surfaces of the stomach
   c. Some oesophageal branches pass through the oesophageal hiatus of the diaphragm and anastomose with branches to the oesophagus from the thoracic aorta.

## The Hepatic Artery

1. The hepatic artery first runs to the right and somewhat downwards on the posterior abdominal wall (29.1) to reach the superior part of the duodenum.
2. It then passes forwards above the first part of the duodenum and below the epiploic foramen.
3. Finally, it turns upwards to enter the free margin of the lesser omentum. It now lies anterior to the foramen epiploicum.
4. Ascending in the lesser omentum it reaches the porta hepatis where it divides into right and left branches for the corresponding lobes of the liver.
5. Within the free margin of the lesser omentum the artery lies in front of the portal vein with the bile duct to its right (29.2).

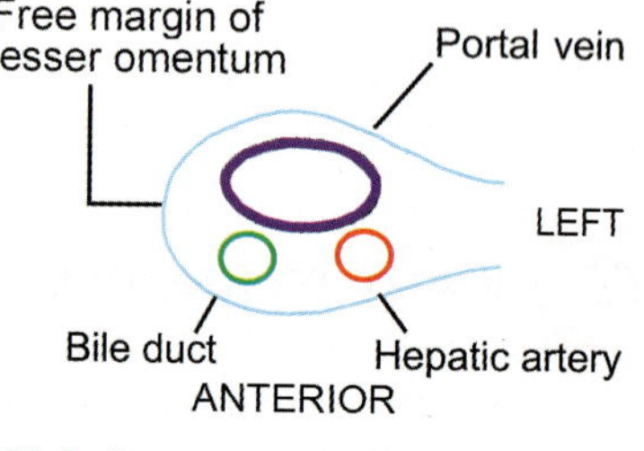


**29.2:** Structures in the free margin of the lesser omentum

Branches of the hepatic artery are as follows:

1. The right gastric artery
2. The gastroduodenal artery
3. The supraduodenal artery (sometimes)
4. The cystic artery
5. Terminal hepatic branches (29.3).

### Right Gastric Artery

1. The right gastric artery arises as the hepatic artery lies above the duodenum.
2. It passes to the left along the lesser curvature of the stomach to anastomose with the left gastric artery.

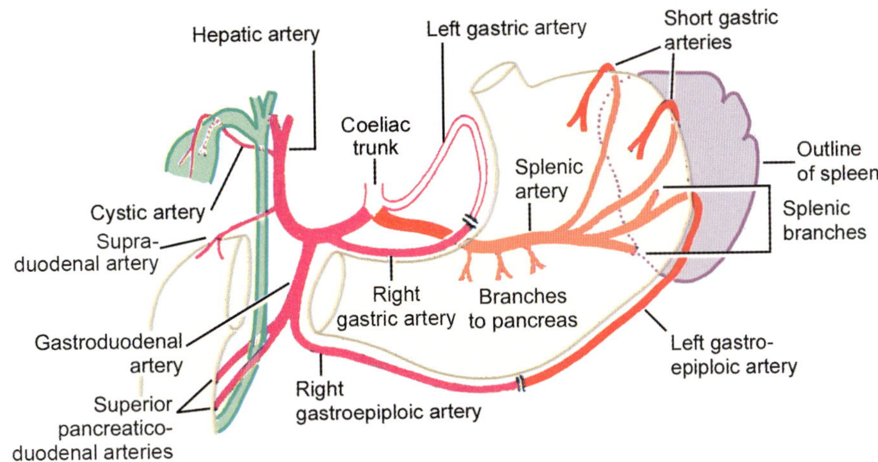


**29.3:** Scheme to show the distribution of the hepatic and splenic arteries

### Gastroduodenal Artery

1. The gastroduodenal artery also arises from the hepatic artery as the latter lies above the duodenum (29.3).
2. It descends ***behind*** the superior part of the duodenum. Here it lies in front of the neck of the pancreas and to the left of the bile duct.
3. It ends by dividing into the right gastroepiploic and superior pancreaticoduodenal arteries (anterior and posterior).
4. The gastroduodenal artery also gives off small branches to the stomach, the pancreas, and the duodenum.
5. It sometimes gives off the supraduodenal artery (See below).

### Right Gastroepiploic Artery

1. The right gastroepiploic artery (29.3) runs to the right along the greater curvature of the stomach (between the two layers of the greater omentum).
2. It ends by anastomosing with the left gastroepiploic artery (a branch of the splenic artery).
3. The right gastroepiploic artery gives branches to the stomach and to the greater omentum.

### Superior Pancreaticoduodenal Arteries

1. There are two superior pancreaticoduodenal arteries: anterior and posterior. They descend respectively anterior and posterior to the junction of the second part of the duodenum with the pancreas.
2. They supply the pancreas, and the duodenum up to the level of the major duodenal papilla. Here, they anastomose with the inferior pancreaticoduodenal artery (branch of superior mesenteric artery).
3. Note that the part of the duodenum above the major duodenal papilla is a derivative of the foregut.
   a. It is, therefore, supplied by branches of the coeliac trunk, which is the artery of the foregut.
   b. The rest of the duodenum is derived from the midgut, the artery of which is the superior mesenteric. The part of the duodenum below the major duodenal papilla is, therefore, supplied by the branches of the superior mesenteric artery.

### Supraduodenal Artery

1. The supraduodenal artery may arise from the gastroduodenal artery (29.3) or directly from the hepatic artery.
2. It supplies the superior part of the duodenum.

### Cystic Artery

1. The cystic artery (29.3) usually arises from the right branch of the hepatic artery.
2. It passes to the right behind the hepatic and cystic ducts to reach the gall bladder that it supplies.

3. It also gives branches to the hepatic ducts and the upper part of the bile duct.
4. Its origin and course are highly variable.

### Hepatic Branches

The right and left hepatic branches enter the corresponding lobe of the liver and divide within them in a fairly constant manner. As a result of this fact the liver can be divided into a number of arterial segments (described in Chapter 28).

## The Splenic Artery

1. The splenic artery arises from the coeliac trunk.
2. Its initial part runs to the left on the posterior abdominal wall along the upper border of the pancreas (29.3). Here, it is separated from the stomach by the lesser sac of peritoneum (29.4).
3. Reaching the front of the left kidney the artery passes into the lienorenal ligament to reach the hilum of the spleen where it divides into several branches. These are as follows (29.3):
   a. Several branches are given off to the pancreas, as the artery runs along this organ.
   b. A number of ***short gastric arteries*** arise near the hilum of the spleen. They pass through the gastrosplenic ligament to supply the fundus of the stomach.
   c. The ***left gastroepiploic artery*** arises near the hilum of the spleen. It passes downwards, forwards and to the right through the gastrosplenic ligament to reach the greater curvature of the stomach. It gives branches to the stomach, and to the greater omentum and ends by anastomosing with the right gastroepiploic artery.
   d. The ***splenic branches*** enter the hilum of the spleen to supply the organ.
      i. From the above account of the coeliac trunk and its branches it will be seen that, apart from the liver, pancreas and spleen, the trunk supplies the infradiaphragmatic part of the gut up to the middle of the descending part of the duodenum (up to the major duodenal papilla).
      ii. This part of the gut is derived from the embryonic foregut. The coeliac trunk is, therefore, described as the ***artery of the foregut*** (29.5).

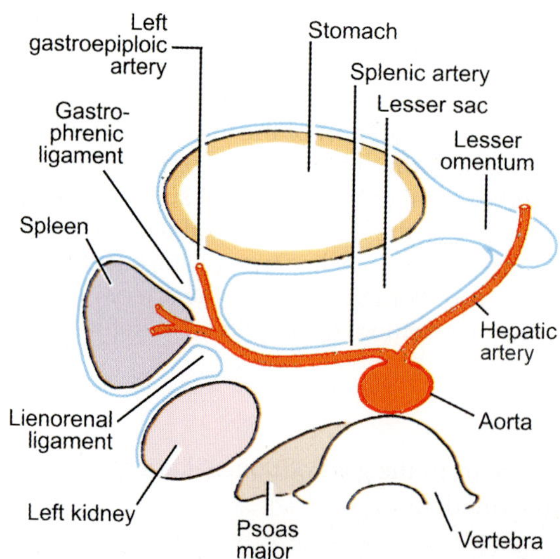


**29.4:** Schematic transverse section to show the course of the splenic artery

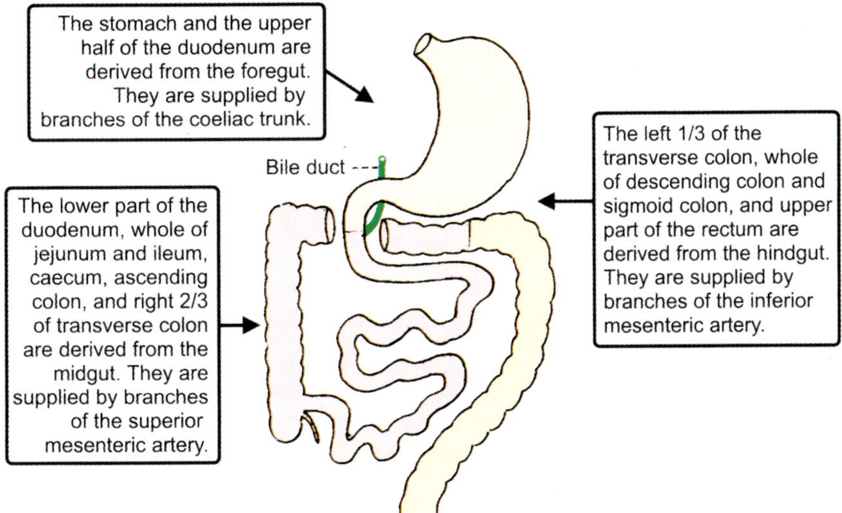


**29.5:** Scheme to show parts of the gut supplied by the coeliac trunk, the superior mesenteric and inferior mesenteric arteries

## SUPERIOR MESENTERIC ARTERY

1. a. The superior mesenteric artery is the artery of the midgut.
   b. Its area of supply extends cranially up to the middle of the descending part of the duodenum, and caudally to the junction of the right two-thirds and left one-third of the transverse colon.
2. The artery arises from the front of the abdominal aorta a little below the coeliac trunk and runs downwards and forwards.
3. Its initial part lies over the posterior abdominal wall.
4. The artery then crosses in front of the horizontal part of the duodenum to enter the root of the mesentery.
5. Passing through the root of the mesentery it runs downwards and to the right to reach the ileocaecal junction.
6. The artery gives off numerous branches to the gut and these are described below.

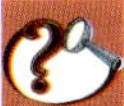

### WANT TO KNOW MORE?

**Relations of Superior Mesenteric Artery**

1. The initial part of the artery lies over the posterior abdominal wall.
   a. This part lies deep to the pancreas and the splenic vein, and superficial to the left renal vein that separates it from the front of the aorta.
   b. The uncinate process of the pancreas also lies deep to it.
2. The next part of the artery passes in front of the horizontal part of the duodenum. It then passes into the root of the mesentery. This part of the artery crosses the following:
   a. Inferior vena cava
   b. Right ureter
   c. Right psoas major.
3. The artery is accompanied by the superior mesenteric vein, which lies to its right side, and by a plexus of nerves.

## Branches of Superior Mesenteric Artery

1. a. The ***inferior pancreaticoduodenal artery*** is the first branch.
   b. It divides into anterior and posterior branches that run upwards on corresponding aspects of the head of the pancreas.
   c. They supply the pancreas and duodenum and anastomose with the branches of the superior pancreaticoduodenal arteries.
2. a. The ***branches to the jejunum and ileum*** are many.
   b. They arise from the left side of the superior mesenteric artery and pass through the mesentery to reach the gut.
   c. The branches anastomose with each other to form a series of arches from which numerous straight arteries arise to supply the gut (29.6).
3. The ***ileocolic artery*** arises from the right side of the lower part of the superior mesenteric artery. It runs on the posterior abdominal wall a little above the parent vessel.
   a. It ends by dividing into superior and inferior branches.
   b. The inferior branch anastomoses with the terminal part of the superior mesenteric artery.
   c. The superior branch anastomoses with the right colic artery.
   d. The ileocolic artery gives off various branches that supply the terminal part of the ileum, the caecum, the appendix and the lower one-third of the ascending colon (29.6).
4. The ***right colic artery*** arises from the right side of the superior mesenteric artery at about its middle.
   a. It passes to the right (on the posterior abdominal wall) to reach the ascending colon.
   b. It terminates by dividing into descending and ascending branches that anastomose with the ileocolic and middle colic arteries, respectively.
   c. The artery supplies the upper two-thirds of the ascending colon.

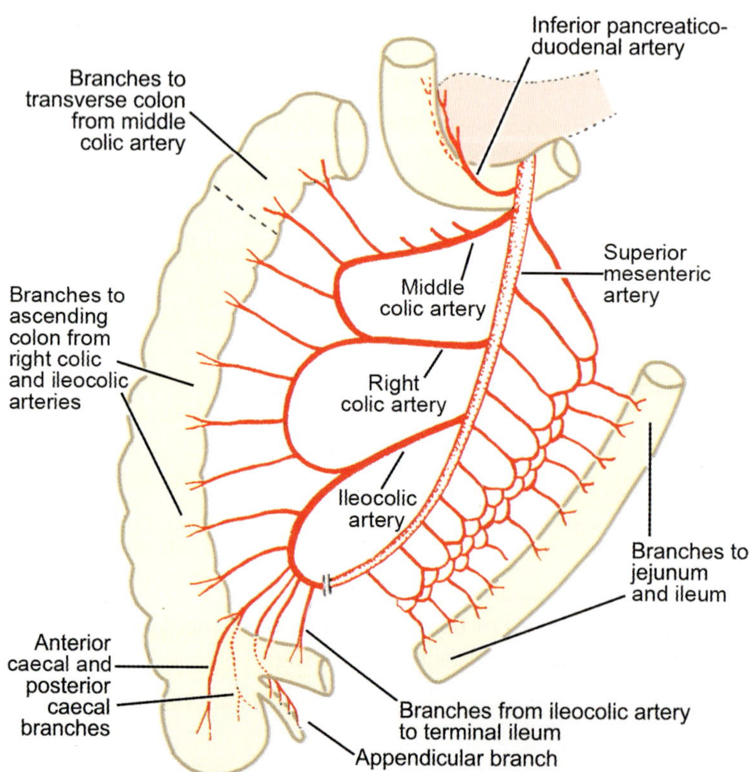


**29.6:** Distribution of superior mesenteric artery

5. The ***middle colic artery*** arises from the right side of the superior mesenteric artery just below the duodenum.
   a. It runs downwards into the transverse mesocolon to reach the transverse colon.
   b. Its branches anastomose (on the right side) with those of the right colic artery, and (on the left side) with those of the left colic artery (a branch of the inferior mesenteric artery).
   c. They supply the right two-thirds of the transverse colon.
      i. Note that the inferior pancreaticoduodenal, right colic and ileocolic branches have a retroperitoneal course (29.7).
      ii. The middle colic artery runs in the transverse mesocolon.
      iii. The jejunal and ileal branches traverse the mesentery of the small intestine.

## INFERIOR MESENTERIC ARTERY

The distribution of inferior mesenteric artery is shown in 29.8.

1. a. The inferior mesenteric artery supplies the hindgut.
   b. Its area of supply extends from the junction of the right two-thirds and left one-third of the transverse colon to the rectum.
2. The artery arises from the front of the aorta about 3 cm above its bifurcation. It runs downwards (and slightly to the left) over the posterior abdominal wall.
3. Beginning over the middle of the aorta (deep to the horizontal part of the duodenum) it gradually crosses to its left side. It then crosses the left common iliac artery below which its continuation is called the ***superior rectal artery***.
4. The branches given off by the inferior mesenteric artery are the left colic, sigmoid and superior rectal arteries.

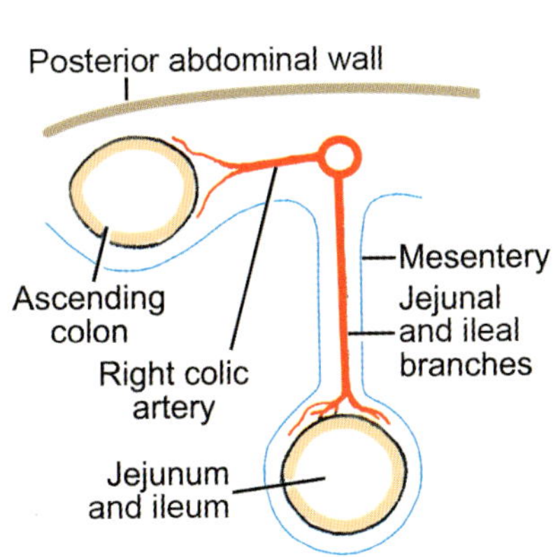


**29.7:** Scheme to show that some branches of the superior mesenteric artery are retroperitoneal while some pass through folds of peritoneum

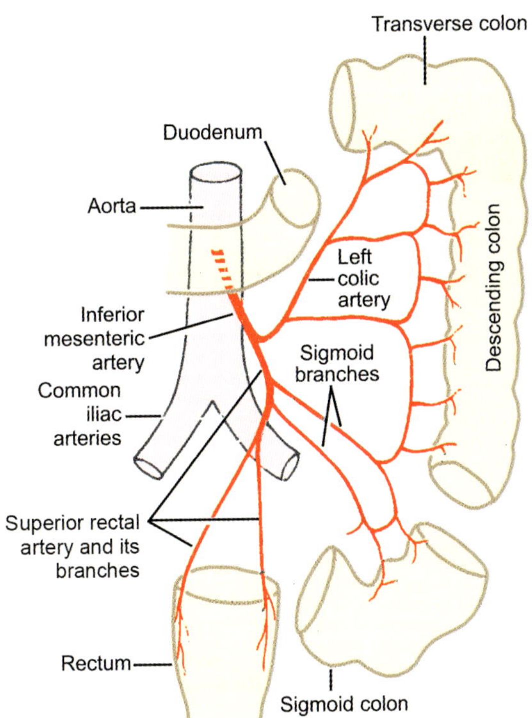


**29.8:** Distribution of inferior mesenteric artery

5. The ***left colic artery*** runs upwards and to the left behind the peritoneum of the posterior abdominal wall and divides into ascending and descending branches.
   a. The ascending branch enters the transverse mesocolon. Here, it anastomoses with the middle colic branch of the superior mesenteric artery.
   b. The various branches of the left colic artery subdivide and form arcades from which straight arteries arise to supply the left one-third of the transverse colon and most of the descending colon.
6. The ***sigmoid branches*** enter the pelvic mesocolon to reach the sigmoid colon. They anastomose with the lower branches of the left colic artery and help to supply the lower part of the descending colon.

### Superior Rectal Artery

1. The superior rectal artery is a continuation of the inferior mesenteric artery into the true pelvis. It runs across the left common iliac artery and vein to reach the rectum.
2. It divides into two main branches one of which descends on either side of the rectum and supplies it.
3. Their area of supply extends up to the sphincter ani externus.
4. They anastomose with the middle rectal artery (branch of internal iliac) and with the inferior rectal artery (branch of internal pudendal artery).

## THE HEPATIC PORTAL SYSTEM

1. a. Normally the arteries supplying an organ end in a set of capillaries from which blood is collected by veins that carry it to the heart (29.9A).
   b. In some cases, however, the veins from an organ enter another organ where they divide into a second set of capillaries (or sinusoids). Such an arrangement is called a ***portal system*** (29.9B).
2. The best example of a portal system is the hepatic portal system.
   a. The arteries supplying the abdominal part of the gastrointestinal tract (excluding the lower part of the anal canal) break up into capillaries in its wall (first set).
   b. Veins draining these capillaries ultimately end in the portal vein that enters the liver. Within the liver the portal vein divides into sinusoids (= second set of capillaries). This blood is returned to the heart through the hepatic veins and the inferior vena cava.
3. The main veins comprising the hepatic portal system are shown in 29.10.
   a. The portal vein is formed by the union of the ***superior mesenteric*** and ***splenic*** veins.
   b. The ***inferior mesenteric vein*** joins the splenic vein.

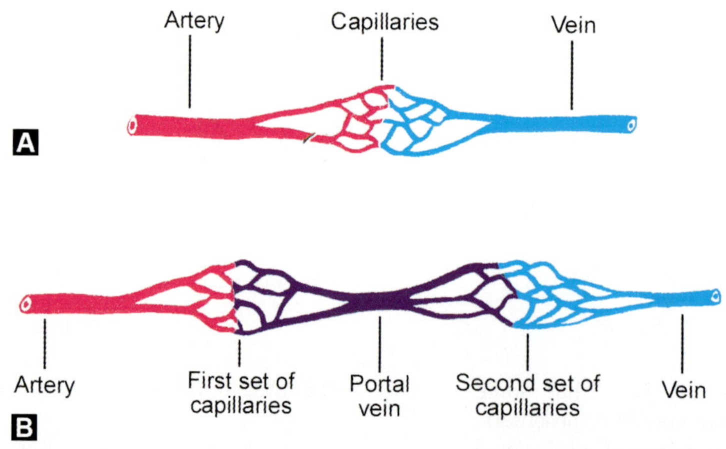


**29.9A and B:** Scheme to compare (A) systemic and (B) portal circulations

c. The right and left ***gastric veins*** drain directly into the portal vein.
d. The ***left gastroepiploic*** and ***short gastric*** veins drain into the splenic vein.
e. The ***right gastroepiploic vein*** drains into the superior mesenteric vein.

4. The splenic vein, the superior and inferior mesenteric veins, and the veins of the stomach accompany the corresponding arteries and have tributaries corresponding to branches of these arteries.
5. Note that veins corresponding to branches of the coeliac trunk end directly in the portal vein.

## Splenic Vein

1. Emerging from the hilum of the spleen, the splenic vein runs through the lienorenal ligament and then runs across the posterior abdominal wall, posterior to the body of the pancreas, and anterior to the left kidney.
2. It ends behind the neck of the pancreas by uniting with the superior mesenteric vein to form the portal vein (29.10).

## Portal Vein

1. The portal vein is formed by the union of the superior mesenteric and splenic veins.
2. The point of union lies at the level of the second lumbar vertebra, behind the neck of the pancreas.

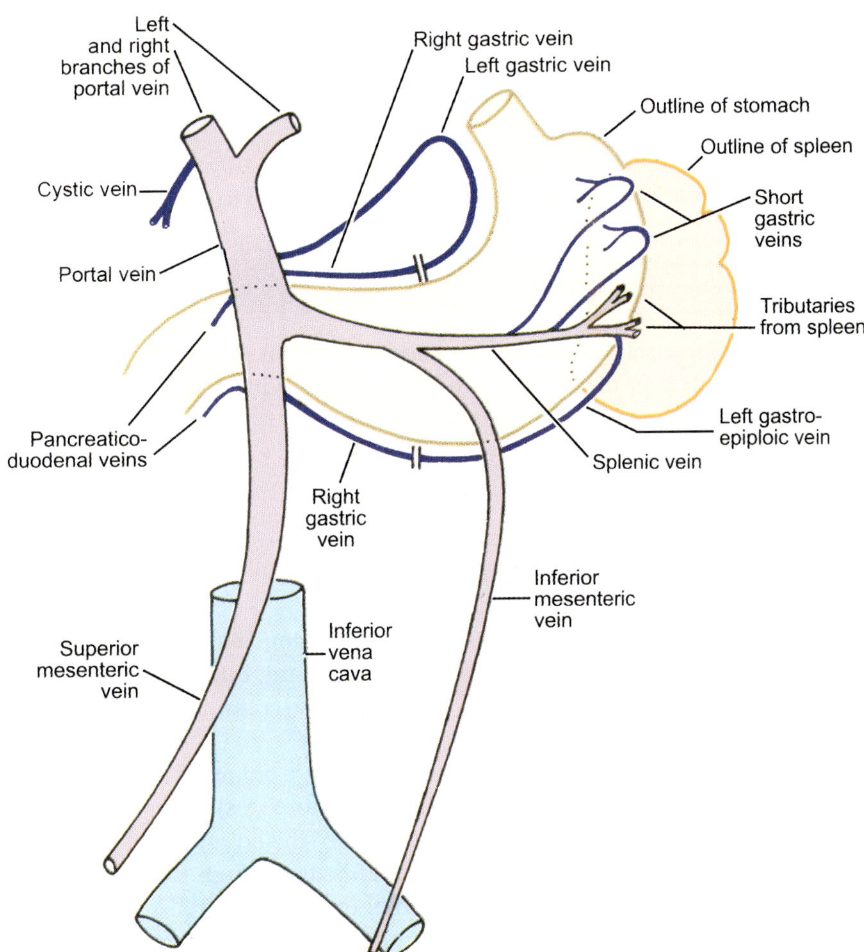


**29.10:** Scheme to show the tributaries of the portal vein

3. The vein passes upwards and to the right to reach the porta hepatis where it ends by dividing into right and left branches.
4. These branches enter the substance of the liver.

## WANT TO KNOW MORE?

*Relations of Portal Vein*

1. The portal vein has important relations (29.11 and 29.12). Its lower part is placed on the posterior abdominal wall, in front of the inferior vena cava.
2. This part lies behind the neck of the pancreas, and higher up behind the superior part of the duodenum.
3. Above the duodenum, the vein enters the free margin of the lesser omentum.
   a. It is now separated from the inferior vena cava by the epiploic foramen (29.11).
   b. As it enters the porta hepatis it is separated from the inferior vena cava by the caudate process of the liver.
4. The following additional relations may now be noted.
   a. The vein is separated from the superior part of the duodenum by the bile duct and the gastroduodenal artery.
   b. Within the free margin of the lesser omentum the bile duct and the hepatic artery are in front of it. The bile duct is to the right of the artery.
5. The right branch of the portal vein receives the cystic vein from the gall bladder. It is distributed to the right lobe of the liver.
6. The left branch of the portal vein is joined by the ligamentum teres (representing the obliterated left umbilical vein).
   a. It is connected to the inferior vena cava by the ligamentum venosum (obliterated ductus venosus).
   b. The left branch is distributed to the left lobe of the liver and also to the caudate and quadrate lobes.

## Hepatic Veins

1. The hepatic veins are terminal parts of an elaborate venous tree that permeates the liver.
2. The hepatic veins emerge from liver tissue that is in close contact with the upper part of the inferior vena cava, and immediately enter the vena cava.

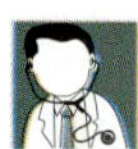

## CLINICAL CORRELATION

### Portosystemic Anastomosis and Associated Conditions

1. At certain sites veins of the portal system anastomose with systemic veins.
2. Normally, the flow through these communications is insignificant, but when there is obstruction to flow of blood in the portal circulation (e.g., by cirrhosis of the liver) these communications enlarge and serve as alternative channels of flow.
3. It is important to know the sites of such communications as these enlarged veins are of clinical significance.
4. The sites of communication (portosystemic or portocaval anastomoses) are as follows:
   a. The ***region of the umbilicus*** is drained by systemic veins of the anterior abdominal wall.
      i. Some small paraumbilical veins pass from the umbilicus through the falciform ligament to reach the liver where they anastomose with the left branch of the portal vein.
      ii. In portal obstruction, blood flows through paraumbilical veins into systemic veins at the umbilicus.
      iii. The superficial veins of the abdominal wall enlarge and are seen radiating from the umbilicus. (The appearance is called ***caput medusae***).

b. The ***lower end of the oesophagus*** drains partly into the left gastric vein (portal) and partly into the accessory hemiazygos vein (systemic).
   i. In portal obstruction, the communications between these two sets of veins enlarge to form swellings called ***oesophageal varices***.
   ii. Such varices may not be confined to the lower end of the oesophagus but may extend for some distance into the stomach.
   iii. Rupture of these varices can cause serious bleeding.
   iv. Oesophageal varices can be demonstrated radiologically (by barium swallow) and can be directly seen through oesophagoscopy.

c. Veins from the ***wall of the anal canal*** drain partly into the superior rectal vein (portal), and partly into the middle and inferior rectal veins (systemic). Enlargement of the communications between these veins can be an important factor predisposing to formation of ***haemorrhoids*** or ***piles***. (See under clinical correlations of anal canal).

d. Other sites of communication between systemic and portal veins are seen in relation to:
   i. The ***bare area of the liver*** (where hepatic veins anastomose with phrenic and intercostal veins).
   ii. The ***posterior abdominal wall*** where veins draining the parts of the gut that are retroperitoneal (i.e., the duodenum, the ascending colon and descending colon) anastomose with systemic veins of the posterior abdominal wall (renal, lumbar and phrenic veins).

e. In fetal life, most of the blood in the portal vein is short circuited to the inferior vena cava through the ***ductus venosus***. This channel may sometimes remain patent after birth forming a natural portocaval shunt.

*Portal Hypertension*

1. We have seen that portosystemic anastomoses undergo enlargement when there is obstruction to flow of blood in the portal vein.
2. Such obstruction can be caused by cirrhosis of liver (a disease in which liver tissue undergoes extensive fibrosis).
3. It can also be caused by thrombosis in the portal vein.
4. Obstruction leads to increased pressure in the portal circulation, the pressure rising from a normal of about 10 mmHg to over 40 mmHg in portal hypertension.
5. Surgical treatment of portal hypertension aims at creating a shunt between the portal vein (or superior mesenteric vein) and the inferior vena cava. Alternatively, the splenic vein is cut and joined to the left renal vein.

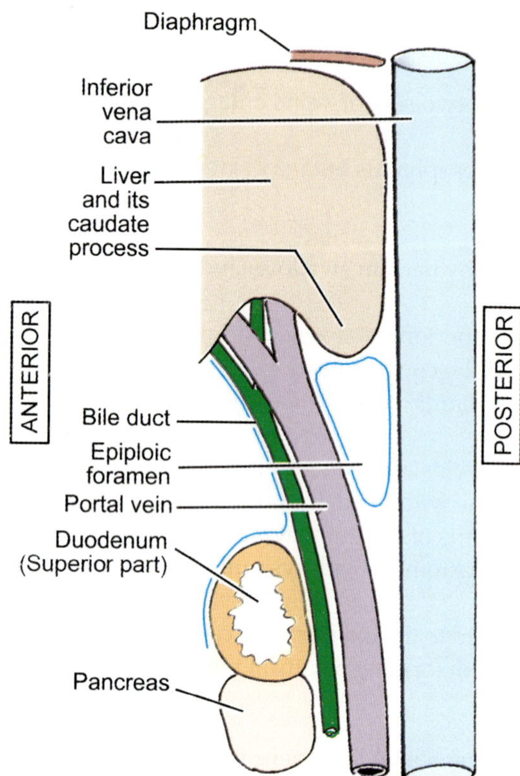


**29.11:** Scheme to show some relations of the portal vein (schematic parasaggital section)

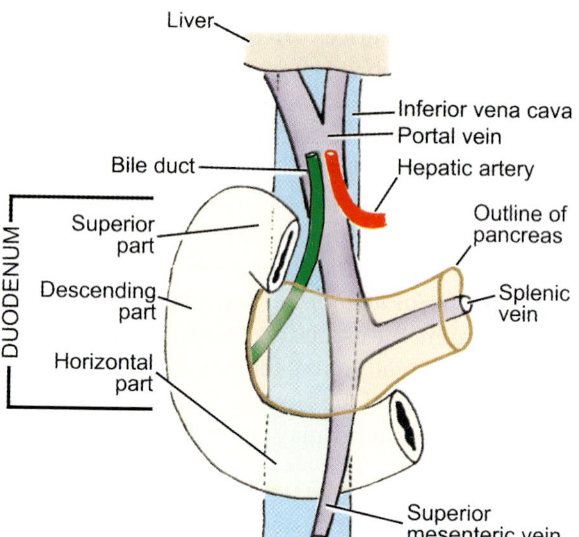


**29.12:** Some relations of the portal vein as seen from the front

# 30 Kidney, Ureter and Suprarenal Gland

CHAPTER

## INTRODUCTION TO THE URINARY SYSTEM

1. The organs of the body that are concerned with the formation of urine and its elimination from the body are referred to as urinary organs.
2. They consist (30.1) of:
   a. The right and left ***kidneys***, in which urine is formed.
   b. The right and left ***ureters***.
   c. The ***urinary bladder***, in which urine is stored temporarily and is also concentrated.
   d. The ***urethra*** which carries urine from the urinary bladder to the exterior.
3. In this chapter, we will consider the kidneys and the abdominal parts of the ureters. The pelvic parts of the ureters, the urinary bladder, and the urethra will be considered in chapter 33.
4. The ***suprarenal glands*** are endocrine organs. It is convenient to consider them here because of their close topographic relationship to the kidneys.

## THE KIDNEYS

1. Each kidney has a characteristic bean-like shape (30.2). It has a convex lateral margin and a concavity on the medial side that is called the ***hilum***.
2. It has upper and lower ends and anterior and posterior surfaces.
3. Terminal branches of the renal artery enter the kidney at the hilum, and the veins emerge from it. The hilum also gives attachment to the upper expanded end of the ureter (called the ***renal pelvis***).
4. The position of the kidneys relative to the anterior abdominal wall is shown in 30.3.
   a. Because of the presence of the liver on the right side, the right kidney lies slightly lower than the left kidney.
   b. The hilum of each kidney lies more or less in the transpyloric plane, a little medial to the tip of the ninth costal cartilage.
   c. The vertical axis of the kidney is placed obliquely (30.2 and 30.3) so that its upper end is nearer the median plane than the lower end.
   d. The upper end is about 2.5 cm (1 inch) from the median plane, while the lower end is about 7.5 cm (3 inches) from it.
5. In relation to the posterior surface of the body:
   a. The hilum of the kidney lies at the level of the first lumbar spine (30.4).
   b. The upper pole lies at the level of the 11th thoracic spine.
   c. The lower pole lies at the level of the third lumbar spine.
6. Keeping these facts in the mind, and also keeping in mind the dimensions of the kidney (shown in 30.2). It is possible to draw the outline of the kidney relative to the surface of the body (30.3 and 30.4).
7. While doing so it has to be remembered that although the width of the kidney is actually about 6 cm it appears to be only 4.5 cm when viewed from the front (or back) because of foreshortening (as explained in 30.5).

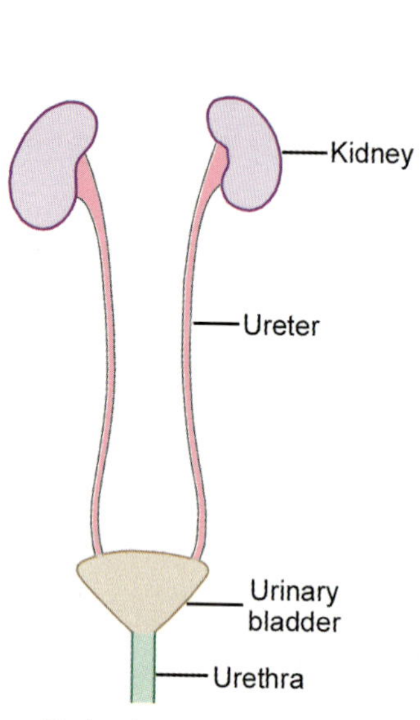


30.1: The urinary organs

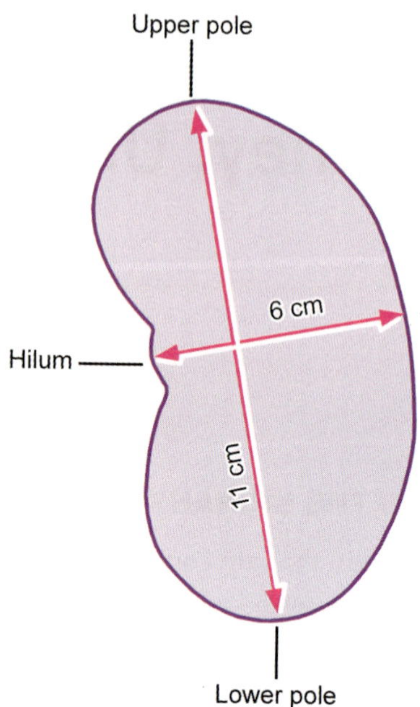


30.2: Approximate dimensions of a kidney. The anteroposterior diameter is about 3 cm

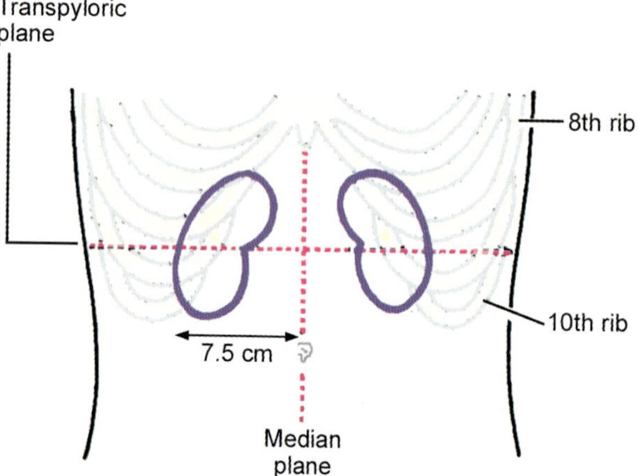


30.3: Projection of the kidney to the front of the body

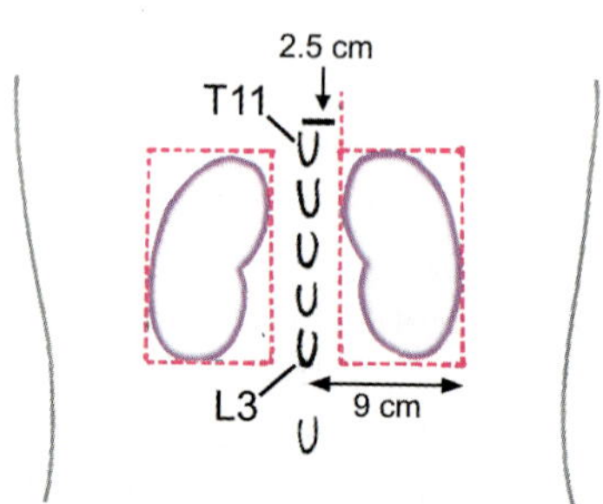


30.4: Surface projection of the kidney on the back of the body

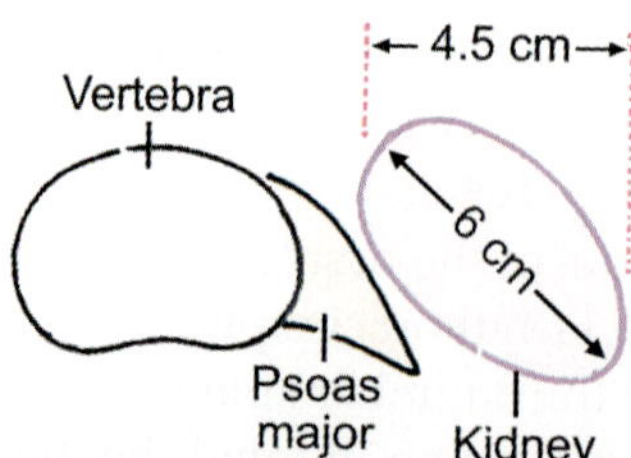


30.5: Scheme to explain the foreshortening of the width of the kidney when viewed from the front or back

8. In 30.4 note that the area in which the kidney lies can be represented as a parallelogram (***Morrison's parallelogram***).
   a. The upper and lower boundaries of this parallelogram are formed by transverse lines drawn through the eleventh thoracic and third lumbar spines.
   b. Its medial and lateral boundaries are formed by vertical lines 2.5 cm and 9 cm from the median plane. Note that the width of the parallelogram is more than that of the kidney as the kidney lies obliquely within it.

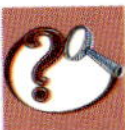

## WANT TO KNOW MORE?

### Relations of the Kidneys

*Posterior Relations*

Each kidney rests on the following (30.6):

1. The diaphragm.
2. The corresponding psoas major.
3. Quadratus lumborum.
4. The origin of the corresponding transversus abdominis muscle.
5. The medial and lateral lumbocostal arches (from which some fibres of the diaphragm take origin) also lie behind the kidney.
6. The diaphragm separates the upper part of the kidney from the pleura and from the twelfth rib. The left kidney being higher, it is also separated by the diaphragm from the eleventh rib.

*Anterior Relations of Right Kidney*

1. The relations of the anterior surface of the right kidney are as follows:
   a. The medial part is overlapped by the duodenum.
   b. The lower part is overlapped by the right colic flexure.
   c. Above the right colic flexure the surface is in contact with the visceral surface of the liver.
   d. A small area on the superomedial part of the anterior surface is in contact with the left suprarenal gland.
   e. Another small area on the inferomedial part of the surface comes in contact with a coil of jejunum.
2. Note that the liver and jejunum are separated from the kidney by peritoneum. The other structures are in direct contact with the kidney.

*Anterior Relations of the Left Kidney*

1. The relations of the anterior surface of the left kidney are as follows (30.7):
   a. The upper lateral part is in contact with the renal impression on the spleen.
   b. The pancreas runs across the middle of the anterior surface.
   c. The splenic artery runs across the kidney immediately above the pancreas.
   d. The left colic flexure comes in contact with the lower lateral part of the anterior surface.
   e. Just above the area for the pancreas the anterior surface of the left kidney comes in contact with the stomach and helps to form the stomach bed.
   f. The upper medial part of the anterior surface is in contact with the left suprarenal gland.
   g. The greater part of the anterior surface below the area for the pancreas is in contact with coils of jejunum.
2. Note that the suprarenal, the pancreas and the colon are in direct contact with the kidney. But the spleen, the stomach and the coils of jejunum are separated from it by peritoneum.
3. The lienorenal ligament is attached to the front of the left kidney along the medial margin of the splenic area.

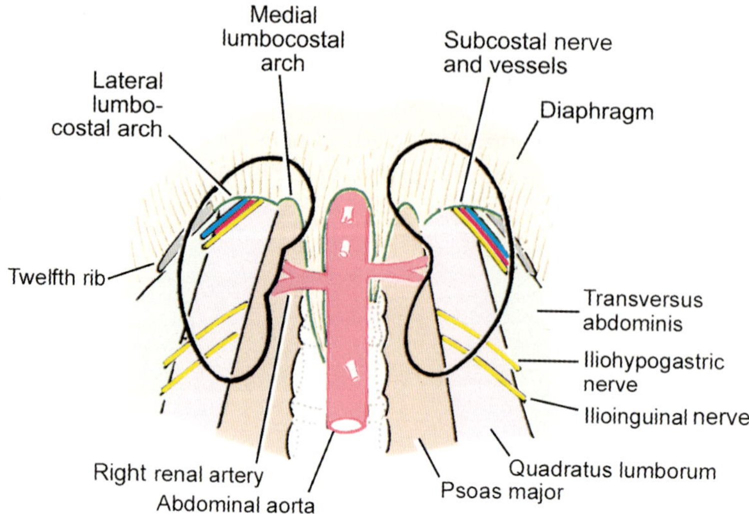


**30.6:** Posterior relations of kidneys

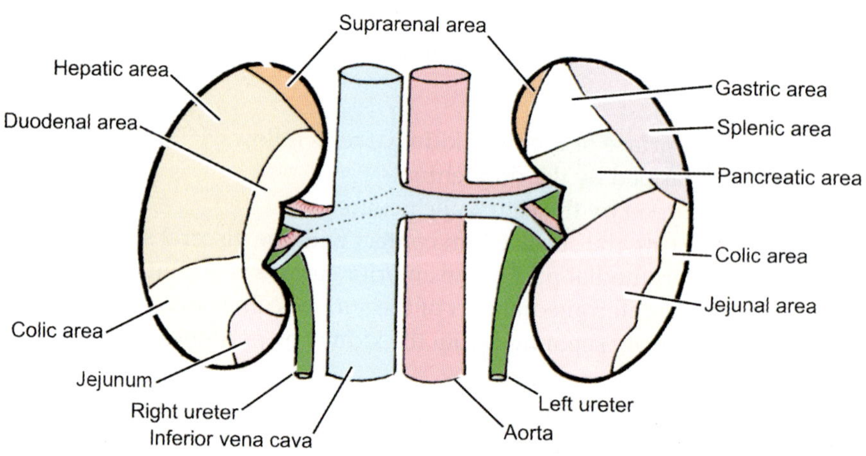


**30.7:** Areas on anterior surfaces of right and left kidneys related to various viscera

## Structures in the Hilum

1. The central part of the medial border of the kidney is marked by the hilum. The renal vein (or its tributaries), the renal artery (or its branches), and the renal pelvis (see below) enter or leave the kidney here. It is important to note the relative position of these structures.
   a. The vein is most anterior.
   b. The artery is in the middle.
   c. The renal pelvis is most posterior.
2. Examination of the hilum therefore, enables one to distinguish between the anterior and posterior aspects of the kidney.
3. The direction of the ureter enables the upper and lower ends of the kidney to be distinguished. In this way it becomes possible to distinguish between isolated right and left kidneys.

4. When we examine a transverse section across a kidney it is seen that the hilum leads into a space called the ***renal sinus*** (30.8).
5. The renal sinus is occupied by:
   a. The upper expanded part of the ureter that is called the ***renal pelvis.***
   b. By renal vessels.
   c. By some fat.
6 a. Within the renal sinus the pelvis divides into two (or three) parts called ***major calyces*** (singular = calyx).
   b. Each major calyx divides into a number of minor calyces (30.9). The end of each minor calyx is shaped like a cup.
   c. A projection of kidney tissue called a ***papilla*** fits into the cup.

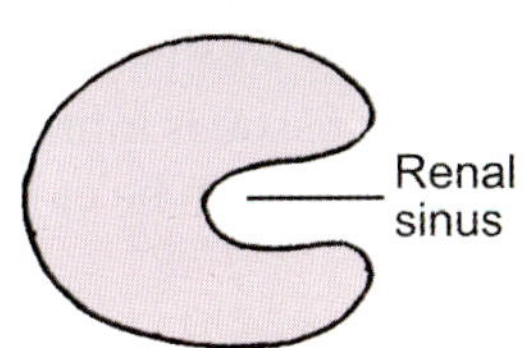


**30.8:** Transverse section through a kidney to show the hilum

## Gross Internal Structure

1. When we examine a coronal section through a kidney we can make out some features of its internal structure (30.10).
2. Firstly, it is seen that the papillae are the apical parts of triangular areas of renal tissue called the ***renal pyramids***.
3. The number of pyramids in a kidney is variable. The average number is about eight.
4. As the apex (or papilla) of one pyramid fits into one minor calyx. The number of pyramids is equal to that of the calices (but the number need not correspond exactly as more than one papilla may invaginate into one calyx).
5. As seen in 30.10, the pyramids occupy the inner part of the kidney and are, therefore, collectively referred to as the ***medulla***.
6. The kidney tissue lying between the bases of the pyramids and the surface of the kidney is referred to as the ***cortex***.
7. Extensions of the cortex occupy the intervals between adjacent pyramids. These extensions are called ***renal columns***.

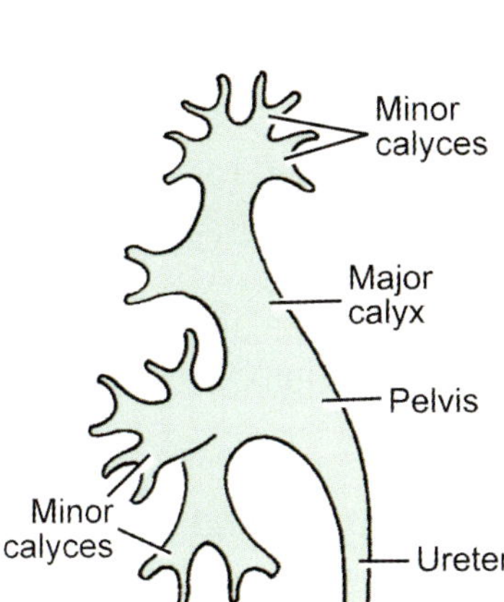


**30.9:** Scheme to show the major and minor calyces

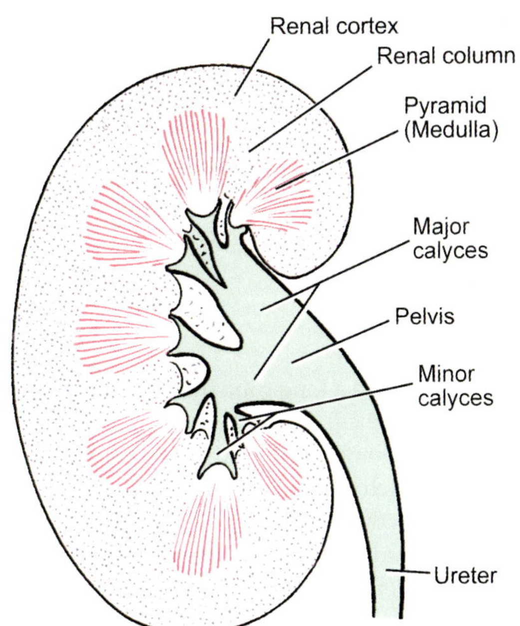


**30.10:** Some features to be seen in a coronal section through the kidney

## Renal Capsule

Kidney tissue is intimately covered by a thin layer of fibrous tissue that is called the capsule. In the healthy kidney the capsule can be easily stripped off. It become adherent in some diseases.

## Renal Fascia

1. Beyond the capsule the kidney is surrounded by a layer of ***perirenal fat*** (also called ***perinephric fat***). Some of this fat extends into the renal sinus.
2. The perinephric fat is surrounded by a layer of fibrous tissue that constitutes the ***renal fascia***.
   a. There are two layers of this fascia: anterior and posterior.
   b. The two layers are continuous with each other around the lateral border of the kidney (30.11).
   c. When traced medially the anterior layer passes in front of the renal vessels and fuses with the connective tissue in front of the aorta and the inferior vena cava.
   d. The posterior layer passes over the quadratus lumborum and the psoas major to fuse with the fascia in front of the lumbar vertebrae.
   e. When traced upwards, the anterior and posterior layers of the renal fascia enclose the suprarenal gland. Above the gland the layers fuse with each other and with the fascia over the diaphragm (30.12).
   f. When traced downwards the two layers do not fuse with each other. The posterior layer fuses with fascia over the iliacus muscle. The anterior layer becomes indistinct some distance below the kidney.
3. Around the renal fascia, there is a layer of ***pararenal fat***.

### WANT TO KNOW MORE?

*Renal Segments*

1. The kidneys are supplied by the renal arteries and are drained by the renal veins (chapter 31).
2. Near the hilum of the kidney, the renal artery divides into anterior and posterior divisions.
3. Within the renal sinus, these divide further into primary branches each of which supplies a specific region of renal tissue, there being no anastomoses between arteries to adjoining regions.
4. These primary branches are called ***segmental arteries***. Based on their distribution the kidney can be divided into five segments as shown in 30.13.
   a. The ***lymphatic drainage*** of the kidneys is into the lateral aortic lymph nodes.
   b. The kidneys are supplied by autonomic nerves that reach them along the renal arteries.
   c. Clinical correlations of the kidneys are considered below along those of the ureters.

## THE URETERS

1 a. The ureter (right or left) is a long tube that connects the lower end of the renal pelvis with the urinary bladder.
   b. It is about 25 cm (10 inches) long.
   c. The upper half of this length lies on the posterior abdominal wall and the lower half in the true pelvis.

2. The abdominal part of each ureter runs downwards (with a slight medial inclination).
   a. Posteriorly, it rests on the psoas major.
   b. Anteriorly, it is covered by the peritoneum of the posterior abdominal wall.
3. At the brim of the pelvis, the ureter crosses the upper end of the external iliac artery (and vein), and comes to lie on the lateral wall of the pelvis.
4. Here, it runs backwards and laterally. Finally, it leaves the pelvic wall and turns medially and forwards to reach the posterolateral part of the urinary bladder.

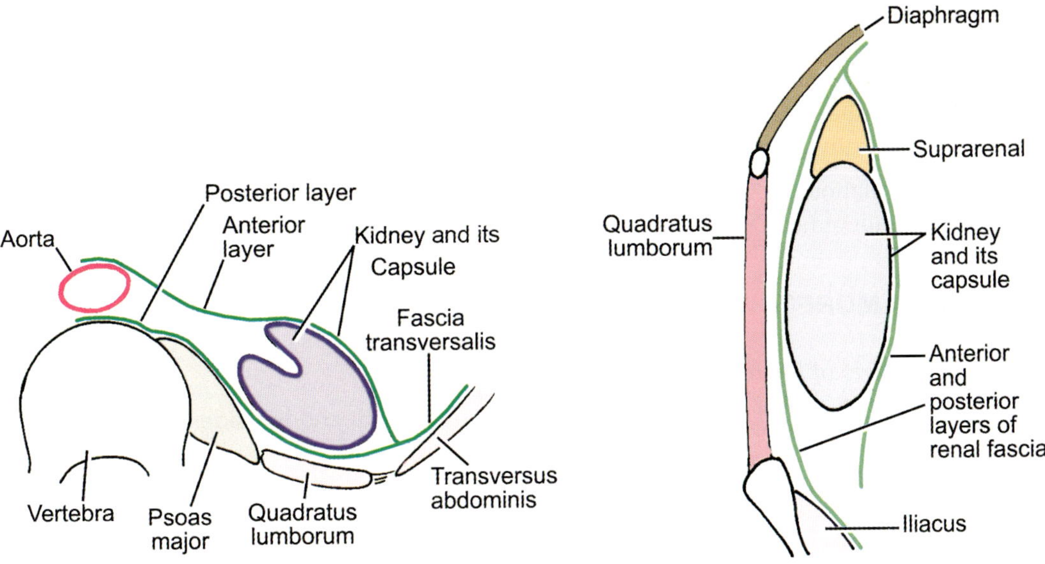


**30.11:** Transverse section through kidney showing the arrangement of the renal fascia

**30.12:** Sagittal section through kidney to show arrangement of renal fascia

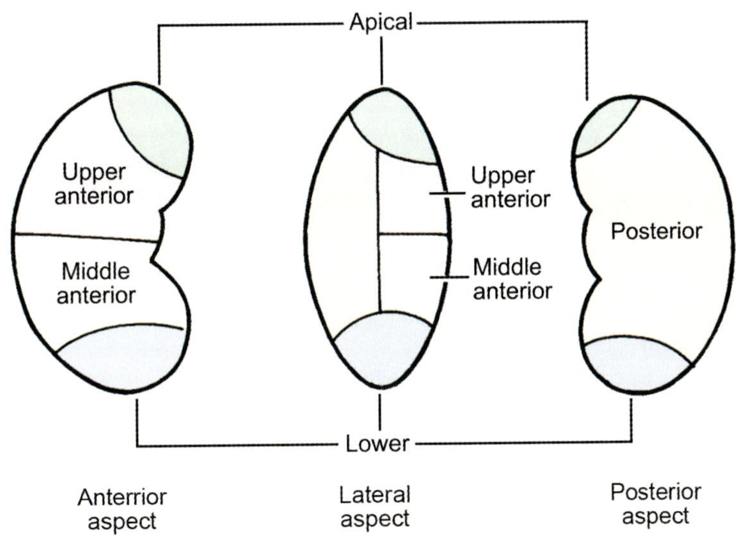


**30.13:** Scheme to show the segments of the kidney

5 a. The renal pelves and the ureters are frequently visualised in the living by taking skiagrams after injecting radio-opaque dye into a vein.
   b. The dye is excreted by the kidney into the urine rendering the pelves, ureters and urinary bladder visible.
   c. The procedure is called ***excretion urography*** (also called intravenous or descending pyelography or urography.).
6. The ureters can also be visualised by direct injection of radio-opaque dyes into them by using an instrument introduced through the urethra and urinary bladder. This procedure is called ***ascending or retrograde pyelography*** (or urography).

7. In interpreting such urograms it is important to know the skeletal relationships of the ureters.
   a. The abdominal part runs downwards in line with the tips of the transverse processes of lumbar vertebrae.
   b. After entering the pelvis the ureter runs across the sacroiliac joint, and the anterior border of the greater sciatic notch to reach the ischial spine.
   c. The ureter turns medially at this spine. Its point of termination corresponds to the pubic tubercle.

   Further details of the relations of the abdominal parts of the ureters are as given below. The relations of the pelvic part will be considered in Chapter 33 along with other pelvic viscera.

## WANT TO KNOW MORE?

*Relations of Abdominal Parts of Ureters*

The relations of the abdominal part of the ureter are different on the right and left sides.

*Relations of Right Ureter*

1. The abdominal part of the right ureter is overlapped at its upper end by the descending part of the duodenum.
2. Lower down it is crossed by the terminal ileum and by the root of the mesentery.
3. Several smaller structures cross the right ureter from medial to lateral side.
4. Crossing in front of the ureter there are:
   a. The testicular or ovarian vessels.
   b. The right colic and ileocolic branches of the superior mesenteric artery.
   c. The terminal part of the superior mesenteric artery, itself (in the root of the mesentery).
   d. The arteries are accompanied by the corresponding veins.
5. The genitofemoral nerve crosses behind the ureter.
6. The inferior vena cava lies a short distance medial to the right ureter.

*Relations of Left Ureter*

1. The abdominal part of the left ureter is crossed (near the brim of the pelvis) by the sigmoid colon.
2. This ureter passes deep to the apex of the V-shaped attachment of the sigmoid mesocolon.
3. As on the right side the ureter is crossed, posteriorly, by the genitofemoral nerve.
4. It is crossed, in front, by:
   a. The testicular or ovarian vessels.
   b. The left colic branches of the inferior mesenteric artery.
5. The inferior mesenteric vein is placed parallel to the left ureter, a little to its medial side.

Further details about the ureter including blood supply, innervation and lymphatic drainage are given in Chapter 33 where the pelvic part is considered. A complete idea of the ureter can be obtained only by study of this chapter and chapter 33.

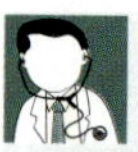

## CLINICAL CORRELATION

**Kidneys and Ureters**

*Congenital Anomalies of the Kidney*

1. Gross anomalies are as follows:
   a. Absence of one or both kidneys.
   b. Underdevelopment (hypoplasia) or over-development (hyperplasia).
   c. Adrenal tissue may be present within the kidney substance.
   d. There may be duplication of a kidney.

2. Anomalies of shape:
   a. The lower poles of the two kidneys may be fused (***horseshoe kidney***).
   b. The two kidneys may form one mass lying in the midline (***pancake kidney***).
   c. The fetal kidney is lobulated. Fetal lobulation may persist.
3. Anomalies of position:
   a. The kidneys may lie in the sacral region, or in the lower lumbar region because of the failure of normal ascent.
   b. Both kidneys may lie on one side of the midline.
4. In the fetal kidney, the hilum faces anteriorly and later rotates to a medial position. The testis may remain ***unrotated***, or may rotate in a reverse direction.
5. The kidney may be full of cysts (***congenital polycystic kidney***).
6. Additional renal arteries, arising from the aorta below the level of the normal renal artery, may be present (***aberrant renal arteries***). Such an artery can press on the ureter leading to obstruction.

*Congenital Anomalies of the Ureters*

1. The ureter may be partially, or completely, duplicated. The duplication may accompany duplication of the kidney or may be independent.
2. The ureter may open at an abnormal site:
   a. Into vagina
   b. Into rectum
   c. Into urethra
   d. Into ductus deferens
   e. Into seminal vesicle.
3. There may be obstruction to the ureter. Obstruction may be a result of stenosis, or presence of valves.
4. a. The upper end may be blind.
   b. The part of the ureter above the obstruction dilates (***hydroureter***).
   c. Obstruction can also lead to dilation of the renal pelvis and kidney (***hydronephrosis***).
5. Sometimes the right ureter may lie behind the vena cava (the real defect being in the position of the vena cava).

*Renal Segments*

1. The kidneys can be divided into a number of segments on the basis of their arterial supply (page 600).
2. Knowledge of the segments is useful in planning partial resection of the kidney.

*Injuries*

1. The kidney may be injured by a fall or a blow on the loin.
2. It can also be injured in crushing injuries.
3. The ureters can be injured in operations on the abdomen.

*Calculi*

1. In many persons, stones may be formed in the renal pelvis.
2. The stones may consist predominantly of calcium oxalate, calcium phosphate, or uric acid and urate.
3. Such calculi may pass into the ureter, and through it into the urinary bladder. Small stones may be discharged to the outside through the urethra.
4. A stone lodged in the kidney may be painless. Sometimes it gives a dull pain that may be felt posteriorly in the renal angle, or anteriorly in the hypochondrium (***fixed renal pain***). Similar pain can arise from other causes.
5. A stone passing through the ureter causes severe pain called ***renal colic***.
   a. The pain starts in the back in the region of the renal angle and radiates downwards and forwards towards the inguinal region (from loin to groin).
   b. This pain is felt in the region that is supplied by spinal segments T11 to L2.

c. When the stone reaches the lower part of the ureter pain may be felt in the scrotum, the tip of the penis, or in the upper part of the thigh.

6. Operations for removal of renal calculi may involve opening of the renal pelvis (***pyelolithotomy***), or an incision into the kidney (***nephrolithotomy***).
7. Incisions into the kidney are usually made along the convex lateral border (***Brodal's line***) as this does not involve cutting of large vessels within the kidney. (However, this is not a blood-less plane as was taught earlier).
8. Sometimes partial removal of the kidney (***partial nephrectomy***) may be necessary.
9. Sometimes a stone may destroy much of the renal substance, and if the other kidney is healthy, the entire kidney may have to be removed (***nephrectomy***).
10. Two recent developments have revolutionised treatment of urinary calculi.
    a. In ***percutaneous removal of stones,*** an instrument called a ***nephroscope*** is passed into the renal pelvis along a needle introduced through the loin. Stones can be seen and can be removed whole or after breaking them into small pieces.
    b. In ***lithotripsy,*** an instrument (***lithotriptor***) generates powerful shock waves that can pass through tissues of the body and can be focused at a given site. Such waves can reduce a stone to sand, or to very small pieces, which can then be flushed out through the urinary passages. Unfortunately, these newer techniques are expensive and not suited to all patients.

11 a. A stone passing down the ureter can get arrested somewhere along its length. This is more likely to occur at places where the ureter is normally constricted (see chapter 33).
    b. Various techniques are used for dislodging such a stone.
    c. In one of these, a ***ureteroscope*** is passed into the ureter (through the urethra and urinary bladder). A stone can be seen and removed through this instrument. Sometimes open surgery is needed (***ureterolithotomy***).

12. Urinary obstruction caused by calculi or other causes can lead to dilatation of the ureter above the site of obstruction (***hydroureter***). It can also lead to dilatation of the renal pelvis and calyces (***hydronephrosis***).

*Infections*

1. Infections of the lower urinary tract are common and they can ascend to the renal pelvis and kidney substance. Infection can also reach the kidneys through the circulation.
2. Infection of the kidney and pelvis is called ***pyelonephritis***. It may be acute or chronic.
3. Sometimes the kidney can be reduced to a bag of pus, most of the kidney tissue being destroyed (***pyonephrosis***).
4. Infection from a kidney can spread to tissues around it leading to a ***perinephric abscess***. A perinephric abscess can also be caused by infection reaching the region through the circulation, or from other organs in the region (e.g., the appendix).

## THE SUPRARENAL GLANDS

1. As implied by the name the right and left suprarenal glands lie in close relationship to the upper poles of the corresponding kidneys.
2. They are enclosed with the kidney in the renal fascia, but lie outside the renal capsule (30.12).
3. Each suprarenal gland is relatively flat and has an anterior and a posterior surface.
4. When seen from the front the right suprarenal gland is triangular. It has medial, lateral and inferior borders (the last being called the base).
5. The left suprarenal gland is semilunar. It has a convex medial margin and a concave lateral margin.
6. Each gland is about 50 mm in vertical diameter, about 30 mm from side to side, and about 10 mm from front to back.

**WANT TO KNOW MORE?**

*Relations of the Suprarenal Glands*

1. Relations common to both glands
   a. The posterior surface of each suprarenal gland rests (in its upper part) on the diaphragm, and (in its lower part) on the superomedial part of the corresponding kidney.
   b. The areas of the kidneys related to the suprarenal glands are shown in 30.7.
   c. Medial to each gland there is the corresponding crus of the diaphragm on which there is the corresponding ***coeliac ganglion***, and the corresponding inferior phrenic artery (a branch of the abdominal aorta).
2. Additional relations of the right suprarenal gland
   a. The anterior surface of the right suprarenal gland can be divided into medial and lateral parts by a vertical line.
   b. The medial part is overlapped by the inferior vena cava.
   c. The lateral part comes into contact with the liver. The upper half of the lateral part is in contact with the bare area of the liver, while its lower part is separated from the visceral surface by peritoneum.
3. Additional relations of the left suprarenal gland
   a. The upper part of the anterior surface is covered by the peritoneum forming the posterior wall of the lesser sac.
   b. It forms part of the stomach bed.
   c. The lower part of the anterior surface is overlapped by the splenic artery and the body of the pancreas. This part is not covered by peritoneum.
   d. In addition to the crus of the diaphragm and the coeliac ganglion (common to both sides) the left gastric artery lies medial to the left suprarenal gland.

## Structure and Functions of the Suprarenal Glands

1. The suprarenal gland is surrounded by a capsule. Septa arising from the capsule extend into the substance of the gland.
   a. The gland is made up of a superficial layer the ***cortex***, and a deeper part called the ***medulla***.
   b. The volume of the medulla is about one tenth of the cortex.
2. Both the medulla and the cortex consist of cords or groups of cells separated by sinusoids. On the basis of the arrangement of its cells the cortex can be divided as follows:
   a. The outermost layer is called the ***zona glomerulosa***. Here, the cells are arranged in the form of inverted U-shaped structures, or acinus-like groups.
   b. The next zone is called the ***zona fasciculata.*** Here, the cells are arranged in straight columns.
   c. The innermost layer of the cortex is called the ***zona reticularis.*** This layer is made up of cords of cells that branch and anastomose with each other forming a kind of reticulum.
3. The medulla is made up of groups of cells, some of which may be arranged in columns. The cell groups or columns are separated by wide sinusoids. Nerve fibres and neurons are also present.
   The hormones produced by the suprarenal glands are as follows:

### *Hormones of the Suprarenal Cortex*

a. The cells of the zona glomerulosa produce the hormone ***aldosterone*** that helps to maintain the water and electrolyte balance of tissues.
b. The cells of the zona fasciculata produce ***hydrocortisone*** (and related compounds). These have widespread effects all over the body, including the maintenance of carbohydrate balance.

c. The cells of the zona reticularis probably produce ***sex hormones*** including progesterone, oestrogens and androgens.

### Hormones of the Suprarenal Medulla

1. Both functionally and embryologically the medulla of the suprarenal gland is distinct from the cortex.
2. When the suprarenal gland is fixed in a solution containing a salt of chromium (e.g., potassium dichromate) the cells of the medulla show yellow granules in their cytoplasm. This is called the ***chromaffin reaction*** and the cells that give a positive reaction are called ***chromaffin cells***.
3. The cells of the cortex do not give this reaction. A similar reaction is also given by cells of sympathetic ganglia.
4. a. The cells of the suprarenal medulla are modified postganglionic sympathetic neurons.
   b. They receive the terminals of preganglionic sympathetic neurons.
   c. Like typical postganglionic sympathetic neurons they secrete noradrenalin and adrenalin into the blood mainly at times of stress (fear, anger etc.) and result in widespread effects similar to those of stimulation of the sympathetic nervous system (e.g., increase in heart rate and blood pressure).

## WANT TO KNOW MORE?

***Blood Vessels and Nerves of the Suprarenal Glands***

1. Each suprarenal gland receives three suprarenal arteries:
   a. Superior from the corresponding inferior phrenic artery.
   b. Middle from the abdominal aorta.
   c. Inferior from the corresponding renal artery.
2. The adrenal is drained by one vein. On the right side it drains into the inferior vena cava, and on the left side into the left renal vein.
3. Lymphatics drain to lateral aortic nodes.
4. The medulla of the suprarenal gland receives numerous preganglionic sympathetic nerves.

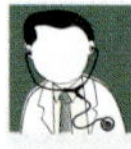

## CLINICAL CORRELATION

***Congenital Anomalies***

1. Adrenal cortical tissue may be present at various ectopic sites including the kidney substance, the ovaries and the broad ligament.
2. The entire adrenal may be ectopic and may be fused to the kidney or to the liver.
3. a. Congenital hyperplasia (over-development) of the cortex in the males leads to the ***adrenogenital syndrome*** marked by very early development of secondary sexual characters.
   b. In the female it may cause enlargement of the clitoris and the child may be mistaken for a male (***pseudo-hermaphroditism***).

***Other Correlations***

1. After puberty hyperplasia of the adrenal cortex, or a cortical tumour, leads to ***Cushing's syndrome***. In this syndrome, seen mostly in females, there is abnormal deposit of fat in the face, neck and trunk but the limbs remain thin and weak.

2. Cortical hyperplasia in infancy has been mentioned under congenital malformations.
3. Chronic deficiency of cortical hormones leads to ***Addison's disease***.
4. a. Acute deficiency of cortical hormones can result from haemorrhage into the cortex.
   b. This may occur in an infant after a difficult child-birth.
   c. In the adult similar haemorrhage may be caused by a meningococcal septicaemia.
   d. Acute deficiency is also be caused by bilateral adrenalectomy.
5. Tumours in the adrenal may arise from sympathetic nervous tissue (***neuroblastoma***) or from chromaffin cells (***phaeochromocytoma***).
6. Adrenal masses can be detected by computerised tomography. (Old techniques like radiological examination after injecting oxygen into retroperitoneal tissues, retrograde venography and arteriography have become obsolete).

31

CHAPTER

# Posterior Abdominal Wall and Some Related Structures

## Skeletal Basis of Posterior Abdominal Wall

1. The bones to be seen in the region of the posterior abdominal wall are:
   a. The five lumbar vertebrae
   b. The sacrum and coccyx
   c. The hip bones which take part in forming the bony pelvis.
2. The lumbar vertebrae have been described in Chapter 24, and the hip-bones in Chapter 9.
3. In studying the posterior abdominal wall, it is important to know the features of the twelfth rib that has been described in an earlier chapter.
4. The main joints in the region are the intervertebral joints. These have been described in Chapter 17.

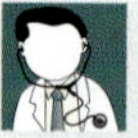

### CLINICAL CORRELATION

#### LUMBAR VERTEBRAE

**Congenital Malformations**

Vertebrae have a complex developmental history, and abnormalities resulting from maldevelopment are frequently seen.

1. The two halves of the neural arch may fail to fuse in the midline. This condition is called ***spina bifida***.
   a. If the gap between the neural arches is small, no obvious deformity may be apparent on the surface (***spina bifida occulta:*** occult = hidden).
   b. When the gap is large, meninges and nerves may bulge out through the gap forming a visible swelling.
   c. When the swelling contains only meninges and CSF it is called a ***meningocoele***.
   d. When neural elements are also present in the swelling the condition is called ***meningomyelocoele***.
2. Two or more vertebrae that are normally separate may be fused to one another. The fifth lumbar vertebra may be partially, or completely fused to the sacrum (***sacralisation of 5th lumbar vertebra***).
3. Alternatively, the first piece of the sacrum may form a separate vertebra (***lumbarisation of first sacral vertebra***).
4. Abnormality in ossification of a vertebra may result in a condition in which the spine, laminae and inferior articular processes are not fused to the rest of the vertebra.
   a. Normally, vertebral bodies do not slip forwards over one another because of the restraining influence of the inferior articular processes.
   b. However, when the abnormality described above is present, body weight can cause the body of the fifth lumbar vertebra to slip forwards over the sacrum. This condition is called ***spondylolisthesis***.
   c. Sometimes, a similar condition may affect the fourth lumbar vertebra that may then slip forwards over the fifth lumbar vertebra.
   d. Spondylolisthesis can be a cause of persistent low back pain.

**Fractures of Lumbar Vertebrae**

1. Like other vertebrae those in the lumbar region can be fractured by direct injury. Such injury usually results in fracture of the spinous process, transverse process or lamina.
2. a. If the lumbar spine is forcibly flexed (as in a fall from a height) the body of a vertebra can be compressed.
   b. In a compression injury, the vertebral arch and the ligaments around the body can remain intact and can prevent the spinal cord from being injured.
3. In more severe injuries compression of the body of a lumbar vertebra may be combined with fracture of the articular processes (***fracture dislocation***). The vertebrae involved become unstable and injury to structures within the spinal canal can result.
4. a. Such injury in the lumbar region leads to the ***cauda equina syndrome***.
   b. The patient has a flaccid paraplegia.
   c. Sensations are lost over the perineum and upper medial area of thighs (the area corresponding to that which comes in contact with a saddle).
   d. There is incontinence of urine and of feces.

***Lumbar Puncture***

1. The term lumbar puncture is applied to a procedure in which a long needle is passed into the subarachnoid space through the interval between the 3rd and 4th lumbar vertebrae, or sometimes through the interval between the 4th and 5th vertebrae.
2. a. In this connection, it is important to note that the lower end of the spinal cord lies at the level of the lower border of the first lumbar vertebra.
   b. The subarachnoid space (containing cerebrospinal fluid) extends down to the level of the lower border of the second sacral vertebra.
   c. Hence, a needle passed into the lower lumbar part of the vertebral canal does not injure the spinal cord.
3. Remember, however, that here the subarachnoid space contains nerve roots forming the cauda equina. They are not injured as they are mobile.
4. Lumbar puncture has several uses as follows:
   a. Samples of cerebrospinal fluid (CSF) can be obtained for examination. Important points to note about CSF are its colour, its cellular content, and its chemical composition (specially the protein and sugar content).
   b. The pressure of CSF can be estimated.
   c. Air or radio-opaque dyes can be introduced into the subarachnoid space for certain investigative procedures. A skiagram taken after injecting iodinized oil into the subarachnoid space outlines the space.
   d. Anaesthetic agents injected into the subarachnoid space act on the lower spinal nerve roots and render the lower part of the body insensitive to pain. This procedure, called ***spinal anaesthesia***, is frequently used for operations on the lower abdomen and on the lower extremities.

**Prolapse of Intervertebral Disc**

1. The intervertebral discs are very strong in the young. With advancing age, however, the annulus fibrosus becomes weak and it then becomes possible for the nucleus pulposus to burst through it.
2. This is called prolapse of the intervertebral disc (though it is really prolapse of the nucleus pulposus).
3. A prolapsed nucleus pulposus usually passes backwards and laterally and may press upon nerve roots attached to the spinal cord at that level.
4. Prolapse results in local pain in the back.
5. When nerves are pressed upon there is shooting pain along the course of the nerve involved.
6. Disc prolapse occurs most frequently in the lumbosacral region and results in pain shooting down the back of the leg and thigh. This is called ***sciatica***.

**Psoas Abscess**

1. Tubercular infection of thoracic or lumbar vertebrae (commonly seen a few decades ago) can lead to formation of pus.

2. As the bodies of lumbar vertebrae are closely related to the psoas major this pus passes into the potential space deep to the fascia enclosing the muscle.
3. It then descends along the fascia to reach the femoral triangle where it forms a swelling.
4. Such a swelling may sometimes be confused with a femoral hernia.
(A tubercular abscess is referred to as a cold abscess because the usual signs of inflammation are missing).

### Thoracolumbar Fascia

1. The thoracolumbar fascia is intimately related to the muscles of the posterior abdominal wall. It has three layers (31.1A).
2. a. The ***posterior layer*** covers the deep muscles of the back. It is attached medially to the lumbar and sacral spines.
   b. Laterally, it blends with the anterior layer. The two layers form an aponeurosis that gives attachment to the internal oblique and transversus muscles.
3. a. The ***middle layer*** separates the erector spinae from the quadratus lumborum.
   b. It is attached medially to the tips of the transverse processes of the lumbar vertebrae.
   c. Laterally, it blends with the posterior layer.
4. a. The ***anterior layer*** covers the anterior surface of the quadratus lumborum.
   b. It is attached medially to the anterior surfaces of the transverse processes of the lumbar vertebrae and merges laterally with the posterior layer as mentioned above.
5. a. The posterior layer can be traced upwards (superficial to the erector spinae) into the thorax at the upper end of which it becomes continuous with the deep cervical fascia.
   b. The serratus posterior inferior, and superior, are superficial to it.
6. Inferiorly, the posterior layer can be traced medially to the sacrum and laterally to the iliac crest.
7. The middle layer is attached to the twelfth rib above, and to the iliac crest below.
8. The anterior layer is also attached below to the iliac crest. Its upper end forms the lateral arcuate ligament that gives origin to the diaphragm.

## MUSCLES OF POSTERIOR ABDOMINAL WALL

The muscles of the posterior abdominal wall are:
1. The psoas major
2. The psoas minor

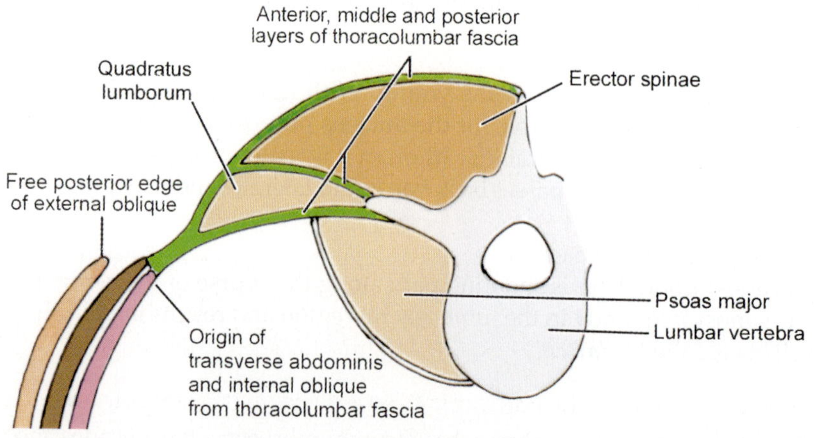


**31.1A:** The lumbodorsal fascia

3. The iliacus
4. The quadratus lumborum.

The attachments of the psoas muscles and of the iliacus are given in Table 31.1B. The quadratus lumborum is described in 31.2A and is shown in 31.2B.

## WANT TO KNOW MORE?

### Relations of the Psoas Major

The psoas major has important relations in the abdomen.

1. Just below its upper end, this muscle is crossed by the medial arcuate ligament.
   a. This ligament gives origin to some fibres of the diaphragm, which, therefore, overlaps the uppermost part of the psoas major.
   b. This part of the muscle lies in the thorax (posterior mediastinum) and may be related to pleura.
2. The upper part of the muscle forms part of the posterior abdominal wall.
   a. The intermediate part crosses the sacroiliac joint and runs along the brim of the true pelvis.
   b. The lower part passes behind the inguinal ligament to enter the thigh.
3. The ***abdominal part*** of the muscle is related anteriorly (on both sides) to the corresponding:
   a. Kidney
   b. Renal vessels
   c. Ureter
   d. Gonadal vessels
   e. Genitofemoral nerve.
4. The medial margin of the muscle is related to the sympathetic trunk.
5. The lumbar arteries and veins lie between the tendinous arches (that give origin to the muscle) and the vertebral bodies.
6. The medial margin of the right psoas major lies a little lateral to the abdominal aorta.
7. The ***pelvic part*** of the muscle is related anteriorly to:
   a. The external iliac artery
   b. Gonadal vessels
   c. The genitofemoral nerve.
8. The femoral nerve is related to the lateral margin of the muscle.
9. The right psoas major is crossed by the terminal part of the ilium.
10. The left psoas major is crossed by the terminal part of the descending colon.
11. The ***femoral part*** of the muscle lies inferiorly to the inguinal ligament.
    a. It lies in front of the hip joint from which it is separated by a huge bursa.
    b. It is related laterally to the iliacus, the femoral nerve intervening between the two; and medially to the pectineus.
    c. The femoral artery lies in front of the muscle.

### Relations of the Iliacus

1. The iliacus passes from the abdomen to the thigh (along with the psoas major) lying behind the inguinal ligament and in front of the hip joint.
2. It is related anteriorly to the lateral cutaneous nerve of the thigh and, by its medial margin, to the femoral nerve.
3. In the abdomen, the muscle of the right side is related anteriorly to the caecum, and the muscle of the left side to the descending colon.

**Notes on Quadratus Lumborum**

1. The quadratus lumborum is so called because of its quadrilateral shape.
2. It forms the posterior abdominal wall between the psoas major medially, and the transversus abdominis laterally.
3. It is enclosed between the anterior and middle layers of the thoracolumbar fascia.

***Relations***

1. a. Just below its upper end, the quadratus lumborum is crossed by the lateral arcuate ligament, which gives origin to part of the diaphragm.
   b. The part of the quadratus lumborum above the ligament is, therefore, covered by the diaphragm.
2. On both sides (right and left), the quadratus lumborum muscle is related anteriorly to:
   a. The lower part of the corresponding kidney.
   b. The subcostal nerves and vessels.
   c. The ilioinguinal nerve and the iliohypogastric nerve which intervenes between the muscle and the kidney.
3. The right and left muscles are related to the ascending and descending colon respectively.

## THE ABDOMINAL AORTA

1. An introduction to the aorta and its subdivisions has been given in Chapter 21. The parts of the aorta lying in the thorax have been described in that chapter. Here, we will consider the abdominal part of the aorta.
2. The abdominal aorta is a continuation of the descending thoracic aorta (21.8).
3. Its upper end lies at the level of the lower border of the twelfth thoracic vertebra, and behind the median arcuate ligament.
4. It descends in front of the upper three lumbar vertebrae and terminates in front of the fourth lumbar vertebra by dividing into the right and left common iliac arteries.

**31.1B: Muscles of the posterior abdominal wall**

| *Muscle* | *Psoas Major* | *Psoas Minor* | *Iliacus* |
|---|---|---|---|
| Origin | Through several slips from the following:<br>1. Transverse process of each lumbar vertebra (anterior surface)<br>2. Intervertebral discs and bodies of vertebrae (lateral parts). Five slips highest between T12 and L1, lowest between L4 and L5<br>3. Tendinous arches along sides of upper four lumbar vertebrae | 1. Intervertebral disc between T12 and L1<br>2. Adjoining parts of bodies of vertebrae | 1. Iliac fossa (on inner side of hip bone)<br>2. Iliac crest, inner lip<br>3. Iliolumbar ligament<br>4. Anterior sacroiliac ligament<br>5. Sacrum: Lateral part of upper surface |
| Insertion | Lesser trochanter of femur | 1. Iliopectineal eminence<br>2. Pecten pubis | 1. Tendon of psoas major<br>2. Lesser trochanter of femur<br>3. Small area below lesser trochanter |
| Nerve supply | Ventral rami of spinal nerves L1, L2, L3 | Branch from spinal nerve L1 | Femoral nerve |
| Action | 1. Flexion of thigh at hip joint<br>2. Flexion of lumbar part of vertebral column<br>3. Balances trunk in standing | Weak flexor of lumbar vertebral column | 1. Flexion of thigh (hip joint)<br>2. Flexion of lumbar part of vertebral column |

| 31.2A: Quadratus lumborum | |
|---|---|
| Origin | The origin lies inferiorly.<br>1. Laterally from iliac crest (posterior 1/3 of inner lip of ventral segment, behind the transversus abdominis).<br>2. Medially from iliolumbar ligament (which passes from the iliac crest to the transverse process of vertebra L5). |
| Insertion | 1. Lower border of 12th rib (medial half).<br>2. Small slips to transverse processes of vertebrae L1 to L4. |
| Nerve supply | Ventral rami of spinal nerves T12, L1 to L4. |
| Action | 1. Fixes the 12th rib allowing the diaphragm to act better during respiration.<br>2. Lateral flexor of vertebral column. |

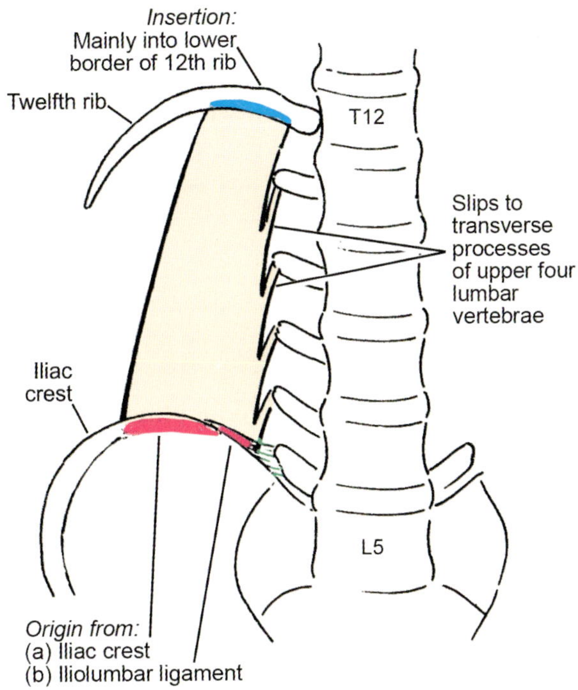


**31.2B:** Scheme to show attachments of the quadratus lumborum muscle

## WANT TO KNOW MORE?

### Relations of Abdominal Aorta

1. The abdominal aorta is related, posteriorly, to the upper four lumbar vertebrae.
2. The lumbar arteries (that arise from the posterior aspect of the aorta), and some lumbar veins, lie between the aorta and the vertebral column.
3. Anteriorly, the aorta is related to some of its own branches. These are:
   a. The coeliac trunk
   b. The superior mesenteric artery
   c. The right and left testicular or ovarian arteries
   d. The inferior mesenteric artery.

4. Anterior to the coeliac trunk, there is a part of the liver called the papillary process, the lesser omentum and part of the cavity of the omental bursa.
5. Anterior to the superior mesenteric artery, there is the pancreas and the splenic vein.
6. The left renal vein runs across the aorta just below the origin of the superior mesenteric artery. A part of the pancreas called the uncinate process lies deep to this artery.
7. Between the origins of the testicular (or ovarian) and inferior mesenteric arteries, the aorta is crossed by the horizontal (or third) part of the duodenum and by the root of the mesentery.
8. The lowest part of the aorta is covered by the peritoneum lining the posterior abdominal wall.
9. On either side of the aorta, there is the corresponding crus of the diaphragm, the coeliac ganglion, and the sympathetic trunk.
10. Additional structures present on the right side are the azygos vein, the thoracic duct and the inferior vena cava.

## BRANCHES OF ABDOMINAL AORTA

The branches of the abdominal aorta can be classified as follows (31.3):

1. ***Ventral branches*** to the gut:
   a. Coeliac
   b. Superior mesenteric
   c. Inferior mesenteric.
2. ***Lateral branches*** to:
   a. Kidneys
   b. Suprarenals
   c. Gonads
   d. Diaphragm (renal, middle suprarenal, gonadal and inferior phrenic).
3. ***Dorsal branches*** to the body wall:
   a. Lumbar arteries.
   b. Median sacral artery.
4. ***Terminal branches***:
   - Common iliac.

The ventral branches of the abdominal aorta have been considered in detail in Chapter 29. The other branches are considered below.

### Lateral Branches of Aorta

1. The most important of these are the ***renal arteries***, and the ***arteries to the testes or ovaries***.
2. In addition, there are two smaller pairs of arteries namely, the ***inferior phrenic*** and the ***middle suprarenal*** arteries (31.2 and 31.4).

#### *Inferior Phrenic Arteries*

1. The right and left inferior phrenic arteries (31.4) arise from the uppermost part of the abdominal aorta. One or both of them may arise from the coeliac trunk.
2. The left artery passes laterally deep to the oesophagus while the right artery passes laterally deep to the inferior vena cava.
3. They divide into a number of branches that ramify on the inferior surface of the diaphragm and supply it.
4. Each artery gives a superior suprarenal branch to the corresponding suprarenal gland.

#### *Middle Suprarenal Arteries*

The middle suprarenal arteries (31.2 and 31.4) arise from the aorta at the level of the origin of the superior mesenteric artery, and end in the corresponding suprarenal gland.

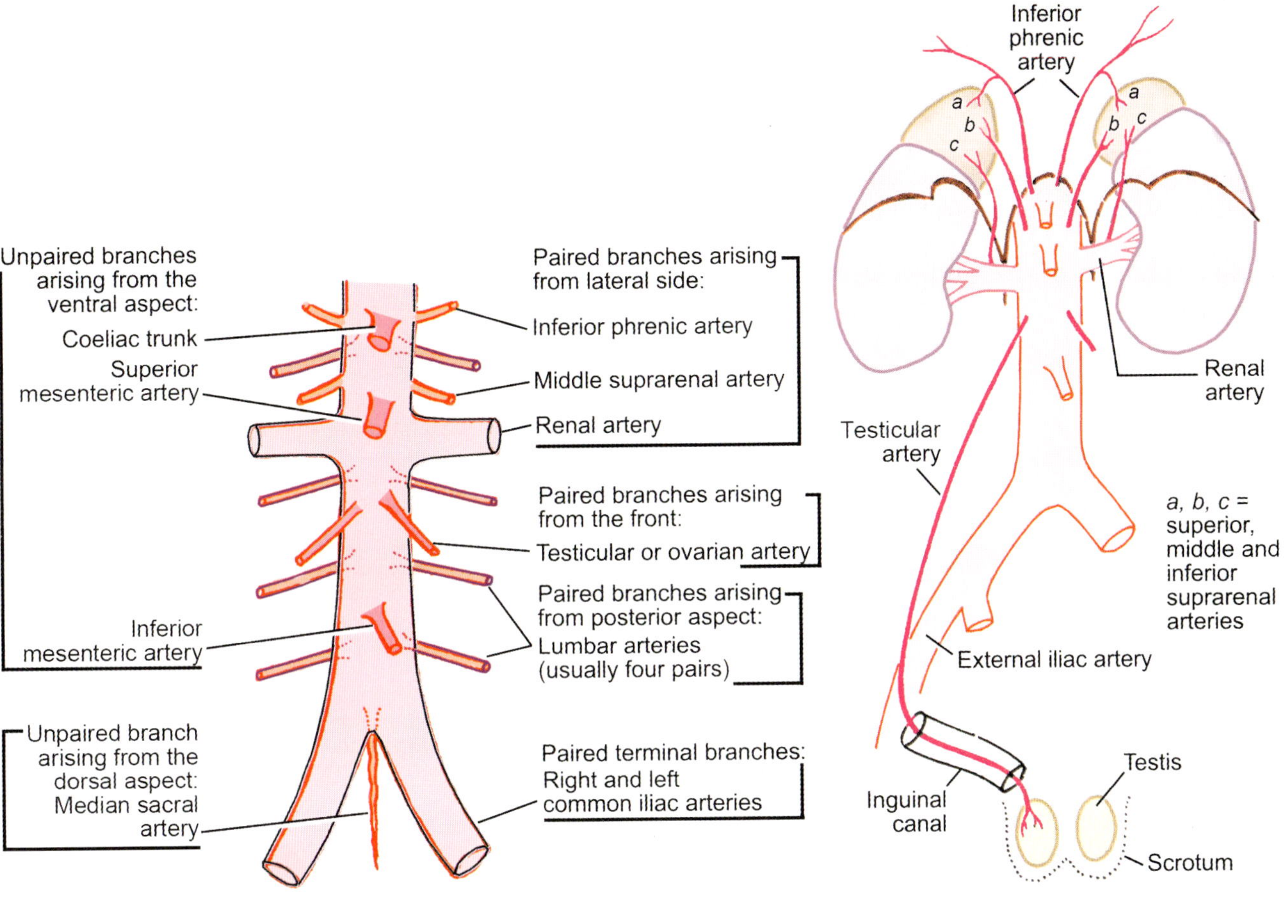


**31.3:** Branches of the abdominal aorta

**31.4:** Scheme to show the lateral branches of the abdominal aorta

## The Renal Arteries

1. The renal arteries arise from the lateral side of the abdominal aorta, a little below the origin of the superior mesenteric artery (31.4).
2. The right artery is a little longer, and a little lower, than the left renal artery.
3. Each artery runs laterally to reach the hilum of the corresponding kidney. Here, it divides into four or five branches that enter the kidney to supply it.
4. Each branch supplies a discrete area of the kidney, and the pattern of distribution is fairly constant. This allows the kidney to be divided into a number of arterial segments.
5. Apart from branches to the kidney each renal artery gives off one or more ***inferior suprarenal arteries*** (31.4) and also supplies the upper part of the ureter.

## The Testicular Arteries

1. The right and left testicular arteries arise from the abdominal aorta a little below the renal arteries.
2. Each artery runs downwards and laterally over the posterior abdominal wall to reach the external iliac artery.
3. The artery runs downwards along the external iliac artery to reach the internal inguinal ring.
4. It passes through the inguinal canal as a constituent of the spermatic cord, and accompanies the cord into the scrotum. Here it divides into branches that supply the testis (31.4).

## The Ovarian Arteries

1. Like the testicular arteries the ovarian arteries arise from the aorta a little below the renal arteries.
2. The upper part of each artery (right and left) runs downwards and laterally over the posterior abdominal wall (formed here by the psoas major) to reach the external iliac artery.
3. The ovarian artery then crosses the external iliac vessels to enter the true pelvis.
4. Leaving the lateral wall of the pelvis the ovarian artery passes successively through the suspensory ligament of the ovary, the broad ligament of uterus and the mesovarium to reach the ovary.

## Dorsal Branches of Abdominal Aorta

These are the ***lumbar arteries*** and the ***median sacral artery***.

### *The Lumbar Arteries*

1. The lumbar arteries are intersegmental arteries that supply the body wall, and are in series with the intercostal and subcostal arteries (31.5).
2. Four pairs of lumbar arteries arise from the back of the aorta. There is one pair opposite each of the upper four lumbar vertebrae.
3. The course of the arteries is variable, but typically each artery runs laterally and backwards on the body of the vertebra.
4. It passes deep to the crus of the diaphragm (upper arteries only), the psoas major and the quadratus lumborum.
5. At the lateral border of the quadratus lumborum, the artery enters the interval between the internal oblique and the transversus abdominis (compare with intercostal arteries).
6. They end by supplying the anterior abdominal wall and anastomose with arteries in the region.

### *Median Sacral Artery*

1. The median sacral artery is small (31.5). It arises from the back of the aorta just above its bifurcation.
2. It descends in the midline over the lower two lumbar vertebrae, the sacrum and the coccyx.
3. It often gives rise to a small pair of ***fifth lumbar arteries***.
4. It also gives off four pairs of small arteries that run over the sacrum to enter the anterior sacral foramina.
5. The lower part of the median sacral artery lies behind the rectum to which it gives some branches.

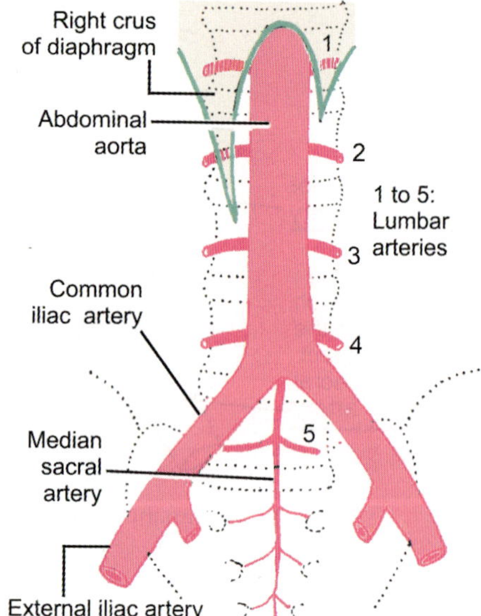


**31.5:** Scheme to show the posterior branches of the abdominal aorta.

1 to 4: Lumbar arteries arising from aorta.
5: Fifth lumbar artery arising from median sacral artery

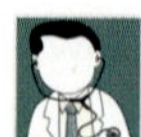

## CLINICAL CORRELATION

**Degenerative Changes in the Aorta**

1. As age advances, the walls of arteries undergo degenerative changes. The walls become thicker because of deposition of fatty substances in them. This process is called ***atheroma***.
2. Prominent atheromatous deposits may take place in the aorta, makings its walls rough and reducing its lumen.
3. Such changes, taking place at the bifurcation of the aorta can greatly reduce blood supply to the lower limbs. The patient then has pain in the legs when trying to walk (***claudication***).
4. Lack of blood flow into the internal iliac arteries can lead to impotence.
5. The bifurcation of the aorta can also be blocked by an embolus.

6. In suitable cases, blockage arising from these causes can be corrected by suitable surgical techniques.
   a. An operation for removal of the thickened lining of an artery is called ***endarterectomy***.
   b. Removal of a thrombus is called ***thrombo-endarterectomy***.
7. In some cases, segments of the aorta may be replaced or bypassed using synthetic grafts.
8. Atheromatous disease can also lead to the formation of an ***aneurysm*** (dilatation of the wall) of the aorta (because of weakening of the wall). The affected segment may require replacement with a graft.

**Angiography**

1. There have been many advances in techniques for visualising blood vessels of different organs.
2. A suitable radio-opaque dye injected into the femoral artery under high pressure enters the aorta (against the direction of blood flow) and outlines the aorta.
3. a. A more sophisticated method is to introduce a catheter into the femoral artery and pass it up into the aorta.
   b. The tip of the catheter can be guided into a large branch e.g., the coeliac trunk and dye can be injected directly into the artery and its branches.
   c. After a short interval, the dye passes into venous blood (venous filling phase) and the veins are then seen.

## Common Iliac Arteries

1. The right and left common iliac arteries are terminal branches of the abdominal aorta (31.5).
2. Each of these arteries is about 4 cm long. The artery of the right side is slightly longer than the left.
3. Each common iliac artery runs downwards and laterally and terminates by dividing into the external and internal iliac arteries. Some important relations of the arteries are considered below.

**WANT TO KNOW MORE?**

*Relations to Skeleton*

1. Each artery begins in front of the body of the fourth lumbar vertebra, a little to the left of the median plane (31.5).
2. It terminates in front of the sacroiliac joint, at the level of the disc between the fifth lumbar vertebra and the sacrum.
3. It is related posteriorly to the bodies of the fourth and fifth lumbar vertebrae and to the disc between them.

*Relation to Common Iliac Veins and Inferior Vena Cava*

1. In 31.6 note that the union of the right and left common iliac veins to form the inferior vena cava lies below and to the right of the bifurcation of the aorta; and that the veins lie posterior to the arteries.
2. It will now be easy to see that:
   a. The right common iliac artery is related posteriorly to both common iliac veins and to the beginning of the inferior vena cava. The vena cava and the right common iliac vein are lateral to its upper part, while the left common iliac vein is medial to its upper part.
   b. The left common iliac vein is partly medial to and partly behind the left common iliac artery.

*Anterior Relations*

1. The arteries are covered in front by peritoneum that separates them from coils of small intestine.
2. Each artery is crossed by the ureter, just near its termination (31.7).
3. The left common iliac artery is crossed by the superior rectal artery.
4. Both (right and left) common iliac arteries are crossed by sympathetic nerve fibres going to the superior hypogastric plexus (31.7).

*Lateral Relations*

The arteries are related laterally to the psoas major.

*Posterior Relations*

Deep in the interval between the fifth lumbar vertebra and the psoas major two important nerves, the lumbosacral trunk and the obturator nerve lie behind the artery.

## External Iliac Arteries

1. The external iliac arteries begin at the bifurcation of the common iliac. They run downwards and laterally and terminate deep to the inguinal ligament.
2. Each artery is continued into the corresponding thigh as the femoral artery.

### WANT TO KNOW MORE?

*Relations Common to both Arteries*

1. Each artery is related posterolaterally to the psoas major muscle, and postero-medially to the corresponding external iliac vein.
2. It is covered anteriorly and medially by peritoneum that separates it from coils of intestine. The artery is crossed by a number of structures as follows:
   a. Near its beginning, the artery may be crossed by the ureter (and in the female by the ovarian artery).
   b. The distal part of the vessel is crossed obliquely by the testicular artery (in the male) and by the genital branch of the genitofemoral nerve.
   c. Near its termination, it is crossed in the male by the ductus deferens; and in the female by the round ligament of the uterus.

*Relations Peculiar to Right or Left Artery*

On the right side the artery is crossed by the terminal ileum and frequently by the vermiform appendix. On the left side it is crossed by the sigmoid colon.

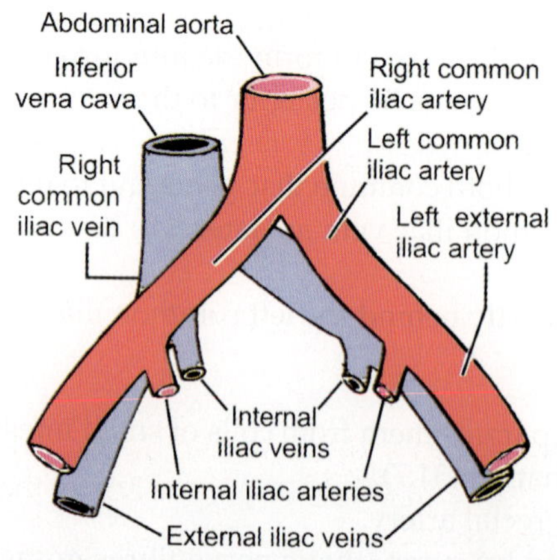


**31.6:** Relationship of right and left common iliac arteries and veins to one another

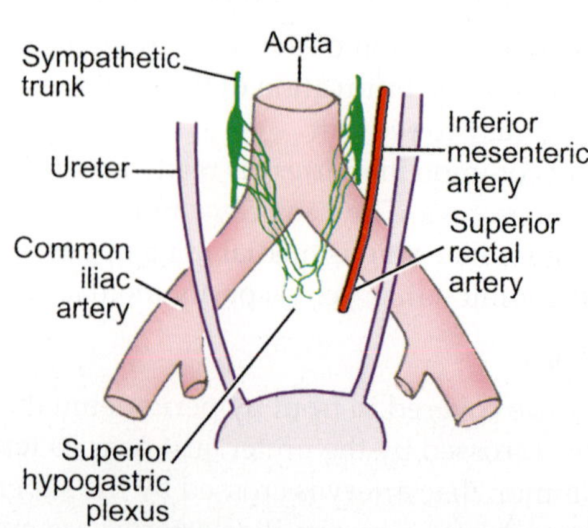


**31.7:** Anterior relations of common iliac arteries

### *Branches of External Iliac Artery*

These are the inferior epigastric and the deep circumflex iliac arteries. They are intimately related to the anterior abdominal wall and have been already described.

## The Internal Iliac Arteries

Each internal iliac artery (right or left) begins as a terminal branch of the common iliac artery, in front of the sacroiliac joint (31.5). The artery is distributed mainly within the pelvis and will be considered in Chapter 32.

## THE INFERIOR VENA CAVA AND ITS MAIN TRIBUTARIES

1. The structures in the abdomen and in the lower limb are drained through the inferior vena cava. This is the largest vein in the body. It lies on the posterior abdominal wall to the right of the abdominal aorta.
2. It is formed by the union of the right and left common iliac veins (31.8). It ends by piercing the diaphragm to open into the right atrium.
3. The common iliac veins are formed by the union of the internal and external veins. These veins run along the corresponding arteries.
4. Each external iliac vein begins behind the inguinal ligament as the continuation of the femoral vein. The femoral vein drains the lower limb and lies alongside the femoral artery.

### WANT TO KNOW MORE?

**Relations of the Inferior Vena Cava**

1. The upper part of the vena cava rests on the right crus of the diaphragm.
2. The lower part of the vena cava lies on the third, fourth and fifth lumbar vertebrae.
3. The diaphragm is separated from the vessel by a part of the right suprarenal gland and by the right coeliac ganglion.
4. Lateral to the 3rd, 4th and 5th lumbar vertebrae the vena cava lies on the medial margin of the right psoas major.
5. The right sympathetic trunk descends behind the vena cava.
6. Several arteries arising from the aorta and passing to the right cross behind the vena cava. These are:
   a. The right renal artery
   b. The right inferior phrenic artery
   c. The right suprarenal artery
   d. The 3rd and 4th right lumbar arteries.
7. The anterior relations of the inferior vena cava are shown in 31.9. The vena cava is overlapped (from above downwards) by:
   a. The liver
   b. The epiploic foramen which separates it from the right free margin of the lesser omentum
   c. The superior part of the duodenum
   d. The head of the pancreas
   e. The horizontal part of the duodenum
   f. The root of the mesentery containing the superior mesenteric artery and vein
   g. The right common iliac artery.
8. Other structures anterior to the vessel are as follows:
   a. The portal vein, and the bile duct, lie between the vena cava and the superior part of the duodenum.
   b. Higher up the portal vein and the bile duct and the hepatic artery lie in the free margin of the lesser omentum. They are separated from the vena cava by the foramen epiploicum.
   c. The right testicular or ovarian artery crosses the vena cava descending obliquely between it and the horizontal part of the duodenum.

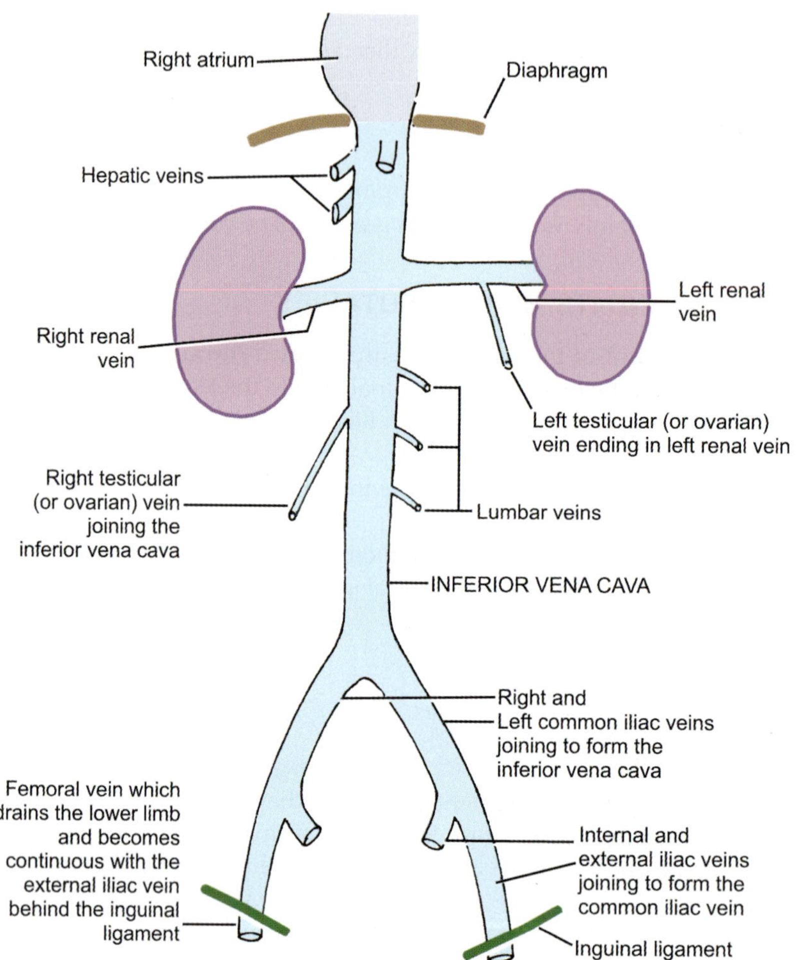


**31.8:** Scheme to show the inferior vena cava and its tributaries

## Direct Tributaries of Inferior Vena Cava

The largest tributaries of the inferior vena cava are the hepatic veins from the liver and the renal veins from the kidneys.

1. The ***hepatic veins*** are terminal parts of an elaborate venous tree that permeates the liver.
   a. The hepatic veins emerge from liver tissue that is in close contact with the upper part of the vena cava, and immediately enter the vena cava.
   b. The cut ends of the veins are seen on the vena cava when the liver is removed. See 31.8.
2. The right or left ***renal vein*** runs horizontally from the hilum of the corresponding kidney to join the inferior vena cava.
   a. The right vein is about 2.5 cm long. It lies behind the descending part of the duodenum.
   b. The left renal vein is much longer (7.5 cm) than the right vein as it has to cross the midline to reach the vena cava.
   c. The left renal vein crosses anterior to the aorta, and posterior to the body of the pancreas and the splenic vein.
3. From a developmental point of view, part of the left renal vein is homologous to a segment of the inferior vena cava near the termination of the renal veins. It, therefore, happens that some veins of the right side open into

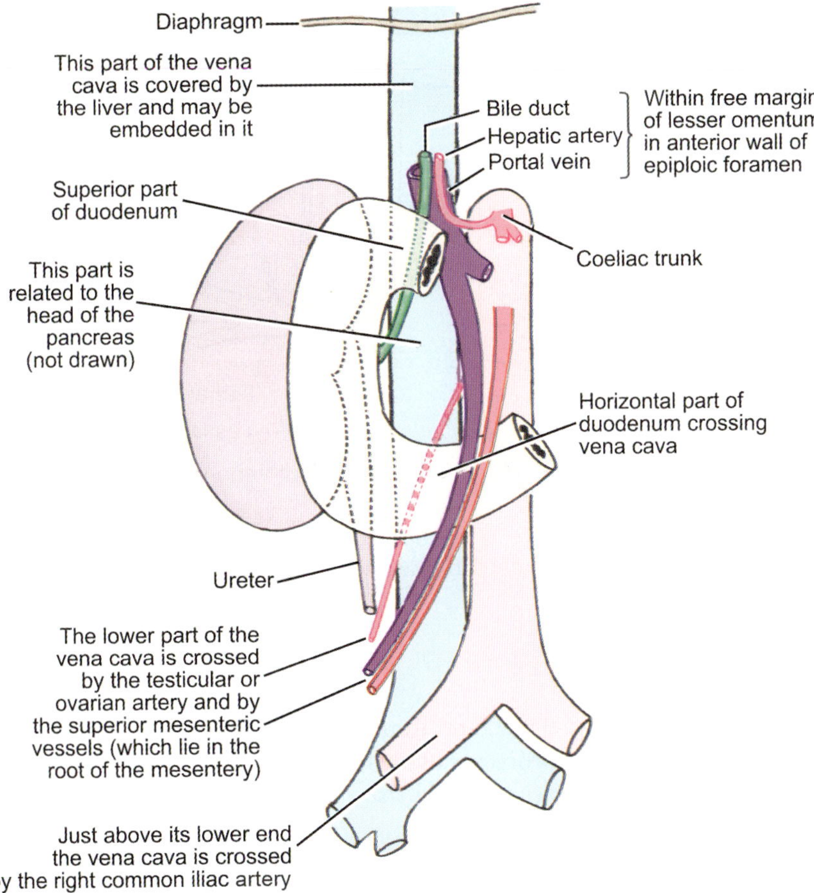


**31.9:** Scheme to show the anterior relations of the inferior vena cava

the inferior vena cava, but the corresponding veins of the left side end in the left renal vein. These veins are as follows (31.10):

a. The ***inferior phrenic veins*** accompany the corresponding arteries.
   i. The vein of the right side ends in the inferior vena cava.
   ii. The vein of the left side usually ends in the left renal vein.
b. On either side, the ***suprarenal vein*** emerges from the hilum of the corresponding suprarenal gland.
   i. The vein of the right side opens into the back of the inferior vena cava.
   ii. That of the left side opens into the left renal vein.
c. In the male the ***testicular vein*** travels through the spermatic cord and the inguinal canal in the form of a plexus (called the ***pampiniform plexus***).
   i. At the deep inguinal ring, two veins emerge from this plexus and run over the lower part of the posterior abdominal wall along with the testicular artery.
   ii. Higher up they unite to form a single trunk that opens on the right side into the inferior vena cava; and on the left side into the left renal vein.
d. In the female the testicular veins are replaced by ***ovarian veins*** that form a plexus in the broad ligament.
   i. Two veins arising from the plexus accompany the ovarian artery.
   ii. Higher up they unite to form one vein that terminates like the testicular vein.

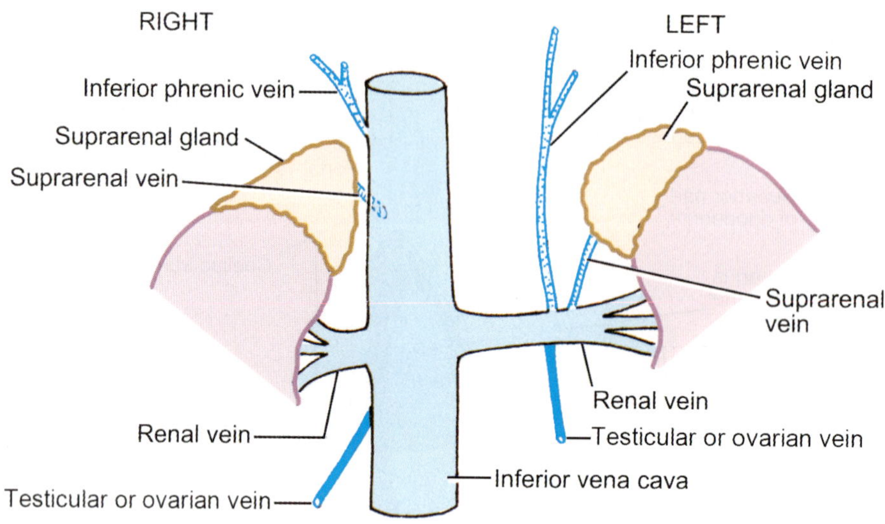


**31.10:** Scheme to show some veins that open, on the right side into the inferior vena cava and on the left side into the left renal vein

4. The ***lumbar veins*** accompany the lumbar arteries (31.11).
   a. There are four of them on either side.
   b. They drain blood from the abdominal wall and from the vertebral venous plexuses.
   c. In front of the roots of the transverse processes of the lumbar vertebrae, the lumbar veins communicate with each other by a vertical venous channel called the ***ascending lumbar vein.***

## WANT TO KNOW MORE?

5. Parallel and medial to the ascending lumbar vein there is another vertical vein called the ***lumbar azygos vein***.
6. a. The 1st and 2nd lumbar veins may end in the ascending lumbar vein or in the lumbar azygos vein; or more rarely in the inferior vena cava.
   b. The 3rd and 4th lumbar veins usually end in the inferior vena cava.
   c. The mode of termination of the lumbar veins is subject to considerable variation (31.11).

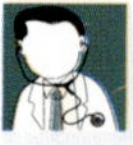

## CLINICAL CORRELATION

### Inferior Vena Cava

*Congenital Anomalies*

1. The inferior vena cava has a complicated developmental history and various anomalies may be seen.
2. In the embryo, the vena cava is a paired structure that normally persists only on the right side.
3. Persistence on both sides results in a ***double inferior vena cava***.
4. a. Generally, the duplication is confined to the part below the level of the renal arteries (infrarenal segment).
   b. Sometimes, the infrarenal segment may persist only on the left side (instead of the right) leading to a ***left inferior vena cava***.

5. Sometimes, the part of the inferior vena cava related to the stomach (hepatic segment) may be missing. The vena cava is then continuous with a much enlarged azygos vein through which it drains into the superior vena cava (***azygos continuation of inferior vena cava***).
6. Normally, the inferior vena cava lies behind the right ureter. However, it may lie in front of the ureter.

*Obstruction*

1. The inferior vena cava may be obstructed by formation of a thrombus. It may also be obstructed by pressure from a malignant growth. Obstruction leads to oedema in the lower limbs.
2. a. When the inferior vena cava is obstructed communications between tributaries of the inferior vena cava with those of the superior vena cava become important, and can undergo considerable enlargement.
   b. From below, the veins involved are:
      i. The inferior epigastric
      ii. Circumflex iliac
      iii. External pudendal.
   c. Blood from them passes into:
      i. The lateral thoracic
      ii. Internal thoracic
      iii. Posterior intercostal veins.
3. Superficial channels of communication become prominent over the abdominal wall. The ***thoracoepigastric*** vein is an important channel of communication.
4. Communications between the superior and inferior venae cavae are also established through the azygos and hemiazygos veins and through the vertebral venous plexus.
5. In pregnancy, the inferior vena cava may be pressed upon by the enlarged uterus, and this may lead to oedema in the dependent parts of the lower limb.

## Common Iliac Veins

1. Each common iliac vein (right and left) is formed by union of the corresponding internal and external iliac veins. This union takes place in front of the sacroiliac joint.
2. From here, the vein passes upwards and medially and ends by joining the vein of the opposite side to form the inferior vena cava (in front of the fifth lumbar vertebra).
3. As the lower end of the inferior vena cava lies to the right of the middle line, the right common iliac vein has to follow a shorter and more vertical course than the vein of the left side.

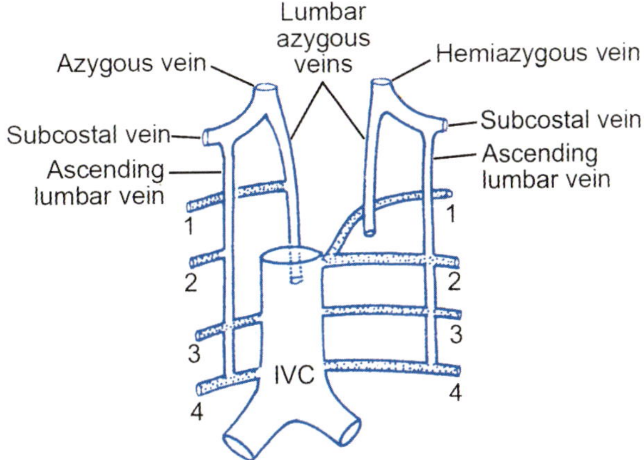


**31.11:** Scheme to show the lumbar veins (1 to 4). They may end in the inferior vena cava (IVC), in the ascending lumbar vein, or in the lumbar azygous vein

**WANT TO KNOW MORE?**

*Relations of Common Iliac Veins*

These are shown in 31.12.

1. The lower part of the right common iliac vein is behind the corresponding artery.
2. Higher up, it becomes lateral to the artery.
3. The left common iliac vein is medial to the corresponding artery over the greater part of its course.
4. Its terminal part is behind the right common iliac artery.
5. The left common iliac vein is crossed by the superior rectal artery and vein as they run through the root of the transverse mesocolon.

   The tributaries of the common iliac veins are shown in 31.13. The iliolumbar and median sacral veins accompany the corresponding arteries.

## External Iliac Veins

1. Each external iliac vein begins behind the corresponding inguinal ligament as a continuation of the femoral vein.
2. It runs upwards and medially, along the brim of the pelvis. It ends in front of the sacroiliac joint by joining the internal iliac vein to form the common iliac vein.
3. The vein is medial to the corresponding artery (e in 31.12), but near its upper end it becomes posterior to the artery and passes behind the internal iliac artery (f).
4. Along with the external iliac artery the vein rests on the psoas major.
5. The right and left veins are crossed by the same structures that cross the corresponding arteries.
6. On both sides, the vein is crossed (from above downwards) by:
   a. The internal iliac artery (31.12)
   b. The ureter
   c. The testicular or ovarian artery
   d. The ductus deferens (or in the female by the round ligament of the uterus).

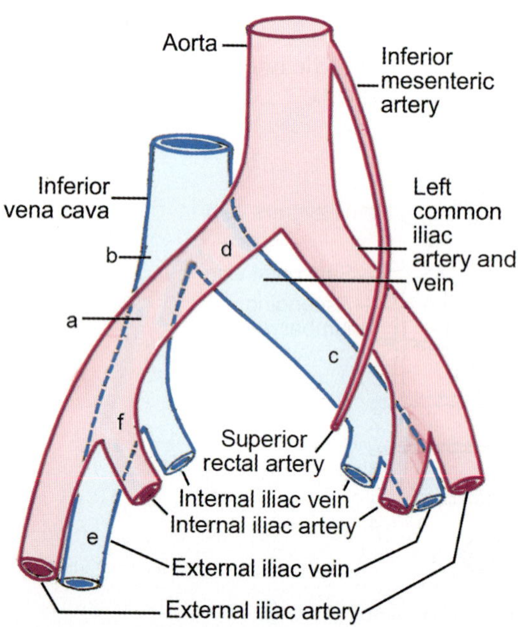


**31.12:** Relations of common iliac veins

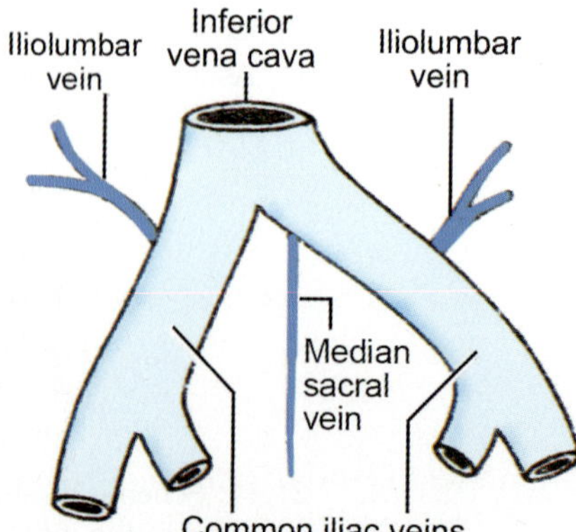


**31.13:** Tributaries of common iliac veins

7. On the right side, it is also crossed (in addition to the above) by the terminal part of the ileum and sometimes by the vermiform appendix.
8. On the left side, the vein is also crossed by the sigmoid colon.
9. The tributaries of the external iliac veins are:
   a. The inferior epigastric vein
   b. The deep circumflex iliac vein
   c. The pubic veins.

   These veins run along the corresponding arteries.

### The Internal Iliac Veins

These will be considered when we discuss the wall of the pelvis (Chapter 32).

## NERVES OF POSTERIOR ABDOMINAL WALL

The main nerves present in relation to the posterior abdominal wall are as follows:

1. Just below the twelfth rib, we see the ***subcostal nerve***. This nerve is a continuation of the ventral ramus of the twelfth thoracic spinal nerve.
2. Most of the other nerves seen are branches of the lumbar plexus. This plexus is formed by ventral rami of lumbar nerves, within the substance of the psoas major muscle. This plexus is concerned mainly with the innervation of the lower limb and has been described in Chapter 10.
3. The branches of the lumbar plexus seen are:
   a. The iliohypogastric nerve
   b. The ilioinguinal nerve
   c. The genitofemoral nerve
   d. The lateral cutaneous nerve of the thigh
   e. The femoral nerve.

   These nerves are described in Chapter 10.

### Autonomic Nerves of Abdomen and Pelvis

1. Autonomic nerves may be sympathetic or parasympathetic.
2. Sympathetic nerves to be seen in the abdomen and pelvis are branches given off by the sympathetic trunk in this region. Some branches given off by the thoracic part of the sympathetic trunk also enter the abdomen.
3. Parasympathetic nerves are derived from two sources.
   a. One source is the vagus nerve that is the tenth cranial nerve. It descends through the neck and thorax into the abdomen.
   b. In addition to the vagus, some abdominal and pelvic organs receive parasympathetic fibres through the sacral parasympathetic outflow.

### Autonomic Ganglia and Plexuses in Abdomen and Pelvis

1. Many autonomic nerve fibres, both sympathetic and parasympathetic, reach viscera after passing through a number of plexuses. Although, they are called plexuses they contain numerous neurons and are, in fact, equivalent to ganglia. The plexuses/ganglia to be seen in the abdomen and pelvis are as follows:
2. The ***coeliac ganglion*** (right or left) is the largest autonomic ganglion in the body. It is irregular in shape.
   a. Its lower part is often separate from the rest of the ganglion and is called the ***aorticorenal ganglion***.
   b. The coeliac ganglion lies on the posterior abdominal wall, in front of the corresponding crus of the diaphragm.
   c. Just medial to it, there is the abdominal aorta (at the level of origin of the coeliac trunk), and just lateral to the ganglion there is the suprarenal gland.
   d. The right coeliac ganglion lies behind the inferior vena cava, and the left ganglion lies behind the splenic vessels.

3. Fibres passing from one ganglion to the other (across the aorta and around the origin of the coeliac trunk) form the ***coeliac plexus***. The ***coeliac ganglion*** and ***coeliac plexus*** lie in relation to the abdominal aorta at the level of the origin of the coeliac trunk. The coeliac plexus is the uppermost part of an extensive ***aortic plexus*** surrounding the abdominal aorta. This is continued into subsidiary plexuses around the branches arising from the vessel.
   a. The part of the aortic plexus between the origins of the superior and inferior mesenteric arteries is called the ***intermesenteric plexus***.
   b. The part overlying the bifurcation of the aorta is called the ***superior hypogastric plexus***.
   c. When traced downwards it divides into the right and left ***inferior hypogastric plexuses*** related to the corresponding internal iliac arteries.
   d. Some other plexuses are present in close relation to viscera, or even within their walls. The ***vesical plexus*** surrounds the urinary bladder. In the gut there is a ***myenteric plexus*** (of Auerbach) between the muscle coats, and a ***submucosal plexus*** (of Meissner).

## Parasympathetic Nerves in Abdomen and Pelvis

1. Parasympathetic nerve fibres are derived from a cranial outflow and a sacral outflow.
2. In the thorax and abdomen, the cranial outflow is represented by the vagus nerve.
   a. In the thorax fibres of the vagus form an anterior and a posterior oesophageal plexus.
   b. Fibres emerging from the lower end of the anterior oesophageal plexus collect to form the ***anterior vagal trunk*** that is made up mainly of fibres of the left vagus nerve.
   c. Similarly, fibres arising from the posterior oesophageal plexus (derived mainly from the right vagus) collect to form the ***posterior vagal trunk***.
   d. These two trunks enter the abdomen through the oesophageal opening in the diaphragm. They are responsible for the parasympathetic supply to the greater part of the gastrointestinal tract and to some other organs.
3. Preganglionic neurons that constitute the ***sacral parasympathetic outflow*** are located in the intermediolateral grey column in spinal segments S2, S3 and S4.
   a. They emerge from the spinal cord through the ventral nerve roots of the corresponding spinal nerves.
   b. They soon leave the spinal nerves through their ***pelvic splanchnic*** branches.
   c. The preganglionic fibres end in relation to postganglionic neurons which are located either in the walls of the viscera supplied or in plexuses related to them.
   d. The organs supplied directly by the pelvic splanchnic nerves are:
      i. The urinary bladder
      ii. The rectum
      iii. The testes or ovaries
      iv. The uterus
      v. The uterine tubes
      vi. The penis or clitoris.
   e. Some fibres of these nerves pass through the hypogastric plexuses to supply the pelvic colon, the descending colon and the left one-third of the transverse colon. (Note that the parts of the gut supplied are hindgut derivatives).

## Sympathetic Nerves in Abdomen and Pelvis

*Branches of Thoracic Part of Sympathetic Trunk Entering the Abdomen*

1. The lower thoracic sympathetic ganglia give origin to prominent medial branches called the ***greater, lesser*** and ***lowest splanchnic nerves***.
2. All these nerves pass through the diaphragm and enter the abdomen.
3. Here the greater splanchnic nerve ends mainly in the coeliac ganglion. Some fibres of the greater splanchnic nerve end in the aorticorenal ganglion.

4. The lesser splanchnic nerve ends in the aorticorenal ganglion.
5. The lowest splanchnic nerve ends in the renal plexus.

### *Lumbar Part of Sympathetic Trunk*

The sympathetic trunk passes from the thorax to the abdomen by passing posterior to the medial arcuate ligament. Sometimes it may pass through the crus of the diaphragm. There are usually four ganglia on the lumbar part of the trunk. Their branches and communications are as follows:

1. The ganglia give off grey rami communicantes to the lumbar nerves.
2. The first two ganglia (sometimes three) receive white rami from the corresponding spinal nerves. These white rami are part of the thoracolumbar outflow carrying preganglionic fibres to the sympathetic trunk.
3. Each ganglion gives off a ***lumbar splanchnic branch***. These branches end in the coeliac, renal, aortic, and superior hypogastric plexuses.
4. Vascular branches reach the aortic plexus. From here, they extend into plexuses on the common iliac, internal iliac, external iliac, and the proximal parts of the femoral arteries.

## Lymphatics of Abdomen

1. The largest lymph vessel in the body is the ***thoracic duct***. This duct begins in the abdomen as an upward continuation of a sac-like structure called the ***cisternal chyli***.
2. The thoracic duct has been described in Chapter 22.
   a. This duct (which is the largest lymph vessel in the body) begins within the abdomen as a continuation of the ***cisterna chyli***.
   b. The cisternal chyli is seen in relation to the posterior abdominal wall. It is an elongated lymphatic sac about 6 cm long. It is placed vertically in front of the first and second lumbar vertebrae.
   c. It lies to the right of the abdominal aorta, and deep to the right crus of the diaphragm.
   d. Superiorly, the cisternal chyli becomes continuous with the thoracic duct.
   e. The connections of the cisterna chyli are considered in Chapter 34 in which the lymphatics of the abdomen are discussed.
3. Most of the lymph from the abdomen drains into the cisternal chyli and from there into the thoracic duct.

### *Chief Lymph Nodes of Abdomen and Pelvis*

1. The entire lymph from the abdomen (and from the lower limbs) ultimately ends in terminal groups of lymph nodes present in relation to the abdominal aorta. These nodes are arranged in three main groups, each having a specific area of drainage.
   a. On either side of the aorta, there are the right and left ***lateral aortic*** nodes. Some outlying members of these groups lying behind the aorta constitute the ***retroaortic nodes***.
   b. In front of the aorta, there are the ***preaortic nodes***.
   c. These are divided into the ***coeliac***, the ***superior mesenteric*** and the ***inferior mesenteric*** nodes lying around the origins of the corresponding arteries.
2. On each side, the efferents from the lateral aortic nodes form the corresponding ***lumbar trunk*** that ends by joining the cisterna chyli.
3. Efferents from the preaortic nodes form the ***intestinal trunk*** that also ends in the cisterna chyli.
4. The coeliac lymph nodes receive lymph from:
   a. The stomach
   b. Part of the duodenum
   c. The liver
   d. The extrahepatic biliary apparatus
   e. The pancreas
   f. The spleen.

5. The superior mesenteric lymph nodes receive lymph from:
   a. The jejunum
   b. The ileum
   c. The caecum
   d. The appendix
   e. The ascending colon
   f. The transverse colon
   g. Part of the duodenum.
6. The inferior mesenteric lymph nodes receive lymph from:
   a. The descending colon
   b. The sigmoid colon
   c. The upper part of the rectum.
7. Numerous groups of outlying nodes are associated with the lymphatic drainage of the organs mentioned above.
8. The ***lateral aortic nodes*** (34.3) receive all the lymph draining through the common iliac nodes. They also receive lymph directly from the:
   a. Posterior abdominal wall
   b. The kidneys and upper part of the ureters
   c. The testes or ovaries
   d. The uterine tubes and part of the uterus
   e. Suprarenal glands.
9. The ***common iliac nodes*** (34.3) lie along the corresponding blood vessels. They receive lymph from the external and internal iliac nodes and send it to the lateral aortic nodes.
10. The ***internal iliac nodes*** (34.3) lie along the corresponding blood vessels. They receive most of the lymph of the pelvic organs and from the deeper tissues of the perineum. They also receive some vessels of the lower limbs that travel along the superior and inferior gluteal blood vessels.
11. The ***external iliac lymph nodes*** (34.3) lie along the external iliac blood vessels. They receive lymph from the lower limb through the inguinal nodes. They also receive direct lymph vessels from the deeper tissues of the infraumbilical part of the anterior abdominal wall and from some pelvic organs.

### *Lymphatic Drainage of Abdominal Wall*

*The skin*

1. The skin above the level of the umbilicus(in front) and above the iliac crest (at the back) drains into the axillary lymph nodes.
2. The skin of the anterior abdominal wall below the umbilicus drains into the superficial inguinal lymph nodes.

*Deeper tissues*

1. Lymph vessels from the posterior abdominal wall travel along the lumbar vessels to the lateral aortic nodes, including the retroaortic nodes.
2. The vessels from the upper part of the anterior and lateral part of the abdominal wall travel along the superior epigastric vessels to the parasternal nodes.
3. The vessels from the lower part of the anterolateral abdominal wall travel along the inferior epigastric and circumflex iliac vessels. Passing through nodes placed along these vessels they reach the external iliac nodes.

# 32 CHAPTER Walls of the Pelvis

In a study of the walls of the pelvis we have to consider the bones and joints, the muscles and fascia; and the blood vessels, nerves and lymphatics of the region.

### Bones and Joints of Pelvis

The bones and joints of the pelvis have already been considered in chapter 24.

## MUSCLES AND FASCIA OF PELVIC WALL

### Preliminary Remarks

The pelvic muscles arise from the inner wall of the bony pelvis. These are:

1. The piriformis
2. The obturator internus
3. The levator ani
4. The coccygeus.
   a. The piriformis and the obturator internus are described in 32.1. The levator ani is described in 32.2. The coccygeus is described in 32.3.
   b. The levator ani and the coccygeus muscles of the two sides form the ***pelvic diaphragm***. They are shown in 32.4.
   c. Present in relation to pelvic muscles (and viscera) there are layers of fascia that are collectively referred to as ***pelvic fascia***.

**32.1: Piriformis and Obturator Internus**

| *Muscle* | *Origin* | *Insertion* | *Action* | *Nerve supply* |
|---|---|---|---|---|
| Piriformis | 1. Anterior (pelvic) surface of sacrum (by three digitations). | Upper border of greater trochanter of femur. | Lateral rotator of femur. | Direct branches from nerves L5, S1, S2. |
| Obturator internus | 1. From pelvic surface of hip bone including the following:<br>a. Body, superior ramus, and inferior ramus of pubis.<br>b. Ramus and body of ischium.<br>c. Part of ilium.<br>2. Obturator membrane. | 1. Tendon leaves the pelvis through the lesser sciatic foramen to appear in the gluteal region.<br>2. Tendon thens runs laterally behind the hip joint to reach the medial surface of greater trochanter of femur (in front of trochanteric fossa). | Lateral rotator of femur | Nerve to obturator internus (L5, S1) |

| 32.2: Levator ani | |
|---|---|
| Origin | (From front to back)<br>1. Pelvic surface of body of pubis<br>2. Obturator fascia<br>3. Spine of ischium. |
| Insertion | The fibres arch backwards and medially.<br>1. In the male the most anterior fibres run across the sides of the prostate to end in the perineal body. These fibres constitute the levator prostate muscle.<br>2. In the female the corresponding fibres pass across the sides of the vagina to end in the perineal body. They form the pubovaginalis muscle.<br>3. The intermediate fibres pass across the sides of the rectum and become continuous with those of the opposite side behind the anorectal junction. They form the puborectalis. They merge with the internal and external sphincters of the anal canal to form the anorectal ring.<br>4. The most posterior fibres are attached to the coccyx, and to a fibrous band called the anococcygeal ligament. |
| Nerve supply | 1. Branch from 4th sacral nerve.<br>2. Branch from inferior rectal nerve or from perineal division of pudendal nerve. |
| Action | 1. Along with coccygeus it forms the pelvic diaphragm.<br>2. Supports pelvic viscera.<br>3. Acts as a sphincter for rectum and vagina. |

| 32.3: Coccygeus | |
|---|---|
| Origin | From ischial spine. |
| Insertion | Lateral margin of:<br>1. Coccyx<br>2. Last piece of sacrum. |
| Nerve supply | Fourth and fifth sacral nerves |
| Actions | 1. Helps to form the pelvic diaphragm.<br>2. Pulls the coccyx forwards after it has been pushed back. |

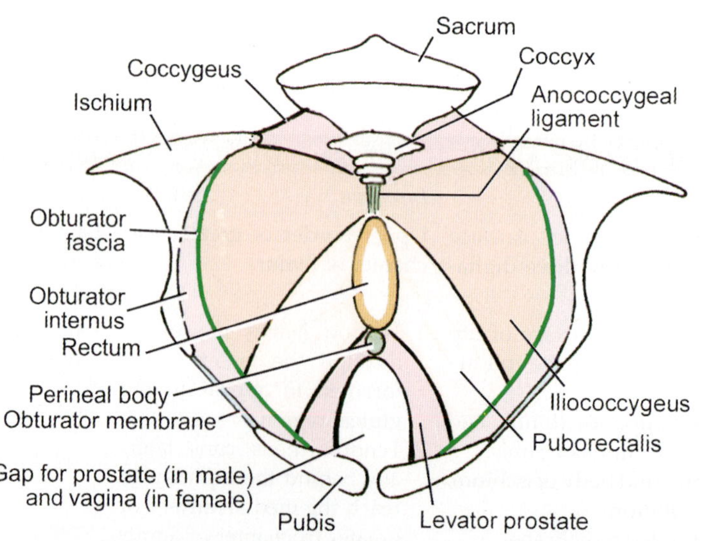


32.4: Scheme to show the arrangement of the levator ani and coccygeus muscles

## Notes on Levator Ani

1. The levator ani is shown schematically in 32.4 in which the pelvis has been cut transversely along a line passing through the upper part of the pubis (in front) and the ischial spine behind. The origin of the muscle from the pelvic aspect of the lower part of the hip-bone is shown in 32.5.
2. The anorectal ring is formed as shown in 33.6 and 33.7. It can be felt by a finger placed in the rectum. Its importance is described in chapter 33.
3. The levator ani is related above to the urinary bladder, prostate or vagina, and rectum. Some part of it is covered by peritoneum.

## Pelvic Diaphragm

1. The levator ani and the coccygeus form a transverse partition across the pelvis which is called the pelvic diaphragm.
2. This diaphragm separates the pelvic viscera (above) from structures in the perineum (32.6) and the ischiorectal fossa (32.7).
3. The pelvic diaphragm is pierced by the rectum (32.7), the urethra (32.6) and in the female by the vagina.
4. The diaphragm supports the pelvic viscera. It acts as a sphincter for the rectum and the vagina.
5. The coccygeus can pull the coccyx forwards after it has been pushed back during defecation or parturition.
6. The relationship of the pelvic fascia to the pelvic diaphragm is described below.

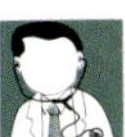

### CLINICAL CORRELATION

1. The pelvic diaphragm is subject to great stress during childbirth. It can be damaged or weakened.
2. A weakened pelvic diaphragm can lead to prolapse of the uterus or of the rectum.

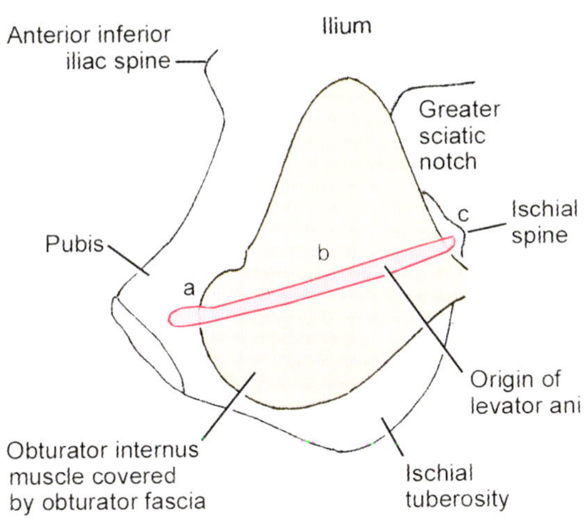


**32.5:** Lower part of hip bone viewed from the pelvic aspect to show the obturator internus and the origin of the levator ani

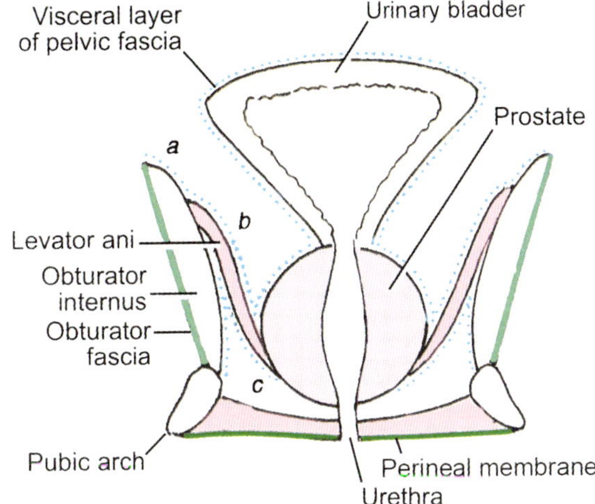


**32.6:** Coronal section through the anterior part of the pelvic diaphragm in the male

## The Pelvic Fascia

1. The pelvic fascia consists of two main parts (32.6 and 32.7).
2. The ***parietal layer*** (shown in interrupted line) lines the pelvic muscles.

3. The ***visceral layer*** (shown in fine dotted line) surrounds individual viscera.
4. The parietal fascia covers the piriformis and the obturator internus.
   a. Over the obturator internus it is thick (specially in its upper part) ('a' in 32.6) and forms the ***obturator fascia***.
   b. The fascia over the piriformis is thin. It separates the internal iliac vessels and their branches from the muscle; but the sacral nerves lie between the muscle and the fascia.
5. The pelvic diaphragm is covered by one layer of fascia above it, and another below it.
   a. When traced medially the upper layer ('b' in 32.6) blends with the fascia of viscera that pierce the diaphragm (32.6 and 32.7).
   b. Laterally the superior layer merges with the obturator fascia and reinforces its upper part.
   c. The fascia below the pelvic diaphragm ('c') lines the medial wall of the ischiorectal fossa (32.7). More anteriorly (32.6) it merges with the superior fascia of the urogenital diaphragm.

## BLOOD VESSELS OF TRUE PELVIS

These are the internal iliac artery and its branches and the corresponding veins.

### Internal Iliac Artery

1. Each internal iliac artery (right or left) begins as a terminal branch of the common iliac artery, in front of the sacroiliac joint (31.12).
2. It runs downwards to reach the upper margin of the greater sciatic foramen.
3. Here, it divides into anterior and posterior trunks (32.9).
4. Some relations of the artery are shown in 32.8.

#### *Branches of Internal Iliac Artery*

*The branches arising from the anterior trunk of the internal iliac artery are as follows:*

1. The ***superior vesical artery*** (32.9 and 32.10) runs forwards and medially to supply the upper part of the urinary bladder.
   a. The artery is crossed by the ductus deferens and may give a branch to it.
   b. The stem of the artery represents the proximal part of the umbilical artery of the fetus. That is why it is continuous with the medial umbilical ligament that represents the distal obliterated part of the umbilical artery.

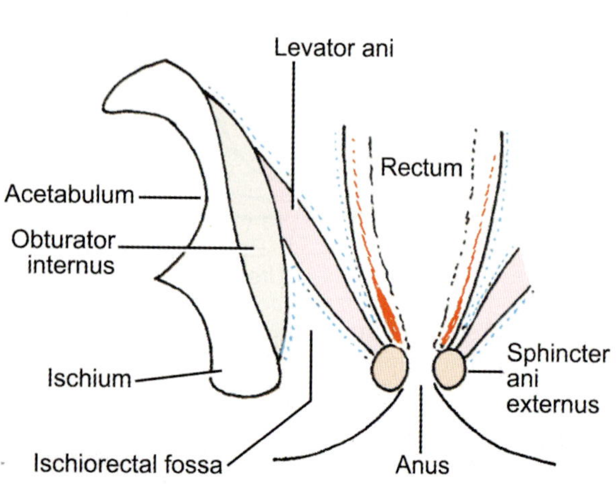


**32.7:** Coronal section through the posterior part of the pelvic diaphragm in the male

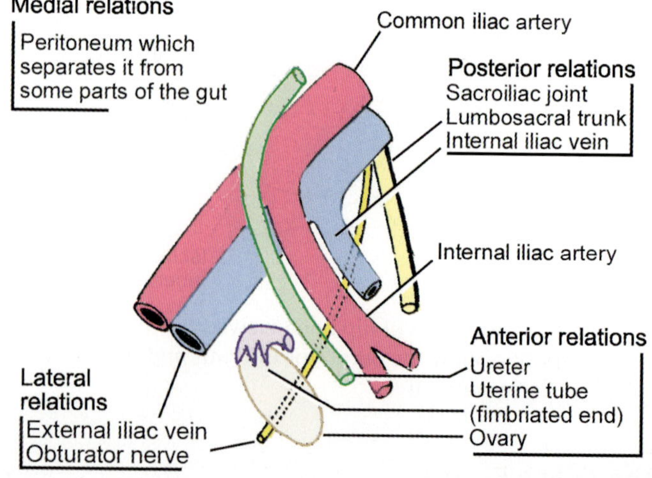


**32.8:** Some relations of the internal iliac artery as seen from the medial side

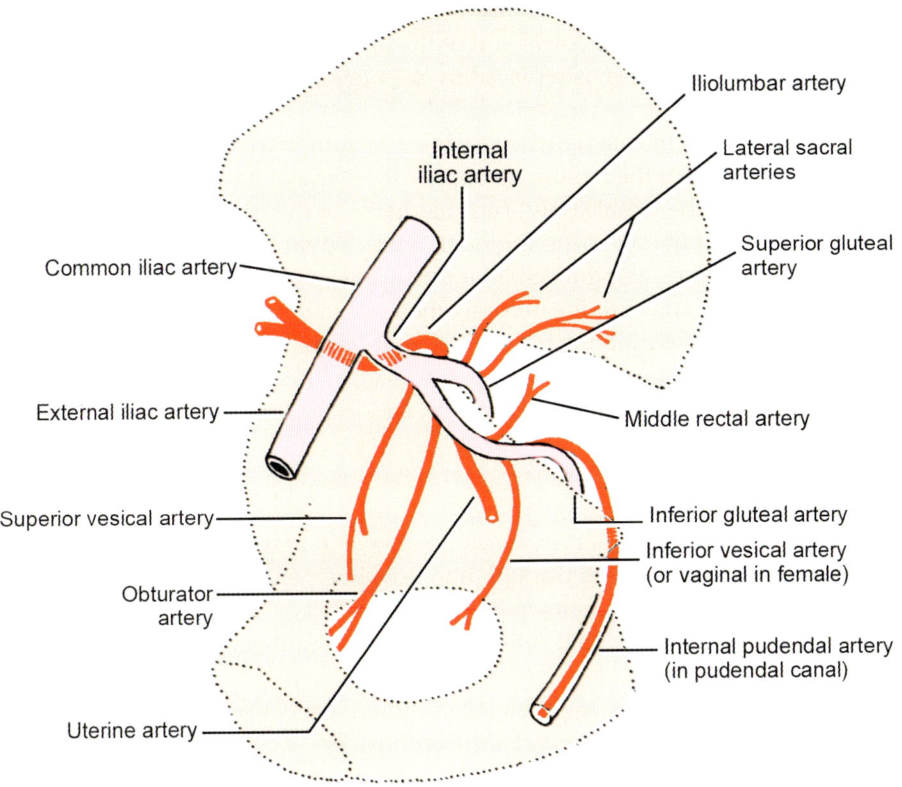


**32.9:** Scheme to show the branches of the internal iliac artery

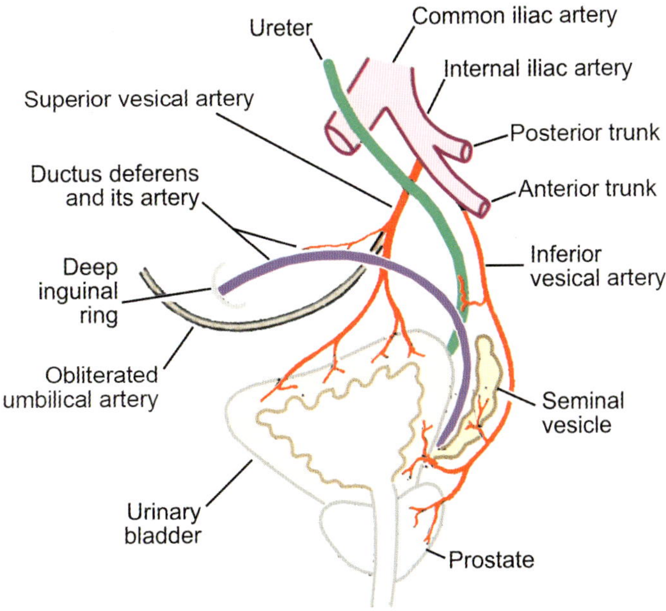


**32.10:** Scheme to show the superior and inferior vesical arteries

2. The ***inferior vesical artery*** (present only in the male) runs forwards and medially to supply the urinary bladder, the prostate, the seminal vesicle and the lower end of the ureter (32.10).
3. In the female the inferior vesical artery is replaced by the ***vaginal artery*** that supplies the vagina, the urinary bladder and part of the rectum.
4. The ***middle rectal artery*** (32.9) runs medially to reach the rectum, where it anastomoses with the superior and inferior rectal arteries. Apart from the rectum it supplies the seminal vesicles and the prostate.
5. The ***uterine artery*** (present in the female only) runs medially on the pelvic floor (formed by the levator ani) to reach the lateral side of the upper end of the vagina (lateral vaginal fornix) (32.11).
   a. Leaving the pelvic wall it runs along the side of the uterus, within the two layers of the broad ligament to reach the junction of the uterus with the uterine tube.
   b. Finally it turns laterally (still within the broad ligament) to reach the hilum of the ovary. Here it anastomoses with the ovarian artery.
   c. Apart from branches to the uterus, the uterine tube, and to the ovary, it gives some branches to the vagina (32.11).
6. The ***obturator artery*** runs forwards and downwards on the lateral pelvic wall (formed here by obturator fascia covering the obturator internus).
   a. It is accompanied by the obturator nerve (which lies above it) and the obturator vein (below it).
   b. Reaching the obturator canal it passes through it to leave the pelvic cavity.
7. The branches of the obturator artery are shown in 32.12 and 32.13.
   a. Note in particular the pubic branch that runs over the pubis and anastomoses with the pubic branch of the inferior epigastric artery.
   b. Sometimes the anastomosis is large and then the obturator artery appears to be a branch of the inferior epigastric artery. It is then called the ***abnormal obturator artery***.
   c. The importance of an abnormal obturator artery lies in the fact that it is closely related to (the neck of the sac of) a femoral hernia. The hernia passes through the femoral canal lying medial to the femoral vein.
   d. In cases of strangulation of the hernia the surgeon may cut the lacunar ligament to enlarge the femoral canal.
   e. Usually the abnormal obturator artery passes lateral to the femoral canal, in contact with the femoral vein and is safe in such an operation.
   f. Sometimes, however, it may lie along the medial margin of the femoral ring i.e., along the free margin of the lacunar ligament. Such an artery is likely to be cut if an attempt is made to enlarge the femoral ring.

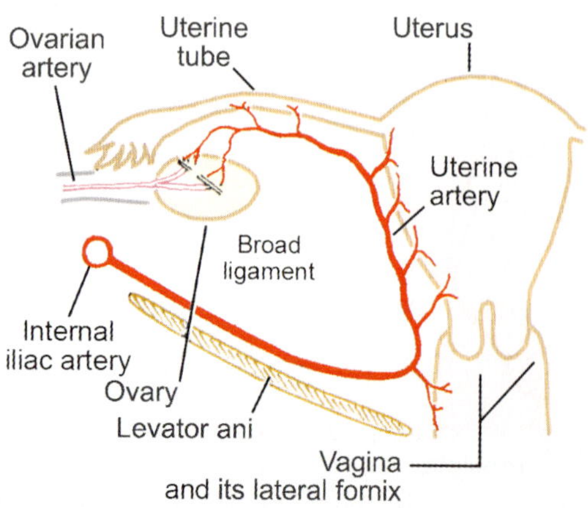


**32.11:** Scheme to show course and branches of the uterine artery

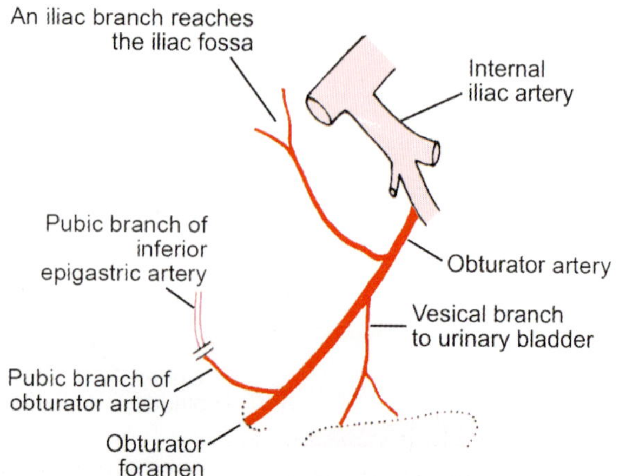


**32.12:** Scheme to show the branches given off by the obturator artery within the pelvis

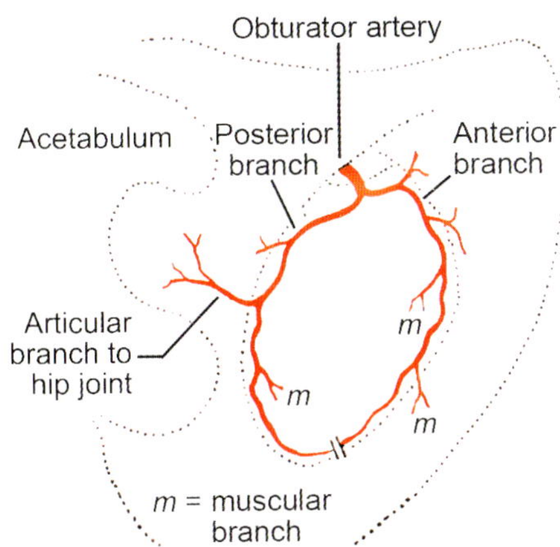


**32.13:** Scheme to show the branches given off by the obturator artery outside the pelvis

8. The ***internal pudendal artery*** supplies the external genitalia. It follows a complicated course.
   a. Starting within the pelvic cavity the artery passes out of it through the greater sciatic foramen to enter the gluteal region.
   b. After a short course in this region the artery passes through the lesser sciatic foramen to reach the lateral wall of the ischiorectal fossa. Its further course lies in the perineum and has been described earlier.
9. The ***inferior gluteal artery*** begins within the pelvis where it lies anterior to the piriformis. It passes through the greater sciatic foramen, below the piriformis, to enter the gluteal region.

*The branches arising from the posterior trunk of the internal iliac artery are as follows:*

1. The ***superior gluteal artery*** is the main continuation of the posterior trunk of the internal iliac artery. It leaves the pelvic cavity by passing through the greater sciatic foramen, above the piriformis muscle.
2. The ***lateral sacral arteries***, superior and inferior, pass medially and divide into branches that pass through the anterior sacral foramina to supply the sacrum and related structures.
3. The ***iliolumbar artery*** arises from the posterior trunk of the internal iliac artery (32.14). It runs upwards and laterally and passes deep to the psoas major. Here it divides into a ***lumbar branch*** that supplies the psoas major and an ***iliac branch*** that supplies the iliacus and can be seen on its surface.

## The Internal Iliac Veins

1. Each internal iliac vein is formed by the confluence of several veins that accompany the branches of the internal iliac artery (with the exception of the iliolumbar veins which end in the common iliac veins).
2. The vein begins near the upper part of the greater sciatic foramen. From here it runs upwards posteromedial to the internal iliac artery.
3. The vein ends by joining the external iliac vein to form the common iliac vein. The termination lies in front of the sacroiliac joint.
4. The pelvic organs are drained through a number of venous plexuses that ultimately drain into the internal iliac vein. These plexuses surround the urinary bladder (vesical plexus), the prostate, the uterus, the vagina and the rectum.
5. The ***prostatic plexus*** of veins receives the deep dorsal vein of the penis.
   a. This vein is placed on the dorsum of the penis, in the middle line, deep to the deep fascia, in between the right and left dorsal arteries.
   b. The prostatic plexus communicates with the vesical plexus and drains into the internal iliac vein through the veins from the urinary bladder.
   c. It also gives origin to the venae comitantes of the internal pudendal artery.

6. The ***rectal venous plexus*** consists of two parts—internal and external.
   a. The internal plexus lies in the submucosa, whereas the external plexus lies outside the muscular coat (In other words the two plexuses are separated by the muscle coat).
   b. The internal plexus drains mainly into the superior rectal vein. This vein becomes continuous with the inferior mesenteric vein.
   c. The external plexus is drained by all three veins of the rectum. These are:
      i. The superior rectal vein (which is continued into the inferior mesenteric vein).
      ii. The middle rectal vein (which is a tributary of the internal iliac).
      iii. The inferior rectal vein (which is a tributary of the internal pudendal vein).
7. The superior rectal vein is a tributary of the portal venous system, while the middle and inferior rectal veins are part of the systemic circulation.
   a. The portal and systemic circulations, therefore, communicate through the rectal venous plexuses.
   b. The internal rectal plexus has a series of dilatations that are placed immediately above the anal orifice. These sometimes get enlarged to form piles.

## Veins of the Vertebral Column

1. These veins are present in relation to the entire length of the vertebral column but it is convenient to consider them here.
2. The vertebrae are surrounded by a dense plexus of veins (32.15).
   a. The plexus is divisible into an external part on the outer surface of the vertebra; and an internal part lining the vertebral canal.
   b. Each of these parts is divided into anterior and posterior divisions.
   c. A basivertebral vein from each vertebral body drains into the anterior internal plexus. It also communicates with the anterior external plexus.
3. Apart from veins draining blood from the vertebrae, the plexus receives veins from the meninges and from the spinal cord.
4. Opposite each intervertebral foramen the plexus drains into an intervertebral vein.
5. The intervertebral veins end in the vertebral, intercostal and lumbar veins.
6. In the pelvis the plexuses communicate with veins from some pelvic viscera.

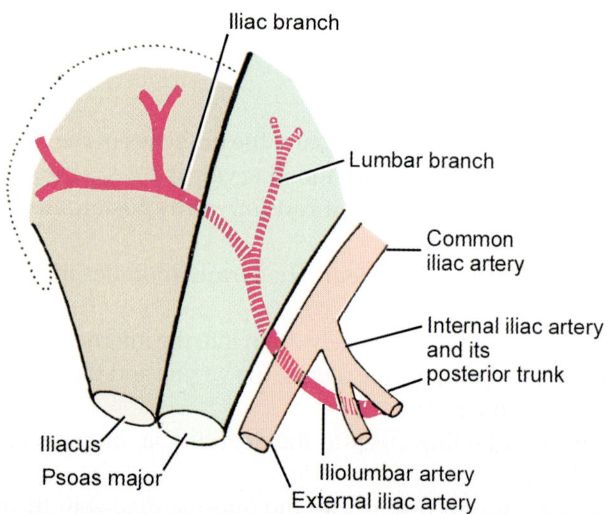


**32.14:** Course and branches of iliolumbar artery

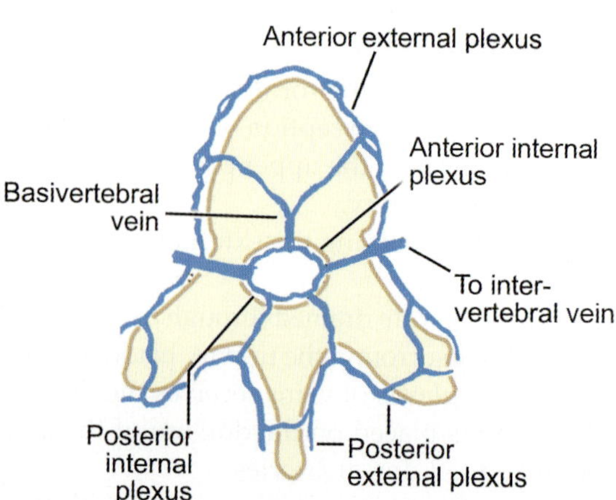


**32.15:** Vertebral venous plexus

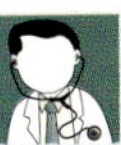

**CLINICAL CORRELATION**

Tumours of pelvic viscera (e.g., of the prostate) may spread to vertebral bodies through communications with the vertebral venous plexus.

## NERVES OF THE PELVIS

The nerves to be seen in relation to the pelvic wall are as follows:

1. The ***genitofemoral nerve*** is a branch of the lumbar plexus. It emerges from the surface of the psoas major muscle and runs downwards over its anterior surface.
2. The ***obturator nerve*** is a branch of the lumbar plexus. It runs forwards over the lateral wall of the true pelvis just above the obturator artery and leaves the pelvis through the obturator canal to reach the thigh.
3. The ***lumbosacral trunk*** is derived from the fourth and fifth lumbar nerves. It descends into the true pelvis by passing over the ala of the sacrum to join the sacral plexus. The lumbosacral trunk lies just behind the common iliac vessels.
4. The ***sacral ventral rami*** and ***sacral plexus*** lie in front of the sacrum. The roots S1, S2 and S3 are large and that of S4 is much smaller. These roots take part in forming the sacral plexus.
5. The main continuation of the sacral plexus is the ***sciatic nerve*** that passes out of the pelvis (into the gluteal region) through the greater sciatic foramen. The sciatic nerve and some other branches of the sacral plexus are described in Chapter 11.
6. The ***pudendal nerve*** is a branch of the sacral plexus.
   a. It receives contributions from nerves S2, S3 and S4. Along with the internal pudendal artery the nerve passes through the greater sciatic foramen to enter the gluteal region.
   b. After a short course in this region the nerve passes through the lesser sciatic foramen to reach the lateral wall of the ischiorectal fossa. The nerve is distributed mainly to the perineum.
7. The lower sacral rami (S4, S5) join the coccygeal nerve to form the ***coccygeal plexus*** that lies over the pelvic surface of the coccygeus muscle. The plexus gives off the ***anococcygeal nerves***. These nerves pass through the sacrotuberous ligament to reach the skin overlying the coccyx.

### Autonomic Nerves

#### *Pelvic Part of Sympathetic Trunk*

1. This part of the sympathetic trunk bears four or five ***sacral ganglia***.
2. In front of the coccyx the right and left sympathetic trunks both end a median ganglion, the ***ganglion impar.***
3. Branches arising from the pelvic part of the sympathetic trunk are distributed mainly to blood vessels of the lower limbs.

#### *Sacral Parasympathetic Outflow*

1. Preganglionic neurons that constitute the sacral parasympathetic outflow are located in segments S2, S3 and S4 of the spinal cord.
2. The nerve fibres pass into corresponding nerves.
3. The sacral nerves concerned give off ***pelvic splanchnic*** branches.
4. Preganglionic neurons end in plexuses related to various pelvic viscera. Postganglionic neurons are located in these plexuses.
5. Some fibres pass through hypogastric plexuses to reach parts of the gut derived from the hindgut (left one-third of transverse colon, descending colon, pelvic colon).

## Lymphatics of Pelvis

Lymph from the pelvis drains into widely separated lymph nodes as follows:

1. Most of the lymph from the pelvic viscera drains to the ***internal iliac nodes***.
2. Some lymph reaches ***sacral nodes*** (lying in front of the sacrum).
3. Lymph from some organs reaches the ***external iliac nodes*** and through them to common iliac nodes.
4. Lymph from the testis (or ovary), part of uterine tube and part of uterus reaches the ***lateral aortic nodes*** directly.
5. The upper part of the rectum drains to the ***inferior mesenteric nodes.***
6. Some structures in the perineum drain into ***superficial or deep inguinal lymph nodes***.

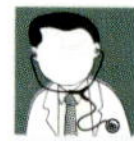

### CLINICAL CORRELATION

As the pelvic wall is closely related to pelvic viscera any pathological condition affecting the viscera can have effects on the pelvic wall. These are considered in chapter 33.

# 33 CHAPTER Pelvic Viscera and Peritoneum

## PELVIC VISCERA

1. The viscera to be seen in the true pelvis belong to the gastrointestinal, urinary and reproductive systems.
2. The viscera belonging to the alimentary system are the sigmoid colon, the rectum and anal canal. In addition, some coils of small intestine are often present in the pelvis.
3. The viscera belonging to the urinary system are the pelvic parts of the ureters, the urinary bladder and the urethra (male or female).
4. The main reproductive organs to be seen in the male pelvis are the pelvic part of the right and left ductus deferens, the seminal vesicles, and the prostate gland.
5. Reproductive organs present in the female pelvis are the uterus, the right and left uterine tubes, and the vagina.
6. The greater part of the gastrointestinal tract has been described in chapter 27 in which the sigmoid colon has also been described. The rectum and anal canal are considered below.

### THE RECTUM

1. The rectum is a wide tube about 12 cm long. It lies in the true pelvis, more or less in the middle line.
2. Its upper end is continuous with the sigmoid colon. The junction lies in front of the third sacral vertebra.
3. The lower end of the rectum lies a little below and in front of the tip of the coccyx. This end becomes continuous with the anal canal.
4. The lower part of the rectum which is wider than the upper part, is called the ***ampula***.

#### Curves of the Rectum

1. The rectum has an anteroposterior curve corresponding to that of the sacrum and coccyx.
2. In addition to its downward direction the upper part of the rectum is directed backwards, and the lower part is directed forwards.
3. The rectum also has three lateral curves (33.1).
   a. The upper end lies in the middle line. In passing downwards the rectum:
      i. Deviates first to the right ('a' in 33.1).
      ii. Then to the left ('b' in 33.1).
      iii. And again to the right ('c' in 33.1).
      iv. Finally returning to the middle line at its lower end.

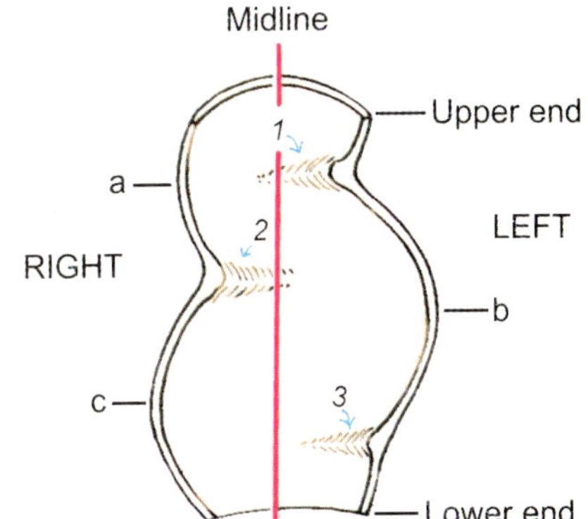

33.1: Scheme to show lateral curvatures and folds of the rectum

##### *Folds in the Rectum*

1. The mucous membrane of the rectum shows a number of transverse folds.

2. Usually three folds are present (1, 2 and 3 in 33.1).
3. The circular and longitudinal muscle coats may extend into these folds.
4. Longitudinal folds are also present.

## Peritoneal Relations

1. The upper one-third of the rectum is covered by peritoneum in front and also on the sides (33.2).
2. The middle one-third is covered by peritoneum only in front.
3. The lower one-third of the rectum is not covered by peritoneum (33.3).
4. In the male, the peritoneum passes from the front of the rectum to the urinary bladder forming the ***rectovesical pouch*** (33.11).
5. In the female (33.13), the peritoneum from the front of the rectum passes to the posterior wall of the vagina forming a pouch erroneously called the ***rectouterine pouch*** (or ***pouch of Douglas***). (This pouch is really rectovaginal).
6. It is important to know that the bottom of the rectovesical pouch (male) is 7.5 cm (3 inches) from the anus; and that of the rectovaginal pouch is about 5 cm (2 inches) from the anus.

### WANT TO KNOW MORE?

***Structure of the Rectum***

1. The structure of the rectum differs from that of the colon in that:
   a. There are no *taenia coli*
   b. No sacculations
   c. No appendices epiploicae.
2. The folds of the rectum have been mentioned above.

***Relations of the Rectum***

1. The rectum rests posteriorly on:
   a. The lower part of the sacrum (33.13 and 33.14)
   b. The coccyx (33.13)
   c. The right and left piriformis muscles (33.2)
   d. The right and left coccygeus muscles.
   e. The right and left levator ani muscles.
2. Several nerves and vessels intervene between the rectum and these structures.
3. Anteriorly, the rectum is related in the male, to:
   a. The urinary bladder (33.3 and 33.11)
   b. The seminal vesicles
   c. The ductus deferentia
   d. The lower ends of the ureters and the prostate (33.3).
4. In the female the rectum is related anteriorly to the vagina and the lower part of the uterus (33.13).
5. In both sexes the upper part of the rectum may be related anteriorly to the sigmoid colon and/or coils of ileum (33.2 and 33.13).
6. These parts of the intestine may also form lateral relations of the upper part of the rectum.
7. Lower down the lateral walls of the rectum are embraced by the right and left coccygei and the right and left levator ani muscles (33.3 and 33.4).

***Supports of the Rectum***

The rectum is held in place by thickenings of fascia or ligaments.

1. The ***fascia of Waldeyer*** connects the posterior aspect of the anorectal junction to the lower part of the sacrum.
2. The ***lateral rectal ligaments*** connect the lateral aspect of the rectum to the posterolateral part of the wall of the pelvis (33.2). The middle rectal vessels pass through them.

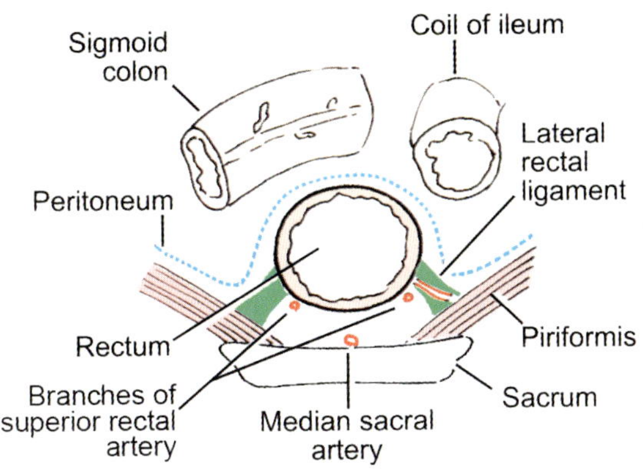


33.2: Transverse section through upper one-third of rectum to show some relations

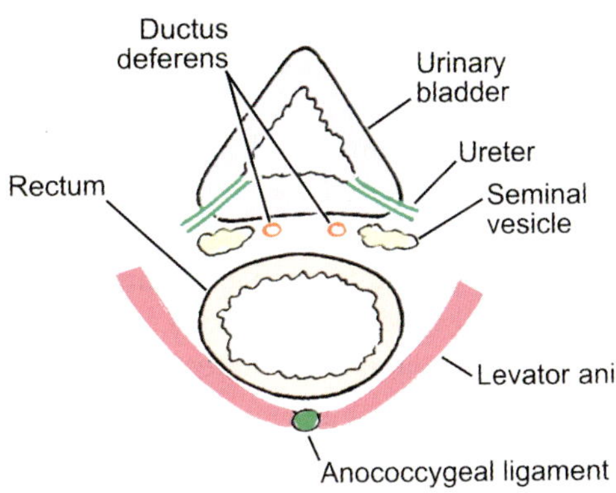


33.3: Transverse section through lower part of rectum in the male

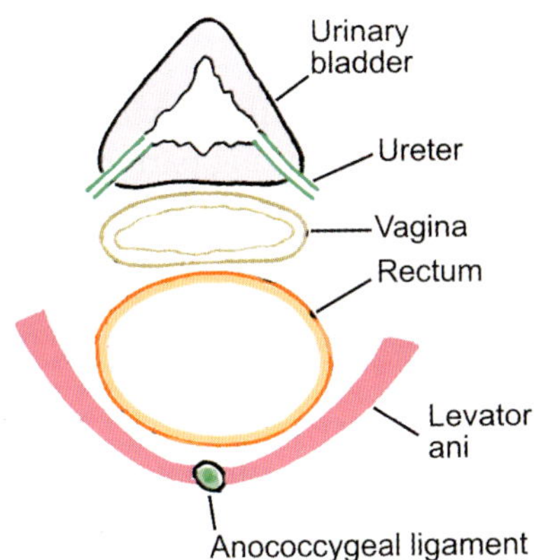


33.4: Transverse section through lower part of rectum in the female

The blood supply, the lymphatic drainage and the nerve supply of the rectum are considered along with those of the anal canal, below.

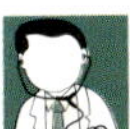

## CLINICAL CORRELATION

***Rectal Examination***

1. Considerable information about the structures surrounding the rectum and anal canal can be obtained, in the living, by palpation with a finger inserted through the anus. This is referred to as rectal examination. (The procedure is often referred to by doctors as "PR" which is an abbreviation for examination 'per rectum').
2. The structures that can be felt through the anterior wall of the rectum and anal canal in the male are (from below upwards):
   a. The bulb of the penis and membranous urethra
   b. The prostate
   c. The seminal vesicles
   d. The base of the urinary bladder.

3. In the female the main structures in front of the anal canal are the vagina and uterus, but as these are directly accessible for examination (through the vagina) a rectal examination is needed for them only when for some reason a vaginal examination is not desirable.
4. Posteriorly, in both the male and female, the coccyx and the lower part of the sacrum can be felt; and laterally, the ischial spine and ischial tuberosity can be palpated.
5. In addition, an experienced surgeon can recognise abnormalities in surrounding viscera (ovary, uterine tube, ureters, a pelvic appendix) such as inflammation or enlargement.
6. Enlarged internal iliac lymph nodes, abnormalities in the rectovesical or rectouterine pouches, or in the ischiorectal fossae can also be detected.

*Proctoscopy and Sigmoidoscopy*

1. A proctoscope is an instrument through which the interior of the anal canal and rectum can be examined.
2. However, it may not be possible to see the upper part of the rectum with a proctoscope.
3. A sigmoidoscope can be used for this purpose.
4. In passing a sigmoidoscope into the rectum the curvatures of the rectum and the presence of transverse folds within it has to be remembered.

*Prolapse of the Rectum*

1. The rectum and other pelvic viscera are supported by the pelvic diaphragm.
2. When this diaphragm is weakened e.g., by damage during parturition, the rectum can ***prolapse*** out of the anus.
   a. Prolapse may be partial in which case the protrusion consists only of mucosa.
   b. Complete in which all layers of the rectal wall are present.
3. Weakening of muscles in old age can be a predisposing factor for prolapse.

*Carcinoma*

1. The rectum is commonly affected by carcinoma.
2. Spread of a rectal carcinoma is usually slow but it can ultimately invade surrounding structures including
   a. The prostate
   b. The seminal vesicles and urinary bladder
   c. The uterus and vagina
   d. The ureters
   e. The sacral plexus.

## THE ANAL CANAL

1. The anal canal is the lowest part of the alimentary canal. Above it is continuous with the lower end of the rectum. Below it opens to the exterior at the *anus*.
2. The anal canal is about 4 cm in length. It is distinctly narrower than the rectum. From 33.11 it will be seen that there is a sudden change in direction of the alimentary canal at the junction of the rectum with the anal canal. While the lower part of the rectum is directed downwards and forwards, the anal canal is directed downwards and backwards.
3. The anorectal junction lies at the level of the pelvic diaphragm (formed here by the levator ani muscles).
4. The rectum lies above the pelvic diaphragm in the true pelvis, whereas the anal canal lies below the diaphragm in the perineum.

### Relations of Anal Canal

Note the following features in 33.5, which is a view of the anal triangle as seen from below.

1. The lower aperture of the anal canal (or anus) is in the form of an anteroposterior slit, the right and left walls being in apposition. The position is the same in the interior of the anal canal also.

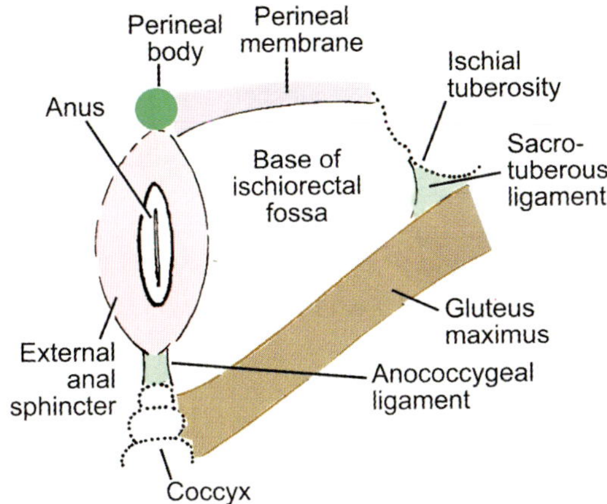


**33.5:** Anal triangle seen after removing overlying skin, to show some relations of the anal canal

2. Posteriorly, the anal canal is separated from the coccyx by a mass of fibromuscular tissue that is called the ***ano-coccygeal ligament*** (or ***body***).
3. In front of the anal canal there is another similar mass called the ***perineal body***.
   a. A number of muscles of the perineum gain attachment to this body and make it a region of importance for maintaining the integrity of the pelvic floor.
   b. The perineal body separates the anal canal from the membranous urethra and the bulb of the penis in the male (33.11); and from the vagina in the female (33.13).
4. Lateral to the anal canal there is a triangular depression called the ***ischiorectal fossa***.

## Interior of the Anal Canal

1. For convenience of description the interior of the anal canal may be considered in three parts.
2. The upper 15 cm or so are lined by mucous membrane. This mucous membrane shows six to ten longitudinal folds. These folds are called ***anal columns*** (33.6A and B).
3. The lower ends of the anal columns are united to each other by short transverse folds of mucous membrane. These folds are called the ***anal valves***.
4. Above each anal valve there is a depression in the mucosa that is called an ***anal sinus***.
5. The anal valves together form a transverse line that runs all round the anal canal. This is called the ***pectinate line***.

## WANT TO KNOW MORE?

6. a. From an embryological point of view the part of the anal canal above the pectinate line is believed to be derived from the cloaca, and its lining epithelium is of endodermal origin.
   b. In contrast, the part below the line is derived from a surface depression called the proctodaeum, and its lining epithelium is ectodermal.
   c. In early fetal life the two parts are separated by the anal membrane which subsequently disappears.
   d. Remnants of this membrane may be present in the form of small projections from the anal valves. These projections are called ***anal papillae***.

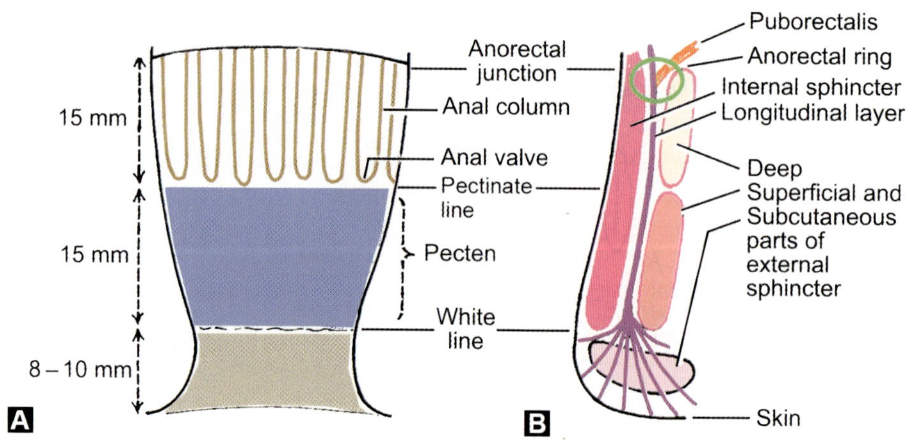


**33.6A and B:** Schemes to show: A. Some landmarks in the anal canal; B. The anal musculature

7. a. The next 15 mm or so of the anal canal is also lined by mucous membrane, but anal columns are not present here.
   b. The mucosa has a bluish appearance because of a dense venous plexus that lies between it and the muscle coat.
   c. The mucosa is less mobile than in the upper part of the anal canal.
   d. This region is referred to as the ***pecten*** or ***transitional zone***.
8. The lower limit of the pecten often has a whitish appearance because of which it is referred to as the ***white line*** (***of Hilton***).
9. The third, or lowest, subdivision of the anal canal is about 8 to 10 cm long. It differs from the upper and middle parts in that it is not lined by mucous membrane, but by skin.
10. a. The epithelium lining the upper 15 mm of the anal canal is columnar (or stratified columnar); that lining the middle part (pecten) is stratified squamous, but is distinguished from skin in that there are no sebaceous or sweat glands, or hair, in relation to it.
    b. The epithelium of the lowest part resembles that of true skin in which sebaceous and sweat glands are present.

### *Anal Glands*

1. Above each anal valve there is a space called the anal sinus.
2. Opening into the sinus there are anal glands that extend into the submucosa.
3. Some of them extend into the muscle layer. The openings of the glands on the anal mucosa are referred to as ***anal crypts***.

### *The Anal Musculature*

The anal canal is surrounded by a number of sphincters that are as follows (33.6B):

1. The ***internal anal sphincter*** is formed by thickening of the circular muscle coat of the gut. It is, therefore, made up of smooth muscle. It extends from the upper end of the anal canal up to the white line.
2. The ***external anal sphincter*** is made up of striated muscle. It is subdivided as follows.
3. The ***subcutaneous part*** lies below the level of the white line i.e., inferior to the level of the internal sphincter.

## WANT TO KNOW MORE?

a. When a finger is placed in the anal canal a distinct ***intersphincteric groove*** can be palpated between the lower end of the internal sphincter and the upper margin of the subcutaneous external sphincter.
b. In section the subcutaneous part of the external sphincter looks like a transverse band (33.6B). A surface view of the sphincter is seen 33.5.
c. Most of fibres of the sphincter are arranged in the form of rings round the anal canal, but some of them join the perineal body anteriorly, and the anococcygeal ligament posteriorly.

4. The ***superficial part*** of the external sphincter lies external to the lower part of the internal sphincter between the levels of the pectinate line and the white line (33.6B). The fibres of this part are attached posteriorly to the coccyx and anteriorly to the perineal body.
5. The ***deep part*** of the external sphincter lies external to the upper half of the internal sphincter (above the level of the pectinate line).

## WANT TO KNOW MORE?

Most of its fibres run circularly around the anal canal, but some of them become continuous anteriorly with the superficial transverse perinei muscles, and posteriorly with the anococcygeal ligament.

*The following additional facts about the musculature of the anal canal are worthy of note.*

1. The anorectal junction is closely related to the puborectalis part of the levator ani muscle (33.7).
   a. The fibres of the puborectalis form a sling that keeps the anorectal junction pulled forwards, thus maintaining the angle between the rectum and the anal canal.
   b. The fibres of the puborectalis mingle intimately with the upper part of the internal anal sphincter, and with the deep part of the external sphincter to form a prominent ring of muscle around the anorectal junction.
   c. This ring, which can be palpated by a finger placed in the anal canal, is called the ***anorectal ring***. The integrity of this ring is of great functional importance as damage to it results in incontinence of feces.
2. a. Some fibres of the puborectalis merge with the longitudinal muscle at the lower end of the rectum.
   b. Together these fibres descend in the wall of the anal canal between the internal sphincter and the deep and superficial parts of the external sphincter (33.6B).
   c. These longitudinal fibres are intermingled with numerous elastic fibres that become more and more numerous as the bundles descend, so that near the lower end of the internal sphincter the fibres in the longitudinal layer are almost entirely elastic.
   d. These fibres fan out into small bundles that penetrate through the subcutaneous part of the external sphincter to gain attachment to the skin surrounding the anus.
   e. They are often said to be responsible for corrugation (folds) in this part of the skin.
   f. Some bundles of these elastic fibres pass through the interval between the lower end of the internal sphincter and the upper edge of the subcutaneous external sphincter to reach the skin lining the anal canal in the region of the intersphincteric groove (33.6B).

### *Blood Vessels of Rectum and Anal Canal*

1. The rectum and anal canal are supplied by:
   a. The superior rectal artery which is a continuation of the inferior mesenteric artery.
   b. By the right and left middle rectal arteries.
   c. By the right and left inferior rectal arteries.
   d. By the median sacral artery.

2. The superior rectal artery supplies:
   a. The full thickness of the upper part of the rectum.
   b. The mucous membrane of the entire rectum.
   c. The mucous membrane of the anal canal up to the anal valves.
3. The middle rectal artery supplies the muscle wall of the lower part of the rectum.
4. The inferior rectal arteries supply:
   a. The anal sphincters
   b. The entire thickness of the anal canal below the anal valves.
5. The median sacral artery gives branches to the posterior part of the anorectal junction and the anal canal.
6. The veins of the rectum and anal canal begin in two plexuses.
   a. The internal rectal plexus lies in the submucosa.
   b. The external rectal plexus lies lateral to the muscle coat.
   c. The internal rectal plexus is drained mainly by the superior rectal vein, which is continued into the inferior mesenteric vein.
   d. The external rectal plexus is drained mainly into the middle and inferior rectal veins.
7. It has to be stressed that the superior rectal vein is a tributary of the portal system, whereas the middle and inferior rectal veins are systemic veins.
   a. These veins anastomose with one another.
   b. Blood from the portal venous system can pass into the systemic circulation through these anastomoses.
   c. These are amongst the most important portocaval anastomoses to be seen in the body. Under certain circumstances pressure in the portal venous system rises and blood then flows across these anastomoses in increasing amounts leading to their dilatation.
   d. This results in production of swellings of the anal mucosa. These swellings are filled with blood and are called ***haemorrhoids*** or ***piles*** (see below).

*Lymphatic Drainage of Rectum and Anal Canal*

1. The upper part of the rectum drains to inferior mesenteric lymph nodes.
2. The lower part of the rectum and the upper part of the anal canal drain into the internal iliac nodes.
3. The lower part of the anal canal drains into the superficial inguinal nodes.
4. For further details see chapter 34.

*Nerve Supply of Rectum and Anal Canal*

1. The nerve supply of the rectum and the upper part of the anal canal is through autonomic nerves.
2. The internal anal sphincter is also supplied by these nerves (sympathetic).
3. The external anal sphincter is supplied by the inferior rectal branch of the pudendal nerve and by the perineal branch of the fourth sacral nerve.
4. The sensory supply to the mucous membrane of the rectum and the upper part of the anal canal is through autonomic nerves.
5. The sensory supply to the lower part of the anal canal is through the inferior rectal nerve.
6. The region supplied by the inferior rectal nerve (somatic) is much more sensitive to pain than the region supplied by autonomic nerves.

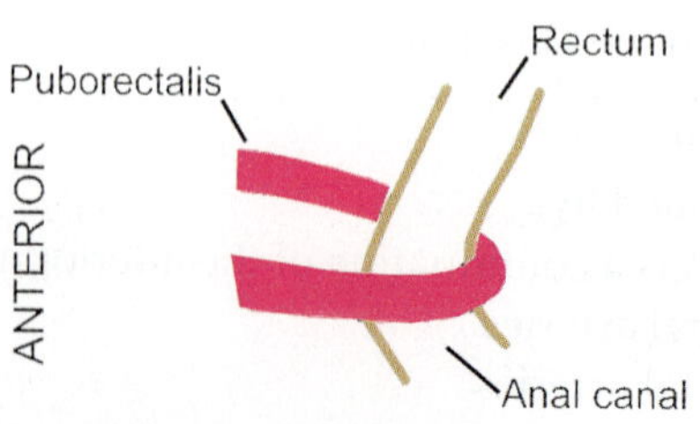


**33.7:** The puborectalis sling

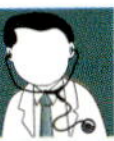

## CLINICAL CORRELATION ANAL CANAL

**Haemorrhoids (or Piles)**

This term is used to describe swellings in the anal canal produced by dilated veins. Haemorrhoids may be internal or external.

***Internal or True Haemorrhoids***

1. Internal or true haemorrhoids are located in the part of the anal canal lined by mucosa. They are therefore painless.
2. They are located in relation to anal columns above the level of anal valves, and are formed by dilatation of radicles of the superior rectal vein.
3. Some anatomical considerations relevant to the formation of internal haemorrhoids are as follows:
   a. There is one tributary of the superior rectal vein in each anal column. However, the tributaries located in the left lateral, right posterior, and right anterior positions are largest and the first to enlarge. These enlargements are called ***primary piles***.
   b. When the anal canal is viewed with the patient lying supine with the thighs raised (lithotomy position) the position of primary piles is often described with reference to a clock. They are said to be located at the 3 o'clock, 7 o'clock and 11 o'clock positions. Secondary piles may form later at other positions.
   c. Submucous connective tissue at the anorectal junction is very loose and the radicles of the superior rectal vein lie unsupported in this tissue.
   d. The veins pierce the muscle coat and are pressed upon when the muscle contracts during defecation. This increases pressure within them.
   e. There are no valves in the superior rectal or inferior mesenteric veins. The tributaries of the these veins in the anal columns, therefore, bear the pressure of the entire column of blood right up to the portal vein.
   f. This explains why haemorrhoids are more liable to occur in persons who have to stand for long periods.
   g. This also explains why the tendency to formation of piles is increased in portal hypertension (as mentioned above).
4. Apart from anatomical factors hereditary factors have also been blamed for causation of haemorrhoids.
   a. It has been observed that persons who have haemorrhoids also frequently have varicose veins, suggesting the possibility of some inherent weakness in the walls of veins.
   b. The relationship of haemorrhoids to portal hypertension has been contested and some authorities believe that there is no such correlation.
   c. In some cases haemorrhoids can be caused by pressure on, or blockage of, veins caused by a rectal carcinoma. During pregnancy haemorrhoids may form because of pressure of the enlarged uterus on the superior rectal vein.
5. The most important clinical feature of piles is painless bleeding which may take place every time the patient passes stools.
6. Surgically, haemorrhoids are classified as follows:
   a. ***First degree*** when the piles do not project out of the anus at any time.
   b. ***Second degree*** when they prolapse out of the anus during defecation, but get reduced by themselves.
   c. ***Third degree*** when reduction is not spontaneous after prolapse.
7. Haemorrhoids cause discomfort when they become large or prolapse.
8. Discomfort becomes much more severe when there is thrombosis within a pile; or when the haemorrhoid gets infected or ulcerated.
9. A prolapsed pile may get gripped by the external anal sphincter leading to strangulation.
10. Treatment of haemorrhoids can be conservative but when this is unsuccessful the haemorrhoids can be removed surgically (***haemorrhoidectomy***).

### *External Haemorrhoids*

1. In contrast to internal haemorrhoids, external haemorrhoids are formed by dilatation of tributaries of the inferior rectal veins.
2. They are placed below the anal valves and are covered by skin.
3. They are highly painful.
4. Some haemorrhoids may extend partly under mucosa and partly under skin (***interno-external haemorrhoids***).
5. Rupture of a small tributary of the inferior rectal vein can give rise to a ***perianal haematoma***.

### *Infections in Anorectal Region*

1. Because of constant contact with fecal material the anal canal is a frequent site of infection.
2. Small glands opening into the anal sinuses are often foci of infection. Infection can lead to the formation of ***abscesses***.
3. In the absence of timely treatment abscesses may burst
   a. Into the anal canal or rectum or
   b. May open to the outside over the skin of the perineum forming sinuses.
4. When an abscess opens in both directions it leads to formation of a ***fistula*** that is a narrow inflamed tract of communication between the lumen of the anal canal and outside.
5. From the point of view of treatment it is necessary to know the locations of perianal abscesses and fistulae as follows.

### *Perianal Abscesses*

A perianal abscess may be seen in the following positions:

1. ***Submucous*** under the mucosa of the anal canal.
2. ***Subcutaneous*** under perianal skin.
3. ***Ischiorectal*** in the ischiorectal fossa.
4. ***Pelvirectal*** in the space lateral to the rectum just above the levator ani.

### *Anal Fistulae*

Fistulae may be present as follows:

1. A fistula lying above the level of the anorectal ring is a ***high level*** anal fistula.
2. Any fistula lying below the anorectal ring is a low level fistula. The track of such a fistula may lie:
   a. Between the deep and superficial parts of the external anal sphincter.
   b. Between the superficial and subcutaneous sphincters.
   c. Superficial to the subcutaneous sphincter.
3. Fistulae do not heal without surgical intervention.
   a. It is necessary to excise the track of the fistula.
   b. In doing so it has to be remembered that excision of a high level fistula requires division of the anorectal ring, and special procedures are necessary to ensure that division of the ring does not result in anal incontinence.

### *Anal Fissure*

1. A hard fecal mass can produce a tear in an anal valve.
2. The tear usually extends to the anus constituting an anal fissure.
3. Anal fissure is a very painful condition.
4. Fissures tend to occur most commonly in the midline anteriorly or posteriorly, probably as these sites are least supported by the external sphincter.

### *Other Conditions Affecting the Anal Canal*

1. In some newborn infants, the anal canal does not open to the outside. This condition is called ***imperforate anus***.
2. A congenital ***stricture*** may develop in the region of the pectineal line. Strictures may also be acquired.
3. The anal canal can be the site of a ***carcinoma***.

## THE URETERS

1. The abdominal part of the ureter has been described earlier. We have seen that about half the length of the ureter lies in the true pelvis.
   a. At the brim of the pelvis the ureter crosses the upper end of the external iliac artery (and vein), and comes to lie on the lateral wall of the pelvis.
   b. Here it runs backwards and laterally.
   c. Finally it leaves the pelvic wall and turns medially and forwards to reach the posterolateral part of the urinary bladder.

### WANT TO KNOW MORE?

2. The skeletal relationships of the pelvic part of the ureter are as follows:
   a. After entering the pelvis the ureter runs across the sacroiliac joint, and the anterior border of the greater sciatic notch to reach the ischial spine.
   b. The ureter turns medially at this spine.
   c. Its point of termination corresponds to the pubic tubercle.

*Relations of Pelvic Part of Ureter*

1. These are similar on the right and left sides.
2. As the ureter runs backwards and laterally on the lateral wall of the pelvis it lies on the fascia covering the obturator internus.
3. Here the ureter crosses several structures that lie between it and the lateral pelvic wall.
4. In the male (33.8) these are:
   a. The superior vesical artery
   b. The obturator nerve, artery and vein
   c. The inferior vesical artery.
5. In the female (33.9) these are:
   a. The superior vesical artery
   b. The obturator nerve, artery and vein
   c. The vaginal artery
   d. The uterine artery.
6. In both the male and female, the ureter is related posteriorly to the internal iliac vessels that separate it from the lumbosacral trunk and from the sacroiliac joint.
7. In the female, the ovary lies immediately in front of the ureter. Here the ureter forms the posterior wall of a depression (ovarian fossa) in which the ovary lies.
8. As the ureter leaves the lateral pelvic wall and turns anteromedially it lies over the levator ani, but is separated from it by a mass of fat. The relations of this part are different in the male and female.
   a. In the male, the ureter is crossed by the ductus deferens (33.8). It passes just above the seminal vesicle to reach the urinary bladder (see 33.12).
   b. In the female, the ureter passes a short distance lateral to the cervix of the uterus (just above the lateral fornix of the vagina), and then passes anterior to the vagina to reach the urinary bladder.
   c. Lateral to the cervix, the ureter is crossed by the uterine artery and the broad ligament. (In 33.9, note the double relationship of the ureter to the uterine artery).

9. The terminal part of the ureter passes obliquely through the thickness of the wall of the urinary bladder to open into its posterior wall. The openings lie at the lateral angles of a triangular area of the posterior wall of the urinary bladder called the ***trigone*** (33.15).

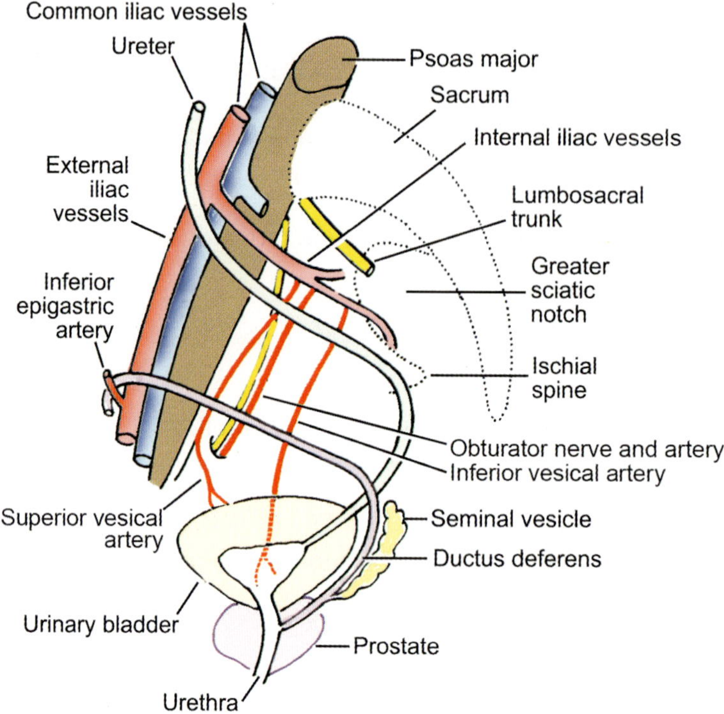


**33.8:** Scheme to show the course and relations of the pelvic part of the ureter in the male

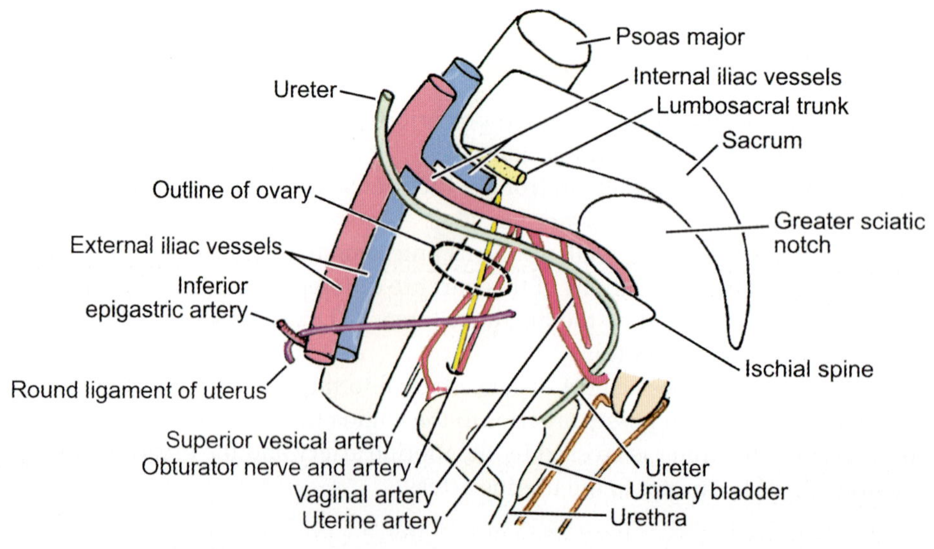


**33.9:** Scheme to show the course and relations of pelvic part of the female ureter

## WANT TO KNOW MORE?

*Constrictions of the Ureter*

The average diameter of the ureter is about 3 mm. It shows three constrictions:

1. One at its upper end (i.e., at the junction with the pelvis).
2. Another at its lower end (i.e., at its junction with the urinary bladder).
3. And a third where it crosses the brim of the pelvis.

*Blood Vessels, Lymphatics and Nerves*

1. Each ureter receives branches from several ***arteries*** that lie near it. These are (from above downwards):
   a. The renal artery
   b. The abdominal aorta
   c. The testicular or ovarian artery
   d. The common iliac artery
   e. The internal iliac artery
   f. Its vesical branches
   g. In the female the ureter also receives branches from the uterine artery.
2. The ***veins*** correspond to the arteries.
3. The ***lymphatic drainage*** of the ureter is as follows:
   a. The upper abdominal part drains to lateral aorta nodes.
   b. The lower abdominal part drains to common iliac nodes.
   c. The pelvic part drains into external iliac and internal iliac nodes.
4. Some points of ***nerve supply*** are as follows:
   a. Autonomic nerves are not essential for peristalsis in the ureter. They may have a modifying effect.
   b. Autonomic nerves are predominantly sensory. Distension of the ureter by a stone causes severe pain (renal colic). Pain is referred to segments T10 to L2. These are the segments in which preganglionic sympathetic neurons are located.
   c. Pain starts on the back over lower ribs and shoots downwards and forwards to the inguinal region, scrotum, and sometimes to front of thigh.
   d. Parasympathetic fibres are derived from the sacral outflow.
   e. For further details see chapter 34.

The clinical correlations of the ureter have been considered in Chapter 30 along with those of the kidneys.

## THE URINARY BLADDER

1. In the adult the urinary bladder lies in the pelvis. However, when distended with urine, part of it extends above the level of the pubic symphysis and comes in contact with the anterior abdominal wall.
2. In the infant the bladder lies above the level of the pubic symphysis i.e., it is an abdominal organ rather than a pelvic one.
3. Urine is formed continuously in the kidneys and is conveyed to the urinary bladder through the ureters.
4. a. The urinary bladder acts as a reservoir.
   b. When it is distended beyond a certain limit the desire for passing urine is felt. This limit is usually reached when the bladder contains about 300 ml of urine.
   c. The maximum capacity of the urinary bladder is about 500 ml.
5. The empty urinary bladder has four surfaces each of which is triangular (33.10). In other words the bladder is shaped like a tetrahedron.
   a. The ***posterior surface*** is also called the ***base*** or ***fundus***. It is broad above and pointed below.
   b. The ***superior surface*** faces upwards. Its posterior end is broad. Anteriorly it narrows to form the ***apex*** of the bladder.

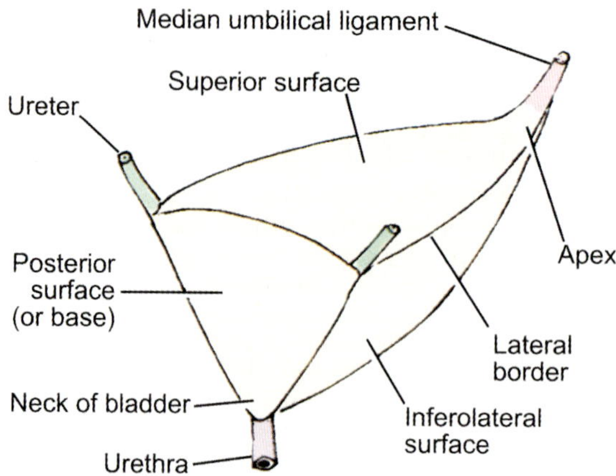


**33.10:** Scheme to show the surfaces of the urinary bladder

   c. The right and left ***inferolateral surfaces*** face downwards, laterally and forwards. They meet the superior surface at the right and left ***lateral borders.*** Posteriorly they meet the lateral margins of the base.
6. The right and left ureters join the urinary bladder at its posterolateral angles.
7. The lowest part of the bladder is called the neck. The urethra emerges from the bladder here.
8. The apex of the bladder gives attachment to the lower end of the median umbilical ligament (33.12).

## WANT TO KNOW MORE?

*Relations of Urinary Bladder in the Male*

1. The superior surface of the bladder is separated by peritoneum from part of the sigmoid colon and from coils of small intestine (33.11).
2. The inferolateral surfaces lie a little behind the pubic bones. They are separated from these bones by a mass of fat and by the puboprostatic ligaments (see below).
3. The base of the bladder lies in front of the rectum, but is partly separated from it by the right and left seminal vesicles and the right and left ductus deferens (33.12).
4. The neck of the bladder rests on the prostate (33.11).
5. The superior surface of the urinary bladder is covered by peritoneum (33.11). Traced anteriorly this peritoneum becomes continuous with that lining the anterior abdominal wall.
   a. In the middle line this peritoneum is raised into a fold called the ***median umbilical fold*** because of the presence here of the median umbilical ligament.
   b. Traced laterally the peritoneum of the superior surface is reflected on to the lateral pelvic wall. This peritoneum is referred to as the ***false lateral ligament*** of the bladder.
   c. Traced posteriorly the peritoneum on the superior surface of the bladder passes on to the upper part of the base. It is then reflected on to the front of the rectum. The peritoneum lined depression between the urinary bladder and the rectum is called the ***rectovesical pouch*** (37.9).
   d. In the fetus the rectovesical pouch is much deeper and extends up to the pelvic floor. The lower part of the pouch is obliterated by fusion of the layers of peritoneum lining it. The remains of this peritoneum persist as the ***rectovesical fascia*** that separates the lower part of the base of the bladder, and lower down the prostate, from the rectum.
6. The inferolateral surfaces of the urinary bladder are not lined by peritoneum.

*Relations of Urinary Bladder in the Female*

1. The greater part of the superior surface of the bladder is lined by peritoneum that separates it from the body of the uterus (33.13).
2. When traced backwards this peritoneum is reflected on to the front of uterus at the junction of the body with the cervix.
3. The posterior part of the superior surface of the bladder is in direct contact with the upper part of the cervix.
4. The relations of the inferolateral surfaces of the bladder are the same as in the male except that the puboprostatic ligaments are replaced by the pubovesical ligaments.
5. The base of the bladder is in contact with the anterior wall of the vagina.
6. The neck of the bladder rests on pelvic fascia.

*Ligaments of the Urinary Bladder*

The urinary bladder is kept in place by a number of so-called ligaments. Some of these are thickenings of fascia and are referred to as 'true' ligaments. Others are folds of peritoneum. These are referred to as the false ligaments.

*True ligaments*

1. The ***median umbilical ligament*** connects the apex of the urinary bladder to the umbilicus. It is the remnant of an embryonic structure the ***urachus*** that is derived from the allantoic diverticulum.
2. The fascia over the upper surface of the levator ani (pelvic fascia) is thickened anteriorly to form the ***medial*** and ***lateral puboprostatic ligaments*** (in the male) or the ***pubovesical ligaments*** (in the female). Laterally the same fascia stretches from the bladder to the fascia covering the obturator internus. This is called the ***lateral true ligament*** of the bladder.
3. The lateral margins of the base of the bladder are joined to the lateral pelvic wall by fascia surrounding the veins that pass from the bladder to the internal iliac veins. This fascia constitutes the ***posterior ligament*** of the bladder.

*False Ligaments (Peritoneal Folds)*

1. The median umbilical ligament raises up a median fold of peritoneum called the ***median umbilical fold*** (33.12).
2. In the fetus the right and left umbilical arteries pass from the internal iliac arteries to the umbilicus (on their way to the placenta).
   a. After birth the proximal parts of these arteries become the superior vesical arteries.
   b. Their distal parts become obliterated and form the ***medial umbilical ligaments*** that connect the superior vesical arteries to the umbilicus. They lie just lateral to the urinary bladder (33.12).
   c. They raise up folds of peritoneum called the ***right*** and ***left medial umbilical folds***. (Distinguish carefully between the 'medial' and the 'median' folds and ligaments.)
3. Peritoneum reflected from the superior surface of the bladder to the lateral wall of the pelvis is referred to as the ***lateral false ligament*** of the bladder.
4. Two folds of peritoneum (right and left) pass backwards from the lateral margin of the base of the bladder to the sacrum. These folds pass lateral to the rectum and form the lateral boundaries of the rectovesical pouch. These folds are called the ***sacrogenital folds*** or the ***posterior ligaments*** of the bladder (33.14).

## Interior of the Urinary Bladder

1. The interior of the bladder is lined by mucous membrane. In the empty bladder the mucosa shows numerous folds. These get stretched out when the bladder distends.
2. On the posterior wall of the bladder, however, there is a triangular area where the mucosa is relatively fixed. This area is called the ***trigone*** (33.15).
3. The ureters open into the urinary bladder at the upper lateral corners of the trigone while the upper end of the urethra opens at the lower angle.

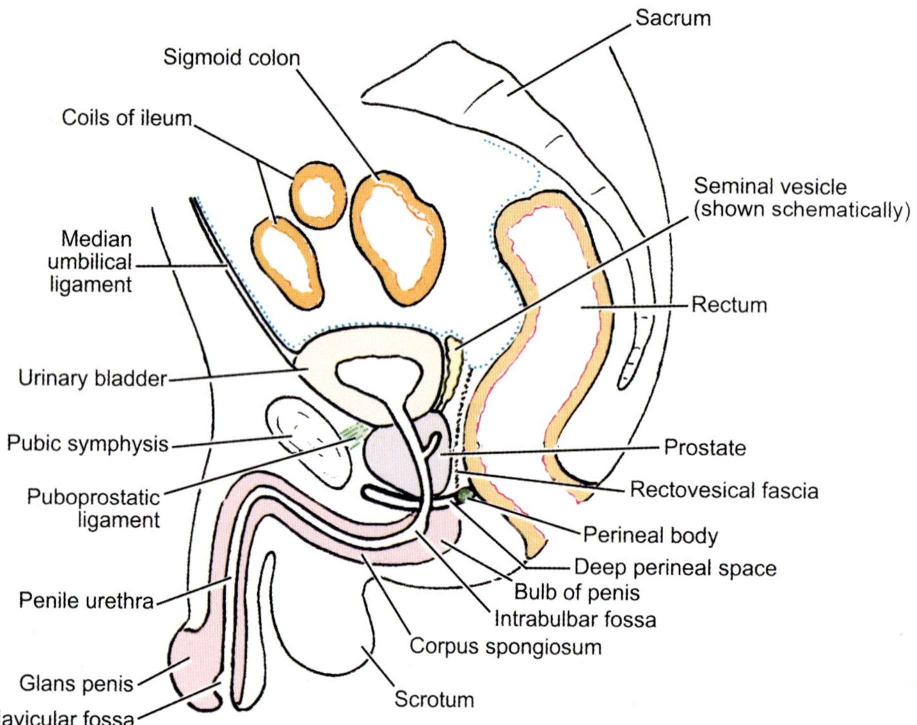


**33.11:** Sagittal section through the male pelvis

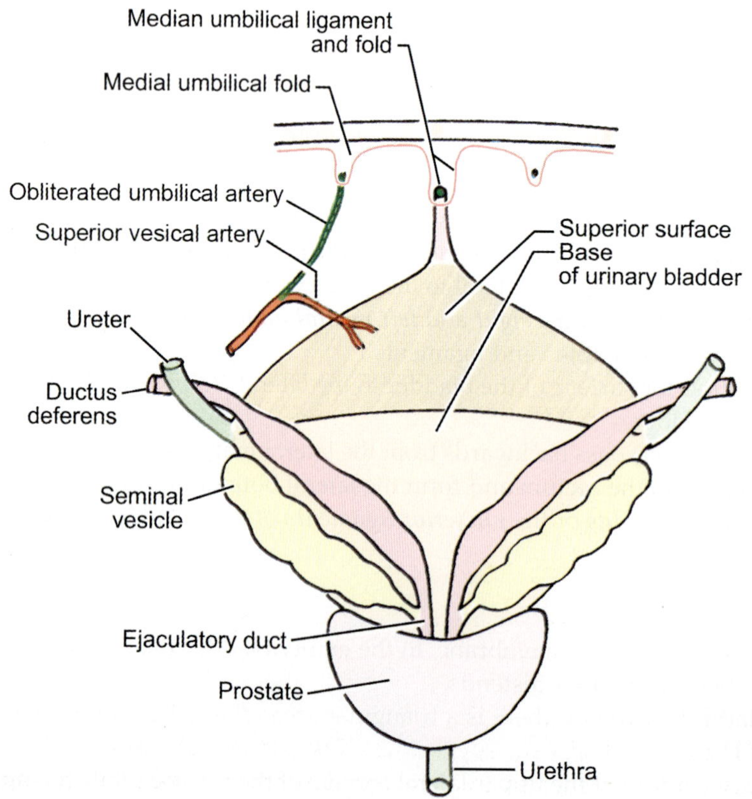


**33.12:** Male urinary bladder and some related structures seen from behind

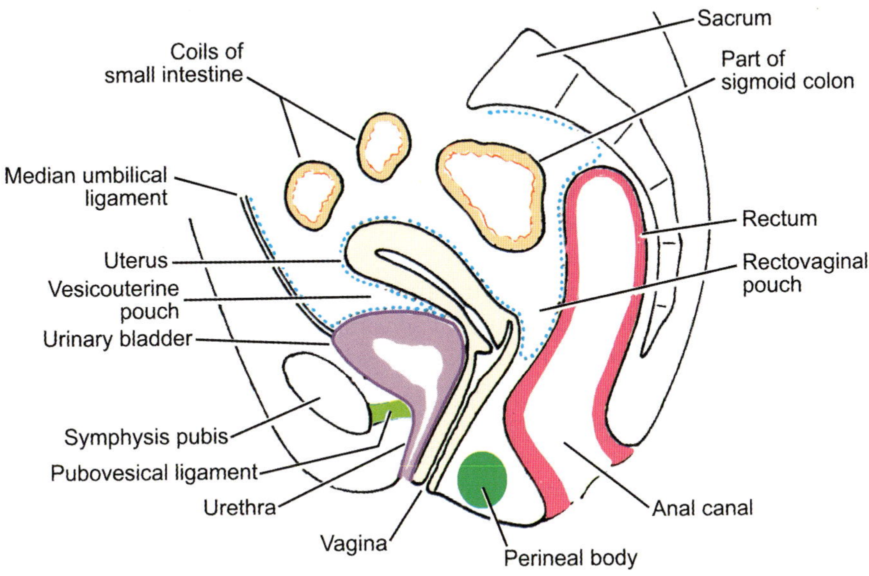


**33.13:** Sagittal section through female pelvis

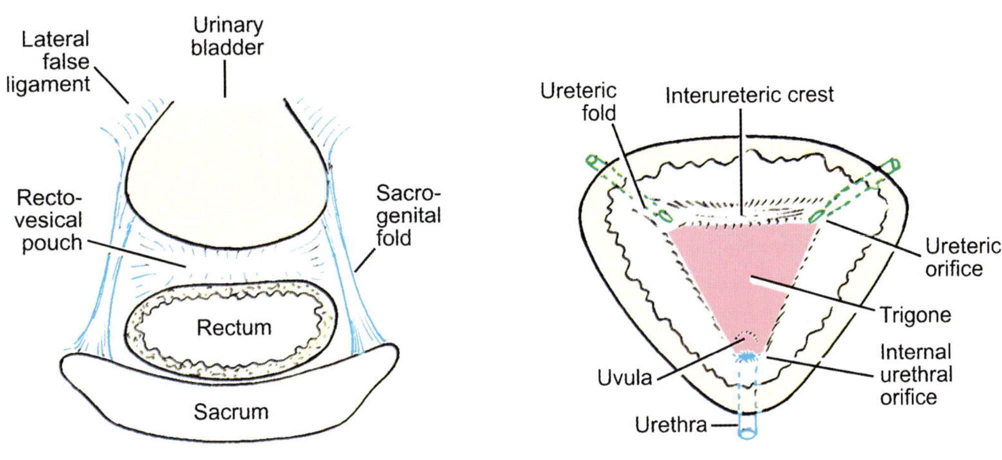


**33.14:** Rectovesical pouch and sacrogenital folds as seen from above

**33.15:** Some features to be seen in the interior of the urinary bladder

4. The urethral opening is called the ***internal urethral orifice***.
5. The upper margin of the trigone forms a ridge stretching between the openings of the two ureters. It is called the ***interureteric crest***. Some additional features are shown in 33.15.

## WANT TO KNOW MORE?

***Vessels and Nerves of the Urinary Bladder***

1. The urinary bladder is supplied (in the male) by the superior and inferior vesical arteries.
2. In the female the inferior vesical artery is replaced by the vaginal artery and the uterine artery also gives branches to the bladder.

3. Veins from the bladder pass backwards in the posterior ligaments of the bladder to reach the internal iliac veins.
4. Lymphatics from the urinary bladder drain into external iliac lymph nodes.
5. The urinary bladder is supplied by autonomic nerves.
   a. Parasympathetic nerves stimulate the detrusor muscles and are inhibitory to sphincters.
   b. Traditionally sympathetic nerves are said to have the opposite effects. However, it is now believed that normal bladder function is controlled only by parasympathetic nerves and that sympathetic nerves only have a vasomotor effect.
   c. Sensations of bladder filling and pain travel through both sympathetic and parasympathetic nerves.
   d. Within the central nervous system pathways for sensations of bladder filling and for pain are different. Pain from the bladder can be abolished by ***anterolateral cordotomy*** without affecting sensations of bladder filling.
   e. Parasympathetic fibres are derived from the sacral outflow. Fibres travel through pelvic splanchnic nerves, inferior hypogastric plexus and vesical plexus.
   f. Sympathetic fibres are derived from spinal segments T10 to L2.
   g. See effects of injury to spinal cord on bladder function, below.

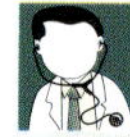

## CLINICAL CORRELATION

### Urinary Bladder

*Congenital Malformations*

1. a. There may be agenesis of the entire bladder or only of the sphincter vesicae.
   b. The anterior wall of the urinary bladder is absent in ***ectopia vesicae***.
   c. The overlying anterior abdominal wall is also absent so that the posterior wall of the bladder (trigone) appears on the surface of the body.
2. The lumen of the bladder may be divided completely (by septa) or partially (by a constriction) into upper and lower compartments. The latter condition is called ***hourglass bladder***.
3. The bladder may communicate with the rectum.
4. Congenital diverticulae may be present.
5. See urinary fistula (chapter 25).

***Relationship to Anterior Abdominal Wall***

1. In an infant the urinary bladder is partially in contact with the anterior abdominal wall.
2. As the pelvis enlarges, the bladder sinks into the true pelvis.
3. In the adult the empty bladder does not come in contact with the anterior abdominal wall. However, when it is distended its upper part is in contact with the abdominal wall above the pubic symphysis.
4. It is important to note that as the distended bladder ascends the fold of peritoneum passing from the anterior abdominal wall to the superior surface of the bladder also rises so that no peritoneum intervenes between a distended bladder and the anterior abdominal wall.
5. This relationship is of practical importance.
   a. In a patient with urinary obstruction, and consequent distension of the bladder, the distension can be relieved by passing a needle into the bladder through the anterior abdominal wall (just above the pubic symphysis).
   b. The bladder can be approached surgically through a suprapubic incision (after distending it). This operation is used for removal of stones from the bladder (***suprapubic lithotomy***).
   c. A distended bladder can be injured by a blow or stab wound in the lower part of the abdomen.

*Effect of Spinal Cord Injury on Bladder*

1. The nerve supply of the urinary bladder is described above. Some effects of spinal cord injury have been mentioned there. The following additional points may be noted.
2. Acute injury to the spinal cord is followed by a state of spinal shock. At this stage muscle in the bladder wall become atonic, but the sphincters remain contracted. This leads to distension of the bladder, the urine dribbling out when pressure rises to a level that cannot be opposed by the sphincters.
3. A few days after injury the bladder begins to contract reflexly when it is full (as in an infant). This is the ***automatic reflex bladder***. It is produced by reflexes mediated by the sacral segments of the spinal cord. If these segments are damaged reflex emptying does not occur, and there is dribbling when the bladder is distended.

*Other Causes of Urinary Retention*

1. Retention of urine can also occur by obstruction to the urethra from any cause.
2. Two important causes are enlargement of the prostate (in the elderly), and a stricture of the urethra.
3. Retention is relieved by passing a suitable catheter into the bladder through the urethra. (See prostate, below).

*Other Correlations*

1. Calculi may form in the bladder.
   a. They are seen much more commonly in males than in females.
   b. They can be of varying chemical composition.
   c. They can be crushed through a lithotrite introduced through the urethra. The procedure is called ***litholapaxy***. They can also be removed by suprapubic lithotomy (see above).
2. Congenital malformations resulting in abnormal communications of the bladder have been mentioned above. Injury during parturition can lead to a ***vesicovaginal fistula***.
3. Infection in the bladder is called ***cystitis***.
4. Neoplasms, both benign (papilloma) and malignant (carcinoma) may be seen.

## THE URETHRA

1. The urethra is a tube that connects the lower end (or neck) of the urinary bladder to the exterior. Urine stored in the bladder is passed out through it.
2. The urethra is much longer in the male (about 20 cm) as compared to the female (4 cm).
3. In both sexes its average diameter is about 6 mm.
4. The course and relations of the urethra are different in the male and female. For an understanding of the relations it is necessary to have a clear conception of the perineal spaces and of structures in the perineum. These have been described in chapter 26.

### The Male Urethra

The male urethra is divisible into three parts (33.11).

1. The first part starts at the internal urethral orifice and descends through the prostate to reach the urogenital diaphragm. This part of the urethra is embedded within the prostate gland and is, therefore, called the ***prostatic part***. It is about 3 cm long. Some features to be seen in its interior are described below.
2. The next (***membranous***) part is about 1.5 cm long. It passes through the deep perineal space. This space is bounded:
   a. Above by the superior fascia of the urogenital diaphragm (part of pelvic fascia).
   b. Below by the inferior fascia of the urogenital diaphragm. This fascia is also called the ***perineal membrane***.
   c. Between the two layers there is the ***sphincter urethrae externus*** that surrounds this part of the urethra.

3. The third part of the urethra runs through the bulb and corpus spongiosum of the penis (33.11). It is, therefore, called the ***penile part*** or the ***spongiose part***.
   a. The bulb of the penis lies in immediate contact with the lower surface of the perineal membrane. The urethra enters the bulb immediately after piercing this membrane.
   b. The bulb is continuous anteriorly with the corpus spongiosum. The initial part of the corpus spongiosum forms part of the 'root' of the penis and is fixed in the perineum, while its subsequent part lies in the 'free' part of the penis. The urethra passes through these parts.
   c. Near the tip of the penis, the corpus spongiosum expands to form the glans penis, which is traversed by the terminal part of the urethra. The total length of the penile part of the urethra is about 15 cm.

### The Female Urethra

The female urethra corresponds to the prostatic and membranous parts of the male urethra, and is about 4 cm long (33.11). Throughout its length the urethra is closely related to the anterior wall of the vagina.

#### WANT TO KNOW MORE?

1. We have seen that the average diameter of the male urethra is about 6 mm. The membranous urethra is the narrowest part. The penile urethra shows a dilatation as it lies in the bulb (called the ***intrabulbar fossa***), and another in the glans penis (called the ***navicular fossa***) (33.11). The male urethra is narrowest at its external orifice.
2. a. Except during the passage of urine, the walls of the urethra are apposed to each other the lumen being a mere slit. The appearances seen in transverse sections through various levels of the male urethra are shown in 33.16.
   b. In cross section the female urethra is a transverse slit, but at its external orifice the slit becomes anteroposterior (as in the male).

### Anatomy of the Male and Female Urethra

#### *Sphincters of the Urethra*

The features of the sphincters of the urethra are as follows:

1. Both in the male and in the female the urethra is surrounded by an internal sphincter, the ***sphincter vesicae***; and
2. By an external sphincter, the ***sphincter urethrae*** (33.17).
3. The sphincter vesicae is usually described as a ring of smooth muscle surrounding the urethra at its junction with the bladder. This sphincter is involuntary and is supplied by autonomic nerves. (However many authorities doubt whether a real sphincter exists here).
4. The sphincter urethrae surrounds the urethra as it passes through the deep perineal space. It is made of striated muscle fibres. It is voluntary and is supplied by the perineal branch of the pudendal nerve.
5. The prostatic part of the male urethra shows the following features (33.18).
   a. On its posterior wall there is a median ridge of mucous membrane that is called the ***urethral crest***.
   b. On either side of the crest there is a depression called the ***prostatic sinus***.
   c. Numerous prostatic ducts open into the prostatic sinuses.
   d. Midway between its upper and lower ends the urethral crest bears a rounded swelling called the ***colliculus seminalis***.
   e. The colliculus shows three openings. In the middle line there is the opening of a small blind sac called the ***prostatic utricle***. On either side of the opening of the utricle there are openings of the right and left ejaculatory ducts.

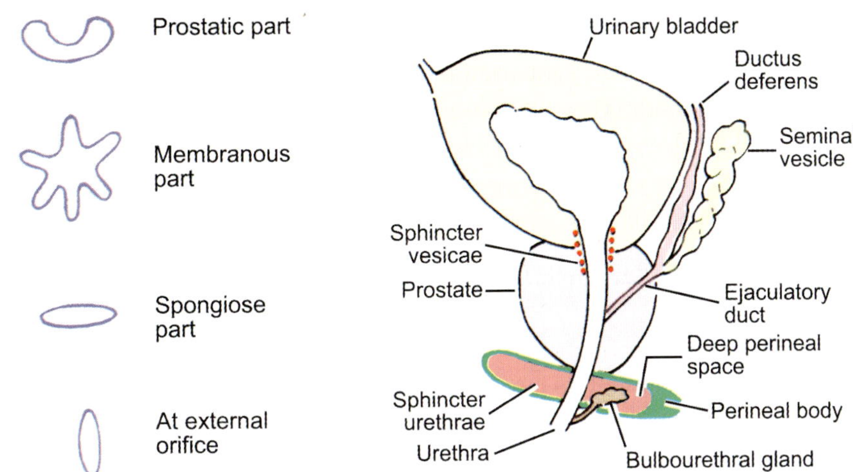


**33.16:** Transverse sections through various parts of the male urethra to show the shape of its lumen

**33.17:** Diagram showing the sphincters of the urethra, and the bulbourethral glands

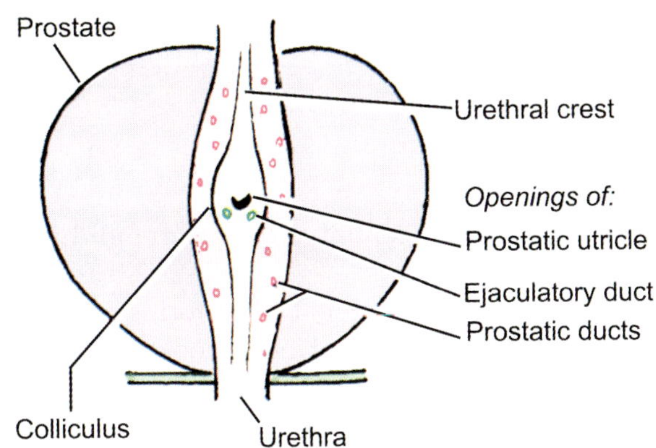


**33.18:** Posterior wall of the prostatic urethra

## WANT TO KNOW MORE?

*Glands and Lacunae Related to the Urethra*

1. The prostate is the largest gland related to the male urethra. It is described below.
2. On either side of the membranous part of the male urethra there is the corresponding bulbourethral gland (33.17).
3. Numerous urethral glands lie in the submucosa of the penile part of the male urethra and open into the urethra.
4. In addition the urethral wall has a number of recesses or lacunae, the largest being present in the navicular fossa (in the glans). The importance of the lacunae is that catheters or other instruments introduced into the urethra may get stuck in them.
5. Urethral glands and lacunae are also present in the female urethra. The female urethral glands are believed to be homologous with the prostate.

*Lymphatic Drainage*

1. The prostatic and membranous parts of the urethra drain to the internal iliac nodes.
2. The penile part drains into the superficial inguinal nodes.
3. Some vessels from the urethra reach the external iliac nodes.

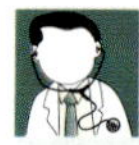

## CLINICAL CORRELATION OF URETHRA

*Congenital Malformations*

1. The urethra may show obstruction (at its junction with the bladder).
2. It may show various types of duplication.
3. There may be abnormal communications with the rectum, vagina or ureter.
4. See hypospadias and epispadias, in chapter 26.

*Other Correlations*

1. Instruments are commonly passed through the urethra to:
   a. Relieve urinary retention (***catheterisation***),
   b. To visualise the interior of the urinary bladder, the ureter, or the urethra itself.
2. Infection in the urethra is called ***urethritis***.
3. Injury or chronic infection can lead to formation of a ***stricture*** that becomes a cause of urinary retention.
4. The urethra can be injured by falls on the perineum or by lack of care in passing an instrument.

## Ductus Deferens

1. The ductus deferens begins in the scrotum (as a continuation of the epididymis). It passes through the inguinal canal to enter the abdomen.
2. The part of the ductus deferens that lies in the inguinal canal forms part of the spermatic cord. At the deep inguinal ring the ductus deferens enters the abdomen. Here it hooks around the lateral side of the inferior epigastric artery (25.26 and 26.5).
3. The ductus then runs backwards (and somewhat downwards). Crossing medial to the external iliac vessels the ductus deferens comes to lie in the lateral wall of the true pelvis (33.8).
4. As it runs backwards over this wall it crosses the following.
   a. The umbilical artery (or superior vesical artery)
   b. The obturator nerve and vessels
   c. The inferior vesical artery
   d. The ureter.
5. The terminal part of the ductus deferens is seen in 33.12. Having crossed the ureter the duct runs downwards and medially behind the base of the urinary bladder, medial to the seminal vesicle.
6. Here the deferent ducts of the two sides approach the middle line.
7. Just above the prostate the ductus deferens ends by joining the duct of the seminal vesicle to form the ejaculatory duct.
8. (Note that the base of the urinary bladder lies immediately in front of the rectum, so that the terminal parts of the right and left deferent ducts lie between these organs along with the seminal vesicles.)
9. The ductus deferens has a very narrow lumen, but has a thick wall. When palpated it feels like a cord.
10. Its initial part (lying behind the testis) is highly convoluted, but the rest of it is straight.
11. The part lying behind the urinary bladder is dilated and is called the ***ampulla;*** but the terminal part of the duct again narrows down before joining the duct of the seminal vesicle (33.12).

## The Seminal Vesicles

1. The right and left seminal vesicles lie posterior to the base of the urinary bladder, between it and the rectum (33.12).
2. Each vesicle is about 5 cm long.
3. The lower ends of the right and left seminal vesicles lie close together near the median plane. From here each vesicle passes upwards and laterally so that the upper ends of the two vesicles are far apart, and lie near the ureters.
4. When dissected out each seminal vesicle is seen to be a long tube convoluted upon itself. One end of this tube is blind. The other end emerges at the lower end of the seminal vesicle as its ***duct.***
5. This duct joins the corresponding ductus deferens to form the ejaculatory duct.
6. Lymphatics from the seminal vesicle drain into the internal and external iliac lymph nodes.

## The Ejaculatory Ducts

1. Each ejaculatory duct is formed by union of the ductus deferens and the duct of the seminal vesicle.
2. It passes downwards and forwards through the substance of the prostate (33.17 and 33.20) to open on the colliculus seminalis (33.18) just lateral to the aperture of the prostatic utricle.

# THE PROSTATE

1. The prostate is a glandular structure. Its position is shown in 33.11.
2. The prostate lies in the space between the lower end of the urinary bladder and the upper surface of the uro-genital diaphragm.
3. It lies behind the lower part of the symphysis pubis, and in front of the rectum.
4. It is traversed by the prostatic part of the urethra, and the ejaculatory ducts. The prostatic utricle also extends into it.
5. From 33.12 it will be seen that the prostate is broadest above (***base***) and narrowest below (***apex***).
   a. Its width at the base is about 4 cm; its vertical diameter is about 3 cm; so that its width is greater than its length.
   b. The anteroposterior diameter is about 2 cm.
6. The prostate has five surfaces.
   a. The ***superior surface,*** or base, is in contact with the neck of the urinary bladder.
   b. The ***posterior surface,*** is in contact with the rectum and can be palpated through the latter.
   c. The ***anterior surface*** is connected to the pubic bones by the right and left puboprostatic ligaments (33.11).
   d. The right and left ***inferolateral surfaces*** are in contact with the corresponding levatores ani muscles. (These parts of the levatores ani muscles are often referred to as the ***levatores prostatae***).
7. The substance of the prostate is often described as being divided into a number of lobes, but this is a subject on which there is considerable controversy. Traditionally five lobes are described.
   a. There are right and left ***lateral lobes.***
   b. These are separated in front by an ***anterior lobe.***
   c. Posteriorly the lateral lobes are separated by a ***posterior lobe*** (33.19).
8. The part of the prostate between the posterior part of the base (above), and the ejaculatory ducts (below), is called the ***middle*** (or ***median***) lobe (33.20).
9. On embryological grounds the prostate can be divided into an ***inner glandular zone*** (derived from mesoderm) and an ***outer glandular zone*** (derived from endoderm). These subdivisions are of clinical significance (see below).
10. The prostate is surrounded by a fibrous ***capsule*** that is closely adherent to the gland.
11. Outside the capsule there is a fibrous ***sheath*** that is part of the pelvic fascia.
12. Between the capsule and the sheath there is a dense venous plexus.
13. The posterior part of the fibrous sheath, which separates the prostate from the rectum is formed by the rectovesical fascia (or fascia of Denonvilliers).

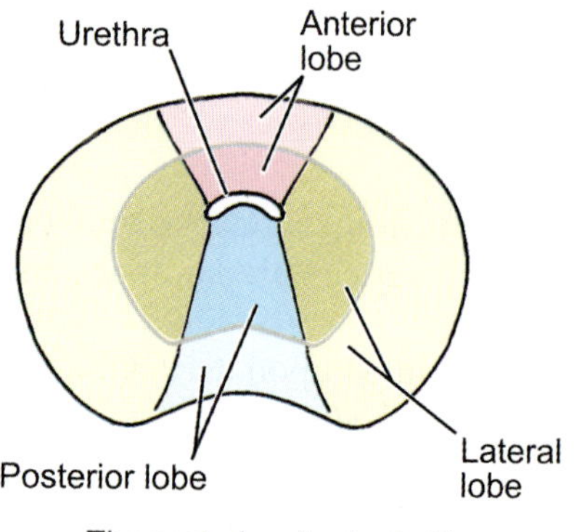


**33.19:** Transverse section through the prostate to show its lobes

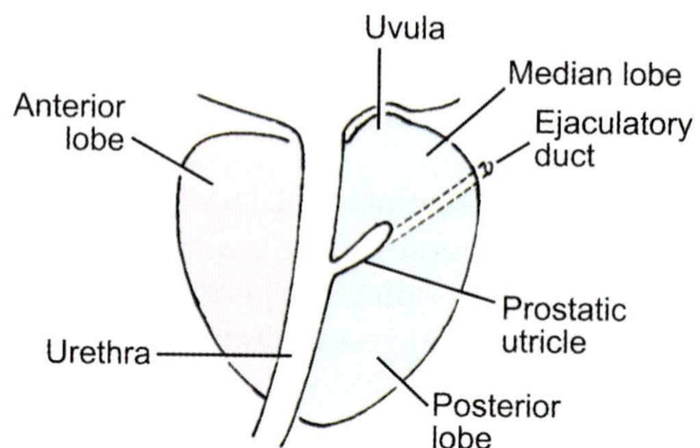


**33.20:** Sagittal section through the prostate to show its lobes

14. Note that the fibrous sheath of the prostate is sometimes referred to as its false capsule. However, this term should be avoided as some authorities use it for a condensation of prostatic tissue deep to the capsule.
15. The substance of the prostate consists of glandular tissue, masses of which are separated by fibromuscular septa.
    a. The glandular tissue is poorly developed at birth.
    b. It gradually undergoes growth, but this growth becomes much faster at the time of puberty.
    c. After the age of fifty years (or so) the prostate may undergo atrophy.
    d. In some persons it undergoes benign hypertrophy (see below).

## WANT TO KNOW MORE?

*Blood Vessels, Lymphatics and Nerves of Prostate*

1. The prostate is supplied by branches of the inferior vesical, middle rectal and internal pudendal arteries.
2. The veins drain through the prostatic venous plexus into the internal iliac veins.
3. The lymphatics drain into the internal and external iliac nodes (Chapter 34).
4. The nerves are autonomic and reach the prostate through the inferior hypogastric plexus (Chapter 34).

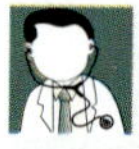

## CLINICAL CORRELATION

### Prostate

1. The two most important clinical conditions affecting the prostate are enlargement in old age (benign hypertrophy, or benign enlargement), and carcinoma.
2. To understand these conditions it is important to know the division of the prostate into lobes and into an inner glandular zone (derived from mesoderm) and an outer glandular zone (derived from endoderm).
3. The prostate can be felt by rectal examination, and its enlargement determined.

*Benign Enlargement of Prostate*

1. Benign hypertrophy of the prostate is due to the formation of an adenoma.
2. This condition occurs most frequently in the median lobe; and somewhat less frequently in the inner parts of the lateral lobes.

3. The region corresponds to the inner glandular zone, which is therefore also called the ***adenomatous zone***. (In contrast, the outer glandular zone is frequently the site of carcinoma and is, therefore, called the ***carcinomatous zone***).
4. Some facts concerning benign enlargement of the prostate are as follows.
5. One of the important symptoms of prostatic enlargement is repeated desire to pass urine but with difficulty in doing so. The condition can also lead to urinary retention. The reasons for these symptoms are as follows.
   a. We have seen that benign hypertrophy most frequently affects the median lobe of the prostate. This lobe enlarges upwards and forwards and can cause obstruction to the flow of urine.
   b. The median lobe produces a projection on the interior of the urinary bladder just behind the internal urethral orifice. This projection is called the uvula (33.20).
   c. With enlargement of the median lobe the uvula also enlarges and may form a flap that covers the internal urethral meatus and obstructs it.
   d. The enlarging uvula may insinuate itself into the internal urethral sphincter and thus make it inefficient. If this happens urine keeps entering the prostatic urethra resulting in a constant desire to micturate.
   e. The enlarged uvula leads to the formation of a pouch that is not emptied during urination leading to stagnation of urine.
6. Obstruction to flow of urine is also caused by distortion of the prostatic urethra produced by enlargement of the prostate.
7. Traditionally an enlarged prostate has been treated by surgical removal (prostatectomy).
   a. The organ can be approached through the urinary bladder (***transvesical prostatectomy***),
   b. Through the retropubic region without entering the bladder (***retropubic prostatectomy***), or
   c. Through the perineum (***perineal prostatectomy***).
8. However, at present the operation of choice is removal through an instrument passed through the urethra. This is called ***transurethral resection*** (TUR).
9. In traditional removal of the prostate it has to be remembered that:
   a. The prostate is surrounded by a fibrous capsule that is closely adherent to the gland.
   b. Outside the capsule there is a fibrous sheath that is part of the pelvic fascia.
   c. Between the capsule and the sheath there is a dense venous plexus.
   d. In operations for removal of the prostate the surgeon often prefers not to disturb the venous plexus; and removes the prostate from within its capsule.
10. The posterior part of the fibrous sheath, which separates the prostate from the rectum is formed by the rectovesical fascia (or fascia of Denonvilliers).
11. Note that the fibrous sheath of the prostate is sometimes referred to as its false capsule. However, this term should be avoided as some authorities use it for a condensation of prostatic tissue deep to the capsule.

*Other Correlations*

1. We have noted that carcinoma of the prostate is common, and that it occurs in the outer glandular zone.
2. Infection of the prostate is called prostatitis, which may be acute or chronic. Prostatitis may sometimes be tubercular.

## WANT TO KNOW MORE?

**The Bulbourethral Glands**

1. The right and left bulbourethral glands (33.17) are located in the deep perineal space on either side of the membranous urethra.
2. They are embedded within the fibres of the sphincter urethrae.
3. Each gland gives off a long duct that pierces the perineal membrane to enter the superficial perineal space. Here it ends by opening into the spongiose (penile) part of the male urethra.

## Female Reproductive Organs

1. The female reproductive organs consist of:
   a. The female internal and external genitalia
   b. The mammary glands.
2. The female external genitalia have been considered along with other structures in the perineum in chapter 26. The mammary glands have described along with the pectoral region in chapter 3.
3. The female internal genitalia consist of:
   a. The ovaries
   b. The uterus and uterine tubes
   c. The vagina. These are described below.

## THE OVARIES

1. The right and left ovaries are the female gonads.
2. Female gametes, called *ova* (singular = Ovum), are produced in them.
3. Each ovary is shaped like an almond. It is approximately 3 cm in length, 1.5 cm in width, and 1 cm in thickness.
4. It is covered by a germinal epithelium that is continuous with the peritoneum.
5. From 33.21 it will be seen that the uterus is attached, on either side, to a fold of peritoneum called the ***broad ligament***.
   a. The broad ligament stretches from the side of the uterus to the sidewall and floor of the pelvis.
   b. The ligament is placed obliquely so that it has one surface directed forwards and downwards, and another directed backwards and upwards.
   c. The ovary is attached to the posterosuperior aspect of the broad ligament by a fold of peritoneum called the *mesovarium*.
   d. The part of the broad ligament between the attachment of the mesovarium and the lateral wall of the pelvis is called the ***suspensory ligament of the ovary***.
6. Because of its peritoneal attachments the ovary has considerable mobility leading to variations in its orientation. The description of the orientation that follows is, therefore, applicable only to women who have not had a pregnancy (nulliparous women).
7. The long axis of the ovary is vertical. It has upper and lower ends, medial and lateral surfaces, and anterior and posterior borders.
   a. The ***anterior border*** gives attachment to the mesovarium and is, therefore, also called the ***mesovarian border***.
   b. The ***posterior border*** is also called the ***free*** border.
   c. The ***lateral surface*** of the ovary lies in contact with the peritoneum covering the lateral wall of the pelvis. It lies in a depression called the ***ovarian fossa***.
   d. This fossa is bounded (33.22) as follows:
      i. Posteriorly by the ureter and internal iliac vessels.
      ii. Anteriorly by the external iliac vessel.
      iii. Inferiorly by the superior vesical artery (persisting proximal part of the umbilical artery).
      iv. The obturator vessels and nerve cross lateral to the ovarian fossa.
   e. The ***medial surface*** is in contact with the terminal part of the uterine tube.
8. The ***upper pole*** is in intimate contact with the uterine tube and is, therefore, also called the ***tubal end***. It is directed upwards, a little forwards and laterally. It lies close to the external iliac vessels.
9. The ***lower pole*** is directed downwards, and somewhat backwards and medially. It gives attachment to the ***ligament of the ovary***. This ligament passes in the interval between the two layers of the broad ligament to reach the uterus (near the attachment of the uterine tube to the latter) (33.21).
10. The substance of the ovary is divisible into an outer ***cortex*** and an inner ***medulla***.

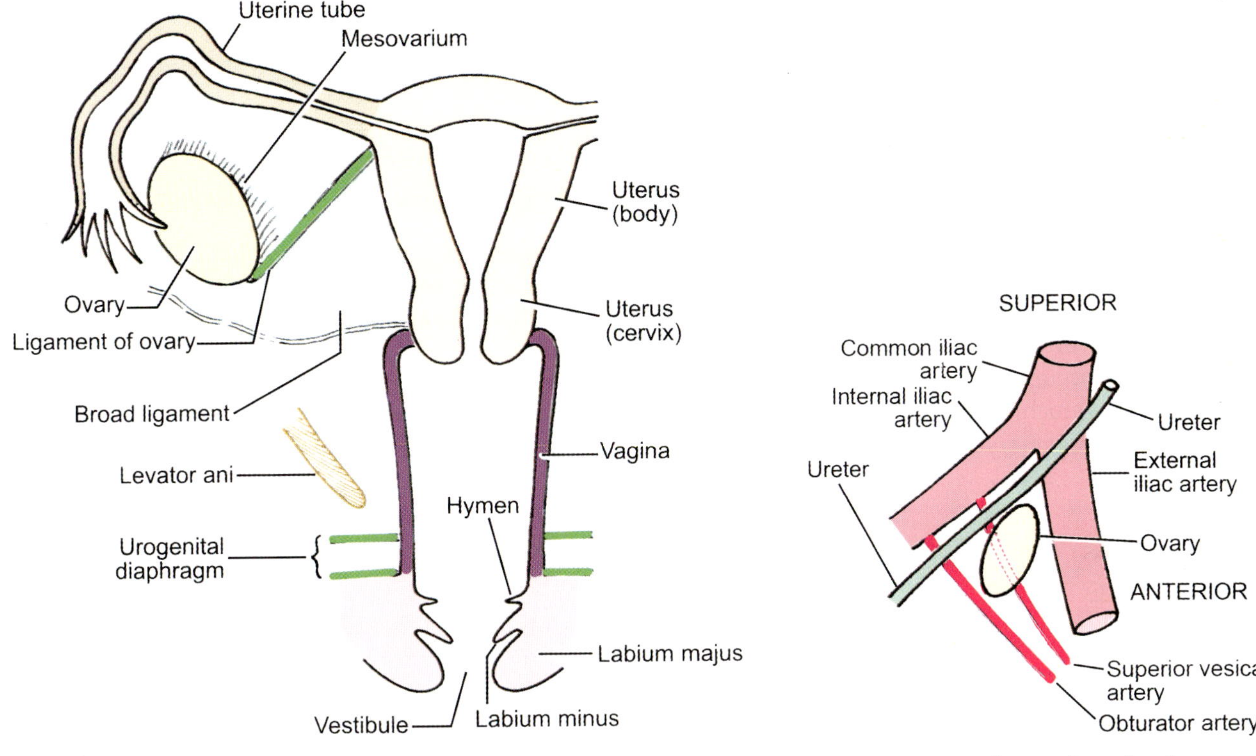


**33.21:** Scheme to show the female reproductive organs

**33.22:** Boundaries of ovarian fossa

11. In the cortex there are rounded structures called ***ovarian follicles*** (also called ***Graafian follicles***).
    a. In relation to the wall of each follicle there is one developing ovum surrounded by supporting follicular cells.
    b. In the reproductive period of a woman's life one ovarian follicle matures every month.
    c. It forms an elevation on the surface of the ovary and with further enlargement, it ruptures shedding the ovum. This is called ***ovulation***.
    d. The region of the developing follicle is overlapped by the fimbriated end of the uterine tube (see below) which receives the ovum discharged from the ovary.
12. After the ovum is discharged the remaining part of the ovarian follicle is converted into a yellowish body called the ***corpus luteum***.

## WANT TO KNOW MORE?

### *Blood Vessels, Lymphatics, and Nerves of the Ovary*

1. The ovary is supplied by the ovarian artery; and by some branches of the uterine artery (32.11).
2. A number of veins arise from the ovary and form a pampiniform plexus (as in the testis). The ovarian veins arise from this plexus.
3. The right vein terminates in the inferior vena cava, but the left vein ends in the left renal vein.
4. Lymph vessels from the ovary pass along the ovarian vessels to the lateral aortic lymph nodes.
5. The ovary is innervated by autonomic nerves that probably reach it along the ovarian vessels.

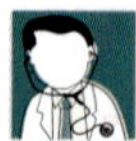

## CLINICAL CORRELATION OF OVARIES

*Congenital Malformations*

1. The ovary may be absent, or may be duplicated.
2. It may undergo abnormal descent into the inguinal canal or even into labium majus.
3. Adrenal or thyroid tissue may be present in it. Also see ***teratoma*** below.

*Other Correlations*

1. The ovary may be the site of carcinoma. Peculiar tumours called ***teratomas*** may occur. They may contain a mixture of various kinds of tissue. They are derived from undifferentiated cells persisting from embryonic life.
2. Cysts may form in the ovary and may reach a very large size.
3. The ovaries occupy the ovarian fossa only up to the time of the first pregnancy. After pregnancy the broad ligament (to which the ovaries are anchored) becomes lax and the ovaries can descend and can even lie in the rectouterine pouch (***prolapse of the ovaries***). An ovary lying in this pouch can be felt on vaginal examination.

## THE UTERINE TUBES

1. Each uterine tube (right or left) lies in the free margin of the corresponding broad ligament. It has medial and lateral ends (33.21).
2. The ***medial end*** is attached to the corresponding side of the uterus. Here its lumen communicates with the cavity of the uterus.
3. The ***lateral end*** of the tube lies near the ovary. At this end it has an opening through which its lumen is in communication with the peritoneal cavity. This opening is called the ***abdominal ostium*** (33.21).
4. The uterine tube is about 10 cm long.
   a. About 1 cm of the tube, near the medial end, is embedded in the muscle wall of the uterus: this is the ***uterine part*** of the tube.
   b. The next 3 cm or so is thick-walled and has a narrow lumen so that it is cord like: this part is called the ***isthmus***.
   c. The next 5 cm or so is thin walled and has a much larger lumen than the rest of the tube. This dilated part is called the ***ampulla***.
5. The lateral end of the uterine tube is funnel shaped and is called the ***infundibulum.***
   a. The walls of the infundibulum are prolonged into a number of irregular processes called ***fimbria***.
   b. One of these fimbria is larger than the others and is in close contact with the ovary. It is called the ***ovarian fimbria***.
6. In the nulliparous woman the uterine tube comes into contact (from medial to lateral side) first with the lower (or medial) pole of the ovary; then ascends along its anterior (or mesovarian) border to reach the superior pole. It finally descends to partially cover the medial surface of the ovary (33.23).
7. Ova discharged from the ovary enter the uterine tube through the infundibulum and pass into the ampulla. They slowly travel towards the uterus.
8. If sexual intercourse takes place at the appropriate time spermatozoa enter the uterine tube through the vagina and uterus and meet the ovum in the ampulla of the tube. Fertilisation normally takes place in the ampulla.
9. The fertilised ovum travels through the uterine tube towards the uterus to enter its cavity. Here it gets implanted in the uterine wall.
10. If fertilisation does not occur the unfertilised ovum enters the uterus and is discharged through the vagina.

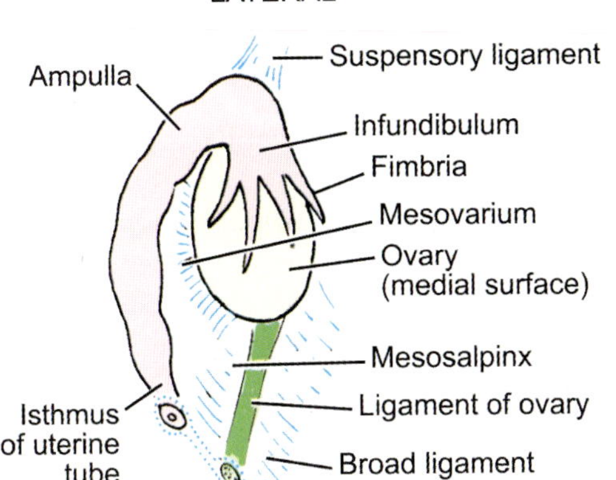


**33.23:** Relationship of uterine tube to ovary as seen from the medial side

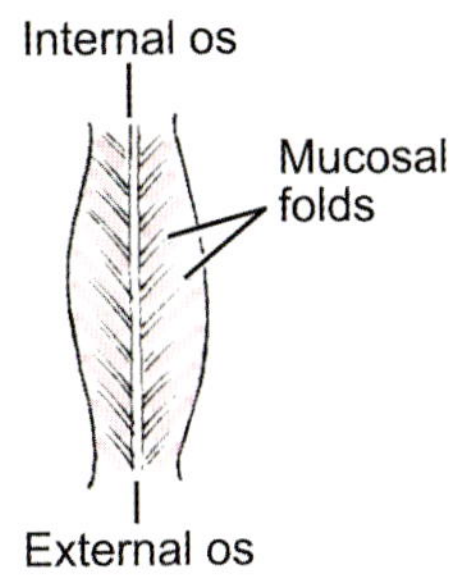


**33.24:** Mucosal folds in the canal of the cervix

## WANT TO KNOW MORE?

### *Blood Vessels, Lymphatics and Nerves of the Uterine Tubes*

1. The medial two-thirds of each uterine tube are supplied by the corresponding uterine artery and its lateral one third by the ovarian artery (32.11). This blood drains through the corresponding veins.
2. Lymph vessels travel along the ovarian vessels to the lateral aortic nodes.
3. Each uterine tube is supplied by autonomic nerves, sympathetic and parasympathetic.
   a. Parasympathetic fibres are partly vagal (along the ovarian artery) and partly from the pelvic splanchnic nerves (along the uterine artery).
   b. Afferents travel through sympathetic nerves along the ovarian vessels. The spinal segments concerned are T10 to L2.

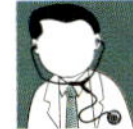

## CLINICAL CORRELATION OF UTERINE TUBES

1. The ovarian tubes may be absent, may be duplicated or may show atresia.
2. Inflammation of the uterine tubes is ***salpingitis***.
   a. This can lead to blockage of the tubes, and this can become a cause of infertility.
   b. Patency of the tubes can be tested by injecting a radio-opaque dye into them (***hysterosalpingography***).
   c. Spillage of dye into the peritoneal cavity (through the lateral end of the tube) is an indication of patency.
3. The uterine tubes can be purposely cut and ligated (***tubectomy***) as a family planning measure (to prevent pregnancy) .
4. If a fertilised ovum gets stuck in the uterine tube (thus failing the reach the uterus) it may start developing there resulting in a ***tubal pregnancy***.
   a. Such a pregnancy seldom goes on to full term.
   b. As pregnancy advances the uterine tube can rupture. This can lead to serious haemorrhage into the peritoneal cavity.

## THE UTERUS

1. A general idea of the form of the uterus is presented in 33.21.
2. The uterus is piriform. It is broader above and narrows down below.
3. The uterus is about 7.5 cm (3 inches) in length. Its maximum width (near its upper end) is about 5 cm (2 inches). Its thickness (anteroposterior) is about 2.5 cm (1 inch).
4. The exterior of the uterus shows a constriction at the junction of its upper two thirds with the lower one third. The part above the constriction is called the ***body***: It is broad above and narrow below. The part below the constriction is called the ***cervix***. This part is more or less cylindrical.
5. Sections across the uterus show that it has a thick wall, and a relatively narrow lumen.
6. The wall is made up of a thick layer of muscle (called the ***myometrium***) and of an inner lining of mucosa (called the ***endometrium***).
7. In a sagittal section through the uterus the lumen is seen as a narrow slit, the anterior and posterior walls being close to each other.
8. In the coronal plane the lumen of the body of the uterus is triangular (33.21). The lumen of each uterine tube joins the lateral angle of this triangle.
9. The part of the body of the uterus that lies above the level of the openings of the uterine tubes is called the ***fundus***.
10. The cavity of the cervix (or ***canal of the cervix***) is roughly cylindrical. However, its upper and lower ends are somewhat narrower than the central part. The upper narrow end is called the ***internal os*** and the narrow lower end is called the ***external os*** (33.24).
11. The cavity of the uterus communicates with that of the vagina through the external os. On both the anterior and posterior walls of the canal of the cervix, the mucosa shows a longitudinal ridge. Shorter folds arising from this ridge pass upwards and laterally like branches from the stem of a tree.
12. The uterus lies in the true pelvis. Its orientation is best appreciated in a sagittal section through the pelvis (33.13).
    a. In the erect posture the long axis of the uterus is oblique. Its so-called 'upper' end (or fundus) is directed forwards and somewhat upwards. The so-called 'lower' end is directed backwards and somewhat downwards.
    b. The long axis of the uterus is more or less at right angles to the long axis of the vagina. The forward bending of the uterus relative to the vagina is referred to as ***anteversion*** of the uterus.
    c. The uterus is also slightly bent forwards on itself. This is referred to as ***anteflexion***.
13. The caudal part of the cervix projects into the upper part of vagina through the anterior wall of the latter. It is separated from the vaginal wall by recesses called the anterior, lateral, and posterior ***fornices*** (singular = fornix) of the vagina. The posterior fornix is deepest.

### *Peritoneum Related to the Uterus*

1. The peritoneum from the anterior abdominal wall passes on to the superior surface of the urinary bladder (33.11). From the posterior part of this surface the peritoneum is reflected on to the 'anterior' (actually anteroinferior) surface of the uterus at the junction of the body with the cervix.
2. It lines the 'anterior' surface of the body, passes over fundus and runs over the 'posterior' (actually posterosuperior) aspect of the uterus reaching the upper part of the vagina from where it is reflected on to the front of the rectum.
3. The peritoneum lined space between the front of the body of the uterus and the superior surface of the urinary bladder is called the ***vesico-uterine pouch***.

4.a. The space between the uterus (and the uppermost part of the vagina) in front, and the rectum behind is called the ***rectouterine pouch*** (or ***pouch of Douglas***).

b. The pouch is really rectovaginal.

c. It is important to know that the bottom of the pouch is only about 5 cm (2 inches) from the anal orifice.

5. When traced laterally the layers of peritoneum lining the front and back of the uterus meet along its lateral margins to form the broad ligament.

*Relations of the Uterus*

1. We have seen that the 'anterior' surface of the uterus is related to the superior surface of the urinary bladder. The body of the uterus is separated from the bladder by peritoneum, but the upper part of the cervix is in direct contact.
2. The lower part of the cervix lies within the vagina. It is separated anteriorly from the uppermost part of the anterior vaginal wall by the anterior fornix of the vagina.
3. The 'posterior' surface of the uterus (both body and cervix) is separated by peritoneum from the sigmoid colon and from coils of small intestine. The lowest part of the uterus (cervix) forms the anterior wall of the posterior fornix of the vagina.
4. On either side the corresponding uterine artery reaches the lateral side of the cervix and then ascends along the lateral margin of the body of the uterus, lying between the two layers of peritoneum forming the broad ligament (32.11).
5. The ureters run downwards and forwards a short distance (about 2 cm) lateral to the cervix (33.9 and 33.25).

**WANT TO KNOW MORE?**

*Variability in Size, Shape and Position of the Uterus*

1. At the time of birth the cervix of the uterus is large and the body small. Thereafter, the body grows more than the cervix so that by puberty the uterus acquires its normal piriform shape.
2. The uterus undergoes slight enlargement at the time of each menstrual period.
3. It undergoes tremendous enlargement in pregnancy, when its upper end reaches the epigastrium.
4. After the end of pregnancy the uterus gradually approaches near its normal size, but the size of its cavity and the thickness of its muscle wall remains larger than they were before pregnancy. The external os also becomes more prominent.
5. The uterus undergoes atrophy in old age.
6. The normal uterus is anteverted and anteflexed (see above). With filling of the urinary bladder the uterus comes more and more in line with the vagina (i.e., it becomes retroverted), but when the bladder empties the uterus resumes its normal anteverted position. However, in certain cases the uterus becomes fixed in the retroverted position and this may give rise to problems.

*Upper and Lower Uterine Segments*

1. The uterus can be divided into an upper part, consisting of the fundus and the greater part of the body; and a lower part consisting of the lower part of the body, and of the cervix.
2. These are called the ***upper uterine segment***, and the ***lower uterine segment*** respectively.
3. Enlargement of the uterus in pregnancy involves mainly the upper uterine segment.
4. The upper one third of the cervix is sometimes referred to as the ***isthmus***. It is 'taken up' into the body of the uterus as pregnancy advances.
5. The placenta is normally attached only to the upper uterine segment.

*Blood Vessels, Lymphatics and Nerves of the Uterus*

1. The uterus is supplied by the uterine arteries.
2. Branches of the right and left arteries anastomose freely across the middle line.
3. Both the myometrium and the endometrium receive a rich blood supply.
4. The main trunk of the uterine artery and many of its branches show marked tortuosity.
5. Branches of the uterine arteries anastomose with those of the ovarian and vaginal arteries. The uterine veins follow the arteries.

6. Lymphatics drainage is as follows:
   a. Vessels from the upper part of the uterus (and uterine tubes) reach the lateral aortic nodes.
   b. The lower part of the body of the uterus drains into external iliac nodes.
   c. The cervix drains into external iliac, internal iliac and sacral nodes (see chapter 34).
7. The uterus is supplied by autonomic nerves, both sympathetic and parasympathetic. The nerves reach the uterus through the hypogastric plexuses and along the ovarian artery (ovarian plexus). The sympathetic fibres are derived from spinal segments T12 to L1. The parasympathetic fibres are derived from the sacral outflow (see chapter 34).

### *Ligaments of the Uterus*

The uterus is attached to surrounding structures through a number of so-called ligaments. Some of these are made up of fibrous tissue (true ligaments), but others are only folds of peritoneum (false ligaments).

#### *Folds of peritoneum*

1. The fold of peritoneum passing from the anterior aspect of the uterus to the urinary bladder is called the ***anterior ligament.***
2. The fold of peritoneum passing from the posterior aspect of the uterus (to the upper part of the vagina and then) to the rectum is called the ***posterior ligament***. This fold forms the floor of the retrouterine pouch (pouch of Douglas).
3. Two folds (right and left) pass from the side of the cervix to the rectum and posterior wall of the pelvis. These are called the ***rectouterine folds***. These folds form the lateral boundaries of the rectouterine pouch.
4. The right and left ***broad ligaments*** connect the sides of the uterus to the lateral wall and floor of the pelvis. Several structures intimately related to the broad ligament have already been mentioned. These are:
   a. The ovary
   b. The uterine tube
   c. The uterine artery
   d. The ovarian artery (in the suspensory ligament)
   e. The ligament of the ovary
   f. The proximal part of the round ligament of the uterus (see below) is also present
   g. Small remnants of some embryonic structures are present in the broad ligament near the ovary. These are the ***epoophoron*** and the ***paroophoron***.

#### *Fibrous ligaments*

1. The ***transverse cervical ligament*** (also called the ***lateral, cardinal*** or ***Mackenrodt's ligament***) passes from the lateral side of the cervix (and the upper end of the vagina) to the lateral wall of the pelvis (33.26). The uterine vessels are embedded in it.
2. The ***pubocervical ligaments*** connect the cervix with the pubic bones (right or left).
3. The ***uterosacral ligaments*** connect the uterus to the sacrum. They lie within the rectouterine peritoneal folds (described above).
4. The ***round ligament*** of the uterus is 10 to 12 cm long.
   a. At one end it is connected to the upper lateral part of the body of the uterus, just below and in front of the uterine tube.
   b. The initial part of the ligament lies within the broad ligament.
   c. The next part runs forwards across the lateral wall of the pelvis (33.9). Crossing the external iliac vessels it hooks round the lateral side of the inferior epigastric artery, and enters the deep inguinal ring. It then passes through the inguinal canal and after emerging from the superficial inguinal ring it ends in the connective tissue of the labium majus.
   d. Note that in its relationship to the inferior epigastric artery, and to the inguinal canal, the round ligament occupies a position similar to that of the ductus deferens in the male. It is, however, not a homologue of the duct.

*Supports of the uterus*

The uterus is maintained in position by various factors. The most important of these are:

a. The pelvic diaphragm including the levator ani muscles and the pelvic fascia lining them.
b. The urogenital diaphragm and the perineal body.
c. The transverse cervical, pubocervical and uterosacral ligaments.

Additional support is provided by the peritoneal folds described above, and by the vagina.

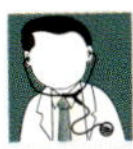

## CLINICAL CORRELATION OF UTERUS

*Congenital Anomalies*

1. The uterus may be duplicated, may be divided by a septum, or may be absent.
2. Only one half of the uterus (and one uterine tube) may be present (***unicornuate uterus***).
3. Sometimes the cervix is absent.
4. There may be atresia of the lumen.
5. Finally, the uterus may remain rudimentary.

*Other Correlations*

1. The uterus undergoes great enlargement (and many other changes) during pregnancy. The uterine mucosa undergoes cyclic alterations as a part of the menstrual cycle.
2. We have seen that the normal uterus is anteverted and anteflexed. The uterus can become ***retroverted***.
3. Weakening of the pelvic diaphragm can lead to ***prolapse*** of the uterus. Retroversion predisposes to prolapse (as the uterus comes into line with the vagina).
4. Neoplasms may take place.
   a. The most common growth is a fibroma (fibroid) which can be multiple.
   b. Carcinoma is common in the cervix.
5. Surgical procedures are commonly performed on the uterus.
   a. In cases in which normal birth of a baby is not possible delivery may be done by opening the uterus (***Caesarean section***).
   b. Any operation for opening of the uterus is called ***hysterotomy***, and removal of the uterus is called ***hysterectomy***.
   c. Instruments may be passed into the uterus after dilating the cervix for termination of pregnancy, or for curetting (scraping) of the endometrium.
6. Intrauterine contraceptive devices (IUCD) made of metal or plastic may be inserted into the uterus to prevent implantation of a fertilised ovum.

## THE VAGINA

1. The vagina is a tubular structure with a muscular wall.
2. Its lower end opens to the exterior through the vestibule (33.21).
3. a. At its upper end it is attached to the cervix of the uterus.
   b. The cervix projects into the upper part of the vagina through the uppermost part of its anterior wall (33.13).
   c. The space between the cervix and the adjoining parts of the vaginal wall is divided (for descriptive purposes) into the anterior, posterior, and lateral fornices.
4. From 33.13 it can be seen that the long axis of the vagina runs upwards and backwards. This axis is approximately at right angles to that of the uterus.

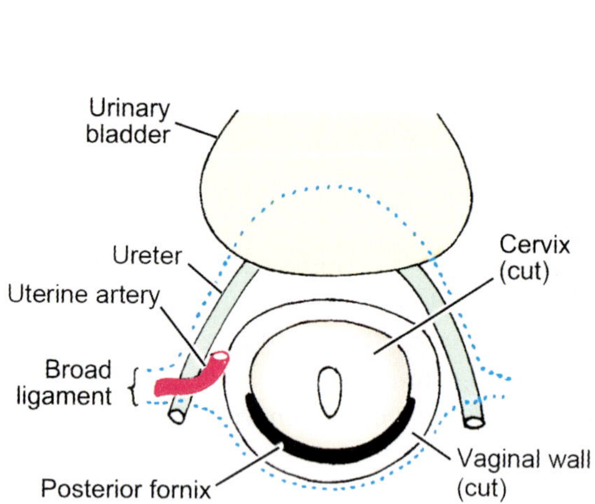


**33.25:** Scheme to show the relationship of the ureters to the cervix of the uterus

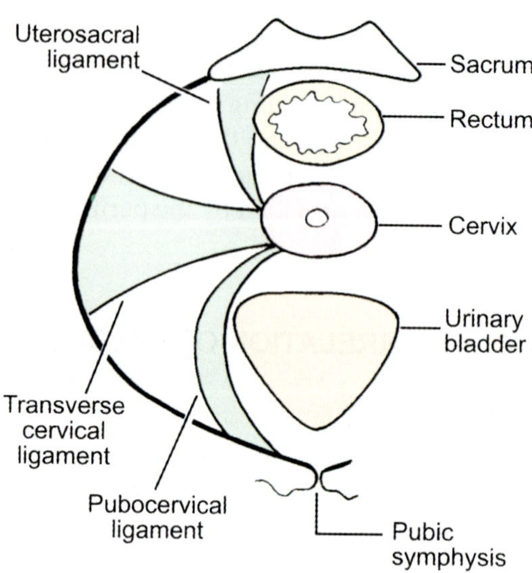


**33.26:** Scheme to show some ligaments of the uterus

5. The vagina has anterior and posterior walls.
   a. The anterior wall is shorter than the posterior.
   b. The anterior wall is about 7.5 cm (3 inches) long.
   c. The posterior wall is about 9 cm long.
6. The anterior wall of the vagina is related above to the base of the urinary bladder, and below to the urethra. The relationship with the urethra is intimate, the latter being embedded in the vaginal wall.
7. The posterior wall of the vagina is related from above downwards to:
   a. The rectouterine pouch
   b. The rectum
   c. The perineal body (which separates it from the anal canal).
8. Laterally, the vagina is related to the following:
   a. The levator ani muscles.
   b. At its upper end the vagina is related laterally to the right and left ureters.
   c. the right and left uterine arteries (33.25).

## WANT TO KNOW MORE?

9. The vagina is supplied mainly by the vaginal branch of the internal iliac artery. It also receives branches from the uterine, internal pudendal and middle rectal arteries.
10. The vaginal veins end in the internal iliac veins.
11. The lymphatic drainage of the vagina is as follows.
    a. Lymph vessels from the upper part of the vagina travel along the uterine artery to the internal and external lymph nodes.
    b. Those from the middle of the vagina run along the vaginal artery to reach the internal iliac nodes.
    c. The lower part of the vagina drains into the superficial inguinal nodes.
12. The vagina receives autonomic nerves that reach it along the vaginal arteries.
13. The lower part of the vagina receives sensory branches from the pudendal nerves (through their inferior rectal and posterior labial branches) (also see chapter 34).

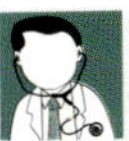

## CLINICAL CORRELATIONS OF VAGINA

*Congenital Anomalies*

1. The vagina may be duplicated, may be subdivided by a septum, or may be absent.
2. The hymen may be imperforate.
3. Abnormal communications may exist with the rectum (***rectovaginal fistula***) or with the urinary bladder (***vesicovaginal fistula***).

*Vaginal Examination*

Most of the structures related to the vagina can be palpated through fingers introduced into the vagina.

1. On the anterior side we can feel the pubic symphysis, the urinary bladder, and the urethra.
2. Posteriorly we can feel the rectum, and any structure lying in the rectouterine pouch. The perineal body can also be felt.
3. On either side the structures that can be felt through the vaginal wall are the ovary, the uterine tube, the ureter, and the urogenital diaphragm. The position and size of the uterus can be determined.

*Other Correlations*

1. Prolapse of the uterus is accompanied by some degree of prolapse of the vagina. There can be ***prolapse of the vagina*** without prolapse of the uterus.
2. The vaginal wall can be weakened by pressure of the fetal head.
   a. Trauma during childbirth can lead to the formation of a fistula between the vagina and the rectum.
   b. The urinary bladder may bulge into the vagina through the weakened anterior wall (***cystocele***).
   c. The rectum may bulge through the posterior wall (***rectocele***).
3. Surgical procedures on the vagina include cutting of its wall (***colpotomy***), or repair of the wall (***colporrhaphy***).
4. Injury to the vagina can be caused by carelessly passed instruments. Perforation of the posterior fornix in this way can lead to peritonitis and death.
5. A collection of pus in the rectouterine fossa can be drained through the posterior fornix of the vagina.

# THE PERITONEUM

## Some Introductory Remarks about the Peritoneum

1. The abdominal cavity and most of the viscera within it are lined by a serous membrane called the ***peritoneum***.
2. Like the pleura the peritoneum is a closed sac that is invaginated by viscera. It, therefore, comes to have a ***parietal*** layer lining the abdominal wall; and a ***visceral*** layer that is in intimate relationship to the viscera.
3. The parietal and visceral layers of peritoneum are separated only by a potential space called the ***peritoneal cavity***. This space contains a thin film of fluid that has a lubricating function. It allows free movement of the viscera against the abdominal wall and against each other.
4. Notice carefully the distinction between the terms 'abdominal cavity' and 'peritoneal cavity'. The abdominal cavity contains all the contents of the abdomen, while the peritoneal cavity is only a potential space.
5. Some viscera project only partially into the peritoneal cavity. As a result they are in contact with the posterior abdominal wall, and are only partly lined by peritoneum. Such viscera and other structures are described as being ***retroperitoneal***. Such a viscus has very limited mobility. Examples of retroperitoneal viscera are:
   a. The duodenum
   b. The ascending colon
   c. The descending colon
   d. The kidneys.

6. In contrast to such viscera others are suspended from the abdominal wall by double layered 'folds' of peritoneum passing from the abdominal wall to the viscera. The best example of such a viscus is the small intestine. The fold of peritoneum by which it is attached to the posterior abdominal wall is called the ***mesentery***.
7. In the embryo the gut is a straight midline tube attached to the posterior abdominal wall by a dorsal 'mesentery' (33.27).
   a. To begin with the attachment of the dorsal mesentery to the body wall is in the midline.
   b. However as the gut increases in length it gets folded on itself and comes to be arranged in a complicated manner.
   c. In particular note that the stomach and the transverse colon come to lie transversely (from their original vertical position).
8. The attachments of the dorsal mesentery corresponding to different parts of the gut also shift along with parts of the gut. Simultaneously some parts of the gut lose their mesenteries and become retroperitoneal. These parts are:
   a. The greater part of the duodenum
   b. The ascending colon
   c. The descending colon
   d. The rectum.
9. The ultimate positions at which these segments of the gut get 'fixed' on the posterior abdominal wall are shown in 33.30.
10. a. We have already noted that the fold of peritoneum that suspends the greater part of the small intestine is called the mesentery.
    b. The fold of peritoneum suspending the transverse colon is called the ***transverse mesocolon,*** and that suspending the pelvic colon is called the ***pelvic mesocolon.***
11. The arrangement of the peritoneum in the cranial part of the gut (including the abdominal part of the oesophagus, the stomach, and the first two centimeters of the duodenum) is somewhat more complicated than elsewhere.
    a. This part of the gut is attached to the abdominal wall by two embryonic folds of peritoneum (33.27 and 33.28).
    b. One of these, the ***dorsal mesogastrium,*** is merely the cranial part of the dorsal mesentery discussed above.
    c. The second fold, the ***ventral mesogastrium*** passes from this part of the gut to the anterior abdominal wall.
12. In later development the liver develops within the ventral mesogastrium so that the peritoneum forming it becomes divided into three parts.
    a. One part passes from the stomach to the liver. This is called the ***lesser omentum*** (33.29).
    b. The second part surrounds the liver forming the visceral peritoneum over it.

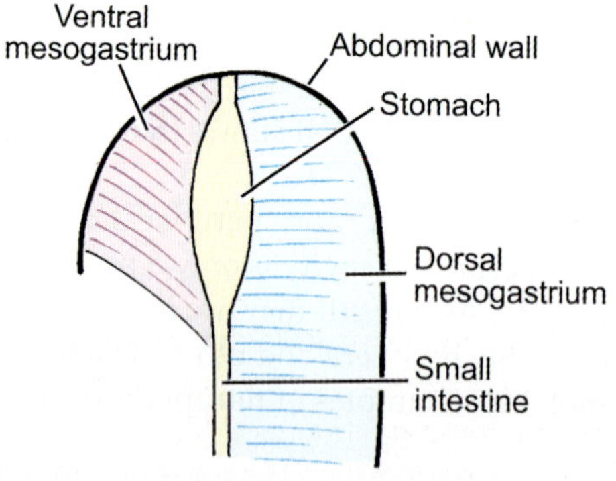


**33.27:** Scheme to show the ventral and dorsal mesogastrium

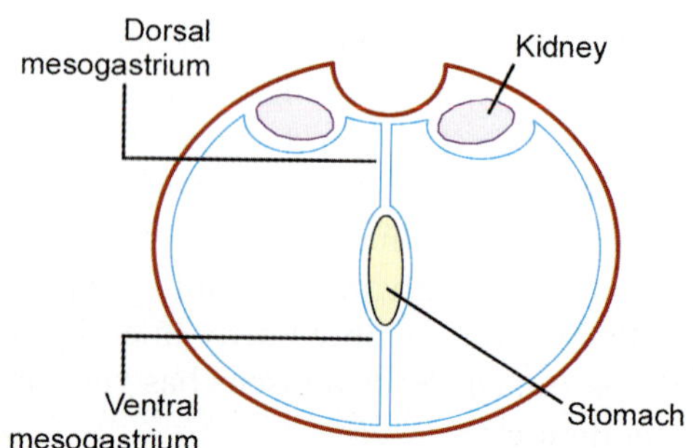


**33.28:** Scheme to show the orientation of the dorsal ventral mesogastrium before rotation of the stomach

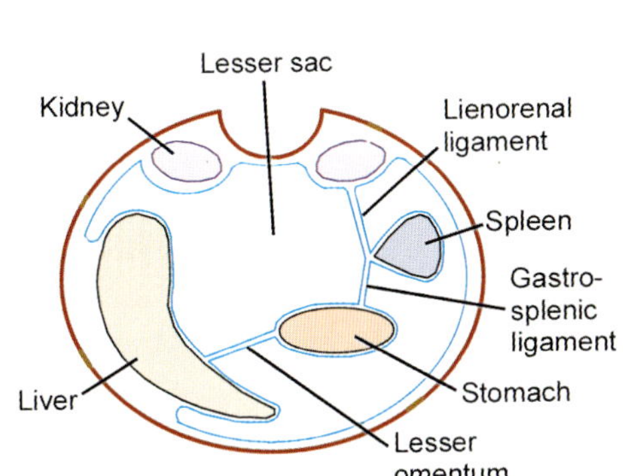


**33.29:** Scheme to show the alterations of the ventral and dorsal mesogastrium as a result of the formation of the liver and spleen

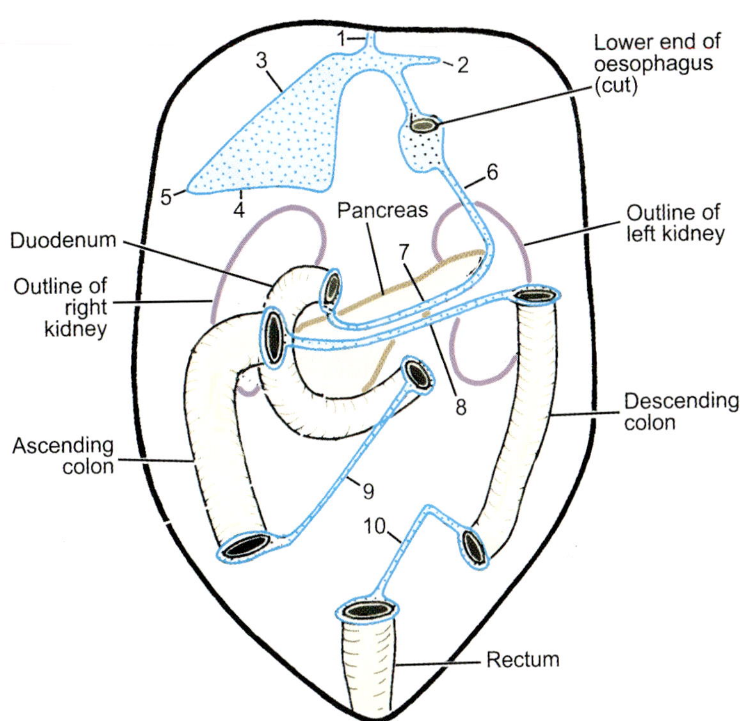


**33.30:** Scheme to show the retroperitoneal parts of the gut, and the attachments of folds to the posterior wall of the abdomen.
1: Falciform ligament; 2: left triangular ligament;
3 and 4: Superior and inferior layers of coronary ligament;
5: Right triangular ligament; 6: Lienorenal ligament;
7: Greater omentum; 8: Transverse mesocolon;
9: Mesentery of jejunum and ileum; 10: Pelvic mesocolon.

c. The third part passes from the liver to the anterior abdominal wall and diaphragm in the form of a number of ligaments (33.29). (These ligaments are merely folds of peritoneum and have no similarity to ligaments of joints).

13. The arrangement of the dorsal mesogastrium also becomes altered. The spleen develops in the cranial part of the dorsal mesogastrium that is thus divided into:
    a. A part passing from the stomach to the spleen, called the ***gastrosplenic ligament.***
    b. A part passing from the spleen to the posterior abdominal wall (33.29).
14. The attachment of this part of the dorsal mesogastrium shifts from the midline to the left side, over the region of the left kidney. As a result the part of the dorsal mesogastrium passing from the spleen to the posterior abdominal wall becomes the ***lienorenal ligament***. (Note: lien = spleen) (also see 33.30).
15. Caudal to the gastrosplenic and lienorenal ligaments, the attachment of the dorsal mesogastrium to the posterior abdominal wall changes from a vertical position to a transverse one. This is in keeping with a change in the orientation of the stomach.
16. Simultaneously, this fold elongates greatly and forms a double layered loop of peritoneum that runs downwards from the stomach, curves on itself, and runs up again to reach the attachment on the posterior abdominal wall. This double-layered fold of peritoneum is called the ***greater omentum*** (see 33.31).
17. 33.30 shows the final position of the attachment of the dorsal mesentery on the posterior abdominal wall.
18. In those parts where the gut has become retroperitoneal, the gut itself is seen.
19. Between these segments of gut there are the attachments of the remnants of the dorsal mesentery.

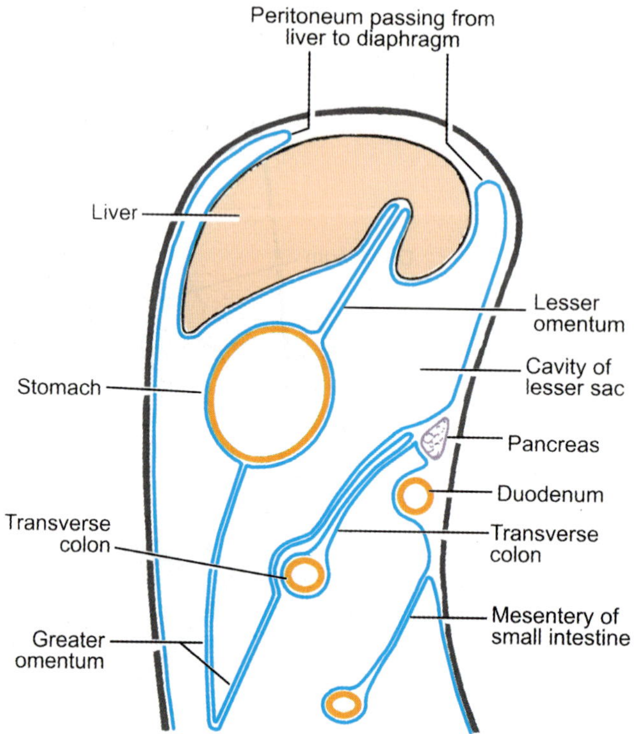


**33.31:** Schematic sagittal section through the abdomen to show some features of peritoneum

20. The two together form one continuous (but complicated) line of attachment that is as follows. Starting at the oesophagus (just below the orifice for it in the diaphragm) there are, in that order
    a. The lienorenal ligament
    b. The greater omentum
    c. The duodenum
    d. The mesentery of the small intestine (jejunum and ileum)
    e. The ascending colon
    f. The transverse mesocolon
    g. The descending colon
    h. The pelvic mesocolon
    i. The rectum.
21. Note that the attachments of the greater ometum and of the transverse mesocolon are both orientated transversely and lie close to each other. Also note that the attachment of the pelvic mesocolon is shaped like an inverted 'V'.
22. A part of the peritoneal cavity, called the ***lesser sac,*** lies behind the lesser omentum and the stomach (33.30 and 33.31). The lesser sac also extends into the interval between the anterior and posterior parts of the greater omentum (also see 33.29).
23. In distinction to the lesser sac the rest of the peritoneal cavity is called the ***greater sac***. The greater and lesser sacs communicate through a narrow opening that lies just above the duodenum. This opening is called the ***aditus to the lesser sac*** (***foramen epiploicum***).

***The peritoneum in some specific situations has already been described as follows:***

1. The mesentery in chapter 27.
2. The transverse mesocolon in chapter 27.
3. The sigmoid mesocolon in chapter 27.

4. The peritoneum relations of the liver including consideration of the lesser omentum, the falciform ligament, the coronary ligament and the peritoneal spaces around the liver in chapter 28.
5. Peritoneal relations of the spleen in chapter 28.

We will now consider the arrangement of peritoneum in some other regions.

### Anterior Abdominal Wall

1. The peritoneum lining the anterior abdominal wall is raised to form a number of short folds. Above the umbilicus, in the middle line, there is the ***falciform ligament*** (33.32). It is produced because of the presence within it of the ligamentum teres (which is a remnant of the left umbilical vein).
2. Below the umbilicus there are a series of vertical folds (33.32).
   a. In the middle line there is the ***median umbilical fold*** raised by the median umbilical ligament (remnant of urachus).
   b. Further laterally, there are right and left ***lateral umbilical folds*** produced by the right and left inferior epigastric arteries.
3. On either side of the median umbilical fold (i.e., between the median and medial folds) there are depressions called the (right and left) ***supravesical fossae***.
4. Between the medial and lateral umbilical folds there are depressions called the ***medial inguinal fossae***. Lateral to the lateral folds there are ***lateral inguinal fossae***. The deep inguinal rings are related to these fossae.

### Urinary Bladder, Rectum, Uterus

1. On either side of the urinary bladder there is a depression called the ***paravesical fossa*** (33.33).
2. It is bounded laterally by a ridge raised by the ductus deferens (in the male) or by the round ligament of the uterus (in the female).
3. On either side of the rectum there is a depression called the ***pararectal fossa*** (33.34). In the male it is bounded laterally by the sacrogenital folds; and in the female by the rectouterine folds.
4. On either side of the uterus the peritoneum passes laterally as the broad ligament.

### Liver

1. The peritoneum lining the anterior part of the diaphragm is reflected onto the liver as the superior layer of the coronary ligament.

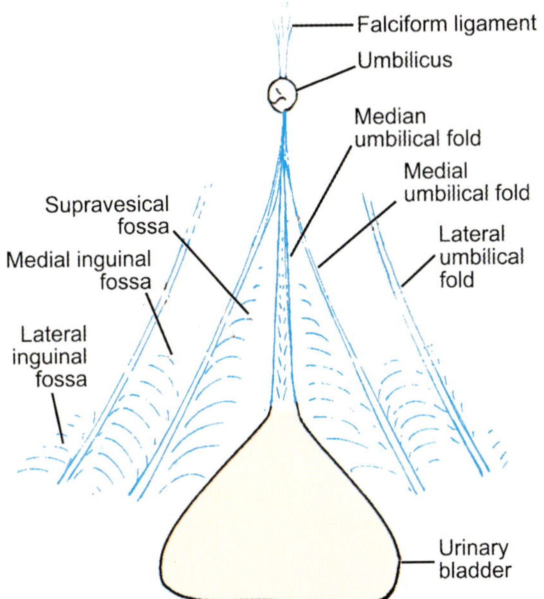


**33.32:** Peritoneal folds on posterior aspect of anterior abdominal wall

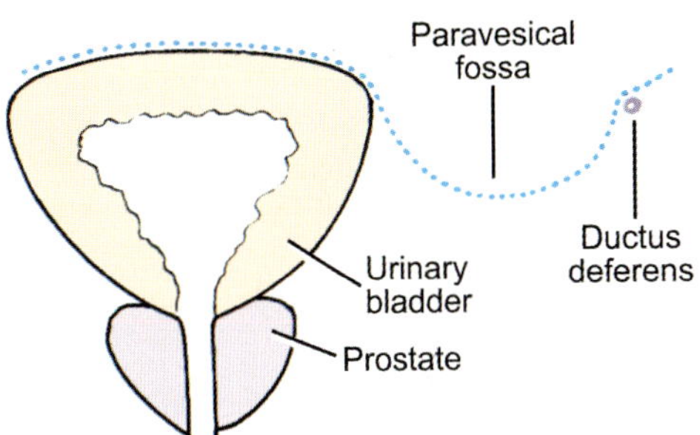


**32.33:** Schematic coronal section through the urinary bladder to show the paravesical fossa

2. After lining the diaphragmatic surface of the liver, it winds round the inferior border to cover the gall bladder and part of the visceral surface.
3. At the posterior end of the visceral surface it gets reflected on to the front of the right suprarenal gland, and from there to the front of the right kidney, forming the inferior layer of the coronary ligament.
4. Between the superior and inferior layers of this ligament the bare area of the liver is in direct contact with the posterior part of the diaphragm.
5. From the front of the kidney the peritoneum descends over the superior part of the duodenum and over the transverse colon.
6. A parasagittal section to the left of the caudate lobe of the liver is shown in 33.35. In this plane the peritoneum from the posterior surface of the fundus of the stomach passes directly to the diaphragm forming the ***gastrophrenic ligament***. This ligament forms the roof of the lesser sac in this situation.

### Duodenum

1. Most of the duodenum is retroperitoneal and is covered by peritoneum only on its anterior aspect.
2. The proximal portion of the superior part of the duodenum is however lined on both its anterior and posterior aspects by peritoneum (continuous with that on the anterior and posterior surfaces of the stomach).
3. The two layers lining the proximal part of the duodenum meet above to form the extreme right part of the lesser omentum. This part of the lesser omentum passes to the liver as the right free margin of the omentum.
4. The right free margin of the lesser omentum encloses the bile duct, the hepatic artery and the portal vein.
5. Immediately posterior to the right free margin of the lesser omentum we see the ***aditus to the lesser sac***. Its boundaries are as follows.
   a. Anteriorly, right free margin of lesser omentum.
   b. Posteriorly, peritoneum over inferior vena cava.
   c. Below, superior part of duodenum.
   d. Above, caudate process of the liver.
6. Peritoneum lining the posterior surface (of the proximal half) of the superior part of the duodenum is reflected onto the front of the pancreas. This reflection forms the right margin of the lesser sac in this position.

### The Lesser Sac (Omental Bursa)

Numerous references have been made to the lesser sac in previous chapters, and in the foregoing descriptions in this chapter. We will now review the boundaries of this sac.

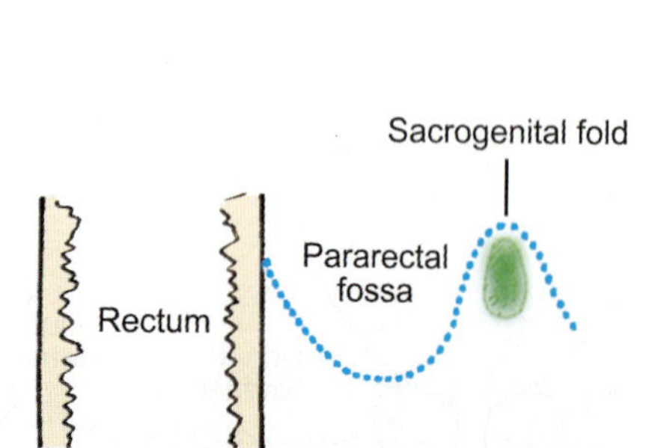


**33.34:** Schematic coronal section through the rectum to show the pararectal fossa

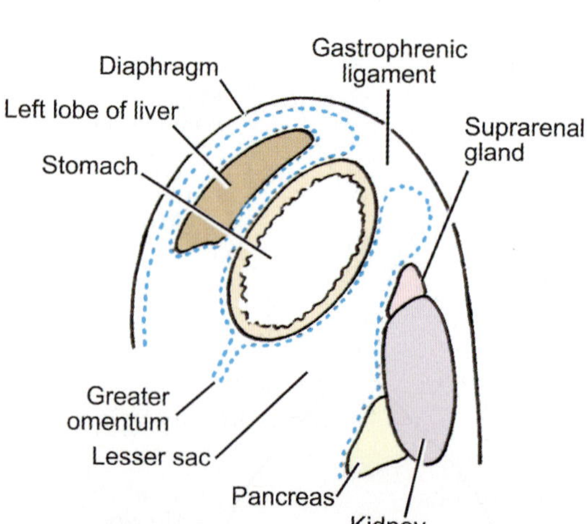


**33.35:** Schematic sagittal section of the upper part of the abdomen to the left of the caudate lobe of the liver, but to the right of the spleen

*Some elementary facts are as follows:*

1. The lesser sac is a fairly large recess of the peritoneal cavity, that communicates with the main peritoneal cavity (or greater sac) only through the foramen epiploicum. The sac has anterior and posterior walls that meet each other at right, left, upper and lower borders.
2. The anterior wall of the lesser sac is formed (from above downwards) by the lesser omentum (posterior layer), the peritoneum lining the posterior surface of the stomach, and the anterior two layers of the greater omentum.
3. The upper part of the posterior wall of the lesser sac is formed by the peritoneum lining several structures on the posterior abdominal wall.
4. The lower part of the posterior wall of the lesser sac is formed by the posterior two layers of the greater omentum.
5. The lower border of the lesser sac is formed by continuity of the anterior two layers of the greater omentum with its posterior two layers.

**WANT TO KNOW MORE?**

Some details of the lesser sac are as follows:

1. The ***retroperitoneal structures*** related to the lesser sac are:
   a. The pancreas (anterior surface of upper part of the head, anterior surface of the neck, and anterior surface of the body)
   b. Part of the left kidney
   c. The left suprarenal gland
   d. The upper part of the abdominal aorta
   e. The diaphragm
   f. The coeliac trunk and its splenic, left gastric and hepatic branches are also situated behind the upper part of the posterior wall of the sac.
2. The ***upper border*** of the lesser sac is formed as follows:
   a. Towards the right side it is formed by the reflection of peritoneum from the upper end of (the posterior surface of) the caudate lobe of the liver to the diaphragm.
   b. To the left of the caudate lobe it is formed by reflection of peritoneum from the back of the upper part of the fundus of the stomach to the diaphragm: this peritoneum forms the ***gastrophrenic ligament*** (33.35).
3. a. The ***left border*** of the lesser sac is formed, in the greater part of its extent, in the same way as the lower border i.e., by continuity of the anterior two layers of the greater omentum with its posterior two layers.
   b. Higher up the left border is formed by the gastrosplenic and lienorenal ligaments (33.36). These ligaments are continuous, below, with the greater omentum; and above with the gastrophrenic ligament.
4. The formation of the right border of the lesser sac can be divided into several parts as follows:
   a. The lower part of the right border is formed by continuity of the anterior two layers with the posterior two layers of the greater omentum.
   b. At the upper end of the greater omentum its anterior two layers pass on to the anterior and posterior aspects of the stomach and the proximal portion of the superior part of the duodenum. The peritoneum on the back of this part of the duodenum gets reflected on to the front of the neck of the pancreas thus forming the right margin of the lesser sac at this level.
   c. Immediately above the duodenum there is a gap in the right border of the sac because of the presence here of the foramen epiploicum (33.36).
   d. Above the foramen epiploicum the caudate lobe of the liver projects into the lesser sac from the right side. Here the right margin of the lesser sac is formed by peritoneum covering the caudate lobe.
   e. The boundaries of the foramen epiploicum (aditus into lesser sac) are described above in relation to the duodenum.

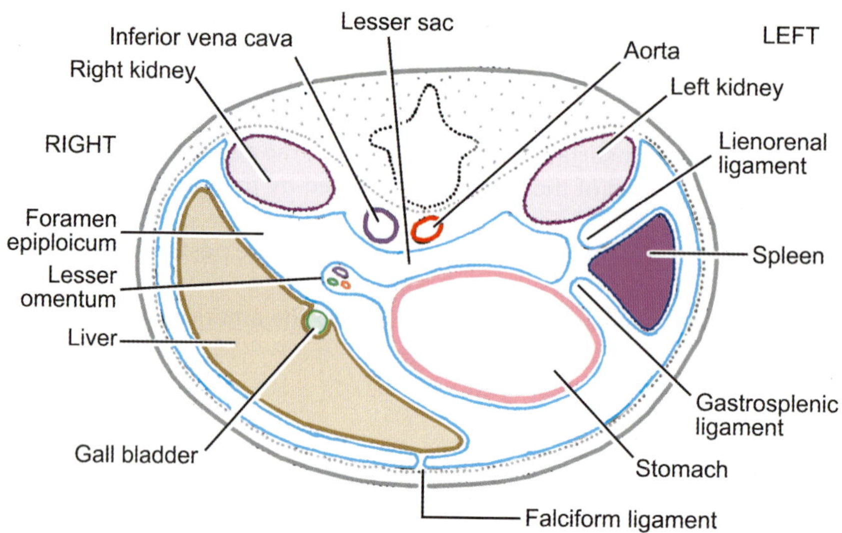


**33.36:** Transverse section across abdomen at the level of the foramen epiploicum to show peritoneal reflections

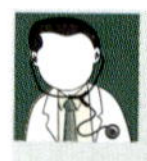

## CLINICAL CORRELATION OF PERITONEUM

### *Peritoneal Fluid*

1. The smoothness of the peritoneal surface, and the presence of a thin film of fluid between adjacent layers of peritoneum, greatly facilitates movements of viscera over one another. Such movements take place as a result of respiration, of peristaltic movements of the intestines, and because of alternate distension and emptying of organs like the stomach, and the urinary bladder.
2. The peritoneal fluid is not static but circulates through the peritoneal cavity and is frequently replaced. In general it tends to flow in an upward direction towards the diaphragm. The fluid can be absorbed from the peritoneal cavity into the blood stream, and most of such absorption takes place in the region below the diaphragm.
3. Advantage of the rapid transfer of substances between peritoneal fluid and blood is taken in the procedure called ***peritoneal dialysis***. In this procedure, a suitable watery solution is made to circulate through the peritoneal cavity before being withdrawn. In this way harmful substances such as urea can be removed from blood. (It may be noted, however, that the technique, used in the past to treat patients with renal failure, has been almost completely replaced by haemodialysis).
4. Under certain conditions there may be great increase in the quantity of peritoneal fluid. This condition is called ***ascites***. However, because of the size of the peritoneal cavity, almost a litre and a half of fluid may collect before its presence can be recognised on clinical examination. Recognition of ascites is more difficult in an obese person.
5. Fluid that has accumulated in the peritoneal cavity can be removed through a canula introduced through the abdominal wall. The procedure is called ***paracentesis***. It may be done through the linea alba or on one flank.
6. The large absorptive area of the peritoneum poses a serious danger when infection develops in the peritoneal cavity (***peritonitis***). Toxins are rapidly absorbed into blood leading to toxaemia. Because of this reason generalised peritonitis can be a life-threatening condition.
7. However, the peritoneum itself tries to combat the spread of infection in various ways.
   a. The peritoneal fluid is rich in antibodies and in cellular elements (like lymphocytes) that counteract infection.
   b. When infection develops in an area (usually by spread from an inflamed viscus like the appendix) the peritoneum tries to localise the infection by formation of adhesions.

   c. The greater omentum plays a special role in this regard. It has the ability to move to a site of infection and tries to wrap itself around the infected region. It is for this reason that the greater omentum has been termed the "policeman of the abdomen".
8. Occasionally surgeons use the greater omentum to close perforations in the gut, or to cover the area of an intestinal anastomosis.
9. It has been mentioned above that the area where maximal absorption of peritoneal fluid takes place is just below the diaphragm.
   a. In a supine position peritoneal fluid tends to gravitate into this region (specially into the right posterior subphrenic space).
   b. Absorption of toxins can be minimised by placing the patient in a position in which the back is raised to an angle of 45 degrees.
   c. In this position the fluid gravitates into the pelvis where absorption is much less pronounced (see rectouterine pouch, below).

***Pain in Peritoneal Infection***

1. Abdominal infections are accompanied by pain.
   a. The visceral peritoneum, supplied by autonomic nerves, is much less sensitive to pain than the parietal peritoneum that is innervated by somatic nerves.
   b. Pain arising in the visceral peritoneum is stimulated mainly by stretching, and tends to poorly localised.
   c. In contrast pain caused by inflammation of an area of parietal peritoneum can be accurately localised.
2. Embryologically, the gut is a midline structure. Because of this, visceral pain arising in the gut is at first felt over the midline.
   a. Pain arising in the stomach and duodenum is referred to the epigastrium,
   b. that from the rest of the small intestine, the appendix and the ascending colon to the area around the umbilicus; and from the rest of the gut to the hypogastrium.
   c. For example in a case of acute appendicitis pain is first felt round the umbilicus. When the parietal peritoneum gets involved pain shifts to the right iliac fossa.
3. Inflammation of the parietal peritoneum also makes it very sensitive to stretching.
   a. This forms the basis of a clinical test called ***rebound tenderness***.
   b. If a finger is pressed over an inflamed area of abdomen and then suddenly removed abrupt stretching of the abdominal wall (as a result of rebound) leads to severe pain.

***Isolated Pockets in Peritoneum***

We have seen that the peritoneal cavity is divided into various parts as a result of the presence of many folds. Because of this infection can occur in localised pockets of peritoneum as follows:

1. Infection may occur in the ***subphrenic spaces*** that surround the liver. The anatomy of these spaces, which has been described earlier is of considerable surgical importance.
   a. The right posterior space (or right subhepatic space) is the most dependent part of the peritoneal cavity (in a supine position).
   b. It is closely related to the right kidney and is therefore also called the ***hepatorenal pouch*** (also called ***Morison's pouch***).
   c. This is the commonest site of a ***subphrenic abscess***.
   d. Infection may spread to this space from the gall bladder, the vermiform appendix or from any other organ in the region.
   e. The peritoneum lining the undersurface of the diaphragm is innervated by the phrenic nerve the fibres of which are derived from the same spinal segments (C3, 4, 5) which supply the skin of the shoulder. Pain arising from a subdiaphragmatic infection can therefore be referred to the shoulder.
   f. It may also be noted that infection can spread through the diaphragm into the pleural cavity.

2. Fluid may accumulate in the lesser sac.
   a. Normally such fluid flows into the hepatorenal pouch through the aditus of the lesser sac, but it remains in the lesser sac if the aditus is obstructed by adhesions.
   b. Entry of fluid into the lesser sac may result from perforation of an ulcer on the posterior wall of the stomach.
   c. Accumulation of fluid in the lesser sac is a frequent complication of inflammation in the pancreas (*pancreatitis*) and such a collection is referred to as a *pseudopancreatic cyst*.
3. *Rectouterine pouch*: Peritoneum on the front of the rectum is reflected on to the upper most part of the vagina forming the so called rectouterine pouch. (The term is sanctified by long usage but the pouch is really rectovaginal).
   a. Clinicians often refer to this pouch as the *pouch of Doughlas*.
   b. In a sitting or standing person this pouch is the most dependent part of the peritoneal cavity and fluid or pus tends to collect here when there is infection.
   c. This pouch is bounded, posteriorly, by the rectum; anteriorly, by the posterior aspect of the uterus and the uppermost part of the vagina (posterior fornix); and inferiorly by the rectovaginal fold of peritoneum.
   d. It is important to know that the floor of pouch lies only 5.5 cm from the anus. It can be palpated, and drained, either through the posterior fornix of the vagina or through the rectum.
   e. In the male the rectouterine pouch is replaced by the rectovesical pouch (which lies between the rectum and the urinary bladder). The floor of this pouch is 7.5 cm from the anus.

### *Internal Hernia*

Abdominal contents can herniate to the outside through areas of weakness in the abdominal wall.

1. In some cases coils of gut, or greater omentum, may herniate into a localised part of the peritoneal cavity itself.
2. This condition is called *internal hernia*.
3. Such herniation can take place through the aditus to the lesser sac.
4. It can also take place into peritoneal recesses present in relation to the duodenum and to the caecum (see below).
5. An internal hernia might get strangulated. A surgeon has to know the positions of the recesses and has to remember that some of the folds of peritoneum bounding the recesses contain blood vessels.

### *Peritoneal Recesses*

1. In addition to the various omenta, ligaments and mesenteries already mentioned in relation to the peritoneum, a number of smaller folds may sometimes be present.
2. They may partially cut off recesses of the peritoneal cavity.
3. Pieces of intestine may get 'caught' in these recesses leading to complications that may require surgical intervention. It is, therefore, necessary to know the location of these spaces.
4. The largest such recess is the lesser sac.
5. Smaller recesses are found mainly in relation to the duodenum, the ileocaecal region and the sigmoid mesocolon.

### *Duodenal Recesses*

1. The *superior duodenal recess* lies to the left of the upper part of the ascending part of the duodenum. It is open downwards. It is closely related to the inferior mesenteric and left renal veins, and to the abdominal aorta.
2. The *inferior duodenal recess* lies a little below the superior recess. It opens upwards.
3. The *paraduodenal recess* lies a little to the left of the ascending part of the duodenum. It extends to the left behind a fold of peritoneum containing the inferior mesenteric vein.
4. The *retroduodenal recess* lies behind the horizontal and ascending parts of the duodenum, in front of the abdominal aorta. Its opening is directed downwards and to the left.
5. The *duodenojejunal recess* lies to the left of the abdominal aorta deep to the transverse mesocolon. The pancreas, the left kidney and the left renal vein are closely related to it.

6. The ***mesenteroparietal recess*** lies below the duodenum, behind the upper part of the mesentery. The superior mesenteric artery lies in the anterior wall of its opening.

***Recesses Present in Relation to the Caecum***

1. The ***superior ileocaecal recess*** lies to the left of the ileocaecal junction in front of the terminal ileum. It is bounded anteriorly by a fold of peritoneum containing the anterior caecal vessels. The recess opens downwards and to the left.
2. The ***inferior ileocaecal recess*** lies to the left of the caecum in front of the mesoappendix and behind the terminal part of the ileum. It is bounded in front by a fold passing from the ileum to the mesoappendix. It opens downwards and to the left.
3. The ***retrocaecal recess*** lies behind the caecum. The vermiform appendix usually lies in this recess.

A recess may also be present deep to the apex of the sigmoid mesocolon. It is related to the left ureter and the left common iliac artery.

***Laparotomy and Laparoscopy***

1. An operation that opens the peritoneal cavity is called ***laparotomy***. The procedure may be preliminary to surgery on any organ, or may be used to inspect the interior of the abdominal cavity in cases where diagnosis is otherwise difficult.
2. However, it is now possible to inspect the interior of the peritoneal cavity by introducing an instrument called a ***laparoscope*** through a small opening in the abdominal wall. The procedure is called ***laparoscopy***. Several abdominal surgical procedures are now being carried out through such instruments.

34

CHAPTER

# Lymphatics and Autonomic Nerves of Abdomen and Pelvis

## LYMPHATICS OF ABDOMEN AND PELVIS

1. The largest lymph vessel in the body is the ***thoracic duct***. This duct begins in the abdomen as an upward continuation of a sac-like structure called the ***cisternal chyli***.
2. Most of the lymph from the abdomen drains into the cisternal chyli and from there into the thoracic duct (through which it is poured into the venous system).

## CHIEF LYMPH NODES OF ABDOMEN AND PELVIS

1. The entire lymph from the abdomen (and from the lower limbs) ultimately ends in terminal groups of lymph nodes present in relation to the abdominal aorta. These nodes are arranged in three main groups, each having a specific area of drainage.
   a. On either side of the aorta there are the right and left ***lateral aortic*** nodes (34.1). Some outlying members of these groups lying behind the aorta constitute the ***retroaortic nodes***.
   b. In front of the aorta there are the ***preaortic nodes***.
   c. These are divided into the ***coeliac***, the ***superior mesenteric*** and the ***inferior mesenteric*** nodes (34.2) lying around the origins of the corresponding arteries.
2. On each side the efferents from the lateral aortic nodes form the corresponding ***lumbar trunk*** that ends by joining the cisterna chyli (34.1).
3. Efferents from the preaortic nodes form the ***intestinal trunk*** that also ends in the cisterna chyli.
4. The area of drainage of the preaortic nodes is shown in 34.2.
5. The coeliac lymph nodes receive lymph from:
   a. The stomach
   b. Most of the duodenum
   c. The liver
   d. The extrahepatic biliary apparatus
   e. The pancreas
   f. The spleen.
6. The superior mesenteric lymph nodes receive lymph from:
   a. Part of the duodenum, and the whole of
   b. The jejunum
   c. The ileum
   d. The caecum
   e. The appendix
   f. The ascending colon
   g. The transverse colon.

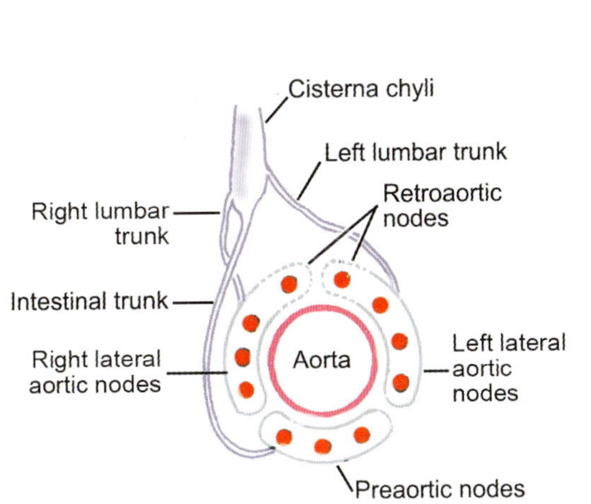


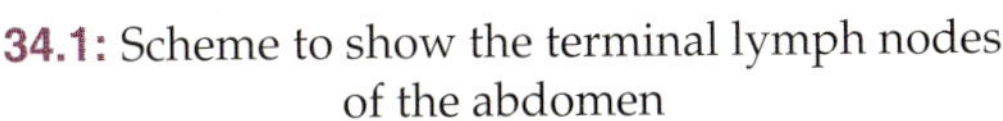
**34.1:** Scheme to show the terminal lymph nodes of the abdomen

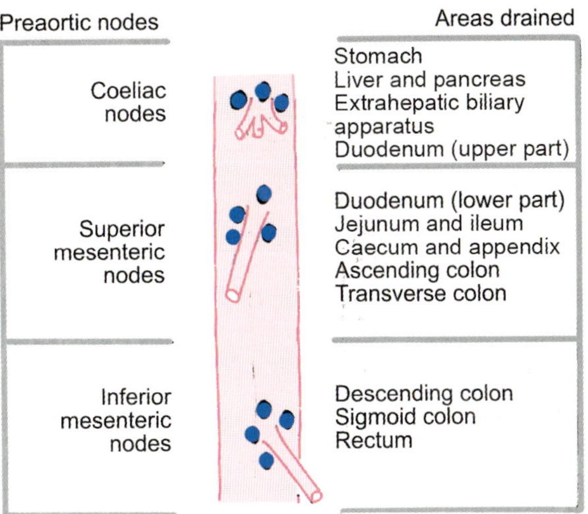


**34.2:** Subgroups of the preaortic lymph nodes, and areas drained by them

7. The inferior mesenteric lymph nodes receive lymph from:
   a. The descending colon
   b. The sigmoid colon
   c. The upper part of the rectum.

   Numerous groups of outlying nodes are associated with the lymphatic drainage of the organs mentioned above. These nodes are referred to while discussing lymphatic drainage of the organs concerned.
8. The ***lateral aortic nodes*** (34.3) receive all the lymph draining through the common iliac nodes. They also receive lymph directly from the
   a. Posterior abdominal wall
   b. Kidneys and upper part of the ureters
   c. Testes or ovaries
   d. Uterine tubes and part of the uterus.
9. a. The ***common iliac nodes*** (34.3) lie along the corresponding blood vessels.
   b. They receive lymph from the external and internal iliac nodes and send it to the lateral aortic nodes.
10. a. The ***internal iliac nodes*** (34.3) lie along the corresponding blood vessels.
    b. They receive most of the lymph of the pelvic organs and from the deeper tissues of the perineum.
    c. They also receive some vessels of the lower limbs that travel along the superior and inferior gluteal blood vessels.
11. a. The ***external iliac lymph nodes*** (34.3) lie along the external iliac blood vessels.
    b. They receive lymph from the lower limb through the inguinal nodes.
    c. They also receive direct lymph vessels from the deeper tissues of the infraumbilical part of the anterior abdominal wall and from some pelvic organs.

## LYMPHATIC DRAINAGE OF ABDOMINAL AND PELVIC VISCERA

### Lymphatic Drainage of the Stomach

For purposes of lymphatic drainage the stomach may be divided into four areas as follows (34.4):

1. Draw a vertical line immediately to the left of the cardio-oesophageal junction. The part to the left of this line is area *A*.
2. Draw another vertical line separating the pyloric part of the stomach (Area *D*) from the body.

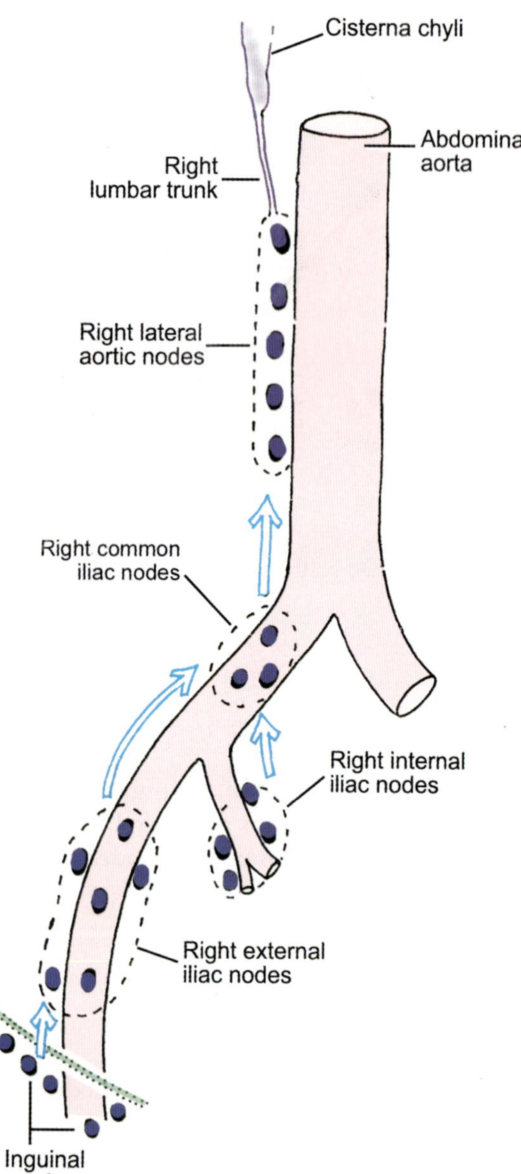


34.3: The lateral aortic lymph nodes

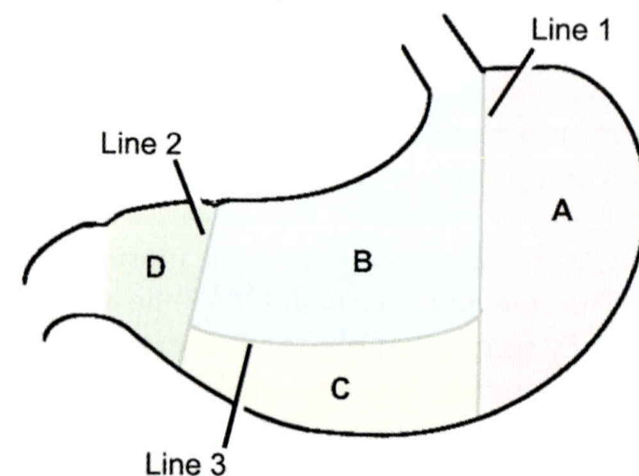


34.4: Areas of stomach having separate lymphatic drainage

3. Divide the area between these two vertical lines into two unequal parts by a curved line drawn parallel to the greater curvature so that the area above it (Area *B*) is larger (2/3rd) than the area (*C*) below it.
   The lymphatic drainage of these areas is shown in 34.5 and is described below:
   a. Area *A* drains into the ***pancreaticosplenic nodes*** lying along the splenic artery (i.e., on the back of the stomach). Lymph vessels from these nodes travel along the splenic artery to reach the coeliac nodes.
   b. Area *B* drains into the ***left gastric nodes*** lying along the artery of the same name. These nodes also drain the abdominal part of the oesophagus. Lymph from these nodes drains into the coeliac nodes.
   c. Area *C* drains into the ***right gastroepiploic nodes*** that lie along the artery of the same name. Lymph vessels arising in these nodes drain into the ***pyloric nodes*** that lie in the angle between the first and second parts

of the duodenum. From here the lymph is drained further into the ***hepatic nodes*** that lie along the hepatic artery; and finally into coeliac nodes.

d. Lymph from area ***D*** drains in different directions into the pyloric, hepatic and left gastric nodes, and passes from all these nodes to the coeliac nodes.

e. Note that lymph from all areas of the stomach ultimately reaches the coeliac nodes. From here it passes through the intestinal lymph trunk to reach the cisterna chyli.

## Lymphatic Drainage of the Duodenum

1. Most of the lymph vessels from the duodenum end in the ***pancreaticoduodenal nodes*** present along the inside of the curve of the duodenum (i.e., at the junction of the pancreas and the duodenum) (34.6).
2. From here the lymph passes partly to the hepatic nodes, and through them to the coeliac nodes and partly to the superior mesenteric nodes.
3. Some vessels from the first part of the duodenum drain into the pyloric nodes, and through them to the hepatic nodes. Some vessels drain into the hepatic nodes directly. All the lymph reaching the hepatic nodes drains into the coeliac nodes.

## Lymphatic Drainage of the Jejunum and Ileum

1. The small intestine has a very rich lymphatic drainage. Some food substances, chiefly fats, are absorbed through them.
2. Mucous membrane of the region is studded with finger like processes called villi.
3. Each villus has a central lymph vessel called a ***lacteal*** (34.7). Lymph from lacteals drains into plexuses in the wall of the gut and from there to vessels in the mesentery (34.8).
4. It ultimately reaches lymph nodes present in front of the aorta at the origin of the superior mesenteric artery.
5. Before reaching these nodes the lymph from the intestines passes through hundreds of lymph nodes located in the mesentery. These nodes are present:
   a. Near the mesenteric border of the gut.
   b. Along the branches of the superior mesenteric artery, including the arcades.
   c. Along the trunk of the superior mesenteric artery itself.

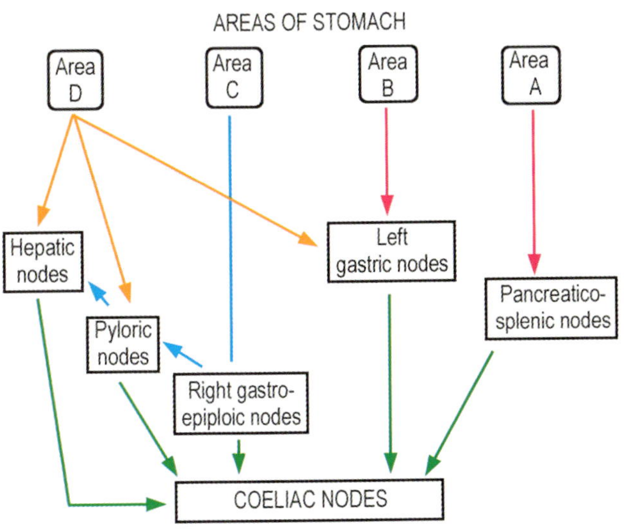


**34.5:** Scheme to show the lymphatic drainage of the stomach

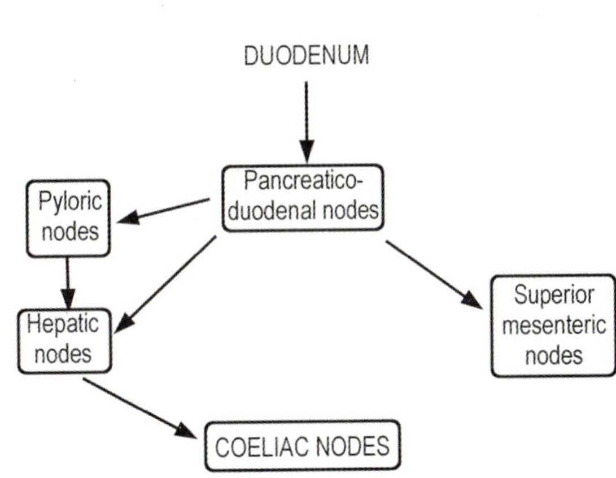


**34.6:** Scheme to show the lymphatic drainage of the duodenum

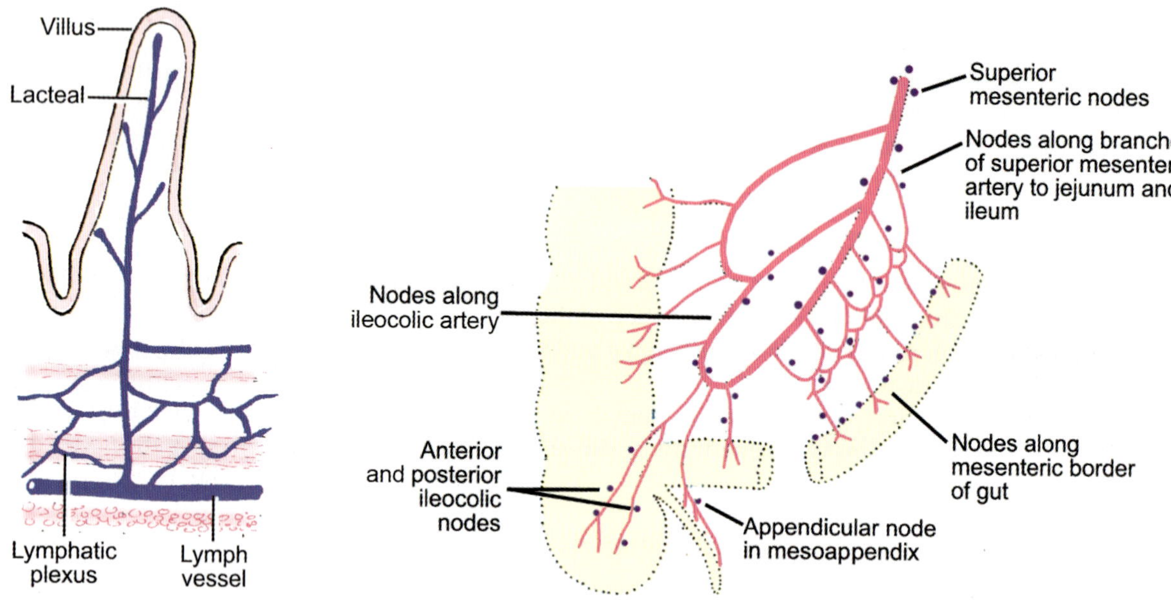


**34.7:** Scheme to show arrangement of lymph vessels within the gut

**34.8:** Lymph nodes draining the jejunum ileum, caecum and appendix

6. The terminal part of the ileum is drained, in a similar manner, by nodes lying along the ileocolic artery and its ileal branch (see 34.8).

## Lymphatic Drainage of Caecum and Appendix

1. The lymph from the caecum and appendix drains into the superior mesenteric lymph nodes after passing through the several outlying nodes.
2. The outlying nodes are present along the ileocolic artery and its anterior caecal, posterior caecal and appendicular branches (***anterior ileocolic nodes; posterior ileocolic nodes*** and ***appendicular nodes*** respectively)(34.8).

## Lymphatic Drainage of Colon

1. The ascending colon and the transverse colon drain into the superior mesenteric group of preaortic nodes.
2. The descending colon and sigmoid colon drain into the inferior mesenteric group of preaortic nodes. On its way to these groups the lymph passes through outlying nodes that lie (34.9):
   a. On the wall of the colon itself (***epicolic nodes*** ).
   b. Along the 'inner' border of the colon (paracolic nodes).
   c. Along the right and middle colic branches of the superior mesenteric artery and the left colic branch of the inferior mesenteric artery.

## Lymphatic Drainage of Rectum and Anal Canal

1. The upper part of the rectum drains to the inferior mesenteric nodes through vessels passing along the inferior mesenteric artery ('1' in 34.10).
2. The lower part of the rectum and the upper part of the anal canal drain into the internal iliac nodes through vessels running along the middle rectal artery.
3. The lower part of the anal canal drains into the superficial inguinal nodes.

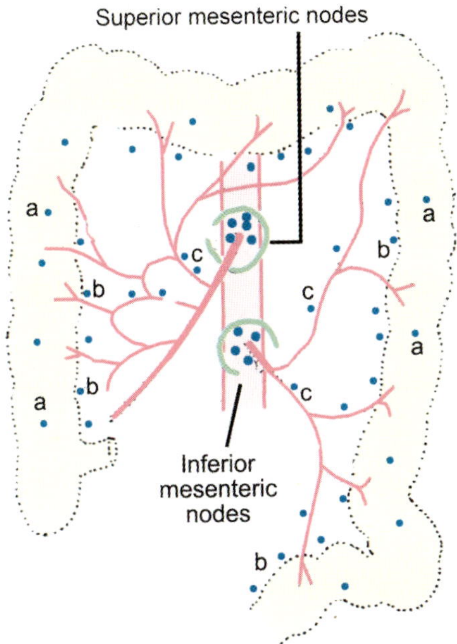


34.9: Lymph nodes draining the colon

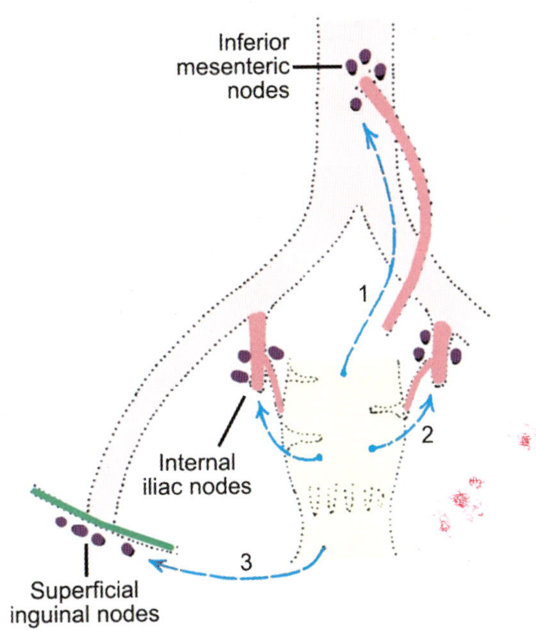


34.10: Scheme to show the lymphatic drainage of the rectum and anal canal

## Lymphatic Drainage of the Liver

The lymphatic vessels of the liver can be divided into a superficial set and a deep set (34.11).

### Superficial Vessels

1. Part of the liver near the inferior vena cava (including parts of the posterior, superior and inferior surfaces) drains to nodes around the upper end of the inferior vena cava ('a' in 34.11).
2. Most of the inferior surface and the adjoining part of the anterior surface drain to nodes in the porta hepatis ('b' in 34.11) and through them to the coeliac nodes.
3. Part of the convex anterosuperior surface drains directly to the coeliac nodes ('c' in 34.11) through vessels running along the inferior phrenic artery.

### Deep Vessels

1. Some vessels ascend along the hepatic veins and end in nodes around the upper end of the inferior vena cava ('d' in 34.11).
2. Some vessels descend to nodes in the porta hepatis ('e' in 34.11).

## Lymphatic Drainage of Gall Bladder and Bile Duct

1. The gall bladder and bile duct drain to the ***hepatic nodes*** (lying along the hepatic artery), and through them to the coeliac nodes (34.12).
2. Two of the hepatic nodes are specially important. One of them, the ***cystic node*** lies near the neck of the gall bladder. Another node lies in the anterior wall of the epiploic foramen.
3. Vessels from the lower end of the bile duct drain into the pancreaticoduodenal nodes.

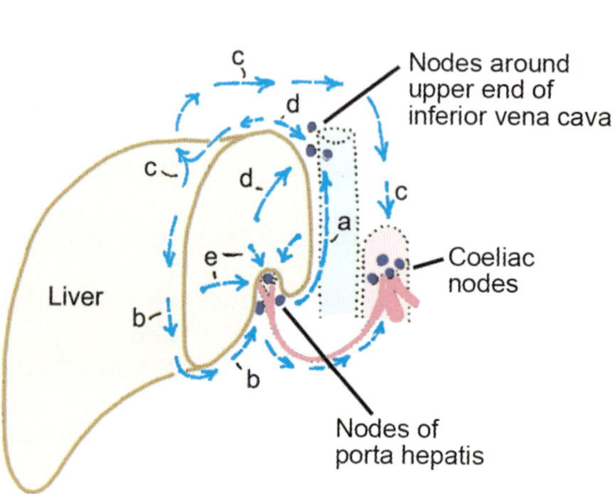


**34.11:** Lymphatic drainage of the liver

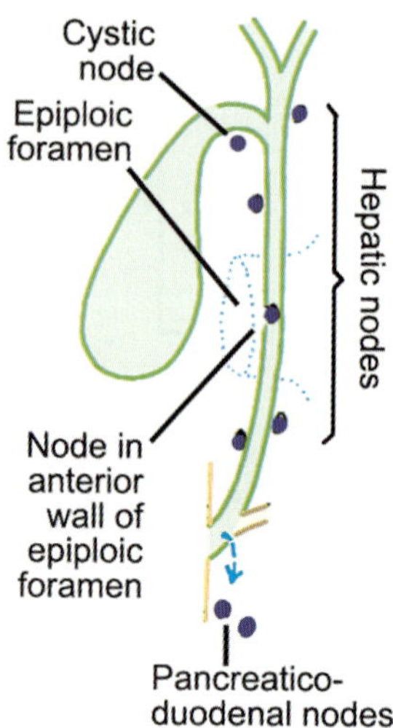


**34.12:** Lymphatic drainage of gall bladder and bile duct

## Lymphatic Drainage of the Pancreas

1. The pancreas drains into:
   a. The pancreaticosplenic nodes lying along the splenic artery.
   b. The pancreaticoduodenal nodes lying at the junction of pancreas and duodenum (both anteriorly and posteriorly) (34.13).
2. From these nodes most of the lymph drain into the coeliac nodes, but some of it drain into the superior mesenteric nodes. Some vessels also reach the superior mesenteric nodes directly (3).

## Lymphatic Drainage of Kidney

All lymph vessels from the kidneys drain directly into the lateral aortic nodes. There are three sets of vessels (34.14).

1. From the perirenal fat ('a').
2. From a superficial plexus under the capsules ('b').
3. Deep vessels from renal tissue ('c').

## Lymphatic Drainage of the Ureter

1. The upper abdominal part of the ureter drains directly to the lateral aortic nodes.
2. The lower abdominal part drains into the common iliac nodes.
3. The pelvic part of the ureter drains into the external iliac and internal iliac nodes .
4. Ultimately all the lymph from the ureter reaches the lateral aortic nodes.

## Lymphatic Drainage of Urinary Bladder

The urinary bladder drains into the external iliac lymph nodes.

## Lymphatic Drainage of Urethra

1. The prostatic and membranous parts of the urethra drain into the internal iliac lymph nodes.
2. The penile part of the male urethra drains to the superficial inguinal nodes.
3. Some vessels pass through the inguinal canal and reach the external iliac nodes.

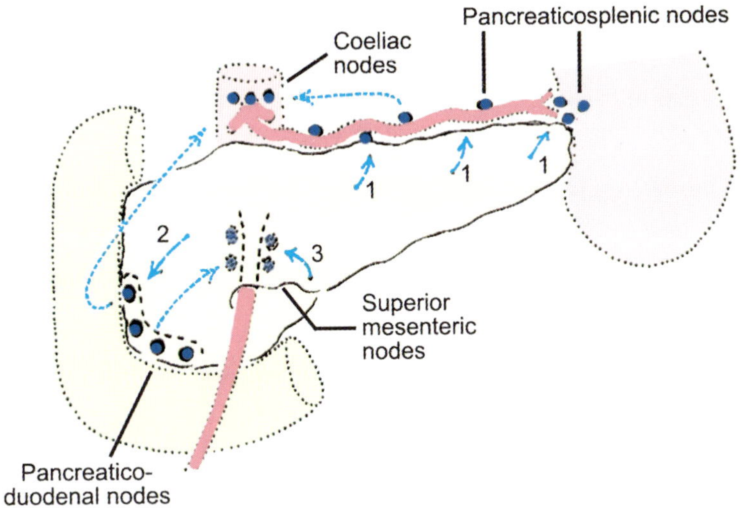


**34.13:** Lymphatic drainage of the pancreas

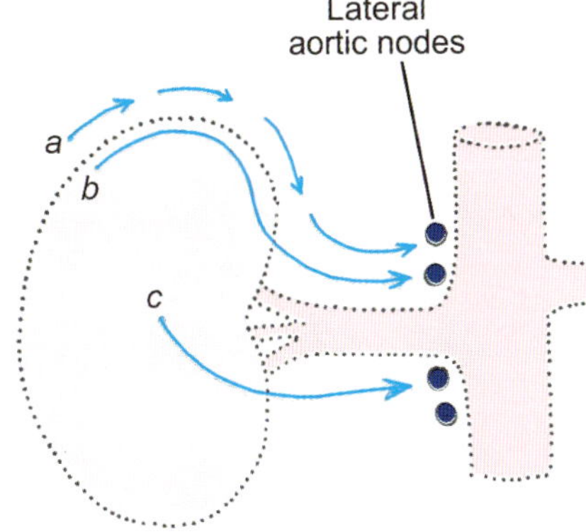


**34.14:** Lymphatic drainage of the kidney

## Lymphatic Drainage of the Prostate and of the Seminal Vesicles

The prostate and seminal vesicles drain to both the internal and external iliac nodes.

## Lymphatic Drainage of Testes and Ovaries

Lymph from the testis or ovary passes along the testicular or ovarian vessels directly to the lateral aortic lymph nodes.

## Lymphatic Drainage of the Perineum

1. Superficial structures in the perineum including the lower part of the anal canal (34.15), the scrotum and penis in the male, and the lower part of the vagina in the female, drain into the upper medial group of superficial inguinal lymph nodes.
2. The glans (penis or clitoris), however, drains into the deep inguinal nodes.
3. Some vessels from the glans reach the external iliac nodes.
4. Deeper tissues of the perineum drain into the internal iliac lymph nodes.

## Lymphatic Drainage of Uterus and Uterine Tube

1. Lymph from the uterine tube ('a' in 34.16) and from the upper part of the uterus; ('b' in 34.16) travels along the ovarian vessels to reach the lateral aortic nodes (34.16).
2. Lymph from the lower part of the body of the uterus ('c' in 34.16) travels to the external iliac nodes.
3. Lymph from the cervix travels (34.17):
   a. Laterally to the external iliac nodes ('d' in 34.17).
   b. Posterolaterally to the internal iliac nodes ('e' in 34.17).
   c. Posteriorly to the ***sacral nodes*** ('f' in 34.17). The sacral nodes lie in front of the sacrum along the median sacral artery.

## Lymphatic Drainage of Abdominal Wall

### *The Skin*

a. The skin above the level of the umbilicus (in front) and above the iliac crest (at the back) drains into the axillary lymph nodes.
b. The skin of the anterior abdominal wall below the umbilicus drains into the superficial inguinal lymph nodes.

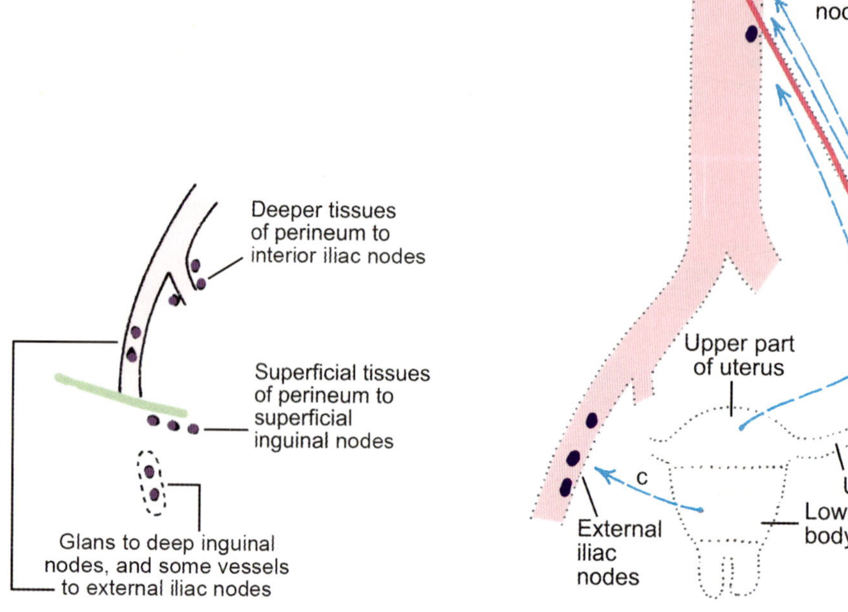


**34.15:** Lymphatic drainage of the perineum

**34.16:** Scheme to show the lymphatic drainage of the uterus

*Deeper Tissues*

a. Lymph vessels from the posterior abdominal wall travel along the lumbar vessels to the lateral aortic nodes, including the retroaortic nodes.
b. The vessels from the upper part of the anterior and lateral part of the abdominal wall travel along the superior epigastric vessels to the parasternal nodes.
c. The vessels from the lower part of the anterolateral abdominal wall travel along the inferior epigastric and circumflex iliac vessels. Passing through nodes placed along these vessels they reach the external iliac nodes.

## AUTONOMIC NERVES OF ABDOMEN AND PELVIS

1. Autonomic nerves may be sympathetic or parasympathetic.
2. Sympathetic nerves to be seen in the abdomen and pelvis are branches given off by the sympathetic trunk in this region. Some branches given off by the thoracic part of the sympathetic trunk also enter the abdomen.
3. Parasympathetic nerves are derived from two sources:
   a. One source is the vagus nerve which is the tenth cranial nerve. It descends through the neck and thorax into the abdomen.
   b. In addition to the vagus some abdominal and pelvic organs receive parasympathetic fibres through the sacral parasympathetic outflow.

### Autonomic Ganglia and Plexuses in Abdomen and Pelvis

1. a. Many autonomic nerve fibres, both sympathetic and parasympathetic, reach viscera after passing through a number of plexuses (34.18).
   b. Although they are called plexuses they contain numerous neurons and are, in fact, equivalent to ganglia.
   c. The plexuses/ganglia to be seen in the abdomen and pelvis are as follows.

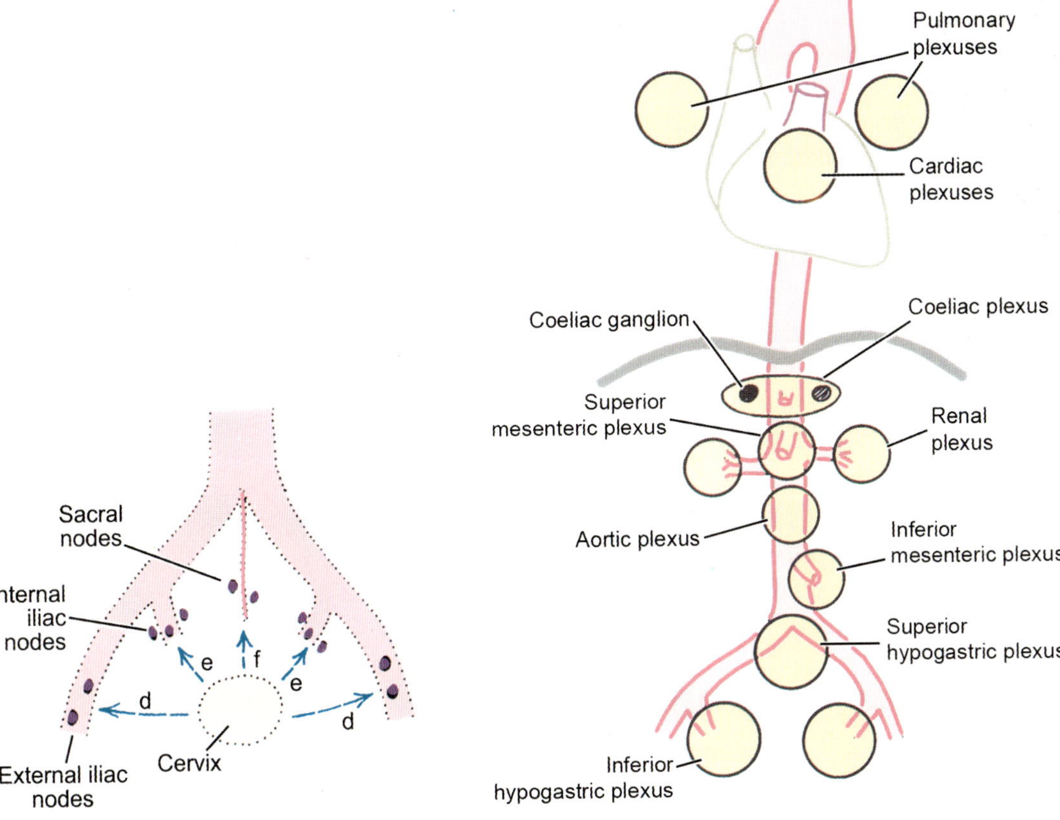


**34.17:** Scheme to show the lymphatic drainage of the cervix of the uterus

**34.18:** Schematic presentation of the location of important autonomic plexuses in the thorax and abdomen

2. The ***coeliac ganglion*** and ***coeliac plexus*** lie in relation to the abdominal aorta at the level of the origin of the coeliac trunk. The coeliac plexus is the uppermost part of an extensive ***aortic plexus*** surrounding the abdominal aorta. This is continued into subsidiary plexuses around the branches arising from the vessel.
   a. The part of the aortic plexus between the origins of the superior and inferior mesenteric arteries is called the ***intermesenteric plexus***.
   b. The part overlying the bifurcation of the aorta is called the ***superior hypogastric plexus***.
   c. When traced downwards it divides into the right and left ***inferior hypogastric plexuses*** related to the corresponding internal iliac arteries.
   d. Some other plexuses are present in close relation to viscera, or even within their walls. The ***vesical plexus*** surrounds the urinary bladder. In the gut there is a ***myenteric plexus*** (of Auerbach) between the muscle coats, and a ***submucous plexus*** (of Meissner).

## PARASYMPATHETIC NERVES IN ABDOMEN AND PELVIS

1. Parasympathetic nerve fibres are derived from a cranial outflow and a sacral outflow.
2. In the thorax and abdomen the cranial outflow is represented by the vagus nerve.
   a. In the thorax fibres of the vagus form an anterior and a posterior oesophageal plexus.
   b. Fibres emerging from the lower end of the anterior oesophageal plexus collect to form the ***anterior vagal trunk*** which is made up mainly of fibres of the left vagus nerve.

c. Similarly, fibres arising from the posterior oesophageal plexus (derived mainly from the right vagus) collect to form the ***posterior vagal trunk***.
d. These two trunks enter the abdomen through the oesophageal opening in the diaphragm. They are responsible for the parasympathetic supply to the greater part of the gastrointestinal tract and to some other organs.

3. Preganglionic neurons that constitute the ***sacral parasympathetic outflow*** are located in the intermediolateral grey column in spinal segments S2, S3 and S4 (34.23).
   a. They emerge from the spinal cord through the ventral nerve roots of the corresponding spinal nerves.
   b. They soon leave the spinal nerves through their ***pelvic splanchnic*** branches.
   c. The preganglionic fibres end in relation to postganglionic neurons which are located either in the walls of the viscera supplied or in plexuses related to them (34.19A and B).
   d. The organs supplied directly by the pelvic splanchnic nerves are:
      i. The urinary bladder
      ii. The rectum
      iii. The testes or ovaries
      iv. The uterus
      v. The uterine tubes
      vi. The penis or clitoris.
   e. Some fibres of these nerves pass through the hypogastric plexuses to supply the pelvic colon, the descending colon and the left one third of the transverse colon. (Note that the parts of the gut supplied are hindgut derivatives).

## SYMPATHETIC NERVES IN ABDOMEN AND PELVIS

### Branches of Thoracic Part of Sympathetic Trunk Entering the Abdomen

1. The lower thoracic sympathetic ganglia give origin to prominent medial branches called the ***greater, lesser*** and ***lowest splanchnic nerves***.
2. All these nerves pass through the diaphragm and enter the abdomen.

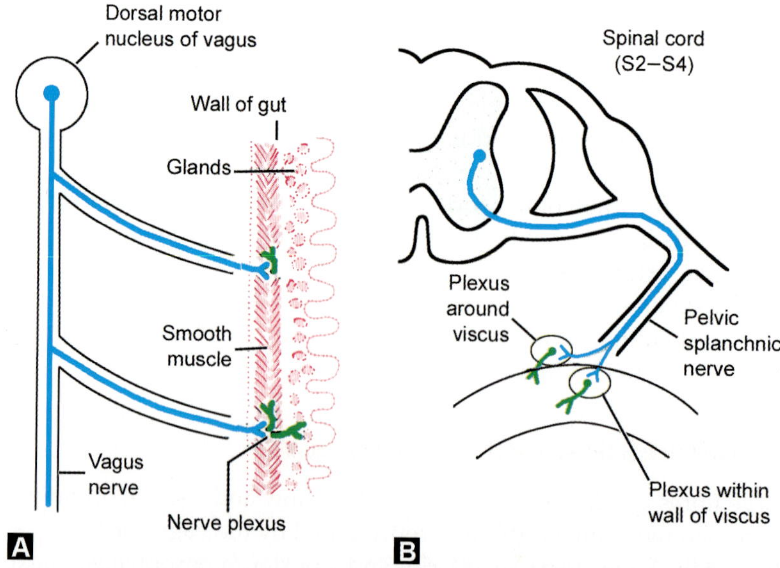


**34.19A and B:** Efferent autonomic neurons. (A) Neurons related to the vagus; (B) Neurons passing through pelvic splanchnic nerves

3. Here the greater splanchnic nerve ends mainly in the coeliac ganglion (34.33). Some fibres of the greater splanchnic nerve end in the aorticorenal ganglion.
4. The lesser splanchnic nerve ends in the aorticorenal ganglion.
5. The lowest splanchnic nerve ends in the renal plexus.

## Lumbar Part of Sympathetic Trunk

The sympathetic trunk passes from the thorax to the abdomen by passing posterior to the medial arcuate ligament. Sometimes it may pass through the crus of the diaphragm. There are usually four ganglia on the lumbar part of the trunk. Their branches and communications are as follows:

1. The ganglia give off grey rami communicantes to the lumbar nerves.
2. The first two ganglia (sometimes three) receive white rami from the corresponding spinal nerves. These white rami are part of the thoracolumbar outflow carrying preganglionic fibres to the sympathetic trunk.
3. Each ganglion gives off a ***lumbar splanchnic branch***. These branches end in the coeliac, renal, aortic, and superior hypogastric plexuses.
4. Vascular branches reach the aortic plexus. From here they extend into plexuses on the common iliac, internal iliac, external iliac, and the proximal parts of the femoral arteries.

## Pelvic Part of Sympathetic Trunk

1. This part of the trunk bears four or five ***sacral ganglia***. In front of the coccyx the right and left sympathetic trunks both end in a median ganglion, the ***ganglion impar***. The branches arising from the pelvic part of the sympathetic trunk are as follows:
   a. Grey rami are given off to the sacral and coccygeal nerves (see below).
   b. Other branches from the ganglia join the inferior hypogastric plexus.
2. The lumbar and sacral sympathetic ganglia are concerned with the sympathetic innervation of the lower limbs.
   a. The preganglionic fibres concerned arise from neurons in the lateral grey column of spinal segments T10 to L2 (or L3).
   b. They pass through the corresponding spinal nerves, and white rami arising from them, into the sympathetic trunk. Postganglionic fibres travel as follows:
      i. Some fibres arising in lumbar ganglia travel through the plexuses on the aorta, the common iliac and external iliac arteries to innervate the proximal part of the femoral artery.
      ii. Some fibres arising in lumbar ganglia pass through grey rami into the lumbar nerves, and through them into the femoral nerve. They pass through the branches of the femoral nerve to supply the distal part of the femoral artery.
      iii. Fibres arising in sacral ganglia pass through grey rami to the sacral nerves, and through them into the tibial nerve. Travelling through this nerve they reach the popliteal artery and its branches.

## Afferent Autonomic Pathways

1. Both sympathetic and parasympathetic nerves carry numerous afferent fibres (These are classified as general visceral afferent).
2. The neurons concerned are located in dorsal nerve root ganglia of spinal nerves, or in sensory ganglia of cranial nerves.
3. They carry impulses arising in viscera and in blood vessels to the central nervous system. The cell bodies of the neurons concerned may be located in one of the following situations.

### *Afferents Related to Cranial Parasympathetic Nerves*

1. In general, these are the general visceral afferent fibres of cranial nerves.
2. All such fibres carrying afferent impulses from the abdomen belong to the vagus nerve.
3. The cell bodies of the neurons concerned are located in the various plexuses already considered above.

4. The central processes of the neurons pass through the vagus nerve to reach the brain (medulla oblongata) where they terminate in the nucleus of the solitary tract.
5. The peripheral processes innervate visceral structures (34.20A). Sensory fibres carried by the vagus innervate all organs to which its efferent fibres are distributed.

### *Afferents Related to Sacral Parasympathetic Nerves*

1. These afferent fibres are peripheral processes of pseudounipolar neurons located in the dorsal root ganglia of the second, third and fourth sacral nerves (34.20B).
2. These fibres run through the pelvic splanchnic nerves to innervate pelvic viscera.
3. The central processes of these neurons enter the spinal cord.
4. The spinal pathways carrying afferent impulses from the viscera are not fully established.

### *Afferents Related to Sympathetic Nerves*

1. Afferent fibres accompany almost all efferent sympathetic fibres. These afferent fibres are peripheral process of pseudounipolar neurons located in the dorsal root ganglia of spinal nerves T1 to L2 or L3 (34.34).
2. Some important points that may be noted about autonomic afferent are as follows:
   a. Autonomic afferents are necessary for various visceral reflexes. Most of these impulses are not consciously perceived.
   b. Some normal visceral sensations that reach consciousness include those of hunger, nausea, rectal distension and sexual sensations.
   c. Under pathological conditions visceral pain is perceived. This is produced by distension, by spasm of smooth muscle, or by anoxia.
   d. Sensory impulses from the same organ may travel along both sympathetic and parasympathetic nerves.

   The nerve supply of individual organs has been described while describing the organs.

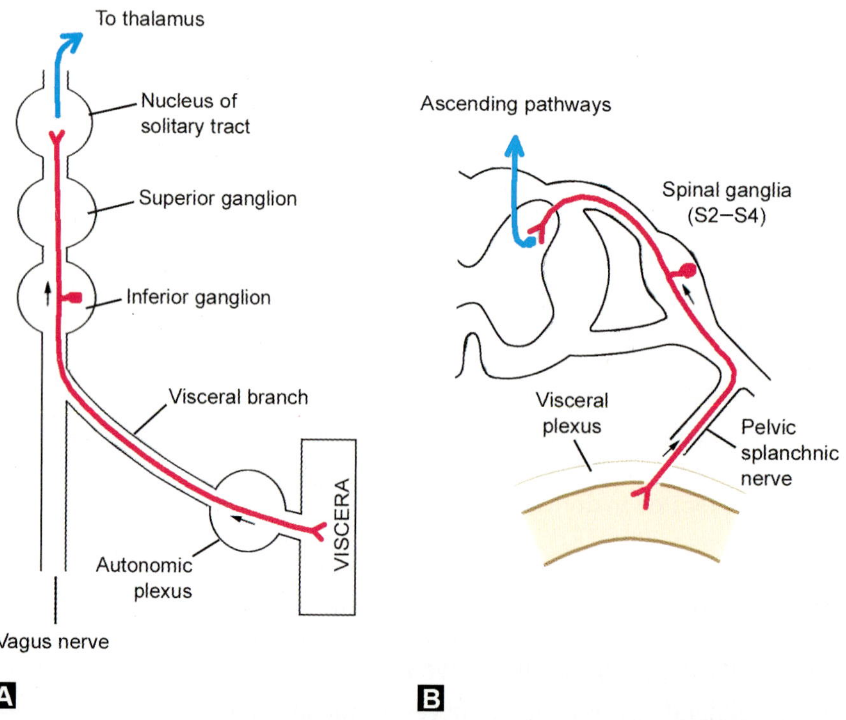


**34.20A and B:** Arrangement of afferent autonomic neurons. (A) Nerve fibres passing through the vagus nerve; (B) Nerve fibres passing through sympathetic nerves

# 35 CHAPTER

# Surface and Radiological Anatomy of the Abdomen

## REGIONS OF THE ABDOMEN

The lines used to divide the abdomen into different regions have been described in Chapter 25 and shown in 25.5.

## RELATIONSHIP OF INGUINAL CANAL TO THE SURFACE OF THE ABDOMINAL WALL

1. The position of the inguinal canal is seen in 35.1. The canal lies above the medial half of the inguinal ligament.
2. The lateral end of the canal lies at the deep inguinal ring and its medial end at the superficial inguinal ring.
   a. To mark the superficial inguinal ring draw a triangle just above the pubic tubercle. For the shape of the triangle see 35.1.
   b. To mark the deep inguinal ring draw a roughly circular area 1 cm above the midinguinal point.
   c. The inguinal canal can now be marked by joining the upper and lower edges of the deep and superficial inguinal rings.
   d. The lines should be about 1 cm apart and about 3.7 cm long.

## SURFACE MARKING OF PARTS OF THE GASTROINTESTINAL TRACT

### Abdominal Part of Oesophagus

See Chapter 23.

### Surface Marking of Stomach

To draw the outline of the stomach first define the cardiac and pyloric ends and then draw the lesser and greater curvatures by joining these ends with curved lines (35.2).

1. The ***cardiac end*** of the stomach lies over the left 7th costal cartilage.
   a. Mark a point on this costal cartilage 2.5 cm to the left of the median plane. This point marks the middle of the cardiac orifice.
   b. The right margin of the orifice lies 1 cm to the right of this point, and the left margin is 1 cm to the left of it.
2. The ***pyloric orifice*** is also about 2 cm broad. Its middle lies on the transpyloric plane about 1.2 cm (half inch) to the right of the median plane.
3. The ***lesser curvature*** can be marked by joining the right border of the cardiac orifice with the left border of the pyloric orifice.
   a. The line is J-shaped.
   b. It is concave upwards, and the lowest part of its curve reaches slightly below the transpyloric plane.
4. The ***fundus*** and ***greater curvature*** can be marked by a much longer line joining the left border of the cardiac orifice with the right border of the pyloric orifice.
   a. The first part of the line is drawn with an upward convexity that reaches the fifth left intercostal space just below the nipple. It then continues to the left and downwards to return to the level of the cardiac orifice (The line up to this point represents the outline of the fundus of the stomach).

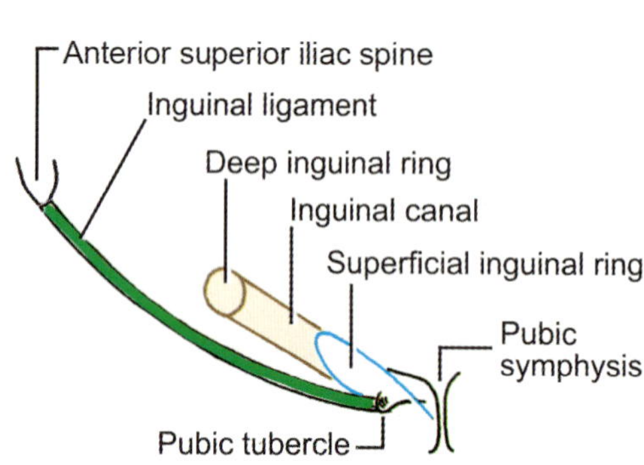


**35.1:** Diagram to show the position of the inguinal canal

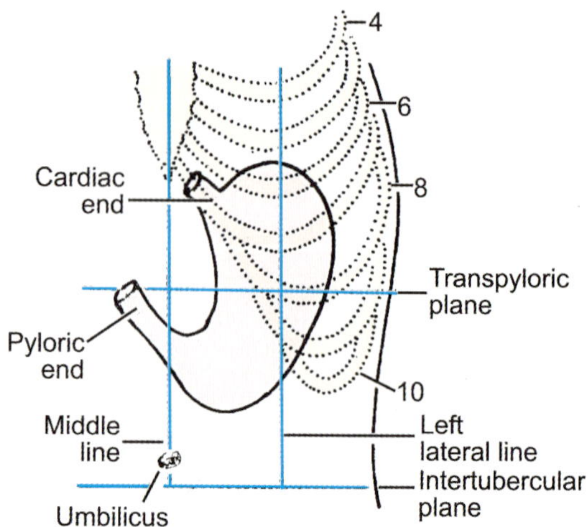


**35.2:** Surface projection of the stomach

b. The second part of the line (representing the margin of the body of the stomach) forms a convexity to the left and downwards, cutting the costal margin between the tips of the 9th and 10th costal cartilages, and extending down to the level of the subcostal plane.
c. It should be remembered that the outline of the stomach as marked above is only approximate, as it changes with distension. The organ moves with respiration.

## Surface Marking of Duodenum

The surface projection of the duodenum is shown in 35.3. The projection of the duodenum is represented by two parallel lines 2.5 cm apart that are drawn as follows:

1. The *first part* of the duodenum begins at the pyloric end of the stomach (transpyloric plane half an inch to the right of the median plane). It is 2.5 cm (1 inch) long. It can be marked by two lines 2.5 cm apart that pass upwards and to the right from the pyloric end of the stomach.
2. The upper end of the *second part* of the duodenum is continuous with the termination of the first part.
   a. The junction lies just below the right costal margin.
   b. From here, the second part descends almost vertically (with a slight curve to the right) for a distance of 7.5 cm.
   c. The right margin of this part of the duodenum lies along the right lateral line (35.3).
   d. The lower end of the second part reaches the subcostal plane.
3. a. The *third part* of the duodenum lies transversely at the level of the subcostal plane.
   b. It is about 10 cm long, and slightly convex downwards. Its right end is continuous with the lower end of the second part.
   c. Traced to the left the third part of the duodenum crosses the median plane, lying above the level of the umbilicus.
4. The *fourth part* of the duodenum is only 2.5 cm long. It is marked by two lines running upwards and to the left from the end of the third part.

## Surface Projection of Root of Mesentery

1. The attachment of the root of the mesentery is given below (35.4).
2. The root of the mesentery can be represented by a broad obliquely placed line 15 cm long (35.4).
3. Its upper end lies to the left of the median plane, about 3 cm below and medial to the tip of the ninth costal cartilage (This point corresponds to the position of the *duodenojejunal junction*).

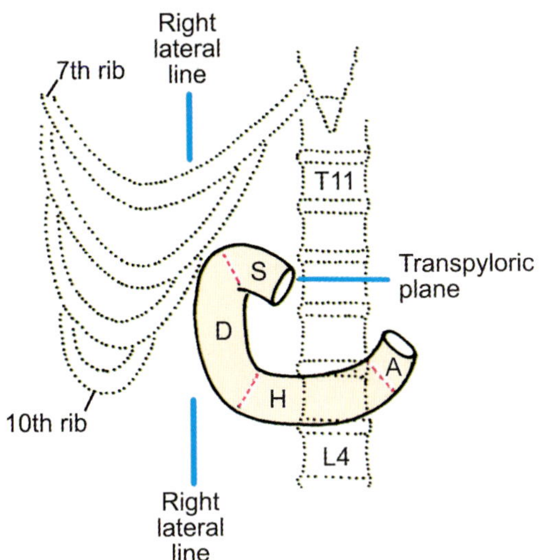


**35.3:** Surface projection of the duodenum. S:superior part; D:descending part; H:horizontal part; A:ascending part

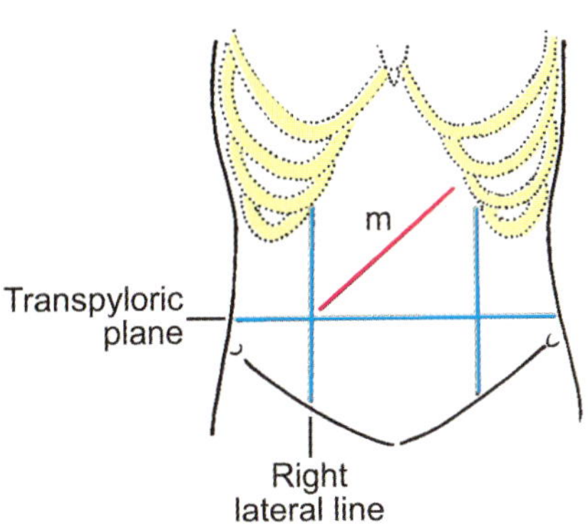


**35.4:** Attachment of the root of the mesentery to posterior abdominal wall

4. The lower end of the root of the mesentery lies to the right of the median plane, at the junction of the right lateral and intertubercular planes (35.4). This point also marks the position of the ***ileocaecal junction*** (35.5).

## Surface Marking of Caecum and Appendix

The ***caecum*** lies in the right iliac fossa. For guidance on how to mark it see 35.5.

1. First draw the right lateral and transtubercular planes.
2. Next note that the caecum is 6 cm long and 7.5 cm broad.
3. Draw a vertical line starting at the intersection of the right lateral and intertubercular planes and carry it down for about 6 cm (This line marks the left margin of the caecum).
4. Draw a second line parallel to the first and 7.5 cm to its right (This line marks the right margin). Join the lower ends of the two lines by a line convex downwards to complete the outline of the caecum.
5. To localise the root of the ***vermiform appendix*** remember that it lies just below the ileocaecal junction.
6. We have seen that this junction lies at the intersection of the right lateral and transtubercular planes. A point 2 cm below the intersection lies over the ***root of the appendix***.
7. Because of the great variability in the position of the appendix there is not much point in trying to mark it on the surface.
8. Just remember that the average length of the appendix is 9 cm, but it can be much shorter or longer.
9. The various positions in which the appendix can lie are shown in 27.17.

## Surface Marking of Large Intestine

The surface projection of various parts of the large intestine is shown in 35.5. The lengths of different parts of the large intestine are shown in 27.19.

### *Ascending Colon*

1. The ascending colon begins at the level of the transtubercular plane (as an upward continuation of the caecum) (35.5).
2. It ascends to a level just below the transpyloric plane, and ends at the level of the 9th right costal cartilage.
3. Here, it becomes continuous with the transverse colon at the right colic flexure.

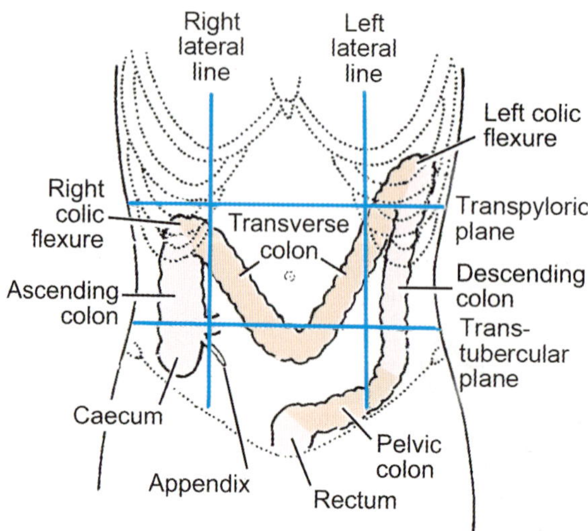


**35.5:** Surface projection of the large intestine

4. It can be marked by two vertical lines, the first drawn along the right lateral line and the second drawn 5 cm to the right of the first line.

### *Transverse Colon*

1. The transverse colon begins at the right colic flexure (i.e, at the level of the upper part of the 9th costal cartilage) (35.5).
2. It runs to the left, with a marked downward curve, to reach the left colic flexure.
3. This flexure lies to the left of the left lateral line, at the level of the left 8th costal cartilage.
   a. Note that the left colic flexure is placed at a higher level than the right flexure.
   b. Between the two colic flexures, the transverse colon hangs downwards to a varying degree (as it is suspended by the transverse mesocolon) and can reach the level of the transtubercular plane or even lower.
4. Using this information, the transverse colon can be marked using two parallel lines that are about 5 cm apart.

### *Descending Colon*

1. The descending colon is somewhat narrower than the ascending or transverse colon (35.5).
2. It is marked by drawing two lines, 2.5 cm apart that begin at the left colic flexure (i.e., over the left eighth costal cartilage) and running downwards a little to the left of the left lateral line.
3. Its lower end lies just above the inguinal ligament.

### *Sigmoid Colon*

The sigmoid colon is in the form of coils that lie predominantly in the true pelvis. No useful purpose is served by trying to mark it on the surface.

1. It begins, as a continuation of the descending colon, just above the left inguinal ligament and descends into the true pelvis.
2. It terminates near the middle line of the pelvis by becoming continuous with the upper end of the rectum (see below).

### *Rectum and Anal Canal*

1. The ***rectum*** lies immediately in front of the sacrum. Its surface projection can be marked over the lower part of the back.

2. To do so first palpate the second sacral spine.
3. Next, locate the posterior superior iliac spines. They may not be palpable but their position is indicated by a dimple about 4 cm lateral to the second sacral spine.
4. Draw two lines joining the posterior superior iliac spines to the anus.
5. The rectum begins over the third piece of the sacrum (i.e., just below the level where the second sacral spine can be palpated).
6. The ***anorectal junction*** lies just below the tip of the coccyx.
7. The parts of the lines drawn above, corresponding to the levels mentioned, enable the rectum and anal canal to be marked.

## SURFACE MARKING OF BILIARY APPARATUS, PANCREAS AND SPLEEN

### Surface Marking of the Liver

1. The position of the liver relative to the regions of the abdomen, and to the lower ribs and costal cartilages has been described earlier. The projection of the liver can be drawn both on the anterior and posterior aspects of the trunk. A projection on the anterior surface is illustrated in 35.6.
2. When seen from the front (or from the back), the liver has a triangular outline. The triangle is bounded by upper, lower and right lateral borders.
3. From 35.6, note that the ***upper border*** lies deep to the lower part of the thoracic cage.
   a. It is convenient to mark the upper border beginning at its left end.
   b. This end lies just below the left nipple, in the ***left fifth intercostal space 9 cm from the median plane***.
   c. Draw a line joining this point to the ***xiphisternal joint***.
   d. This line will have a slight downward slope. Carry the line to the right of the middle line (with a slight upward convexity) till it reaches the place where the upper border of the right ***fifth costal cartilage*** is crossed by the ***right lateral line***.
   e. Carry the line further to the right, more or less horizontally, and note that on reaching the midaxillary line the projection of the upper border lies over the ***sixth rib***.

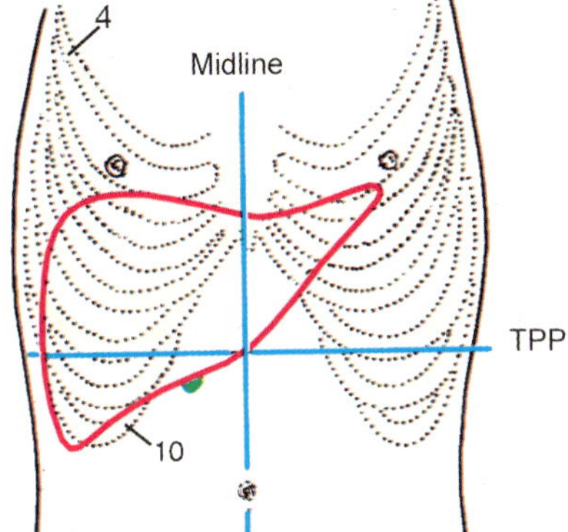


**35.6:** Surface projection of the liver

   f. Continue the line across the side of the thorax to the back and continue it to the ***inferior angle of the scapula***.
   g. Finally extend the line so that it reaches the middle line at the back, at the level of the ***8th thoracic spine***.
4. To mark the ***lower border*** of the liver return to the front of the trunk and go back to the left end of the superior border (i.e., ***left fifth intercostal space 9 cm from the median plane***).
   a. This is also the starting point for marking the lower border of the liver. From here draw a line running downwards and to the right so that it cuts the left costal margin over the ***tip of the left eighth costal cartilage***.
   b. Carry the line downwards and to the right to the ***intersection of the transpyloric plane with the median plane***.
   c. Crossing the median plane carry the line to the right costal margin which it should cut at the level of the ***tip of the ninth costal cartilage***.
   d. Continue the line to the midaxillary line where it should lie over the ***tip of the tenth costal cartilage***.
   e. Finally carry the line across the back of the trunk to reach the median plane (at the back) at the level of the ***11th thoracic spine***.

### Fundus of Gall Bladder

The fundus of the gall bladder projects from just below the lower border of the liver (seen as a large black dot in 35.6 but not labelled) and comes into contact with the anterior abdominal wall.

To mark the fundus of the gall bladder proceed as follows:

1. Ask the subject (on whom you are doing the marking) to draw his abdomen inwards. This will make the rectus abdominis prominent. The lateral margin of the muscle can then be seen as a line (linea semilunaris). Trace this line upwards to the point where it meets the costal margin.
2. Draw the lower border of the liver as described above and mark the gall bladder as a small convex area just below the border, over the place where the right linea semilunaris meets the costal margin.

### Bile Duct

1. To mark the position of the bile duct draw the transpyloric plane.
2. Also draw the projection of the second part of the duodenum (as described above).
3. Take a point 5 cm above the transpyloric plane, and 2 cm to the right of the median plane.
4. Draw a vertical line downwards from this point for 4 cm.
5. From here continue the line with an inclination to the right till it reaches the medial border of the second part of the duodenum, at about its middle.

### Surface Marking of Pancreas

We have seen that the pancreas is divisible into the head, the body and the tail. We have also noted that the head lies within the C-shaped curve of the duodenum.

1. To mark the projection of the head of the pancreas, first mark the duodenum as described above. Also mark the transpyloric and subcostal planes.
   a. The 'inner' border of the C-shaped curve of the duodenum demarcates the head of the pancreas.
   b. Draw two lines about 3 cm apart that pass upwards and to the left from the head. The initial 1 cm of these lines should lie over the transpyloric plane. This part represents the neck of the pancreas (which lies behind the pylorus).
2. Continue the two lines upwards and to the left till they reach the subcostal plane. This continuation of the lines which should be about 10 cm long represents the body of the pancreas.
3. The terminal part of the same lines represents the tail.
4. The overall shape of the pancreas should be drawn as shown in 28.29.

### Surface Marking of the Spleen

1. Begin by studying 28.23 that shows the relationship of the spleen to the 9th, 10th and 11th ribs. This relationship is the key to the surface marking of the spleen.
2. Remember that the spleen lies on the left side of the abdomen, in contact with the posterior part of the thoracic cage. So the spleen is marked on the back of the trunk on the left side.
3. The long axis of the spleen lies along the long axis of the 10th rib.
   a. The medial end lies over the 10th rib, about 5 cm from the median plane.
   b. The lateral end lies over the 10th rib in the midaxillary line.
4. The upper border of the spleen is drawn by joining the medial and lateral ends by a line convex upwards so that its uppermost part reaches the upper border of the 9th rib.
5. The lower border of the spleen is drawn by joining its medial and lateral ends by a line convex downwards and reaching the lower border of the 11th rib.

## SURFACE MARKING OF URINARY ORGANS

### Surface Marking of Kidneys

The following facts are relevant to surface marking of the kidneys:

1. The vertical diameter of the kidney is about 11 cm. The transverse diameter is actually about 6 cm. It appears to be only 4.5 cm when viewed from the front (or back) because of foreshortening.

2. Because of the presence of the liver on the right side, the right kidney lies slightly lower than the left kidney.
3. The vertical axis of the kidney is placed obliquely (30.2 and 30.3) so that its upper end is nearer the median plane than the lower end.
4. The upper end is about 2.5 cm (one inch) from the median plane, while the lower end is about 7.5 cm (three inches) from it.

### *Surface Marking from the Front*

1. The position of the kidneys relative to the anterior abdominal wall is shown in 35.7.
2. The hilum of each kidney lies more or less in the transpyloric plane, a little medial to the tip of the ninth costal cartilage.
3. Keeping in mind the points 'a' to 'd' given above the outline of the kidney can be drawn.

### *Surface Marking from Behind*

1. In relation to the posterior surface of the body:
   a. The hilum of the kidney lies at the level of the first lumbar spine (35.8).
   b. The upper pole at the level of the 11th thoracic spine.
   c. The lower pole at the level of the third lumbar spine.
2. In 35.8 note that the area in which the kidney lies can be represented as a parallelogram (***Morrison's parallelogram***).
   a. The upper and lower boundaries of this parallelogram are formed by transverse lines drawn through the eleventh thoracic and third lumbar spines.
   b. Its medial and lateral boundaries are formed by vertical lines 2.5 cm and 9 cm from the median plane.
3. The outline of the kidney can be drawn within the parallelogram keeping in mind points 'a' to 'd' given above.

## Surface Marking of Ureter (Abdominal Part)

1. Like the marking of the kidney the abdominal part of the ureter can also be marked from the front or from the back.
2. To mark the ureter on the front of the abdomen locate (a) the tip of the 9th costal cartilage, and (b) the pubic tubercle. A line joining these two points marks the position of the abdominal part of the ureter.
3. To mark the ureter on the back, locate the second lumbar spine. Take a point about 4 cm lateral to the spine. From here draw a line downwards to reach the posterior superior iliac spine.

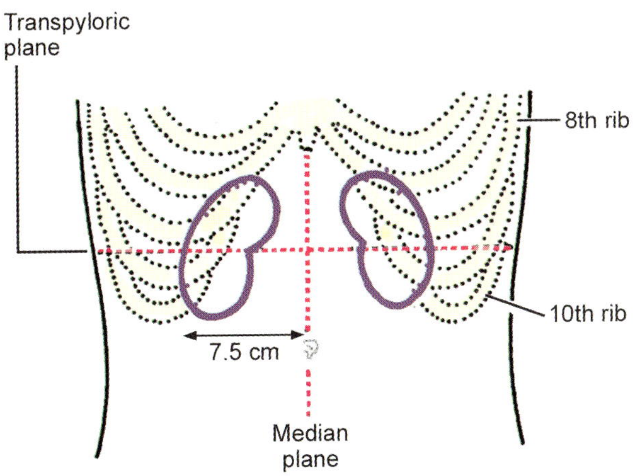


**35.7:** Projection of the kidney to the front of the body

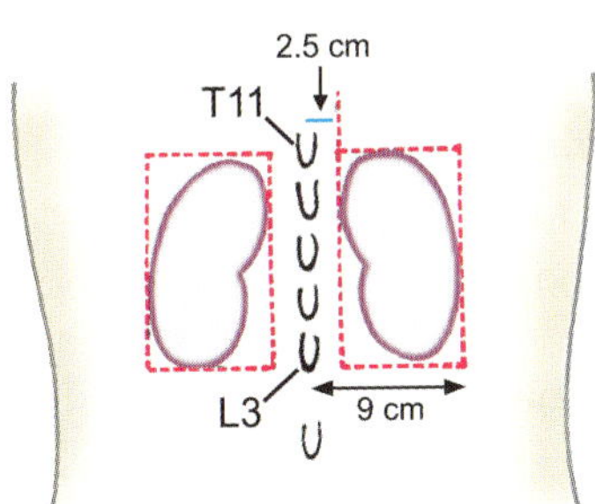


**35.8:** Surface projection of the kidney on the back of the body

## SURFACE MARKING OF SOME ARTERIES

### Surface Marking of Abdominal Aorta

1. Remember that the abdominal aorta lies more or less in the median plane and is about 2 cm broad.
2. Its upper end lies in front of the lower border of vertebral body T12, and its lower end in front of L4.
3. The lower end inclines slightly to the left.
4. On the front of the abdomen, the level of the upper end lies 2.5 cm above the transpyloric plane.
5. The lower end lies over a point about 1 cm below and to the left of the umbilicus.
6. The aorta can be marked by drawing two vertical lines 2 cm apart between these levels.

### Surface Marking of Some Branches of Aorta

#### *Coeliac Trunk*

1. We have seen that the upper end of the abdominal aorta lies in the middle line about 2.5 cm above the transpyloric plane.
2. The coeliac trunk can be represented as a small circle drawn in front of the aorta 1 cm below its upper end.

#### *Left Gastric Artery*

1. First mark the coeliac trunk (as described above).
2. Mark the cardiac end of the stomach (described earlier in this chapter).
3. A line joining these two gives the position of the left gastric artery.

#### *Splenic Artery*

1. Draw a broad line starting at the position of the coeliac trunk and passing upwards and to the left for about 10 cm.
2. If you also mark the pancreas it will be seen that the artery lies behind it.

#### *Hepatic Artery*

1. This artery follows a course that is somewhat V-shaped.
2. Draw a line 2.5 cm long starting from the coeliac trunk (see above) and running downwards and to the right.
3. From here draw a vertical line 2.5 cm long.

#### *Superior Mesenteric Artery*

1. You can remember the marking of this artery easily if you remember that:
   a. The artery arises from the abdominal aorta a short distance below the origin of the coeliac trunk.
   b. It runs to the ileocaecal junction.
2. The upper end of the artery lies in the median plane just above the transpyloric plane.
3. The lower end lies at the point where the right lateral line cuts the transtubercular plane.
4. The line representing the artery should be drawn with a slight convexity to the left.

#### *Inferior Mesenteric Artery*

1. This artery takes origin from the abdominal aorta and runs downwards and to the left.
2. Its upper end lies in the median plane 4 cm below the transpyloric plane.
3. The lower end lies 4 cm below the umbilicus, and 4 cm to the left of the median plane.
4. The artery should be drawn with a slight convexity to the left.

#### *Surface Marking of Common Iliac and External Iliac Arteries*

1. We have seen that the projection of the lower end of the abdominal aorta lies about 1 cm below and to the left of the umbilicus.

2. Draw a broad line from here to the midinguinal point (i.e., midway between the anterior superior iliac spine and the pubic symphysis).
3. The upper one-third of this line gives the surface marking of the common iliac artery, while its lower two-thirds give the marking of the external iliac artery.

## SURFACE MARKING OF SOME LARGE VEINS

### Inferior Vena Cava

1. The inferior vena cava is about 2.5 cm broad.
2. Remember that it lies to the right of the abdominal aorta, and so its marking has to be to the right of the median plane.
3. Its left edge should be about 1 cm to the right of the median plane and its right edge 2.5 cm further to the right.
4. It begins just below the transtubercular plane and ends opposite the sternal end of the right sixth costal cartilage.
5. Note that in marking the aorta we proceeded from above downwards, but in marking the vena cava we started at the lower end and went upwards. In each case, we have followed the direction of blood flow.

### Common and External Iliac Veins

1. Draw a line from the lower end of the inferior vena cava to a point a little medial to the midinguinal point. The line should have a convexity laterally.
2. The upper one-third of this line represents the common iliac vein, while its lower two-thirds represent the external iliac vein.

### Portal Vein

1. First mark the transpyloric plane.
2. Mark a point on it a little to the right of the median plane.
3. Mark a second point about 1 cm further to the right.
4. From each of these points draw lines 8 cm long and running upwards and to the right. These two lines will give you the right and left margins of the portal vein.

## RADIOLOGICAL ANATOMY OF THE ABDOMEN AND PELVIS

Radiographs illustrating the appearances using different imaging techniques are presented in 35.9 to 35.15.

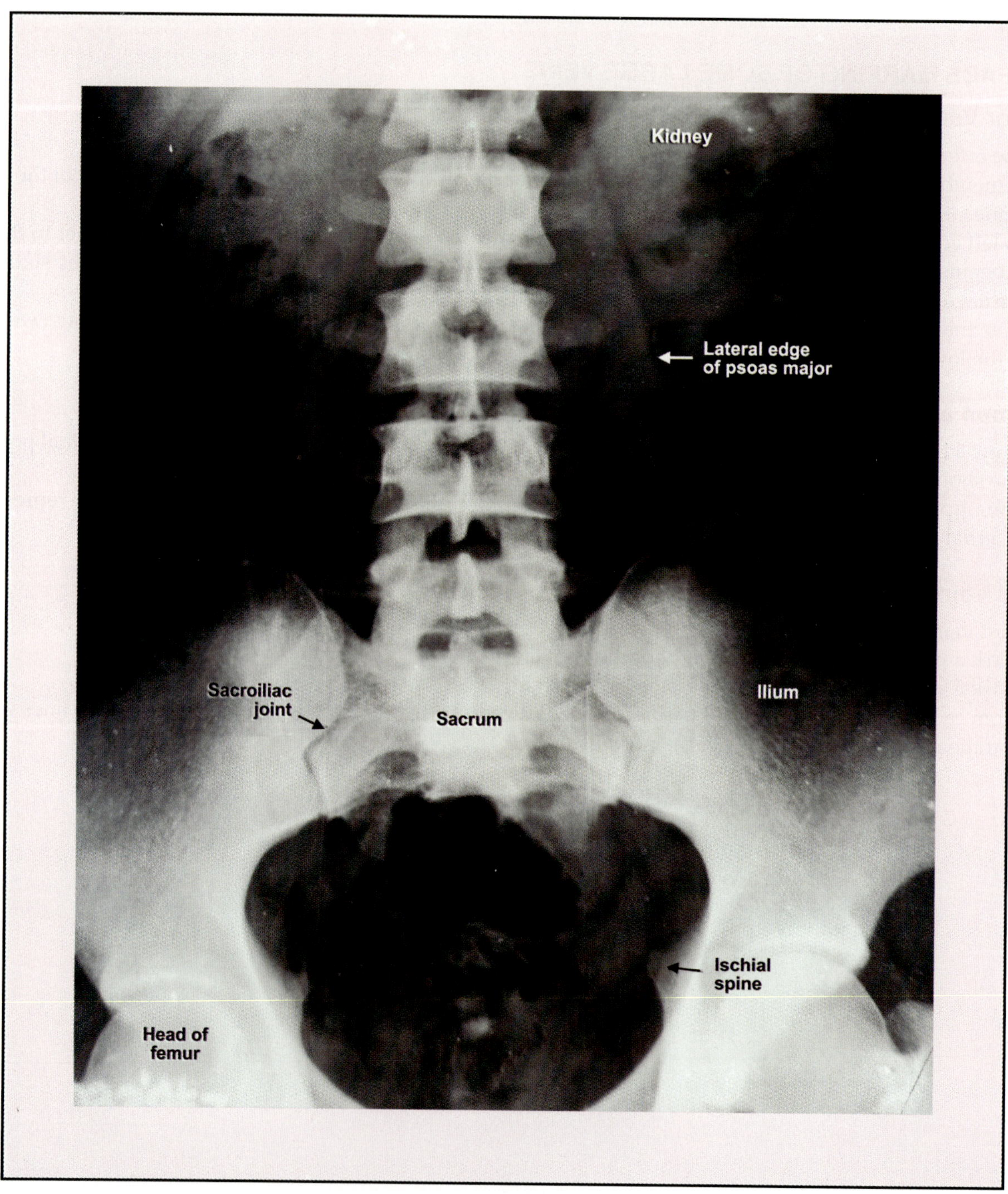


**35.9:** Plain radiograph of the abdomen. Note the shadows of lumbar vertebrae. In each vertebra identify the vertebral bodies. The gaps between them represent areas occupied by intervertebral discs. Also note the spinous and transverse processes. The sacrum is seen articulating with the hip bones at the sacroiliac joints. The upper parts of the heads of the right and left femur are seen. Soft tissues that can be identified are the lateral edges of the psoas major muscles, and the kidneys. The irregular black areas over the kidney region, and in the pelvis are caused by gas present in the intestines

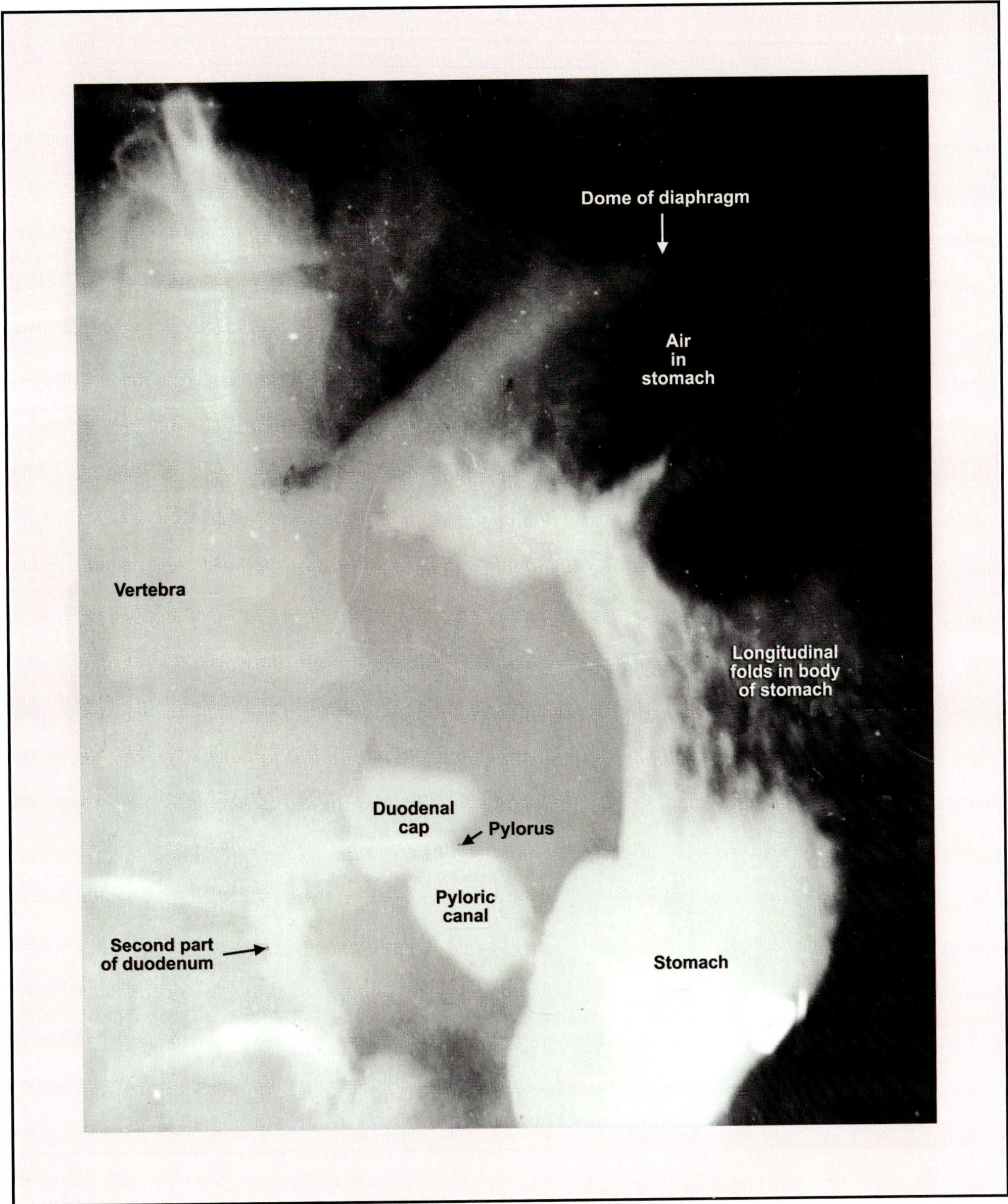


**35.10:** Radiograph of upper abdomen (oblique view) after a barium meal. The lower part of the stomach, and part of the duodenum, are outlined. Note the characteristic shape of the duodenal cap

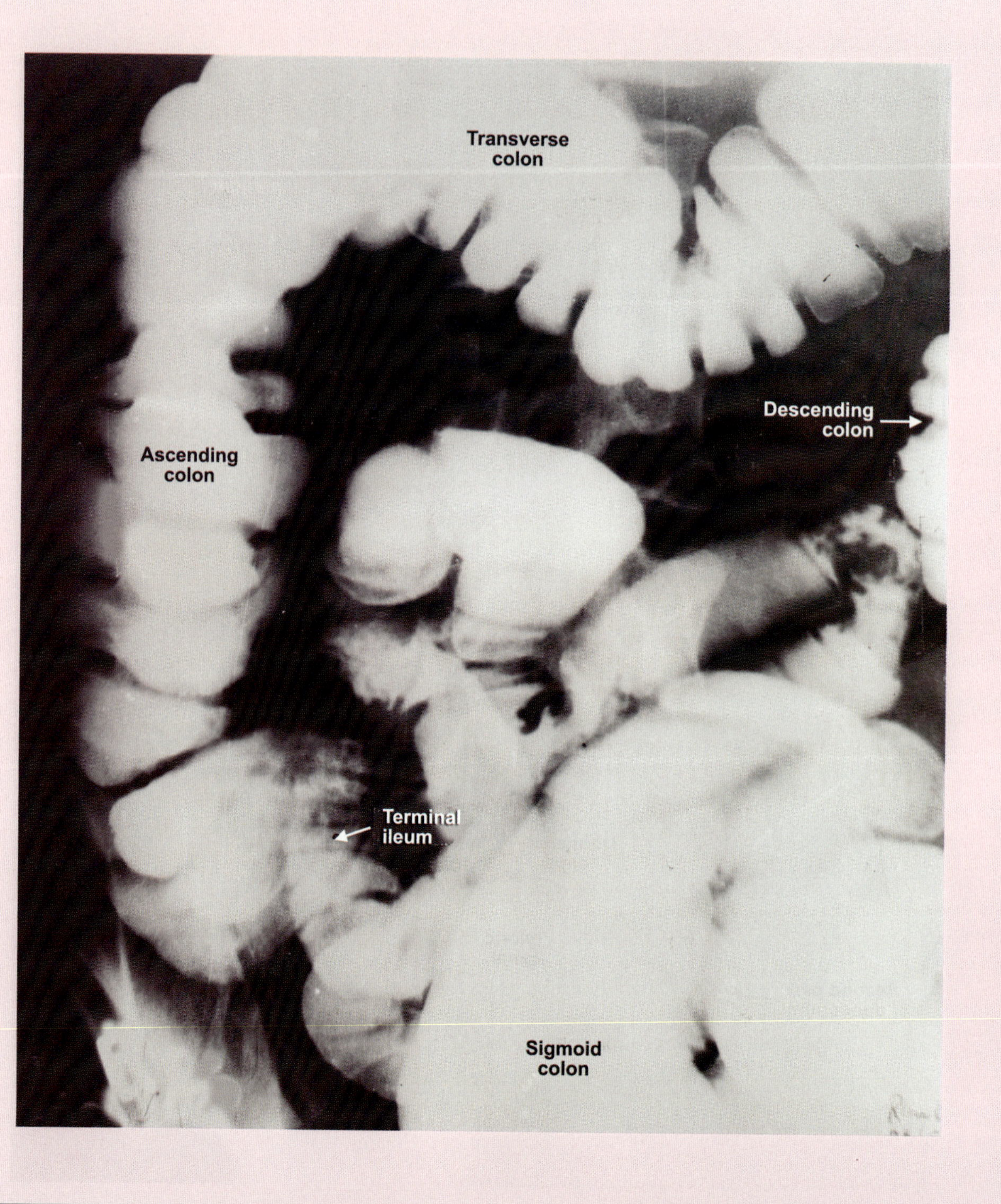


**35.11:** Radiograph of abdomen after a barium enema. The colon is outlined

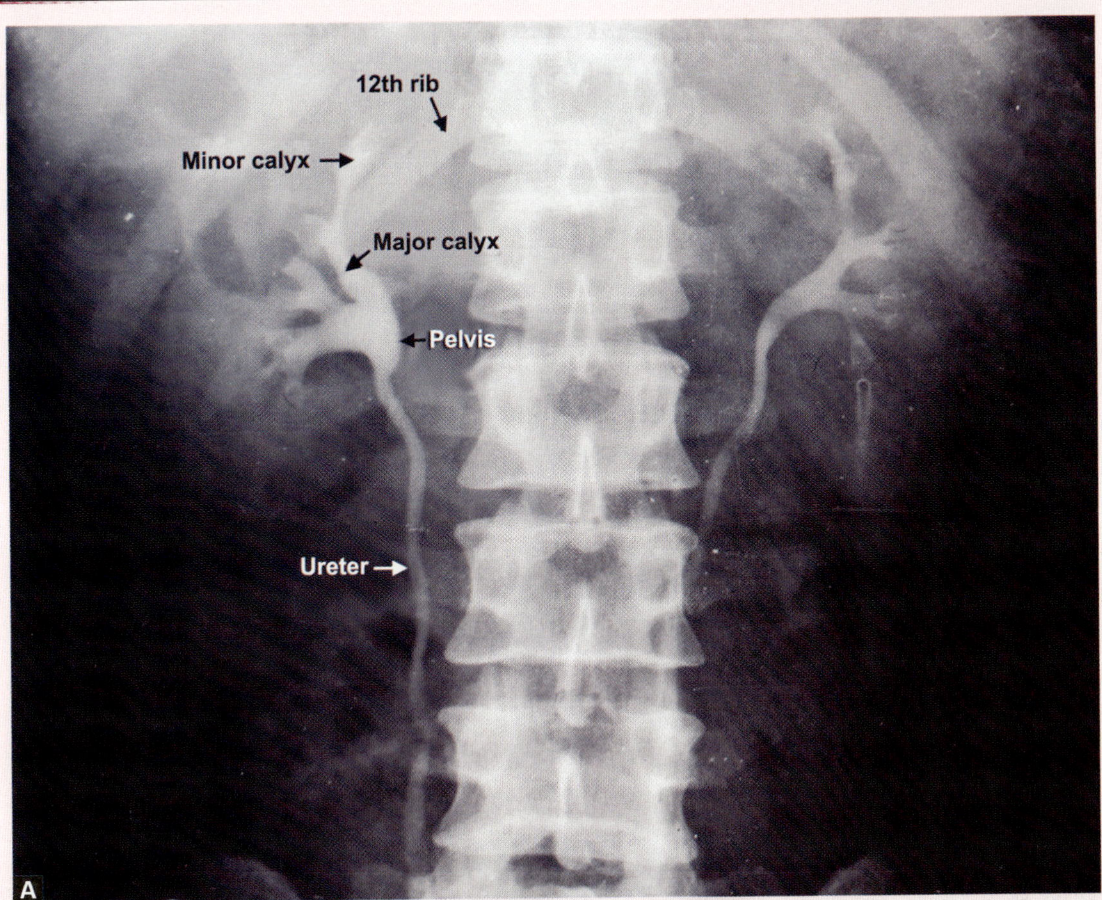


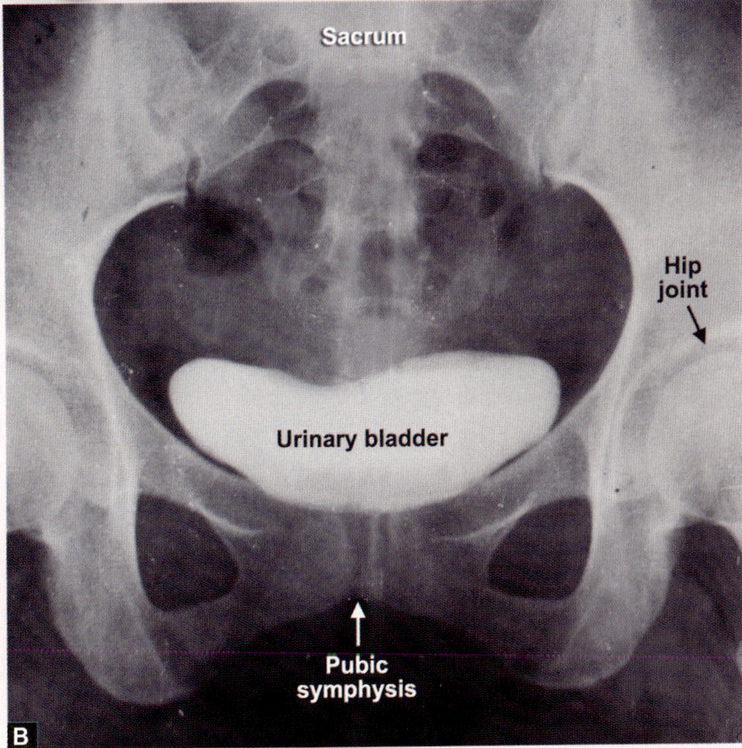


**35.12A and B:** Radiographs taken after intravenous injection of a contrast medium that is excreted by the kidneys (intravenous pyelography). In radiograph 'A' taken soon after injection, the calyces, and part of the ureters are seen. In radiograph 'B' taken some time later, the urinary bladder is outlined

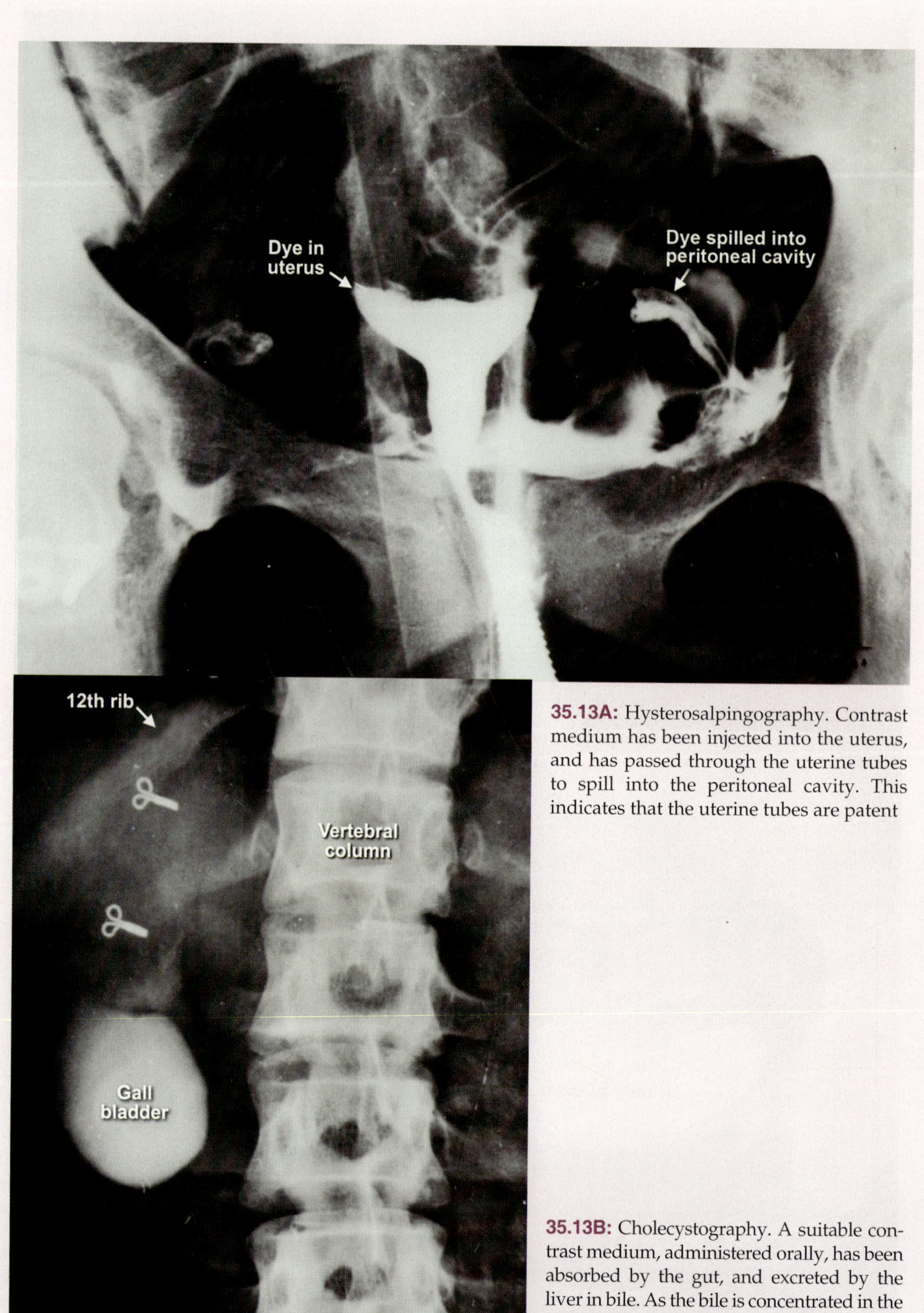


**35.13A:** Hysterosalpingography. Contrast medium has been injected into the uterus, and has passed through the uterine tubes to spill into the peritoneal cavity. This indicates that the uterine tubes are patent

**35.13B:** Cholecystography. A suitable contrast medium, administered orally, has been absorbed by the gut, and excreted by the liver in bile. As the bile is concentrated in the gall bladder the organ is outlined

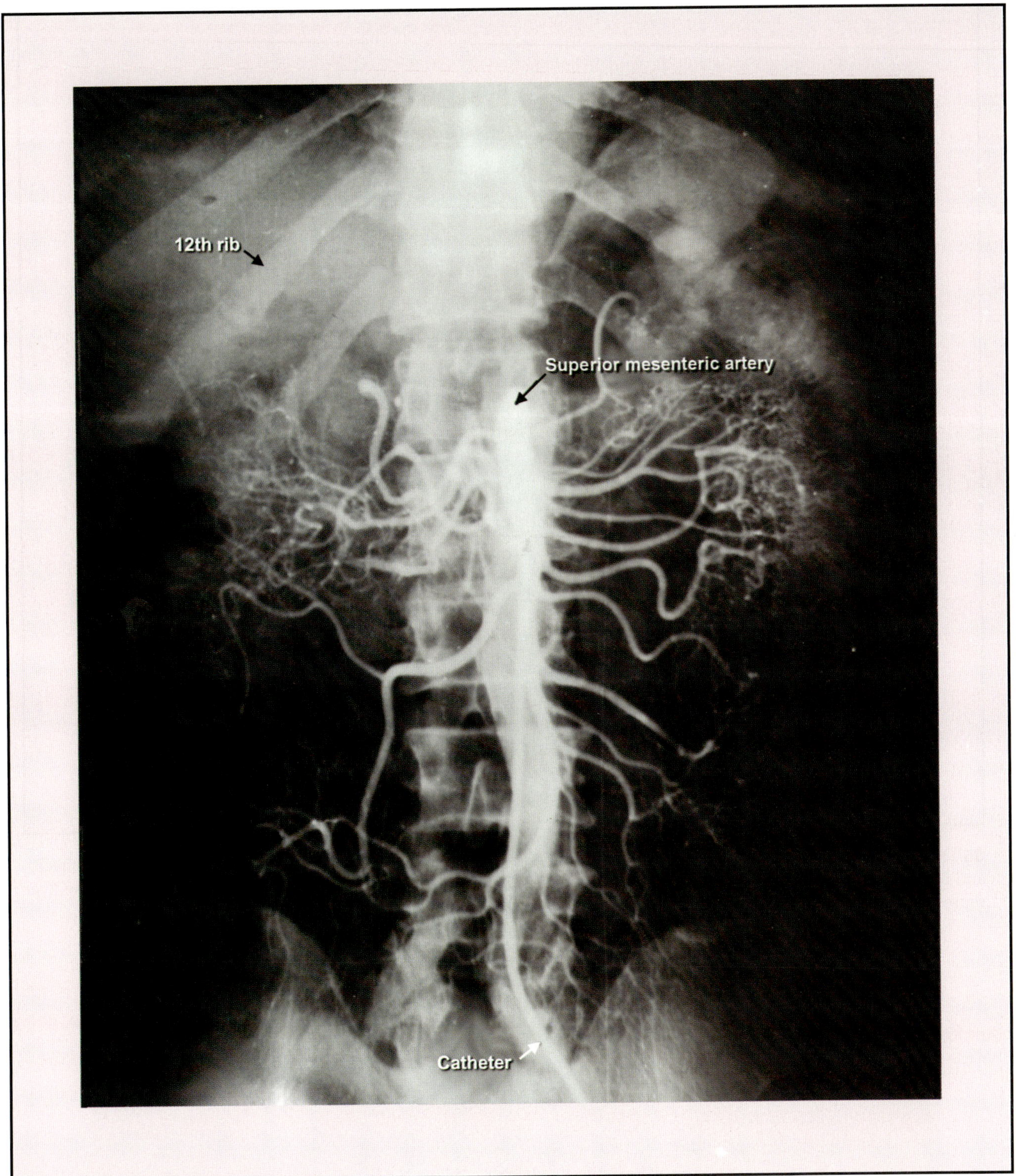


**35.14:** Selective superior mesenteric arteriography. A catheter was introduced into the femoral artery, passed up the aorta, and manipulated to the enter the opening into the superior mesenteric artery. Contrast medium was injected and a radiograph taken

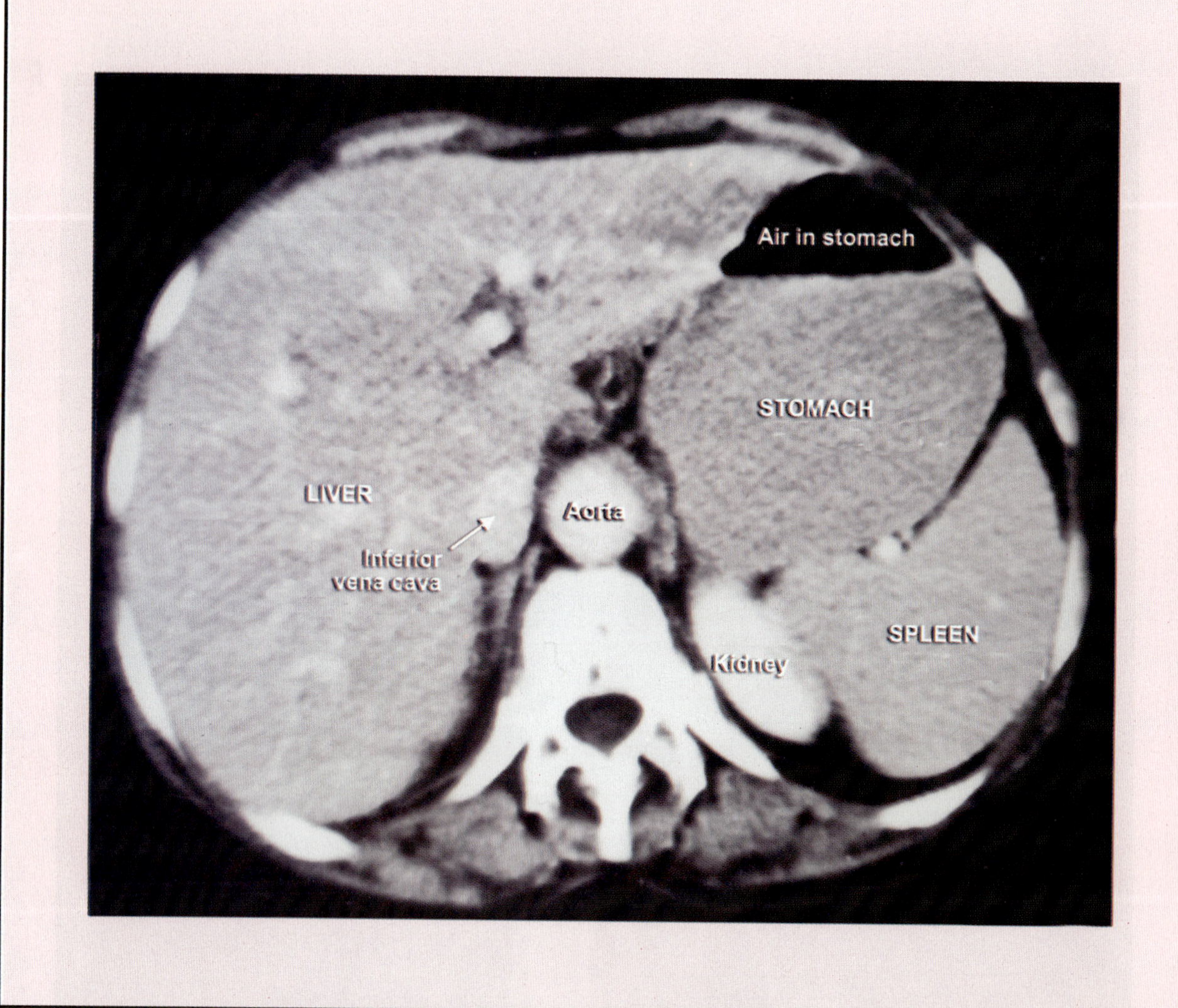


**35.15 :** Cross section of upper abdomen obtained by CT scan. Contrast media were administered orally (for stomach), and intravenously (for blood vessels). See labelling for identification of organs seen. The radiating shadows in the liver represent blood vessels. Part of the stomach lumen in filled by air

# PART 5

# Head and Neck

36

CHAPTER

# Bones and Joints of the Head and Neck

## VERTEBRAL COLUMN

The structure of a typical vertebra has been considered in chapter 16. Here we will consider some additional features of typical cervical vertebrae, and also some atypical cervical vertebrae.

### Typical Cervical Vertebrae

1. a. Each ***transverse process*** of a typical cervical vertebra is pierced by a foramen transversarium (36.1).
   b. It is relatively short.
   c. The part of the process in front of the foramen is called the anterior root; and the part behind it is called the posterior root (36.2).
   d. The part lateral to the foramen is usually called the costotransverse bar, but it is more correct to call it the intertubercular bar.
   e. The anterior and posterior roots end in thickenings called the anterior and posterior tubercles respectively.
   f. When viewed from the lateral side the transverse process is seen to be grooved. One cervical nerve lies in this groove after it passes out of the intervertebral foramen.
   g. In the cervical region the costal element forms the anterior root, the costotransverse bar, and both the anterior and posterior tubercles.
2. a. The ***vertebral bodies*** are small in the cervical vertebrae.
   b. In shape the body is oval.

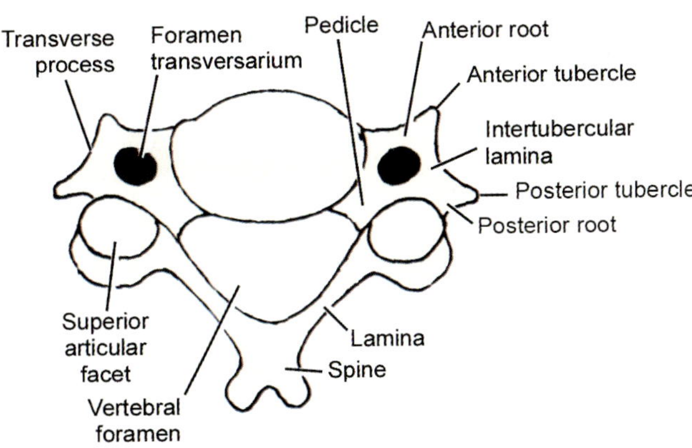


36.1: Typical cervical vertebra seen from above

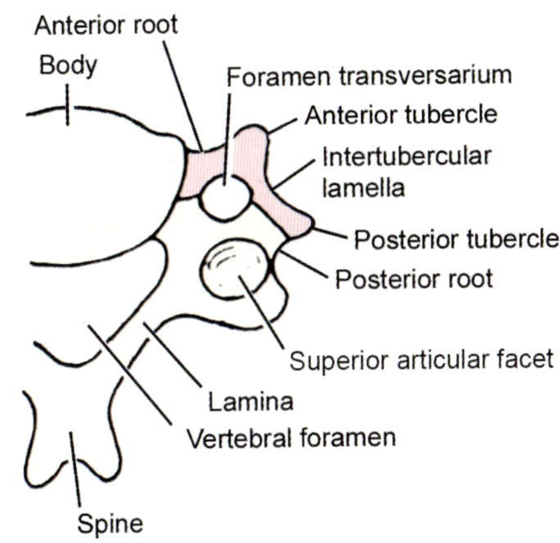


36.2: Cervical transverse processes showing the parts derived from the costal elements (pink shading)

   c. The upper surface of the body is concave from side-to-side. The posterolateral parts of its edge are raised to form distinct lips. As a result of this the superior vertebral notch is prominent.
3. The ***pedicles*** are long and directed backwards and laterally.
4. The ***laminae*** of cervical vertebrae are long (transversely) and narrow (vertically).
5. The ***spinous processes*** are short and bifid.
6. a. In the cervical region the ***articular facets*** are flat. The superior facets are directed equally backwards and upwards. The inferior facets are directed forwards and downwards.
   b. The superior and inferior articular processes form a solid articular pillar that helps to transmit some weight from one vertebra to the next lower one.

## ATYPICAL CERVICAL VERTEBRAE

### The Atlas (First Cervical) Vertebra

1. The first cervical vertebra is called the atlas. It looks very different from a typical cervical vertebra as it has no body, and no spine (36.3 and 36.4).
2. It consists of two ***lateral masses*** joined, anteriorly, by a short ***anterior arch***; and, posteriorly, by a much longer ***posterior arch***. The arches give the atlas a ring-like appearance.
3. A large transverse process, pierced by a foramen transversarium, projects laterally from the lateral mass.
4. The superior aspect of each lateral mass shows an elongated concave facet that articulates with the corresponding condyle of the occipital bone (to form an ***atlanto-occipital joint***). Nodding and lateral movements of the head take place at the two (right and left) atlanto-occipital joints.
5. The inferior aspect of each lateral mass (36.4) shows a large oval facet for articulation with the corresponding superior articular facet of the axis (second cervical vertebra) to form a ***lateral atlanto-axial joint***.
6. The medial side of the lateral mass shows a tubercle that gives attachment to the transverse ligament of the atlas (shown in dotted line in 36.3).
   a. This ligament divides the large foramen (bounded by the lateral masses and the arches) into anterior and posterior parts.
   b. The posterior part corresponds to the vertebral foramen of a typical vertebra. The spinal cord passes through it.
   c. The anterior part is occupied by the dens (which is an upward projection from the body of the axis).

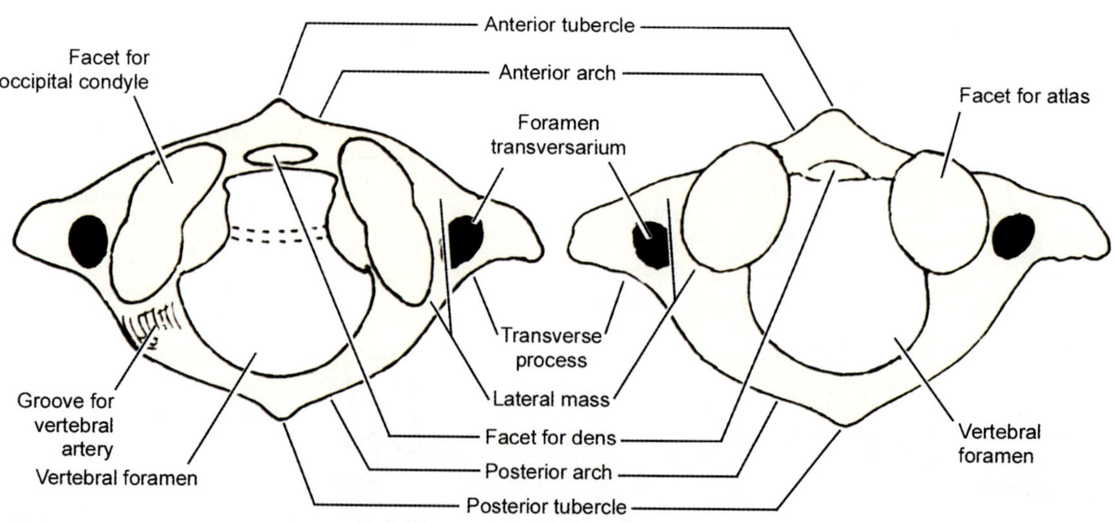


**36.3:** The atlas (first cervical vertebra) seen from above

**36.4:** The atlas (first cervical vertebra) seen from below

7. a. The dens articulates with the posterior aspect of the anterior arch, that bears a circular facet for it.
   b. The dens also articulates with the transverse ligament, these two articulations collectively forming the ***median atlanto-occipital joint***.
   c. In side-to-side movements of the head the atlas moves with the skull around the pivot formed by the dens.
8. The anterior arch bears a small midline projection called the ***anterior tubercle***.
9. The posterior arch bears a similar projection, the ***posterior tubercle***, which may be regarded as a rudimentary spine.
   a. The upper surface of the posterior arch has a groove for the vertebral artery.
   b. The groove is continuous laterally with the foramen transversarium.

### *Some Relations of the Atlas*

1. The vertebral artery passes upwards through the foramen transversarium and then runs medially on the groove over the posterior arch.
2. The first cervical nerve crosses the posterior arch deep to the vertebral artery and divides here into anterior and posterior primary rami.
3. Structures passing through the vertebral canal include:
   a. The spinal cord
   b. The meninges
   c. The spinal part of the accessory nerve
   d. The anterior and posterior spinal arteries.

## The Axis (Second Cervical) Vertebra

1. The most conspicuous feature of the axis, that distinguishes it from all other vertebrae, is the presence of a thick finger-like projection arising from the upper part of the body. This projection is called the ***dens***, or ***odontoid process*** (36.5).
2. a. The dens fits into the space between the anterior arch of the atlas and its transverse ligament to form the median atlanto-occipital joint.
   b. The anterior aspect of the dens bears a convex oval facet for articulation with the anterior arch.
   c. Its posterior aspect shows a transverse groove for the transverse ligament.
3. On either side of the dens, the axis vertebra bears a large oval facet for articulation with the corresponding facet on the inferior aspect of the atlas.

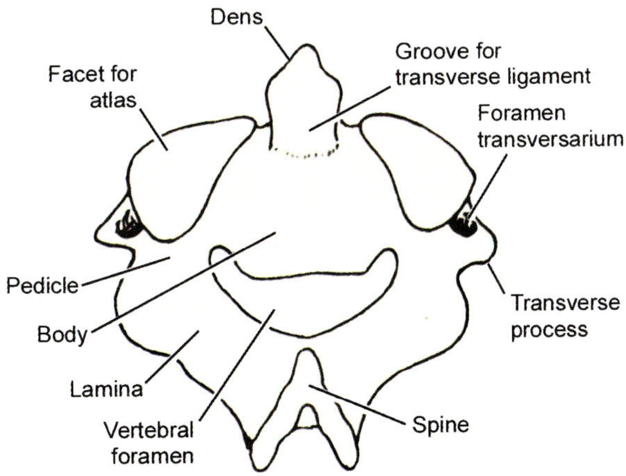


**36.5:** The second cervical vertebra (axis) seen from the posterosuperior aspect

4. The transverse process of the axis lies lateral to this facet.
   a. It is small and ends in a single tubercle corresponding to the posterior tubercle of a typical cervical vertebra.
   b. The transverse process is pierced by a foramen transversarium.

## The Seventh Cervical Vertebra

1. The seventh cervical vertebra differs from a typical vertebra in having a long thick spinous process that ends in a single tubercle (36.6).
2. The tip of the process forms a prominent surface landmark. Because of this fact this vertebra is referred to as the ***vertebra prominens***.
3. The transverse processes are also large and have prominent posterior tubercles.
4. Note that the vertebral artery and vein ***do not*** traverse the foramen transversarium of this vertebra.

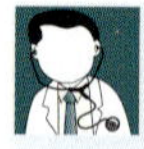

## CLINICAL CORRELATION OF CERVICAL SPINE

**Congenital Malformations**

1. See congenital malformations of the vertebral column described in chapter 24.
2. The two halves of the neural arch may fail to fuse in the midline. This condition is called ***spina bifida***. If the gap between the neural arches is small no obvious deformity may be apparent on the surface (***spina bifida occulta:*** occult = hidden).
3. Two or more cervical vertebrae may be fused to one another resulting in a short neck (***Klippel-Feil syndrome***).
   a. The atlas vertebra may be fused to the occipital bone (***occipitalisation of atlas***).
   b. The dens may not be fused to the body of the axis vertebra.
4. See cervical spondylolisthesis, below.
5. Congenital torticolis: See infantile torticolis, below.

**Other Correlations**

1. In the condition called infantile torticolis, the mastoid process of one side is pulled towards the sternoclavicular joint of the same side (i.e., the two attachments of the sternocleidomastoid are pulled towards each other).
   a. As a result the head is tilted to one side and rotated to the opposite side.
   b. The condition (previously regarded as congenital) is now believed to be a result of injury to the sternocleidomastoid muscle during birth, and its gradual fibrosis.
   c. The altered position of the neck leads to deformity of cervical vertebrae that may become wedge shaped.
   d. The face can also become asymmetrical.
   e. The torticolis is often preceeded by a swelling (tumour) on the sternocleidomastoid.
2. Degenerative changes taking place in the cervical spine, with age, often lead to stiffness and pain in the neck (***cervical spondylosis***).
   a. The intervertebral joints undergo inflammation that is associated with the formation of bony outgrowths (osteophytes).
   b. The outgrowths can encroach on intervertebral foramina narrowing them so that cervical nerves may be pressed upon.
   c. Such pressure (accentuated by the presence of oedema) can lead to pain that often radiates into the upper limb.
3. Prolapse of an intervertebral disc can occur in the cervical region. The symptoms are similar to those of cervical spondylosis.
4. Cervical vertebrae can be dislocated or fractured by falls on the head. This is because such falls cause acute flexion of the neck.

5. a. In the thoracic and lumbar regions of the vertebral column adjoining vertebrae are maintained in position by close interlocking of the articular processes. Dislocation of the vertebral column can take place only after fracture of the articular processes.
   b. However, in the cervical region the articular surfaces are flat and almost horizontal, so that dislocation is possible without fracture.
   c. Dislocation and fracture of the vertebral column are very serious because of damage to the spinal cord.
   d. In death by hanging, the dens (of the axis) dislocates backwards (by tearing through the transverse ligament of the atlas), and crushes the lower medulla and the spinal cord. Sometimes there is fracture of the axis vertebra.
6. A cervical vertebra (usually the atlas) may slip forwards over the next vertebra even in the absence of injury (***cervical spondylolisthesis***). This may be caused:
   a. By failure of the dens to fuse with the body of the axis.
   b. By weakness of the transverse ligament of the atlas caused by inflammation.

## THE SKULL

1. The skull forms the skeleton of the head. It is a difficult part of the skeleton to study as there is a very large number of named features on it, and many of these are difficult to identify.
2. Here we will confine ourselves only to the most important features. Students interested in further details and more illustrations should see the author's HUMAN OSTEOLOGY.
3. As the skull is rounded we have to examine it from all sides. For the same reason many features are seen from more than one side.
4. The bone forming the lower jaw is called the ***mandible***.
5. The other bones of the skull are firmly united to one another at joints called ***sutures***. These bones collectively form the ***cranium***. (Cranium = skull minus mandible).
6. The cranium consists of two main parts:
   a. Its upper and posterior part contains a large ***cranial cavity*** in which the brain lies.
   b. Anteriorly, and inferiorly, the cranium forms the skeleton of the face including the walls of the ***orbits*** (in which the eyeballs lie), the cavity of the nose, and the upper part of the cavity of the mouth.

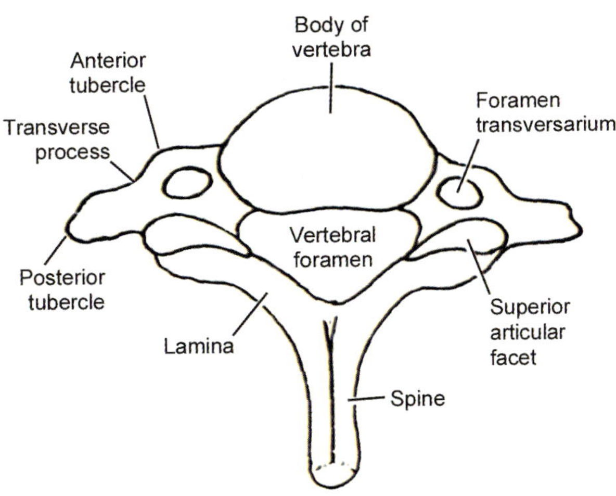


**36.6:** Seventh cervical vertebra seen from above

7. The upper dome-like part of the skull is called the ***vault*** or ***skull-cap***. It forms the upper, lateral, anterior and posterior walls of the cranial cavity. Note that its anterior wall forms the forehead.
8. The part of the skull forming the floor of the cranial cavity is called the ***base***.

## Skull Seen from Above

Looking at the skull from above (36.7) we see four bones.

1. The bone forming the anterior part of the vault is the ***frontal bone***.
2. The greater part of the roof and side walls of the cranial cavity are formed by the right and left ***parietal bones***.
   a. The two parietal bones meet in the midline at the ***sagittal suture***.
   b. Their anterior margins join the frontal bone at the ***coronal suture*** that runs transversely across the vault.
3. The posterior part of the vault is formed by the ***occipital bone***. The occipital bone is joined to the parietal bone at the ***lambdoid suture***. It is so called as it is shaped like the Greek letter 'lambda' (that is like an inverted 'Y').
4. The point where the coronal and sagittal sutures meet is called the ***bregma***, while the point where the sagittal suture meets the lambdoid suture is called the ***lambda***.
5. In the fetal skull (and for a few months after birth) there are gaps in the bones of the skull in these situations, these being filled by membranes. These gaps are called the ***anterior*** and ***posterior fontanelles***.
6. Examination of the parietal bone shows that in one area it is more convex than at other places. This area is called the ***parietal tuber*** (or ***parietal eminence***).

## Skull Seen from Behind

When we view the skull from behind we see many features seen from the top (36.8).

1. Now we see more of the occipital bone, and lateral to it we see a small part of the temporal bone.
2. Near the middle of the occipital bone we see a median projection called the ***external occipital protuberance***.
3. Extending laterally from the protuberance we see a curved ridge called the ***superior nuchal line***.

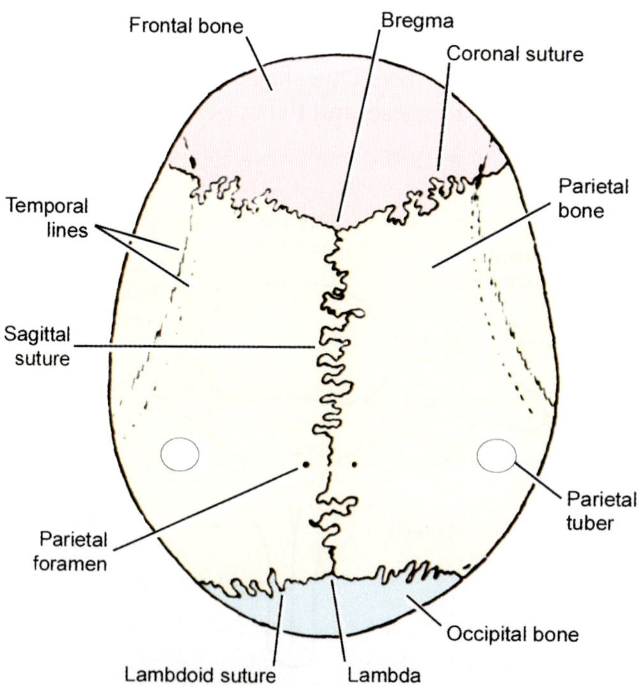


**36.7:** Skull viewed from above

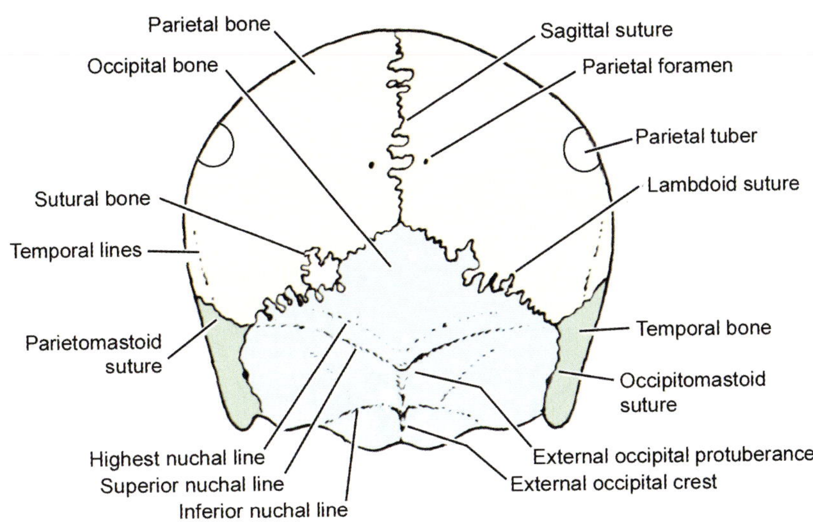


**36.8:** Features seen on the skull when viewed from behind

4. Extending downwards (and forwards) from the protuberance we see a median ridge called the ***external occipital crest***.
5. Extending laterally from the crest we see the ***inferior nuchal line***.
6. A little above the superior nuchal lines we see the ***highest nuchal lines*** (running parallel to the former).

## Skull Seen from the Front

The skull is viewed from the front in figure 36.9A. (The mandible is not included).

1. The region of the forehead is formed by the anterior part of the frontal bone. A small part of the parietal bone can be seen lateral to the frontal bone.
2. Just below the frontal bone we see the opening into the orbit (shaded grey).
3. Lateral to the orbit we see a part of the temporal bone (purple) and the zygomatic bone (blue).
4. Inferior to the orbit there is the maxilla (upper jaw) bearing the upper teeth.
5. Near the middle line we see the nasal aperture that leads into the nasal cavity.
6. Just above the nasal aperture we see the right and left nasal bones.

Some other features to be seen on the front of the skull are as follows:

1. A little above the orbit the frontal bone is more convex than elsewhere. This area is the ***frontal eminence***.
2. The upper margin of the orbit is formed by the frontal bone. Near its medial end the margin shows the ***supraorbital notch***. Medial to it, there is a smaller ***frontal notch*** (or foramen).
3. The lateral margin of the orbit is formed by the ***zygomatic process of the frontal bone***, above; and by the ***frontal process of the zygomatic bone***, below.
4. The medial margin of the orbit is formed by the ***nasal process of the frontal bone***, above; and by the ***frontal process of the maxilla***, inferiorly.
5. The inferior margin of the orbit is formed by the zygomatic bone that is joined by the ***zygomatic process of the maxilla***.
6. A little below the orbital margin, the anterior surface of the maxilla shows the ***infraorbital foramen***. On the lateral surface of the zygomatic bone we see a ***zygomaticofacial foramen***.
7. Through the nasal aperture we can see some bones that lie within the nasal cavity. In the midline note the ***ethmoid bone*** and the ***vomer***. These form part of the ***nasal septum***. Laterally we see two curved plates, the ***middle and inferior nasal conchae*** projecting into the nasal cavity.

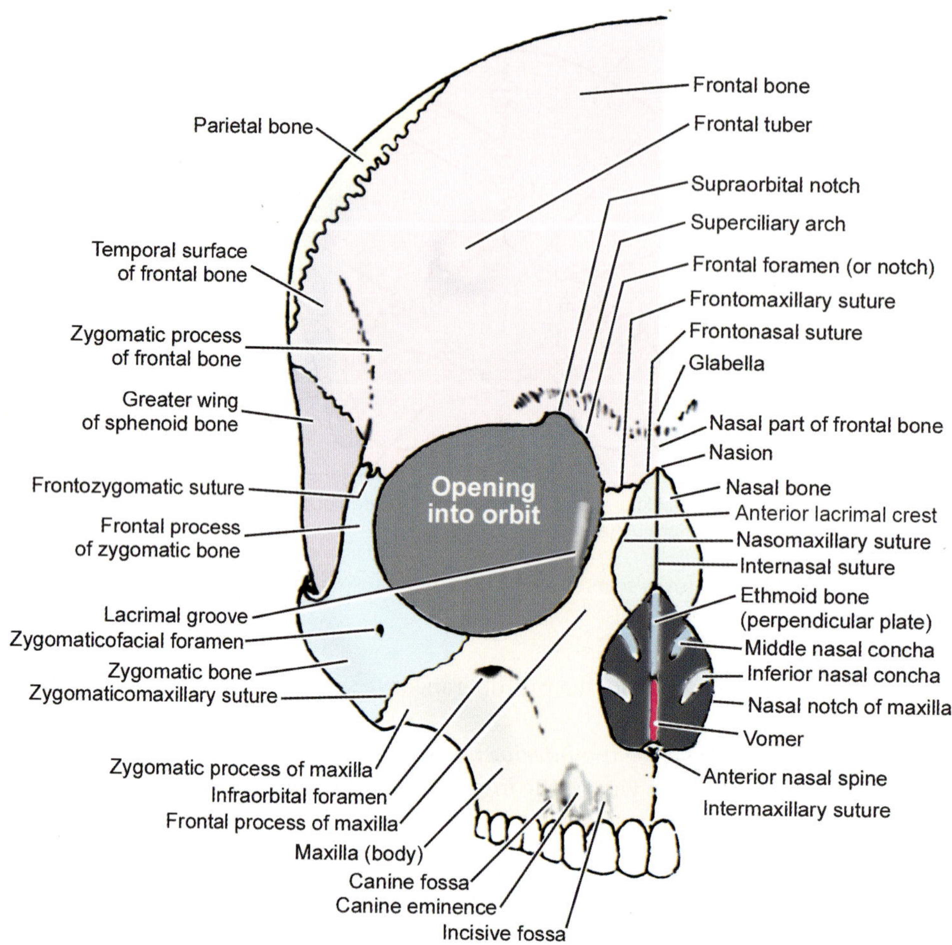


**36.9A:** Skull seen from the front

8. Each maxilla bears eight ***teeth***. Beginning from the midline there are:
   a. Two incisors
   b. One canine
   c. Two premolars
   d. Three molars.
9. The part of the maxilla that bears the teeth is called the ***alveolar process***.

## The Orbit

The interior of the orbit is shown in 36.9B. Confirm the facts mentioned above, about the orbital margin.

### *Walls of the Orbit*

1. Each orbit is shaped like a pyramid. The orbital opening represents the base of the pyramid, while the apex lies at the posterior end.
2. The orbit has a roof, a floor, a medial wall and a lateral wall; but these are not sharply marked off from one another.
3. a. The ***roof*** is formed mainly by the orbital plate of the frontal bone.
   b. Posteriorly, a small part of the roof is formed by the lesser wing of the sphenoid.

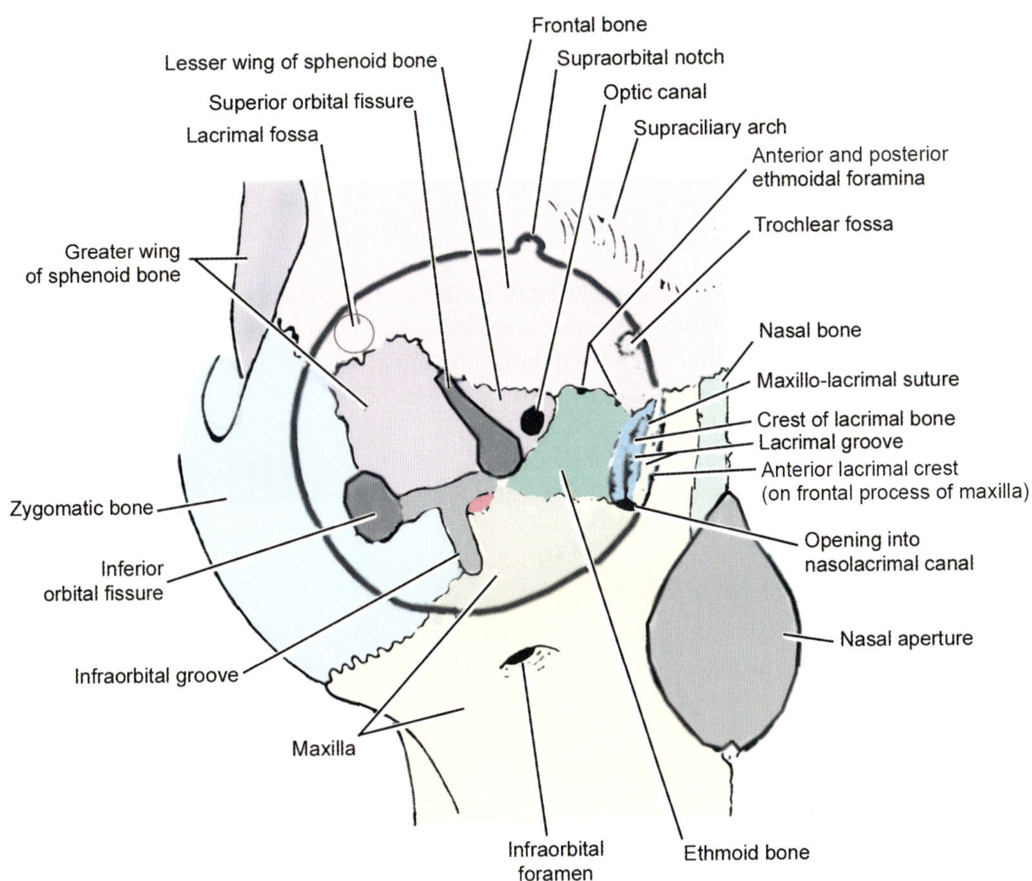


**36.9B:** Orbit and surrounding structures

c. The anterolateral part of the roof has a depression called the lacrimal fossa.
d. Close to the orbital margin, at the junction of the roof and medial wall, there is a small depression called the trochlear fossa.

4. a. The ***floor*** is formed mainly by the maxilla. (This part of the maxilla is its orbital surface).
   b. The anterolateral part of the floor is formed by the zygomatic bone.
5. The ***lateral wall*** is formed–
   a. In its anterior part by the zygomatic bone.
   b. In its posterior part by the greater wing of the sphenoid.
6. a. The ***medial wall*** is formed mainly by the orbital plate of the ethmoid.
   b. Anterior to the ethmoid the medial wall is formed by the lacrimal bone, and by the frontal process of the maxilla.
   c. The region of the medial wall formed by the lacrimal bone and by the maxilla shows a deep ***lacrimal groove*** (for the lacrimal sac). The groove is continuous, inferiorly, with the ***nasolacrimal canal***, the lower end of which opens into the nasal cavity.

### *Apertures in the Orbit*

1. The ***superior orbital fissure*** is a prominent cleft that separates the posterior parts of the roof and lateral wall. It is bounded above and medially by the lesser wing of the sphenoid, and below and laterally by the greater wing.
2. Medial to the superior orbital fissure, at the apex of the orbit, there is the opening of the ***optic canal***.

3. The ***inferior orbital fissure*** intervenes between the posterior parts of the floor and the lateral wall of the orbit.
   a. It is bounded above and laterally by the greater wing of the sphenoid.
   b. Below and medially by the orbital surface of the maxilla.
4. The fissure is continuous anteriorly with the ***infraorbital groove*** on the maxilla. Anteriorly, the groove ends in a canal that passes through the bony substance of the maxilla to open on its surface through the ***infraorbital foramen***.

## Skull Seen from Lateral Side

1. First identify the various bones seen in 36.10. Most of them have already been seen from other aspects.
   a. Identify the frontal bone forming the region of the forehead.
   b. The parietal bone forming the vault behind the frontal bone.
   c. The occipital bone at the posterior end of the skull.
   d. The maxilla bearing the upper teeth.
   e. Below the parietal bone we see the temporal bone.
   f. Just in front of the temporal bone we see the greater wing of the sphenoid bone, and further anteriorly we see the zygomatic bone.

*Additional features to be identified are as follows:*

2. Running across the frontal, parietal and temporal bones we see two C-shaped ***temporal lines***.
   a. Anteriorly, there is only one line, but over the parietal bone superior and inferior lines can be distinguished.

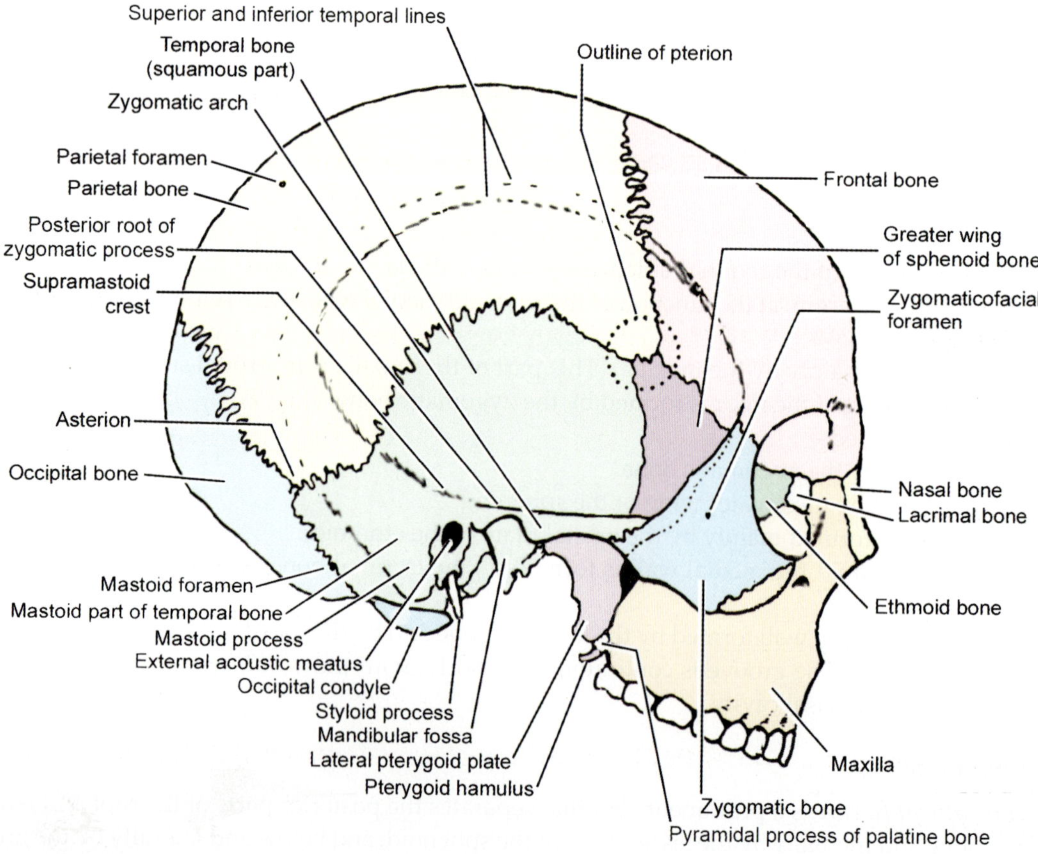


**36.10:** Skull seen from lateral side

   b. At its anterior end the temporal line becomes continuous with the sharp lateral edge of the zygomatic process of the frontal bone.
   c. The superior temporal line fades away over the posterior part of the parietal bone.
   d. The inferior line curves forwards and reaches the zygomatic arch (see below).
3. The oval area enclosed by the temporal line is called the ***temporal fossa***. Its floor is formed by:
   a. The temporal bone
   b. The parietal bone
   c. The frontal bones
   d. The greater wing of the sphenoid bone.
4. These four bones meet within a small area (shown as a circle) that is called the ***pterion***.
5. The ***zygomatic arch*** is a bar of bone lying horizontally over the lateral aspect of the skull. There is a gap between it and the floor of the temporal fossa.
   a. The posterior part of the arch is formed by the zygomatic process of the temporal bone.
   b. The anterior part by the temporal process of the zygomatic bone.
6. Just below the posterior end of the zygomatic arch there is a large oval aperture. This is the ***external acoustic meatus***. It leads into the ear.
   a. The meatus is surrounded by a plate of bone with an irregular surface.
   b. This plate belongs to the tympanic part of the temporal bone.
7. Just behind the external acoustic meatus there is a thick downward projection called the ***mastoid process***. This process forms the mastoid part of the temporal bone.
8. A little below the external acoustic meatus there is a pin-like process directed downwards and forwards. This is the ***styloid process***, which is also a part of the temporal bone.
9. Running medially into the base of the skull (seen from below) we see yet another part of the temporal bone. This is called the ***petrous part***, as it is stone like.
10. The greater part of the ear lies within the petrous part of the temporal bone.
11. A little in front of the external acoustic meatus there is a depression, the ***mandibular fossa***, into which the head of the mandible fits, to form the ***temporomandibular joint***.
12. The shape of the ***zygomatic bone*** is best appreciated from the lateral side.
    a. Note its articulations with the frontal bone, the temporal bone and the maxilla.
    b. In addition to the lateral surface the bone also has a temporal surface directed towards the temporal fossa.
13. When we view the skull from the lateral side we see some parts of the ***sphenoid bone***.
    a. The greater part of the bone lies in the base of the skull. Here we see the ***greater wing*** forming part of the floor of the temporal fossa. (We have already seen that the greater wing takes part in forming the lateral wall of the orbit).
    b. Another part of the sphenoid bone that is seen from the lateral side is the ***pterygoid process***, which is made up of medial and lateral ***pterygoid plates***. The pterygoid process comes into contact with the posterior aspect of the maxilla.
14. The ***infratemporal fossa*** is a space that lies lateral to the pterygoid process.
    a. Its roof is formed by the infratemporal surface of the greater wing of the sphenoid.
    b. The infratemporal fossa communicates with the temporal fossa through the gap between the zygomatic arch and the side of the skull.
    c. The anterior wall of the infratemporal fossa is formed by the posterior surface of the maxilla.

### Skull Seen from below (Base of Skull)

1. When the skull is viewed from below (36.11) we see parts of several bones already identified. These are:
   a. The maxilla (pink)
   b. The sphenoid bone (purple)
   c. The temporal bone (green)
   d. The occipital bone (blue)

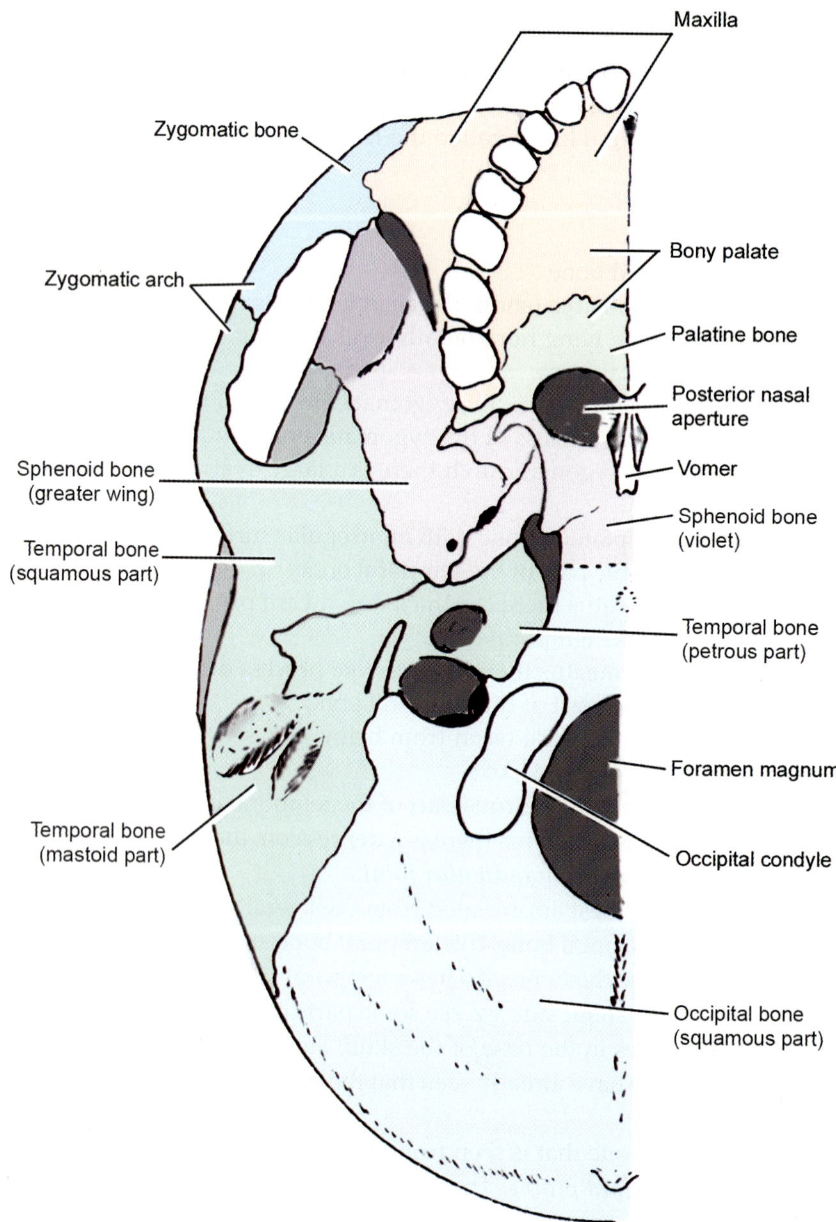


**36.11:** Skull as seen from below

   e. We also see parts of the zygomatic bone of the vomer.
   f. The palatine bone (yellow) that is seen for the first time.
2. The maxillae bear the upper teeth.
   a. Lateral to the teeth a part of the maxilla is seen articulating with the zygomatic bone.
   b. Medial to the teeth the maxilla forms the anterior part of the bony palate.
   c. The posterior part of the palate is formed by the right and left ***palatine bones***.
   d. Above the posterior edge of the palate we see the posterior openings of the right and left nasal cavities that are separated by the vomer.

3. Behind the vomer we see the sphenoid, which is an unpaired bone.
   a. It has a median part, the body.
   b. On either side of the body, there is a greater wing (that is seen partly on the base of the skull and partly on the lateral wall).
4. Posteriorly, the body of the sphenoid is continuous with the basilar part of the occipital bone.
5. Just behind the basilar part the occipital bone has a large foramen, the ***foramen magnum*** through which the cranial cavity communicates with the vertebral canal.
6. Posterior to the foramen magnum the occipital bone forms a large part of the base of the skull.
7. The lateral part of the base of the skull is formed by the temporal bone that is wedged in between the sphenoid and occipital bones. Portions of the petrous part, the squamous part and the mastoid part of the temporal are seen on the base of the skull.
8. The zygomatic arch is seen from below. Note the gap between it and the side of the skull.

   We shall now examine the features to be seen on each of these bones when the skull is viewed from below.

*Note the following in 36.12:*

1. a. The alveolar process of the maxilla projects downwards and provides attachment to the upper teeth.
   b. The posterior end of each alveolar process forms a backward projection called the ***maxillary tuberosity***.
   c. Within the concavity of the arch formed by the alveolar process we see the ***bony palate*** that separates the nasal cavities (above) from the cavity of the mouth (below).
   d. The anterior part of the palate is formed by the ***palatal processes*** of the right and left maxillae.
   e. The part of the alveolar process bearing the incisor teeth, and including the adjoining part of the palate is called the ***pre-maxilla***.
2. Lateral to the alveolar arch we see the inferior aspect of the ***zygomatic process*** of the maxilla as it passes laterally to meet the zygomatic bone.

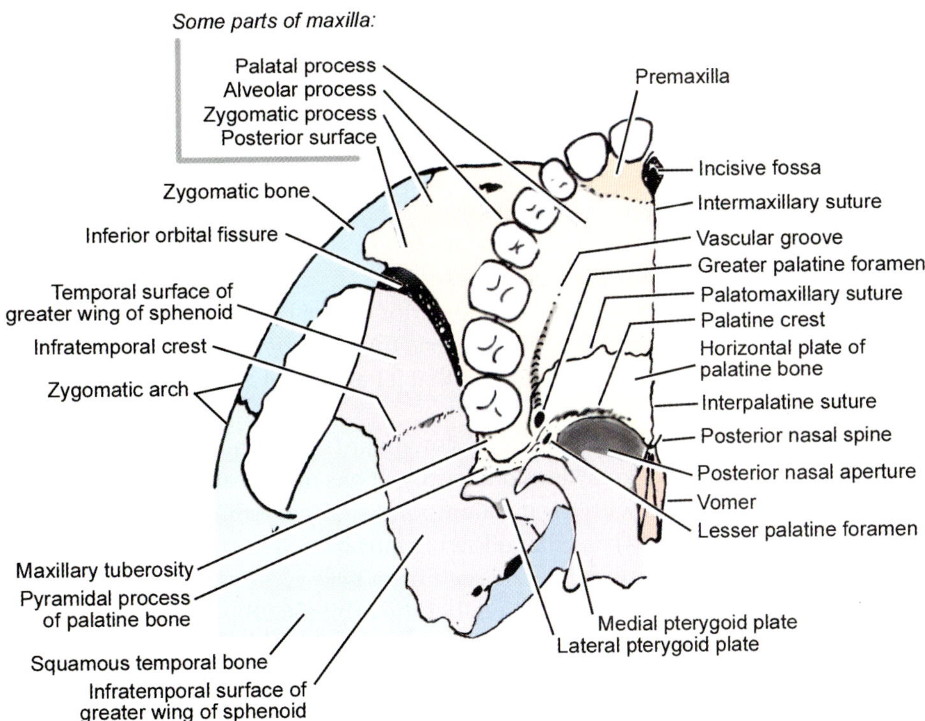


**36.12:** Anterior part of skull seen from below

3. We also see the posterior surface of the maxilla that is separated (posterolaterally) from the greater wing of the sphenoid by the ***inferior orbital fissure***.
4. The posterior part of the palate is formed by the ***palatine bones***.
   a. This part of each palatine bone is called the ***horizontal plate***.
   b. The posterior borders of the horizontal plates of the palatine bones are free and form the posterior margin of the hard palate.
   c. A little in front of the posterior border we see a curved ridge called the ***palatine crest***.
5. The part of the palate formed by the palatine bone shows the ***greater*** and ***lesser palatine foramina***.
   a. The greater palatine foramen lies on the most lateral part of the horizontal plate, just medial to the last molar tooth. It is the lower opening of the canal of the same name.
   b. The lesser palatine foramina, usually two, are present just behind the greater palatine foramen.
6. Just above the posterior margin of the hard palate there are two ***posterior nasal apertures***.
   a. Each aperture is bounded, below, by the posterior edge of the horizontal plate of the palatine bone.
   b. The lateral wall of the aperture is formed by another part of the palatine bone that is called the ***perpendicular plate***.
   c. The perpendicular plate of the palatine bone and the ***medial pterygoid plate*** of the sphenoid bone together form the lateral wall of the region where the nose and pharynx meet.
7. The vomer is a flat plate of bone that forms part of the nasal septum. It has been seen through the anterior nasal aperture (36.9A).

*Note the following features to be seen on the sphenoid bone in 36.12 to 36.14.*

1. The sphenoid bone is large, extending across the entire width of the base of the skull and extending also onto the lateral wall of the vault.
2. It is made up of several parts that have already been encountered. These are:
   a. The body (that is median in position).
   b. The right and left greater and lesser wings.
   c. The right and left pterygoid processes.
3. When viewed from below the body of the sphenoid is seen in the roof of the posterior part of the nasal cavity and of the adjoining nasopharynx.
4. Posteriorly, the body of the sphenoid is directly continuous with the basilar part (or body) of the occipital bone.
5. The pterygoid process projects downwards from the junction of the body of the sphenoid with the greater wing.
   a. It consists of ***medial*** and ***lateral pterygoid plates***.
   b. These plates meet anteriorly, but posteriorly they are free.
   c. The space between them is called the ***pterygoid fossa***.
   d. Anteriorly, the pterygoid process is fused to the posterior aspect of the maxilla in its middle part.
   e. Higher up it is separated from the maxilla by the ***pterygomaxillary fissure***.
6. a. The medial pterygoid plate is directed backwards so that it has medial and lateral surfaces, and a free posterior border.
   b. The lower end of the posterior border is prolonged downwards and laterally to form the ***pterygoid hamulus***.
7. The lateral pterygoid plate projects backwards and laterally. It has medial and lateral surfaces. At its upper end its lateral surface becomes continuous with the infratemporal surface of the greater wing (36.13 and 36.14).
8. The greater wing of the sphenoid (36.14) has the following surfaces:
   a. The infratemporal and temporal surfaces can be seen from below.
   b. The orbital surface has been seen in the lateral wall of the orbit (36.9B).
9. a. The anterior margin of the infratemporal surface of the sphenoid bone is separated from the maxilla by the inferior orbital fissure.
   b. Laterally, the infratemporal surface is separated from the temporal surface by the ***infratemporal crest***.
   c. The posterior margin of the lateral part of the infratemporal surface articulates with the infratemporal surface of the squamous part of the temporal bone.

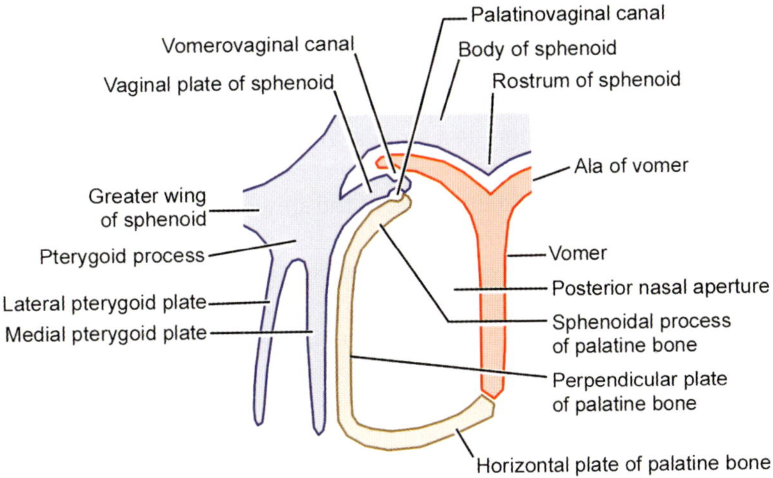


**36.13:** Schematic coronal section to show relationship of pterygoid process to the rest of the sphenoid bone

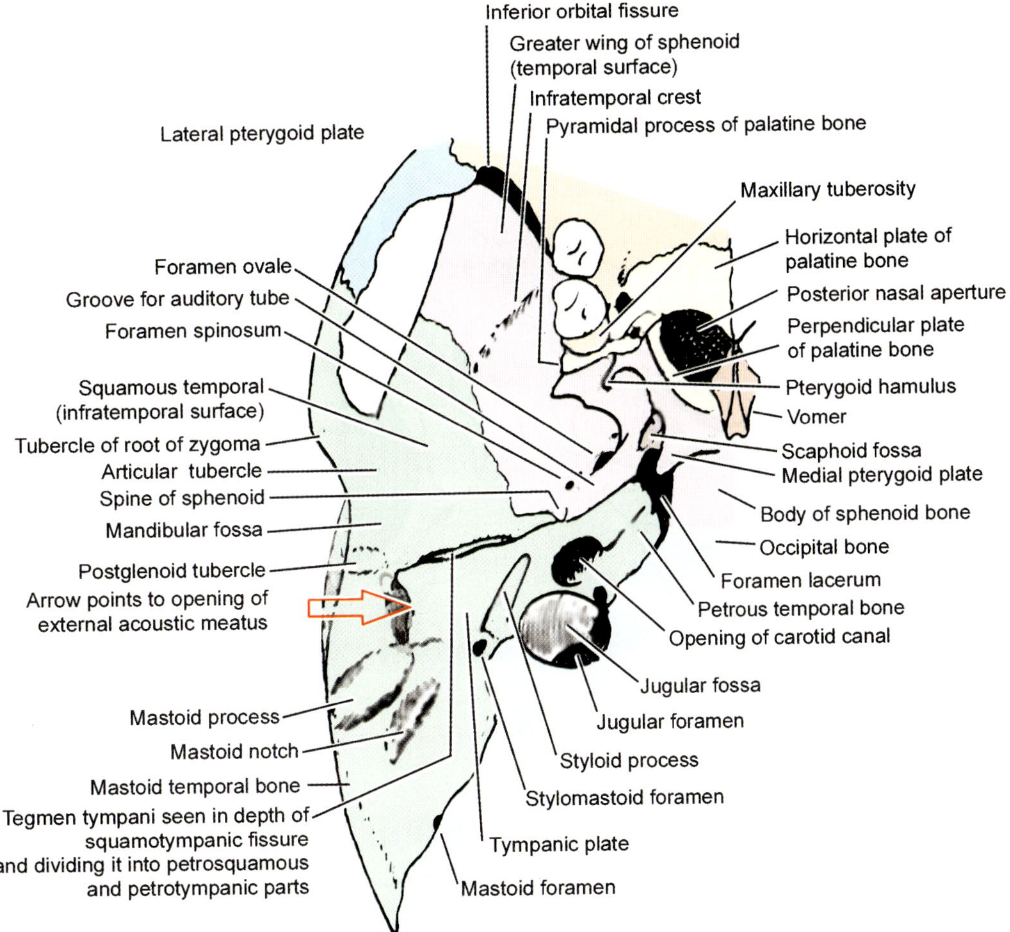


**36.14:** Part of base of skull formed by temporal and sphenoid bones

10. Medially, the infratemporal surface of the greater wing is continuous with the body of the sphenoid.
11. Posteriorly, the greater wing meets the anterior margin of the petrous temporal bone.
12. Two important foramina are seen near the posterior border of the greater wing.
    a. The ***foramen ovale*** lies posterolateral to the upper end of the lateral pterygoid plate.
    b. Posterolateral to the foramen ovale there is a smaller round foramen called the ***foramen spinosum***. It is so called because it lies just in front of a downward projection called the ***spine of the sphenoid***.
13. a. Posteromedial to these foramina, and to the spine of the sphenoid, the posterior margin of the greater wing forms the anterior wall of a prominent groove.
    b. The posterior wall of this groove is formed by the petrous temporal bone.
    c. The two bones meet in the floor of the groove that is meant for the cartilaginous part of the ***auditory tube***.
    d. Traced laterally, the groove ends in relation to the opening of the bony part of the auditory tube.

### *Additional Features on the Temporal Bone*

Additional features on the temporal bone are illustrated in 36.14 and 36.15

1. The squamous part of the temporal bone has a ***temporal surface*** that has been seen from the lateral aspect. Part of it can be seen from below.
2. Inferior and medial to the temporal surface, the squamous part of the temporal bone has an ***infratemporal surface*** that takes part in forming the roof of the infratemporal fossa (along with the infratemporal surface of the greater wing of the sphenoid).

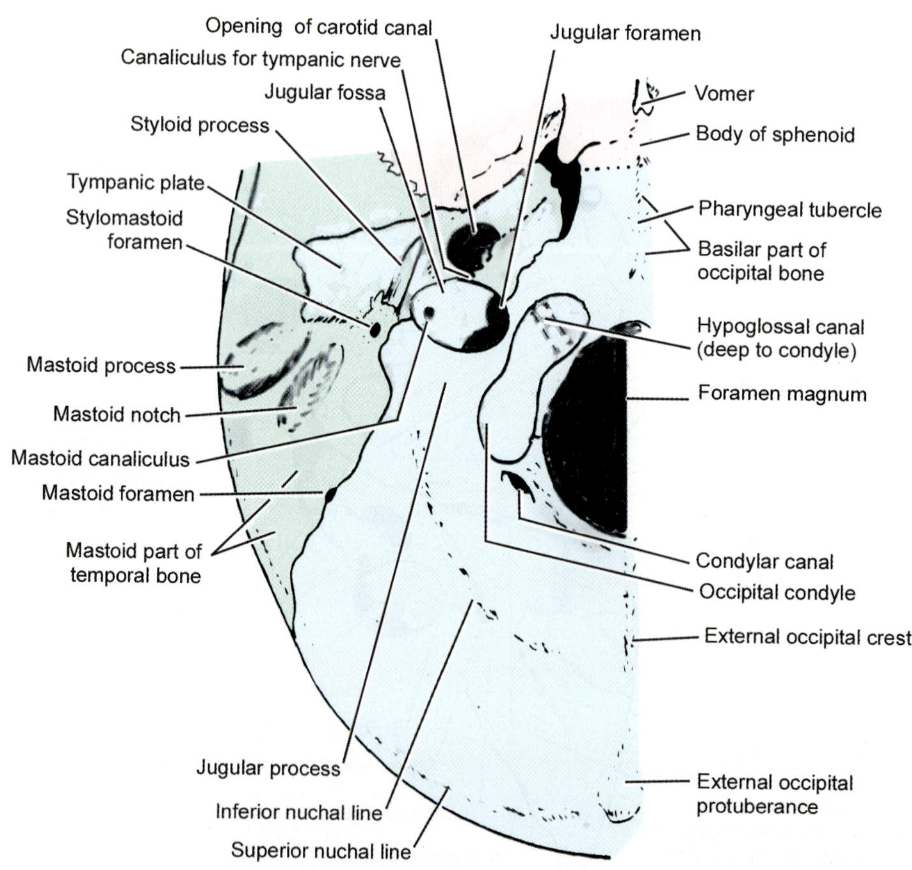


**36.15:** Posterior part of the base of the skull formed by the temporal and occipital bones

3. Behind its infratemporal surface, the squamous part of the temporal bone bears the ***mandibular fossa***.
   a. This fossa is bounded anteriorly by a rounded eminence called the ***articular tubercle***.
   b. The ***articular area for the mandible*** extends onto the tubercle.
4. The tympanic plate separates the mandibular fossa from the external acoustic meatus. (The arrow in figure 36.14 points to the opening of the meatus that cannot be seen from below).
5. The junction of the mandibular fossa (squamous part of temporal bone) with the tympanic plate is marked by the ***squamotympanic fissure***.
6. Projecting through the fissure we sometimes see the lower edge of a plate of bone called the ***tegmen tympani***.
7. The posterior part of the tympanic plate partially surrounds the base of the ***styloid process***.
8. The petrous part of the temporal bone runs forwards and medially between the greater wing of the sphenoid (anterolaterally), and the occipital bone (posteromedially).
   a. Its apex is separated from the body of the sphenoid, the root of the pterygoid process, and the basilar part of the occipital bone by a very irregular aperture called the ***foramen lacerum***.
   b. The inferior surface of the petrous temporal bone is marked by a large round aperture. This is the lower opening of the ***carotid canal*** through which the internal carotid artery enters the cranial cavity.
   c. The canal passes medially, through the substance of the petrous temporal bone and opens into the posterior wall of the foramen lacerum.
9. Behind the opening of the carotid canal there is another large depression, the ***jugular fossa***. This fossa leads posteriorly into the ***jugular foramen***. This foramen is bounded posteriorly and below by the occipital bone, and opens into the posterior cranial fossa.
10. In the mastoid part of the temporal bone we have already noted the presence of the mastoid process.
   a. Medial to the mastoid process there is a deep ***mastoid notch***.
   b. Near the anterior end of the notch, and just behind the styloid process we see the ***stylomastoid foramen***.

### *Additional Features on the Occipital Bone*

The greater part of the occipital bone is seen when the skull is viewed from below.

1. The most conspicuous feature on it is the large ***foramen magnum*** through which the cranial cavity communicates with the vertebral canal.
2. The part of the bone anterior to the foramen magnum is the ***basilar part***.
   a. Anteriorly, the basilar part of the occipital bone is directly continuous with the body of the sphenoid bone.
   b. These two bones are separated by a plate of cartilage in the young, but fuse with each other in the adult.
3. The parts of the occipital bone lateral to each side of the foramen magnum are its lateral (or ***condylar***) parts. Here we see the prominent ***occipital condyles***.
   a. Each condyle (right or left) articulates with the corresponding superior articular facet on the atlas vertebra to form an ***atlanto-occipital joint***.
   b. There are two canals closely related to the occipital condyles.
   c. The ***hypoglossal*** (or anterior condylar) ***canal*** opens on the surface of the skull just above the lateral border of the anterior part of the condyle, and is hidden from view by the condyle. The canal runs backwards to open into the posterior cranial fossa.
   d. Behind the condyle there is a depression, the ***condylar fossa*** in which the opening of the ***posterior condylar canal*** is sometimes seen.
4. a. The part of the occipital bone lateral to the condyle is called the ***jugular process***.
   b. It forms the posterior (and inferior) wall of the jugular fossa and foramen.
   c. The ***jugular foramen*** passes backwards and medially from the fossa. It is often partially divided into anterior, middle and posterior parts.
5. The part of the occipital bone behind the foramen magnum is the ***squamous part***.
   a. Posteriorly, the squamous part forms the posterior part of the vault of the skull.
   b. Its external surface is marked by:
      i. The external occipital protuberance.
      ii. The external occipital crest.

iii. The inferior, superior and highest nuchal lines.
iv. Numerous unnamed ridges that give it a rough surface for muscular attachments.

## The Cranial Fossae

1. When the top of the skull (skull cap) is removed by a transverse cut we can view the floor of the cranial cavity.
2. It is seen to be divided into three depressions called the ***cranial fossae***, anterior, middle, and posterior.

### *Anterior Cranial Fossa*

1. a. The floor of the anterior cranial fossa (36.16) is formed mainly by the orbital plates (right and left) of the frontal bone.
   b. Anteriorly, the right and left halves of the frontal bone are separated by a median projection called the ***frontal crest***.
   c. Just behind the crest there is a depression called the ***foramen caecum***.
2. Between the right and left orbital plates of the frontal bone there is a notch occupied by the ***cribriform plate of the ethmoid bone***.
   a. This plate has numerous foramina.
   b. It also bears a median vertical projection called the ***crista galli*** that lies immediately behind the foramen caecum.
3. The posterior part of the floor of the anterior cranial fossa is formed by the sphenoid bone. This part is called the ***jugum sphenoidale.***
   a. In the median part it is formed by the anterior part of the superior surface of the body of the sphenoid.
   b. Laterally, the floor is formed by the ***lesser wing*** of the sphenoid.

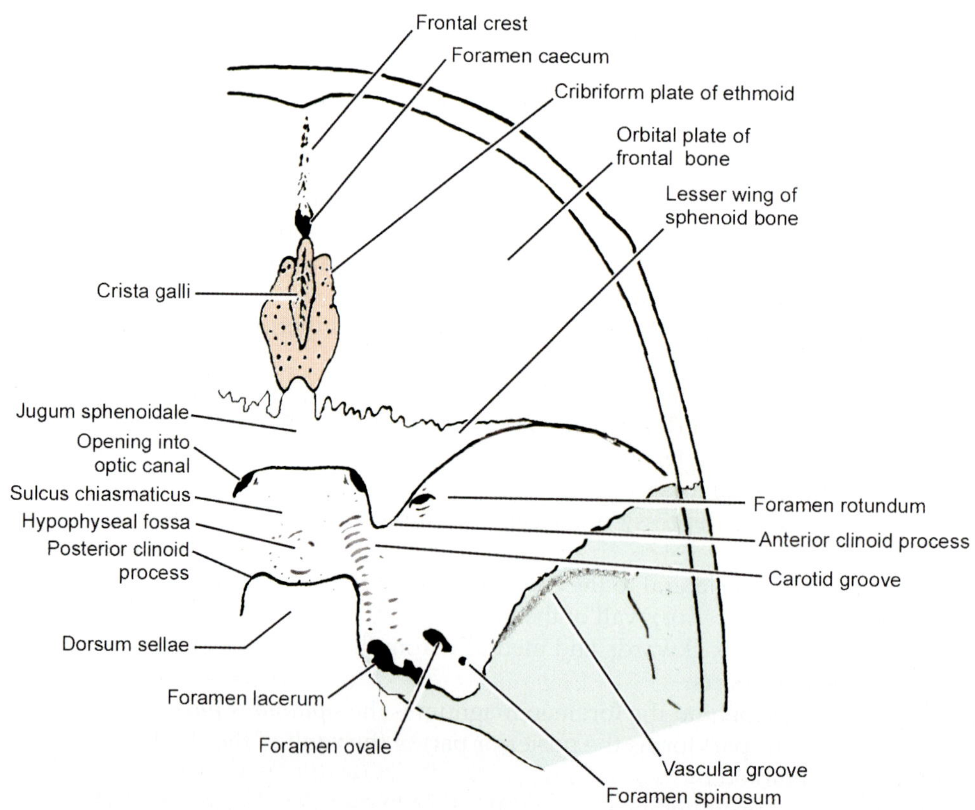


**36.16:** Parts of the anterior and middle cranial fossae seen from above

c. The lesser wing also forms the sharp posterior edge of the floor of the anterior cranial fossa.
d. The medial edge of each lesser wing projects backwards as the ***anterior clinoid process***.

### *Middle cranial fossa*

1. The middle cranial fossa (36.16 and 36.17) has a raised median part formed by the body of the sphenoid bone, and two large deep hollow areas on either side.
2. The features to be seen in relation to the body of the sphenoid are as follows:
   a. Immediately behind the jugum sphenoidale the body of the sphenoid is crossed by a transverse shallow groove that connects the two optic canals. It is called the ***sulcus chiasmaticus*** (even though the optic chiasma does not lie over the sulcus).
   b. Behind the sulcus the superior surface of the body of the sphenoid shows a median elevation, the ***tuberculum sellae***; and behind the tuberculum there is a depression called the ***hypophyseal fossa***.
   c. Posterior to the hypophyseal fossa there is a vertical plate of bone called the ***dorsum sellae***.
   d. The deep hollow bounded anteriorly by the tuberculum sellae, and posteriorly by the dorsum sellae is called the ***sella turcica***.

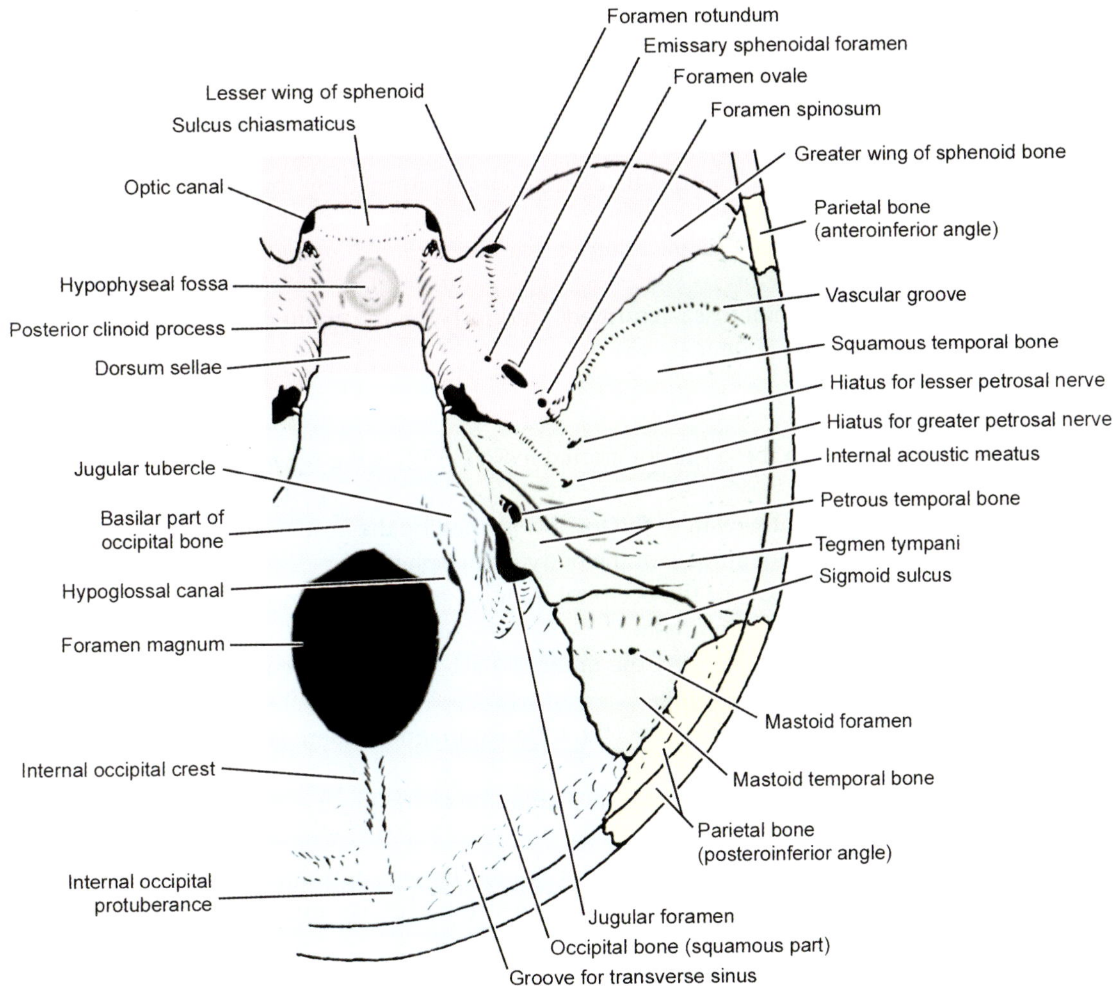


**36.17:** Floor of middle and posterior cranial fossae

   e. The superolateral angles of the dorsum sellae are called the ***posterior clinoid processes.***
   f. On each side the body of the sphenoid slopes downwards into the floor of the deep lateral part of the middle cranial fossa. In this situation each side of the body of the sphenoid is marked by a shallow ***carotid groove.***
   g. Posteriorly, the carotid groove becomes continuous with the foramen lacerum.
   h. Anteriorly, the carotid groove turns upwards medial to the anterior clinoid process.
3. On either side, the anterior wall of the middle cranial fossa is formed by the greater and lesser wings of the sphenoid.
   a. The lesser wings are attached to the sides of the body of the sphenoid by two roots; anterior (or upper), and posterior (or lower).
   b. The optic canal passes forwards and laterally between the body of the sphenoid and the two roots of the lesser wing.
   c. The greater and lesser wings are separated by the ***superior orbital fissure*** that leads into the orbit.
   d. Just below the medial end of this fissure, and just lateral to the carotid groove we see the ***foramen rotundum.*** This foramen opens anteriorly into the pterygopalatine fossa.
4. The posterior wall of the middle cranial fossa is formed, on either side, by the anterior sloping surface of the petrous temporal bone.
   a. The apex of the bone is separated from the body of the sphenoid by the ***foramen lacerum*** already seen from below.
   b. A little above and lateral to the foramen the surface of the petrous temporal bone shows a shallow depression called the ***trigeminal impression.***
   c. The anterior surface of the petrous temporal bone is formed by a thin plate of bone that separates the middle cranial fossa from the cavities of the middle ear, the auditory tube and the mastoid antrum. This plate is called the ***tegmen tympani.***
5. The floor of the deep lateral part of the middle cranial fossa is formed by the greater wing of the sphenoid, medially, and by the squamous part of the temporal bone, laterally.
   a. Near the posterior margin of the greater wing we see the ***foramen ovale,*** and the ***foramen spinosum*** that have already been seen from below.
6. The lateral wall of the middle cranial fossa is formed, anteriorly, by the greater wing of the sphenoid, and posteriorly by the squamous temporal bone.

### *Posterior Cranial Fossa*

1. The most prominent landmark in the posterior cranial fossa (36.17) is the ***foramen magnum*** already seen from below.
2. Anterior to the foramen magnum the wall of the fossa is formed by the basilar part of the occipital bone that is continuous above with the posterior surface of the body of the sphenoid.
3. The lateral margin of the basilar part of the occipital bone is separated from the petrous temporal bone by a fissure that ends below in the jugular foramen.
4. Between the jugular foramen, laterally, and the anterior part of the foramen magnum, medially, there is a rounded elevation called the ***jugular tubercle.***
5. In the interval between the jugular tubercle and the foramen magnum there is a fossa. The ***hypoglossal canal*** opens into this fossa.
6. When present, the ***posterior condylar canal*** opens just lateral to the jugular tubercle immediately behind the jugular foramen.
7. The lateral part of the anterior wall of the posterior cranial fossa is formed by the posterior surface of the petrous temporal bone. A little above the jugular foramen this surface presents the opening of the ***internal acoustic meatus.***
8. The floor and lateral walls of the posterior cranial fossa are formed, posteriorly, by the squamous part of the occipital bone; and in the anterolateral part by the mastoid part of the temporal bone.

9. Behind the foramen magnum the two halves of the fossa are separated by a ridge called the ***internal occipital crest***.
   a. Posteriorly, the crest ends in an elevation called the ***internal occipital protuberance***.
   b. Running laterally from the protuberance, in the transverse plane, we see a prominent wide groove (***transverse sulcus***) in which the transverse sinus is lodged.
   c. The groove first lies on the occipital bone, and near its lateral (or anterior) end it crosses the posteroinferior angle of the parietal bone.
   d. It then runs downwards and medially with an S-shaped curve to reach the jugular foramen.
   e. This S-shaped part of the groove is called the ***sigmoid sulcus***.
   f. The terminal part of the groove lies on the occipital bone just behind the jugular foramen.

## Foramina of the Skull

The bones of the skull show numerous foramina, small and large. The most important foramina are those that give passage to very important structures like cranial nerves, large blood vessels, etc. These are listed below.

1. The lower end of the medulla oblongata passes through the ***foramen magnum*** to become continuous with the spinal cord. Other important structures passing through the foramen magnum are the vertebral arteries and the spinal part of the accessory nerve.
2. The internal carotid artery enters the skull by passing through the ***carotid canal***.
3. The junction of the upper end of the internal jugular vein with the sigmoid sinus lies in the ***jugular foramen***.
4. Bundles of nerve fibres that constitute the olfactory nerve pass through minute apertures in the cribriform plate of the ethmoid bone. This plate intervenes between the nasal cavity and the anterior cranial fossa.
5. The optic nerve passes from the middle cranial fossa into the orbit through the ***optic canal***.
6. The oculomotor, trochlear and abducent nerves enter the orbit through the ***superior orbital fissure***.
7. The trigeminal nerve has three divisions each of which leaves the middle cranial fossa through a different foramen.
   a. The ophthalmic division enters the orbit through the ***superior orbital fissure***.
   b. The maxillary division passes into the ***foramen rotundum***.
   c. The mandibular division passes through the ***foramen ovale*** to reach the infratemporal region.
8. The facial nerve leaves the posterior cranial fossa by passing into the ***internal acoustic meatus***. After a complicated course through the petrous part of the temporal bone, it emerges on the external surface of the skull through the ***stylomastoid foramen***.
9. The vestibulocochlear nerve leaves the posterior cranial fossa by passing through the ***internal acoustic meatus***, to reach the internal ear. The internal ear lies within the substance of the petrous part of the temporal bone.
10. The glossopharyngeal, vagus and accessory nerves leave the posterior cranial fossa through the ***jugular foramen***, to enter the neck.
11. The hypoglossal nerve leaves the posterior cranial fossa through the ***hypoglossal canal***.

## The Nasal Cavity

1. The nasal cavity consists of right and left halves that are separated by a ***nasal septum*** (36.18 and 36.19).
2. The cavity opens, anteriorly, on the front of the skull through the ***anterior nasal aperture***; and, posteriorly, on the base of the skull just above the posterior edge of the bony palate, through the right and left ***posterior nasal apertures***.
3. Each half of the cavity has a lateral wall, a medial wall formed by the nasal septum, a floor formed by the upper surface of the palate, and a roof.
4. The formation of the ***lateral wall*** is complicated and we will not go into details. The bones taking part in forming it are:
   a. The medial surface of the maxilla
   b. The palatine bone (perpendicular plate)
   c. The lacrimal bone

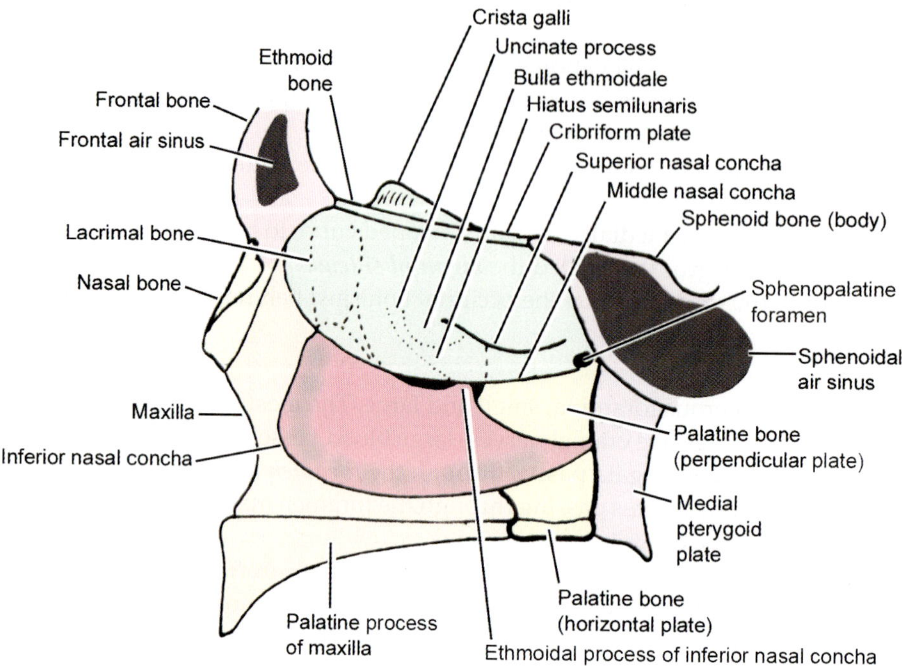


**36.18:** Lateral wall of nasal cavity

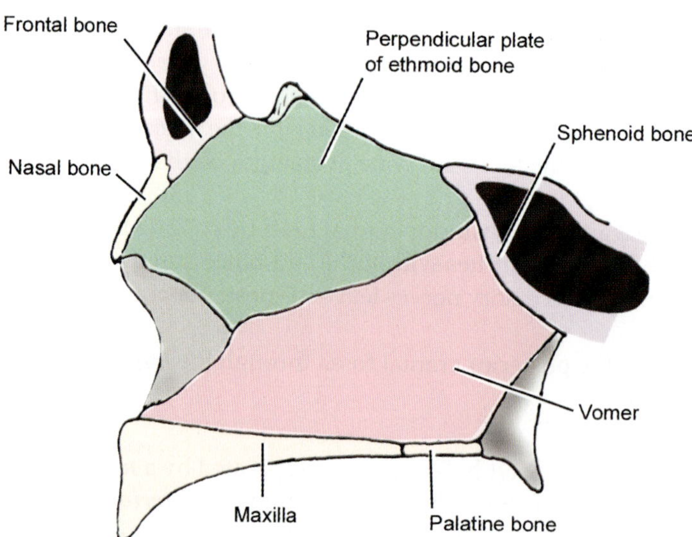


**36.19:** Main bones taking part in forming the nasal septum

   d. The inferior nasal concha
   e. The ethmoid bone.

5. The ***floor*** of the nasal cavity is formed by the upper surface of the bony palate. Each half of the palate is formed anteriorly by the palatine process of the maxilla, and posteriorly by the horizontal plate of the palatine bone.

6. Several bones take part in forming the *roof* of the nasal cavity. From front to back these are parts of:
   a. The nasal bone
   b. The frontal bone
   c. The cribriform plate of the ethmoid
   d. The anterior surface of the body of the sphenoid bone.
7. The ***medial wall*** or ***nasal septum*** (36.19) is formed as follows:
   a. Its upper part is formed by the perpendicular plate of the ethmoid bone.
   b. Its lower part is formed by the vomer.
   c. Anteriorly, there is a gap in the septum that is filled in by cartilage.
   d. Around the edges of the septum there are small contributions to the septum from the nasal, frontal, sphenoid, maxillary and palatine bones.
8. The openings into the nasal cavity are described along with those of the paranasal sinuses (see below).

## The Paranasal Sinuses

1. The paranasal sinuses are spaces present in bones around the nasal cavity, and into which they open (36.20).
2. The ***maxillary sinus*** lies within the maxilla. It opens into the middle meatus of the nasal cavity.
3. The right and left ***frontal sinuses*** are present in the frontal bone. Each sinus lies deep to a triangular area the angles of which lie:
   a. At the nasion
   b. At a point about 3 cm above the nasion
   c. At a point on the supraorbital margin at the junction of the medial one-third with the lateral two-thirds.
4. The frontal sinus extends for some distance into the orbital plate of the frontal bone between the roof of the orbit and the floor of the anterior cranial fossa.
5. Each frontal sinus usually opens into the middle meatus through a funnel-like space, the ***ethmoidal infundibulum*** (36.20) that is continuous with the upper end of the ***hiatus semilunaris***.
6. The right and left ***sphenoidal sinuses*** are present in the body of the sphenoid bone.
   a. Each sinus opens into the corresponding half of the nasal cavity through an aperture on the anterior aspect of the body of the sphenoid.

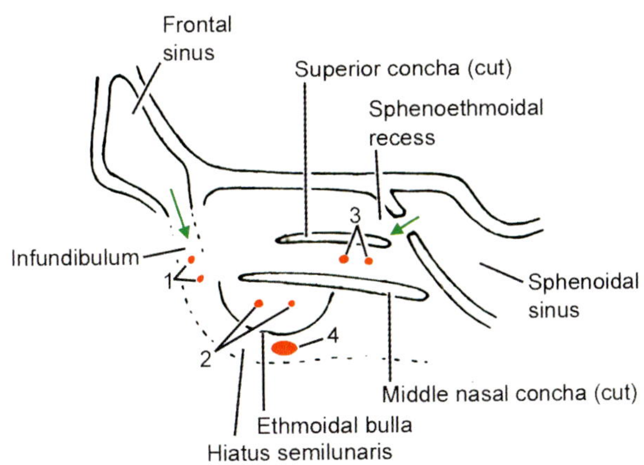


**36.20:** Position of the openings of paranasal sinuses into the nasal cavity

b. The part of the nasal cavity into which the sinus opens lies above the superior nasal concha and is called ***sphenoethmoidal recess*** (36.20).

7. The ***ethmoidal air sinuses*** are located within the lateral part (or labyrinth) of the ethmoid bone.
   a. Each labyrinth (right or left) is bounded medially by the medial plate of the ethmoid, and laterally by the orbital plate.
   b. The ethmoidal air sinuses lie between these plates.
   c. They can be divided into anterior, middle and posterior groups.
8. a. The anterior ethmoidal sinuses open into the ethmoidal infundibulum, or into the upper part of the hiatus semilunaris.
   b. The middle ethmoidal sinuses open on or near the bulla ethmoidalis.
   c. The posterior ethmoidal sinuses open into the superior meatus of the nasal cavity.

#### *Other Apertures in the Nasal Cavity*

In addition to the anterior and posterior nasal apertures, and the openings of the paranasal sinuses, we see the following openings in the nasal cavity.

1. The ***nasolacrimal canal*** opens into the inferior meatus. The upper end of this canal is seen in the orbit.
2. The ***sphenopalatine foramen*** opens behind the superior meatus, just above the posterior end of the middle concha (36.18). This foramen lies in the medial wall of the pterygopalatine fossa.
3. The nasal cavity communicates with the anterior cranial fossa through numerous apertures in the cribriform plate of the ethmoid bone.
4. In the anterior part of the floor of the nasal cavity there is a funnel-shaped opening that leads into the incisive canals that open on the lower surface of the palate.

### The Fontanelles

1. In the skull of the newborn, there are some gaps in the vault of the skull that are filled by membrane. These gaps are called ***fontanelles*** or fonticuli. They are located in relation to the angles of the parietal bone as follows:
   a. The ***anterior fontanelle*** lies at the junction of the sagittal, coronal and frontal sutures. (Note that at birth the frontal bone is in two halves that are separated by a frontal suture).
   b. The ***posterior fontanelle*** is triangular. It lies at the junction of the sagittal and lambdoid sutures.
   c. The ***sphenoidal (anterolateral) fontanelle*** is present in relation to the anteroinferior angle of the parietal bone, where it meets the greater wing of the sphenoid.
   d. The ***mastoid fontanelle (posterolateral)*** is present in relation to the posteroinferior angle of the parietal bone (that meets the mastoid bone).
2. The fontanelles disappear (by growth of the bones around them) at different ages after birth.

## THE MANDIBLE

1. The mandible is the bone of the lower jaw and bears the lower teeth (36.21 to 36.24).
   a. It consists of an anterior U-shaped ***body***.
   b. Two ***rami*** (right and left) that project upwards from the posterior part of the body.
2. The bone has internal (or medial) and external (or lateral) surfaces.
3. The body of the bone has an upper part that bears the teeth (***alveolar process***), and a lower border that is called the ***base***.
4. The ramus has a posterior border, a sharp anterior border, and a lower border that is continuous with the base of the body.
   a. The posterior and inferior borders of the ramus meet at the ***angle*** of the mandible.
   b. The anterior border of the ramus is continued downwards and forwards on the lateral surface of the body as the ***oblique line***. This line ends anteriorly near the ***mental tubercle***.

c. A little above the anterior part of the oblique line we see the ***mental foramen*** that lies vertically below the second premolar tooth.
d. Just below the incisor teeth the external surface of the ramus shows a shallow ***incisive fossa***.

5. Arising from the upper part of the ramus there are two processes.
6. The anterior of these is the ***coronoid process***. It is flat (from side to side) and triangular.
7. The posterior or ***condylar process*** is separated from the coronoid process by the ***mandibular notch***.
8. The upper end of the condylar process is expanded to form the ***head*** of the mandible.
   a. The head is elongated transversely and is convex both transversely and in an anteroposterior direction.
   b. It bears a smooth articular surface that articulates with the mandibular fossa of the temporal bone to form the temporomandibular joint.
9. The part immediately below the head is constricted and forms the ***neck***. Its anterior surface has a rough depression called the ***pterygoid fovea***.
10. In 36.22 the mandible is seen from the medial side.
    a. A little above the centre of the medial surface of the ramus we see the ***mandibular foramen***. It leads into the mandibular canal that runs forwards in the substance of the mandible.
    b. The medial margin of the foramen is formed by a projection called the ***lingula***.
    c. Beginning just behind the lingula and running downwards and forwards we see the ***mylohyoid groove***.
    d. A little above and anterior to the mylohyoid groove, the inner surface of the body of the mandible is marked by a ridge called the ***mylohyoid line***.
    e. The posterior end of this line is located a little below and behind the third molar tooth. From here the line runs downwards and forwards to reach the symphysis menti (see below).
    f. The mylohyoid line divides the inner surface of the body of the mandible into a ***sublingual fossa*** (lying above the line), and a ***submandibular fossa*** (lying below the line).
11. Just below the anterior end of the mylohyoid line the base of the mandible is marked by a deep ***digastric fossa***.
12. In the newborn, the mandible consists of right and left halves that are joined to each other at the ***symphysis menti***; but in later life the two halves fuse to form one bone.

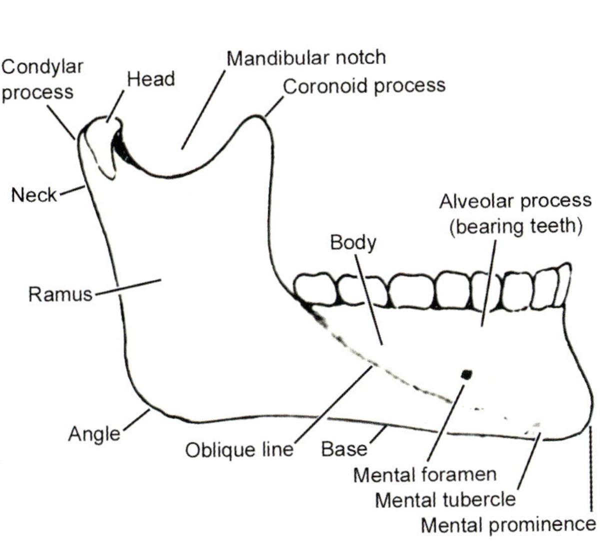


**36.21:** Mandible seen from lateral side

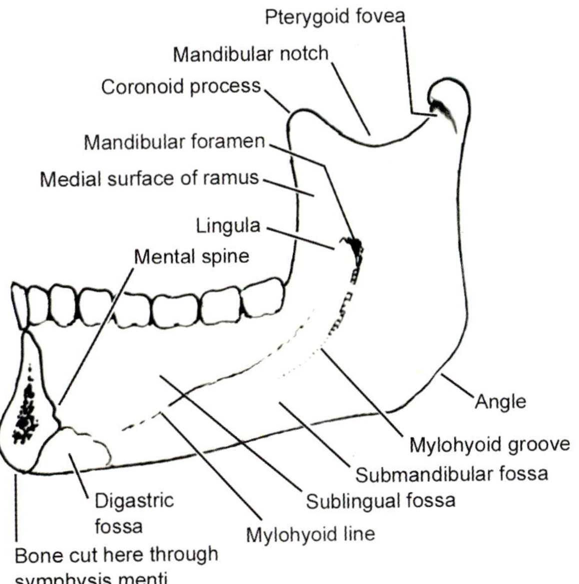


**36.22:** Right half of the mandible seen from the medial side

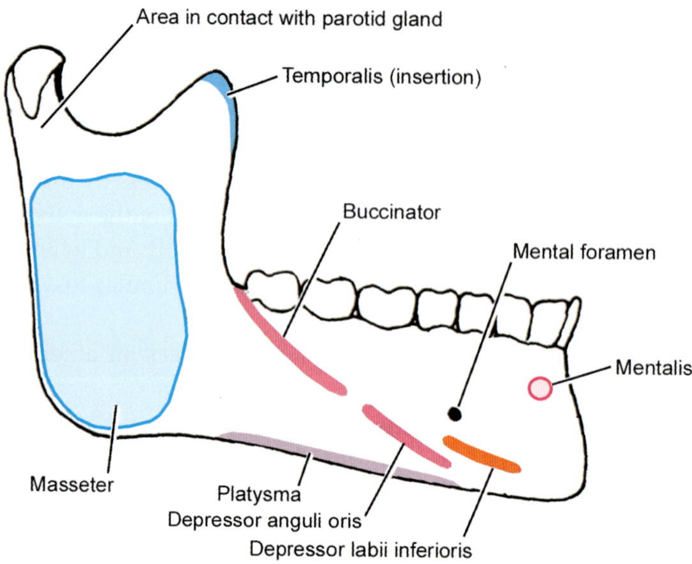


**36.23:** Attachments on mandible seen from lateral side

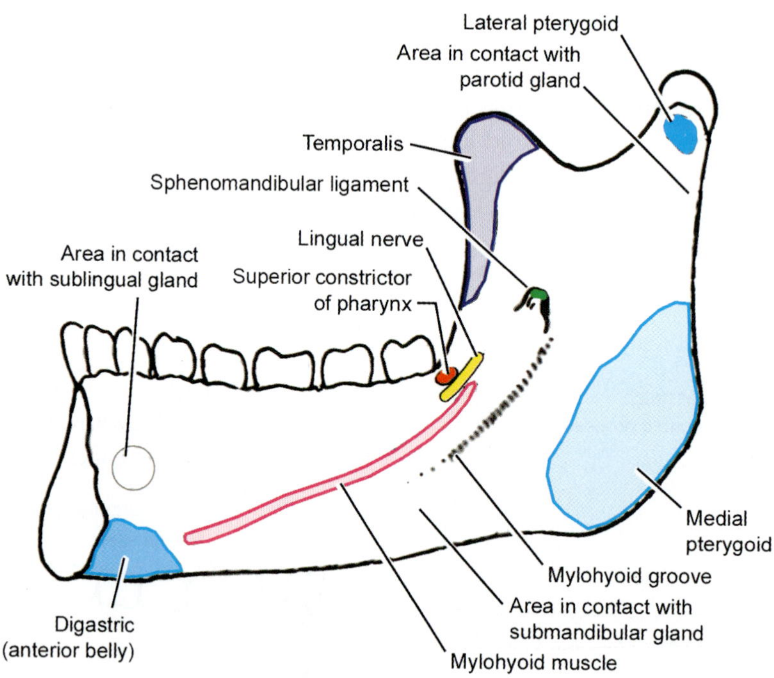


**36.24:** Attachments on mandible seen from medial side

a. When seen from the front, the region of the symphysis menti is usually marked by a slight ridge. Inferiorly, the ridge expands to form a triangular raised area called the ***mental protuberance***.
b. The lateral angles of the protuberance are prominent and constitute the ***mental tubercles***.

13. The posterior aspect of the symphysis menti also shows a median ridge the lower part of which is enlarged and may be divided into upper and lower parts called the ***mental spines*** or ***genial tubercles***.

### *Some Attachments and Relations of the Mandible*

1. The ***masseter*** is inserted into the lateral surface of the ramus and of the angle.
2. The ***buccinator*** arises from the outer surface of the body just below the molar teeth.
3. The ***temporalis*** is inserted into the medial surface of the coronoid process including its apex, and its anterior and posterior borders.
4. The ***lateral pterygoid*** is inserted into the fovea on the anterior aspect of the neck.
5. The ***medial pterygoid*** is inserted into the medial surface of the angle and the adjoining part of the ramus.
6. The ***anterior belly of the digastric*** arises from the digastric fossa (on the anterior part of the base near the midline).
7. The ***mylohyoid*** muscle arises from the mylohyoid line.
8. The ***capsule of the temporomandibular joint*** is attached along the margins of the articular surface.
9. The inferior alveolar nerve and vessels enter the mandibular canal (that lies within the bone) through the mandibular foramen.
10. The mylohyoid nerve and vessels run forwards in the mylohyoid groove.
11. The facial artery is closely related to the mandible.
    a. Its initial part lies deep to the ramus, near the angle.
    b. The artery then runs downwards and forwards deep to the ramus.
    c. It reaches the lower border of the body of the mandible at the anteroinferior angle of the masseter.
    d. The artery then runs upwards and forwards superficial to the body of the mandible.
12. The lingual nerve is closely related to the medial aspect of the body of the mandible just above the posterior end of the mylohyoid line.
13. The sublingual gland lies over the sublingual fossa; and the submandibular gland over the submandibular fossa. The parotid gland is related to the upper part of the posterior border of the ramus.

## THE HYOID BONE

The hyoid bone is not a part of the skull, but is considered here for sake of convenience.

1. The hyoid bone is present in the front of the upper part of the neck.
    a. It is not attached to any other bone directly; but is held in place by muscles and ligaments that are attached to it.
    b. The most important of these are the stylohyoid ligaments by which it is suspended from the base of the skull.
2. The bone consists of a central part called the body, and of two cornua (greater and lesser) on either side (36.25 and 36.26).
3. The ***body*** is roughly quadrilateral. It has an anterior surface and a posterior surface.
4. The ***greater cornua*** are attached to the lateral part of the body, from which they project backwards and laterally.
5. The ***lesser cornua*** are small and conical. They project upwards and laterally from the junction of the body and the greater cornua.

### WANT TO KNOW MORE?

**Some Attachments on the Hyoid Bone**

1. The lowest fibres of the ***genioglossus*** muscle are inserted into the upper border of the body of the bone.
2. The ***geniohyoid*** muscle is inserted on the anterior surface of the body.
3. The ***mylohyoid*** muscle is inserted on the anterior surface of the body below the insertion of the geniohyoid.
4. The ***sternohyoid*** muscle is inserted into the medial part of the inferior border of the body.
5. The ***superior belly of the omohyoid*** muscle is attached to the lateral part of the inferior border of the body.
6. The ***hyoglossus*** muscle arises from the upper surface of the greater cornu (lateral to the origin of the middle constrictor), and from the lateral part of the body.

7. The ***stylohyoid*** muscle is inserted into the upper surface of the greater cornu near its junction with the body.
8. The ***thyrohyoid*** muscle is inserted into the anterior part of the lateral border of the greater cornu.

*Fracture of the Hyoid Bone*

The hyoid bone can be fractured when the neck is forcibly pressed upon as in strangulation, or in hanging. Such a fracture is of considerable medicolegal significance.

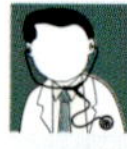

## CLINICAL CORRELATION OF THE SKULL

**Congenital Malformations**

1. ***Anencephaly*** is a malformation in which the greater part of the vault of the skull is missing.
   a. It is caused by failure of the neural tube to close in the region where the brain is to be formed.
   b. Neural tissue, which is exposed to the surface degenerates.
   c. The condition is fairly frequent and is not compatible with life.
2. Establishment of the normal shape of the skull depends on orderly closure of sutures.
   a. Premature union of the sagittal suture gives rise to a boat-shaped skull (***scaphocephaly***).
   b. Early union of the coronal suture results in a skull that is pointed upwards (***acrocephaly***).
   c. Asymmetrical union of sutures (on the right and left sides) results in a twisted skull (***plagiocephaly***).
3. ***Congenital hydrocephalus*** is a condition in which there is obstruction to the flow of cerebrospinal fluid.
   a. As a result, pressure in the ventricular system of the brain increases and leads to its dilatation.
   b. In turn, this leads to enlargement of the head, and wide separation of the bones of the skull.
4. The maxilla, the mandible and the zygomatic bone are derived from the first branchial arch. Occasionally, growth of this arch is defective so that the bones concerned remain underdeveloped, and the face is deformed. The condition is called ***mandibulofacial dysostosis***.
5. Many bones of the skull are formed by intramembranous ossification. The clavicle is also formed in membrane. In the condition called ***cleidocranial dysostosis*** formation of membrane bones is interfered with. Deformities of the skull are seen in association with absence of the clavicle.

**Fractures of the Skull**

Fractures of the skull are serious because of the likelihood of damage to the brain. Some facts of interest regarding these fractures are as follows:

1. The skull of a child is highly elastic and is seldom fractured.
   a. A localized blow on the skull of a child produces a depression on the area struck (pond fracture), the rest of the skull remaining unaffected.
   b. In contrast a blow on the skull of an adult can shatter it, with cracks running in various directions from the area that is hit.
2. The fractures run along lines that are weak.
   a. Injury on the vault of the skull can thus result in fractures of the base of the skull (cranial fossae).
   b. A blow over the parietal bone can lead to a fracture that extends into the squamous part of the temporal bone and into the middle cranial fossa.
   c. In the cranial fossae the fracture line often runs across foramina (which represent sites of weakness).
3. Large bones of the skull are lined on both sides by compact bone. These are called inner and outer tables.The inner table of the skull is more brittle than the outer table, and so a fracture may involve the inner table more extensively than the outer. Sometimes, injury to the head may fracture the inner table leaving the outside of the skull intact.
4. Apart from its elasticity (in the young) other factors that tend to protect the skull from fractures are its rounded shape, and the presence of muscles over the temporal fossa and the occipital region (where the skull wall is thin).

*Fractures of Middle Cranial Fossa*

1. The body and greater wing of the sphenoid are closely related to the middle cranial fossa. A fracture involving the body of the sphenoid bone can lead to leakage of blood and CSF into the sphenoidal air sinuses, and through them into the nose and mouth.
2. The 3rd, 4th and 6th cranial nerves lie in relation to the cavernous sinus (which lies against the body of the sphenoid bone). These nerves can be involved in fractures of the middle cranial fossa.
3. Posteriorly, the middle cranial fossa is bounded by the petrous temporal bone. Involvement of this bone can lead to bleeding and discharge of CSF into the middle ear and external acoustic meatus.
4. The 7th and 8th cranial nerves (which pass through the internal acoustic meatus) can also be injured in a fracture through the petrous temporal bone.

*Fractures of the Anterior Cranial Fossa*

1. This fossa is closely related to the nasal cavity and to the orbits.
2. Fracture through the fossa can lead to bleeding or leakage of CSF through the nose (the blood flowing directly into nose through its roof, or through the frontal air sinus).
3. Bleeding into the orbit can push the eyeball forwards (exophthalmos).
4. Blood in the orbit can seep into the eyelids resulting in a 'black eye'.

*Fractures of the Posterior Cranial Fossa*

1. Fractures through this fossa can lead to bleeding, the blood seeping into the muscles of the back of the neck.
2. The blood often appears superficially over the mastoid process and the sternomastoid muscle.
3. If the fracture passes through the jugular foramen there can be injury to the 9th, 10th and 11th cranial nerves.
4. The walls of the hypoglossal canal are strong and so the 12th cranial nerve usually escapes injury.
5. Injuries (e.g., blows) on the face can lead to fracture of the mandible, the zygomatic bone, the maxilla or the nasal bones.
6. The mandible is commonly fractured.
   a. The fracture can involve the neck, the body, the angle, the symphysis menti or the ramus of the bone.
   b. The fracture can be bilateral.
   c. A fracture through the body of the bone often takes place at the level of the canine socket (the deep socket making the bone weak here). Such a fracture can involve the inferior alveolar nerve.
7. a. A fracture of the maxilla can deform the floor of the orbit causing ocular displacement.
   b. Involvement of the infraorbital nerve can produce anaesthesia over the cheek and upper lip.
8. Fractures of the maxilla, or of the mandible, can cause malocclusion of teeth.

## JOINTS OF HEAD AND NECK

The various types of joints to be seen in the body are classified and described in chapter 7. The joints to be seen in the head and neck are as follows:

### Joints between Bones of the Skull

1. Adjoining edges of bones of the skull are united to each other by fibrous joints called ***sutures***. The structure of sutures is described in chapter 7. The names of individual sutures have been mentioned while describing the skull.
2. Some bones of the skull are united by ***synchondroses***. The structure of a synchondrosis is described in Chapter 7. At such a joint the two articulating surfaces are united by a plate of hyaline cartilage. As age increases the cartilage is gradually invaded by bone and the union becomes bony.

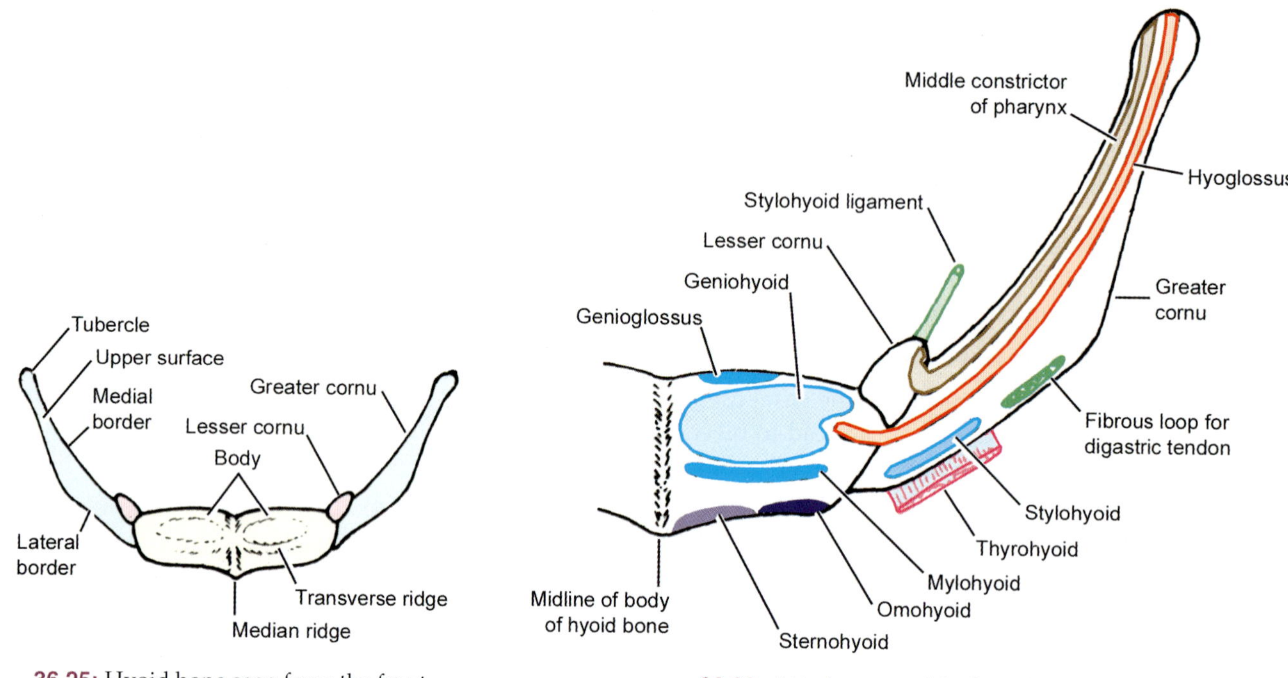


**36.25:** Hyoid bone seen from the front

**36.26:** Attachments of the hyoid bone

3. The bodies of the occipital and sphenoid bones are united by a ***synchondrosis***.
4. A synchondrosis is also present between the body of the sphenoid bone and the apex of the petrous temporal bone.

## The Temporomandibular Joint

At this joint the head of the mandible articulates with the articular fossa present on the temporal bone. This joint is described in chapter 38.

## The Atlanto-occipital Joints

These are the joints between the occipital bone and the atlas. They are described below.

## Joints between Cervical Vertebrae

Of these the joints between the atlas and axis vertebrae are atypical, and are described below. The remaining intervertebral joints are similar to typical intervertebral joints.

## Other Joints

Highly specialised joints are present between ossicles of the middle ear, and between the cartilages of the larynx. These will be considered along with the respective organs.

# THE ATLANTO-AXIAL JOINTS

1. The atlas and axis vertebrae articulate with each other at three joints, one median, and two that are lateral (36.27).

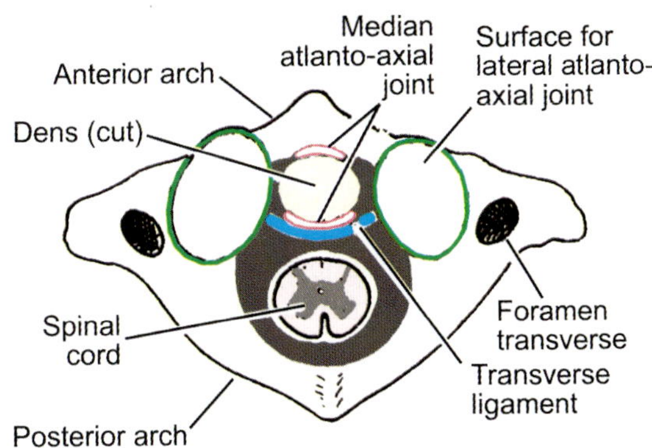


**36.27:** Inferior aspect of atlas to show the atlanto-axial joints

2. The ***median atlanto-axial joint*** is a synovial joint of the pivot variety.
   a. The dens of the axis (the pivot) is placed in the ring formed by the anterior arch of the atlas and its transverse ligament.
   b. In this situation there are really two synovial joints with independent capsules. There is one between the anterior surface of the dens and the posterior aspect of the anterior arch, and the other between the posterior surface of the dens and the transverse ligament.
   c. The transverse ligament is attached at each end to the medial surface of the lateral mass of the atlas.
3. The ***lateral atlanto-axial joints*** are synovial joints of the plane variety.
4. The ligaments connecting the atlas and axis, and the movements at the atlanto-axial joints are considered below along with those of the atlanto-occipital joints.

## THE ATLANTO-OCCIPITAL JOINTS

1. On either side of the foramen magnum, there is a large convex occipital condyle (36.15).
   a. The long axis of the condyle is directed forwards and medially.
   b. The condyle is convex both anteroposteriorly and from side to side.
   c. Each condyle articulates with a facet on the upper surface of the lateral mass of the atlas (36.4). This facet is concave and corresponds in size and direction to the occipital condyle.
2. These articular surfaces are enclosed in capsules to form synovial joints. From a functional point of view, the right and left atlanto-occipital joints together form an ellipsoid joint.

### Ligaments Uniting the Atlas, the Axis and the Occipital Bone

Apart from the capsules of the atlanto-occipital joints, the atlas and axis are united to each other and to the occipital bone by a number of ligaments that are considered below.

1. The ***anterior longitudinal ligament*** (continued upwards from lower vertebrae) is attached to the front of the body of the axis; to the anterior arch of the atlas; and to the basilar part of the occipital bone (36.28A).
2. Between the atlas and the occipital bone, the anterior longitudinal ligament is incorporated in the ***anterior atlanto-occipital membrane*** (36.28A). This membrane is attached below to the upper border of the anterior arch of the atlas, and above to the anterior part of the margin of the foramen magnum.
3. The ***posterior atlanto-occipital membrane*** is attached above to the posterior margin of the foramen magnum, and below to the upper border of the posterior arch of the atlas (36.28B). [The ligament has a free inferolateral margin. The vertebral artery enters the vertebral canal by passing deep to this edge].
4. The highest ***ligamentum flavum*** connects the posterior arch of the atlas to the laminae of the axis vertebra (36.28B).

5. The ***membrana tectoria*** (36.28C) is an upward continuation of the posterior longitudinal ligament (which connects the posterior surfaces of the bodies of adjacent vertebrae).
   a. The membrana tectoria lies posterior to the transverse ligament of the atlas (36.28C).
   b. Its lower end is attached to the posterior surface of the body of the axis.
   c. Its upper end is attached to the occipital bone (basiocciput) above the attachment of the upper band of the cruciform ligament (36.28C).
6. The dens (of the axis) is connected to the occipital bone by the following:
   a. The ***apical ligament*** passes upwards from the tip of the dens to the anterior margin of the foramen magnum (36.28C).
   b. The right and left ***alar ligaments*** are attached below to the upper part of the dens lateral to the apical ligament, and above to the occipital bone on the medial side of the condyle.
7. We have seen that the ***transverse ligament of the atlas*** stretches between the two lateral masses of the bone, behind the dens of the axis.

## Movements at the Atlanto-occipital and Atlanto-axial Joints

1. Being a pivot joint the median atlanto-axial joint allows the atlas (and with it the skull) to rotate around the axis provided by the dens.
   a. This is accompanied by gliding movements at the lateral atlantoaxial joints.
   b. The extent of rotation at this joint is limited by the alar ligaments.
2. From a functional point of view the two atlanto-occipital joints together form an ellipsoid joint.
   a. The main movements allowed by it are those of flexion and extension (of the head) as in nodding.
   b. Slight lateral movements are also allowed, but no rotation is possible.
3. The muscles responsible for these movements are as follows. (See chapter 41 for details of muscles).
4. ***Side-to-side movements*** (at the atlantoaxial joint) are produced by:
   a. The sternocleidomastoid (of the opposite side)
   b. The obliquus capitis inferior
   c. The rectus capitis posterior major
   d. The splenius capitis (of the same side).
5. ***Flexion*** of the head, at the atlanto-occipital joints is produced by:
   a. The longus capitis
   b. The rectus capitis anterior
   c. The range of flexion is increased by movement at cervical intervertebral joints produced by the sternocleidomastoid, the scaleni and the longus cervicis.
6. ***Extension*** of the head, at the atlanto-occipital joint is produced by:
   a. The rectus capitis posterior major and minor
   b. The obliquus capitis superior
   c. The erector spinae
   d. The splenius capitis
   e. The semispinalis capitis
   f. The upper fibres of the trapezius
   g. The range of movement is increased by movements produced between cervical vertebrae by some of these muscles.
7. ***Lateral flexion of the head at the atlanto-occipital joint is produced by:***
   a. The splenius capitis
   b. The semispinalis capitis
   c. The upper fibres of the trapezius
   d. The rectus capitis lateralis
   e. The larger muscles also produce movements between cervical vertebrae. These are assisted by the sternocleidomastoid.

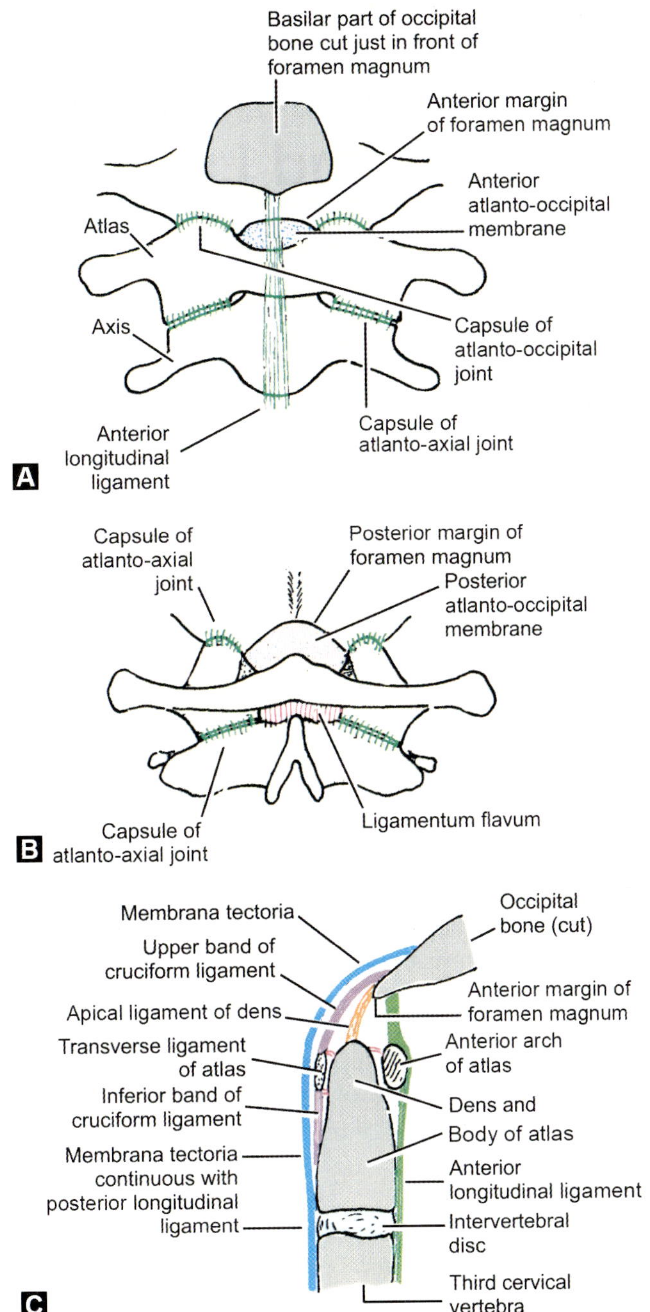


**36.28A to C:** Region of atlanto-occipital and atlanto-axial joints. (A) Seen from the front; (B) Seen from behind; (C) Median section

# 37 CHAPTER

# Scalp, Face, Parotid Region and Lacrimal Apparatus

## THE SCALP

1. The term scalp is applied to the soft tissues covering the vault of the skull.
2. This region extends anteriorly up to the eyebrows (and, therefore, includes the forehead), posteriorly up to the superior nuchal lines, and laterally up to the superior temporal lines.

### Layers of the Scalp

These are shown in 37.1 and are as follows:

1. The most superficial layer is ***skin***. Being hairy, it contains numerous sebaceous glands. The skin is closely adherent to underlying tissues.
2. The ***superficial fascia*** is represented by dense connective tissue that is firmly united to the skin and to the underlying epicranial aponeurosis. Fibrous strands divide the superficial fascia into numerous small pockets.
3. The third layer of the scalp is partly muscular and partly fibrous. It corresponds to deep fascia.
   a. The greater part of this layer is formed by the ***epicranial aponeurosis*** (or galea aponeurotica).
   b. The muscular part is formed by a muscle called the ***occipitofrontalis*** (see below).
4. The three layers of the scalp described above are firmly united to one another. All the three layers move together over the fourth layer that is made up of ***loose areolar tissue***.
   a. The extent of the layer of loose connective tissue corresponds to the extent of the scalp itself.
   b. Loose areolar tissue is traversed by emissary veins passing from the scalp to intracranial venous sinuses.
5. The deepest layer of the scalp is the ***pericranium*** (which is the periosteum over the bones of the vault of the skull). It is important to note that at the edge of each bone of the skull the pericranium is fixed because it is attached to sutural ligaments that are present in sutures of the skull.

### Occipitofrontalis

1. The occipitofrontalis covers the upper curved roof of the skull (37.2)
2. It consists of a posterior ***occipital part*** (or ***occipitalis***), and an anterior ***frontal part*** (or ***frontalis***).
3. Each of these is divided into a right half and a left half.
4. These four parts are continuous with each other through the epicranial aponeurosis.
5. Each ***occipital part*** arises from the occipital bone (lateral two-thirds of the highest nuchal line).
   a. Laterally, the line of origin extends onto the mastoid part of the temporal bone.
   b. The fibres of the occipitalis run upwards and forwards to end in the epicranial aponeurosis.
   c. The occipital parts of the two sides are separated from each other by a part of the epicranial aponeurosis that gains attachment to the external occipital protuberance, and to the medial parts of the highest nuchal lines.
6. a. The ***frontal parts*** are attached posteriorly to the epicranial aponeurosis.
   b. Anteriorly, the fibres have no bony attachment.
   c. The majority of the fibres of the frontalis merge with the upper edge of the orbicularis oculi.

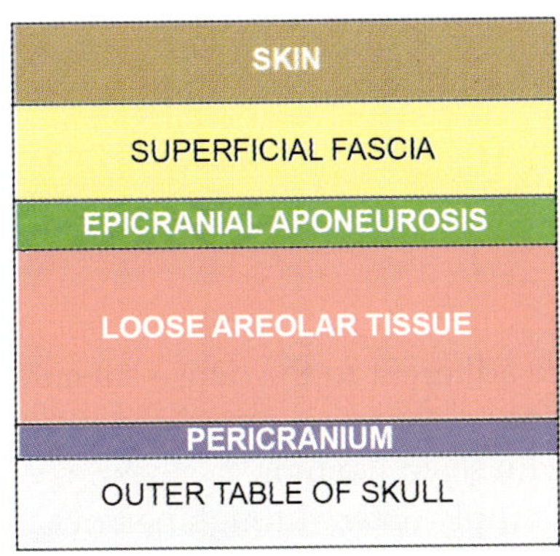


**37.1:** Layers of the scalp (schematic)

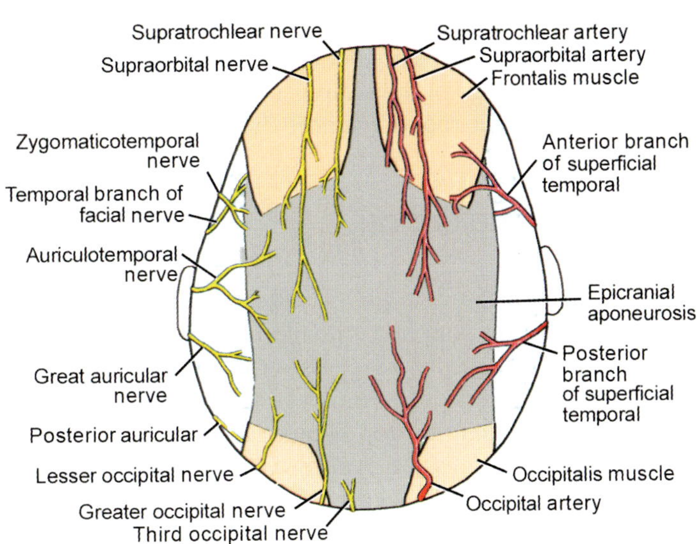


**37.2:** Nerves and arteries of the scalp

d. The medial-most fibres merge with the procerus, which is a small muscle overlying the upper part of the nose.

e. More laterally, the deeper fibres merge with the corrugator supercilii, which is a small muscle underlying the medial part of the eyebrow.

(The procerus, the corrugator supercilii and the orbicularis oculi are considered later in this chapter under muscles of the face).

### *Nerve Supply*

1. The occipital part of the frontooccipitalis is supplied by the posterior auricular branch of the facial nerve.
2. The frontal part by the temporal branches of the same nerve.

### *Action*

1. Acting alternatively, the frontal and occipital parts can move the scalp forwards and backwards over the vault of the skull.
2. The frontal parts raise the eyebrows (as in surprise).
3. Acting from below, they produce transverse wrinkles of the forehead.

## Blood Vessels and Nerves of the Scalp

1. The ***arteries*** that supply the scalp are seen in 37.2. These are:
   a. The supratrochlear and supraorbital branches of the ophthalmic artery in front.
   b. The anterior and posterior branches of the superficial temporal artery laterally.
   c. The occipital artery posteriorly.
2. The ***veins*** of the scalp accompany the corresponding arteries.
3. The ***nerves*** of the scalp may be divided into motor nerves that supply the occipitofrontalis and sensory nerves that supply skin and other tissues of the scalp (37.2).
4. The motor nerves are the temporal and posterior auricular branches of the facial nerve.
5. The sensory nerves are as follows:
   a. In front there are the supratrochlear and supraorbital nerves, which are branches of the frontal nerve (which is itself derived from the ophthalmic division of the trigeminal nerve).

   b. Laterally, there are the zygomatico-temporal, the auriculo-temporal, and great auricular nerves.
   c. Posteriorly, there are the greater occipital, lesser occipital, and third occipital nerves.
6. The ***lymphatic drainage*** of the scalp is into occipital, retroauricular and superficial parotid nodes. Part of the forehead just above the root of the nose drains to the submandibular nodes (see Chapter 47).

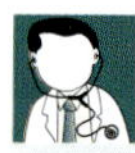

## CLINICAL CORRELATION

### Wounds of the Scalp

1. The scalp is profusely supplied with blood, the arteries entering it from the sides, from the front and from the behind.
2. Because of rich blood supply wounds of the scalp bleed profusely.
3. Bleeding can be difficult to stop because the walls of blood vessels are adherent to the dense subcutaneous fibrous tissue. Direct pressure over the wound is needed to stop bleeding.
4. The profuse blood supply also provides some advantages in dealing with scalp wounds.
   a. Portions of scalp that are torn off (evulsed) retain adequate blood supply (even through narrow areas of attachment), and heal well when stitched back into position.
   b. However, if a portion of scalp is completely detached the surgeon finds it difficult to fill the gap. Hence, the surgeon makes it a point not to cut away parts of the scalp unless absolutely necessary.
5. a. In relation to wounds of the scalp, it is necessary to remember that the skin and the epicranial aponeurosis are firmly united to each other by the layer of dense connective tissue.
   b. Also, remember that the fibres of the aponeurosis run predominantly in an anteroposterior direction.
   c. A wound on the scalp does not gape (i.e., the edges do not separate) unless the epicranial aponeurosis is divided.
   d. Even if the aponeurosis is divided in an anteroposterior cut the wound will not gape because of the predominant direction of the fibres.
   e. It is only when the aponeurosis is cut transversely that the wound can gape widely.
6. Injuries on the head can lead to bleeding into various layers of the scalp.
   a. Bleeding into the superficial fascia is never extensive as the region is divided into small pockets by fibrous tissue.
   b. Bleeding into the layer of loose areolar tissue spreads widely reaching the orbital margin anteriorly, the nuchal lines posteriorly, and the temporal lines laterally.
   c. Bleeding deep to the pericranium (periosteum) does not extend beyond the margins of the bone as the pericranium is adherent to sutural ligaments which limit the spread of blood. The shape of the haematoma, therefore, corresponds to that of the underlying bone (***cephalhaematoma***).

### Infections of the Scalp

1. An infection in the subcutaneous tissue is limited to a small area as the tissue is divided into small pockets by dense fibrous tissue.
2. For the same reason, pressure on nerves in the area is high and leads to severe pain.
3. An infection in the layer of loose areolar tissue can spread to the limits of the space (see above).
4. As this layer is traversed by emissary veins, infection can pass through these veins to intracranial venous sinuses.
5. That is why the layer of loose areolar tissue is called the ***dangerous area of the scalp***.
6. Osteomyelitis of the skull bones can also be caused by spread of infection through emissary veins.

### Swellings on the Scalp

#### *Sebaceous Cysts*

1. Because of the presence of numerous hair follicles, and the sebaceous glands associated with them, the scalp is a common site for sebaceous cysts. The cysts are often multiple.

2. A sebaceous cyst is caused by blockage to the discharge of secretion of a sebaceous gland. The secretion accumulates and leads to formation of the cyst. The interior of the cyst is lined with epithelial cells.

*Dermoid Cysts*

1. Dermoid cysts are formed by multiplication of epithelial cells that get buried under the skin surface.
2. The cysts may be congenital, or may be caused by pricks.
3. A dermoid cyst can lead to erosion of underlying bone.

*Neoplasms*

Various types of tumours, benign and malignant, may occur in the scalp.

## THE FACE

### The External Nose

1. The prominence on the face that the layman refers to as the nose is strictly speaking the external nose. (The nasal cavities constitute the internal nose.)
2. Certain descriptive terms applied to parts of the external nose are as follows:
   a. The upper end (where the nose becomes continuous with the forehead) is called the ***angle.***
   b. The ridge-like free border passing down from the angle is called the ***dorsum nasi.***
   c. The dorsum nasi ends below in a rounded prominence that forms the tip, or ***apex***, of the nose.
   d. On either side, the external nose has lateral surfaces that are continuous behind with the cheeks. The lowest parts of the lateral surfaces are rounded and mobile. These are called the ***alae nasi.***
   e. The upper parts of both lateral surfaces (just below the angle) together form the ***bridge*** of the nose.
3. The shape of the nose is maintained by the presence of a skeleton made up partly of bone and partly of cartilage.
   a. The upper part of the lateral wall is formed by (1) the nasal bone and (2) the frontal process of the maxilla.
   b. The anteroinferior part is reinforced by pieces of cartilage.
      i. There is an upper nasal cartilage.
      ii. A lower nasal cartlage.
      iii. Some minor cartilages are also present.
   c. The wall of the ala nasi is formed by fibro-fatty tissue.
4. The ***external nares*** (or anterior nares) are the external openings of the nasal cavities. They are located on the inferior aspect of the nose. They are bounded laterally by the alae nasi and medially by the lowest part of the nasal septum.

### Lips and Cheeks

Some facts worth noting about the lips and cheeks are as follows:

1. The ***lips***, upper and lower, are lined on the outside by skin and on the inside by mucous membrane.
2. The junction between the two forms the 'edge' of each lip.
3. The substance of the lip is formed by the orbicularis oris muscle and by numerous smaller muscles that blend with it (See 37.10).
4. The points, on either side, where the upper and lower lips meet are called the ***angles of the mouth***.
5. The deep surface of each lip is connected to the gum by a median fold of mucous membrane called the ***frenulum***.
6. The ***cheeks*** are, like the lips, made up of an outer layer of skin, an inner layer of mucous membrane and an intervening layer of muscle, connective tissue and fat.
   a. The muscle layer is formed chiefly by the buccinator (37.12).
   b. The fat is especially prominent in infants and is responsible for the rounded appearance of the cheeks.

c. Numerous glands are present in relationship to the lips and cheeks. They open into the vestibule of the mouth.

## The Eyelids and Conjunctiva

The parts of the eyeball will be studied in detail later (Chapter 44). Here, we will look at the eyes as part of the face.

1. The part of the eye seen on the face consists of a part that is white, and a circular area in front that looks dark.
2. The so-called 'white of the eye' is formed by a layer of the eyeball that is called the ***sclera*** (37.3).
3. The sclera is lined (on the outside) by a thin transparent membrane the ***ocular conjunctiva***.
4. The circular dark part seen in the centre of the eye is the ***iris*** . The iris is seen through a transparent disc-like structure—the ***cornea*** which covers it.
5. At the centre of the iris, there is an aperture called the ***pupil***. The pupil appears black because the interior of the eye (which we see through the pupil) is dark.
6. When we view the 'eyes', we see only a small part of the eyeball in the interval between the upper and lower eyelids. This interval is called the ***palpebral fissure*** (37.4).
7. The upper and lower eyelids (or palpebrae) protect the eyeball, especially the cornea, from injury in several ways.
   a. Firstly, they provide protection against mechanical injury by reflex closure when any object suddenly approaches the eye.
   b. The same happens when the cornea is touched (***corneal reflex***).
   c. Secondly, they help to keep the cornea moist as follows. When the eyelids are closed (i.e., when the upper and lower eyelids meet) a capillary space separates the posterior surfaces of the lids from the cornea and the anterior part of the sclera. This space is the ***conjunctival sac*** (37.3). It contains a thin film of lacrimal fluid, which keeps the cornea and conjunctiva moist.

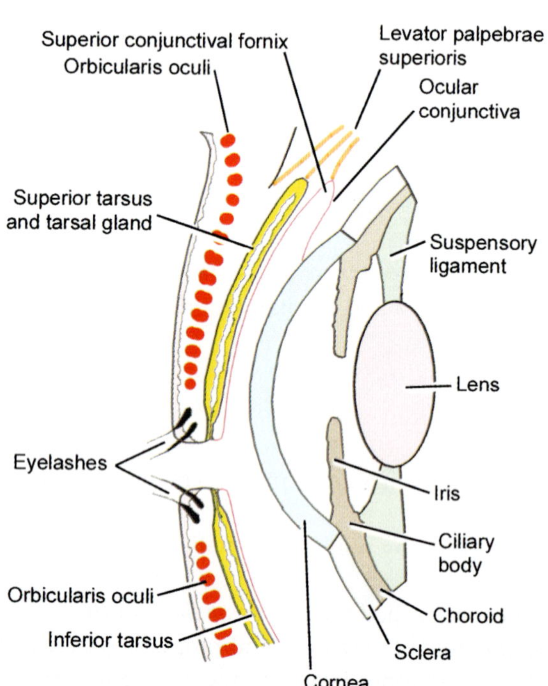


**37.3:** Schematic sagittal section through the eyelids and anterior part of the eyeball

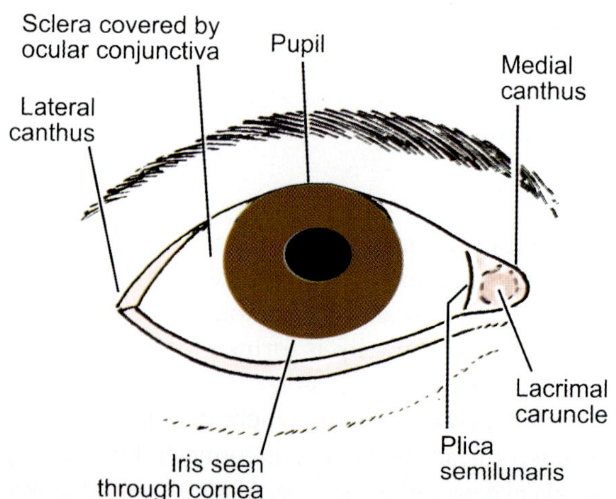


**37.4:** Some features of the eye as seen on the face. The eyelashes are omitted. The interval between the two eyelids is the palpebral fissure

  d. With the 'eyes' open the cornea has a tendency to dry up, but this is prevented by periodic, unconscious closure of the lids (blinking). Every time this happens the film of lacrimal fluid over the cornea is replenished.
  e. Thirdly, lids protect the eyes from sudden exposure to bright light by reflex closure. In bright light, partial closure of the lids may assist the pupils in regulating the light falling on the retina.
8. We have seen above that the space separating the upper and lower eyelids is called the palpebral fissure. The medial and lateral ends of the fissure are called the ***angles*** of the eye. Each angle is also called the ***canthus*** (37.4).
9. The lateral canthus is in contact with the sclera.
10. At the medial canthus, the upper and lower lids are separated by a triangular interval called the ***lacus lacrimalis***.
  a. In the floor of this area, there is a rounded pink elevation called the ***lacrimal caruncle***.
  b. Just lateral to the caruncle, there is a fold of conjunctiva called the ***plica semilunaris***. It represents the third eyelid present in some lower animals (in whom it is called the ***nictitating membrane)***.
11. Each eyelid has a free edge to which eyelashes are attached,
12. Just lateral to the lacrimal caruncle, each lid margin has a slight elevation called the ***lacrimal papilla***.
13. On the summit of the papilla, there is a small aperture called the ***lacrimal punctum***. It is important to note that the punctum is normally in direct contact with the ocular conjunctiva.

## WANT TO KNOW MORE?

The basic structure of an eyelid is shown in 37.5. The various structures forming the eyelid are as follows:
1. Anteriorly, there is a layer of true skin with which a few small hair and sweat glands are associated. The skin is thin.
2. Deeply to the skin, there is a layer of delicate connective tissue, which normally does not contain fat.
3. Considerable thickness of the lid is formed by fasciculi of the palpebral part of the orbicularis oculi muscle (described below).
4. The 'skeleton' of each eyelid is formed by a mass of fibrous tissue called the ***tarsus***, or ***tarsal plate***.
  a. The shape of the tarsi corresponds to that of the lids. They are semi-oval having a straight edge directed towards the margin of the lid and a convex margin directed towards the orbital margin (37.6).
  b. The 'height' of the tarsus is greatest midway between the medial and lateral ends of the tarsus. It is about 10 mm in the upper lid and about 5 mm in the lower lid.
  c. The tarsi narrow down laterally and medially and become continuous with the ***lateral*** and ***medial palpebral ligaments*** through which they are attached to the walls of the orbit, just inside the orbital margin.
  d. The medial palpebral ligament is better developed than the lateral ligament. It gains attachment to the maxilla (lacrimal crest and adjoining part of frontal process).
  e. The lateral ligament is attached to the zygomatic bone.
  f. The upper and lower tarsi are attached to the corresponding part of the orbital margin by a membrane called the ***orbital septum.***
5. On the deep surface of the tarsi, there are a series of vertical grooves in which ***tarsal glands*** (or ***Meibomian glands***) are placed (37.5).
  a. These glands may occasionally be embedded within the tarsal plates.
  b. Each gland has a duct that opens on the free margin of the lid.
  c. The tarsal glands are modified sebaceous glands. They produce an oily secretion a thin film of which spreads over the lacrimal fluid and delays its evaporation.
  d. In addition to tarsal glands, modified sweat glands called ***ciliary glands***, are present in the lids near their free edge.
6. The inner surface of the eyelid is lined by ***palpebral conjunctiva***.
  a. This is a thin transparent membrane continuous with the ***ocular conjunctiva*** lining the anterior part of the sclera.

b. The sharp line of reflection (of the conjunctiva) from the lid to the sclera is called the ***conjunctival fornix*** (superior or inferior) (37.3).

7. The levator palpebrae superioris extends into the upper eyelid anterior to the tarsal plate to gain insertion into it.
   a. This muscle elevates the upper eyelid, in opening the palpebral fissure.
   b. Some fibres of the muscle, which are inserted into the superior conjunctival fornix, pull the fornix up during this movement (37.3 and 37.5).
   c. The palpebral fissure is closed by contraction of the orbicularis oculi.

***Blood Vessels of the Eyelids***

1. The eyelids are supplied by:
   a. The medial palpebral branches of the ophthalmic artery.
   b. The lateral palpebral branches of the lacrimal artery.

***Nerves Supplying the Eyelids***

1. The upper eyelid receives branches from the following nerves (all branches of the ophthalmic division of the trigeminal nerve):
   a. Lacrimal
   b. Supraorbital
   c. Supratrochlear
   d. Infratrochlear nerves.
2. The lower eyelid receives branches from the infraorbital and infratrochlear nerves.

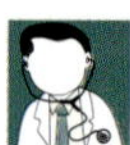

**CLINICAL CORRELATION**

1. Infections are common in the eyelids (***blepharitis***).
2. A pus-filled swelling near the edge of the eyelid is a ***stye***. It is caused by infection in large sebaceous glands present here.
3. Inflammation of a tarsal gland results in a localised swelling called ***chalazion***.
4. Inflammation of the conjunctiva is called ***conjunctivitis***. It may be caused either by infection or by allergy.

## The Lacrimal Apparatus

We have seen that the cornea is kept moist by the lacrimal fluid. The lacrimal apparatus consists of the organs concerned with the secretion and drainage of this fluid.

1. Lacrimal fluid is secreted by the ***lacrimal gland*** and is poured into the conjunctival sac at the superior conjunctival fornix.
2. The fluid passes downwards and medially to reach the lacus lacrimalis. Here it passes through the lacrimal puncta into narrow tubes called the ***lacrimal canaliculi***.
3. These canaliculi open into the ***lacrimal sac***.
4. The lacrimal sac drains into the inferior meatus of the nasal cavity through the ***nasolacrimal duct***.
5. The lacrimal gland will be described when we study the orbit (Chapter 44).
   a. For the time being note that the lacrimal gland lies in relation to the upper lateral part of the wall of the orbit.
   b. An extension of the gland, that passes into the upper eyelid, is called its ***palpebral part*** (37.5 and 37.7).
   c. The lacrimal gland drains into the superior conjunctival fornix through about twelve ducts.
6. The other parts of the lacrimal apparatus are described below. To understand some of the details, you will need to know some features of the bony orbit and the bony nasal cavity (described in Chapter 36).

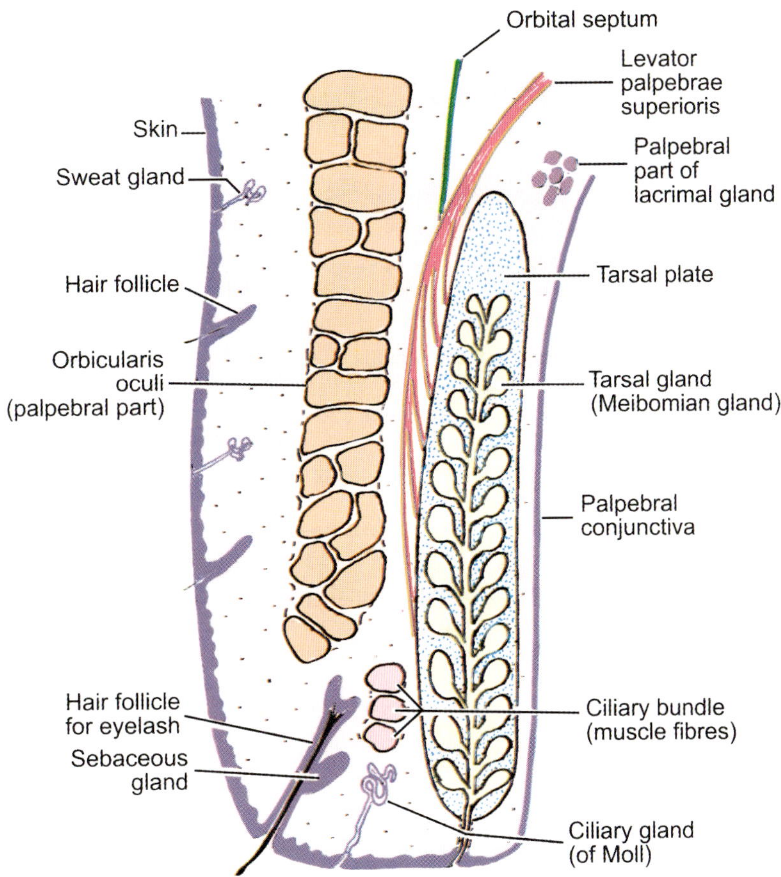


**37.5:** Schematic sagittal section through the upper eyelid

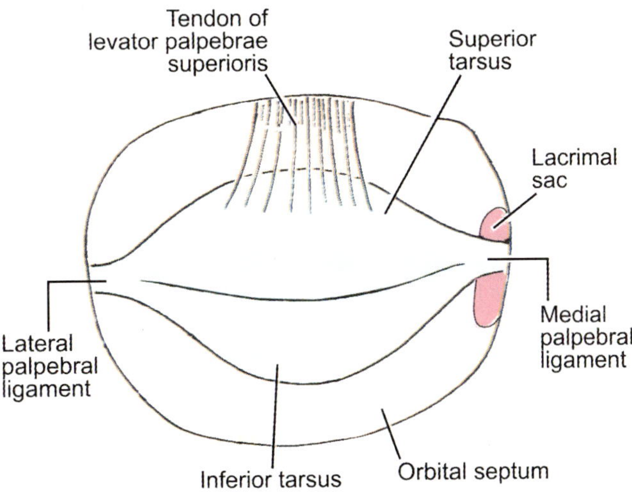


**37.6:** Scheme to show the tarsal plate and the palpebral ligament as seen from the front

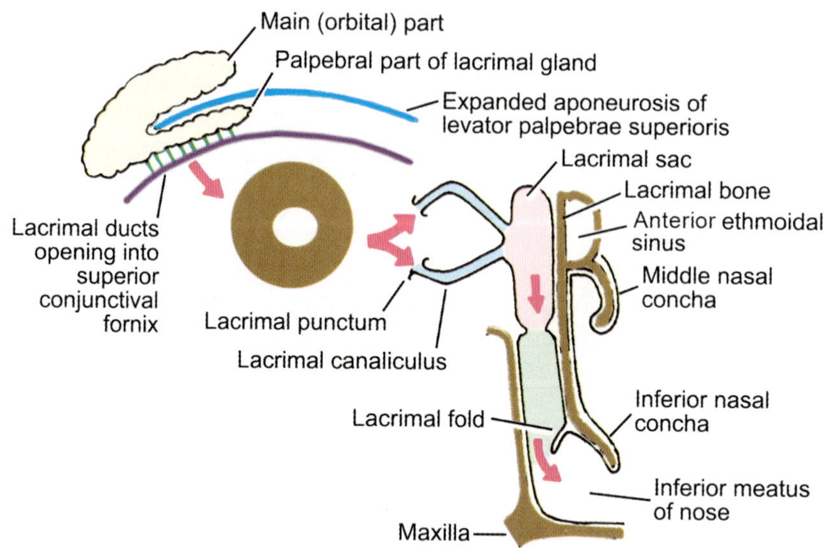


**37.7:** Scheme to show the parts of the lacrimal apparatus. The pink arrows indicate the direction of flow of lacrimal fluid

 **WANT TO KNOW MORE?**

**The Lacrimal Canaliculi**

1. There are two lacrimal canaliculi; upper and lower, in relation to each eye.
2. Each canaliculus is about 10 mm long.
3. It is a narrow tube that starts at the lacrimal punctum and ends by joining the lacrimal sac.
4. Note the direction of each canaliculus as shown in 37.7.

### *The Lacrimal Sac*

1. The lacrimal sac lies in the lacrimal groove on the medial wall of the orbit (37.6 and 37.7).
2. The lacrimal sac is blind at its upper end.
3. Inferiorly, the sac is continuous with the nasolacrimal duct.
4. Laterally, it receives the lacrimal canaliculi near its upper end.

 **WANT TO KNOW MORE?**

5. a. The floor of the lacrimal groove is formed by the lacrimal bone (posteriorly) and the frontal process of the maxilla (anteriorly).
   b. The groove is bounded anteriorly by the anterior lacrimal crest, and behind by the crest of the lacrimal bone.
6. Some relationship of the lacrimal sac can be seen in 37.8 that is a schematic transverse section across the sac.
   a. Note the bones forming the floor of the lacrimal groove.
   b. Medially, the sac is separated by a thin partition of bone from the anterior ethmoidal sinus and lower down from the middle meatus of the nasal cavity (37.7).
   c. Laterally, the lacrimal sac is covered by lacrimal fascia that is attached to the anterior and posterior margins of the lacrimal groove.

d. The medial palpebral ligament is placed in front of the lacrimal sac and is separated from it only by the lacrimal fascia (37.5 and 37.7).
e. The lacrimal part of the orbicularis oculi muscle (see above) takes origin partly from the lacrimal fascia. Every time the muscle contracts, there is pull on this fascia causing the lacrimal sac to expand and helping to suck lacrimal fluid into it.

### *The Nasolacrimal Duct*

1. The nasolacrimal duct (37.8) is a tube about 18 mm long.
2. It may be regarded as the downward continuation of the lacrimal sac.
3. It is closely related to the lateral wall of the nasal cavity, and opens below into the inferior meatus of the nose.
4. The wall of the nasolacrimal duct is made up of bone lined by mucous membrane.
5. The lower end of the nasolacrimal duct is separated from the inferior meatus of the nose by a fold of mucous membrane called the ***lacrimal fold***.

### WANT TO KNOW MORE?

6. The bones helping to form the wall of the duct are the maxilla (laterally); and the lacrimal bone and the inferior nasal concha (medially).

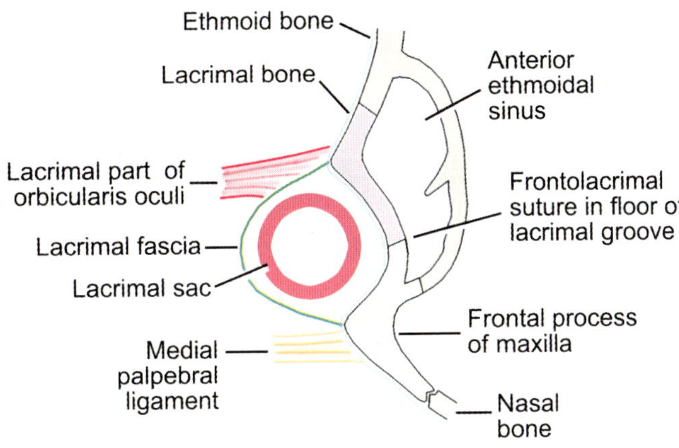


**37.8:** Transverse section through lacrimal sac and some surrounding structures

## MUSCLES OF THE FACE

1. Deep to the skin of the face, there are several muscles that produce varying facial expressions. Many of them are in the form of small slips or narrow bundles. These are named and briefly described in 37.9A. Some of them have bony attachments that are shown in 37.9B.
2. There are three relatively large muscles in the face. These are:
   a. ***Orbicularis oris*** surrounding the opening of the mouth.
   b. ***Orbicularis oculi*** present around the orbital aperture.
   c. The ***buccinator*** that forms the muscular basis of the cheeks.

   These are described in 37.10A. Some features are shown in 37.10B, 37.11 and 37.12.

   All the muscles of the face are supplied by the facial nerve.

| 37.9A: Some muscles of the face | | | |
|---|---|---|---|
| *Name* | *Location* | *Action* | *Bony Attachment* |
| Corrugator supercillii | Above eyebrow, deep to frontalis | Produces vertical wrinkles on forehead | |
| Depressor supercillii | Near eyebrow, merging with orbicularis oculi | Depresses eyebrow | |
| Procerus | Over bridge of nose | Produces transverse wrinkles over bridge of nose | |
| Nasalis (constrictor and dilator) | Over lower part of nose | Constricts or dilates anterior nares | Maxilla |
| Depressor septi | Just below nasal septum | Pulls nasal septum down and helps to dilate anterior nares | Maxilla |
| Levator labii superioris alaeque nasi | From upper part of nose<br>1. One slip to nose<br>2. One slip to upper lip | Raises ala nasi and upper lip | Maxilla, frontal process |
| Levator labii superioris | Above upper lip | Raises uper lip | Maxilla and zygomatic bone |
| Levator anguli oris | Deep to levator labii superioris | Raises angle of mouth | Maxilla below infraorbital for |
| Zygomaticus major | Above lateral angle of upper lip | Pulls angle of mouth upwards and laterally as in laughing | Zygomatic bone |
| Zygomaticus minor | Above lateral angle of upper lip | Pulls up upper lip | Zygomatic bone |
| Risorius | Merges with orbicularis oris at lateral angle of mouth | Retracts angle of mouth | |
| Depressor anguli oris | Below angle of mouth | Depresses angle of mouth | Mandible |
| Depressor labii inferioris | Merges with orbicularis from below | Depresses lower lip | Mandible |
| Mentalis | Over chin | Produces wrinkles on chin | Mandible |
| Incisivus labii superioris | Above upper lip near midline | Anchors upper lip to maxilla | Maxilla |
| Incisivus labii inferioris | Below lower lip near midline | Anchors lower lip to mandible | Mandible |

## WANT TO KNOW MORE?

**Note on Buccinator muscle**

1. Literally, the word buccinator means one who blows a trumpet.
2. The muscle is lined on the inside by the mucous membrane of the mouth.
3. It is related to the following:
   a. Its outer aspect is related to the parotid duct that pierces it opposite the third upper molar tooth.
   b. It comes into relationship with the superficial muscles inserted into the angle of the mouth.
   c. It is also related to the facial artery and vein; and to branches of the facial and buccal nerves.

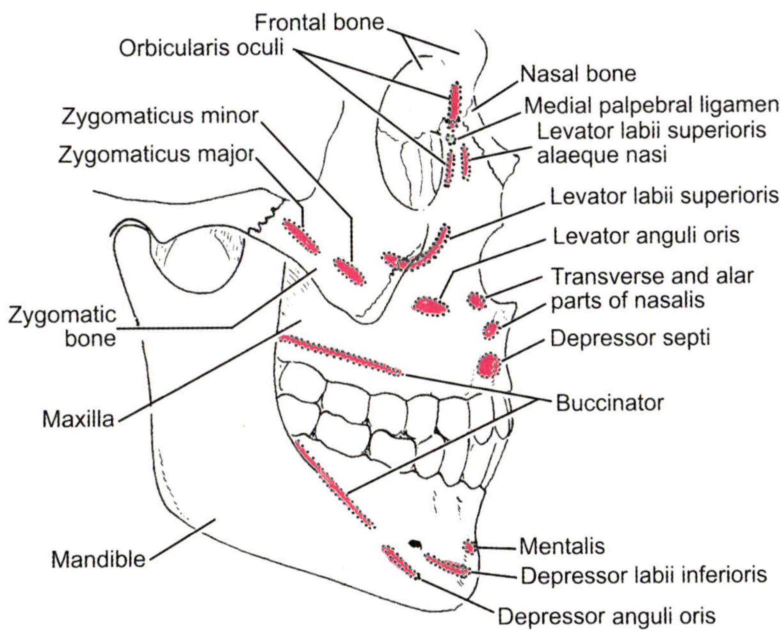


**37.9B:** Facial skeleton seen from the side to show some muscle attachments

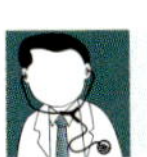

## CLINICAL CORRELATION

### Face

1. The mouth is always examined as part of a general physical examination. Hence, a doctor must be aware of common conditions affecting the region.
   a. The lips are blue in cyanosis.
   b. Inflammation at the angles of the mouth (angular stomatitis) occurs in vitamin deficiencies.
   c. Conjunctiva becomes pale in anaemia, yellow in jaundice, reddish in conjunctivitis.
   d. Conditions affecting the teeth and gums are considered later.
2. a. Hypothyroidism in infants leads to ***cretinism***. A child with cretinism has a puffed face with a protruding tongue, a bulky belly, and sometimes an umbilical hernia.
   b. Hypothyroidism in adults leads to deposition of mucopolysaccharides in subcutaneous tissue. The face is bloated. The lips are thick and protuberant and the expression is dull.
3. In hyperthyroidism, the eyes become prominent (exophthalmos).
4. Interruption of sympathetic supply to the head and neck results in ***Horner's syndrome***. The features of this syndrome are as follows:
   a. There is constriction of the pupil because of paralysis of the dilator pupillae. Unopposed action of the sphincter pupillae leads to constriction.
   b. There is drooping of the upper eyelid (ptosis) because of paralysis of smooth muscle fibres present in the levator palpebrae superioris.
   c. The eyeball is less prominent than normal (enophthalmos).
   d. There is absence of sweating on the affected side of the face. (Remember that secretomotor supply to sweat glands is through sympathetic nerves).
5. a. There is a collection of lymphoid tissue present in relation to the roof of the nasopharynx. It is called the ***nasopharyngeal tonsil***.
   b. When enlarged (because of chronic infection) the pharyngeal tonsils are referred to as ***adenoids***.
   c. Adenoids lead to obstruction in the nasopharynx forcing the child to breathe through the mouth.

   d. A constantly open mouth can lead to deformities of the teeth and palate (as normal pressure of the tongue on the palate is not present).
   e. Infection frequently spreads to the middle ear (through the auditory tube).
   f. Removal of adenoids is called ***adenoidectomy***.
6. ***Injuries*** (e.g., blows) on the face can lead to fracture of the mandible, the zygomatic bone, the maxilla or the nasal bones. The mandible is commonly fractured.
7. The maxilla, the mandible and the zygomatic bone are derived from the first branchial arch. Occasionally, growth of this arch is defective so that the bones concerned remain underdeveloped, and the face is deformed. The condition is called ***mandibulofacial dysostosis***.

*Dangerous Area of Face*

1. Near the medial angle of the eye the supraorbital vein, which is a tributary of the facial vein, communicates with the superior ophthalmic vein (lying in the orbit).
2. The superior ophthalmic vein drains into the cavernous sinus. In this way, the facial vein is brought into communication with the cavernous sinus.
3. The facial vein also communicates with the cavernous sinus through the deep facial vein and the pterygoid plexus.
4. Because of these communications, an infection in the face can spread to the cavernous sinus leading to cavernous sinus thrombosis.
5. It has been observed that such spread of infection is most likely to take place if the infection is over the upper lip or the lower part of the nose. That is why, this region is called the ***dangerous area of the face***.

*Harelip*

1. Embryologically, the upper lip (and the palate) are derived from three elements. These are the right and left ***maxillary processes***, and the ***frontonasal process*** that is a median structure.
2. The frontonasal process forms the median part of the upper lip. This part is called the ***philtrum***. On each side, the frontonasal process fuses with the corresponding maxillary process.
3. Abnormalities in fusion of these processes lead to clefts in the upper lip (called ***harelip*** because the hare normally has an upper lip with a cleft).
4. The defect may be unilateral or bilateral.
5. When defect in fusion is minimal only a small indentation may be seen in the margin of the lip.
6. When non-union is complete the defect extends into the nostril, and is continuous with a defect in the palate.

## PAROTID GLAND

1. The parotid gland is one of the salivary glands. It lies on the lateral side of the face in a depression below the external acoustic meatus, behind the mandible, and in front of the sternocleidomastoid muscle (37.13).
2. It is roughly triangular on cross-section.
   a. It has a lateral or superficial surface
   b. An anteromedial surface
   c. A posteromedial surface (37.13)
   d. At its upper end, it has a small superior surface (37.14)
   e. Its lower end is rounded and is called the apex.
3. a. The superficial surface of the parotid gland extends upwards to the zygomatic arch.
   b. Its lower end (apex) lies behind and below the angle of the mandible.
   c. Anteriorly, it is prolonged forwards superficial to the masseter.
   d. Posteriorly, it overlaps the anterior margin of the sternocleidomastoid (37.13). This surface is covered by skin and fascia. Lymph nodes of the superficial parotid group lie over it.

**37.10A: Large muscles of the face**

| | *Orbicularis oris* | *Orbicularis oculi* | *Buccinator* |
|---|---|---|---|
| Arrangement of fibres | 1. The fibres surround the opening of the mouth<br>2. They form the muscular basis of the lips<br>3. Many facial muscles merge with it (37.10B)<br>4. The muscle is anchored to the maxilla by the incisivus superior and to the mandible by the incisivus inferior | 1. Muscle fasciculi arranged concentrically around palpebral fissure<br>2. The innermost rings lie in the eyelids and form the palpebral part<br>3. Succeeding rings surround the margin of the orbit. They form the orbital part<br>4. Fibres closely related to the lacrimal sac form the lacrimal part<br>5. Fibres of orbital part are attached on the medial side to:<br>a. Nasal part of frontal bone<br>b. Medial palpebral ligament<br>c. Frontal process of maxilla<br>6. The fibres of the palpebralpart are attached medially to the medial palpebral ligament<br>7. They decussate on the lateral side to form the lateral palpebral raphe | 1. The buccinator has a C-shaped line of origin from (37.12)<br>a. Maxilla just above molar teeth<br>b. Pterygomandibular raphe<br>c. Mandible below molar teeth. (The pterygomandibular raphe is raphe of a fibrous band attached above to the ptergoid hamulus and below the mandible)<br>2. Fibres run forwards and become continuous with orbicularis oris |
| Nerve supply | Lower buccal and mandibular branches of facial nerve | Temporal and zygomatic branches of facial nerve | Lower buccal branches of facial nerve |
| Action | 1. Closes the lips<br>2. Performs complex movements required in speech, eating, drinking | 1. Closes palpebral fissure<br>2. The lacrimal part helps to suck lacrimal fluid into the lacrimal sac | 1. Aids mastication by pushing food between the teeth<br>2. Increases air pressure in the mouth as in blowing |

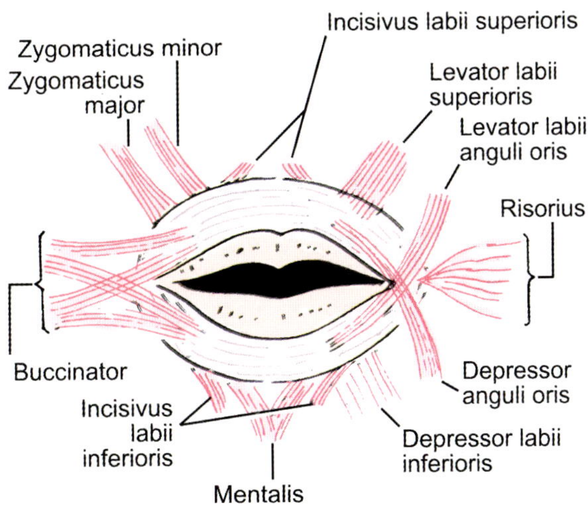


**37.10B:** The orbicularis oris and its relationship to various muscles attached to the lips

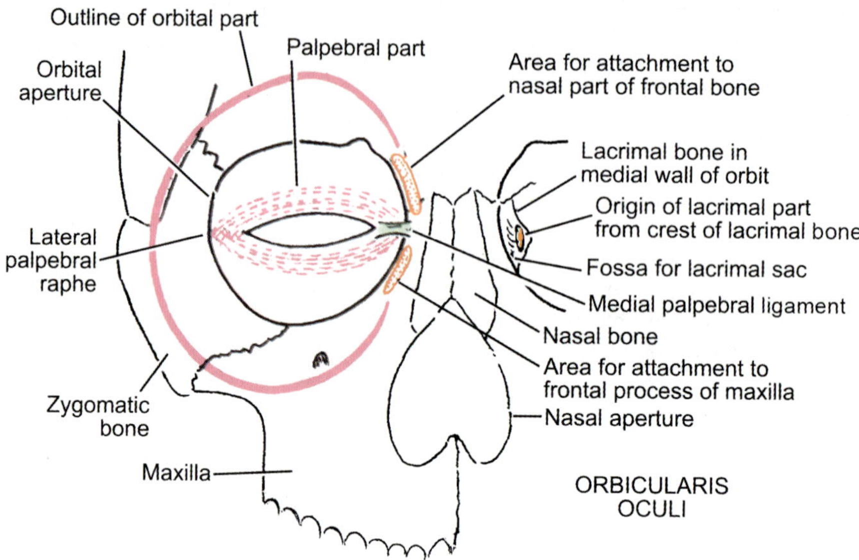


**37.11:** Scheme to show the attachments of the orbicularis oculi muscle

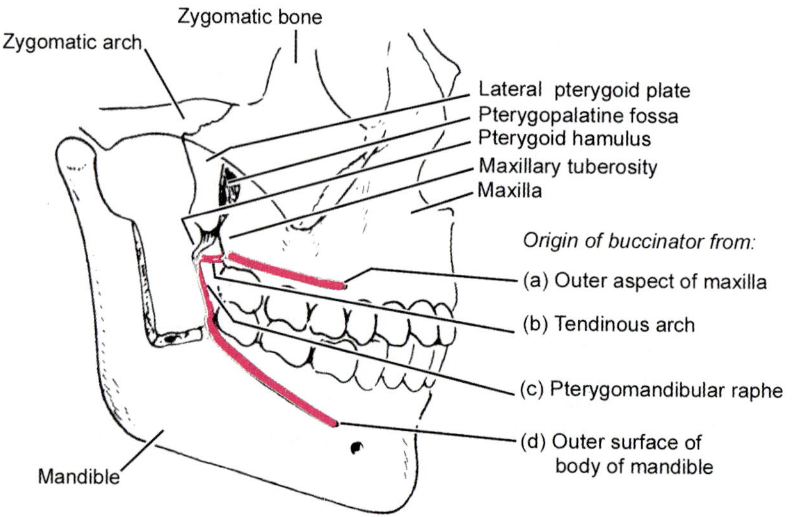


**37.12:** Origin of the buccinator muscle

4. The superior surface of the parotid is concave and fits under the external acoustic meatus. It is also in contact with the posterior surface of the temporomandibular joint (37.14).
5. The anteromedial surface is in contact with the posterior border of the ramus of the mandible (37.13).
   a. Lateral to the ramus, there is the masseter muscle, and deep to it there is the medial pterygoid.
   b. The anteromedial surface is related to all these structures.
6. The posteromedial surface is in contact with the following:
   a. Its upper part is in contact with the mastoid process.
   b. Lower down, it is in contact with the sternocleidomastoid superficially (37.13) and the posterior belly of the digastric deeply.

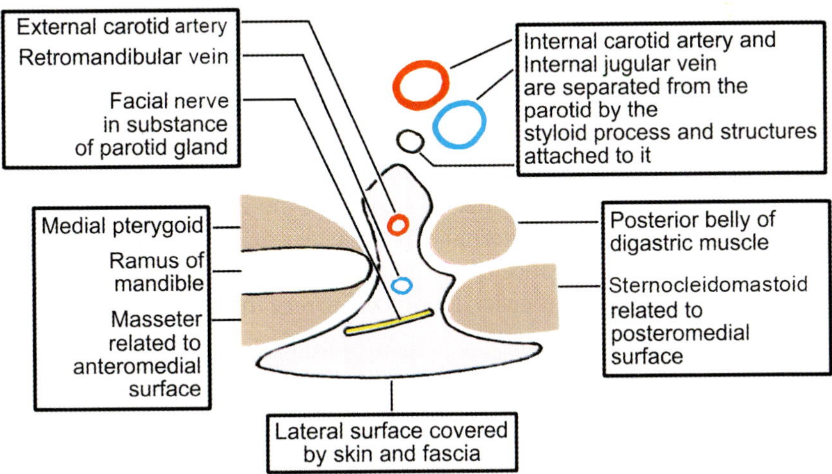


**37.13:** Schematic transverse section through parotid gland to show its relations

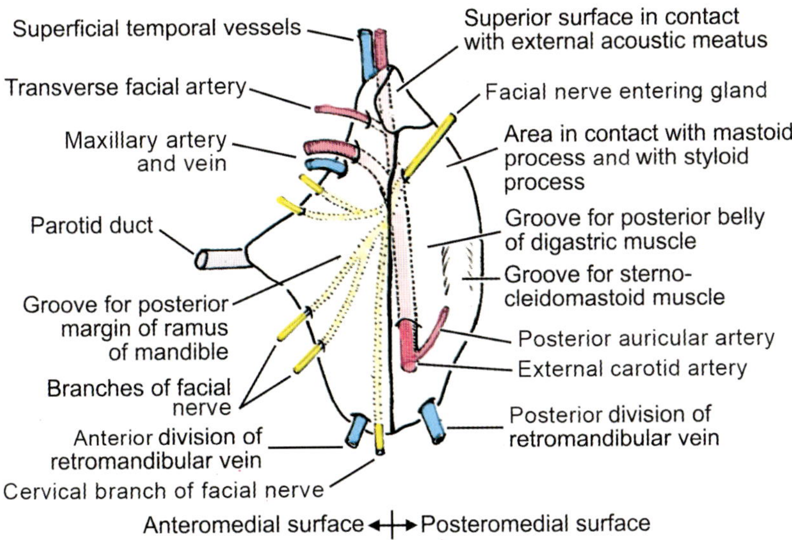


**37.14:** Schematic view of parotid gland as seen from the medial side. Note the structures entering or leaving the gland

c. The deepest part of the gland reaches the styloid process and the structures attached to it. These separate the gland from the internal carotid artery and the internal jugular vein (37.13 and 37.14).

7. Secretions of the parotid gland are collected by a system of ducts that unite to form the ***parotid duct.***
   a. This duct emerges at the anterior margin of the gland and runs forwards across the masseter.
   b. At the anterior border of the masseter, the duct turns medially and pierces the buccinator.
   c. The terminal part of the duct runs forwards deep to the mucous membrane of the cheek.
   d. It opens into the vestibule of the mouth opposite the crown of the upper second molar tooth.
8. A detached part of the parotid gland present just above the parotid duct is called the ***accessory part*** of the parotid gland.

## WANT TO KNOW MORE?

9. The parotid gland is related to several nerves and vessels as follows.
10. The ***external carotid artery*** enters the lower part of the posteromedial surface (37.14).
    a. Ascending within the substance of the gland, it divides into its terminal branches (superficial temporal and maxillary) that emerge on the anteromedial surface of the gland.
    b. The posterior auricular branch of the external carotid artery arises just before the latter enters the gland. Sometimes, it arises within the substance of the gland and emerges on the posteromedial surface.
    c. The transverse facial branch of the superficial temporal artery may arise within the substance of the gland (37.14).
11. The ***retromandibular vein*** lies in the substance of the parotid superficial to the external carotid artery (37.13) (See below).
12. The trunk of the ***facial nerve*** enters the upper part of the posteromedial surface.
    a. Within the gland, it divides into its terminal branches that emerge from the anteromedial surface near its anterior margin (37.14).
    b. The cervical branch of the nerve emerges from the lower end of the gland (37.14).
    c. The facial nerve is often described as dividing the parotid gland into superficial and deep parts.
13. The ***auriculotemporal nerve*** passes laterally between the neck of the mandible and the superior surface of the gland. It gives branches to the gland.
14. The anterior (facial) branch of the great auricular nerve passes forwards over the superficial surface of the gland and supplies the overlying skin.
15. The parotid gland is enclosed in a fibrous capsule derived from the deep cervical fascia as follows:
    a. At the lower end of the gland, the investing layer of the deep cervical fascia splits into two layers.
    b. One layer ascends superficial to the parotid gland to reach the zygomatic arch to which it is attached. This fascia is thick and strong and is called the ***parotid fascia***.
    c. The other layer ascends deep to the gland.
    d. Part of this layer forms a thickened band extending from the posterior margin of the ramus of the mandible to the styloid process. This band is the ***stylomandibular ligament.*** It separates the parotid gland from the submandibular gland.
16. a. The parotid gland is supplied by small branches of the external carotid artery or of its terminal divisions.
    b. The veins drain into the retromandibular and external jugular veins.
17. The lymph vessels from the gland drain into the deep cervical nodes after passing through the superficial parotid nodes (lying on the lateral surface of the gland) and the deep parotid nodes (lying in the substance of the gland).
18. Secretomotor nerves reach the gland through branches from the auriculotemporal nerve. The gland also receives sympathetic nerves.

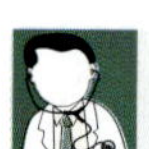

## CLINICAL CORRELATION

### Parotid Gland

1. The salivary glands (including the parotid gland) are commonly infected with a virus that causes mumps. It causes swelling and pain in the gland affected. It can involve more than one gland. The parotid is the most commonly infected salivary gland.
2. The salivary glands can also be infected by spread of infection from the mouth. An abscess may form in the gland.
3. The parotid fascia is very dense and allows very little expansion of the gland. Swellings of the parotid are therefore very painful.
4. Tumours may form in a salivary gland. They may be benign or malignant.

5. Facial paralysis (see below) can occur by involvement of the facial nerve in a malignant growth of the parotid gland, or by injury during removal of the gland. The surgeon tries to protect the nerve by removing the superficial and deep parts separately.

## VESSELS OF THE FACE AND PAROTID REGION

### Arteries

1. The arteries to be seen in the face are the facial artery and the transverse facial branch of the superficial temporal artery.
2. We have seen that the external carotid artery runs through the parotid gland and gives off a number of branches in the region.

#### *Facial Artery in the Face*

1. The facial artery runs part of its course in the neck, and in the submandibular region.
2. It then enters the face by passing round the lower border of the body of the mandible just in front of the masseter muscle.
3. From here, it runs upwards and forwards across the body of the mandible and the buccinator to reach the angle of the mouth.
4. Finally, it ascends along the side of the nose to reach the medial angle of the eye.
5. In the face, the artery gives off branches to:
   a. The lower lip (***inferior labial artery***)
   b. The upper lip (***superior labial artery***)
   c. To the nose (***lateral nasal artery***)
   d. The terminal part of the facial artery is called the ***angular artery***.

#### *Superficial Temporal Artery*

1. The superficial temporal artery arises from the external carotid artery within the parotid gland.
2. It runs upwards behind the temporomandibular joint and ends by dividing into frontal and parietal branches that supply the scalp.
3. It also gives off the ***transverse facial artery*** that runs forwards across the masseter muscle.

### Veins

The veins to be seen in the face and parotid region are the facial vein, the superficial temporal vein, and the retromandibular vein.

1. a. The ***retromandibular vein*** is formed within the upper part of the parotid gland by the union of the superficial temporal and maxillary veins.
   b. Its lower end divides, within the gland, into anterior and posterior divisions that emerge from the gland near its lower end.
   c. The posterior division, which is the main continuation of the retromandibular vein, joins the posterior auricular vein to form the external jugular vein.
   d. The anterior division joins the facial vein to form the common facial vein.
2. a. The ***facial vein*** runs downwards and backwards just behind the facial artery, and receives tributaries corresponding to branches of the artery.
   b. It ends by joining the anterior division of the retromandibular vein to form the ***common facial vein***.
   c. The common facial vein ends in the internal jugular vein.

## LYMPH NODES OF HEAD AND NECK

1. Numerous groups of lymph nodes are present in the head and neck.
2. Some of them are placed superficially:
   a. In the occipital region (***occipital nodes***)
   b. Behind the auricle (***retroauricular nodes***)
   c. In relation to the parotid gland (***superficial and deep parotid nodes***)
   d. In relation to the submandibular gland (***submandibular nodes***)
   e. Below the chin (***submental nodes***).
3. Lymph nodes are also present along some veins.
   a. The ***buccal nodes*** lie along the facial vein.
   b. The ***superficial cervical nodes*** along the external jugular vein.
   c. The ***anterior cervical nodes*** along the anterior jugular vein.
4. Lymph from all these nodes ultimately drains into the ***deep cervical lymph nodes*** that lie along the internal jugular vein.
5. The deep cervical nodes drain into a jugular lymph trunk which joins the thoracic duct (on the left side), or the right lymphatic duct (on the right side).

### Lymphatics of Face

1. The lymphatics of the face drain into:
   a. The superficial and deep parotid lymph nodes
   b. Into the submental nodes
   c. Into the submandibular lymph nodes.
2. As mentioned above, the parotid gland drains into the superficial and deep parotid nodes.

## NERVES OF THE FACE

1. The nerves seen on the face are motor and sensory.
2. The motor nerves are terminal branches of the ***facial nerve***. We have seen that after emerging from the skull, the facial nerve enters the parotid gland and divides within it into several branches that emerge along the borders of the gland (37.14).
3. The facial nerve gives off:
   a. A ***temporal*** branch
   b. A ***zygomatic*** branch
   c. Upper and lower ***buccal*** branches
   d. A ***marginal mandibular*** branch
   e. A ***cervical*** branch.

   These branches supply the various muscles of the face.
4. The sensory nerves seen on the face are terminal ramifications of the ***trigeminal nerve***.
5. Branches arising from the ophthalmic division are:
   a. The ***supratrochlear***
   b. ***Supraorbital***
   c. ***Infratrochlear***
   d. ***External nasal*** nerves.
   e. Some branches are also given off to the upper eyelid.
6. Branches of the maxillary division of the trigeminal nerve to be seen on the face are:
   a. The ***infraorbital*** nerve
   b. The ***zygomaticofacial***
   c. ***Zygomatico-temporal*** nerves.

7. Branches of the mandibular division seen on the face are:
   a. The ***auriculotemporal***
   b. ***Buccal***
   c. ***Mental*** nerves.
8. The area of skin of the face supplied by the three divisions of the trigeminal nerve are showing in 37.15.

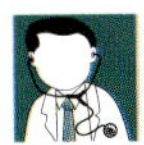

## CLINICAL CORRELATION

### Nerves of the Face

1. The ***trigeminal nerve*** is responsible for sensory supply of most of the face. When a lesion of the nerve is suspected, it is tested as follows:
   a. The sensation of touch in the area of distribution of the nerve can be tested by touching different areas of skin with a wisp of cottonwool.
   b. The sensation of pain can be tested by gentle pressure with a pin.
   c. Motor function is tested by asking the patient to clench his teeth firmly. Contraction of the masseter can be felt by palpation when the teeth are clenched.
2. The ***facial nerve*** supplies the muscles of the face including the muscles that close the eyelids, and the mouth. The nerve is tested as follows:
   a. Ask the patient to close his eyes firmly. In complete paralysis of the facial nerve the patient will not be able to close the eye on the affected side. In partial paralysis, the closure is weak and the examiner can easily open the closed eye with his fingers (which is very difficult in a normal person).
   b. Ask the person to smile. In smiling the normal mouth is more or less symmetrical, the two angles moving upwards and outwards. In facial paralysis, the angle fails to move on the paralysed side.
   c. Ask the patient to fill his mouth with air. Press the cheek with your finger and compare the resistance (by the buccinator muscle) on the two sides. The resistance is less on the paralysed side. On pressing the cheek air may leak out of the mouth because the muscles closing the mouth are weak.
   d. The sensation of taste should be tested on the anterior two-thirds of the tongue by applying substances of different tastes.
3. ***Paralysis of facial nerve***
   The effects of paralysis are due to the failure of the muscles concerned to perform their normal actions. Some effects are as follows:
   a. The normal face is more or less symmetrical. When the facial nerve is paralysed on one side, the most noticeable feature is the loss of symmetry.
   b. Normal furrows on the forehead are lost because of paralysis of the occipitofrontalis.
   c. There is drooping of the eyelid and the palpebral fissure is wider on the paralysed side because of paralysis of the orbicularis oculi. The conjunctival reflex is lost for the same reason.
   d. There is marked asymmetry of the mouth because of paralysis of the orbicularis oris and of muscles inserted into the angle of the mouth. This is most obvious when a smile is attempted. As a result of asymmetry, the protruded tongue appears to deviate to one side, but is in fact in the midline.
   e. During mastication food tends to accumulate between the cheek and the teeth. (This is normally prevented by the buccinator).
   
   Also see testing of the nerve described above.

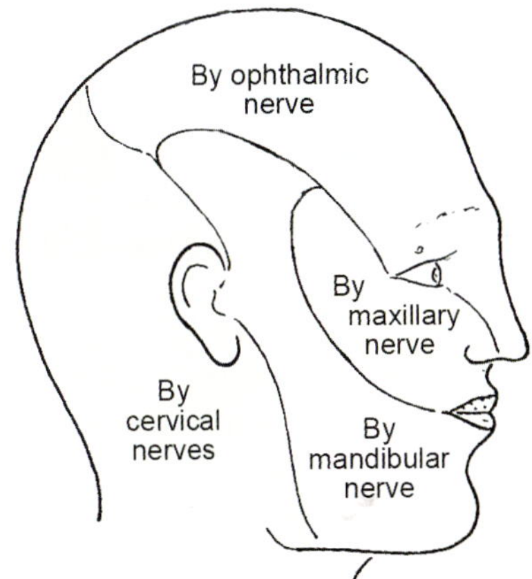


37.15: Areas of skin supplied by the ophthalmic, maxillary and mandibular divisions of the trigeminal nerve

# 38 Temporal and Infratemporal Regions

CHAPTER

## TEMPORAL REGION

### Superficial Structures to be Seen in the Temporal Region

1. The temporal region overlies the ***temporal fossa*** present on the lateral aspect of the skull.
2. The fossa is bounded above by the temporal line and inferiorly by the zygomatic arch.
3. Its floor is formed by:
   a. Part of frontal bone
   b. Part of parietal bone
   c. Part of the squamous temporal bone
   d. Part of the greater wing of the sphenoid bone.
4. The wall has an anterior wall made up mainly by the temporal surface of the zygomatic bone with contributions from the greater wing of the sphenoid and from the frontal bone.
5. A thick fibrous membrane, the ***temporal fascia*** covers the region. This fascia is attached superiorly to the temporal lines, and inferiorly to the zygomatic arch.
   a. Placed over the superficial aspect of the temporal fascia we see some subcutaneous muscles attached to the auricle. These are the ***auricularis superior***, the ***auricularis posterior*** and the ***auricularis anterior***.
   b. A few scattered muscle fibres that run vertically over the upper part of the region are given the name ***temporo-parietalis***. (These are all vestigial muscles of no functional importance).
6. We also see a number of nerves and vessels such as:
   a. Immediately in front of the external acoustic meatus we see the ***auriculotemporal nerve*** emerging from under cover of the upper end of the parotid gland. The nerve ascends into the temporal region and scalp and divides into branches that supply them.
   b. Just in front of the auriculotemporal nerve we see the superficial temporal vessels. The ***superficial temporal artery*** is a terminal branch of the external carotid artery. It divides into branches that supply the temporal region and scalp (named in 38.1A).
7. The ***superficial temporal vein*** is a tributary of the retromandibular vein.

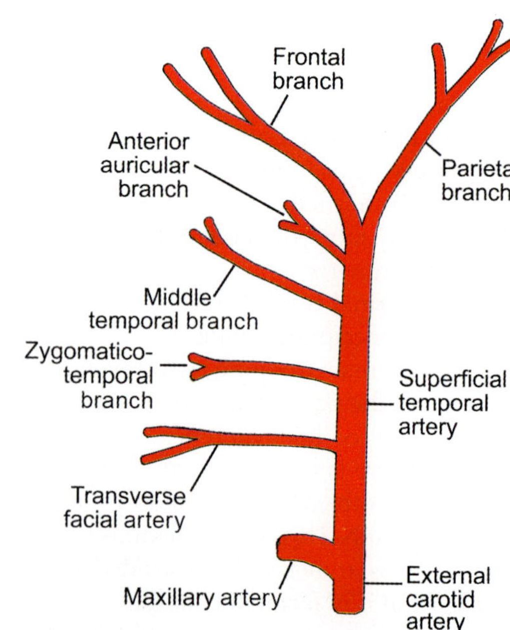


**38.1A:** Branches of superficial temporal artery

8. Some other nerves seen in the region are as follows:
   a. The ***temporal branch of the facial nerve*** runs upwards and forwards to reach the frontalis muscle that it supplies. It also helps to supply the orbicularis oculi and the auricular muscles.
   b. The ***posterior auricular branch of the facial nerve*** lies behind the auricle in the lower part of the temporal region. It runs backwards to reach and supply the occipitalis muscle. It also helps to supply the auricular muscles.
   c. The ***zygomaticofacial nerve*** and the ***zygomaticotemporal nerve*** are derived from the zygomatic branch of the maxillary division of the trigeminal nerve. They help to supply the skin of the region.

#### *Deeper Structures in Temporal Region*

1. The ***temporalis muscle*** is the main content of the temporal fossa.
2. It is covered by temporal fascia.
3. The temporalis is one of the muscles that are responsible for chewing movements (mastication).
4. Deep to this muscle we see the (anterior, middle and posterior) ***deep temporal nerves*** and vessels. The arteries are branches of the maxillary artery, while the nerves arise from the anterior division of the mandibular nerve.
5. The deep temporal nerves supply the temporalis muscle.
   The temporalis muscle is described in 38.2C and is shown in 38.2A and B.

## INFRATEMPORAL FOSSA

### Relationship to the Skull

1. The term infratemporal fossa is applied to an irregular space lying below the lateral part of the base of the skull.
2. The roof of the fossa is formed mainly by the greater wing of the sphenoid bone, with a small contribution from the squamous temporal bone.
3. The fossa is bounded medially by the pterygoid process (of the sphenoid bone). The medial and lateral pterygoid plates arising from the process are intimately related to structures in the fossa.
4. The anterior wall of the infratemporal fossa is formed by the posterior surface of the maxilla.
5. Superiorly, the lateral part of the infratemporal fossa communicates with the temporal fossa through the gap between the zygomatic arch and the rest of the skull.
6. The infratemporal fossa communicates with the pterygopalatine fossa through the pterygomaxillary fissure.
7. Anteriorly, the infratemporal fossa communicates with the orbit through the inferior orbital fissure.

### Some Structures to be Seen Near the Infratemporal Fossa

1. Structures in the fossa (or near it) are exposed by removing the parotid gland and the zygomatic arch.
2. The external carotid artery ascends a short distance behind the ramus of the mandible and terminates by dividing into the superficial temporal and maxillary arteries.
3. The auriculotemporal nerve passes backwards deep to the neck of the mandible and then turns upwards to enter the temporal region.
4. The masseteric branch of the mandibular nerve passes laterally through the mandibular notch to enter the masseter muscle.
5. The buccal nerve and artery emerging from under the anterior margin of the ramus of the mandible to run forwards on the buccinator muscle.

### Superficial Contents of the Infratemporal Fossa

#### *The Pterygoid Muscles*

1. The ***lateral pterygoid muscle*** has two heads: upper and lower. Their fibres run more or less horizontally and converge posteriorly to reach the neck of the mandible.
2. Anteriorly, the two heads diverge and an interval can be seen between them.

3. Inferior to the lateral pterygoid muscle we see the ***medial pterygoid muscle***.
   a. The fibres of this muscle run downwards and backwards. Anteriorly, some fibres of the muscle lie superficial to the lower head of the lateral pterygoid muscle. These fibres constitute the superficial head of the medial pterygoid muscle.
   b. The medial and lateral pterygoid muscles lie deep to the ramus of the mandible. The ramus separates the medial pterygoid muscle from the masseter.
   c. The medial pterygoid muscle overlaps the posterior part of the buccinator muscle.
4. The medial and lateral pterygoid muscles, the masseter, and the temporalis are muscles of mastication and are described in 38.2A to C.

### *Maxillary Artery*

1. The ***maxillary artery*** arises from the external carotid artery just behind the ramus of the mandible.
   a. The artery runs forwards deep to the neck of the mandible to enter the infratemporal fossa (38.1B).
   b. It first runs forwards along the lower border of the lateral pterygoid muscle (first part) and then runs upwards and forwards across the lower head of the muscle (second part).
   c. Finally, it enters the interval between the two heads of the lateral pterygoid and disappears into the pterygomaxillary fissure.
2. Some branches of the artery are as follows (38.1C):
   a. While still posterior to the mandible, the maxillary artery gives off the ***anterior tympanic*** and ***deep auricular*** arteries.
   b. Within the infratemporal fossa the maxillary artery gives off:
      i. The middle meningeal artery
      ii. The inferior alveolar artery
      iii. The buccal artery
      iv. The deep temporal arteries.
   c. Just before entering the pterygomaxillary fissure it gives off the ***posterior superior alveolar artery***.

### *Mandibular Nerve*

1. The main nerve of the infratemporal fossa is the ***mandibular nerve***.
   a. The nerve enters the fossa through the foramen ovale (38.1D).
   b. The upper part of the mandibular nerve lies under cover of the lateral pterygoid muscle.
   c. After a very short course, the trunk of the nerve divides into a thin anterior division and a much thicker posterior division.

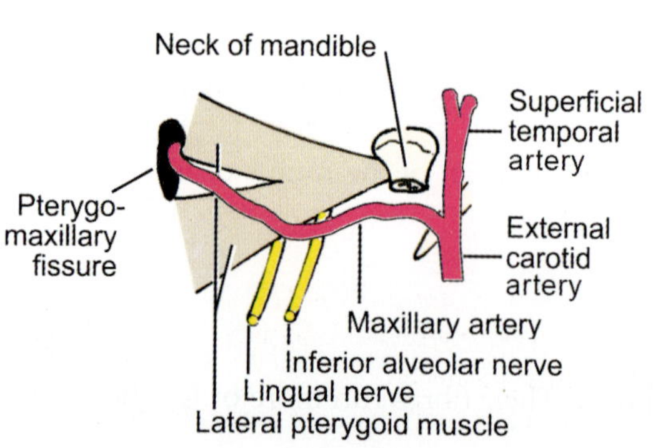


**38.1B:** Course of maxillary artery

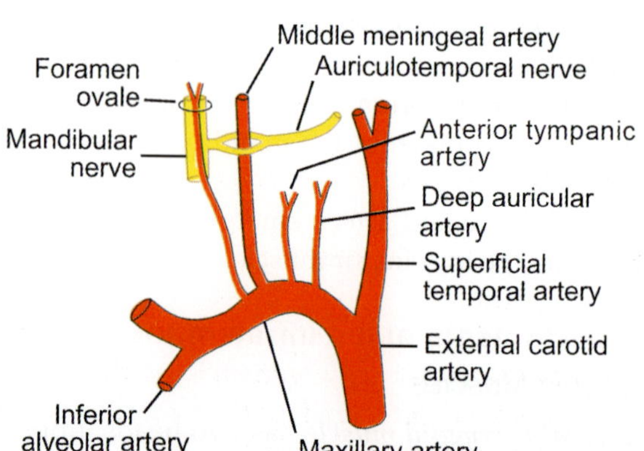


**38.1C:** Branches of first part of maxillary artery in infratemporal region

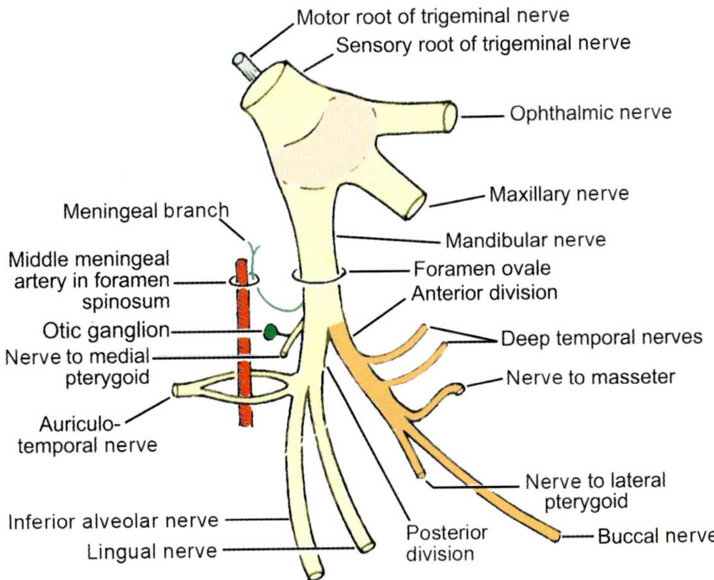


38.1D: Scheme to show branches of mandibular nerve

2. The *anterior division gives off* the following (38.1D):
   a. Deep temporal nerves
   b. Branch to the masseter
   c. Branch to the lateral pterygoid
   d. Finally the anterior division continues onto the surface of the buccinator muscle as the buccal nerve.
3. a. The masseteric nerve and the deep temporal nerves become superficial by passing above the lateral pterygoid muscle.
   b. The buccal nerve emerges through the gap between the two heads of the lateral pterygoid.
4. The *posterior division gives off*:
   a. The ***auriculotemporal nerve*** which arises by two roots that are separated by the middle meningeal artery (38.1D).
   b. The posterior division then divides into two main branches: the ***lingual nerve*** (anteriorly), and the ***inferior alveolar nerve*** (posteriorly)
   c. The lingual nerve is joined (posteriorly) by the ***chorda tympani*** (a branch of the facial nerve).
5. a. The lingual and inferior alveolar nerves emerge from under the lower border of the lateral pterygoid muscle and descend over the surface of the medial pterygoid.
   b. The inferior alveolar nerve is separated from the medial pterygoid muscle by a broad ***sphenomandibular ligament***.
6. The lingual nerve leaves the infratemporal region to pass through the submandibular region on its way to the tongue.
7. a. The inferior alveolar nerve enters the mandibular canal and passes through it to supply the mandible and the lower teeth.
   b. It gives a branch, the ***mental nerve***, which emerges through the mental foramen.
   c. The ***mylohyoid nerve*** is given off from the inferior alveolar nerve just before it enters the mandibular canal.
   d. The mylohyoid nerve pierces through the sphenomandibular ligament.
   e. The mylohyoid nerve descends into the submandibular region to reach some muscles there.

*For further details of arteries and nerves see chapters 42 and 43.*

## MUSCLES OF MASTICATION

The muscles of mastication are:

1. Temporalis
2. Masseter
3. Lateral pterygoid
4. Medial pterygoid.

They are described in 38.2C and shown in 38.2A and B and 38.3 to 38.6.

 **WANT TO KNOW MORE?**

### Notes on Temporalis

1. The anterior fibres of the muscle run vertically downwards; the posterior fibres run horizontally forwards; while the intermediate fibres run obliquely to converge in a tendon (38.3A and B). The tendon passes deep to the zygomatic arch.
2. The movements of elevation and depression of the mandible have two components.
   a. Firstly, there is a hinge-like movement between the condyle of the mandible and the inferior surface of the articular disc of the temporomandibular joint.
   b. The second component is a gliding movement of the disc (along with the head of the mandible).
   c. In wide opening of the mouth the disc glides forwards so that the head of the mandible comes to lie below the articular eminence.
   d. In closing the mouth the posterior horizontal fibres of the temporalis pull the mandible backwards (along with the intra-articular disc), whereas the anterior vertical fibres produce the angular hinge-like movement.

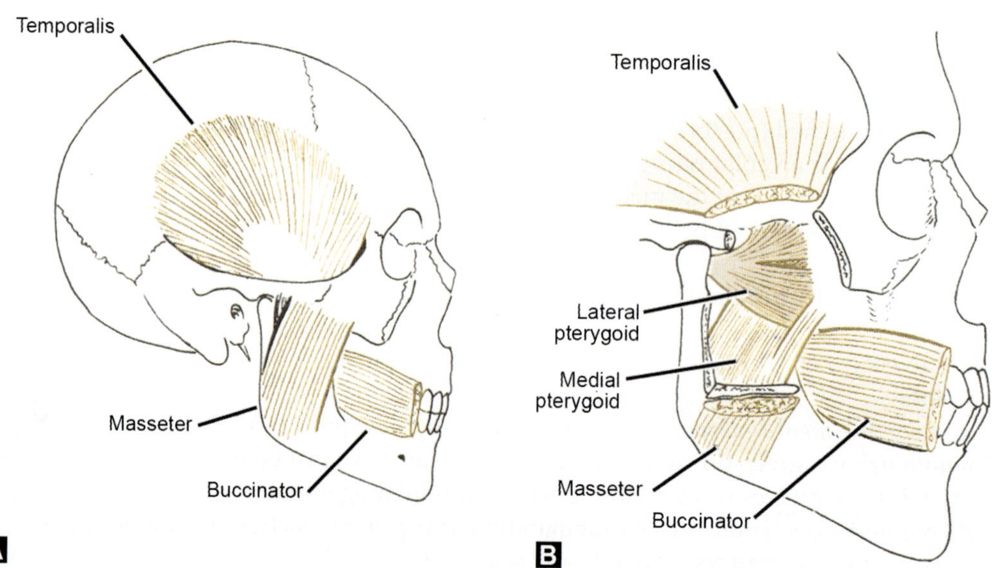


**38.2A and B:** Overall views of the muscles of mastication

| 38.2C: Muscles of mastication | | | | |
|---|---|---|---|---|
| *Muscle* | *Origin* | *Insertion* | *Action* | *Nerve supply* |
| TEMPORALIS | Temporal fossa (on lateral side of skull). Includes parts of frontal, parietal, and squamous temporal bones | Tendon passes deep to zygomatic arch and is inserted to coronoid process of mandible (medial aspect) | Elevates mandible and closes the mouth | Deep temporal branches of mandibular nerve |
| MASSETER | 1. Zygomatic arch:<br>a. Superficial fibres from anterior 2/3 of lower border<br>b. Deep fibres from deep surface and posterior 1/3 of lower border | 1. Mandible on lateral surface of:<br>a. Ramus<br>b. Angle | 1. Elevates mandible to close the mouth<br>2. Anterior fibres protract jaw | Branch from anterior division of mandibular nerve |
| LATERAL PTERYGOID | 1. Upper head:<br>a. Infratemporal surface and<br>b. Infratemporal crest of greater wing of sphenoid bone<br>2. Lower head:<br>Lateral pterygoid plate (lateral surface) | 1. Neck of mandible (fovea on anterior surface)<br>2. Intra-articular disc and capsule of tempo-romandibular joint | 1. Pulls mandible forwards and medially<br>2. Chin moves to opposite side<br>3. Helps to open mouth by pulling head of mandible forwards | Mandibular nerve (anterior division) |
| MEDIAL PTERYGOID | 1. Lateral pterygoid plate (medial surface)<br>2. Palatine bone (pyramidal process)<br>3. Superficial slip from:<br>a. Palatine bone (pyramidal process)<br>b. Maxillary tuberosity | 1. Medial surface of angle of mandible<br>2. Adjoining part of ramus | 1. Pulls mandible forwards and medially<br>2. Moves chin to opposite side<br>3. Elevates jaw to close mouth | Mandibular nerve |

## WANT TO KNOW MORE?

### Temporal Fascia

The temporalis is covered by a thick temporal fascia. The fascia is attached above to the (superior) temporal line, and below to the zygomatic arch.

#### *Notes on Masseter*

1. The masseter is overlapped by:
   a. Skin and some superficial muscles of the face
   b. Anterior part of the parotid gland
   c. The parotid duct
   d. The branches of the facial nerve
   e. The transverse facial vessels.
2. Deep to the masseter, there are:
   a. The ramus of the mandible
   b. The lower part of the temporalis
   c. The posterior part of the buccinator.

**Note on Actions of Pterygoid Muscles**

1. In analysing the actions of these muscles it may be remembered that the pull of a muscle is opposite to the direction of its fibres.
    a. The fibres of the lateral pterygoid pass backwards and laterally. They can, therefore, pull the mandible forwards (protraction) and medially. The effect of the medial pull is that the chin moves to the opposite side.
    b. The fibres of the medial pterygoid also pass backward and laterally (38.5). This muscle can therefore, perform the same actions as described for the lateral pterygoid. However, its fibres also pass downward. Hence, the muscle can elevate the mandible.
2. Now note the following corollaries:
    a. The medial and lateral pterygoids of both sides acting together protract the mandible (38.6).
    b. The medial and lateral pterygoids of one side, acting together, pull the mandibular condyle of that side forwards (and medially). As a result the chin moves forwards and ***to the opposite side***. This movement is facilitated by slight rotation of the head of the mandible of the opposite side. Alternate action of the muscles of the two sides results in side-to-side chewing movements.
    c. The two pterygoid muscles have opposite actions as far as opening and closing of the mouth is concerned.

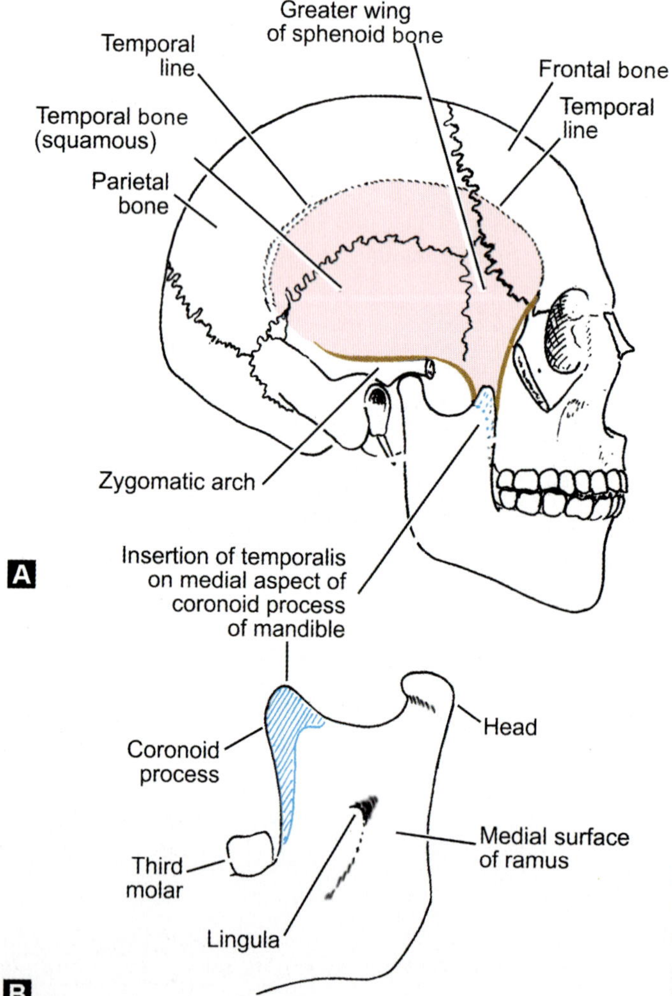


**38.3A and B:** (A) Lateral view of the skull showing the origin of the temporalis muscle from the temporal fossa. Note the bones involved; (B) Ramus of mandible seen from the medial side to show the insertion of the temporalis

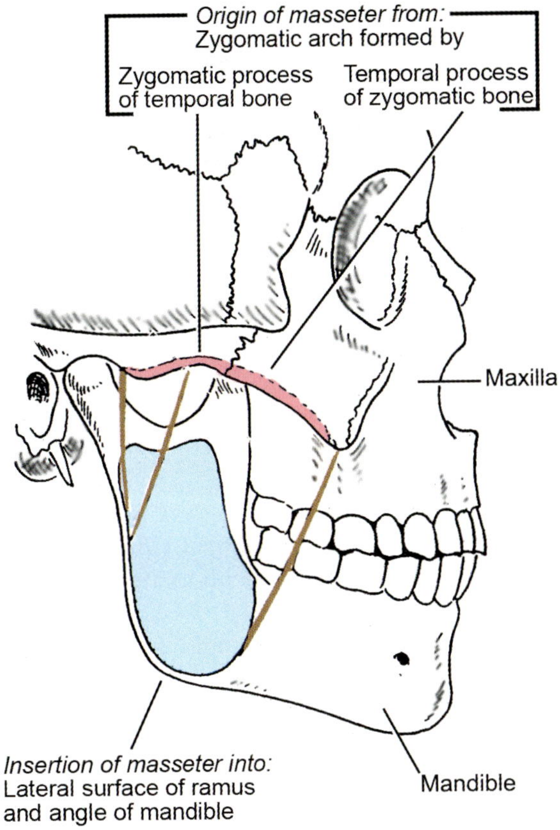

Origin of masseter from:
Zygomatic arch formed by
Zygomatic process of temporal bone
Temporal process of zygomatic bone
Maxilla
Insertion of masseter into:
Lateral surface of ramus and angle of mandible
Mandible

**38.4:** Attachments of the masseter muscle

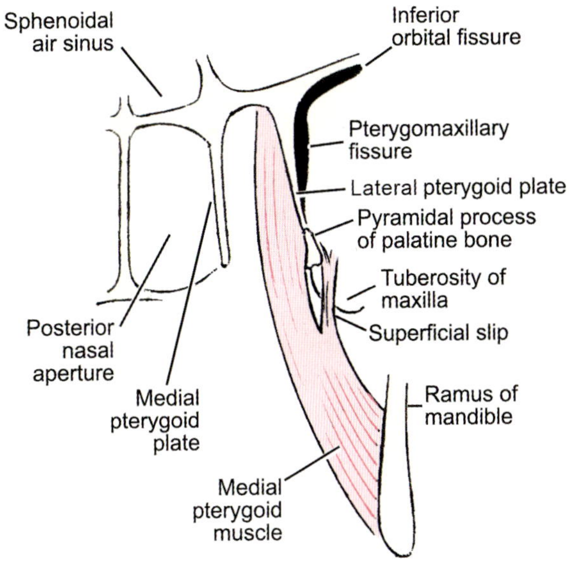

Sphenoidal air sinus
Inferior orbital fissure
Pterygomaxillary fissure
Lateral pterygoid plate
Pyramidal process of palatine bone
Tuberosity of maxilla
Superficial slip
Posterior nasal aperture
Medial pterygoid plate
Ramus of mandible
Medial pterygoid muscle

**38.5:** Scheme to show the arrangement of the medial pterygoid muscle

Coronoid process
Head
Insertion of lateral pterygoid into pterygoid fovea on anterior aspect of neck of mandible
Medial surface of ramus
Insertion of medial pterygoid into medial surface of angle of mandible and adjoining part of ramus
Lingula

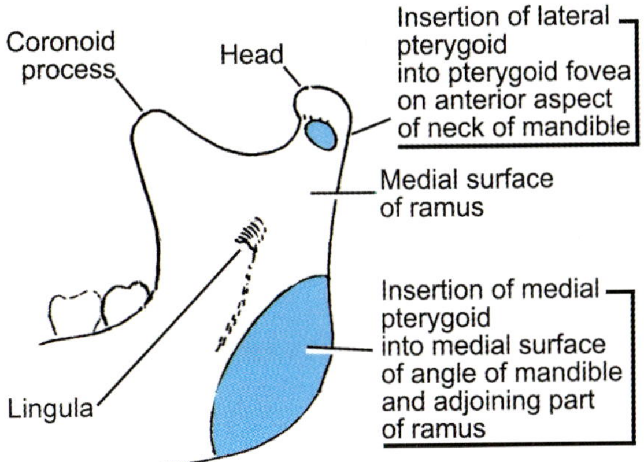

**38.6:** Medial aspect, of the ramus of the mandible, showing areas for insertion of the lateral and medial pterygoid muscles

The medial pterygoid elevates the jaw. The lateral pterygoid helps in opening the mouth by pulling the head of the mandible forwards along with the intra-articular disc (as explained above under actions of temporalis).

## THE TEMPOROMANDIBULAR JOINT

1. This is a synovial joint of the condylar variety. It is a complex joint as its cavity is divided into upper and lower parts by an intra-articular disc.
2. The ***upper articular surface*** of the joint is formed by the mandibular fossa of the temporal bone.
   a. Anteriorly, the surface extends onto the articular tubercle.
   b. The posterior part of the surface is, therefore, concave downwards; and the anterior part is convex.
3. The ***inferior articular surface*** of the joint is formed by the head of the mandible.
   a. The head of the mandible is markedly convex anteroposteriorly, and more gently convex from side-to-side.
   b. The articular surfaces are covered with white fibrocartilage (and not hyaline cartilage as in most other synovial joints; this is because the bones concerned ossify in membrane).
4. The ***articular disc*** is made of fibrocartilage.
   a. Its upper surface is concavoconvex to fit the upper articular surface of the joint.
   b. Its lower surface is concave, the head of the mandible fitting into the concavity.
5. The ***capsule*** of the joint is attached to the margins of the articular surfaces.
6. The inside of the capsule is lined by synovial membrane.
7. The lateral part of the capsule is strengthened by the ***lateral temporomandibular ligament*** (38.7). The upper end of this ligament is attached to the tubercle of the root of the zygoma and its lower end to the lateral aspect of the neck of the mandible.
8. In addition, the joint has two accessory ligaments (that are independent of the capsule and lie some distance away from it).

### WANT TO KNOW MORE?

a. The ***sphenomandibular ligament*** (38.8) is attached above to the spine of the sphenoid, and below to the lingula of the mandible.
b. The ***stylomandibular ligament*** (38.7 and 38.8) extends from the apex of the styloid process to the angle and posterior border of the ramus of the mandible. It is formed by a thickening of the deep fascia of the region.

### Movements at the Temporomandibular Joint

1. The movements at the joint can be divided into those between the upper articular surface and the articular disc, and those between the disc and the head of the mandible.
2. Most movements occur simultaneously at the right and left temporomandibular joints.
3. In forward movement or ***protraction*** of the mandible the articular disc glides forwards over the upper articular surface, the head of the mandible moving with it.
4. The reversal of this movement is called ***retraction***.
5. In slight opening of the mouth (depression of the mandible) the head of the mandible moves on the under-surface of the disc-like a hinge.
6. In wide opening of the mouth, this hinge-like movement is followed by a forward gliding of the disc and the head of the mandible, as in protraction. At the end of this movement the head comes to lie under the articular tubercle. These movements are reversed in closing the mouth (or ***elevation*** of the mandible).
7. ***Chewing movements*** involve side-to-side movements of the mandible.
   a. In these movements, the head of the mandible of one side glides forwards along with the articular disc (as in protraction) but the head of the opposite side merely rotates on a vertical axis.
   b. As a result of this the chin moves forwards and to one side (the side on which no gliding has occurred).
   c. Alternate movements of this kind on the two sides result in side-to-side movements of the lower jaw.
8. These movements are produced chiefly by the muscles of mastication described above. The muscles responsible for these movements are summarised in 38.9. Note that in side-to-side movements the medial and lateral pterygoids of the two sides act alternately. Depression is produced mainly by gravity and is a weak movement compared to elevation.

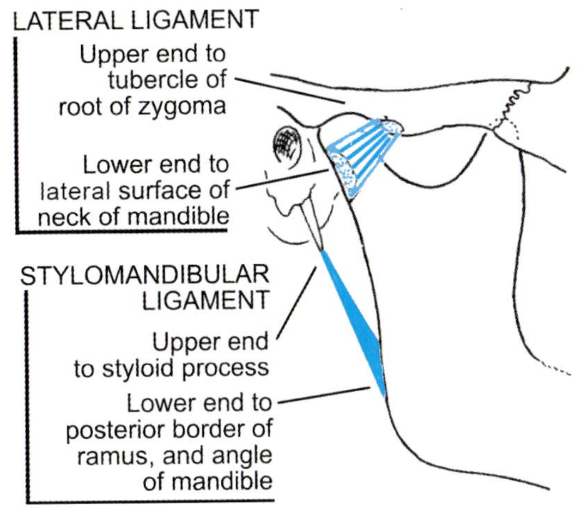


**38.7:** Ligaments of the temporomandibular joint, as seen from the lateral side

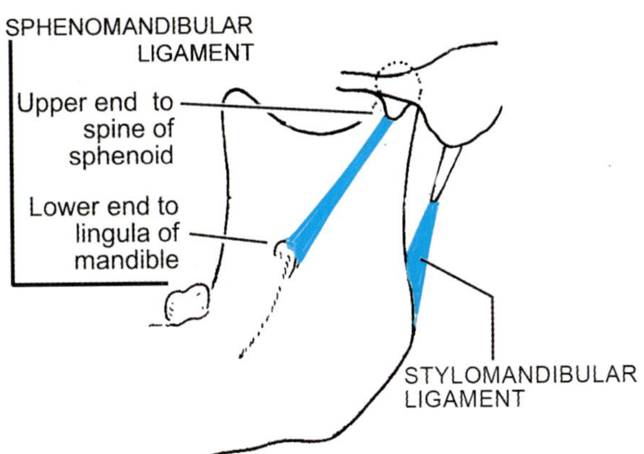


**38.8:** Ligaments of temporomandibular joint as seen from the medial side

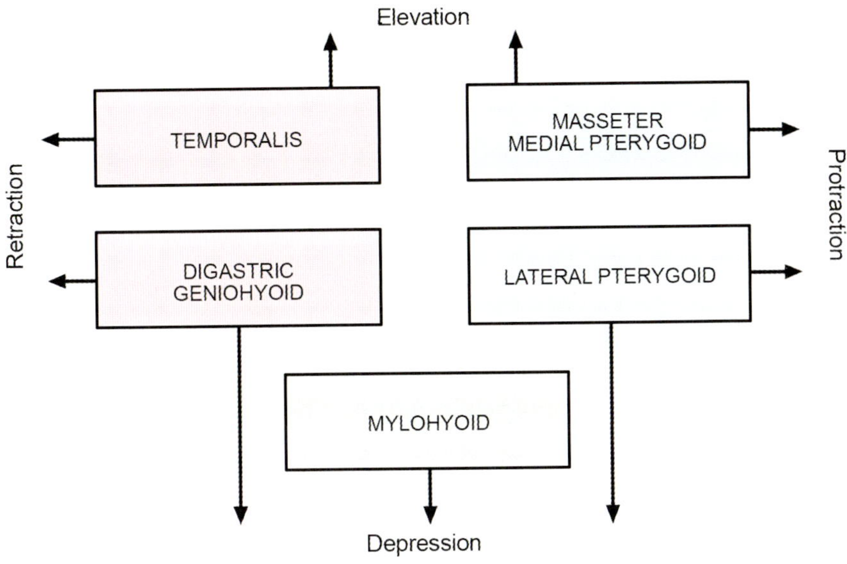


**38.9:** Scheme to show the muscles responsible for movements at the temporomandibular joint

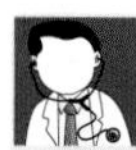

## CLINICAL CORRELATION

1. The movements at the temporomandibular joint have been described above. We have seen that when the mouth is closed, or is slightly open, the head of the mandible lies in the articular fossa.
2. In this position the joint is stable, and a blow on the chin causes fracture of the mandible rather than dislocation. Backwards dislocation (towards the external acoustic meatus) is also prevented by the strong lateral temporomandibular ligament.
3. When the mouth is opened wide the head of the mandible moves forwards and comes to lie just below the articular tubercle. In this position, the temporomandibular joint is highly unstable.
   a. A blow on the chin, or even sudden opening of the mouth as in yawning (involving sudden contraction of the lateral pterygoid muscle) can cause the head of the mandible to slip forwards to the front of the articular tubercle.
   b. Once the joint is thus dislocated the mouth cannot be closed.
   c. To reduce the dislocation, the surgeon inserts both his thumbs into the mouth and exerts downward pressure over the lower molar teeth. Simultaneously, the mandible is pressed backwards.
4. The term derangement of the temporomandibular joint is applied to a condition in which part of the articular disc gets detached from the joint capsule.
   a. This happens after injury.
   b. Movements of the jaw become painful, and clicking sounds may be produced while opening and closing the mouth.

# 39 CHAPTER

# Submandibular Region and Tongue

## INTRODUCTION

1. The structures to be studied in the submandibular region are as follows:
   a. Submandibular salivary gland.
   b. Sublingual salivary gland.
   c. Suprahyoid muscles: Digastric, stylohyoid, mylohyoid and genioglossus. Along with them we will also consider the stylohyoid ligament.
   d. Tongue and its muscles.
2. The blood vessels to be seen in the region are the lingual artery and lingual vein. Nerve supply involves the lingual nerve, the submandibular ganglion, the glossopharyngeal nerve and the hypoglossal nerve.

## THE SUBMANDIBULAR GLAND

1. The submandibular gland is located partly below, and partly deep to the body of the mandible. The part below the mandible lies in the digastric triangle.
2. The gland has three surfaces: Inferior, lateral and medial (39.1).
   a. The ***inferior surface*** is superficial, and is the one seen in the digastric triangle. It is directed downwards and somewhat laterally.
   b. The ***lateral surface*** is hidden from view by the body of the mandible. It lies in contact with the medial surface of the body of the mandible, below the attachment of the mylohyoid muscle (39.5). The posterior part of the lateral surface is separated from the mandible by the medial pterygoid muscle.
   c. The ***medial surface*** rests on several structures (39.2). The most important of these are the mylohyoid muscle (in front), the hyoglossus (in the middle) and the wall of the pharynx (posteriorly).
3. At the posterior margin of the mylohyoid muscle a prolongation of the submandibular gland called the ***deep part*** passes forward in the interval between the mylohyoid (laterally) and the hyoglossus (medially).
4. The following additional relationships may now be noted:
   a. The submandibular gland is enclosed by two layers of fascia formed by splitting of the investing layer of deep cervical fascia. The superficial layer covers the inferior surface of the gland and is attached to the lower border of the mandible. The deeper layer covers the medial surface and is attached above to the mylohyoid line of the mandible.

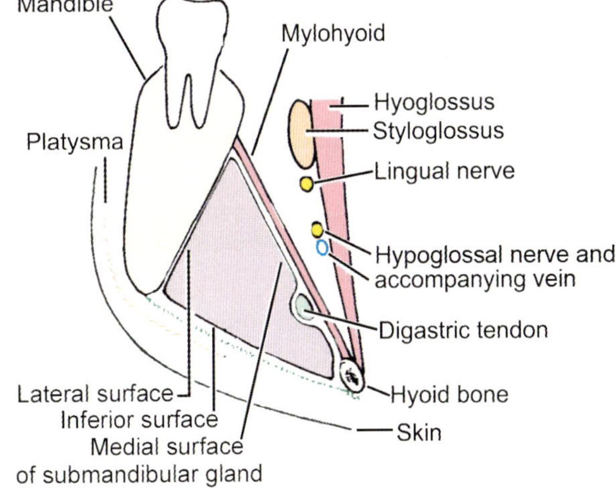


**39.1:** Coronal section through the submandibular region to show the surfaces of the submandibular gland and their relations

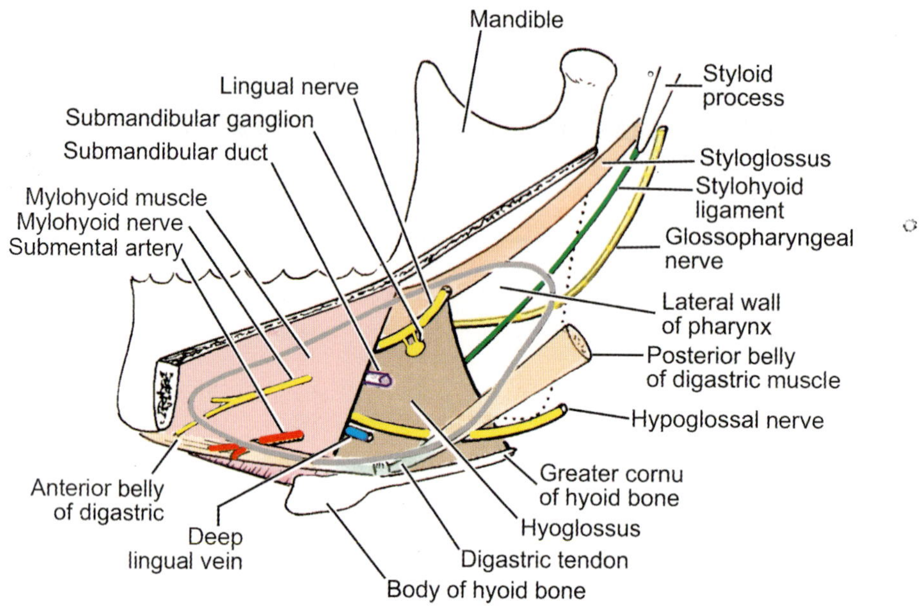


**39.2:** Scheme to show structures deep to the submandibular gland. The outline of the area covered by the gland is shown in grey line

   b. Apart from skin and fascia the inferior surface is overlapped by the platysma. It is crossed by the facial vein, and by the cervical branch of the facial nerve. The submandibular lymph nodes lie over it. Some of the nodes may be embedded within the gland.
   c. The relationship of the facial artery to the gland is worthy of note. The artery first runs upwards along the posterior end of the gland (grooving it). It then runs downwards and forwards between the lateral surface of the gland (deep to the artery) and the medial pterygoid muscle (superficial to it).
   d. The posterior end of the gland reaches as far as the stylomandibular ligament which separates it from the parotid gland.
5. The following additional relations of the medial surface may be noted (39.2):
   a. The anterior part of this surface is separated from the mylohyoid muscle by the mylohyoid nerve and vessels and by the submental vessels.
   b. The intermediate part of the medial surface is separated from the hyoglossus by the styloglossus, the lingual nerve, the submandibular ganglion, the hypoglossal nerve and the deep lingual vein.
   c. Behind the posterior margin of the hyoglossus the gland is related to the styloglossus, the stylohyoid ligament and the glossopharyngeal nerve.

## The Submandibular Duct

1. The submandibular duct emerges from the medial surface of the submandibular gland near the posterior margin of the mylohyoid.
2. In company with the deep part of the submandibular gland it runs forwards in the interval between the mylohyoid (laterally) and the hyoglossus (medially).
3. Its anterior part lies between the sublingual gland (laterally) and the genioglossus (medially).
4. The duct opens into the oral cavity on the sublingual papilla (located below the anterior part of the tongue: 39.11).

## WANT TO KNOW MORE?

### Blood Vessels, Nerves, Lymphatics of Submandibular Gland

1. The *arteries* supplying the submandibular gland are branches of the facial and lingual arteries. The *veins* accompany the arteries.
2. The *secretomotor (parasympathetic) nerve supply* of the gland follows a complex pathway.
   a. Preganglionic fibres arise from the superior salivatory nucleus located in the pons. The fibres pass through the facial nerve, its chorda tympani branch, and the lingual nerve. They end in the submandibular ganglion. Postganglionic fibres begin from the cells of the ganglion and reach the submandibular gland (details in chapter 43).
   b. The gland also receives sympathetic fibres.
3. *Lymphatics* from the submandibular gland drain into the submandibular lymph nodes and through them into the deep cervical nodes, particularly the jugulo-omohyoid node.

## THE SUBLINGUAL GLAND

1. The sublingual gland is present in relation to the floor of the anterior part of the oral cavity. It is placed just deep to the oral mucous membrane and is responsible for raising up the sublingual fold (39.11).
2. Inferiorly, the gland rests on the mylohyoid muscle.
3. Laterally it is in contact with the anterior part of the mandible above the mylohyoid line (39.5).
4. These relationships are best appreciated in a coronal section through the gland (39.3).
5. The anterior end of the gland lies near the midline, close to the gland of the opposite side.
6. Posteriorly the gland is near the deep part of the submandibular gland.
7. The submandibular duct intervenes between the sublingual gland and the genioglossus.
8. Secretions of the sublingual gland leave it through a number of small ducts that open into the oral cavity on the sublingual fold (39.11).

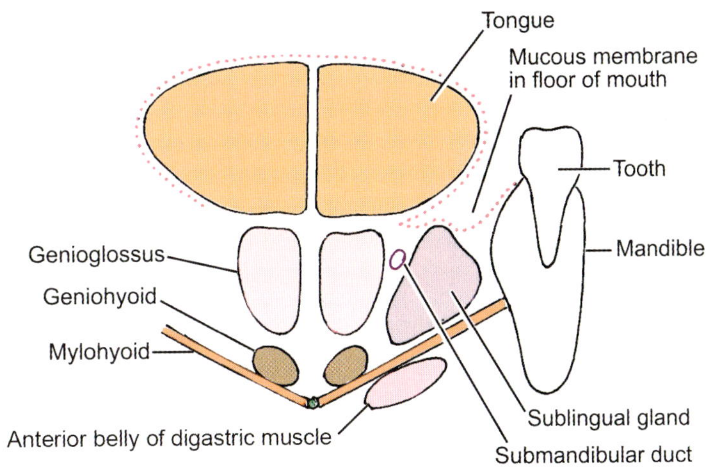


**39.3:** Schematic coronal section through anterior part of tongue and mouth to show relationships of the sublingual salivary gland, and the oral diaphragm

**39.4: Suprahyoid muscles**

| *Muscle* | *Origin* | *Insertion* | *Action* | *Nerve supply* |
|---|---|---|---|---|
| DIGASTRIC | 1. Posterior belly from base of skull deep to mastoid process (mastoid notch of temporal bone)<br>2. Anterior belly from anterior part of base of mandible near midline | The two bellies join the intermediate tendon which is anchored to the hyoid bone through a fibrous pulley | 1. Elevates hyoid bone.<br>2. Fixes the hyoid bone (along with other muscles) | Anterior belly by mylohyoid branch of inferior alveolar nerve<br>Posterior belly by facial nerve |
| STYLOHYOID | Styloid process (posterior aspect) | 1. Tendon splits into two to enclose the intermediate tendon of the digastric muscle<br>2. Tendon is then attached to hyoid bone (at junction of body and greater cornu) | Elevates and retracts hyoid bone | Facial nerve |
| GENIOHYOID | Posterior aspect of symphysis menti (mandible) (below origin of genioglossus) | Hyoid bone (anterior aspect) | 1. Pulls hyoid bone upwards and forwards.<br>2. When hyoid bone is fixed, it can depress mandible | Fibres of nerve C1 travelling through hypoglossal nerve |
| MYLOHYOID | Mylohyoid line on medial surface of the body of the mandible | The fibres pass medially.<br>1. Most posterior fibres are attached to body of hyoid bone (anterior aspect)<br>2. Remaining fibres are inserted into a median raphe extending from hyoid bone to mandible | The muscles of the two sides form the oral diaphragm. They help in deglutition by raising the floor of the mouth | Mylohyoid branch of inferior alveolar nerve |

## WANT TO KNOW MORE?

9. The *secretomotor nerve supply* (parasympathetic) is similar to that of the submandibular gland (see above). Some postganglionic fibres beginning in the submandibular ganglion re-enter the lingual nerve and reach the sublingual gland through the distal part of the lingual nerve (details in chapter 43).
10. The gland receives its blood supply through the sublingual branch of the lingual artery and the submental branch of the facial artery (39.17).

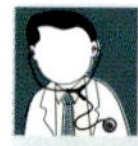

## CLINICAL CORRELATION

### Salivary Glands

1. The salivary glands are commonly infected with a virus that causes ***mumps***. It causes swelling and pain in the gland affected. It can involve more than one gland. The parotid is the most commonly infected salivary gland.
2. The salivary glands can also be infected by spread of infection from the mouth. An abscess may form in the gland.

3. The parotid fascia is very dense and allows very little expansion of the gland. Swellings of the parotid are therefore very painful.
4. Tumours may form in a salivary gland. They may be benign or malignant.
   a. Facial paralysis can occur by involvement in a malignant growth of the parotid gland, or by injury during removal of the gland.
   b. The surgeon tries to protect the nerve by removing the superficial and deep parts separately.
5. A calculus may form in the submandibular gland.
6. In operations on the submandibular gland the close relation of the facial artery to it has to be remembered.

## SUPRAHYOID MUSCLES

These are the digastric, stylohyoid, mylohyoid and geniohyoid muscles. They are described in 39.4. They are shown in 39.1 to 39.9.

### Oral Diaphragm

1. The mylohyoid muscles of the two sides bridge the gap between the two halves of the mandible.
2. In the median plane the two muscles become continuous with each other at a median raphe.
3. In this way the right and left muscles form the floor of the mouth. This floor is called the oral diaphragm (or diaphragma oris) (39.3 and 39.8).

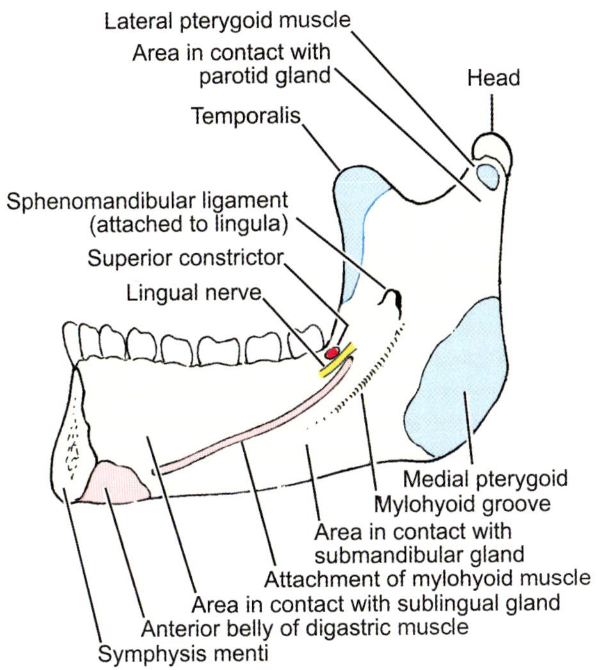


**39.5:** Attachments on one-half of the mandible seen from the medial side

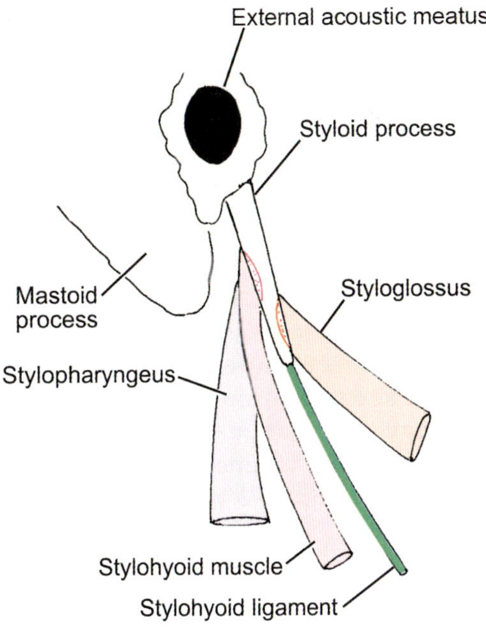


**39.6:** Structures attached to the styloid process. The stylohyoid ligament is attached to the tip, the styloglossus muscle to the anterior aspect (lower part), the stylohyoid muscle to the posterior aspect (upper part), and the stylopharyngeus to the medial aspect

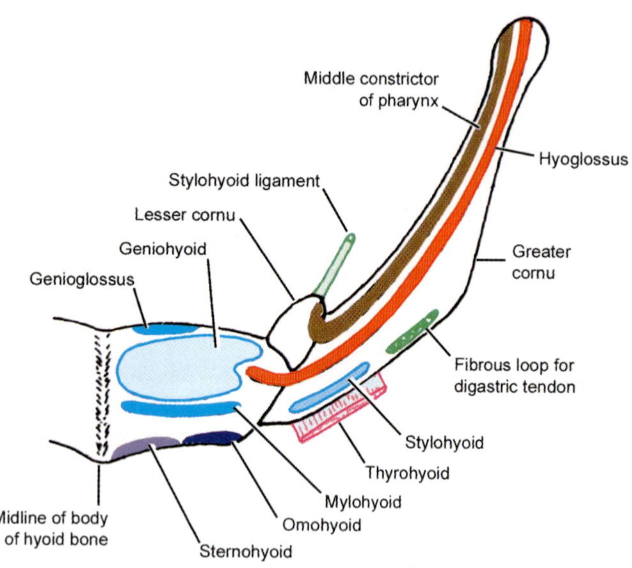


**39.7:** Attachments on hyoid bone: Anterosuperior aspect

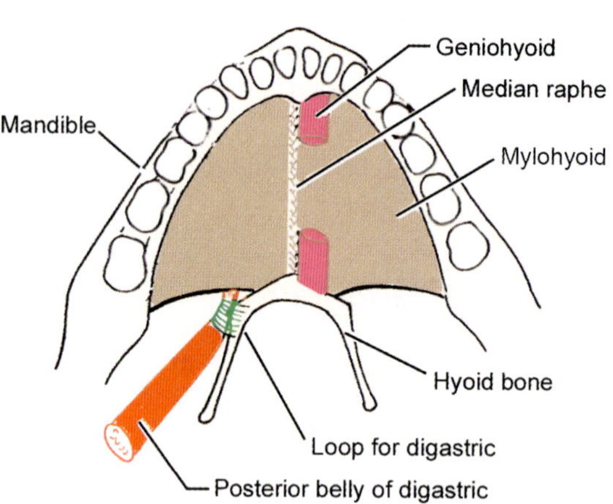


**39.8:** Schematic diagram of floor of mouth seen from above. Note the layout of the mylohyoid and geniohyoid muscles

4. This diaphragm is strengthened, above, by the geniohyoid muscle; and below by the anterior belly of the digastric muscle.

## WANT TO KNOW MORE?

**Relations of Mylohyoid Muscle**

1. The mylohyoid muscle has numerous relations. These are summarised in 39.9 that is a coronal section through the submandibular region.

## THE TONGUE

1. The tongue lies in the oral cavity. The anterior part of the tongue (or ***apex***) can be protruded out of the mouth. It has free upper and lower surfaces.
2. The greater part of the tongue is attached below to the floor of the mouth. The attached part is called the ***root*** of the tongue. This part of the tongue has a free upper surface or ***dorsum***.
3. On either side, the tongue has ***lateral edges*** that are also free. The free surfaces of the tongue are lined by mucous membrane.
4. The substance of the tongue is made up mainly of muscle.
   a. Some of the muscles of the tongue are ***intrinsic*** i.e., they are confined to the tongue.
   b. The ***extrinsic*** enter the tongue from outside.
5. It is through the root that the various extrinsic muscles enter the substance of the tongue. Through these muscles the tongue is anchored to the hyoid bone behind (through the hyoglossus muscle) and to the mandible in front (through the genioglossus muscle).

### Features on the Dorsum of the Tongue

1. The features, seen when the tongue is viewed from above, are shown in 39.10. The upper surface (or dorsum) is seen. Identify the anterior end or apex, and the lateral edges.

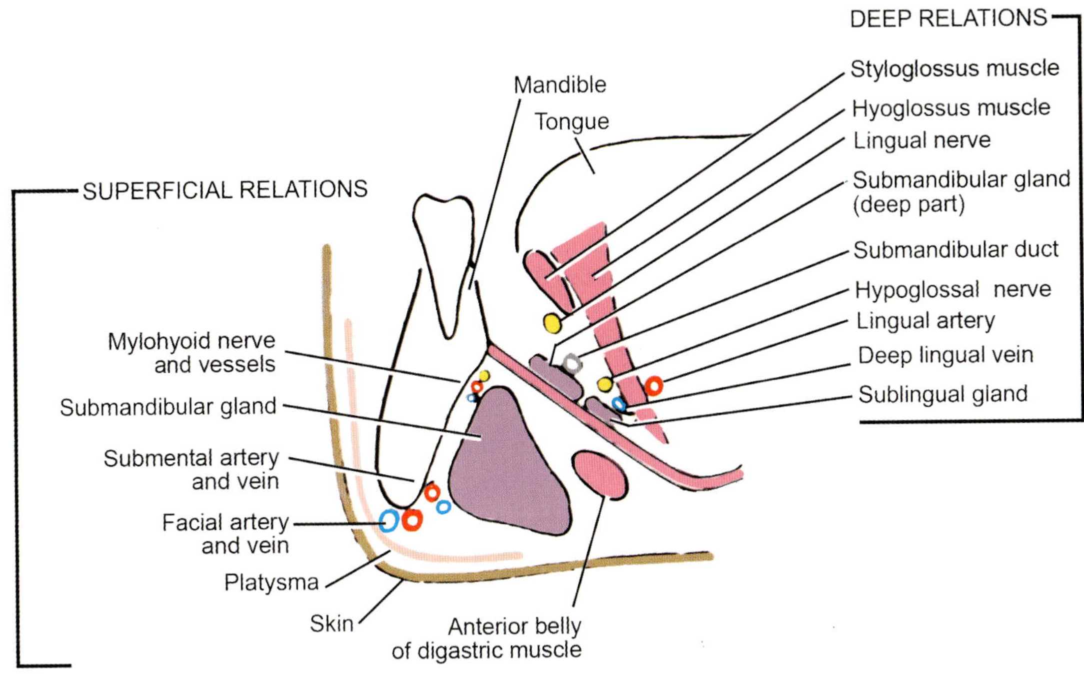


**39.9:** Schematic coronal section of the submandibular region to show the relations of the mylohyoid muscle

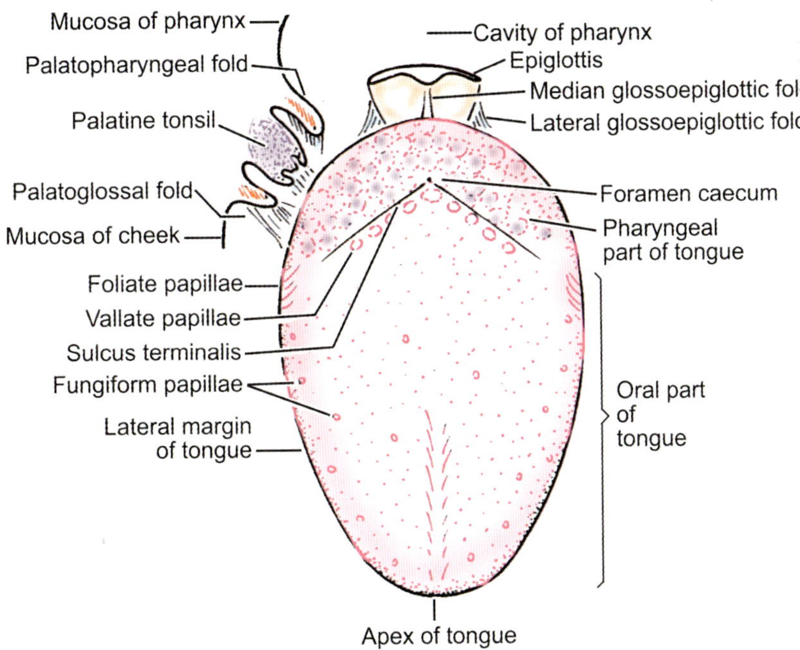


**39.10:** Tongue and some related structures seen from above

2. Near its posterior end the dorsum of the tongue is marked by a V-shaped groove called the ***sulcus terminalis***.
   a. The apex of the 'V' points backwards and is marked by a depression called the ***foramen caecum***.
   b. The limbs of the sulcus terminalis runs forwards and laterally to the lateral margin of the tongue.
3. The sulcus terminalis divides the dorsum of the tongue into an anterior larger part (two-thirds) and a posterior smaller part (one-third).
4. The anterior part lies in the oral cavity and is, therefore, called the ***oral part***. It faces upwards and comes into contact with the palate.
5. The posterior one-third faces backwards and is called the ***pharyngeal part***.
6. The mucous membrane covering the oral part of the dorsum of the tongue is rough because of the presence of numerous finger-like projections or ***papillae***.
   a. The largest of these papillae are seen in a row just in front of the sulcus limitans. These are the ***vallate*** papillae.
   b. Other papillae present on the tongue are described as ***fungiform***. They are present at the apex and along the sides of the tongue.
   c. The most numerous papillae are small and conical in shape. They are called ***filiform*** papillae (39.12).
   d. On the posterior part of the lateral margin of the tongue, there are vertical folds that are called the ***foliate*** papillae (because they look like papillae on section: they are not true papillae).
   e. Another type of papillae sometimes mentioned in relation to the tongue are the papillae ***simplex***. Unlike the other papillae, which can be seen by naked eye, these are microscopic and are quite different from the other papillae. They are not surface projections but are present at the junction of the lining epithelium with underlying tissues (see 39.12). They are the equivalent of dermal papillae seen in the skin.
7. The ***pharyngeal part of the tongue*** faces backwards and forms part of the anterior wall of the oropharynx. Its surface is not covered by papillae. However, it shows a number of rounded elevations that are produced by collections of lymphoid tissue lying deep to the mucosa. This lymphoid tissue is referred to, collectively, as the ***lingual tonsil***.
8. The posterior part of the tongue is connected to the palate (on either side) by a fold of mucous membrane called the ***palatoglossal fold***.
9. Immediately posterior to this fold, we see the palatine tonsil (39.10).
10. The mucous membrane lining the pharyngeal part of the tongue is continuous laterally with the mucosa covering the palatoglossal folds, and with the mucosa covering the palatine tonsils.
11. Posteriorly, the tongue is closely related to the epiglottis (a part of the larynx).
    a. The mucosa of the tongue is connected to the anterior aspect of the epiglottis by a ***median glossoepiglottic fold***; and to its lateral edges by two ***lateral glossoepiglottic folds***.
    b. The space between the tongue and epiglottis on either side of the median glossoepiglottic fold is called the ***vallecula***.
12. Some features to be seen on the lower surface of the anterior part of the tongue are shown in 39.11.
    a. This part of the tongue is not attached to the floor of the mouth, and that is why it can be protruded out of the mouth.
    b. In 39.11 note the ***frenulum linguae*** lying in the middle line. It is a delicate fold of mucosa passing from the tongue to the floor of the mouth.
    c. On either side of the posterior end of the frenulum notice a rounded projection. This is the ***sublingual papilla***.
    d. The submandibular duct opens on the summit of the papilla.
    e. Running laterally from the papilla we see the ***sublingual fold***. This fold is produced by the underlying sublingual salivary gland.
    f. A little lateral to the frenulum a darkish line can be seen running towards the tip of the tongue. The deep lingual vein (that is seen through the mucosa) lies deep to this line.
    g. Further laterally, we see an irregular fold of mucosa called the ***fimbriated fold***.

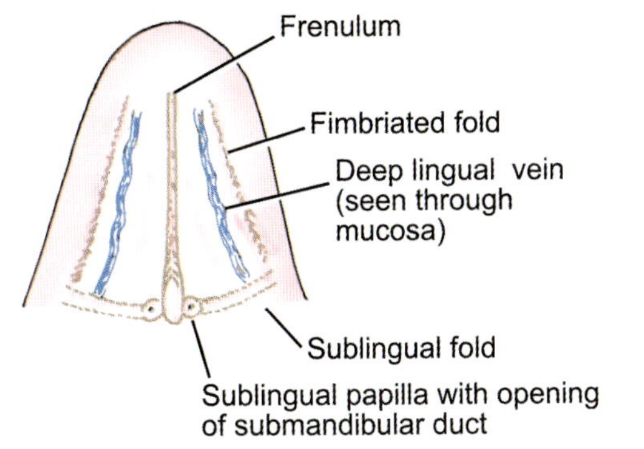


**39.11:** Some structures seen on the undersurface of the anterior part of the tongue

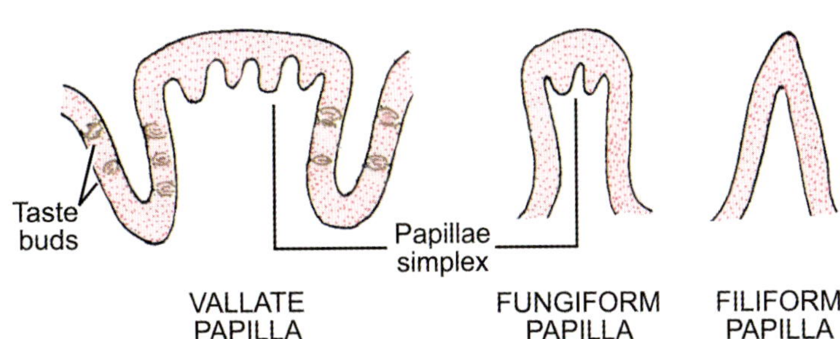


**39.12:** Various kinds of papillae to be seen on the surface of the tongue

## MUSCLES OF THE TONGUE

1. The ***intrinsic muscles*** lie within the substance of the tongue.
2. The ***extrinsic muscles*** of the tongue enter it from the outside. They are the styloglossus, the palatoglossus, the genioglossus, and the hyoglossus. The extrinsic muscles are described in 39.14 and are shown in 39.13.
3. The hyoglossus is related to a large number of important structures. These are listed in 39.15.

### Intrinsic Muscles

Apart from the muscles entering the tongue from the outside the tongue contains intrinsic fibres that are arranged in several groups viz., ***superior longitudinal***, ***inferior longitudinal***, ***transverse*** and ***vertical***.

## BLOOD VESSELS, LYMPHATICS, AND NERVES OF THE TONGUE

### Lingual Artery

1. The lingual artery arises from the external carotid artery opposite the tip of the greater cornu of the hyoid bone (39.16).
2. The ***first part*** of the artery lies in the carotid triangle, superficial to the middle constrictor of the pharynx. It forms a characteristic upward loop that is crossed by the hypoglossal nerve.
3. The ***second part*** of the artery lies deep to the hyoglossus muscle that separates the artery from the hypoglossal nerve. This part of the artery also lies on the middle constrictor.
4. The ***third or deep part*** of the artery runs upwards along the anterior margin of the hyoglossus; and then forwards to the tip of the tongue. This part lies on the genioglossus muscle. The branches of the lingual artery are shown in 39.16.

### Venous Drainage

1. The venous drainage of the tongue is shown in 39.16.
2. ***Dorsal lingual veins*** from the dorsum and sides of the tongue end in the ***lingual vein*** that accompanies the lingual artery and ends in the internal jugular vein.
3. Other veins including the ***deep lingual vein*** (see above) drain through veins that accompany the hypoglossal nerve. These veins may join the lingual vein, or the facial vein, or may enter the internal jugular veins directly.

### Nerves Supplying the Tongue

The ***nerves supplying the tongue*** are of the three functional types:

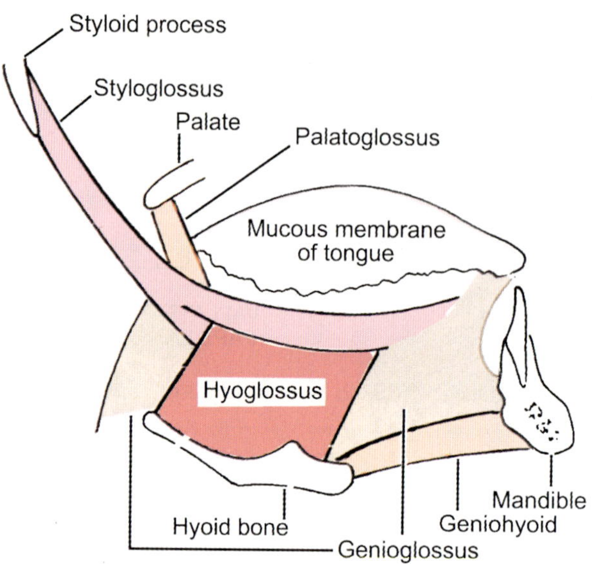


**39.13:** Drawing to show the extrinsic muscles of the tongue

**39.14: Extrinsic muscles of tongue**

| *Muscle* | *Origin* | *Insertion* | *Action* | *Nerve supply* |
|---|---|---|---|---|
| Styloglossus | Styloid process (anterior and lateral aspect) | Merges with side of tongue | Pulls tongue upwards and backwards | Hypoglossal nerve |
| Palatoglossus | Palatine aponeurosis (oral aspect) | Side of tongue | Muscles of both sides acting together bring the palatoglossal arches together closing the aperture from oral cavity to pharynx | Cranial part of accessory nerve |
| Genioglossus | Mandible (Posterior surface of symphysis menti, upper genial tubercles) | Ventral aspect of tongue (whole length) | Protrudes tongue out of mouth by pulling posterior part forwards | Hypoglossal nerve |
| Hyoglossus | Hyoid bone (greater cornu and lateral part of body) | Side of tongue | Depresses tongue | Hypoglossal nerve |

### *Nerves of Ordinary Sensation*

Sensations like touch, pain and temperature are carried from the anterior two-thirds of the tongue by the ***lingual nerve***, and from the posterior one-third by the ***glossopharyngeal nerve***.

### *Nerves of Taste*

Sensations of taste from the anterior two-thirds of the tongue are carried by fibres that are peripheral processes of cells in the geniculate ganglion of the facial nerve. The fibres pass through the facial nerve, its chorda tympani branch and the lingual nerve.

| 39.15: Relations of hyoglossus muscle | |
|---|---|
| Structures passing deep to posterior border | 1. Glossopharyngeal nerve<br>2. Stylohyoid ligament<br>3. Lingual artery |
| Structures superficial to muscle | 1. Lingual nerve<br>2. Hypoglossal nerve<br>3. Submandibular ganglion<br>4. Deep lingual vein<br>5. Submandibular gland (deep part)<br>6. Submandibular duct<br>7. Sublingual gland (part of)<br>8. Styloglossus muscle<br>9. Mylohyoid muscle<br>10. Digastric tendon and pulley<br>11. Stylohyoid muscle |
| Structures deep to muscle | 1. Glossopharyngeal nerve<br>2. Lingual artery and it dorsal lingual branches<br>3. Genioglossus muscle<br>4. Middle constrictor of pharynx<br>5. Inferior longitudinal muscle of tongue<br>6. Stylohyoid ligament |

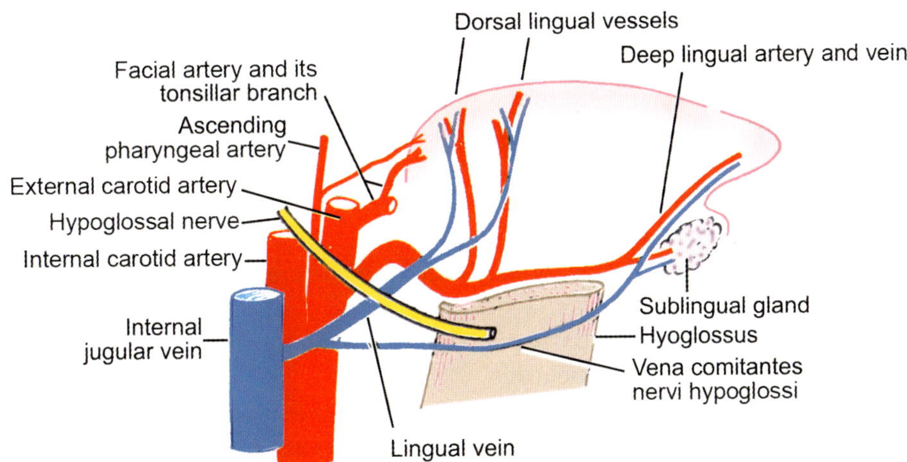


**39.16:** Scheme to show the arteries and veins that supply the tongue

Sensations of taste from the posterior one-third of the tongue are carried by the glossopharyngeal nerve. Taste fibres from the posteriormost part of the tongue (just in front of the epiglottis) are carried by the ***superior laryngeal branch of the vagus nerve***.

### *Nerves Supplying Muscles*

The musculature of the tongue is supplied by the ***hypoglossal nerve***.

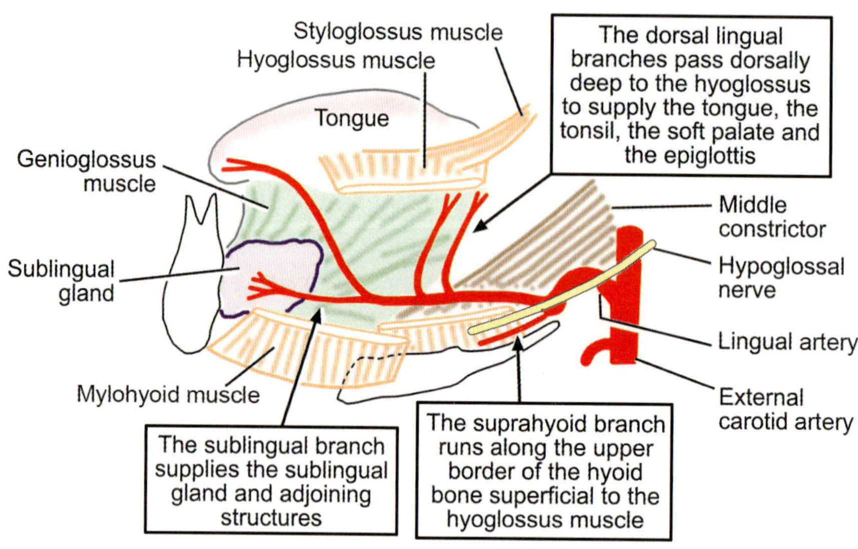


**39.17:** Lingual artery and branches

## The Lingual Nerve

1. The lingual nerve arises from the posterior division of the mandibular nerve (39.18).
2. Its upper part runs downward deep to the lateral pterygoid muscle. It is joined here by the ***chorda tympani*** nerve (a branch of the facial nerve).
3. Lower down, the lingual nerve runs downwards and forwards between the medial pterygoid (deep to it) and the ramus of the mandible (superficial to it).
4. It then enters the mouth (by passing deep to the mandibular attachment of the superior constrictor of the pharynx).
5. Within the mouth the nerve lies deep to the mucous membrane overlying the medial surface of the mandible just below the third molar tooth. It can be felt here.
6. Leaving the gum the nerve enters the side of the tongue.
7. The nerve crosses the styloglossus and runs forwards across the lateral surface of the hyoglossus (i.e., between the hyoglossus and the mylohyoid).
8. At the anterior margin of the hyoglossus, the nerve passes onto the genioglossus and divides into a number of branches that are distributed as described below.
9. While running across the hyoglossus, the lingual nerve lies above the submandibular duct. Continuing forwards the nerve crosses superficial to the duct and then hooks round it to reach its medial side.
10. Lying on the hyoglossus, a little below the lingual nerve, there is the submandibular ganglion.
11. The lingual nerve is connected to the ganglion by two or three branches. Still lower down the hypoglossal nerve runs across the hyoglossus.
12. The lingual nerve carries three types of the fibres that are distributed as follows:
    a. Most of the fibres of the lingual nerve are those of ordinary sensation. They carry the sensations of touch, pain and temperature from the anterior two-thirds of the tongue. They also supply the mucous membrane of the floor of the mouth and the gums related to the lower teeth.
    b. The part of the lingual nerve distal to the attachment of the chorda tympani carries the ***fibres for taste*** from the part of the tongue in front of the sulcus terminalis, but excluding the vallate papillae.
    These fibres pass from the lingual nerve into the chorda tympani.
    c. ***Secretomotor fibres*** for the submandibular and sublingual glands reach the lingual nerve through the chorda tympani. They end in the submandibular ganglion. Postganglionic fibres reach the submandibular gland

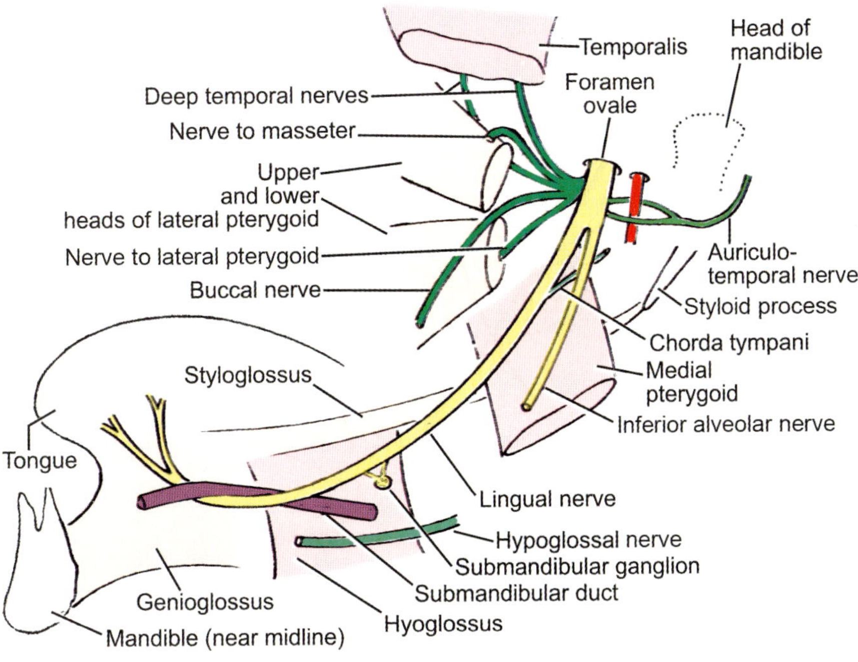


**39.18:** Lingual nerve

through branches to it from the ganglion. The fibres for the sublingual gland re-enter the lingual nerve and pass through its distal part to reach the gland.

## The Submandibular Ganglion

This ganglion lies over the hyoglossus muscle, suspended from the lingual nerve by two or more roots. It is an autonomic ganglion connected with the cranial parasympathetic outflow. The fibres passing through it are as follows:

1. Functionally, the ganglion is concerned with the secretomotor innervation of the submandibular and sublingual salivary glands. These fibres are parasympathetic.
2. The ganglion receives sympathetic fibres from the plexus on the facial artery. These are postganglionic fibres arising in the superior cervical sympathetic ganglion. They pass through the ganglion without relay and supply the blood vessels of the submandibular and sublingual glands.

## The Glossopharyngeal Nerve

1. This is the ninth cranial nerve. It leaves the cranial cavity by passing through the jugular foramen 39.19.
2. It descends in close relation to the internal carotid artery, passing deep to the styloid process and the structures attached to it.
3. Reaching the posterior border of the stylopharyngeus muscle, it curves forwards passing lateral to the muscle.
4. Passing forwards, the nerve reaches the side of the tongue. Here it lies deep to the hyoglossus muscle, superficial to the genioglossus and terminates by dividing into branches to the tongue. The nerve gives many branches that will be studied later.
5. The ***lingual branches*** supply the part of the tongue (mucous membrane) behind the sulcus terminalis. They also supply the vallate papillae. These branches carry fibres for both general sensation and taste.

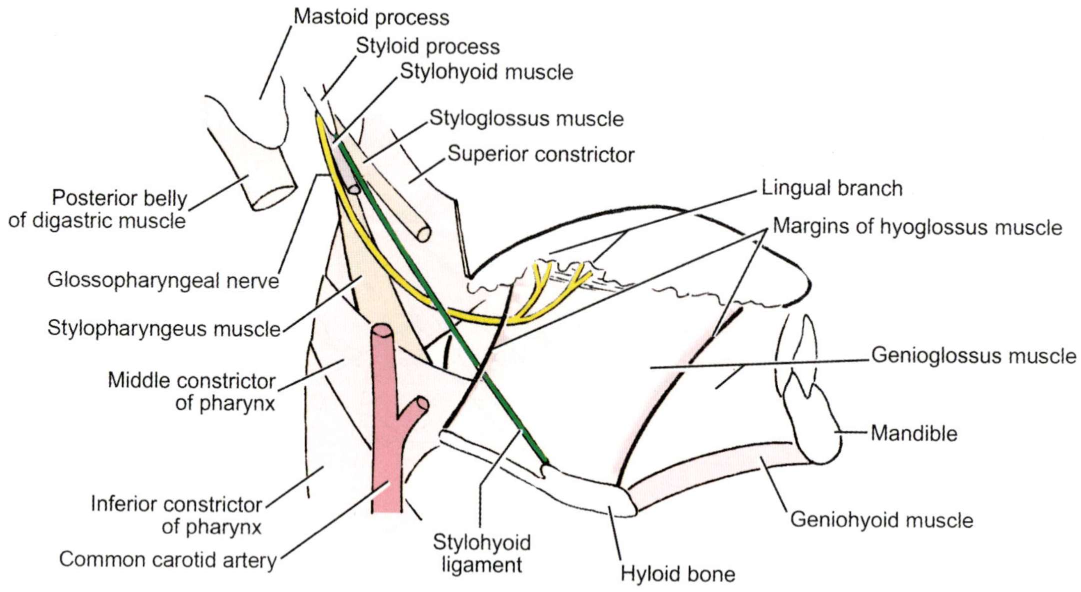


**39.19:** Glossopharyngeal nerve

## The Hypoglossal Nerve

1. This is the twelfth cranial nerve. Its fibres are purely motor. They supply the muscles of the tongue.
2. The hypoglossal nerve arises from the medulla. It leaves the cranial cavity through the hypoglossal canal (or anterior condylar) canal.
3. The nerve descends close to the internal jugular vein and internal carotid artery up to the level of the angle of the mandible. Here the nerve passes forwards crossing the internal and external carotid arteries, and enters the submandibular region (39.20).
4. In the submandibular region, the hypoglossal nerve at first lies superficial to the hyoglossus muscle and then to the genioglossus.
5. It ends by dividing into its terminal branches. These supply all the intrinsic and extrinsic muscles of the tongue (except the palatoglossus which is supplied, along with other muscles of the palate, by the cranial accessory nerve).
6. Some relations of the hypoglossal nerve are as follows:
   a. As the nerve runs forwards in the neck it crosses the internal carotid artery, the external carotid artery and the loop formed by the lingual artery. The loop of the lingual artery is crossed just above the tip of the greater cornu of the hyoid bone.
   b. As the nerve runs forwards above the greater cornu of the hyoid bone it is crossed by the digastric tendon and the stylohyoid.
   c. The relations of the nerve as it crosses the hyoglossus are shown in 39.20. The lingual nerve, the submandibular duct and the deep part of the submandibular gland lie above it. This part of the nerve is deep to the mylohyoid muscle.

## Lymphatic Drainage of the Tongue

1. The tongue is a frequent site of carcinoma and hence a knowledge of its lymphatic drainage is of special importance.

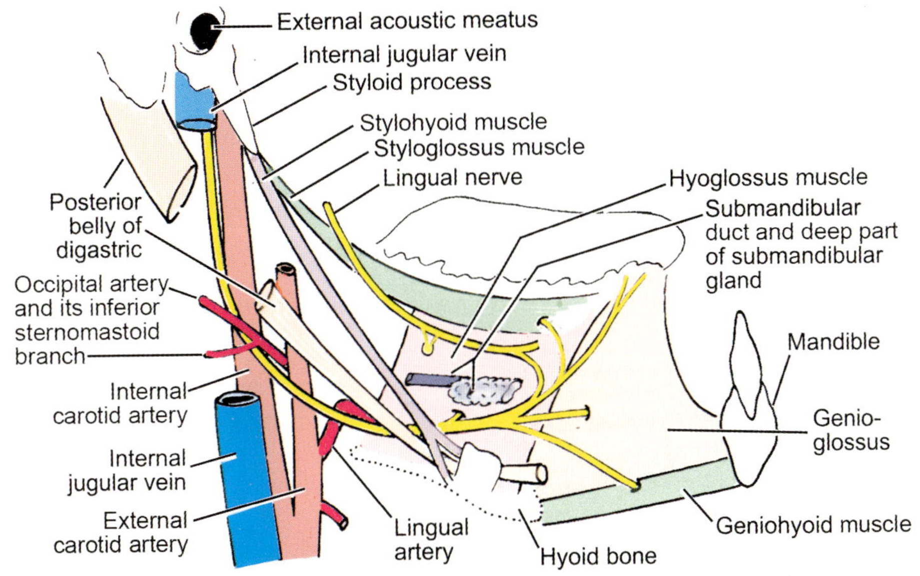


**39.20:** Hypoglossal nerve

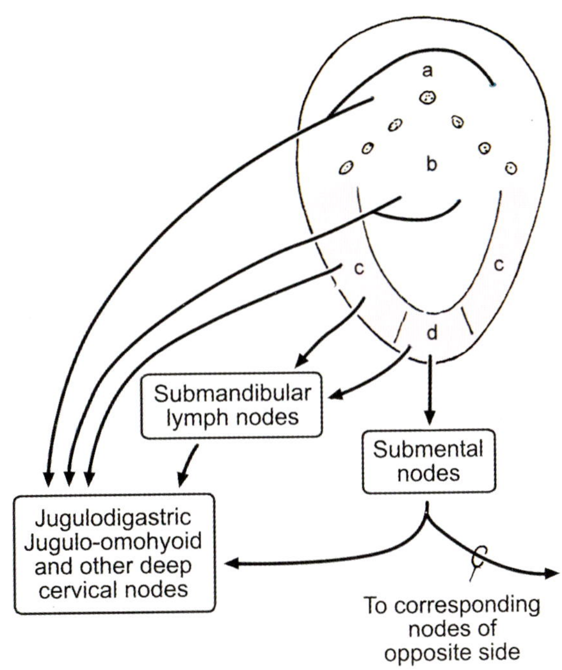


**39.21:** Lymphatic drainage of the tongue

2. From this point of view the tongue may be divided into a part behind the vallate papillae (*'a'* in 39.21); and a part in front of them. The latter is further divided into a central area (*'b'* in 39.21) and a marginal area (*'c'* in 39.21) that includes the tip (*'d'* in 39.21).

3. Lymph from area 'a', area 'b', and the posterior part of area 'c' drains directly into the jugulodigastric, jugulo-omohyoid and other deep cervical nodes.
4. Lymph from the anterior part of area 'c' and from the tip of the tongue (area 'd') reaches the same nodes after passing through the submandibular nodes.
5. Lymph from the tip of the tongue also passes into the submental nodes, and from there into the submandibular and deep cervical nodes.
6. Lymph from areas of the tongue near the middle line can pass to lymph nodes of either the right or left side.

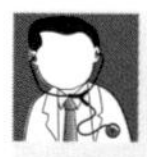

## CLINICAL CORRELATION

### THE TONGUE

**Congenital Malformations**

1. The tongue may be too large (***macroglossia***), or too small (***microglossia***).
2. Very rarely the tongue may be absent (***aglossia***).
3. The tongue may be ***bifid***.
4. The apical part of the tongue may be anchored to the floor of the mouth by a very short frenulum. The condition, which is called ***ankyloglossia*** or tongue tie, interferes with speech.
5. Other rare anomalies include:
   a. The presence of fissures on the tongue.
   b. The presence (within the tongue) of a lingual thyroid.
   c. The presence (within the tongue) of remnants of the thyroglossal duct in the form of cysts.

**Laceration of the Tongue**

1. Laceration of the tongue can occur if the tongue gets caught between the teeth. This is likely to occur while eating, during epileptic attacks, and in injuries leading to fractures of the jaw.
2. Because of the vascularity of the tongue lacerations can cause serious bleeding.
   a. To stop bleeding pressure is applied posterior to the area of laceration (as the lingual artery runs forwards).
   b. Pressure is applied either by holding the tongue between the thumb and index finger; or by placing the thumb on the tongue and the index finger in the submental region.

**Other Correlations**

1. Muscles of the tongue are paralysed in lesions of the hypoglossal nerve.
2. a. Sensations of taste are lost from the anterior two-thirds of the tongue in facial nerve paralysis.
   b. From the posterior one-third in lesions of the glossopharyngeal nerve.
   c. In some cases, taste sensations over the anterior two-thirds of the tongue may be affected in lesions of the trigeminal nerve.
3. The mucosa below the anterior part of the tongue is highly vascular. A drug placed here enters the blood stream faster than it does after an intramuscular injection. (Patients suffering from angina commonly find relief by placing a suitable tablet here).
4. In an unconscious patient, care has to be taken that the tongue does not fall backwards towards the pharynx as this would obstruct respiration. The head is placed on one side and made to hang down.
5. Carcinoma of the tongue (and other parts of the mouth) is common in India because of tobacco chewing.

# 40 CHAPTER Cranial Cavity and Vertebral Canal

## THE CRANIAL CAVITY

### Contents of the Cranial Cavity and Vertebral Canal

1. The most important content of the cranial cavity is the brain; and that of the vertebral canal is the spinal cord.
2. The brain and spinal cord are surrounded by three membranes called the ***meninges***.
3. The meninges are:
   a. The ***dura mater***
   b. The ***arachnoid mater***
   c. The ***pia mater***.
4. Between the arachnoid mater and the pia mater, there is the ***subarachnoid space*** that contains ***cerebrospinal fluid***.
5. In relation to the dura mater, there are a series of venous sinuses that drain intracranial structures including the brain.
6. The cranial cavity is lined on the inside by a periosteum-like membrane called the ***endocranium***.
7. The segment of the vertebral canal lying within each vertebra is lined by periosteum. Some intervertebral ligaments take part in forming the walls of the vertebral canal.
8. In addition to the brain and meninges, the cranial cavity contains the proximal parts of ***cranial nerves.*** They travel from their attachment to the surface of the brain to foramina in the skull through which they leave the cranial cavity.
9. The cranial cavity also contains ***blood vessels*** that supply the brain, the meninges and other intracranial structures.
10. Lying in close relationship to the brain, there are two endocrine glands of great importance. These are:
    a. The hypophysis cerebri
    b. The pineal gland.
11. Apart from the spinal cord, meninges and cerebrospinal fluid, the vertebral canal contains the roots of spinal nerves. It also contains blood vessels. The veins form an elaborate ***vertebral venous plexus***. Some ligaments of intervertebral joints are also present over the walls of the vertebral canal.
12. The brain will be considered in chapter 50 onwards. The hypophysis cerebri and the pineal gland are considered in chapter 46.

#### *The Endocranium*

1. This a fibrous membrane (similar to periosteum) lining the inside of the cranial cavity.
2. At the foramen magnum, and at smaller apertures in the skull, it becomes continuous with periosteum lining the exterior of the skull.
3. At the superior orbital fissure, it becomes continuous with the periosteum lining the orbit.
4. The endocranium is adherent to skull bones, the degree of adherence being variable. The union is better over the cranial fossae rather than over the vault of the skull.

5. At places where cranial nerves leave the cranial cavity, the endocranium extends over them for some distance in the form of a tubular sheath. (However, the optic nerve is covered by sheaths derived from the meninges).
6. At sites of sutures the endocranium blends with sutural ligaments. It is, therefore, firmly anchored here. (The sutural ligaments connect the endocranium with the pericranium).

## THE MENINGES

### The Cerebral Dura Mater

1. The dura mater is a thick fibrous membrane.
   a. It can be divided into a ***cerebral part*** lying in the cranial cavity.
   b. A ***spinal part*** lying in the vertebral canal.
   In this section we will consider the cerebral dura mater.
2. Over the greater part of its extent, the cerebral dura mater is closely adherent to the endocranium (and through the latter to the skull).
3. At places the dura mater separates from endocranium, and forms double layered folds that play an essential role in supporting brain tissue (see below).
4. At places where such folds are formed triangular spaces are left between the endocranium and the dura mater.
   a. These spaces are lined by endothelium, and form venous sinuses. (See superior sagittal sinus and transverse sinus in 40.3).
   b. As we shall see below, all venous sinuses are not triangular in section, and some of them are bounded only by dura mater, the endocranium not taking part.
5. The two largest folds of dura mater are seen in 40.1. These are:
   a. The ***falx cerebri***
   b. The ***tentorium cerebelli***.
6. Two smaller folds are also present. These are:
   a. The falx cerebelli
   b. The diaphragma sellae.
   These folds are described below.

#### *The Falx Cerebri*

1. The falx cerebri lies in the sagittal plane. It is sickle shaped.
2. It has a convex upper edge that is attached to the vault of the skull, in the middle line (i.e., along the sagittal suture).
3. Its lower edge, which is free, is markedly concave downwards.
4. The anterior end of the falx cerebri is narrow and pointed. It is attached to the crista galli.
5. At its posterior end, the falx cerebri has a straight lower edge that is attached to the upper surface of the tentorium cerebelli (40.1). This edge slopes backward and downward.
6. A coronal section through the falx cerebri near its middle is shown in 40.2.
   a. Note that near its upper attachment the two layers of dura mater that form it diverge to enclose a triangular space. The third side of the triangle is formed by endocranium. This space is the ***superior sagittal sinus***.
   b. It is an example of a sinus walled partly by dura mater and partly by endocranium.
   c. At the lower end of the falx cerebri, the dura mater folds on itself to form the free lower edge. An oval space is left in the fold along the lower edge. This space is the ***inferior sagittal sinus***.
   d. The wall of this sinus is formed all round by dura mater (there being no participation of endocranium).
7. In 40.3, we see a coronal section through the posterior part of the falx cerebri.
   a. Here, the lower edge of the falx is attached to the upper surface of the tentorium cerebelli.
   b. At this junction, we have a triangular space that is occupied by the ***straight sinus***.
8. The falx cerebri occupies the longitudinal fissure that (partially) separates the right and left cerebral hemispheres.

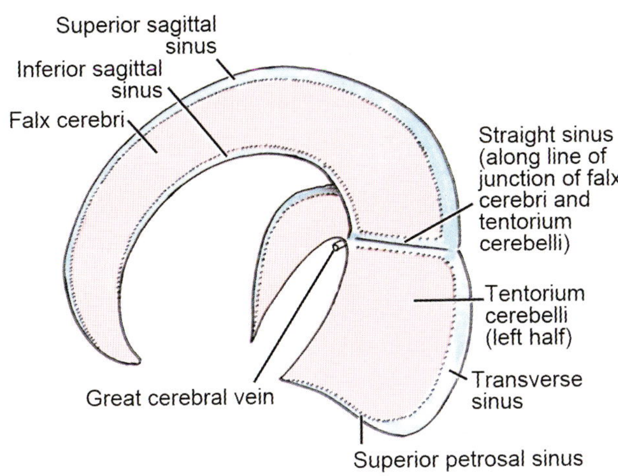


**40.1:** The falx cerebri and tentorium cerebelli

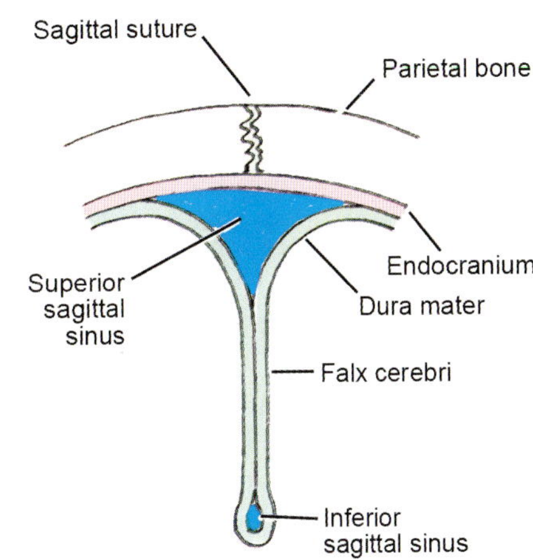


**40.2:** Coronal section through falx cerebri midway between its anterior and posterior ends

### *The Tentorium Cerebelli*

1. In 40.1 and 40.3 observe that, on the whole, the tentorium cerebelli is placed more or less transversely i.e., in a plane that is at right angles to that of the falx cerebri.
2. Its central part is higher than its right and left margins. It, therefore, forms a tent-like roof over the posterior cranial fossa in which the cerebellum lies. That is why this fold of dura mater is called the tentorium cerebelli.
3. When the tentorium cerebelli is viewed from above it has the appearance shown in 40.4. (Also see 40.8 in which part of the tentorium has been removed). Observe the following:
   a. The anterior part of the tentorium cerebelli is marked by a deep ***tentorial notch***. The U-shaped edge of this notch is called the ***free margin*** of the tentorium cerebelli. Traced anteriorly, the free margin extends into the middle cranial fossa and gains attachment to the ***anterior*** clinoid process.
   b. Anteriorly and laterally, each half of the tentorium cerebelli is attached to the superior border of the petrous temporal bone. Medially, this edge is prolonged to reach the ***posterior*** clinoid process.
   c. Posterolaterally, the tentorium cerebelli has a curved edge. Along this edge, the two layers of dura mater forming the tentorium separate and gain attachment to the lips of a broad groove (transverse sulcus) present over the internal surface of the occipital bone. The anterior part of this groove extends on to the internal aspect of the posteroinferior angle of the parietal bone. From 40.3, it will be seen that along this attachment the two layers of dura mater forming the tentorium cerebelli separate to leave a triangular interval that forms the transverse sinus.

**WANT TO KNOW MORE?**

4. A few additional facts about the tentorium cerebelli may now be noted.
   a. The tentorium cerebelli divides the cranial cavity into an ***infratentorial compartment*** that is occupied by the cerebellum and brainstem. The rest of the cranial cavity is the ***supratentorial compartment***. It is occupied mainly by the cerebral hemispheres.
   b. The tentorial notch is the only communication between the two compartments. It is occupied by the midbrain and surrounding meninges. The narrow gap between the midbrain and the edge of the tentorial notch is a site at which flow of CSF through the subarachnoid space can be obstructed following inflammation.

c. In 40.3 we see that anteriorly, the free margin of the tentorium cerebelli crosses above the attached margin. Just in front of the crossing, we see a triangular depression of dura mater.
d. The ***superior petrosal sinus*** is situated along the anterolateral attachment of the tentorium cerebelli.
e. Near the medial part of this attachment, the dura mater forming the lower layer of the tentorium cerebelli is prolonged forwards onto the anterior surface of the petrous temporal bone to form a pouch-like extension. This pouch is called the ***trigeminal cave***, because the trigeminal ganglion lies in it.

### *Falx Cerebelli*

1. In 40.3 note that in the median plane, over the floor of the posterior cranial fossa, there is a short fold of dura mater called the falx cerebelli.
2. The fold is crescentic in shape and is placed in the sagittal plane.
3. It has an anterior edge that is free and a posterior edge that is attached to the occipital bone in the middle line.
4. At its upper end (or base), it is attached to the undersurface of the tentorium cerebelli.
5. Its lower end (or apex) reaches the posterior edge of the foramen magnum. Here is may divide into two parts that pass forwards on either side of the foramen.
6. The occipital sinus lies along the posterior attachment of the falx cerebelli.
7. The falx cerebelli occupies the median groove (vallecula cerebelli) that separates the lower part of the right and left cerebellar hemispheres.

### *Diaphragma Sellae*

1. The body of the sphenoid bone occupies the median region of the middle cranial fossa. The hypophyseal fossa is a depression over this bone.

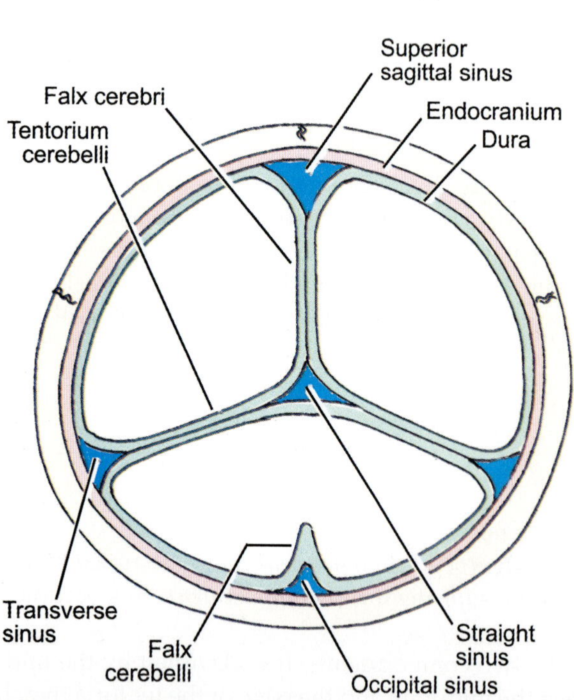


**40.3:** Coronal section through posterior part of falx cerebri and tentorium cerebelli. The falx cerebelli is also shown

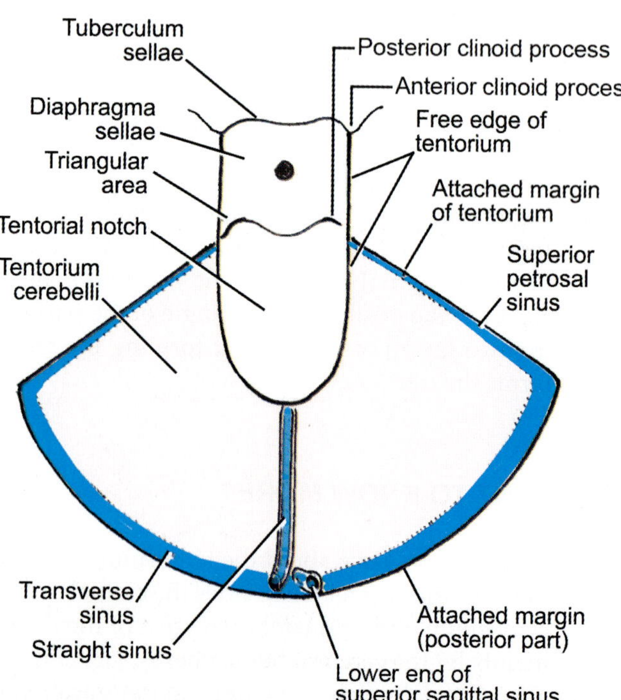


**40.4:** Scheme to show the tentorium cerebelli and its attachments

2. The diaphragma sellae is a horizontal fold of dura mater that roofs over the hypophyseal fossa.
3. There is an aperture at the centre of the diaphargma.
4. Anteriorly, the diaphragma is attached to the tuberculum sellae, and posteriorly to the dorsum sellae.

## WANT TO KNOW MORE?

5. The manner of formation of this fold is shown in 40.5 that is a coronal section across the median part of the middle cranial fossa.
   a. Observe that on either side of the body of the sphenoid bone the dura mater is widely separated from the endocranium to form a space that is occupied by the ***cavernous sinus***.
   b. The dura mater forming the lateral wall of the sinus turns medially to form the roof of the sinus, and then continues medially over the hypophyseal fossa to form the upper layer of the diaphragma sellae.
   c. Reaching the central aperture in the diaphragma sellae the dura mater curves on itself to form the lower layer of the diaphragma.
   d. The dura then descends forming the upper part of the medial wall of the cavernous sinus, and passes medially lining the hypophyseal fossa.
   e. In this way, the dura forms a sac within which the hypophysis cerebri lies. The stalk of the organ passes through the aperture in the diaphragma sellae.

### *Blood Supply and Nerve Supply of Cerebral Dura Mater*

1. A large number of meningeal arteries take part in supplying the cerebral dura mater. They also supply the endocranium and the skull bones (specially the marrow within them). Although, they are called meningeal artery ***they do not supply*** the arachnoid mater and pia mater.
2. The largest meningeal artery is the middle meningeal branch of the maxillary artery. It is responsible for supplying the dura lining the vault of the skull.
3. The nerves to the dura mater are derived from various branches of the trigeminal nerve, and by some branches from the glossopharyngeal, vagus and upper three spinal nerves.

## Arachnoid mater and Pia mater

1. The ***arachnoid mater*** is a thin membrane. There are no blood vessels in it.

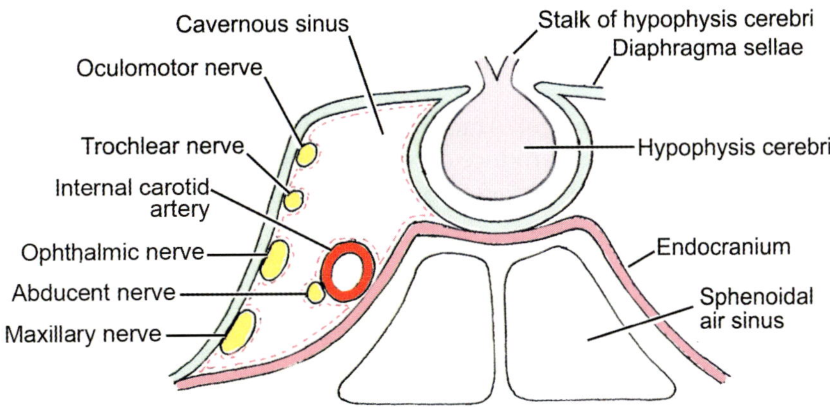


**40.5:** Coronal section through hypophyseal fossa, cavernous sinus and diaphragma sellae

2. The arachnoid mater is separated from the dura mater by the ***subdural space***.
   a. On both sides (dural and arachnoid), the surface lining this capillary interval is smooth.
   b. This facilitates slight movement between the dura and arachnoid.
3. The ***pia mater*** is thicker than the arachnoid mater.
4. In contrast to the arachnoid mater, it is highly vascular, and the blood vessels in it are important for supply of the underlying brain.
5. The pia and arachnoid are separated by the ***subarachnoid space***.
6. This space is filled in by ***cerebrospinal fluid***.
7. Traversing the subarachnoid space there are numerous trabeculae that connect the pia and arachnoid, so that at many places the space resembles a sponge.
8. We have seen that the falx cerebri extends into the longitudinal fissure separating the right and left cerebral hemispheres; and that the tentorium cerebelli extends into the space between the posterior parts of the cerebral hemispheres and the cerebellum. The arachnoid mater also extends into these intervals along with the folds of dura.
9. The surface of the brain is marked by several grooves or ***sulci*** that are of varying depth.
   a. At such sites, the pia mater extends into the sulci lining them, but the arachnoid does not do so.
   b. In other words, the pia mater is closely adherent to the brain surface at all places, but the arachnoid jumps across the sulci.
   c. This means that the subarachnoid space extends into the sulci.
10. a. At places where pial blood vessels penetrate the brain substance, tube like extensions of pia are carried along them for some distance.
    b. Between these pial extensions and the blood vessels these are narrow ***perivascular spaces*** into which cerebrospinal fluid extends. The perivascular spaces are extensions of the subarachnoid space.
11. At some sites where there are deep depressions on the brain surface, the arachnoid mater is separated from the floor of these depressions by relatively large spaces. Such spaces, filled with cerebrospinal fluid, are called ***cisterns***.
12. Like the dura mater, the arachnoid mater and the pia mater are prolonged for some distance on to cranial nerves emerging from the brain.

### *Arachnoid Villi and Granulations*

1. At several sites related to intracranial venous sinuses, the arachnoid mater passes through minute apertures in dura mater to project into the sinuses (40.7).
   a. Here the arachnoid mater is separated from blood in the sinus only by endothelium.
   b. At places such projections are microscopic and are referred to as ***arachnoid villi***.
   c. At other places, these villi form aggregations that are visible to the naked eye and are then called ***arachnoid granulations***.
   d. Arachnoid villi can be identified in all intracranial sinuses. Arachnoid granulations are most numerous in relation to the superior sagittal sinus. They may also be seen in lateral extensions (lateral lacunae) present in relation to this sinus.
   e. In children only arachnoid villi are present. Arachnoid granulations appear later in life and are most prominent in old persons in which they may produce depressions on the skull bones.
   f. The importance of arachnoid villi is that these are sites at which cerebrospinal fluid is absorbed into the blood stream.

### *Choroid Plexuses*

1. At certain sites in relation to the ventricles of the brain, folds of pia mater (or ***tela choroidea***) project into the ventricles. Enclosed within the fold there are tufts of capillaries.
2. This highly vascular pia mater is covered by ***ependyma*** that lines the inside of each ventricle.
3. The masses of vascular pia mater covered by ependyma are referred to as ***choroid plexuses***. They are sites at which cerebrospinal fluid is secreted into the ventricles of the brain.

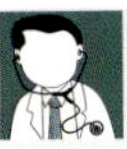

## CLINICAL CORRELATION

**Meninges and Cerebrospinal Fluid**

1. Inflammation of pia and arachnoid is called meningitis.
   a. The condition is characterised by fever and severe headache.
   b. Spasm of extensor muscles leads to rigidity of the neck.
   c. The spasm is a result of irritation of cervical nerve roots as they pass through the subarachnoid space.
   d. CSF pressure and chemical composition show alterations.
2. Samples of CSF may be obtained for examination by lumbar puncture (also see below).
   a. In some cases, lumbar puncture may fail to yield CSF.
   b. In such cases, CSF may be obtained by cisternal puncture.
   c. A needle is introduced from behind, through the interval between the atlas and axis vertebrae.
   d. The needle passes through the posterior atlanto-occipital membrane and enters the cisterna magna.
3. Hydrocephalus extradural and subdural haemorrhage and intracranial venous sinuses (chapter 42) have also been explained.
4. For more details of cerebrospinal fluid see chapter 55.

## Meninges in the Vertebral Canal

1. The dura mater, arachnoid mater and pia mater that surround the brain continue through the foramen magnum into the vertebral canal where they surround the spinal cord.
2. The epidural space, the subdural space, and the subarachnoid space containing cerebrospinal fluid, also continue into the vertebral canal.
3. The spinal dura mater forms a loose tubular covering for the spinal cord.
   a. It extends downwards up to the level of the lower border of the second sacral vertebra.
   b. The arachnoid mater also extends to the same level.
   c. The pia mater is coextensive with the spinal cord that ends at the level of the lower part of the first lumbar vertebra.
4. From 40.6, it will be seen that opposite vertebrae L2 to S2 the vertebral canal contains cerebrospinal fluid (CSF), but not the spinal cord.
   a. A needle can, therefore, be introduced into the subarachnoid space (to withdraw CSF or to inject substances) without danger of damage to the spinal cord.
   b. For this procedure, called ***lumbar puncture***, the needle is most often introduced through the interval between vertebrae L3 and L4.
5. The part of the vertebral canal below the level of the spinal cord contains several roots of spinal nerves that collectively form the ***cauda equina***. These nerve roots are not injured during lumbar puncture as they are easily pushed aside by the needle.
6. The spinal dura mater is separated from the wall of the vertebral canal by the ***epidural space***. Apart from some connective tissue and fat this space contains the ***internal vertebral venous plexus***. Spinal arteries entering the vertebral canal also traverse this space.

## WANT TO KNOW MORE?

**Filum Terminale**

Below the level of the spinal cord pia mater becomes continuous with a fibrous cord called the filum terminale.

### Ligamentum Denticulatum

1. Running longitudinally along each lateral margin of the spinal cord, there is a thickening of pia mater that projects laterally. This thickening is the ligamentum denticulatum.
2. A number of pointed projections extend laterally from this ligament i.e., why it is called the ligamentum denticulatum.
3. The ligamentum denticulatum helps to keep the spinal cord at the centre of the vertebral canal.

#### *Linea Splendens*

This term is applied to a narrow thickening of pia mater present over the anterior median line of the spinal cord.

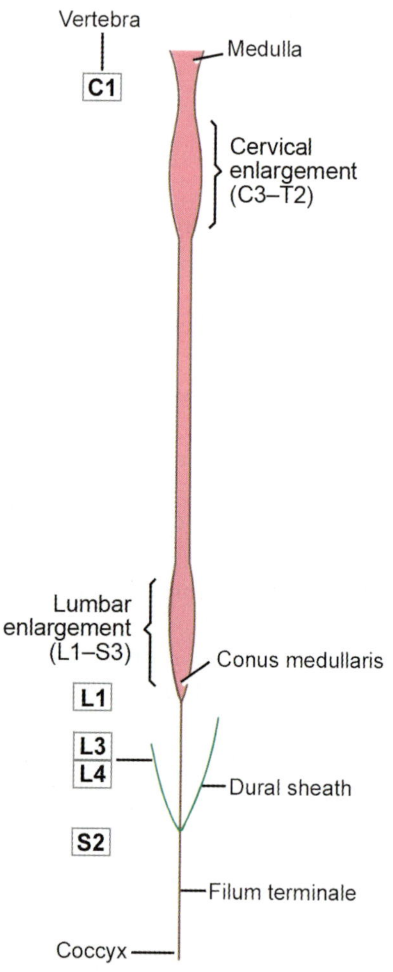


**40.6:** Important vertebral levels in relation to the spinal cord

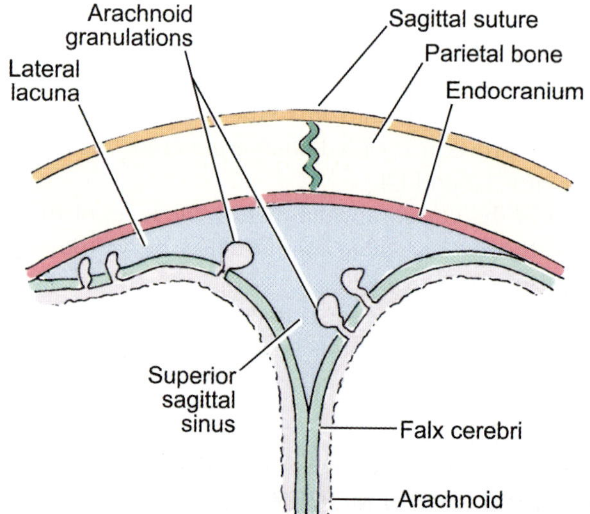


**40.7:** Coronal section to show arachnoid granulations present in relation to the superior sagittal sinus

## Intracranial Venous Sinuses

See chapter 42.

## NERVES AND ARTERIES IN THE CRANIAL CAVITY

### Cranial nerves

The brain gives attachment to 12 pair of ***cranial nerves***. Parts of these nerves traverse the cranial cavity. They are shown in 40.8.

1. In the anterior cranial fossa, there is a median bony projection called the ***crista galli***.
   a. To its right side, we see the ***cribriform plate*** of the ethmoid bone bearing numerous foramina. Bundles of olfactory nerve fibres enter the cranial cavity through these foramina and end in the ***olfactory bulb***.
   b. Posteriorly, the olfactory bulb continues into the ***olfactory tract*** that is attached to the cerebral hemisphere.
2. Medial to the anterior clinoid process we see the ***optic nerve***.
   a. It reaches the cranial cavity from the orbit by passing through the optic canal.
   b. The terminal part of the internal carotid artery is posterolateral to the optic nerve.
3. The ***oculomotor nerve*** emerges from the anterior aspect of the midbrain and passes forwards through the subarachnoid space.
   a. It penetrates the dura in the triangular interval between the free and attached margins of the tentorium cerebelli, and enters the lateral wall of the cavernous sinus.
   b. It runs forwards and enters the orbit through the superior orbital fissure.
4. The ***trochlear nerve*** lies a short distance posterior to the oculomotor nerve.
   a. This nerve emerges from the ***posterior aspect*** of the midbrain, and winds around its lateral side to reach the front of the midbrain.
   b. The nerve runs forwards and penetrates the dura mater just below the free margin of the tentorium cerebelli, a little behind the posterior clinoid process.
   c. The nerve then enters the lateral wall of the cavernous sinus and runs in it up to the superior orbital fissure. It enters the orbit through this fissure.

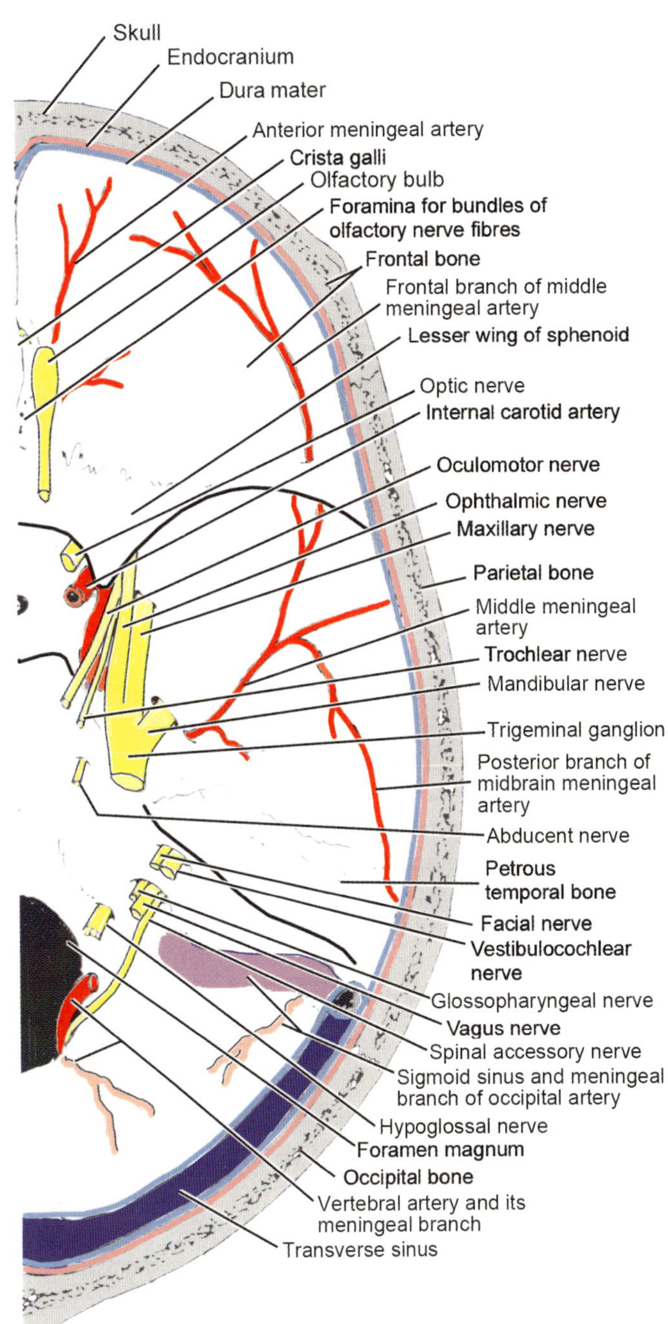


**40.8:** Some structures to be seen in the floor of cranial fossae

5. The ***trigeminal ganglion*** lies in a depression over the anterior aspect of the petrous temporal bone, near its apex.
   a. The ganglion lies within a recess of dura called the ***trigeminal cave***.
   b. Posteriorly, the ganglion is continuous with the sensory root of the ***trigeminal nerve***.
   c. Anteriorly, it is continuous with the ophthalmic, maxillary and mandibular divisions of the same nerve.
   d. The trigeminal ganglion (and cave) are closely related to the posterior end of the cavernous sinus.
6. The ***ophthalmic nerve*** runs forwards in the lateral wall of the cavernous sinus, below the trochlear nerve (40.5). It divides into three branches (lacrimal, frontal, nasociliary) that enter the orbit by passing through the superior orbital fissure.
7. The ***maxillary nerve*** pierces the distal edge of the trigeminal cave and comes to lie in the lowest part of the lateral wall of the cavernous sinus (40.5). It runs forwards and enters the foramen rotundum through which it leaves the cranial cavity.
8. The ***mandibular nerve*** is formed by the union of two roots.
   a. The sensory root arises from the lateral part of the trigeminal ganglion and leaves the cranial cavity through the foramen ovale.
   b. The motor root passes forwards deep to the trigeminal ganglion, passes through the foramen ovale, and then joins the sensory root outside the skull.
9. The ***abducent nerve*** runs upwards and laterally over the anterior wall of the floor of the posterior cranial fossa.
   a. It pierces the dura a little lateral to the dorsum sellae of the sphenoid bone.
   b. It then runs upwards to reach the upper border of the petrous temporal bone and bends round it to enter the middle cranial fossa.
   c. The nerve now comes to lie within the cavernous sinus where it is closely related to the internal carotid artery (40.5).
   d. At the anterior end of the cavernous sinus, the nerve passes through the superior orbital fissure to enter the orbit.
10. The ***facial nerve*** and the ***vestibulocochlear nerves*** enter the internal acoustic meatus located on the posterior aspect of the petrous temporal bone.
11. A short distance below and medial to the internal acoustic meatus we see the jugular foramen.
    a. Passing into it, we see the ***glossopharyngeal nerve*** (medially).
    b. The ***vagus nerve*** (in the middle) and
    c. The ***spinal part of the accessory nerve*** (laterally).
    d. The spinal part of the accessory nerve is formed by union of a number of rootlets that emerge from the lateral aspect of the upper part of the spinal cord. The nerve ascends through the upper part of the vertebral canal, lateral to the spinal cord. It enters the cranial cavity through the foramen magnum and leaves it through the jugular foramen.
12. The hypoglossal nerve passes through the hypoglossal (anterior condylar canal) a little above the lateral margin of the foramen magnum.

**WANT TO KNOW MORE?**

***Other Nerves to be Seen in the Cranial Fossae***

1. Running downwards and medially over the anterior surface of the petrous temporal bone we see:
   a. The greater and lesser petrosal nerves.
   b. The deep petrosal nerve lies in the foramen lacerum.
2. In addition to these, we have already seen that a number of small meningeal branches are given off by some cranial nerves.

All the nerves mentioned are considered completely in chapter 43.

## Arteries to be Seen in the Cranial Cavity

### *Intracranial Part of Internal Carotid Artery*

1. The internal carotid artery enters the skull through the carotid canal (opening on the base of the skull and passing through the petrous temporal bone).
2. After passing through the carotid canal, the artery enters the foramen lacerum through which it enters the cranial cavity.
3. As the foramen lacerum is closely related to the posterior end of the cavernous sinus the artery enters this sinus directly and runs forwards within it (40.8).
4. Near the anterior end of the cavernous sinus the artery turns upwards, pierces the dura mater forming the roof the cavernous sinus and comes into relationship with the cerebrum.
5. The artery now lies medial to the anterior clinoid process, lateral to the optic nerve and optic chiasma.
6. The artery ends here by dividing into the anterior and middle cerebral arteries that supply the brain. It also gives off the ophthalmic artery that runs forwards into the orbit through the optic canal.

### *Vertebral Artery*

1. In 40.8 the vertebral artery is seen ascending into the cranial cavity through the foramen magnum.
2. This artery arises from the subclavian artery in the lower part of the neck, ascends through the foramina transversaria of the upper six cervical vertebrae, passes through the suboccipital region and then enters the upper part of the vertebral canal.
3. After entering the cranial cavity, the vertebral arteries of both sides anastomose in the middle line to form the basilar artery.
4. The vertebral and basilar give branches that supply the brain and spinal cord.

### *The Meningeal Arteries*

1. These are the middle meningeal artery, and several other small arteries.
2. All the arteries mentioned above are described completely in chapter 42.

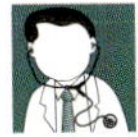

## CLINICAL CORRELATION

### *Congenital Malformations of Skull*

1. a. ***Anencephaly*** is a malformation of the skull in which the greater part of the vault is missing.
   b. It is caused by failure of the neural tube to close in the region where the brain is to be formed.
   c. Neural tissue, which is exposed to the surface degenerates.
   d. The condition is fairly frequent and is not compatible with life.
2. Establishment of the normal shape of the skull depends on orderly closure of sutures.
   a. Premature union of the sagittal suture gives rise to a boat shaped skull (***scaphocephaly***).
   b. Early union of the coronal suture results in a skull that is pointed upwards (***acrocephaly***).
   c. Asymmetrical union of sutures (on the right and left sides) results in a twisted skull (***plagiocephaly***).
3. ***Congenital hydrocephalus*** is a condition in which there is obstruction to the flow of cerebrospinal fluid. As a result pressure in the ventricular system of the brain increases and leads to its dilatation. In turn this leads to enlargement of the head, and wide separation of the bones of the skull.
4. The maxilla, the mandible and the zygomatic bone are derived from the first branchial arch. Occasionally growth of this arch is defective so that the bones concerned remain underdeveloped, and the face is deformed. The condition is called ***mandibulofacial dysostosis***.
5. Many bones of the skull are formed by intramembranous ossification. The clavicle is also formed in membrane. In the condition called ***cleidocranial dysostosis*** formation of membrane bones is interfered with. Deformities of the skull are seen in association with absence of the clavicle.

### *Fractures of the Skull*

Fractures of the skull have been considered in chapter 36. Some additional facts are as follows.

### *Fractures Through the Middle Cranial Fossa*

1. The body and greater wing of the sphenoid are closely related to the middle cranial fossa.
2. A fracture involving the body of the sphenoid bone can lead to leakage of blood and CSF into the sphenoidal air sinuses, and through them into the nose and mouth.
3. The 3rd, 4th and 6th cranial nerves lie in relation to the cavernous sinus (which lies against the body of the sphenoid bone). These nerves can be involved in fractures of the middle cranial fossa.
4. Posteriorly, the middle cranial fossa is bounded by the petrous temporal bone. Involvement of this bone can lead to bleeding and discharge of CSF into the middle ear and external acoustic meatus.
5. The 7th and 8th cranial nerves (which pass through the internal acoustic meatus) can also be injured in a fracture through the petrous temporal bone.

### *Fractures Through the Anterior Cranial Fossa*

1. This fossa is closely related to the nasal cavity and to the orbits. Fracture through the fossa can lead to bleeding or leakage of CSF through the nose (the blood flowing directly into nose through its roof, or through the frontal air sinus).
2. Bleeding into the orbit can push the eyeball forwards (exophthalmos). Blood in the orbit can seep into the eyelids resulting in a 'black eye'.

### *Fractures Through the Posterior Cranial Fossa*

1. Fractures through this fossa can lead to bleeding, the blood seeping into the muscles of the back of the neck.
2. The blood often appears superficially over the mastoid process and the sternomastoid muscle.
3. If the fracture passes through the jugular foramen there can be injury to the 9th, 10th and 11th cranial nerves. The walls of the hypoglossal canal are strong and so the 12th cranial nerve usually escapes injury.

### *Injuries to the Brain Following Injury to the Skull*

1. Fractures of the skull often lead to injury to the brain. An impact on the head can damage the brain even in the absence of a fracture.
2. In this connection, it is to be remembered that the brain is a very delicate tissue. However, it is not damaged by normal bodily movements because:
   a. It is surrounded by a cushion of CSF.
   b. Its displacement is prevented by folds of dura mater (falx cerebri, tentorium cerebelli, falx cerebelli).
   c. Veins passing from the brain to the dural venous sinuses (specially the superior cerebral veins passing to the superior sagittal sinus) also help to keep the brain in position.
3. The cushion of CSF prevents the brain from striking against the inner wall of the skull.
4. A strong impact on the head can shake up the brain.
   a. When this shaking up leaves no apparent physical damage the condition is called ***cerebral concussion***.
   b. It is usually followed by a variable period of unconsciousness.
   c. On regaining consciousness, the patient may suffer from headaches and loss of memory.
5. An injury in which there is superficial injury to brain tissue (but without any break on its surface) is called ***cerebral contusion***; and when there is tearing of brain tissue it is a ***cerebral laceration***.
   a. Severe damage to be brain, specially the brain stem, can lead to prolonged periods of deep unconsciousness (coma) and to death.
   b. Patients who come out of coma may show various neurological symptoms depending on the part of the brain injured.

6. Apart from direct injury to the brain, injury to the skull can affect the brain by causing haemorrhage. Such bleeding can be of various types.
   a. **Extradural haemorrhage**: Injury to meningeal vessels can cause bleeding into the potential space between the dura mater and the skull. The haematoma can press upon the brain surface and produce symptoms. Extradural haemorrhage is often caused by injury to the anterior division of the middle meningeal artery, resulting in pressure over the motor area of the brain.
   b. **Subdural haemorrhage**: Blood accumulates in the space between the dura and arachnoid. It is often caused by rupture of superior cerebral veins at their entry into the superior sagittal sinus. Such injury is most likely to be caused by a blow on the front or back of the head (as such injury causes anteroposterior displacement of the brain stretching the veins).
   c. **Subarachnoid haemorrhage**: Blood flows into the subarachnoid space and mixes with CSF. Such haemorrhage can be caused by rupture of aneurysms that are not uncommon on arteries forming the circulus arteriosus.

## THE SPINAL CORD

1. The spinal cord (or spinal medulla) is the most important content of the vertebral canal. Many facts of importance about the spinal cord will be considered in the section on the brain. Here, we will consider its gross anatomy in relation to other structures within the vertebral canal.
2. The upper end of the spinal cord becomes continuous with the medulla oblongata at the level of the upper border of the first cervical vertebra.
3. It is the medulla oblongata that passes through the foramen magnum, not the spinal cord.
4. The lower end of the spinal cord lies at the level of the lower border of the first lumbar vertebra.
   a. The level is, however, variable and the cord may terminate one vertebra higher or lower than this level.
   b. The level also varies with flexion or extension of the spine.
5. The lowest part of the spinal cord is conical and is called the ***conus medullaris***. The conus is continuous with the filum terminale.
6. When seen in transverse section, the grey matter of the spinal cord forms an H-shaped mass (40.9).
   a. In each half of the cord, the grey matter is divisible into a larger ventral mass, the ***anterior (or ventral) grey column***, and a narrow elongated ***posterior (or dorsal ) grey column***.
   b. In some parts of the spinal cord, a small lateral projection of grey matter is seen between the ventral and dorsal grey columns. This is the ***lateral grey column***.
   c. The grey matter of the right and left halves of the spinal cord is connected across the middle line by the ***grey commissure***.
   d. The grey commissure is traversed by the ***central canal***.
7. The lower end of the central canal expands to form the ***terminal ventricle*** that lies in the conus medullaris.
8. The white matter of the spinal cord is divided into right and left halves, in front by a deep ***anterior median fissure***, and behind by the ***posterior median septum***.
   a. In each half of the cord, the white matter medial to the dorsal grey column forms the ***posterior funiculus*** (or ***posterior white column***).
   b. The white matter medial and ventral to the anterior grey column forms the ***anterior funiculus*** (or ***anterior white column***).
   c. The white matter lateral to the anterior and posterior grey columns forms the ***lateral funiculus***.
   d. The anterior and lateral funiculi are collectively referred to as the ***anterolateral funiculus***.
   e. The white matter of the right and left halves of the spinal cord is continuous across the middle line through the ***ventral white commissure*** that lies anterior to the grey commissure.

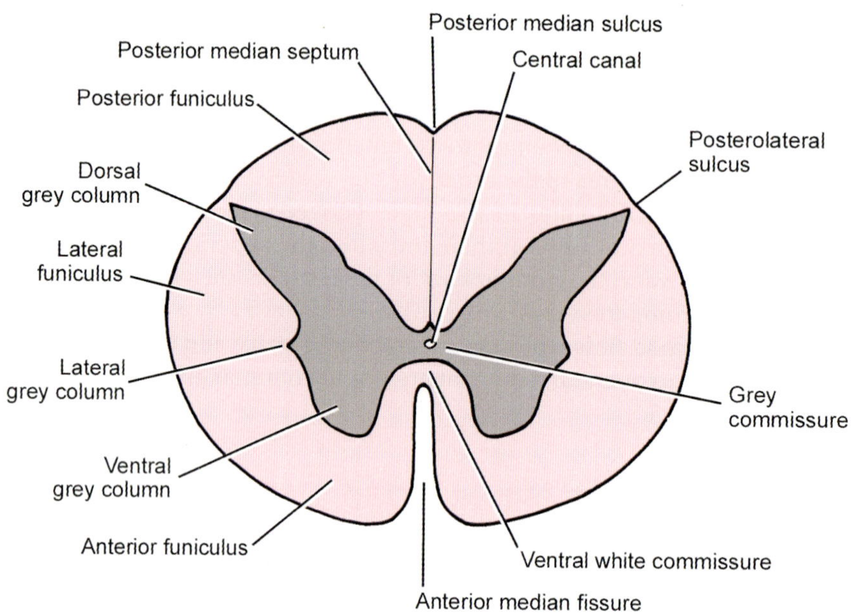


**40.9:** Main features to be seen in a transverse section through the spinal cord

## Spinal Nerves and Spinal Segments

1. The spinal cord gives attachment, on either side, to a series of spinal nerves.
2. Each spinal nerve arises by two roots, anterior (or ventral) and posterior (or dorsal) (40.11).
3. Each root is formed by aggregation of a number of rootlets that arise from the cord over a certain length (40.10). The length of the spinal cord giving origin to the rootlets of one spinal nerve constitutes one ***spinal segment***.
4. The spinal cord is made up of thirty-one segments: 8 cervical, 12 thoracic, 5 lumbar, 5 sacral and one coccygeal. (Note that in the cervical and coccygeal regions the number of spinal segments, and of spinal nerves, does not correspond to the number of vertebrae).
5. The rootlets that make up the dorsal nerve roots are attached to the surface of the spinal cord along a vertical groove (called the posterolateral sulcus) opposite the tip of the posterior grey column (40.9).
6. The rootlets of the ventral nerve roots are attached to the anterolateral aspect of the cord opposite the anterior grey column.
7. The ventral and dorsal nerve roots join each other to form a spinal nerve.
8. Just proximal to their junction the dorsal root is marked by a swelling called the ***dorsal nerve root ganglion***, or ***spinal ganglion*** (40.11).
9. The dorsal and ventral roots of spinal nerves pass through the spinal dura mater separately.
10. Sheaths derived from dura extend over the nerve roots (40.12).

**WANT TO KNOW MORE?**

11. The dorsal and ventral nerve roots unite ***in the intervertebral foramina*** to form the trunks of spinal nerves.
12. The pia mater and arachnoid mater also extend on to the roots of spinal nerves as sheaths.

13. In early fetal life the spinal cord is as long as the vertebral canal, and each spinal nerve arises from the cord at the level of the corresponding intervertebral foramen.
    a. In subsequent development, the spinal cord does not grow as much as the vertebral column and its lower end, therefore, gradually ascends to reach the level of the third lumbar vertebra at the time of birth, and the lower border of the first lumbar vertebra in the adult.
    b. As a result of this upward migration of the cord, the roots of spinal nerves have to follow an oblique downward course to reach the appropriate intervertebral foramen (40.13).
    c. This also makes the roots longer.
    d. The obliquity and length of the roots is most marked in the lower nerves and many of these roots occupy the vertebral canal below the level of the spinal cord. These roots constitute the ***cauda equina***.
    e. Another result of the upward recession of the spinal cord is that the spinal segments do not lie opposite the corresponding vertebrae. This fact is clinically important.
    f. For estimating the position of a spinal segment in relation to the surface of the body, it is important to remember that a vertebral spine is ***always lower*** than the corresponding spinal segment.
    g. As a rough guide, it may be stated that in the cervical region there is a difference of one segment (e.g., the 5th cervical spine overlies the 6th cervical segment); in the upper thoracic region there is a difference of two segments (e.g., the 4th thoracic spine overlies the 6th thoracic segment); and in the lower thoracic region there is a difference of three segments (e.g., the 9th thoracic spine lies opposite the 12th thoracic segment).

14. The spinal cord is not of uniform thickness.
    a. The spinal segments that contribute to the nerves of the upper limbs are enlarged to form the ***cervical enlargement*** of the cord.
    b. Similarly, the segments innervating the lower limbs forms the ***lumbar enlargement*** (40.6).
15. In addition to spinal nerves, the upper five or six cervical segments of the spinal cord give origin to a series of rootlets that emerge on the lateral aspect (midway between the anterior and posterior nerve roots of spinal nerves). These rootlets join to form the ***spinal root of the accessory nerve***.
16. The meninges surrounding the spinal cord have been described above.

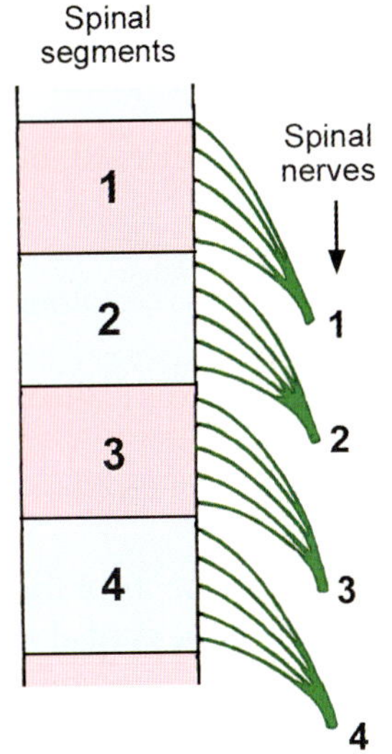


**40.10:** Scheme to illustrate the concept of spinal segments

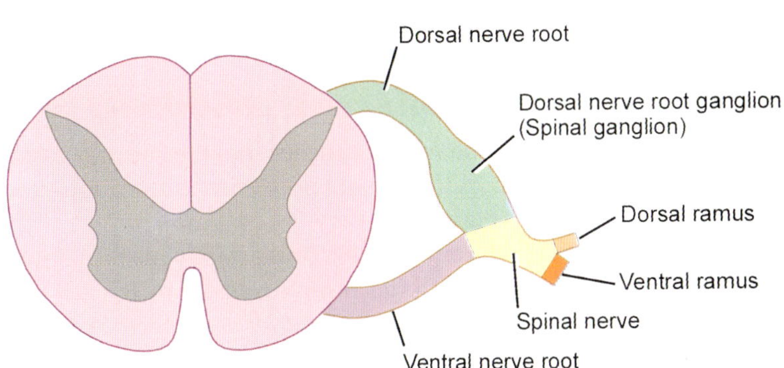


**40.11:** Relationship of a spinal nerve to the spinal cord

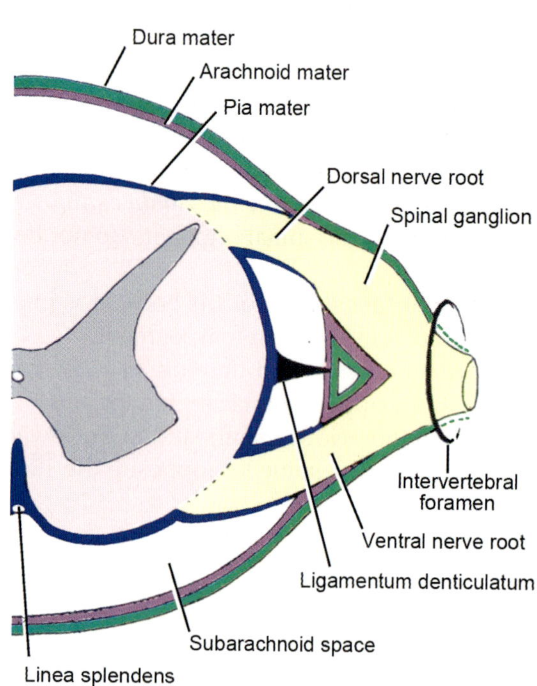


**40.12:** Transverse section through spinal cord to show formation of meningeal sheaths over the roots of a spinal nerve

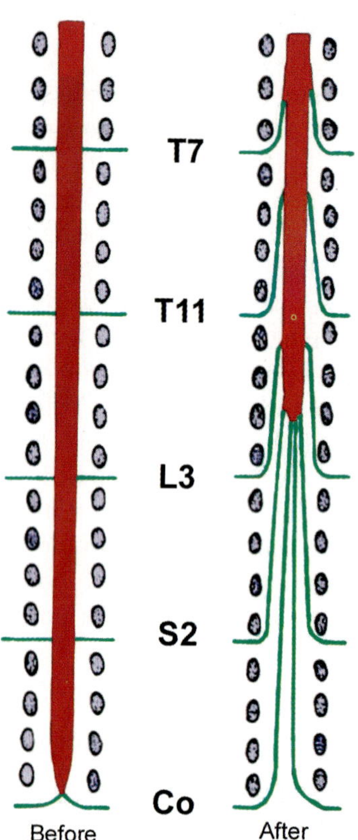


**40.13:** Scheme to show the effect of recession of the spinal cord on course and length of the roots of spinal nerves

## WANT TO KNOW MORE?

*Blood Supply of the Spinal Cord*

1. The spinal cord receives its blood supply from three longitudinal arterial channels that extend along the length of the spinal cord (40.14).
   a. The ***anterior spinal artery*** is present in relation to the anterior median fissure.
   b. Two ***posterior spinal arteries*** (one on each side) run along the posterolateral sulcus (i.e., along the line of attachment of the dorsal nerve roots).
   c. In addition to these channels the pia mater covering the spinal cord has an arterial plexus (called the ***arterial vasocorona***) which also sends branches into the substance of the cord.
2. The main source of blood to the spinal arteries is from the vertebral arteries (from which the anterior and posterior spinal arteries take origin).
   a. However, the blood from the vertebral arteries reaches only up to the cervical segments of the cord.
   b. Lower down the spinal arteries receive blood through ***radicular arteries*** that reach the cord along the roots of spinal nerves. These radicular arteries arise from spinal branches of the vertebral, ascending cervical, deep cervical, intercostal, lumbar and sacral arteries (40.15).
   c. Many of these radicular arteries are small and end by supplying the nerve roots.
   d. A few of them, which are larger, join the spinal arteries and contribute blood to them.

e. Frequently, one of the anterior radicular branches is very large and is called the ***arteria radicularis magna***. Its position is variable. This artery may be responsible for supplying blood to as much as the lower two-thirds of the spinal cord.

3. The greater part of (the cross sectional area of) the spinal cord is supplied by branches of the anterior spinal artery (40.14, left half).
   a. These branches enter the anterior median fissure (or sulcus) and are, therefore, called ***sulcal branches.***
   b. Alternate sulcal branches pass to the right and left sides. They supply the anterior and lateral grey columns and the central grey matter. They also supply the anterior and lateral funiculi.
   c. The remaining cross sectional area of the spinal cord is supplied by the posterior spinal arteries. Branches from the arterial vasocorona also supply the cord.
4. The veins draining the spinal cord are arranged in the form of six longitudinal channels.
   a. These are ***anteromedian*** and ***posteromedian*** channels that lie in the midline.
   b. ***Anterolateral*** and ***posterolateral*** channels that are paired (40.14).
   c. These venous channels are connected to one another by a plexus of veins that form a ***venous vasocorona.***
   d. The blood from these veins is drained into radicular veins that open into a venous plexus lying between the dura mater and the bony vertebral canal (***epidural*** or ***internal vertebral venous plexus***) and through it into various segmental veins.

## Vertebral Venous Plexus

1. Each vertebra is surrounded by a dense plexus of veins (40.16).
   a. The plexus is divisible into an ***external part*** lying on the outer surface.
   b. An ***internal part*** lining the vertebral canal.
2. Each of these parts is divided into anterior and posterior divisions.
3. A ***basivertebral vein*** from each vertebral body drains into the anterior internal plexus. It also communicates with the anterior external plexus.

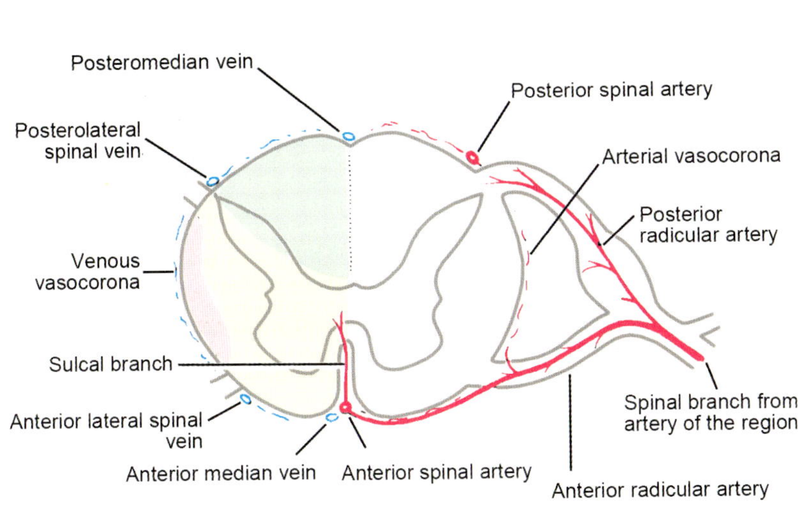


**40.14:** Blood vessels supplying the spinal cord. In the left half of the figure, the area shaded green is supplied by the posterior spinal artery; the areas shaded pink is supplied by the arterial vasocorona; and the area shaded yellow is supplied by the anterior spinal artery

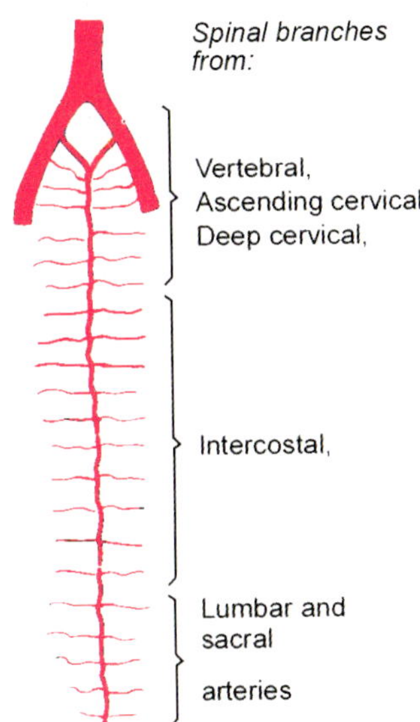


**40.15:** Radicular arteries that contribute blood to spinal arteries

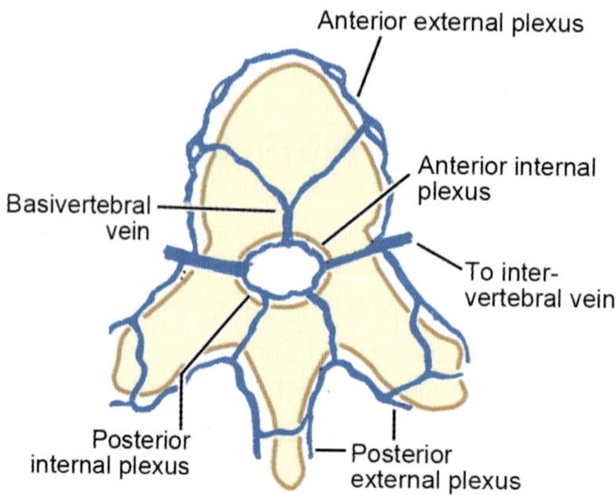


**40.16:** The vertebral venous plexus

4. Apart from veins draining blood from the vertebrae, the plexus receives veins from the meninges and from the spinal cord.
5. Opposite each intervertebral foramen the plexus drains into an ***intervertebral vein***. The intervertebral veins end in the vertebral, intercostal and lumbar veins.
6. In the pelvis the plexuses communicate with veins from some pelvic viscera.
7. The veins of the vertebral plexus do not have valves, and direction of blood flow in them is controlled by differences in venous pressure in different regions.

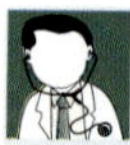

## CLINICAL CORRELATION

Tumours of some viscera (e.g., of the prostate) may spread to vertebral bodies, and even into the skull through communications with visceral venous plexuses.

# 41 CHAPTER

# Muscles of the Neck, Triangles of the Neck, Deep Cervical Fascia and Lymph Nodes

## MUSCLES OF THE NECK

The muscles of the neck are arranged in a number of groups. These are given in 41.1 and 41.2.

### THE PLATYSMA

1. This is the most superficial muscle in the neck. Like the muscles of the face it lies in the superficial fascia (41.21).
2. It is a remnant of an extensive sheet of subcutaneous muscle (called the ***pannulus carnosus***) to be seen in some animals.
3. The muscle is described in 41.3 and shown in 41.4.

### THE STERNOMASTOID AND TRAPEZIUS

1. From 41.2, it will be seen that deeper tissues in the neck are overlapped by two large muscles, the sternocleidomastoid and the trapezius.
2. These two muscles lie between the two layers of the investing fascia of the neck.
3. The trapezius is a muscle of the upper limb (part of which lies in the neck) and has been described on page 70.
4. The sternocleidomastoid is described in 41.3 and is shown in 41.5. It has several important relations that are listed in 41.6.

### INFRAHYOID MUSCLES

These are:

a. The sternohyoid
b. The sternothyroid
c. The thyrohyoid
d. The omohyoid muscles (41.8).

For details of these muscles see 41.7 and 41.8.

**41.1: Groups of muscles of neck**

| | |
|---|---|
| *Subcutaneous* | *Platysma* |
| Superficial (anterior) | Sternocleidomastoid |
| Superficial (posterior) | Trapezius<br>Levator scapulae |
| Infrahyoid | Sternohyoid<br>Sternothyroid<br>Thyrohyoid<br>Omohyoid |
| Lateral vertebral | Scalenus anterior<br>Scalenus medius<br>Scalenus posterior<br>Scalenus minimus |
| Anterior vertebral | Rectus capitis anterior<br>Rectus capitis lateralis<br>Longus colli<br>Longus capitis |
| *Deep muscles of back* | |
| Splenius group | Splenius capitis<br>Splenius cervicis |
| Erector spinae | Spinalis<br>(capitis, cervicis, thoracis)<br>Longissimus<br>(capitis, cervicis, thoracis)<br>Iliocostocervicalis<br>(cervicis, thoracis, lumborum) |
| Transverso-spinalis | Semispinalis<br>(capitis, cervicis, and thoracis)<br>Multifidus<br>Rotatores |
| Suboccipital | Rectus capitis posterior minor<br>Rectus capitis posterior major<br>Obliquus capitis inferior<br>Obliquus capitis superior |

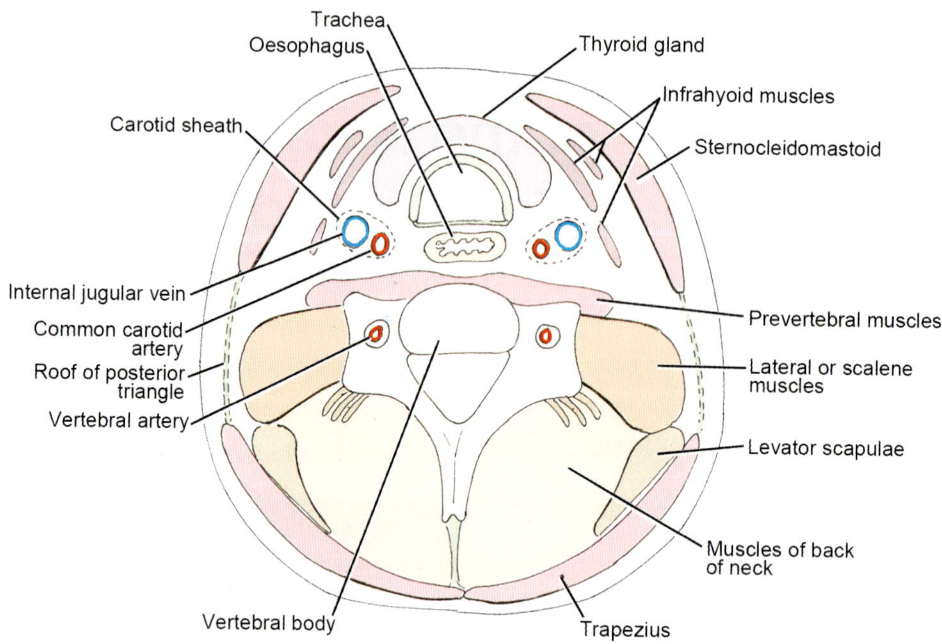


**41.2:** Schematic transverse section through the lower part of the neck. Note the relative position of various groups of muscles present

**41.3: Platysma and Sternocleidomastoid**

| *Muscle* | *Origin* | *Insertion* | *Action* | *Nerve supply* |
|---|---|---|---|---|
| PLATYSMA | Deep fascia over upper part of pectoralis major and anterior part of deltoid muscle | 1. Most anterior fibres interlace with those of opposite side<br>2. Other fibres cross lower border of mandible and merge with muscles at angle of mouth | Produces wrinkles over skin of neck | Cervical branch of facial nerve |
| STERNOCLEIDO-MASTOID | 1. Sternal head from anterior surface of manubrium sterni<br>2. Clavicular head from upper surface of medial part of clavicle | 1. Lateral half of superior nuchal line<br>2. Lateral surface of mastoid process from apex to upper border | 1. When muscle of one side contracts, the head is tilted to the same side<br>2. When muscles of both sides contract the head and neck are flexed | 1. Accessory nerve (spinal part)<br>2. Spinal nerves C2, C3 (ventral rami) |

## THE LATERAL VERTEBRAL MUSCLES

1. These are:
   a. The ***scalenus anterior***
   b. The ***scalenus medius***
   c. The ***scalenus posterior***
   d. The ***scalenus minimus***.

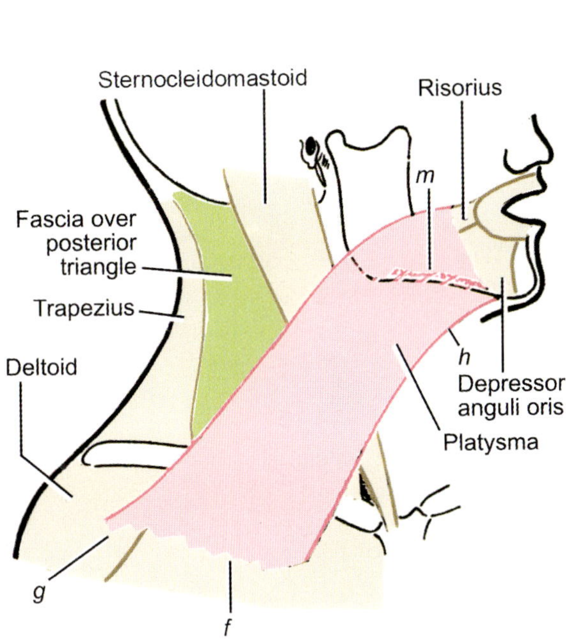


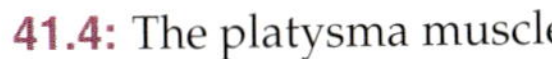
**41.4:** The platysma muscle

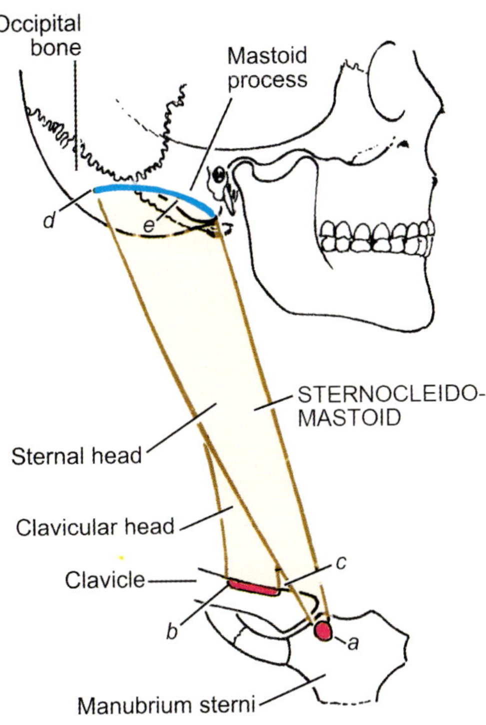


**41.5:** Scheme to show the attachments of the sternocleidomastoid muscle

2. Each muscle is attached at one end to the transverse processes of one or more cervical vertebrae, and at the other end to the first or second rib.
3. For details see 41.9 to 41.11.

## ANTERIOR VERTEBRAL MUSCLES (PREVERTEBRAL MUSCLES)

1. These are:
   a. The ***rectus capitis anterior***
   b. The ***rectus capitis lateralis***
   c. The ***longus capitis***
   d. The ***longus colli***.
2. For details see 41.12 and 41.13.

## DEEP MUSCLES OF THE BACK

### Deep Muscles of the Back and their Layout

1. The deep muscles of the back come into view after the superficial muscles that cover them are removed.
2. They are arranged in layers (from superficial to deep) as shown in 41.15 and 41.21. The upper parts of these muscles are seen in the back of the neck.
3. The muscles are listed in 41.1. Many muscles are in the form of slips that are confined to the back of the thorax and abdomen. It is enough to know their names. Some important members of this group are described in 41.14. Also see 41.16 and 41.17.

**41.6: Relations of sternocleidomastoid muscle**

**SUPERFICIAL RELATIONS**

Parotid gland
Lesser occipital nerve
Great auricular nerve
Platysma
Transverse cervical nerve
External jugular vein
Medial supraclavicular nerve

**DEEP RELATIONS**

***Muscles***

Digastric, post, belly
Splenius capitis
Levator scapulae
Scalenus anterior
Omohyoid, inferior belly
Omohyoid, superior belly
Sternohyoid
Sternothyroid

***Arteries***

Occipital
internal carotid
External carotid
Transverse cervical
Suprascapular
Sternomastoid branch of superior thyroid artery
Common carotid

***Veins***

Internal jugular
Lingual
Common facial

Nerves

Accessory
Roots of cervical plexus
Ansa cervicalis
Phrenic
Roots of brachial plexus
Vagus

Others

Sternoclavicular joint
Deep cervical lymph nodes

**41.7: Infrahyoid muscles**

| *Muscle* | *Origin* | *Insertion* | *Action* | *Nerve supply* |
|---|---|---|---|---|
| STERNOHYOID | 1. Posterior aspect of manubrium sterni (upper part)<br>2. Clavicle medial end (posterior aspect<br>3. Capsule of sternoclavicular joint | Body of hyoid bone | Depresses hyoid bone | Branch from ansa cervicalis |
| THYROHYOID | Oblique line on lamina of thyroid cartilage | Greater cornu of hyoid bone (lower border) | 1. Depresses hyoid bone.<br>2. Can raise larynx if hyoid bone is fixed | Fibres of nerve T1 travelling through hypoglossal nerve |
| STERNO-THYROID | 1. Posterior aspect of manubrium sterni<br>2. Medial end of first costal cartilage | Oblique line on lamina of thyroid cartilage | Pulls larynx downwards | Branch from ansa cervicalis |

*Contd..*

*Contd..*

| *Muscle* | *Origin* | *Insertion* | *Action* | *Nerve supply* |
|---|---|---|---|---|
| OMOHYOID | 1. Inferior belly from upper border of scapula (near scapular notch)<br>2. Superior belly from intermediate tendon | 1. Inferior passes upwards and medially across the floor of the posterior triangle. It joins the intermediate tendon (deep to sterno-cleid-omastoid)<br>2. Superior belly passes upwards to be inserted into hyoid bone (lower border of body) | Depresses hyoid bone | Branch from ansa cervicalis |

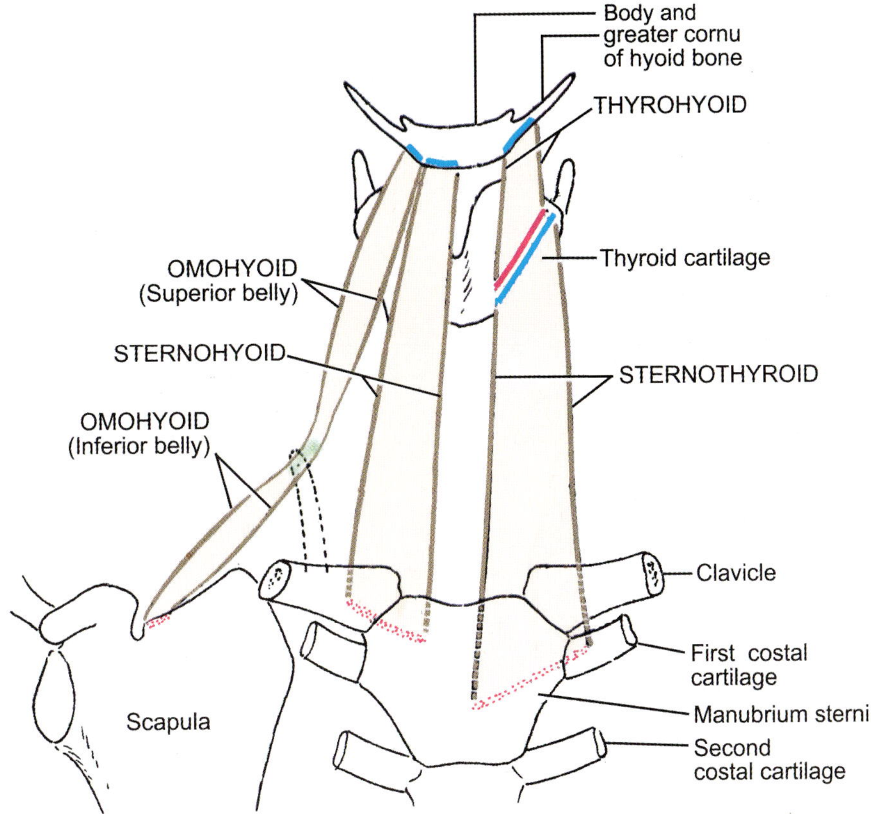


**41.8:** Scheme to show the attachments of the infrahyoid muscles

**41.9: Lateral vertebral muscles**

| *Muscle* | *Origin* | *Insertion* | *Action* | *Nerve supply* |
|---|---|---|---|---|
| SCALENUS ANTERIOR | Vertebrae C3 to C6 (transverse processes) | First rib (inner border, on scalene tubercle) | 1. Bends neck forwards and laterally<br>2. Turns face to opposite side | Spinal nerves C4, 5, 6 (ventral rami) |
| SCALENUS MEDIUS | Vertebrae axis, C3 to C7 (transverse processes) | First rib (upper surface between tubercle and groove for subclavian artery) | 1. Bends cervical spine to its own side<br>2. Can raise first rib in forced inspiration | Spinal nerves C3 to C8 (ventral rami) |
| SCALENUS POSTERIOR | Vertebrae C4 to C6 (transverse process) | Second rib (outer surface, behind attachment of serratus anterior) | 1. Bends cervical spine to its own side<br>2. Can raise second rib | Spinal nerves C6 to C8 (ventral rami) |
| SCALENUS MINIMUS | Vertebra C7 (transverse process) | First rib (inner border, posterior part). Some fibres continuous with suprapleural membrane | Not significant | Spinal nerve C7 |

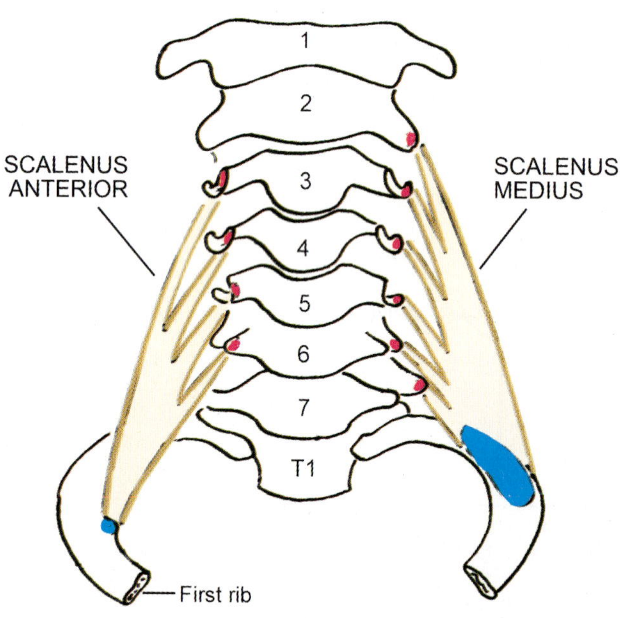


**41.10:** Attachments of the scalenus anterior and scalenus medius muscles

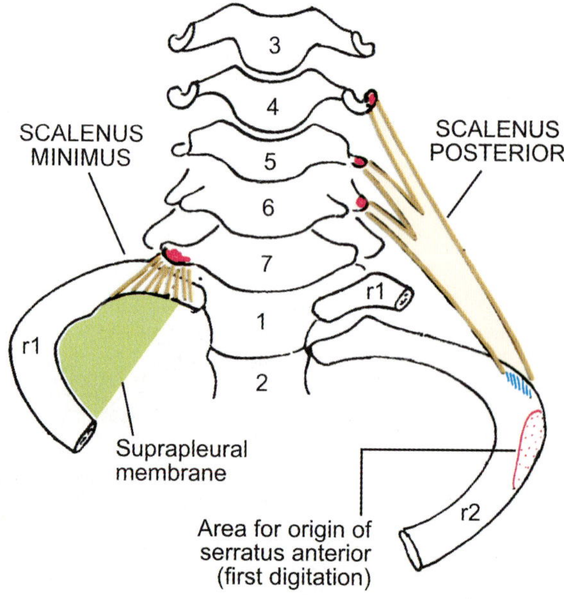


**41.11:** Attachments of the scalenus posterior and scalenus minimus muscles

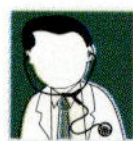

## CLINICAL CORRELATION

1. It may be noted that all the deep muscles of the back are supplied by dorsal primary rami of the spinal nerves of the levels concerned.
2. The muscles can be cut transversely, without denervating parts above or below the incision.

| 41.12: Anterior vertebral muscles | | | | |
|---|---|---|---|---|
| *Muscle* | *Origin* | *Insertion* | *Action* | *Nerve supply* |
| Rectus capitis anterior | Atlas vertebra (lateral mass and transverse process) | Occipital bone (basilar part) | Flexion of head | Spinal nerves C1, C2 ventral rami |
| Rectus capitis lateralis | Atlas vertebra (transverse process) | Occipital bone (jugular process) | Bends head to its own side | Spinal nerves C1, C2 ventral rami |
| Longus colli Upper oblique part: | Vertebrae C3, C4, C5 (transverse process) | Atlas vertebra (anterior arch) | 1. Flexor of neck 2. Lateral flexion and rotation of neck | Spinal nerves C2 to C6 ventral rami |
| Vertical part | Vertebrae C5 to T3 (bodies) | Vertebrae C2, C3, C4 (bodies) | | |
| Inferior oblique part | Vertebrae, upper thoracic (bodies) | Vertebrae C5, C6 (transverse process) | | |
| Longus capitis | Vertebrae C3 to C6 (transverse process) | Occipital bone (basilar part) | Flexor of head | Spinal nerves C1, C2, C3 ventral rami |

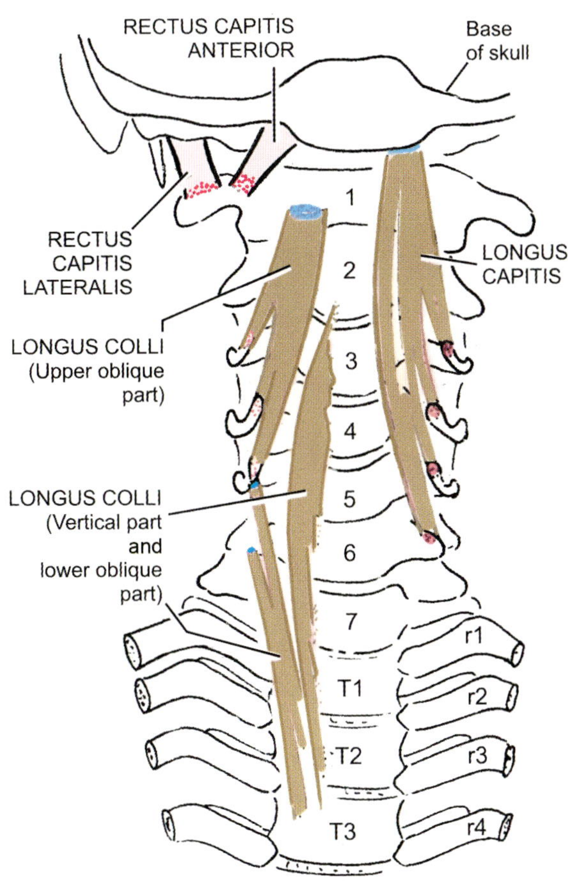


**41.13:** The anterior vertebral (prevertebral) muscles

| 41.14: Some deep muscles of the back | | | | |
|---|---|---|---|---|
| *Muscle* | *Origin* | *Insertion* | *Action* | *Nerve supply* |
| Splenius capitis | 1. Ligamentum nuchae (lower half)<br>2. Vertebral spines C7 to T3 | Back of skull (temporal bone on back of mastoid process and occipital bone below lateral 1/3 of superior nuchal line) | 1. When these two muscles of both sides contract the head is pulled backwards<br>2. When muscles of one side contract the face is rotated to the same side | Dorsal rami of cervical nerves |
| Splenius cervicis | Vertebral spines T3 to T6 | Vertebrate C1, C2, C3(?) contransverse process | | Dorsal rami of cervical nerves |
| Erector spinae | Back of sacrum through a U-shaped tendon. | 1. The muscle divides into three main parts:<br>a. Spinalis<br>b. Longissimus<br>c. Iliocostocervicalis<br>2. Only three slips reach the neck<br>a. Iliocostalis cervicis reaches lower cervical transverse processes<br>b. Longissimus cervicis reaches transverse processes of cervical vertebrae<br>c. Longissimus capitis reaches the skull (mastoid process) | 1. Extensor and lateral flexor of vertebral column<br>2. Keeps the spine erect<br>3. Longissimus capitis turns face to its own side | Dorsal rami of cervical nerves |
| Semispinalis capitus | 1. Transverse processes of upper thoracic vertebrae, and vertebra C7<br>2. Articular processes of vertebrae C4, C5, C6 | Occipital bone (medial part of area between superior and inferior nuchal lines) | 1. Extension of head<br>2. Slightly rotates face to opposite side | 1. Extension of head<br>2. Slightly rotates face to opposite side |

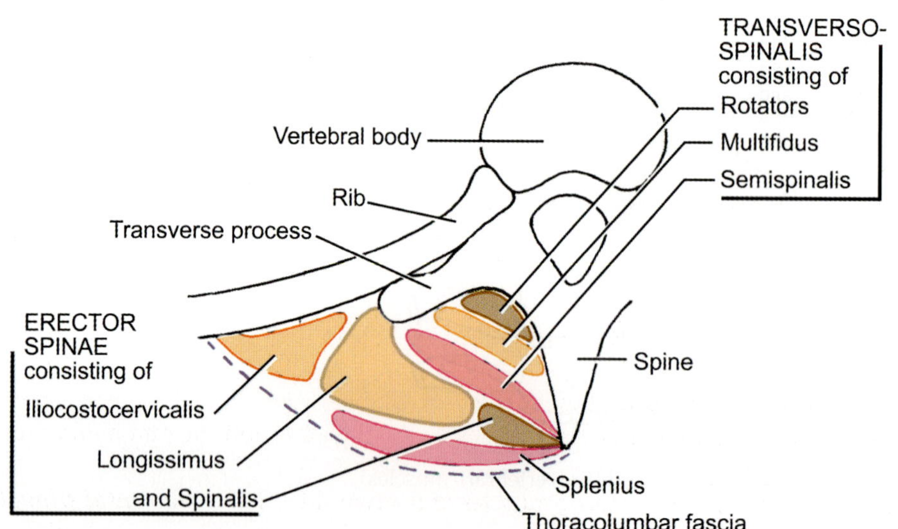


**41.15:** Schematic transverse section to show the arrangement of deep muscles of the back

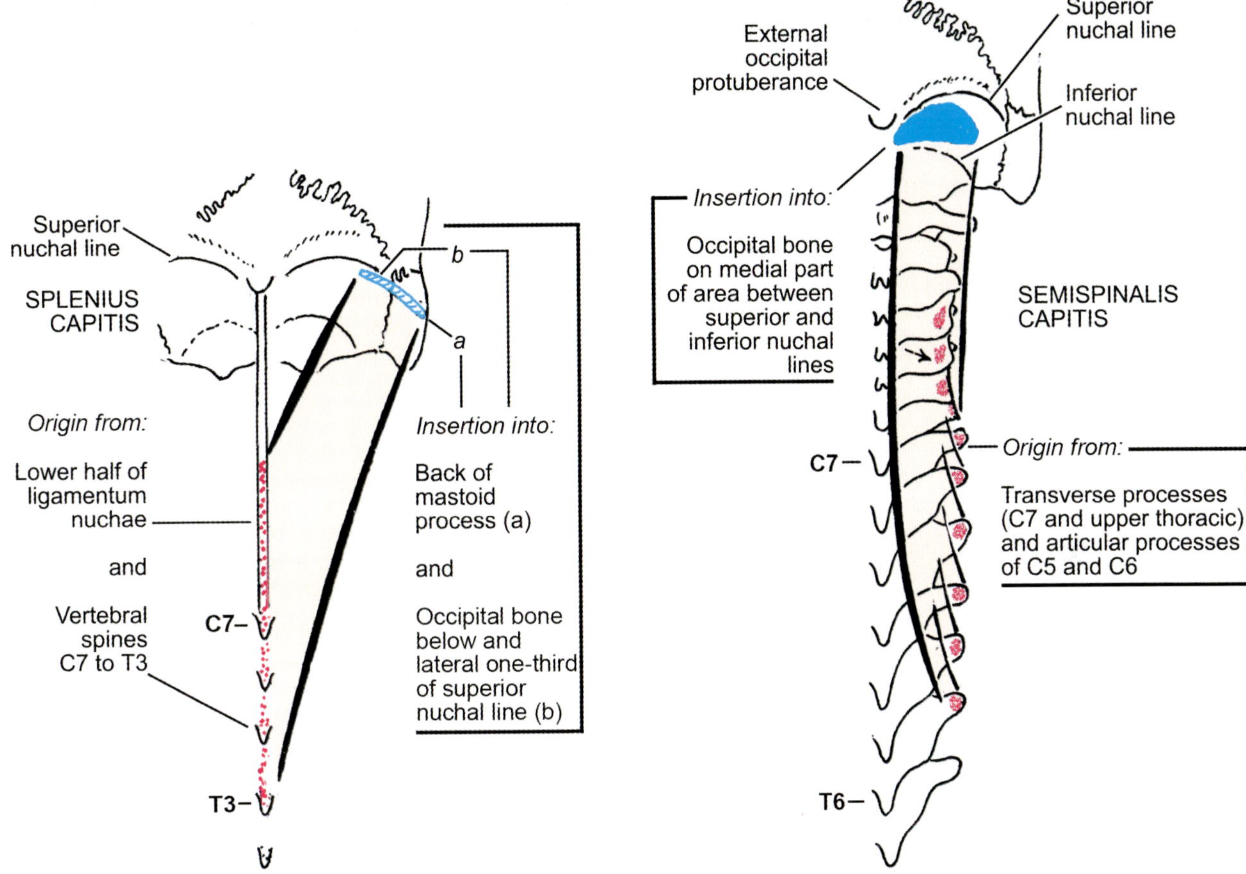


**41.16:** Attachments of the splenius capitis muscle

**41.17:** Scheme to show the attachments of the semispinalis capitis muscle

## Suboccipital Muscles

1. This is a group of small muscles placed in the uppermost part of the back of the neck, deep to the semispinalis capitis.
2. The muscles form the boundaries of the suboccipital triangle.
3. They are described in 41.18 and shown in 41.19.

# TRIANGLES OF THE NECK

1. The ***posterior triangle*** is bounded:
   a. Anteriorly by the posterior border of the sternocleidomastoid.
   b. Posteriorly by the anterior border of the trapezius.
   c. Inferiorly (base) by the clavicle.
2. The ***anterior triangle*** is bounded:
   a. Posteriorly by the anterior border of the sternocleidomastoid.
   b. Medially by the midline of the front of the neck.
   c. Its third (upper) boundary is formed by the base of the mandible.
3. The anterior triangle is further divided into four smaller triangles by the digastric and the omohyoid muscles as follows:
   a. The space between the anterior bellies of the digastric muscles of the two sides is the ***submental triangle***.
   b. The ***digastric triangle*** is bounded:

**41.18: Suboccipital muscles**

| *Muscle* | *Origin* | *Insertion* | *Action* | *Nerve supply* |
|---|---|---|---|---|
| Rectus capitus posterior minor | Atlas (posterior arch) | Occipital bone (medial part of area below inferior nuchal line) | 1. Collectively, these muscles maintain position of the head<br>2. The two recti and the superior oblique extend the head (against gravity)<br>3. The obliquus capitis inferior rotates the head turning the face to its own side<br>4. The rectus capitis posterior major can also produce slight rotation to its own side<br>5. The superior oblique tilts the head to its own side | Dorsal ramus of first cervical nerve |
| Rectus capitis posterior major | Axis vertebra (from spine) | Occipital bone (lateral part of area below inferior nuchal line) | | |
| Obliquus capitis inferior | Axis vertebra (from spine) | Atlas vertebra (transverse process) | | |
| Obliquus capitis superior | Atlas vertebra (transverse process) | Occipital bone (lateral part of area between superior and inferior nuchal lines) | | |

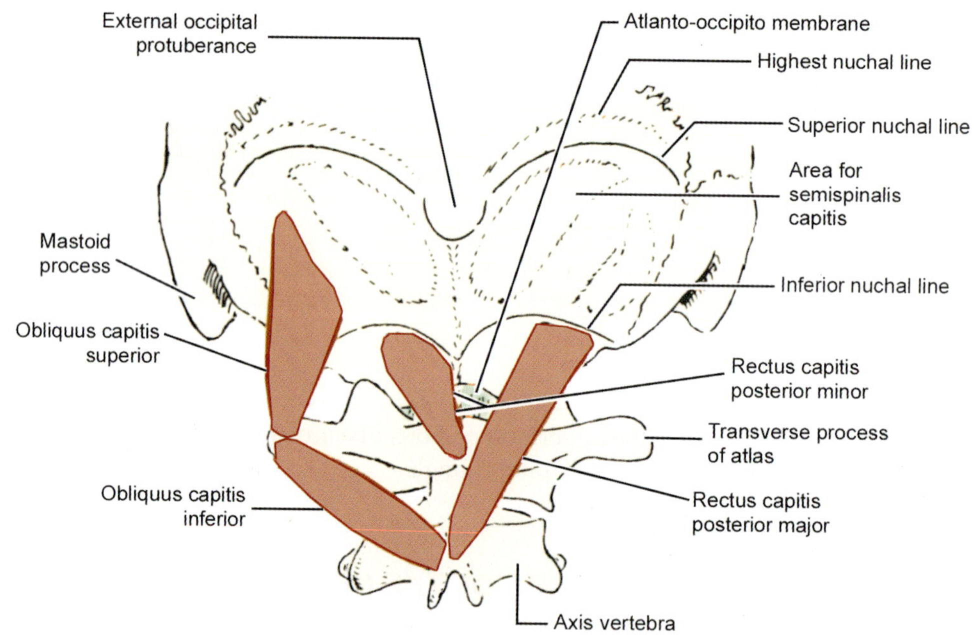


**41.19:** Schematic diagram to show the attachments of the suboccipital muscles

   i. Above by the base of the mandible.
   ii. Behind by the posterior belly of the digastric muscle.
   iii. In front by its anterior belly.

c. The ***carotid triangle*** is bounded:
   i. Behind by the anterior border of the sternocleidomastoid.
   ii. Above and in front by the posterior belly of the digastric.
   iii. Below and in front by the superior belly of the omohyoid muscle.

d. The ***muscular triangle*** is bounded:
   i. Medially (and in front) by the midline of the neck.

ii. Behind and above by the superior belly of the omohyoid.
iii. Behind and below by the lower part of the sterno-cleidomastoid.

e. In addition to the above, the ***suboccipital triangle*** is present deep in the upper part of the back of the neck, and is bounded by the suboccipital muscles.

## THE POSTERIOR TRIANGLE

### Boundaries

As stated above, the posterior triangle is bounded:

a. Anteriorly by the posterior border of the sterno-cleidomastoid.
b. Posteriorly by the anterior border of the trapezius.
c. Inferiorly (base) by the clavicle.

### Floor

1. The floor of this triangle is formed mainly by:
   a. The splenius capitis
   b. The levator scapulae
   c. The scalenus medius.
2. Other muscles that may occasionally be seen in the floor are:
   a. The semispinalis capitis
   b. The scalenus posterior
   c. The scalenus anterior.
3. The lower part of the posterior triangle is crossed by the inferior belly of the omohyoid muscle that divides the triangle into:
   a. An upper part (also called the ***occipital triangle***)
   b. A lower part (also called the ***supraclavicular triangle***).
4. The muscles forming the floor are covered by the prevertebral layer of deep cervical fascia.

### Roof

1. The roof of the posterior triangle is formed by the investing layer of deep cervical fascia. This is best appreciated by examining a transverse section through the neck (41.21).
2. Superficial to the deep cervical fascia the posterior triangle is covered by superficial fascia and skin.
3. Several nerves and vessels are present in relation to the roof of the posterior triangle. These include:
   a. The supraclavicular
   b. Lesser occipital
   c. Great auricular
   d. Transverse cutaneous nerves
   e. The external jugular vein and some of its tributaries
   f. Several unnamed arteries
   g. Lymph vessels.

### Contents

1. Cutaneous branches of the cervical plexus (supraclavicular, lesser occipital, great auricular and transverse cutaneous) enter the posterior triangle by piercing the fascia over its floor, and run for some distance between the floor and roof, before piercing the latter to become subcutaneous.
2. Muscular branches arising from the cervical plexus for the levator scapulae and trapezius run deep to the fascia of the floor.
3. The spinal accessory nerve runs downwards and laterally across the triangle lying between the two layers of the fascia forming the roof.

4. The trunks of the brachial plexus are seen in the lower part of the triangle. A number of branches arising from the plexus are related to the triangle. These are:
   a. The nerve to the rhomboids
   b. The nerve to the serratus anterior
   c. The nerve to the subclavius
   d. The suprascapular nerve.
5. a. The subclavian artery (surrounded by the axillary sheath) runs across the lowest part of the posterior triangle.
   b. The transverse cervical artery runs backwards a little above the posterior belly of the omohyoid muscle.
   c. The occipital artery crosses the apex of the posterior triangle.

## SUBDIVISIONS OF THE ANTERIOR TRIANGLE

### Submental Triangle

*Note that this is an unpaired triangle, half of it lying on each side of the middle line of the neck.*

1. Boundaries:
   a. Above and laterally, this triangle is bounded on each side (right and left) by the anterior belly of the digastric muscle.
   b. The third side of the triangle (base) is formed by the hyoid bone.
2. Floor:
   The floor of the triangle is formed by the mylohyoid muscle.
3. The only contents of the triangle are the submental lymph nodes, and some small blood vessels.

### Digastric Triangle

1. Boundaries:
   a. Above by the base of the mandible
   b. Below by the anterior and posterior bellies of the digastric muscle.
2. Floor is formed by:
   a. Mylohyoid muscle
   b. Hyoglossus muscle
   c. Anterior part of the middle constrictor of the pharynx.
3. Roof is formed by:
   a. Skin, superficial fascia (containing the platysma, the cervical branch of the facial nerve and some cutaneous nerves).
   b. The investing layer of deep fascia.
4. The main content of this triangle is the submandibular gland.
5. The contents of this triangle have been studied in detail in the submandibular region (Chapter 39).

### Carotid Triangle

1. Boundaries:
   a. Posteriorly by the anterior margin of the sternocleidomastoid muscle.
   b. Superiorly by the posterior belly of the digastric muscle.
   c. Anteroinferiorly by the superior belly of the omohyoid muscle (41.20).
2. Its roof is formed by skin, superficial and deep fascia.
3. The floor of the triangle is formed by:
   a. The thyrohyoid muscle
   b. The hyoglossus muscle
   c. The middle and inferior constrictors of the pharynx.

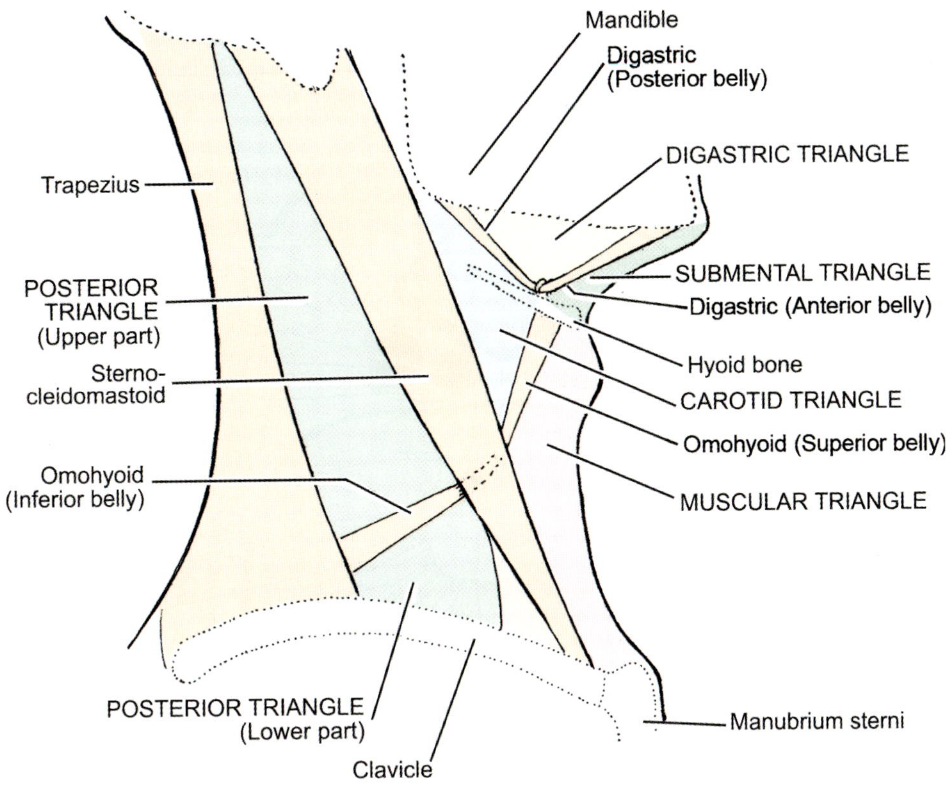


**41.20:** Triangles of the neck (lateral view)

4. The carotid triangle contains several important blood vessels and nerves. These are as follows:
   a. Common carotid artery, along with carotid sinus and carotid body.
   b. Internal carotid artery.
   c. External carotid artery and the following branches arising from it:
      i. Superior thyroid artery
      ii. Lingual artery
      iii. Facial artery
      iv. Ascending pharyngeal artery
      v. Occipital artery.
   d. Internal jugular vein, and some tributaries draining into it.
   e. Vagus nerve and its superior laryngeal branch dividing into external and internal laryngeal nerves.
   f. Spinal accessory nerve.
   g. Hypoglossal nerve and upper root of ansa cervicalis.
   h. Sympathetic trunk.
5. The common carotid and internal carotid arteries, the internal jugular vein and the vagus nerve are surrounded by the carotid sheath.

## Muscular Triangle

1. This triangle is bounded:
   a. Posteroinferiorly by the sternocleidomastoid muscle.
   b. Posterosuperiorly by the superior belly of the omohyoid muscle.
   c. Anteriorly (or medially) by the anterior middle line of the neck.

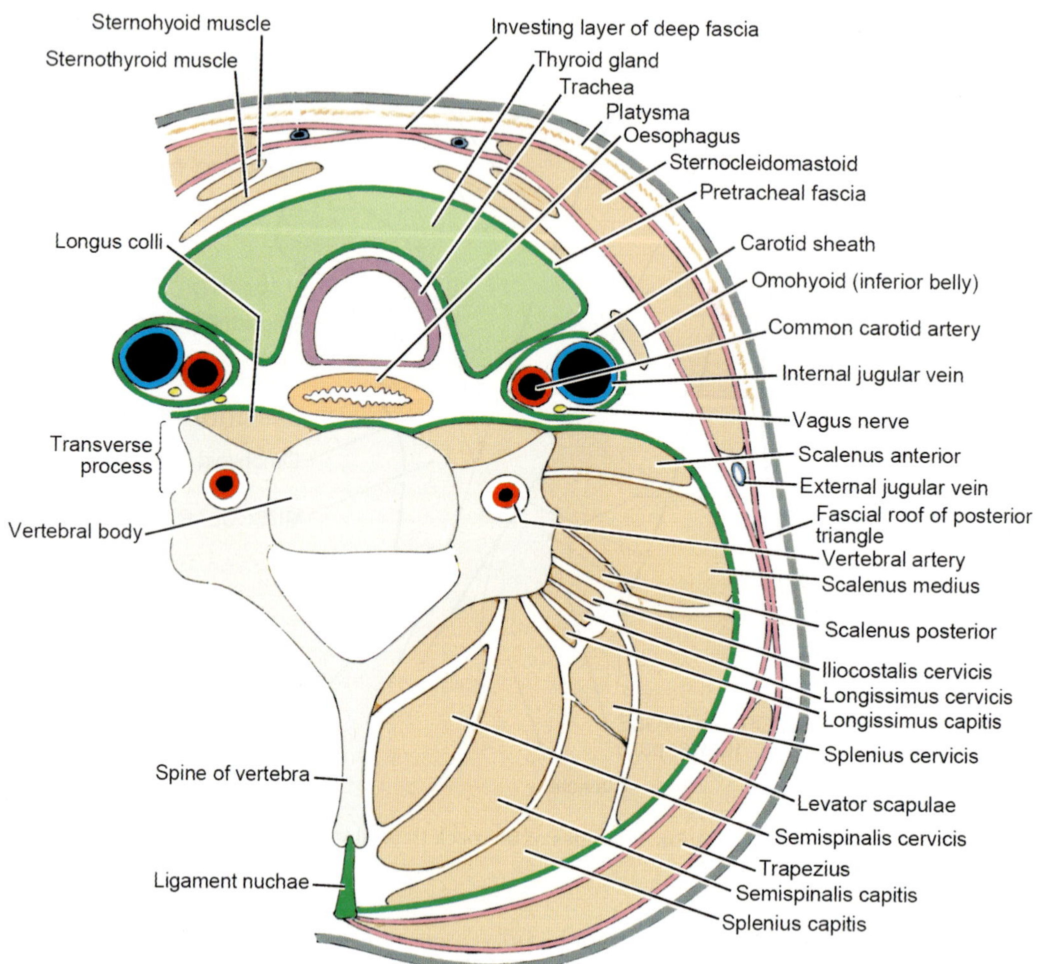


**41.21:** Transverse section through lower part of neck to show various muscles and parts of the deep cervical fascia

2. Contents of triangle:
   a. The triangle contains the infrahyoid muscles.
   b. Deep to these muscles it contains the thyroid gland, the larynx and the trachea.
   c. On either side of the trachea, we see the carotid sheath and its contents.
   d. Part of the brachiocephalic artery may occasionally be present in front of the trachea just above the manubrium sterni.

## SUBOCCIPITAL TRIANGLE

### Boundaries

The suboccipital muscles have been described earlier in this chapter. They form the boundaries of the suboccipital triangle as follows (41.19):

1. Medially and above, there are the rectus capitis posterior major and minor muscles.
2. Laterally and above, there is the obliquus capitis superior.
3. Inferiorly, there is the obliquus capitis inferior.

### Roof

1. The roof of the suboccipital triangle is formed by the semispinalis capitis muscle.
2. Deep to the semispinalis capitis the triangle is covered by dense fascia.
3. To reach the suboccipital triangle we have to remove:
   a. The trapezius
   b. The splenius capitis
   c. The semispinalis capitis muscles
   d. The longissimus capitis, that lies over the lateral part of the triangle.

### Floor

The floor of the suboccipital triangle is formed by:
1. The posterior arch of the atlas.
2. The posterior atlantooccipital membrane.

### Contents

1. Vertebral artery:
   a. The third part of the vertebral artery enters the suboccipital region after emerging from the foramen transversarium of the atlas.
   b. It then runs medially over the posterior arch of the atlas.
   c. Disappears under the lateral free edge of the posterior atlanto-occipital membrane.
2. The dorsal ramus of the first cervical nerve:
   a. It runs backwards above the posterior arch of the atlas, lying below the vertebral artery.
   b. It gives branches to the suboccipital muscles and to the semispinalis capitis.
3. The greater occipital nerve:
   a. Winds round the lower border of the obliquus capitis inferior.
   b. It then runs upwards (and slightly medially) across the suboccipital triangle.
   c. It leaves the triangle by piercing the semispinalis capitis.

## DEEP CERVICAL FASCIA

1. As in other parts of the body, all muscles, blood vessels and nerves of the neck are surrounded by some connective tissue.
2. However, we find that in several planes in the neck the connective tissue is condensed to form recognisable sheets that are collectively referred to as deep cervical fascia.
3. A good idea of the layers of the deep cervical fascia can be obtained by examining a transverse section through the neck (41.21). The layers are as follows.

## INVESTING LAYER

1. Deep to the skin, superficial fascia and platysma we see the investing layer of deep fascia.
2. This layer is made up of two laminae (shown in pink in 41.21) that go right round the neck enclosing all structures deep to them.
3. Anteriorly, near the middle line of the neck the two laminae are fused to each other.
4. Traced laterally, the laminae separate to enclose the sternocleidomastoid muscle.
5. At the posterior edge of this muscle, the layers meet again and form the roof of the posterior triangle.
6. Passing posteriorly they again separate to enclose the trapezius, and end by gaining attachment to the ligamentum nuchae.
7. The vertical extent of the investing layer is as follows:
   a. When traced upwards over the front of the neck, the fascia gets attached to the hyoid bone, and then passes over the submental triangle to reach the lower border of the body of the mandible.

   b. When traced upwards over the sternocleidomastoid muscle the fascia reaches the mastoid process.
   c. When traced upwards over the trapezius it reaches the superior nuchal line and the external occipital protuberance.
   d. In other words, the investing layer extends as far up as the muscles it covers.
   e. Traced downwards on the front of the neck the investing layer of fascia reaches the manubrium sterni. More laterally it reaches the clavicle.
   f. Traced downwards over the trapezius the fascia reaches the lateral part of the clavicle, the acromion, and the spine of the scapula (again being coextensive with the muscles).

8. Note the following additional points about the investing layer of deep cervical fascia.
   a. When traced upwards over the submandibular region the two laminae separate to enclose the submandibular gland.
   b. In the interval between the mandible and the mastoid process the two laminae enclose the parotid gland.
   c. Here the superficial lamina is thick and forms the parotid fascia.
   d. The deep lamina forms the ***stylomandibular ligament*** which intervenes between the parotid gland and the submandibular gland.
   e. Just above the manubrium sterni, the two laminae enclose the ***suprasternal space***. This space contains the sternal heads of the right and left sternocleidomastoid muscles, the interclavicular ligament, the jugular arch joining the right and left anterior jugular veins, and a lymph node.
   f. Above the clavicle (near the base of the posterior triangle), the two laminae of the investing layer enclose the ***supraclavicular space***. This space contains a part of the external jugular vein and the supraclavicular nerves.
   g. The accessory nerve runs across the posterior triangle lying between the two laminae.

## PRETRACHEAL FASCIA

1. In 41.21 note that the thyroid gland is enclosed in a layer of fascia (shown in green). When traced downwards this fascia lies in front of the trachea and is, therefore, called the pretracheal fascia.
2. It passes along the trachea into the superior mediastinum of the thorax to reach the arch of the aorta.
3. When traced upwards the pretracheal fascia is attached to the hyoid bone, and more laterally to the oblique line of the thyroid cartilage. [Note that this line is also the upper limit of the lobe of the thyroid gland].
4. Laterally, the pretracheal fascia fuses with the carotid sheath.

## PREVERTEBRAL FASCIA

1. This layer of deep cervical fascia lies behind the oesophagus and pharynx. It covers the prevertebral muscles.
2. Traced laterally, it passes onto the scalene muscles and levator scapulae, and then over the deep muscles of the back to reach the ligamentum nuchae.
3. The prevertebral fascia covers the floor of the posterior triangle.
4. When traced upwards the prevertebral fascia reaches the base of the skull.
5. Inferiorly, it passes into the thorax in front of the upper thoracic vertebrae.
6. Some additional features of interest about the prevertebral fascia are as follows:
   a. The cervical nerves emerging from intervertebral foramina lie deep to the prevertebral fascia.
   b. The cervical and brachial plexuses formed by union of the ventral rami of these nerves are also deep to this fascia.
   c. Branches from these plexuses to muscles remain deep to the fascia, but cutaneous nerves have to pierce it to become superficial.
   d. The axillary sheath is an extension of this fascia around the subclavian artery and brachial plexus. The sheath extends into the axilla.

## CAROTID SHEATH

1. The tubular sheath of fascia surrounding the common and internal carotid arteries, and the internal jugular vein, is also described as part of the deep cervical fascia.

2. It extends from the lower end of the neck to the base of the skull.
3. The vagus nerve lies within the sheath behind the interval between the common (or internal) carotid artery and the internal jugular vein.
4. The sympathetic trunk descends just outside the sheath posterior to the arteries.
5. The ansa cervicalis is closely related to the front of the carotid sheath.

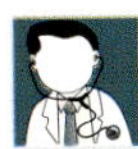

## CLINICAL CORRELATION OF DEEP CERVICAL FASCIA

1. The arrangement of fascial layers in the neck determines the direction of spread of infections as follows:
   a. In tuberculosis of the cervical vertebrae pus is formed and collects between the vertebral column and the prevertebral fascia. The pus can produce a swelling in the posterior wall of the pharynx, and such a swelling is in the midline. The swelling is referred to as a ***chronic retropharyngeal abscess*** (because of the chronic nature of tubercular infection).
   b. The pus from such an abscess can pass downwards (in front of the prevertebral muscles) and can appear under the skin of the posterior triangle of the neck. It can also descend into the axilla along the axillary sheath.
   c. The retropharyngeal lymph nodes are located between the prevertebral fascia (behind) and the buccopharyngeal fascia (in front). In infection of these nodes, an ***acute retropharyngeal abscess*** is formed. It is acute because of the nature of the infection. Unlike a chronic abscess that is situated in the midline, an acute abscess lies to one side of the midline. This is so because the prevertebral fascia and buccopharyngeal fascia are adherent to each other along the midline.
   d. The pus can pass downwards behind the pharynx and oesophagus to reach the superior mediastinum, or even the posterior mediastinum.
   e. An infection in the submandibular region is limited to a triangular area bounded by the two halves of the mandible and (posteriorly) by the hyoid bone. This is so because the investing layer of deep fascia is attached to these bones. Infection here produces a triangular swelling (***Ludwig's angina***). Collection of fluid here can push the tongue upwards.
   f. The deep cervical lymph nodes are often sites of tubercular infection. The pus formed may pierce through a small area of deep fascia and form a swelling under the skin. There is one collection of pus deep to the deep fascia, and another superficial to the fascia the two being in communication through the narrow opening (***collar stud abscess***).
   g. The fascia covering the parotid gland (parotid fascia) is very strong. In infections of the parotid gland (e.g., mumps) the organ can, therefore, not expand. Nerves are pressed upon causing much pain.

## LYMPH NODES OF HEAD AND NECK

### Superficial Lymph Nodes

The lymph nodes that drain the superficial tissues of the head and neck are shown in 41.22. They are as follows:

1. The nodes of the ***occipital group*** lie along the attachment of the trapezius to the occipital bone.
2. The nodes of the ***retroauricular group*** (or mastoid group) lie superficial to the upper attachment of the sternocleidomastoid muscle.
3. The parotid lymph nodes nodes are in two groups, superficial and deep. The nodes of the ***superficial parotid group*** lie over the parotid gland. Those of the ***deep parotid group*** ) are embedded in the gland.
4. The nodes of the ***submandibular group*** lie over the submandibular gland. Some of them are embedded within the gland.
5. The ***submental nodes*** lie below the chin overlying the mylohyoid muscle, between the anterior bellies of the right and left digastric muscles.

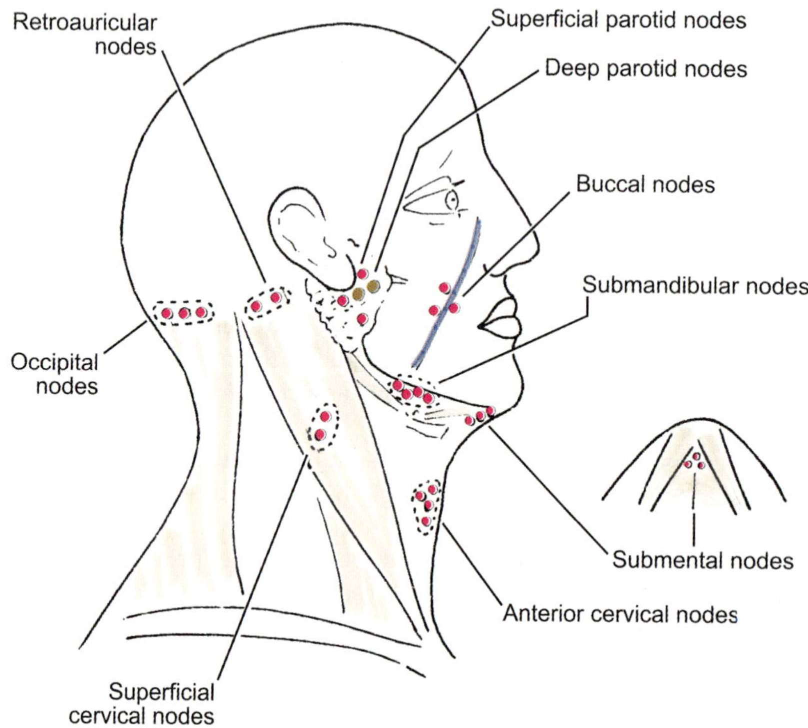


**41.22:** Lymph nodes draining superficial tissues of the head and neck

6. The ***buccal nodes*** lie along the facial vein.
7. The ***superficial cervical nodes*** lie along the external jugular vein, superficial to the sternocleidomastoid muscle.
8. The ***anterior cervical nodes*** lie along the anterior jugular vein.

## Deep Cervical Nodes

1. Lymph from all the superficial nodes described above drains into the deep cervical lymph nodes which lie along the internal jugular vein (41.23).
2. Most of the deep cervical nodes lie deep to the sternocleidomastoid muscle. They are divided (rather arbitrarily) into a ***superior group*** and an ***inferior group.***
3. Some nodes of the superior group lie in a triangle bounded behind by the internal jugular vein, above and in front by the posterior belly of the digastric muscle, and below and in front by the facial vein. These are called the ***jugulodigastric nodes***.
4. One node of the inferior group lies just above the intermediate tendon of the omohyoid muscle. This is the ***jugulo-omohyoid node.***
5. The deeper tissues of the head and neck drain into the deep cervical nodes. Some of these vessels pass through outlying groups of lymph nodes. These are:
   a. Lingual
   b. Infrahyoid
   c. Retropharyngeal
   d. Prelaryngeal
   e. Pretracheal
   f. Paratracheal nodes.
6. They are shown and are briefly described in 41.24.

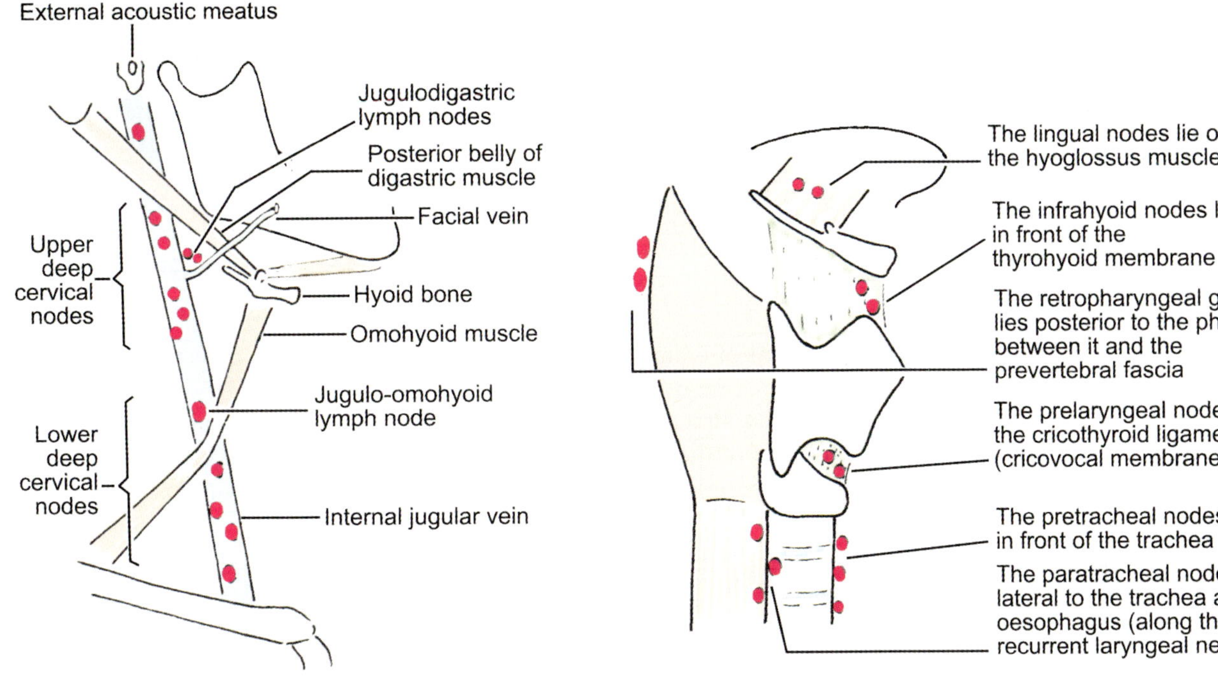


**41.23:** Scheme to show the deep cervical lymph nodes

**41.24:** Outlying members of the deep cervical group of lymph nodes

*Lymphatic Drainage of The Neck*

1. Some of the superficial tissues of the neck drain directly into the deep cervical lymph nodes.
2. Lymph from areas near the occipital nodes, the superficial cervical nodes, the submandibular nodes and the anterior cervical nodes drains first into these nodes and through them to the deep cervical nodes.
3. Lymph from the anterior cervical nodes passes to the infrahyoid, prelaryngeal and pretracheal nodes.
4. Deeper tissues in the neck mostly drain direct into the deep cervical nodes. Some of this lymph reaches them through the following nodes:
   a. Infrahyoid
   b. Prelaryngeal
   c. Pretracheal
   d Paratracheal
   e. Lingual
   f. Retropharyngeal lymph nodes.
5. For lymphatic drainage of individual organs located in the neck see appropriate chapters.

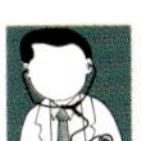

**CLINICAL CORRELATION**

## Enlarged Lymph Nodes

1. Lymph nodes in the head and neck may be enlarged in various diseases. The most important of these are tuberculosis and malignancy.
2. Physical examination of the neck involves systematic palpation of the nodes.
   a. The surgeon stands behind the patient whose neck is slightly flexed (to relax the muscles).

b. Beginning with the suboccipital region the surgeon palpates:
   i. The occipital nodes
   ii. The retroauricular or mastoid nodes
   iii. The parotid nodes
   iv. The submandibular
   v. Submental nodes
   vi. The anterior cervical nodes
   vii. The deep cervical nodes
   viii. The suprasternal nodes
   ix. The supraclavicular nodes.
3. In block dissection of the neck for removal of enlarged lymph nodes (in tuberculosis or malignancy), the submandibular gland is also removed.
4. A segment of the internal jugular vein may also have to be removed. Removal of the vein on one side is compensated by drainage through the vein of the other side. However, if bilateral removal is required, an interval of a few weeks is given between operations on the two sides to allow collateral venous channels to open up.
5. In block dissection special care is taken not to injure the carotid arteries, the vagus nerve, the spinal accessory nerve, the mandibular branch of the facial nerve and the hypoglosssal nerve.
6. However, sometimes the vagus and hypoglossal nerves may have to be removed.
7. Nerves lying deep to the prevertebral fascia (cervical and brachial plexus and their branches) remain intact. If necessary the sternocleidomastoid muscle is divided for better access.

## Tumours of the Neck

1. The lymph nodes in the neck may be involved in carcinoma at various sites.
2. The primary growth may lie in the:
   a. The thyroid
   b. The larynx
   c. The base of the tongue
   d. The laryngopharynx
   e. The paranasal sinuses.
3. Rarely secondaries from carcinoma of the breast, the bronchi the stomach or testis can reach these nodes.
4. Various other tumours may be seen in the neck.
   a. In infancy a swelling of the sternomastoid may be seen and later leads to torticolis.
   b. Tumours may form in remnants of the thyroglossal duct, or in the carotid body.

## Other Swellings

1. Midline swellings may be caused by enlarged submental or suprasternal nodes, thyroglossal cysts, enlargements of thyroid gland, and carcinoma of the larynx.
2. A branchial cyst may form a swelling along the anterior border of the sternocleidomastoid. Rupture of the cyst leads to formation of a branchial fistula. Treatment needs the excision of the tract of the fistula.

# 42 CHAPTER Blood Vessels of Head and Neck

## ARTERIES

### THE COMMON CAROTID ARTERIES

1. On the right side, the common carotid artery is a branch of the brachiocephalic trunk, while on the left side it is a direct branch of the arch of the aorta.
2. It follows that the left common carotid artery runs parts of its course in the thorax where it has been described on page 466.
3. The courses and relations of the cervical parts of the right and left common carotid arteries are similar.
4. Starting behind the corresponding sternoclavicular joint each artery runs upwards and somewhat laterally up to the level of the upper border of the thyroid cartilage (42.1).
5. Here, it terminates by dividing into the internal and external carotid arteries. It (normally) gives no other branches.
6. In its upward course, each common carotid artery lies in a triangular area bounded:
   a. Behind by the transverse processes of the cervical vertebrae (fourth to sixth)
   b. Medially in the lower part, by the oesophagus and trachea
   c. Higher up by the pharynx and larynx
   d. Anterolaterally by the sternocleidomastoid muscle (42.3).
7. The artery is enclosed in a fibrous ***carotid sheath*** that also encloses the internal jugular vein (lateral to the artery) and the vagus nerve (lying posterior to the interval between the artery and the vein).
8. Additional relations of the artery are as follows. Running vertically behind the carotid sheath there are:
   a. The sympathetic trunk (42.3)
   b. The ascending cervical artery (42.1)
   c. The vertebral artery
   d. A part of the subclavian artery
   e. The thoracic duct (on the left side only)
   f. The inferior thyroid artery runs transversely behind the lower part of the artery (42.1).
9. On the right side only, the artery is crossed posteriorly by the recurrent laryngeal nerve; and on the left side only, by the thoracic duct.
10. Apart from the sternocleidomastoid muscle the structures covering the artery anterolaterally are:
    a. The sternohyoid and sternothyroid muscles (in its lower part, deep to the sternocleidomastoid)
    b. The deep cervical fascia, platysma and skin
    c. Deep to the sternocleidomastoid the artery is crossed superficially by (42.2):
       i. The superior belly of the omohyoid muscle (at the level of the cricoid cartilage)
       ii. The sternomastoid branch of the superior thyroid artery (above the omohyoid)

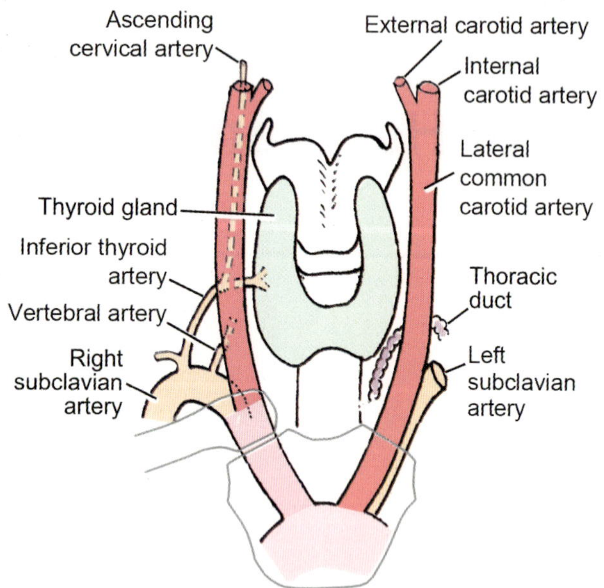


42.1: Relationship of common carotid artery to the larynx, trachea and thyroid. Some structures deep to the artery are also shown

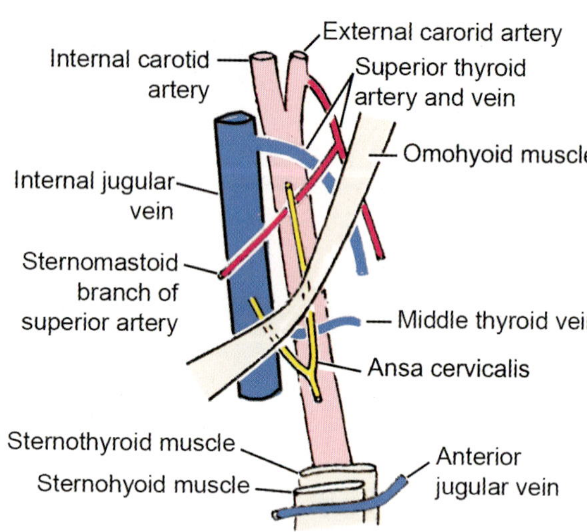


42.2: Right lateral view showing structures crossing superficial to the common carotid artery

iii. The ansa cervicalis (a nerve loop)
iv. The superior thyroid vein (near the upper end of the artery)
v. The middle thyroid vein (below the omohyoid)
vi. The anterior jugular vein (just above the clavicle).

11. Other structures on the medial side of the artery are:
    a. The recurrent laryngeal nerve (running vertically between the trachea and the oesophagus)
    b. The corresponding lobe of the thyroid gland
    c. A part of the inferior thyroid artery.

## INTERNAL CAROTID ARTERY

### Internal Carotid Artery in the Neck

1. The internal carotid artery begins at the upper border of the thyroid cartilage and ascends to reach the base of the skull where it enters the carotid canal.
2. Each artery may be considered as the main upward continuation of the common carotid artery and occupies a similar position (Compare 42.3 and 42.4).
3. a. Like the latter, it is surrounded by a carotid sheath along with the internal jugular vein and the vagus nerve.
   b. It lies on the transverse processes of the upper cervical vertebrae being separated from them by the longus capitis and the superior cervical sympathetic ganglion.
   c. On the medial side, the artery is related to the pharynx.
4. Additional relations are as follows:
   a. At its upper end, the internal jugular vein lies posterior to the artery.
   b. The glossopharyngeal, vagus, accessory and hypoglossal nerves lie between them.
   c. The artery is crossed posteriorly by the superior laryngeal nerve (42.5).
   d. Medially, it is related to the same nerve, the ascending pharyngeal artery and pharyngeal veins as they lie on the pharynx.
   e. Superficially, the artery is crossed by a large number of structures that are listed in 42.5.

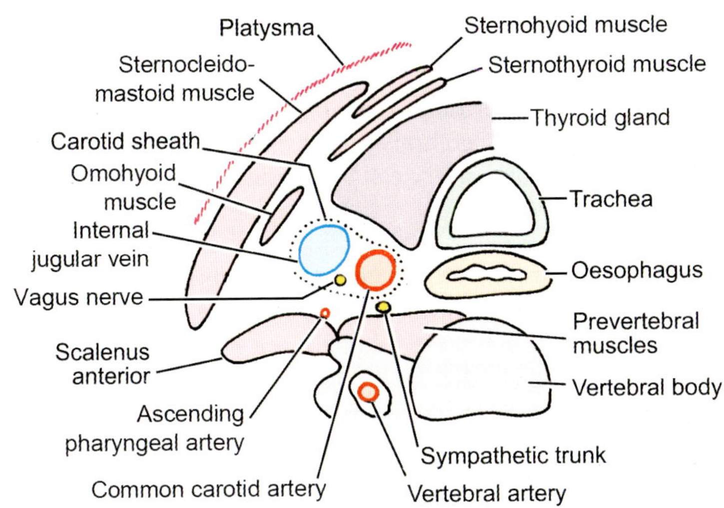


**42.3:** Right lateral view showing structures crossing superficial to the common carotid artery

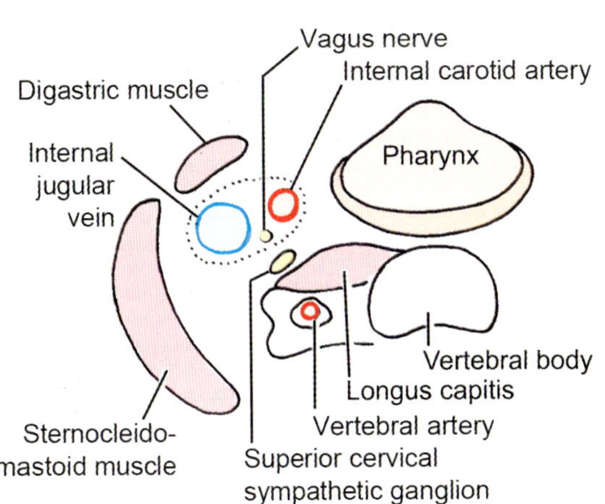


**42.4:** TS neck to show some relations of the internal carotid artery

**42.5: Some structures crossing internal carotid artery**

*Superficial to artery*
1. Styloid process
2. Stylohyoid muscle
3. Stylopharyngeus muscle
4. Digastric, posterior belly
5. Glossopharyngeal nerve
6. Pharyngeal branch of vagus nerve
7. Hypoglossal nerve
8. Ansa cervicalis, superior root
9. Posterior auricular artery
10. Occipital artery
11. Sternomastoid branch of occipital artery
12. Facial vein
13. Lingual vein

*Deep to artery*
14. Superior laryngeal branch of vagus nerve.

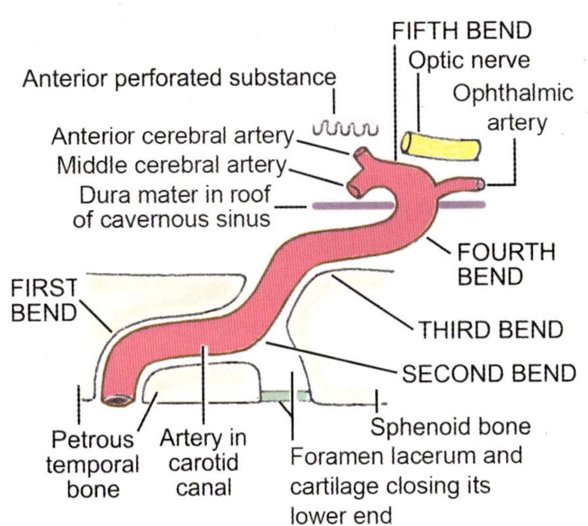


**42.6:** Scheme to show the intracranial course of the internal carotid artery

## Cranial Part of the Internal Carotid Arteries

1. The cranial part of the internal carotid artery has a complicated course.
2. Successive parts of the artery run vertically and horizontally (42.6).
3. On reaching the base of the skull, the artery enters the petrous part of the temporal bone through the external opening of the carotid canal.
4. It then bends sharply (42.6, first bend) to run horizontally forwards and medially through the carotid canal to reach the foramen lacerum.
5. It now undergoes a second bend to run vertically through the upper part of this foramen to enter the cranial cavity.
6. It then lies within the cavernous sinus.
7. Here, it undergoes a third bend to run forwards on the side of the body of the sphenoid bone.

8. Near the anterior end of the body of the sphenoid bone it again bends upwards (fourth bend) on the medial side of the anterior clinoid process. Here, it pierces through the dura mater forming the roof of the cavernous sinus and comes into relationship with the cerebrum.
9. The artery now turns backwards (fifth bend) to reach the anterior perforated substance of the brain.
10. The artery terminates here by dividing into the anterior and middle cerebral arteries.
11. From the above, it is seen that the cranial part of the internal carotid artery can be divided into a ***petrous part***, a ***cavernous part*** and a ***cerebral part***.
12. Additional relations of importance are as follows:
    a. Throughout its course the artery is surrounded by a plexus of sympathetic nerves derived from the superior cervical sympathetic ganglion, and by a plexus of veins that connect the intracranial veins to those outside the skull.
    b. As it lies in the carotid canal, the artery is closely related to the middle ear, the auditory tube and the cochlea.
    c. As the artery passes through the cavernous sinus, it is related to several cranial nerves that are embedded in the lateral wall of the sinus (42.7). From above downwards these are:
        i. The oculomotor, trochlear, and ophthalmic division of the trigeminal nerve
        ii. The maxillary division of the same nerve
        iii. The artery has a more intimate relationship with the abducent nerve that runs in close contact with the inferolateral side of the artery.
    d. After piercing the dura mater, the artery has the optic nerve above it and the oculomotor nerve below it.
13. The internal carotid artery gives off three large branches. These are:
    a. The ***ophthalmic artery*** to the orbit
    b. The ***anterior*** and ***middle cerebral arteries*** to the brain.

    The ophthalmic artery is described in detail below. The cerebral arteries will be considered in the section on the brain (Chapter 56).
14. In addition to these, the internal carotid artery gives off several smaller branches that are shown in 42.8. The posterior communicating and the anterior choroidal artery are intimated related to the brain and will be described in Chapter 56. The other arteries are as follows:

## The Ophthalmic Artery

1. The ophthalmic artery passes forwards to enter the cavity of the orbit through the optic canal.

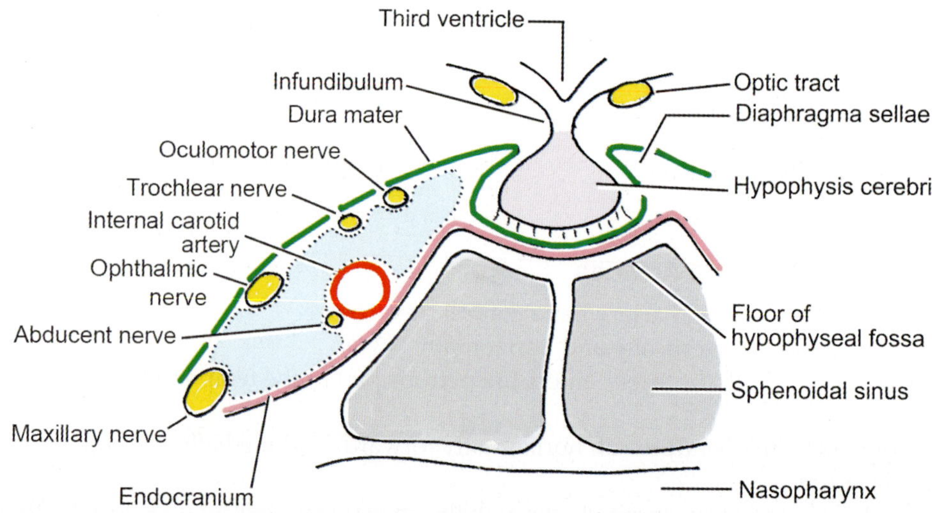


**42.7:** Coronal section through the cavernous sinus showing the internal carotid artery and related structures

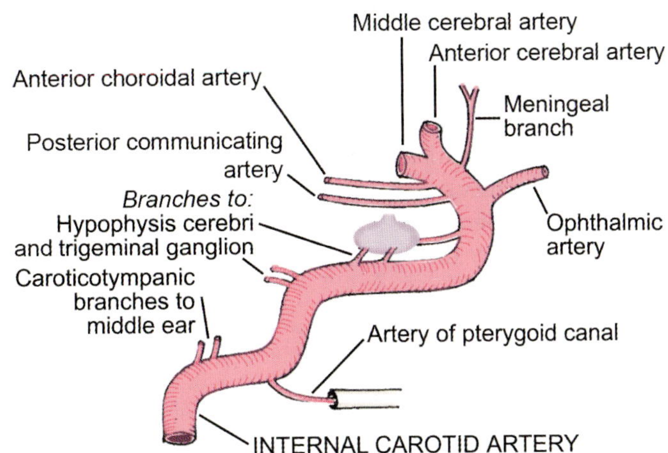


**42.8:** Scheme to show the branches given off by the internal carotid artery

2. In this canal, it lies inferolateral to the optic nerve.
   a. Having entered the orbit the artery is at first lateral to the optic nerve (42.9).
   b. It then crosses above the nerve to reach the medial wall of the orbit and runs forwards along this wall.

### *Branches of the Ophthalmic Artery*

The branches of the ophthalmic artery are shown in 42.9.

1. The ***central artery of the retina*** is the first branch of the ophthalmic artery.
   a. It arises from the ophthalmic artery when the latter is still within the optic canal.
   b. It first lies below the optic nerve.
   c. It pierces the dural sheath of the nerve and runs forwards for a short distance between these two.
   d. It then enters the substance of the nerve and runs forwards in its centre to reach the optic disc.
   e. Here, it divides into branches that supply the retina (42.10).
2. The largest branch of the ophthalmic artery is the ***lacrimal artery*** that runs forwards along the lateral wall of the orbit. The further branches given off by the lacrimal artery are as follows:

**WANT TO KNOW MORE?**

   a. Just near its origin from the ophthalmic artery, the lacrimal artery gives off a ***recurrent meningeal*** branch that runs backwards to enter the middle cranial fossa through the superior orbital fissure.
   b. The lacrimal artery gives off two ***zygomatic*** branches that enter canals in the zygomatic bone. One branch appears on the face through the zygomaticofacial foramen. The other appears on the temporal surface of the bone through the zygomaticotemporal foramen.
   c. Terminal ramifications of the lacrimal artery supply the lacrimal gland.
   d. The lateral palpebral branches supply the eyelids.

   The other branches of the ophthalmic artery arise from the main stem of the artery (42.9).
3. The ***posterior ciliary arteries*** arise as the ophthalmic artery crosses the optic nerve. They run forwards around the optic nerve and supply the eyeball.
4. The ***supraorbital*** branch supplies the skin of the forehead.
5. The ***anterior*** and ***posterior ethmoidal*** branches:
   a. Enter foramina in the medial wall of the orbit to supply the ethmoidal air sinuses.

b. They then enter the anterior cranial fossa.
c. Their terminal branches (specially of the anterior artery) enter the nose and supply part of it.

6. The ***anterior ciliary arteries*** arise from the ophthalmic artery near the anterior part of the eyeball and supply it.
7. The ***medial palpebral*** branches supply the eyelids.
8. The ***supratrochlear artery*** is one of the terminal branches of the ophthalmic artery. It supplies the skin of the forehead (along with the supraorbital artery).
9. The ***dorsal nasal branch*** supplies the upper part of the nose.

In addition to the branches shown in 42.9 the ophthalmic artery and its branches give off several ***muscular*** branches to muscles of the orbit.

## THE EXTERNAL CAROTID ARTERIES

1. Each external carotid artery arises from the common carotid at the level of the upper border of the thyroid cartilage (or the level of the disc between the third and fourth cervical vertebrae) (42.11).
2. It gives off several branches through which it is widely distributed to structures of the head and neck outside the cranial cavity.
3. From its origin, the artery runs upwards and terminates behind the neck of the mandible.
4. The lower part of the artery is anterior and medial to the internal carotid. Its upper part is lateral to the internal carotid.
5. The lower part of the artery is located within the carotid triangle. (The boundaries of the triangle are shown in 42.11). Here, it is relatively superficial being covered by skin, superficial and deep fascia and by the anterior margin of the sternocleidomastoid muscle.

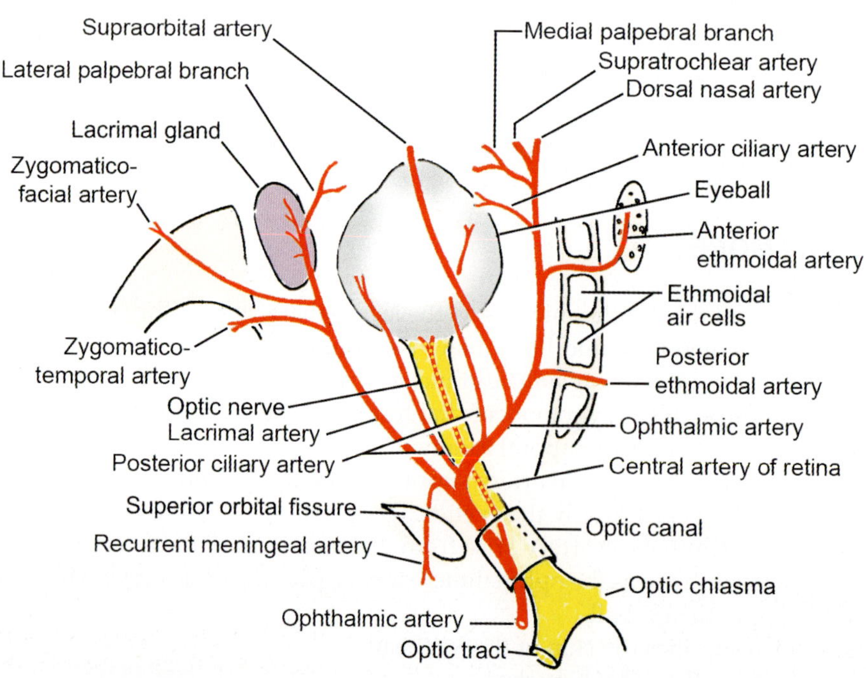


**42.9:** Scheme to show the branches of the ophthalmic artery

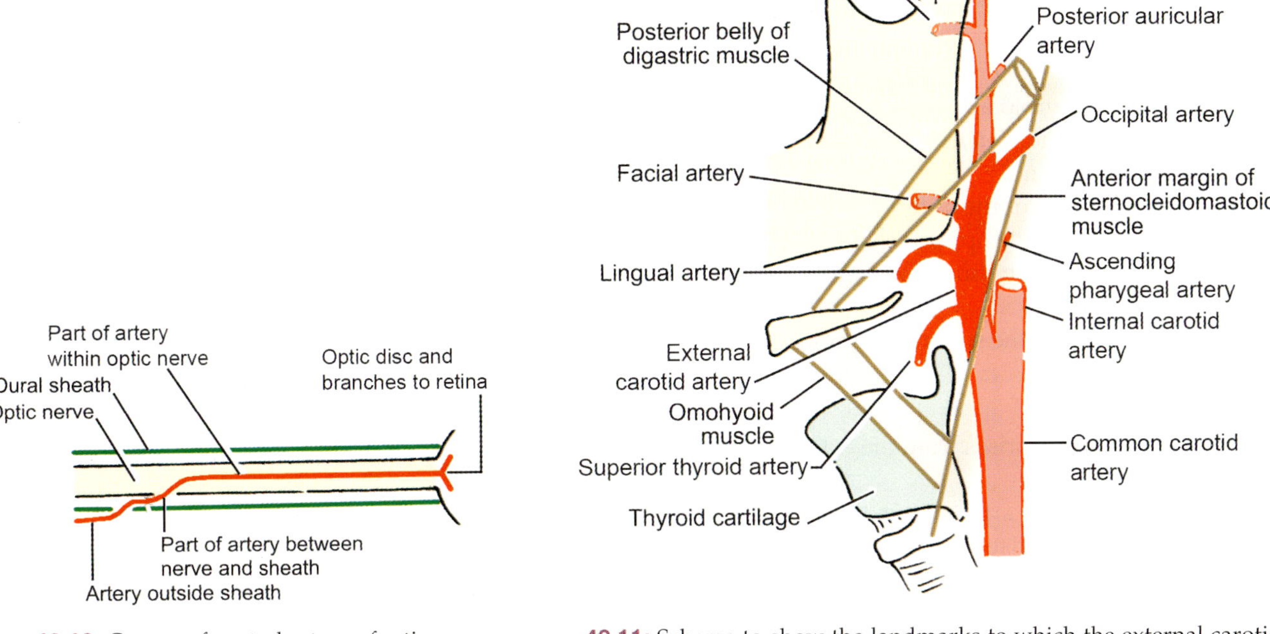


**42.10:** Course of central artery of retina

**42.11:** Scheme to show the landmarks to which the external carotid artery, and its branches, are related. The boundaries of the carotid triangle are shown

6. Above the triangle, the artery lies deep to the posterior belly of the digastric muscle and the parotid gland.
7. Deep to the artery, there is the pharynx. The pharynx is separated from the upper part of the artery by the styloid process (and some muscles attached to it) and by the internal carotid artery.
8. In addition to the relations mentioned above the external carotid artery is crossed by several structures that pass superficial or deep to it. These are listed in 42.12.

## Branches of External Carotid Artery

The branches of the external carotid artery and their levels of origin are as follows (in order of origin) (42.11 and 42.12):

1. The ***ascending pharyngeal*** artery arises from the deep aspect of the external carotid artery just above its lower end.
2. The ***superior thyroid*** artery arises from the front of the external carotid just below the level of the greater cornu of the hyoid bone.
3. The ***lingual*** artery arises from the front of the external carotid artery opposite the tip of the greater cornu of the hyoid bone.
4. The ***facial*** artery arises from the front of the external carotid a little above the origin of the lingual artery.
5. The ***occipital*** artery arises from the back of the external carotid opposite the origin of the facial artery.
6. The ***posterior auricular*** artery arises from the back of the external carotid just above the level at which the latter is crossed by the posterior belly of the digastric muscle.
7. The ***superficial temporal*** artery and the ***maxillary*** artery are terminal branches of the external carotid artery. They begin behind the neck of the mandible, in the substance of the parotid gland.
8. These branches will be considered one by one.

### Ascending Pharyngeal Artery

1. The ascending pharyngeal artery runs upwards to the base of the skull, lying between the pharynx and the internal carotid artery.
2. Its distribution is shown in 42.13

### Superior Thyroid Artery

1. The superior thyroid artery runs downwards and medially to reach the upper pole of the thyroid gland.
2. Here, it divides into ***anterior*** and ***posterior thyroid branches*** (42.14). These branches ramify over the corresponding surfaces of the gland.
3. The terminal part of the anterior branch runs across the upper part of the isthmus of the gland to anastomose with the artery of the opposite side.
4. The posterior branch runs downwards along the posterior border of the thyroid to anastomose with the inferior thyroid artery.
5. Other branches of the superior thyroid artery are shown in 42.14.

### Lingual Artery

1. The lingual artery arises from the external carotid artery opposite the tip of the greater cornu of the hyoid bone (42.11).
2. The ***first part*** of the artery lies in the carotid triangle, superficial to the middle constrictor of the pharynx (42.15). It forms a characteristic upward loop that is crossed by the hypoglossal nerve.
3. The ***second part*** of the artery lies deep to the hyoglossus muscle that separates the artery from the hypoglossal nerve. This part of the artery also lies on the middle constrictor.
4. The ***third or deep part*** of the artery runs upwards along the anterior margin of the hyoglossus; and then forwards to the tip of the tongue. This part lies on the genioglossus muscle.
5. The branches of the lingual artery are shown in 42.15.

| 42.12: Structures crossing external carotid artery |
|---|
| *Superficial to artery* |
| Stylohyoid muscle |
| Posterior belly digastric muscle |
| Facial nerve (in parotid gland) |
| Hypoglossal nerve |
| Common facial vein |
| Superior thyroid vein (sometimes) |
| Veins along hypoglossal nerve |
| *Deep to artery* |
| Styloid process |
| Stylopharyngeus |
| Glossopharyngeal nerve |
| Pharyngeal branch of vagus nerve |
| Superior laryngeal branch of vagus nerve |

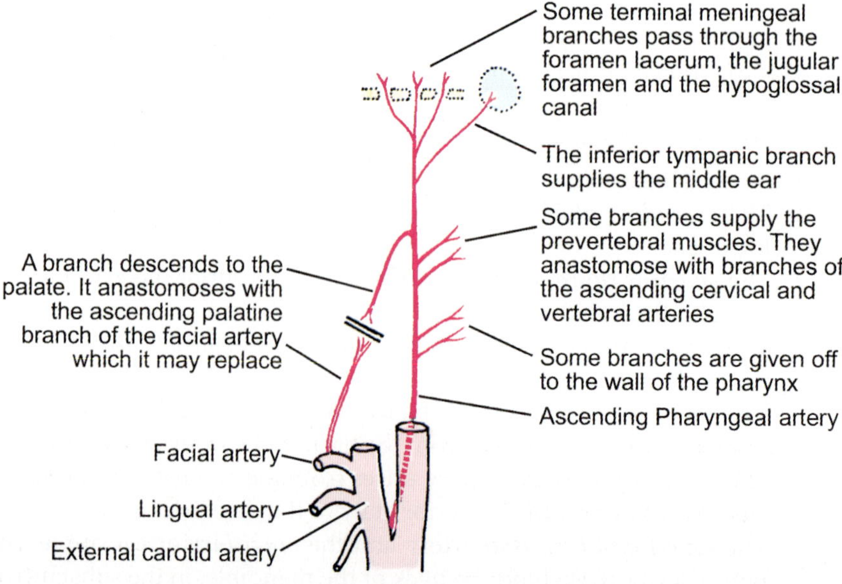


**42.13:** Scheme to show the distribution of the ascending pharyngeal artery

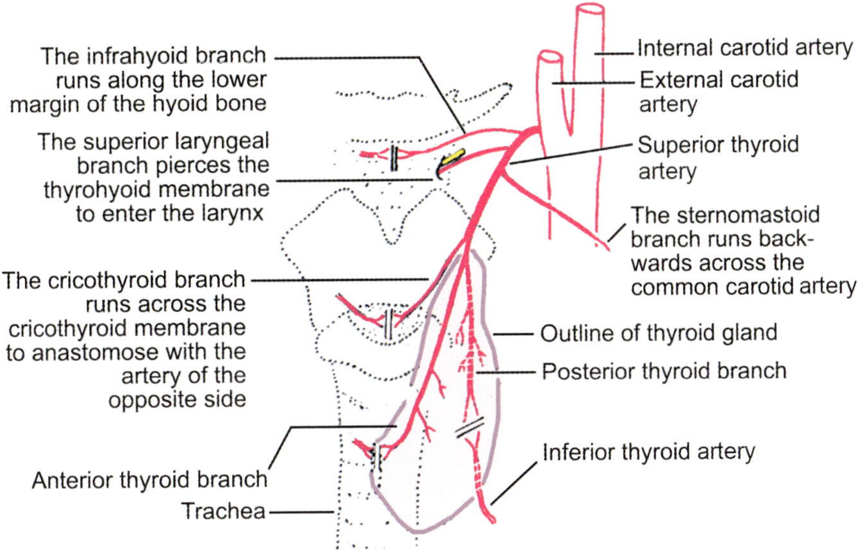


**42.14:** Scheme to show the distribution of the superior thyroid artery

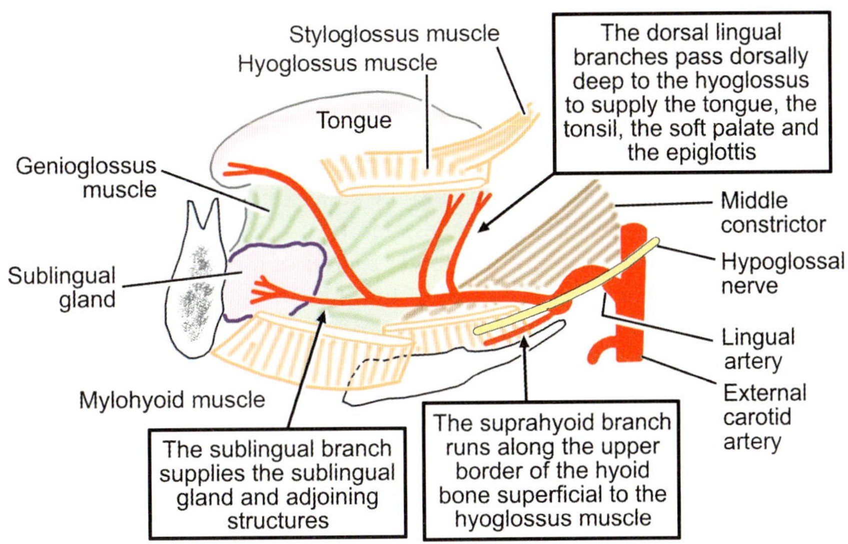


**42.15:** Scheme to show the branches of the lingual artery

### *The Facial Artery*

1. The facial artery arises from the external carotid just above the greater cornu of the hyoid bone (42.17).
2. Its initial part lies deep to the ramus of the mandible, near the angle. This part is closely related to the submandibular gland (42.16).
   a. The artery first runs upwards along the posterior border of the gland and then downwards and forwards between the gland (deep to it) and the medial pterygoid muscle (superficial to it) (42.16).
   b. It reaches the lower border of the mandible at the anterior edge of the masseter (42.17).

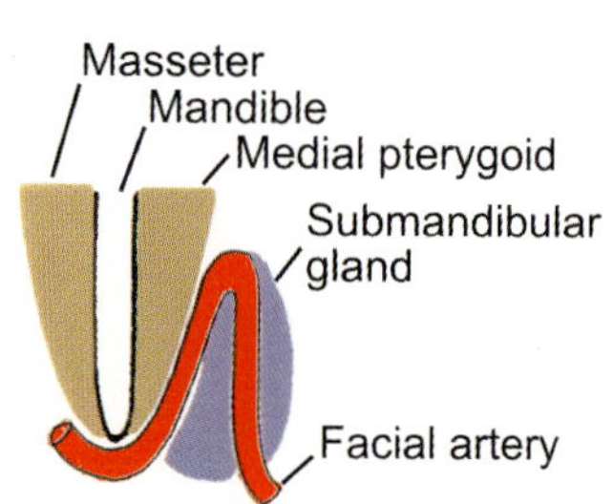


**42.16:** Scheme to show the relationship of the facial artery to the submandibular gland

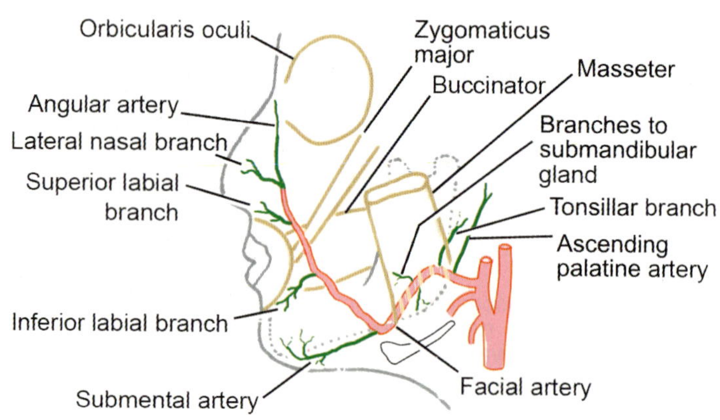


**42.17:** Scheme to show branches of the facial artery

c. Curving round this border the artery runs upwards and forwards across the superficial aspect of the body of the mandible, and across the buccinator muscle to reach the angle of the mouth. It then runs upwards along the side of the nose to reach the medial angle of the palpebral fissure.

3. The branches of the facial artery are shown in 42.17. They are as follows:

**WANT TO KNOW MORE?**

a. The ***ascending palatine*** artery ascends on the lateral side of the pharynx. It supplies the pharynx, the palate, the tonsil and the auditory tube.
b. The ***tonsillar*** branch reaches the tonsil by piercing the superior constrictor muscle.
c. Some branches are given off to the submandibular gland.
d. The ***submental*** artery runs forwards along the lower border of the mandible (over the mylohyoid muscle). It supplies muscles of the region including those of the chin and the lower lip.
e. The ***superior*** and ***inferior labial*** branches supply the lips.
f. The ***lateral nasal*** branch supplies the side of the nose.
g. The terminal part of the facial artery is called the ***angular*** artery.

### *The Occipital Artery*

1. This artery arises from the posterior aspect of the external carotid opposite the origin of the facial artery.
2. It runs backwards along the lower border of the posterior belly of the digastric muscle (42.11) to reach the skull medial to the mastoid process. Here, it lies deep to the sternocleidomastoid, the digastric and some other muscles.
3. It then runs medially, and becoming superficial supplies the posterior part of the scalp. Here the artery is accompanied by the greater occipital nerve.

**WANT TO KNOW MORE?**

4. The occipital artery gives off several branches. These are as follows:
   a. Two branches ***to the sternocleidomastoid*** run backwards across the carotid sheath.
   b. The ***stylomastoid branch*** enters the stylomastoid foramen to supply the middle ear and related structures.

c. The ***auricular branch*** supplies the pinna.
d. The ***mastoid branch*** passes through the mastoid foramen.
e. ***Meningeal branches*** enter the skull through the jugular foramen and the carotid canal.
f. The ***descending branch*** runs down through the deep muscles of the back of the neck. It divides into:
   i. A superficial branch which anastomoses with the transverse cervical artery.
   ii. A deep branch which anastomoses with branches of the vertebral and deep cervical arteries.
g. The ***occipital branches*** supply the posterior part of the scalp.
h. A ***meningeal branch*** may enter the cranium through the parietal foramen.

*The Posterior Auricular Artery*

1. This artery arises from the external carotid just above the posterior belly of the digastric muscle (and stylohyoid muscle).
2. It passes backwards and upwards deep to the parotid gland to reach the mastoid process.
3. The branches of the artery are shown in 42.18.

## *The Maxillary Artery*

1. This is one of the terminal branches of the external carotid artery. It begins behind the neck of the mandible, within the substance of the parotid gland.
2. For convenience of description, it is divided into three parts.
3. The ***first part*** passes forwards deep to the neck of the mandible to reach the infratemporal fossa. Here, it runs forwards along the lower border of the lateral pterygoid muscle (42.19).
4. The ***second part*** of the artery runs forwards and upwards superficial to the lower head of the lateral pterygoid muscle. Frequently, the artery lies deep to the lower head and in that case it may form a loop that projects laterally between the two heads.
5. The ***third part*** of the artery passes between the upper and lower heads of the lateral pterygoid muscle to pass through the pterygomaxillary fissure thus entering the pterygopalatine fossa.

*Branches of first part*

The branches of the first part of the maxillary artery are shown in 42.20. They are described below.

1. The ***deep auricular artery*** supplies the external acoustic meatus, the tympanic membrane and the temporomandibular joint.

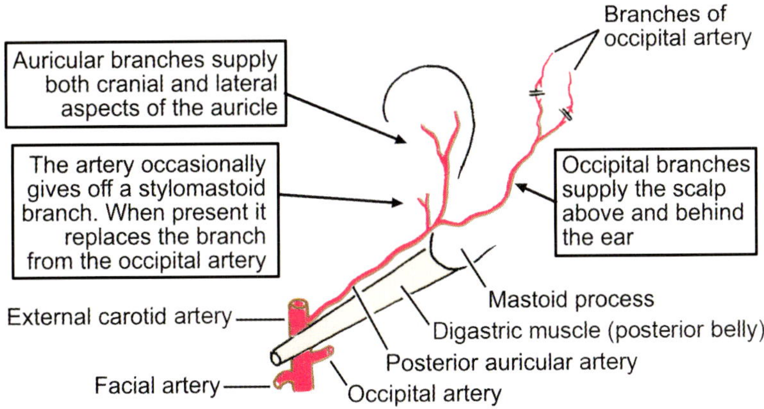


**42.18:** Distribution of the posterior auricular artery

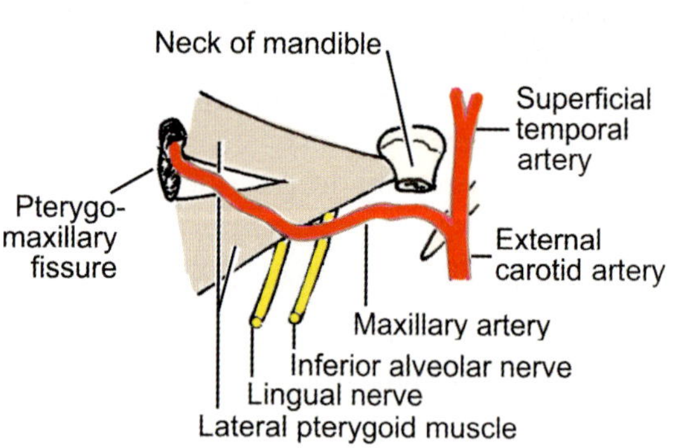


**42.19:** Diagram to show the course of the maxillary artery

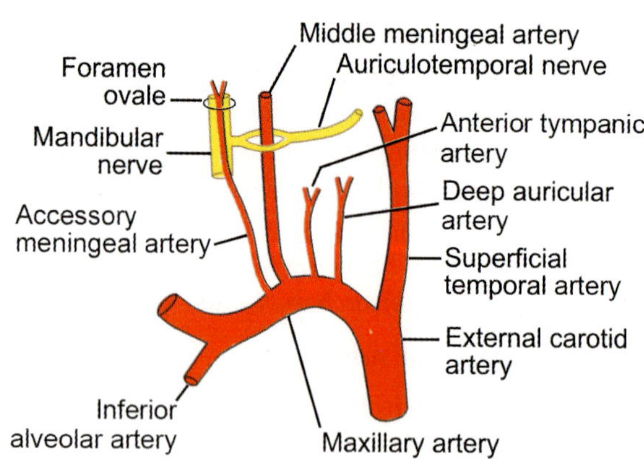


**42.20:** Branches of the first part of the maxillary artery

2. The ***anterior tympanic branch*** supplies the middle ear including the medial surface of the tympanic membrane.
3. a. The ***middle meningeal artery*** runs upwards deep to the lateral pterygoid muscle.
   i. Here it passes between the two roots of the auriculotemporal nerve (42.20).
   ii. The artery enters the cranial cavity through the foramen spinosum.
   iii. It runs forwards and laterally over the floor of the middle cranial fossa and divides into frontal and parietal branches (42.21).
   iv. The ***frontal branch*** runs forwards and upwards across the squamous temporal bone, the greater wing of the sphenoid and the anteroinferior angle of the parietal bone. It divides into branches that run predominantly upwards or backwards over the inner surface of the parietal bone.
   v. The ***parietal branch*** first runs backwards on the squamous temporal bone and then over the parietal bone.

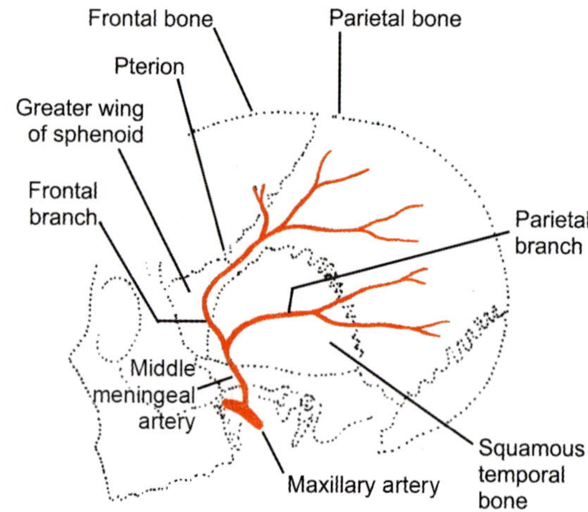


**42.21:** Schematic diagram showing the course of the middle meningeal artery as projected on to the lateral aspect of the skull

## WANT TO KNOW MORE?

b. The following additional points about the middle meningeal artery are worth noting.
   i. It is the largest artery supplying the meninges.
   ii. In 42.21 note that the frontal branch of the artery lies deep to the pterion (circular area at which the frontal, parietal, temporal and sphenoid bones meet); and it can be approached surgically by drilling a hole in the skull in this situation.
   iii. Apart from the meninges the artery supplies the skull bones over which it ramifies, the middle ear (and related structures: the facial nerve, the tensor tympani, the auditory tube) and the trigeminal ganglion.

iv. A branch of the artery passes through the inferior orbital fissure to anastomose with the recurrent meningeal branch of the lacrimal artery. Occasionally, this anastomosis may be large and the lacrimal artery may then appear to be a branch of the middle meningeal.

4. The ***accessory meningeal, branch*** (of the maxillary artery) enters the cranial cavity through the foramen ovale. Apart from the meninges it supplies structures in the infratemporal fossa (42.20).

5. The ***inferior alveolar artery*** (42.22) runs downwards and forwards medial to the ramus of the mandible to reach the mandibular foramen.
   a. Passing through this foramen the artery enters the mandibular canal (within the body of the mandible) in which it runs downwards and then forwards.
   b. Before entering the mandibular canal the artery gives off:
      i. A ***lingual branch*** to the tongue
      ii. A ***mylohyoid branch*** that descends in the mylohyoid groove (on the medial aspect of the mandible) and runs forwards above the mylohyoid muscle.
   c. Within the mandibular canal, the artery gives branches to the mandible and to the roots of each tooth attached to the bone.
   d. It also gives off a ***mental branch*** that passes through the mental foramen to supply the chin.

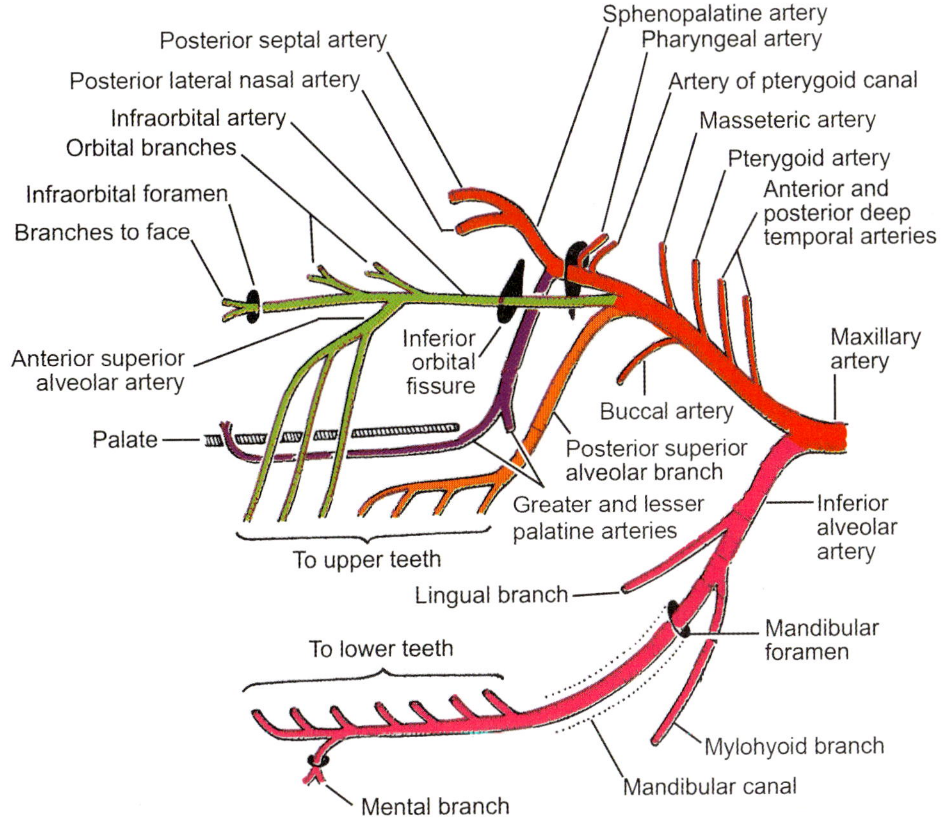


**42.22:** Branches of the maxillary artery

*Branches of second part*

**WANT TO KNOW MORE?**

The branches of the second part of the maxillary artery (42.22) are mainly muscular.

1. The ***deep temporal*** branches (anterior and posterior) ascend on the lateral aspect of the skull deep to the temporalis muscle.
2. Branches are also given off to the ***pterygoid muscles*** and to the ***masseter***.
3. A ***buccal branch*** suplies the buccinator muscle.

*Branches of third part*

The branches of the third part of the maxillary artery are shown in 42.22. They are as follows:

**WANT TO KNOW MORE?**

1. The ***posterior superior alveolar artery*** arises just before the maxillary artery enters the pterygomaxillary fissure. It descends on the posterior surface of the maxilla and gives branches that enter canals in the bone to supply:
   a. The molar and premolar teeth
   b. The maxillary air sinus.
2. The ***infraorbital artery*** also arises just before the maxillary artery enters the pterygomaxillary fissure.
   a. It enters the orbit through the inferior orbital fissure.
   b. It runs forwards in relation to the floor of the orbit, first in the infraorbital groove and then in the infraorbital canal to emerge on the face through the infraorbital foramen.
   c. It gives off some orbital branches to structures in the orbit.
   d. ***Anterior superior alveolar*** branches that enter apertures in the maxilla to reach the incisor and canine teeth attached to the bone.
   e. After emerging on the face, the infraorbital artery gives branches to:
      i. The lacrimal sac
      ii. The nose
      iii. The upper lip.

   *The remaining branches of the third part of the maxillary artery arise within the pterygopalatine fossa.*
3. The ***greater palatine artery*** runs downwards in the greater palatine canal to emerge on the posterolateral part of the hard palate through the greater palatine foramen.
   a. It then runs forwards near the lateral margin of the palate to reach the incisive canal (near the midline) through which some terminal branches enter the nasal cavity.
   b. Branches of the artery supply the palate and gums.
   c. While still within the greater palatine canal, it gives off the ***lesser palatine arteries*** that emerge on the palate through lesser palatine foramina and run backwards into the soft palate and tonsil.
4. The ***pharyngeal branch*** runs backwards through a canal related to the inferior aspect of the body of the sphenoid bone (pharyngeal or palatinovaginal canal). It supplies:
   a. Part of the nasopharynx
   b. The auditory tube
   c. The sphenoidal air sinus.
5. The ***artery of the pterygoid canal*** runs backwards in the canal of the same name and helps to supply the pharynx, the auditory tube and the tympanic cavity.

6. The ***sphenopalatine artery*** passes medially through the sphenopalatine foramen to enter the cavity of the nose.
   a. It gives off ***posterolateral nasal*** branches to the lateral wall of the nose and the paranasal sinuses
   b. ***Posterior septal branches*** to the nasal septum.

### *The Superficial Temporal Artery*

1. This is the second terminal branch of the external carotid artery.
2. It begins behind the neck of the mandible in the substance of the parotid gland.
3. It runs upwards behind the temporomandibular joint and ramifies in the scalp over the temporal region.
4. The artery is accompanied by the auriculotemporal nerve.

*The branches of the artery are shown in 42.23.*

**WANT TO KNOW MORE?**

1. The ***frontal branch*** runs upwards and forwards in the part of the scalp overlying the temporal and frontal bones.
2. The ***parietal branch*** runs backwards in the scalp overlying the temporal and parietal bones.
3. The ***anterior auricular branch*** supplies part of the auricle and the external acoustic meatus.
4. The ***middle temporal artery*** supplies the temporalis.
5. The ***zygomatico-orbital branch*** runs forwards along the upper border of the zygomatic arch up to the lateral angle of the eye.
6. The ***transverse facial branch*** arises within the substance of the parotid gland. It runs forwards across the masseter above the parotid duct.

## THE SUBCLAVIAN ARTERIES

1. The right subclavian artery is a branch of the brachiocephalic trunk and begins behind the right sternoclavicular joint.
2. The left subclavian artery is a direct branch of the aorta.
   a. It has a thoracic part (already considered on page 466) which ends behind the left sternoclavicular joint.
   b. Thereafter, the course and relations of the right and left subclavian arteries are similar (with minor exceptions).
3. Each subclavian artery is the initial part of a long channel that supplies the upper limb.
4. Entering the neck behind the corresponding sternoclavicular joint, the artery loops upwards into the neck.
5. It leaves the neck by passing into the axilla, where it becomes the axillary artery.
6. The subclavian artery (whole of right, and cervical part of left) extends from the sternoclavicular joint to the outer border of the first rib.
7. The artery has numerous relationships as follows.

### Relations of Subclavian Arteries

1. The subclavian artery lies in front of the following structures as it arches across the lower part of the neck:
   a. The apex of the lung
   b. The cervical pleura
   c. The suprapleural membrane.

2. The artery is crossed anteriorly by (42.24) the lower part of the scalenus anterior muscle (which gains insertion into the first rib just in front of the artery).
   a. It divides the artery into the first part, medial to the muscle
   b. The second part deep to it
   c. The third part lateral to it.
3. Some other structures covering the subclavian artery are as follows:
   a. The medial-most part of the subclavian artery lies behind the common carotid artery.
   b. Immediately lateral to the latter, the internal jugular vein runs vertically across the subclavian artery to join the subclavian vein.
   c. The subclavian vein lies below and in front of the artery separated from it by the scalenus anterior muscle.
   d. The artery is also crossed vertically by the vagus nerve (42.25) which lies behind the internal jugular vein.
   e. In other words, the medial part of the subclavian artery is crossed by all structures enclosed by the carotid sheath.
   f. The right vagus nerve gives off its recurrent laryngeal branch just as it reaches the lower margin of the subclavian artery (42.25).
      i. The recurrent laryngeal nerve curves around the inferior and posterior aspects of the artery and runs medially to reach the groove between the trachea and the oesophagus.
      ii. Note that the left recurrent laryngeal nerve arises from the vagus below the arch of the aorta, winds round the ligamentum arteriosum and ascends in the groove between the trachea and the oesophagus. It is not closely related to the left subclavian artery in the neck.
4. The relationship of the right and left phrenic nerves to the subclavian arteries is shown in 42.25A.
   a. The nerves descend across the corresponding scalenus anterior muscle.
   b. On the left side, the nerve passes across the medial border of the scalenus anterior onto the front of the first part of the subclavian artery.
   c. On the right side, the nerve usually crosses the medial border of the scalenus anterior lower down so that the nerve does not come into direct contact with the first part of the subclavian artery, but is separated from the second part by the scalenus anterior. Occasionally, however, the relationship may be the same as on the left side.
5. The relationship of the subclavian artery to the brachial plexus is as follows:

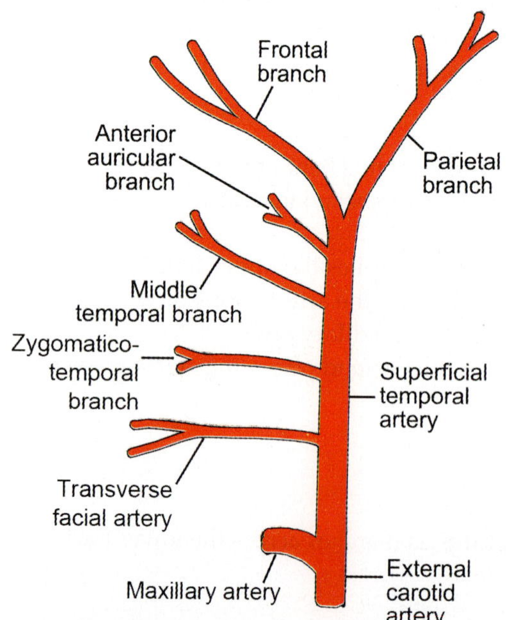


**42.23:** Scheme to show the branches of the superficial temporal artery

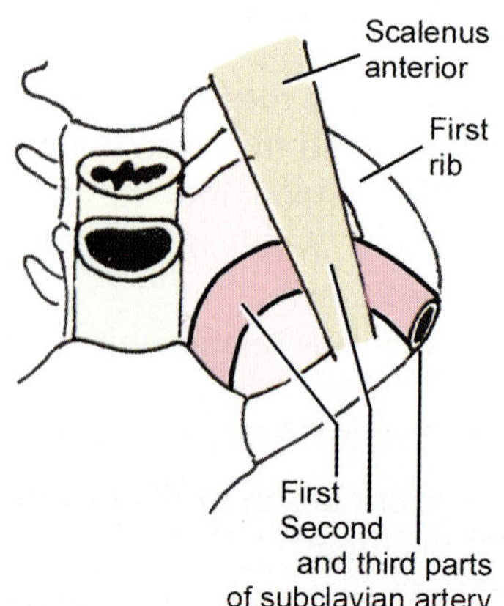


**42.24:** Relationship of the subclavian artery to the scalenus anterior

   a. The first part of the artery lies below the level of the plexus, but the second and third parts come into relationship with the trunks of the plexus.
   b. The lower trunk lies behind and below the second and third parts of the artery.
   c. The upper and middle trunks lie above the second part of the artery, and above and lateral to its third part.
6. The ansa subclavia is a nerve cord that descends from the middle cervical sympathetic ganglion to the front of the first part of the artery, and looping round it ascends behind it to reach the inferior cervical (cervicothoracic) sympathetic ganglion.
7. The terminal part of the thoracic duct comes into relationship with the first part of the left subclavian artery.
   a. After ascending into the neck along the lateral side of the oesophagus the duct turns laterally forming a wide loop that is convex upwards.
   b. The terminal part of this loop descends in front of the artery (near the medial border of the scalenus anterior) to terminate by joining the junction of the left internal jugular and subclavian veins.
8. The relationship of the subclavian artery to the internal jugular and subclavian veins has already been noted. Some other veins related to the subclavian artery are as follows:
   a. The vertebral vein descends across the first part of the subclavian artery to end in the brachiocephalic vein.
   b. The external jugular vein descends across the third part of the subclavian artery to end in the subclavian vein.
   c. In front of the artery the external jugular vein is joined by the transverse cervical, suprascapular and anterior jugular veins.
9. The relations of the subclavian artery explained above are summarised in 42.25B.

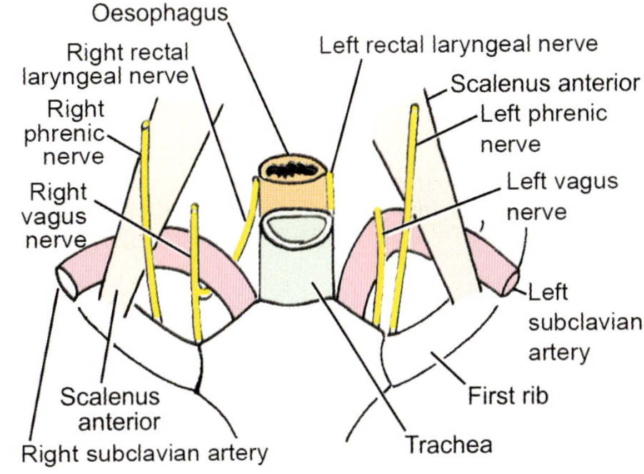


**42.25A:** Relationship of the subclavian artery to the vagus nerve. The phrenic nerve is also shown

**42.25B: Relations of subclavian artery**

*Anterior relations of first part:*
1. Phrenic nerve
2. Thoracic duct
3. Vagus nerve
4. Vertebral artery
5. Ansa subclavia
6. Common carotid artery
7. Internal jugular vein
8. Sternothyroid muscle
9. Sternohyoid muscle
10. Anterior jugular vein
11. Sternocleidomastoid muscle

*Anterior relations of second part:*
1. Sternocleidomastoid
2. Anterior jugular vein
3. Scalenus anterior

*Anterior relations of third part:*
1. Transverse cervical vein
2. Suprascapular vein
3. External jugular vein
4. Anterior jugular vein
5. Clavicle

*Additional anterior relations common to all three parts:*
1. Deep fascia
2. Platysma and superficial fascia
3. Skin

*Posterior relations common to all three parts:*
1. Lung
2. Cervical pleura
3. Suprapleural membrane

*Other posterior relations:*
1. Ansa subclavia behind first part
2. Costocervical trunk behind second part
3. Lower trunk of brachial plexus behind second and third parts

## Branches of The Subclavian Artery

The subclavian artery gives origin to several branches that are shown in 42.26. A brief introduction to these branches is given below. Each branch is considered in detail in subsequent pages.

1. The ***vertebral artery*** arises from the first part. It runs upwards to enter the foramen transversarium of the sixth cervical vertebra.
2. The ***internal thoracic*** artery arises from the first part and runs downwards into the thorax.
3. The ***thyrocervical trunk*** is a short vessel arising just medial to the scalenus anterior muscle i.e., from the first part. On the right side, it usually arises behind the scalenus anterior (then being a branch of the second part). It divides into the inferior thyroid, suprascapular and transverse cervical arteries.
4. The ***costocervical trunk*** arises either from the first or second part. It runs backwards to reach the neck of the first rib. Here, it divides into the deep cervical and superior intercostal arteries.
5. The ***dorsal scapular artery*** is an occasional branch of the third part. When present, it replaces the deep branch of the transverse cervical artery.

   The internal thoracic artery has been dealt with in the thorax and is described on page 464. The other arteries are considered one by one below.

### *The Vertebral Artery*

1. The vertebral artery arises from the first part of the subclavian artery (42.26).
2. It ascends to enter the foramen transversarium of the sixth cervical vertebra (not the seventh) and then continues upwards through the foramina of higher vertebrae.
3. Emerging through the foramen transversarium of the atlas:
   a. The artery winds round the lateral mass of this bone (42.28).
   b. It then lies in the groove on the upper surface of the posterior arch of the atlas.
4. Finally, it passes forwards into the vertebral canal and running upwards passes through the foramen magnum to enter the cranial cavity.
   a. Here it lies lateral to the lower end of the medulla oblongata.
   b. It gradually passes forwards and medially over the medulla and ends at the lower border of the pons by anastomosing with the opposite vertebral artery to form the ***basilar artery***.

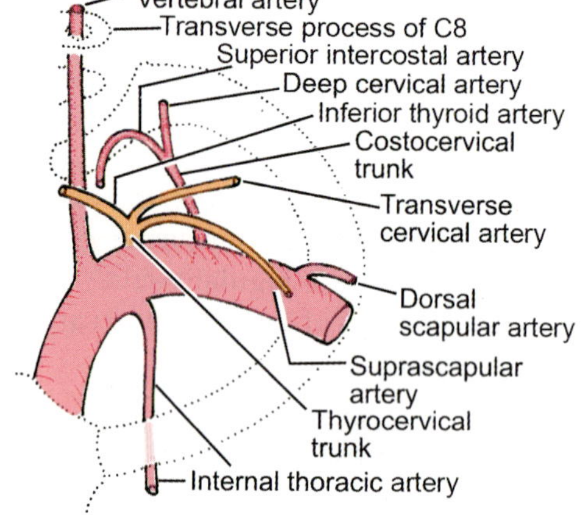


**42.26:** Scheme to show the branches of the subclavian artery

**WANT TO KNOW MORE?**

5. The following additional points about the vertebral artery may now be noted:
   a. The part of the artery between its origin from the subclavian artery and its entry into the foramen transversarium of vertebra C6 constitutes its first part (42.27).
   b. This part lies deep in the lower part of the neck in a triangular interval bounded laterally by the scalenus anterior, medially by the longus colli, and inferiorly by the subclavian artery. This part of the artery lies deep to the common carotid artery.
   c. The part of the artery passing through the foramina transversaria constitutes its second part.

   It is surrounded by a plexus of veins that unite to form the vertebral vein (42.46); and by a plexus of sympathetic nerves derived from the cervicothoracic (or stellate) ganglion.
   d. The part of the vertebral artery winding round the lateral mass of the atlas is its third part.
   e. This part lies in the suboccipital triangle. Its most important relation is the first cervical nerve. The dorsal ramus of the nerve runs backwards between the artery and the posterior arch of the atlas (42.29).

f. The ventral ramus runs forwards round the lateral mass of the atlas, where it lies medial to the artery.
g. The vertebral artery enters the vertebral canal through an aperture bounded laterally by the lateral mass of the atlas and medially by the free lateral margin of the posterior atlanto-occipital membrane (42.28).

6. The branches of the vertebral artery that supply structures in the neck are shown in 42.30. They are as follows:
   a. Some ***muscular branches*** arise from the vertebral artery in the suboccipital triangle.
   b. ***Spinal branches*** pass through the intervertebral foramina to reach the vertebral canal. They help to supply the spinal cord and the vertebrae.
   c. The ***anterior spinal arteries*** of the two sides join to form a single trunk that descends on the anterior aspect of the spinal cord, in the midline.
   d. The ***posterior spinal artery*** descends along the posterolateral aspect of the spinal cord. It divides into two branches, one lying in front of the dorsal nerve roots (a) and one lying behind them (b).
7. The anterior and posterior spinal arteries are joined by spinal branches arising from the vertebral artery itself and from various other arteries.
8. In addition to the branches described above, the vertebral artery gives off the ***posterior inferior cerebellar artery*** that takes part in supplying the brain. It will be considered in the section on the blood supply of the brain. The basilar artery and its branches will also be considered therein.

### *The Thyrocervical Trunk*

1. The thyrocervical trunk is a short artery that arises near the junction of the first and second parts of the subclavian artery.
2. On the left side, it usually arises just medial to the scalenus anterior muscle i.e., from the first part of the subclavian artery.
3. On the right side, the trunk usually arises deep to the scalenus anterior, being a branch of the second part of the subclavian artery.
4. After a short course, the trunk divides into three branches, namely:
   a. The ***inferior thyroid*** artery
   b. The ***suprascapular artery***
   c. The ***transverse cervical*** artery. The transverse cervical artery further divides into a ***superficial*** and a ***deep*** branch.

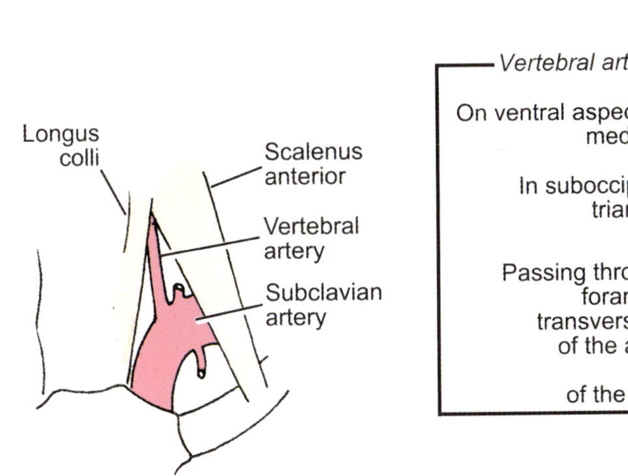


**42.27:** Position of the first part of the vertebral artery

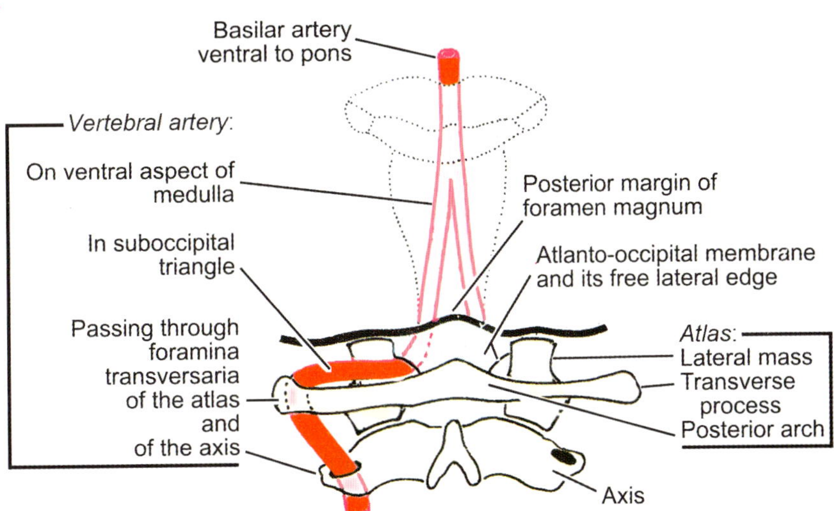


**42.28:** Scheme to show the course of the upper part of the vertebral artery

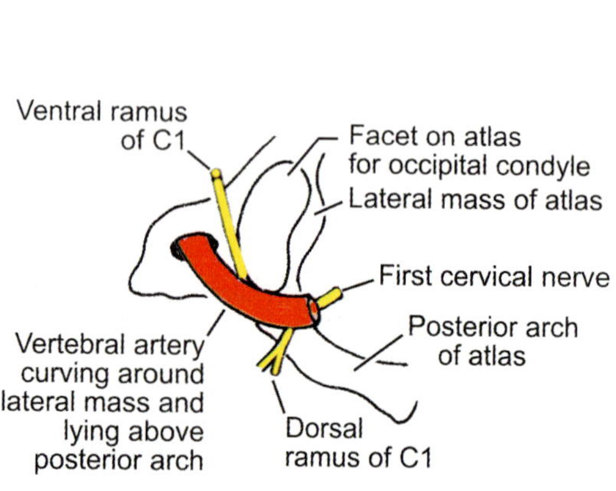


**42.29:** Relationship of the vertebral artery to the atlas vertebra

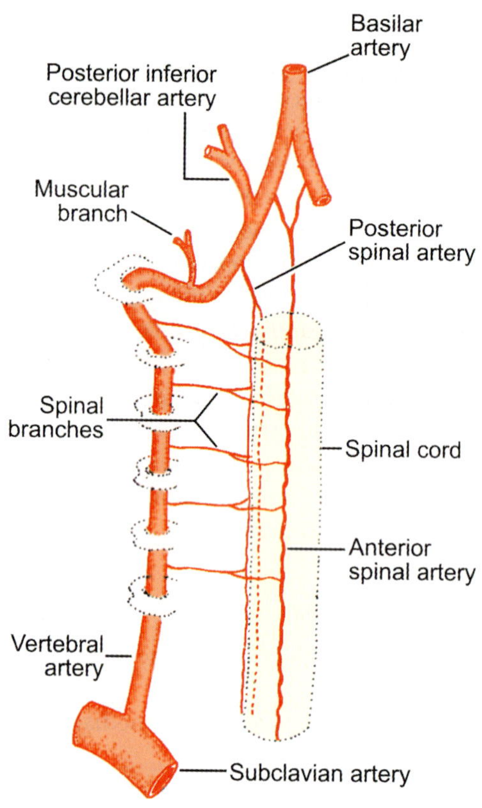


**42.30:** Scheme to show the branches of the vertebral artery

5. Quite frequently, the deep branch arises directly from the third part of the subclavian artery.
   a. In that case, the transverse cervical artery is represented only by its superficial branch and is called the ***superficial cervical*** artery.
   b. The deep branch, arising directly from the subclavian artery is called the ***dorsal scapular*** artery.
6. The transverse cervical artery and the suprascapular artery are concerned mainly in supply of structures in the upper extremity, and are described in Chapter 4. The inferior thyroid artery is described below.

### *The Inferior Thyroid Artery*

1. This artery is a branch of the thyrocervical trunk. It runs upwards for some distance and then turns medially to reach the thyroid gland. The artery is distributed mainly to this gland through an ascending and a descending ***glandular branch.***

**WANT TO KNOW MORE?**

2. Other named branches arising from the inferior thyroid artery are:
   a. The ascending cervical artery
   b. The inferior laryngeal artery (42.31)
   c. Several small branches are also given off to the pharynx, trachea, oesophagus and the infrahyoid muscles.

3. The horizontal part of the artery is crossed by several important structures. They include:
   a. Carotid sheath and its contents
   b. Recurrent laryngeal nerve
   c. Vertebral artery
   d. Thoracic duct
   e. Sympathetic trunk

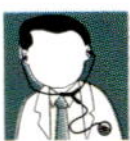

## CLINICAL CORRELATION

4. The relationship of the inferior thyroid artery to the recurrent laryngeal nerve is particularly important.
   a. During the operation for removal of the thyroid (called thyroidectomy), the surgeon has to ligate the artery, and has to be careful that the nerve is not injured.
   b. In this connection, it is important to remember that the nerve may
      i. Cross in front of the terminal branches of the artery
      ii. May pass behind them
      iii. May have some branches in front of the nerve and some behind it.
   c. Note that the artery comes into relationship with the nerve only near the thyroid gland and that it can be ligated safely some distance away from the gland. (In contrast the superior thyroid artery is closely related to the external laryngeal nerve some distance away from the gland and is safely ligated close to the gland).

### *The Costocervical Trunk*

1. The costocervical trunk takes origin from the posterior aspect of the subclavian artery (42.32).
2. On the left side, it arises from the first part, but on the right side, the origin is from the second part.
3. It runs backwards with an upward convexity following the curve of the cervical pleura to reach the neck of the first rib. Here, it divides into the deep cervical and superior intercostal arteries.

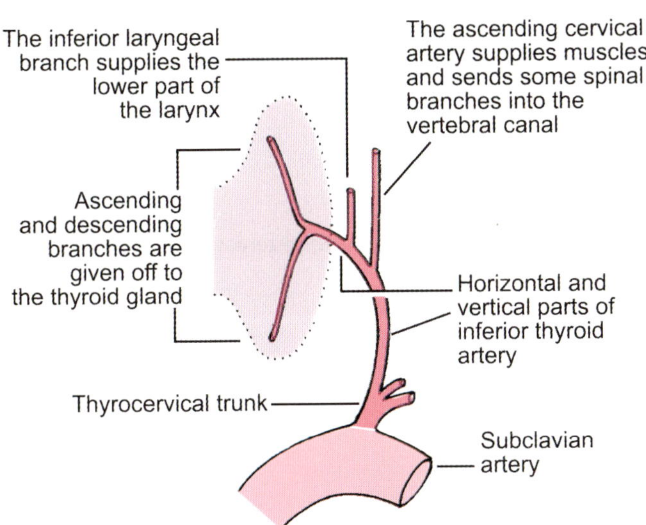


**42.31:** Scheme to show the branches of the inferior thyroid artery

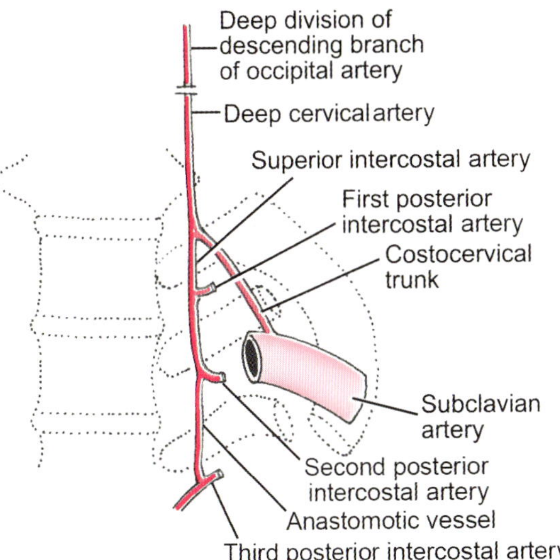


**42.32:** Scheme to show the branches of the costocervical trunk

**WANT TO KNOW MORE?**

4. The ***deep cervical artery*** passes backwards above the neck of the first rib to reach the back of the neck.
   a. Here, it ascends through the deep muscles supplying them.
   b. It anastomoses with the deep division of the descending branch of the occipital artery.
5. The ***superior intercostal artery*** descends across the neck of the first rib to reach the first intercostal space.

**The Dorsal Scapular Artery**

The dorsal scapular artery is an occasional branch arising from the third part of the subclavian artery. When present it replaces the deep branch of the transverse cervical artery.

# VEINS

## THE INTERNAL JUGULAR VEINS

1. The right and left internal jugular veins are the chief veins of the head and neck.
2. On either side, the upper end of the vein lies in the jugular foramen on the base of the skull. Here the internal jugular vein becomes continuous with the sigmoid sinus.
3. The lower end of the vein lies behind the sternal end of the clavicle where the internal jugular joins the subclavian vein to form the corresponding brachiocephalic vein.
4. In its course through the neck, the internal jugular vein lies alongside the internal carotid and common carotid arteries being enclosed along with them in the carotid sheath.
   a. These arteries are medial to the vein, but just below the skull the internal carotid artery is in front of the vein.
   b. The vagus nerve that is also within the carotid sheath lies posteromedial to the vein.
5. The internal jugular vein is related superficially and posteriorly to a number of structures. These are listed in 42.33.

**42.33: Structures superficial and deep to internal jugular vein**

| *Superficial* | *Deep* |
|---|---|
| *Muscles* | *From above downwards* |
| 1. Sternocleidomastoid (in entire length of vein) | 1. Rectus capitis lateralis muscle |
| 2. Posterior belly, digastric | 2. Transverse process of atlas |
| 3. Superior belly, omohyoid, cross the vein | 3. Levator scapulae muscle |
| 4. Sternohyoid | 4. Scalenus medius muscle |
| 5. Sternothyroid over lower part | 5. Scalenus anterior muscle, with phrenic nerve over it |
| | 6. Vertebral artery and vein |
| | 7. Subclavian arery (first part) |
| *Other than muscles* | |
| 1. Accessory nerve | |
| 2. Styloid process | |
| 3. Posterior auricular | |
| 4. Occipital branches of external carotid artery | |
| 5. Descendens cervicalis nerve | |
| 6. Anterior jugular vein (Superficial to sternohyoid and sternothyroid) | |
| 7. Parotid gland (in upper part) | |

6. The upper end of the vein is enlarged to form the ***superior bulb*** that occupies the jugular fossa on the base of the skull. The inferior end of the vein may also show an enlargement called the ***inferior bulb***.

### Tributaries of the Internal Jugular Vein

The tributaries of the internal jugular vein include the intracranial venous sinuses (42.37) and several other veins that are shown in 42.34. They will be described after we have considered the subclavian vein that is the second largest vein of the neck.

## THE SUBCLAVIAN VEINS

1. Each subclavian vein (right and left) begins at the outer border of the first rib, as a continuation of the axillary vein.
2. It runs medially parallel to the subclavian artery, but lies anterior and inferior to the artery. The two vessels are separated by the scalenus anterior.
3. The subclavian vein ends at the medial margin of this muscle by joining the internal jugular vein (42.35).
4. Anteriorly, the subclavian vein is related to the clavicle. Below, the vein rests on the first rib and on the cervical pleura.
   The tributaries of the subclavian vein are shown in 42.36. The external jugular vein and the anterior jugular vein are described later in this Chapter.

## THE INTRACRANIAL VENOUS SINUSES

1. Within the cranial cavity, there are venous channels of a special kind. Their walls are formed of endocranium and dura mater.
2. The endocranium is also called the outer layer of dura mater. It closely lines the inner wall of the cranial cavity.

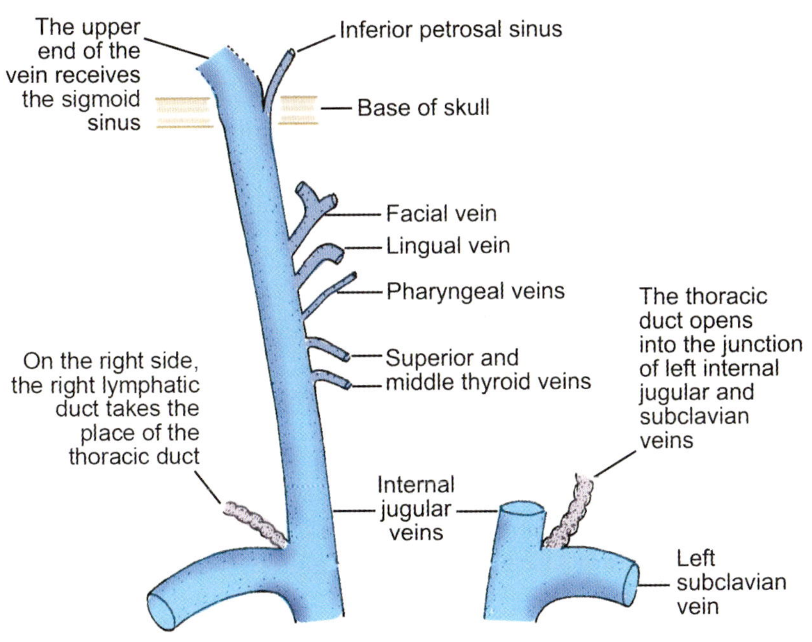


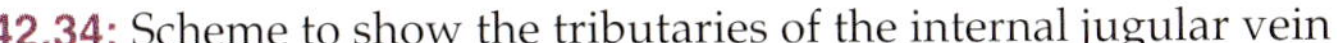
42.34: Scheme to show the tributaries of the internal jugular vein

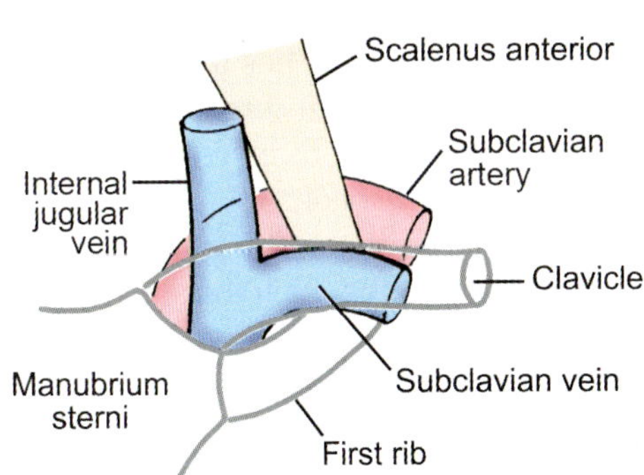


42.35: Some relations of the subclavian vein

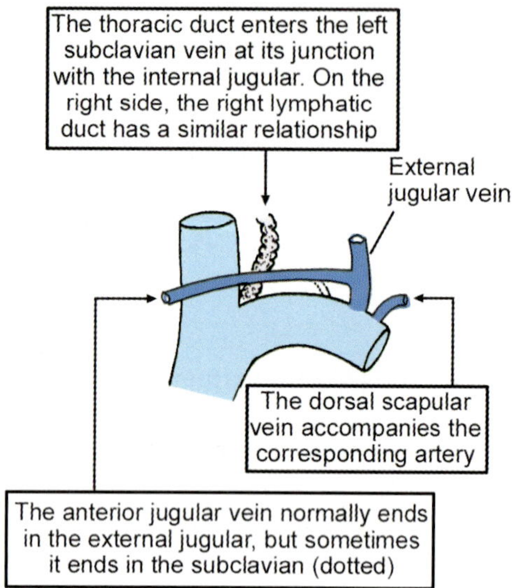


**42.36:** Tributaries of the subclavian vein

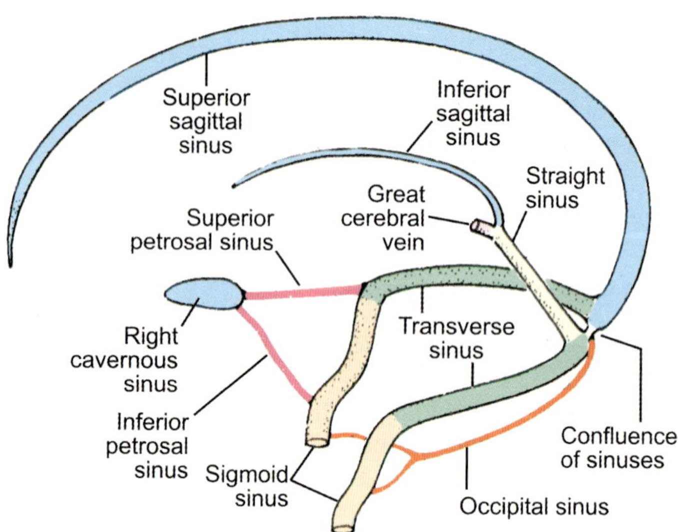


**42.37:** Scheme to show the intracranial venous sinuses. The cavernous and petrosal sinuses are paired, but are shown only on one side for sake of clarity

3. The dura mater (also called the inner layer of dura mater) is closely united to the endocranium over most of its extent. However, at some places the two layers are separated by spaces lined by endothelium. These spaces constitute the intracranial venous sinuses or dural venous sinuses.
4. Various ways in which such a sinus may be formed are evident in 42.38 and 42.39. The main intracranial venous sinuses are shown schematically in 42.37 that is a left anterolateral view. They are also seen in 42.38 and 42.39 that are coronal sections through the cranial cavity.

## Unpaired Sinuses Lying in the Midline

1. The ***superior sagittal sinus*** occupies the triangular space produced by the reflection of the inner layer of dura mater to form the falx cerebri (42.38).
   a. It begins anteriorly in front of crista galli. It then runs backwards deeply grooving the frontal bone (in the midline); the two parietal bones (where they join at the sagittal suture); and the occipital bone (again in the midline).
   b. The sinus ends at the internal occipital protuberance where it becomes continuous (usually) with the right transverse sinus (See below). Sometimes, it is continuous with the left transverse sinus.
2. The ***inferior sagittal sinus*** lies within the lower free margin of the falx cerebri as shown in 42.38. It begins anteriorly and ends posteriorly by joining the straight sinus (42.37).
3. The ***straight sinus*** lies in the triangular interval where the lower edge of the posterior part of the falx cerebri joins the tentorium cerebelli.
   a. Anteriorly, it receives the inferior sagittal sinus, and a vein from the interior of the brain called the ***great cerebral vein*** (42.37).
   b. Posteriorly, the straight sinus ends by becoming continuous with the transverse sinus of the side opposite to that with which the superior sagittal sinus is continuous i.e., usually the left side.
   c. Note that several sinuses meet at the internal occipital protuberance. These are the superior sagittal sinus, the straight sinus and the right and left transverse sinuses (see below). This region is, therefore, called the ***confluence of sinuses***.
4. The ***occipital sinus*** lies in the midline in relation to the floor of the posterior cranial fossa.
   a. Here the dura is raised into a fold called the falx cerebelli; and the sinus lies within this fold.

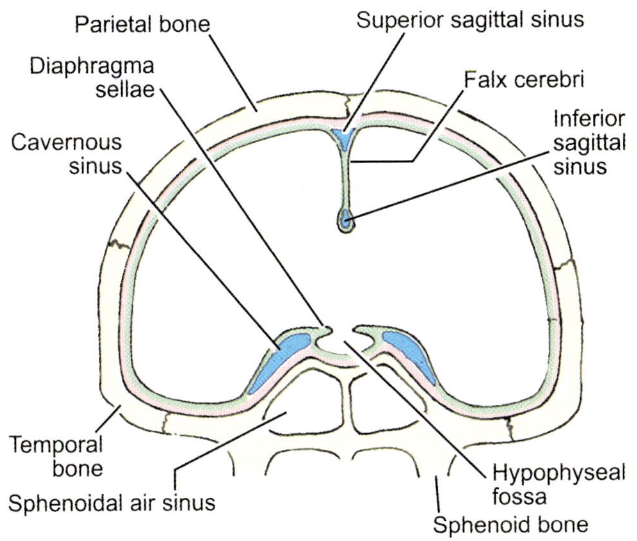


**42.38:** Coronal section through middle cranial fossa to show the position of some intracranial venous sinuses

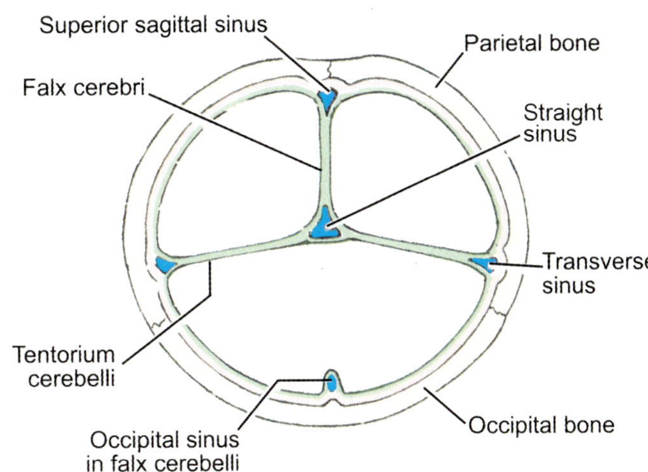


**42.39:** Coronal section through the posterior cranial fossa (behind the foramen magnum) to show the position of some intracranial venous sinuses

b. The anterior end of the occipital sinus bifurcates into two channels that pass round either side of the foramen magnum to join the corresponding sigmoid sinus.
c. The occipital sinus ends posteriorly in the confluence of sinuses (42.40).

## Large Paired Sinuses

1. The right and left ***transverse sinuses*** (42.37 and 42.40) lie horizontally as indicated by their names.
   a. Each sinus begins posteriorly at the internal occipital protuberance. The right sinus is usually a continuation of the superior sagittal sinus and the left sinus is usually a continuation of the straight sinus, but this arrangement is sometimes reversed.
   b. Each sinus runs in a curve at first laterally and then forwards, along the line of attachment of the tentorium cerebelli.
   c. The sinus produces a transverse groove on the inner surface of the occipital bone, and on the posteroinferior angle of the parietal bone.
   d. Finally, it reaches the petrous part of the temporal bone where it becomes continuous with the sigmoid sinus.
2. The right and left ***sigmoid sinuses*** are continuations of the corresponding transverse sinuses.
   a. As indicated by the name each sigmoid sinus is S-shaped.
   b. It first runs downwards and medially in a deep groove on the mastoid part of the temporal bone, and then across the jugular process of the occipital bone.
   c. Finally, it runs forwards to reach the jugular foramen where it ends by becoming continuous with the upper end of the internal jugular vein.

 **WANT TO KNOW MORE?**

d. The upper part of the sinus is related anteriorly to the mastoid antrum from which it is separated only by a thin plate of bone. Infection can, therefore, travel from the mastoid antrum into the sigmoid sinus.

3. The right and left ***cavernous sinuses*** are so called because their cavities are traversed by delicate strands of tissue that appear to subdivide each sinus into a number of smaller spaces (or caverns).
   a. The sinuses lie in the middle cranial fossa.
   b. They are placed anteroposteriorly on either side of the body of the sphenoid bone.
   c. Anteriorly, each sinus reaches the superior orbital fissure. Posteriorly, it reaches the apex of the petrous part of the temporal bone (42.40).
4. The cavernous sinus has important relations (42.41).
   a. The internal carotid artery passes anteriorly within the cavity of the sinus.
   b. The artery is accompanied by the abducent nerve that lies below and lateral to it.
   c. Three cranial nerves are embedded in the lateral wall of the sinus. From above downwards, these are the oculomotor nerve, the trochlear nerve, and the ophthalmic division of the trigeminal nerve.
   d. The maxillary division of the trigeminal nerve runs along the inferior angle of the sinus.
   e. Medially, the sinus is related above to the hypophysis cerebri, and below it is separated from the sphenoidal air sinus by a plate of bone .
   f. A pouch like extension of dura mater containing the trigeminal ganglion (***trigeminal cave***) projects into the posterior part of the sinus.
   g. The tributaries and other communications of the cavernous sinus are shown in 42.40. Note the intercavernous sinuses that connect the right and left cavernous sinuses.

 **WANT TO KNOW MORE?**

**Other Intracranial Sinuses and Veins**

We have now completed the consideration of the major intracranial venous sinuses. Brief mention will now be made of some smaller intracranial sinuses and veins.

1. Each ***sphenoparietal sinus*** (right or left) runs medially along the sharp posterior edge of the floor of the anterior cranial fossa (formed by the lesser wing of the sphenoid). The sinus ends by joining the anterior end of the cavernous sinus (42.40).
2. Each ***superior petrosal sinus*** (right or left) begins at the posterior end of the cavernous sinus.
   a. It runs backwards and laterally along the sharp upper margin of the petrous temporal bone (i.e., along the attached margin of the tentorium cerebelli).
   b. It terminates by joining the junction of the sigmoid sinus and transverse sinus (42.40).
3. Each ***inferior petrosal sinus*** (right or left) begins at the posterior end of the cavernous sinus.
   a. It runs downwards and somewhat laterally in the groove between the petrous temporal bone and the basilar part of the occipital bone.
   b. It passes through the anterior part of the jugular foramen and terminates by joining the upper end of the internal jugular vein (42.40).
   c. The inferior petrosal sinuses of the right and left sides are connected by a ***basilar plexus of veins*** lying on the basal parts of the sphenoid and occipital bones (42.40).
4. The vein accompanying the middle meningeal artery is called the ***middle meningeal sinus.*** The sinus has frontal and parietal tributaries corresponding to those of the artery.

## Veins Draining the Eyeball and Orbit

1. The ***superior ophthalmic vein*** accompanies the ophthalmic artery.
   a. Anteriorly, it communicates with the facial vein.
   b. Posteriorly, it passes through the superior orbital fissure and ends in the cavernous sinus.
   c. The vein acts as a communication between the facial vein and the cavernous sinus. Infections on the face can spread to the cavernous sinus through this route.

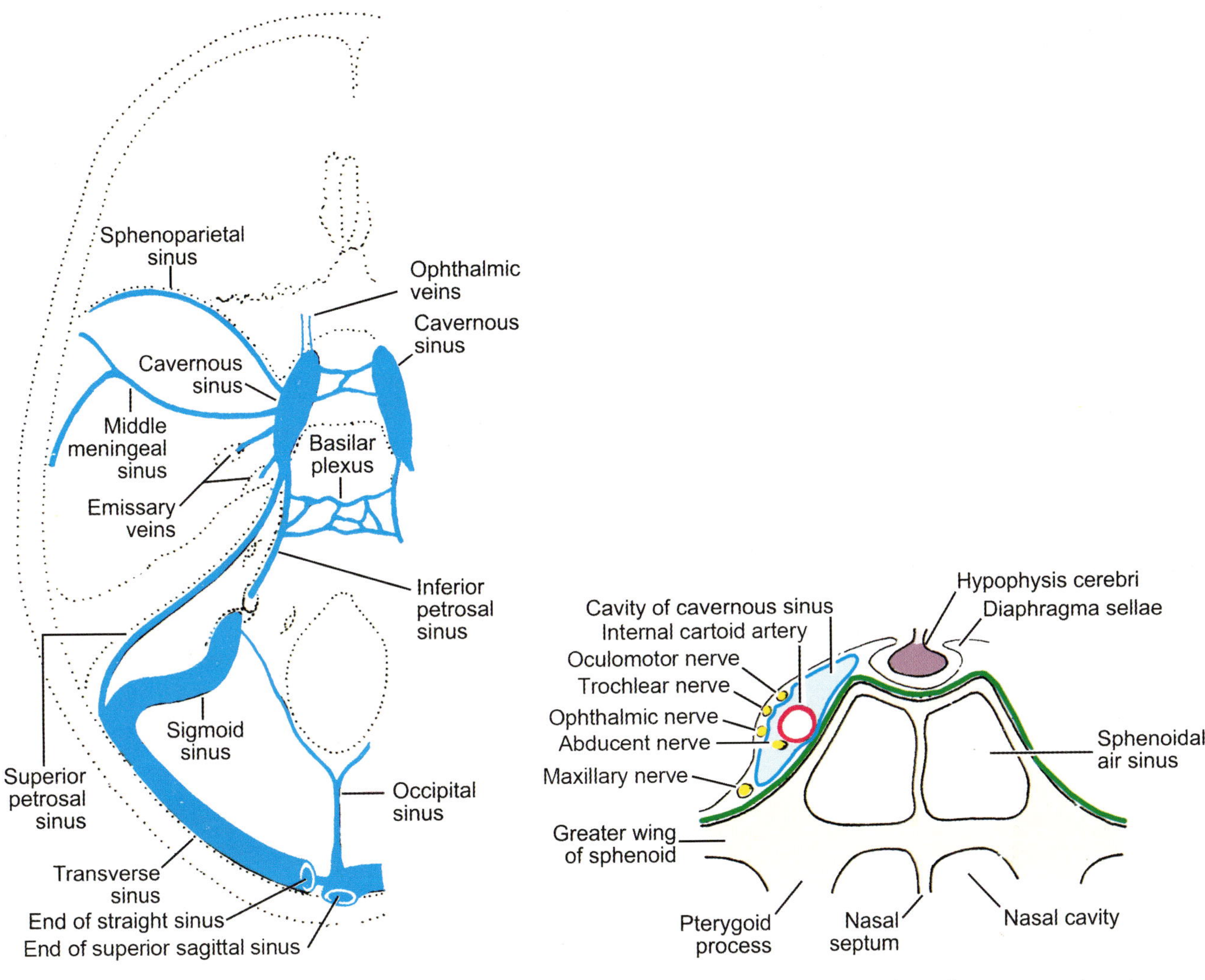


**42.40:** Relationship of the cranial venous sinuses to the floor of the cranial cavity

**42.41:** Coronal section through cavernous sinus to show its relations

2. The ***inferior ophthalmic vein*** lies below the eyeball. It terminates in the cavernous sinus either directly or by joining the superior ophthalmic vein.
3. The ***central vein of the retina*** accompanies the artery of the same name. It ends in the cavernous sinus directly or through the superior ophthalmic vein.

## WANT TO KNOW MORE?

### Some Other Veins in the Head

1. Some venous channels are present within the thickness of the skull bones. They are called ***diploic veins.*** They drain mostly into the intracranial sinuses, but some end in the veins of the scalp.
2. Some ***meningeal veins*** lie in the dura mater. The largest of these are the middle meningeal sinuses. Like the veins from the brain the meningeal veins also drain into the intracranial venous sinuses.

3. The ***emissary veins*** connect the intracranial venous sinuses to veins outside the skull. They are numerous and pass through various foramina of the skull.

## TRIBUTARIES OF INTERNAL JUGULAR VEINS IN THE NECK

### The Facial Vein

1. The facial vein begins near the medial angle of the eye by the union of two superficial veins of the forehead, namely, the ***supratrochlear*** and the ***supraorbital*** veins (42.42).
2. The vein runs downwards and backwards across the face and terminates by joining the anterior branch of the retromandibular vein to form the ***common facial vein*** that ends in the internal jugular vein.
3. Sometimes, the common facial vein is described as part of the facial vein, which is then described as ending in the internal jugular vein.

**WANT TO KNOW MORE?**

4. While running across the face, the facial vein lies over the buccinator muscle (42.42), the body of the mandible and the lower part of the masseter. Below the mandible it crosses the submandibular gland, the posterior belly of the digastric and the stylohyoid muscles.
5. The terminal part of the vein (including the common facial part) crosses the internal and external carotid arteries, the hypoglossal nerve and the loop formed by the lingual artery (42.43).
6. The tributaries of the facial vein are shown in 42.42. The vein communicates with the superior ophthalmic veins and through them with the cavernous sinus.

### The Lingual Vein

1. The lingual vein accompanies the lingual artery and joins the internal jugular vein near the greater cornu of the hyoid bone.

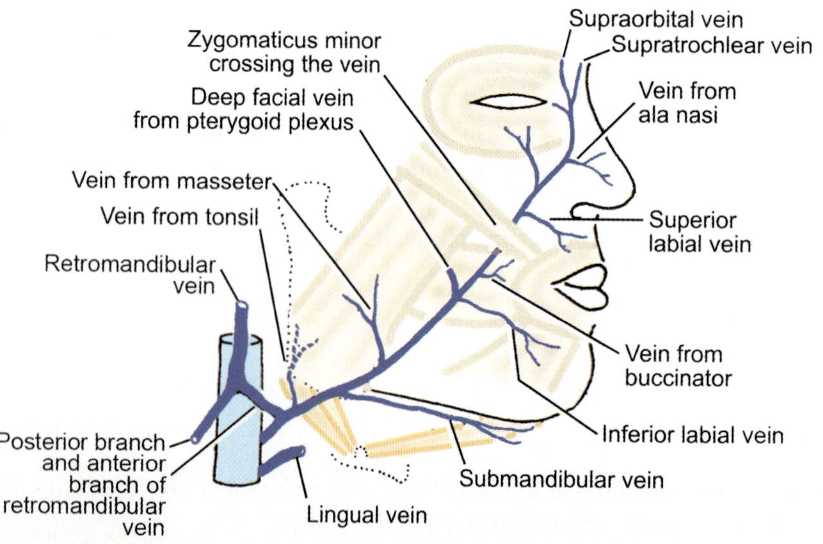


**42.42:** Scheme to show the course and tributaries of the facial vein

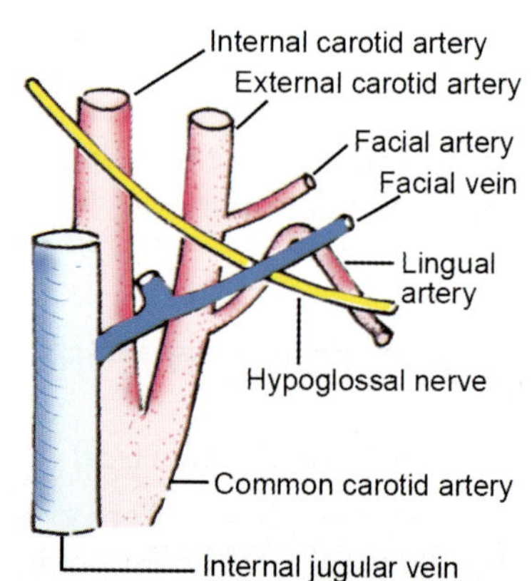


**42.43:** Some relations of the terminal part of the facial vein

2. Some veins of the tongue run along the hypoglossal nerve. They may join the lingual vein or the facial vein or may terminate directly in the internal jugular vein.

## The Superior Thyroid Vein

The superior thyroid vein corresponds in its course and tributaries with the superior thyroid artery (42.44 and 42.14).

## The Middle Thyroid Vein

The middle thyroid vein drains the lower part of the gland. It crosses the common carotid artery to enter the internal jugular vein (42.44).

## The Inferior Thyroid Veins

1. The inferior thyroid veins are not tributaries of the internal jugular, but are described here for sake of convenience.
2. They arise from the lower part of the thyroid gland and descend over the front of the trachea forming a plexus over it.
3. The right and left veins end in the corresponding brachiocephalic veins (42.44).

## Some other Tributaries

In addition to the tributaries described above the internal jugular vein also receives some veins from the pharynx.

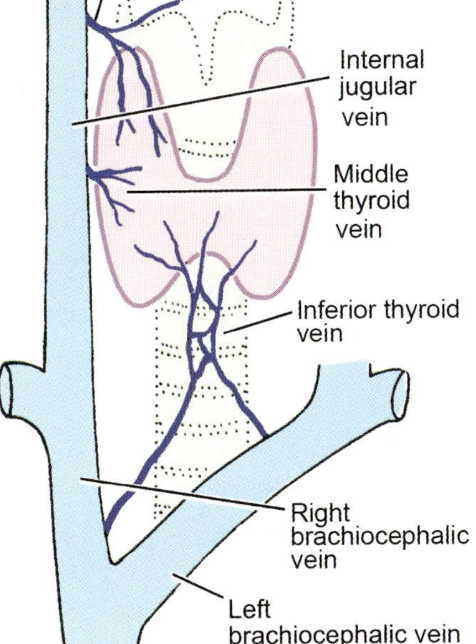


**42.44:** Scheme to show the veins draining the thyroid gland

## OTHER VEINS OF THE HEAD AND NECK

### WANT TO KNOW MORE?

**Superficial Temporal Vein**

1. The superficial temporal vein accompanies the corresponding artery. The vein is formed a little above the zygomatic arch by the union of numerous tributaries present in the scalp.
2. A little below its formation it receives the ***middle temporal vein.***
3. After descending superficial to the zygomatic arch, it is joined by the maxillary vein to form the ***retromandibular vein***. The tributaries of the superficial temporal vein are shown in 42.45.

**The Maxillary Vein and Pterygoid Plexus**

1. The maxillary vein runs alongside the first part of the maxillary artery.
2. It has its origin in the ***pterygoid plexus*** of veins that is present in the infratemporal fossa.
   a. The veins corresponding to the branches of the maxillary artery drain into this plexus.
   b. The plexus is connected to the facial vein through the deep facial vein (42.42).
   c. It is connected to the cavernous sinus by a number of emissary veins.
   d. The plexus is drained by the maxillary vein that ends by joining the superficial temporal vein to form the retromandibular vein.

**The Retromandibular Vein**

1. The retromandibular vein lies behind the ramus of the mandible (as implied by its name).
2. It is formed by union of the superficial temporal and maxillary veins.

3. It is embedded in the parotid gland.
   a. Within the gland, the vein is superficial to the external carotid artery and deep to the facial nerve.
   b. Descending within the substance of the gland, the vein divides into anterior and posterior branches.
4. The anterior branch joins the facial vein.
5. The posterior branch joins the posterior auricular vein (see below) to form the external jugular vein.

**The Posterior Auricular Vein**

1. The posterior auricular vein begins by union of tributaries present in the posterior part of the scalp.
2. It passes downwards and forwards behind the auricle and receives veins from its cranial surface.
3. Finally, it ends by joining the posterior division of the retromandibular vein.

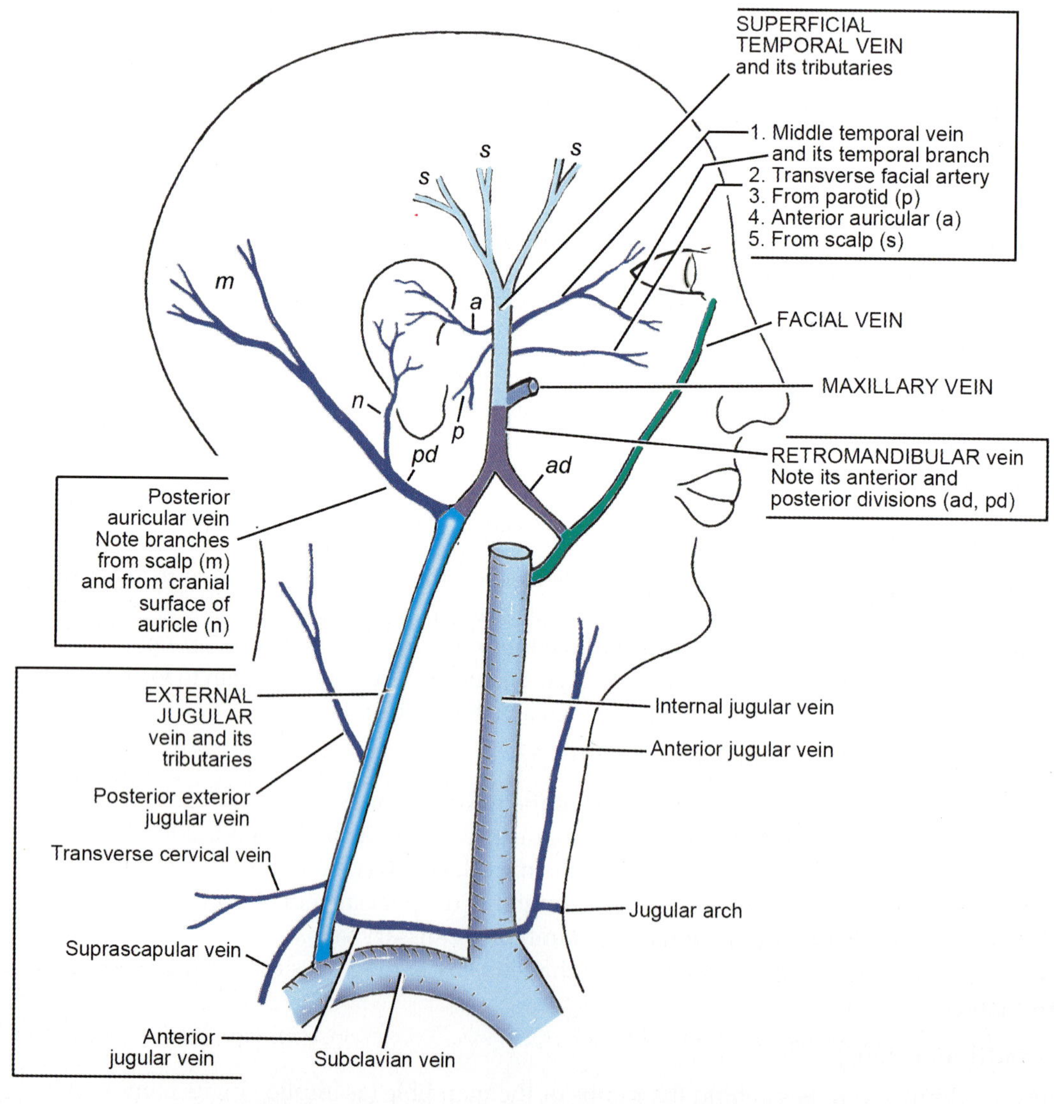


**42.45:** Scheme to show some veins of the head and neck

## The External Jugular Vein

1. The external jugular vein is formed by union of the posterior division of the retromandibular vein with the posterior auricular vein (42.45).
2. The origin lies within the lower part of the parotid gland or just below it. The level corresponds to the angle of the mandible.
3. From here, the vein runs downwards and somewhat backwards and ends by joining the subclavian vein. The termination lies behind the middle of the clavicle, near the lateral margin of the scalenus anterior muscle.
4. The greater part of the vein is superficial being covered by skin, superficial fascia and platysma. As a result, the vein can be clearly seen in the living.
5. It pierces the deep fascia near its termination to reach the subclavian vein.
6. The vein crosses the sternocleidomastoid obliquely running downwards and backwards across it.

**WANT TO KNOW MORE?**

7. Apart from the veins that form it, the external jugular vein receives a number of tributaries. These are:
   a. The ***posterior external jugular vein*** from the upper and posterior part of the neck
   b. The ***transverse cervical vein***
   c. ***Suprascapular veins*** that accompany the corresponding arteries
   d. The anterior jugular vein (42.45).

### The Anterior Jugular Vein

1. The anterior jugular vein runs down the front of the neck a short distance from the midline (42.45).
2. It begins near the hyoid bone and extends downwards to a point a little above the sternoclavicular joint.
3. Here, the vein turns laterally deep to the sternocleidomastoid, but superficial to the sternohyoid and sternothyroid muscles (42.34), and ends by joining the lower end of the external jugular vein.
4. Sometimes, it may end in the subclavian vein (42.36).
5. Just above the sternum, the right and left anterior jugular veins are united by a transverse vein called the ***jugular arch*** (42.45).

### The Occipital Vein

1. The occipital vein begins by union of some veins draining the posterior part of the scalp (42.46).
2. It descends in the scalp a few centimetres behind the auricle.
3. Reaching the attachment of the trapezius to the superior nuchal line it pierces it and becomes deep.
4. It then reaches the suboccipital triangle where it ends in a plexus from which the deep cervical and vertebral veins begin.

### The Deep Cervical Vein

1. The deep cervical vein begins in the venous plexus present in the suboccipital region.
2. It accompanies the corresponding artery through the deep muscles of the back of the neck and ends by joining the lower part of the vertebral vein (42.46).

## The Vertebral Vein

1. The vertebral vein also begins in the suboccipital venous plexus (42.46).
2. It enters the foramen transversarium of the atlas and runs downwards in the form of a dense plexus around the vertebral artery.
3. It is only at the foramen transversarium of the sixth cervical vertebra that the plexus takes the form of a single vessel.
4. The vein runs downwards behind the internal jugular vein and ends in the upper part of the corresponding brachiocephalic vein.

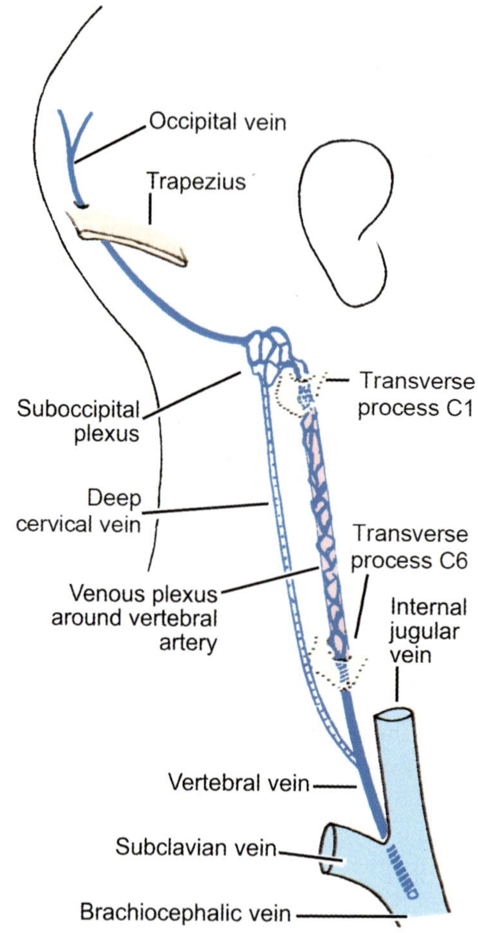


**42.46:** Scheme to show the occipital, vertebral and deep cervical veins

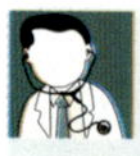

## CLINICAL CORRELATION

### BLOOD VESSELS OF HEAD AND NECK

**The Arteries**

1. In considering the arteries of the head and neck, it must always be remembered that the common and internal carotid arteries, and the vertebral arteries, convey blood to the brain.
2. Similarly, although the subclavian arteries lie in the neck they are the main channels of supply to the upper extremities.
3. Therefore, any form of obstruction to these arteries of the neck can produce symptoms referable to the brain, and to the upper limb.

***Congenital anomalies***

The large arteries of the head and neck develop from a series of aortic arch arteries that lie in the embryonic pharyngeal arches. Some anomalies that can be produced by maldevelopment are given below:

1. Normally, the left common carotid artery is a direct branch of the arch of the aorta.
   a. Sometimes, it may arise as a branch of the brachiocephalic trunk. [The brachiocephalic trunk then divides into three branches viz., right subclavian, right common carotid, and left common carotid].

   b. Sometimes, the left common carotid and left subclavian arteries may arise from the arch of the aorta by a common stem (which is then called the left brachiocephalic trunk).
2. The right subclavian artery may arise as the last branch of the arch of the aorta (or of the descending thoracic aorta).
   a. To reach the neck, the artery has to run upwards behind the oesophagus.
   b. Along with the arch of the aorta, the artery forms an arterial ring enclosing the trachea and oesophagus.
   c. The ring may obstruct the oesophagus leading to dysphagia (***dysphagia lusoria***). The ring can also be a cause of obstruction of the trachea.
3. The left vertebral artery may arise as a direct branch of the arch of the aorta (instead of arising from the subclavian artery).

*Other correlations*

1. During surgical operations, the anaesthetist sits at the head end of the patient and often feels for the pulse in the superficial temporal artery near the zygomatic arch, or in the facial artery as it crosses the lower border of the mandible (near the anterior border of the masseter). Pulsation of the common carotid artery (carotid pulse) can be felt at the level of the superior border of the thyroid cartilage, beneath the anterior border of the sternocleidomastoid muscle.
2. Weakening of the wall of any artery can lead to dilatation of the artery (aneurysm) at that site.
   a. Aneurysms on any intracranial artery can burst and can be a cause of bleeding into the subarachnoid space (see above).
   b. An aneurysm of the third part of the subclavian artery can press on the brachial plexus leading to motor and sensory symptoms in the upper extremity.
3. With age any artery of the body can undergo degenerative changes associated with deposition of fatty substances in the arterial wall (atheromatosis).
   a. Blockage of the common carotid or internal carotid arteries in this way can interfere with blood supply of the brain and of the eyeball.
   b. In suspected cases of blockage, the carotid system of arteries is investigated by ***carotid angiography***.
   c. A radioopaque dye is injected into the common carotid artery either directly or through a catheter (passed up through the femoral artery to reach the arch of the aorta).
   d. Skiagrams taken after the injection reveal the site of blockage. In such skiagrams the petrous, cavernous and cerebral parts of the internal carotid artery cast a typical S-shaped shadow to which the term ***carotid syphon*** is applied.
   e. Atheroma may affect the vertebral arteries, specially their first and fourth parts. These arteries may also be pressed upon by osteophytes in cervical spondylosis. Inadequacy in blood flow through the vertebral and basilar arteries can give rise to attacks of transient ischaemia in which the patient complains of dizziness.
   f. Obstruction of one vertebral artery usually does not produce symptoms because of blood flow through the contralateral vertebral artery. Collateral anastomoses also exist through the ascending cervical, thyrocervical and occipital arteries.
   g. One cause of possible obstruction to flow of blood in the subclavian artery is the presence of a cervical rib. The artery has to loop over the cervical rib to enter the axilla and is therefore pressed upon.
4. Pressure on arteries can be used to stop haemorrhage in the area of its distribution.
   a. The common carotid artery can be compressed against the carotid tubercle (which is the anterior tubercle of transverse process of the sixth cervical vertebra).
   b. It should be remembered that pressure on the carotid sinus causes slowing of heart rate and fall of blood pressure.
   c. Also note that when the neck is extended the carotid sheath is retracted. It is because of this fact that in suicidal attempts at slitting the neck the cut often fails to reach the carotid arteries.

d. Bleeding caused by severe injuries in the proximal part of the upper extremity can be controlled by pressure over the subclavian artery. Pressure is directed downwards and backwards (and somewhat medially). The artery gets compressed against the first rib.

5. We have seen that injury to the middle meningeal artery is an important cause of an extradural haemorrhage.
   a. To reach a bleeding anterior branch of this artery, the surgeon takes a point 4 cm above the middle of the zygomatic arch and bores a hole through the skull. The region corresponds to the pterion.
   b. Extradural haemorrhage from an injured posterior division of the middle meningeal artery is less common. The blood can press upon the superior temporal gyrus and lead to deafness in the ear of the opposite side. To approach this branch, the surgeon makes a hole in the skull over a point 4 cm above and 4 cm behind the external acoustic meatus.

**The Veins**

***Variability***

1. As in other parts of the body the arrangement of veins, specially that of superficial veins, is highly variable. In particular note that the anterior jugular vein (which is normally paired) may be represented by a single median vein, or may be absent on one side.
2. ***Injury to veins***
   Superficial veins are liable to be involved in injuries to the neck.
   a. The external jugular vein is particularly vulnerable.
   b. Normally, when a vein is cut its walls retract thus limiting the amount of bleeding. However, near its lower end the external jugular vein pierces the deep fascia. Here the wall of the vein is adherent to fascia, and this prevents the wall from retracting if the vein is injured.
   c. Also remember that during inspiration pressure in the vein can be negative and air can be sucked into the vein. This can have very serious consequences if it leads to air embolism.

***Dangerous Area of Face***

1. Near the medial angle of the eye the supraorbital vein, which is a tributary of the facial vein, communicates with the superior ophthalmic vein (lying in the orbit).
2. The superior ophthalmic vein drains into the cavernous sinus. In this way the facial vein is brought into communication with the cavernous sinus. The facial vein also communicates with the cavernous sinus through the deep facial vein and the pterygoid plexus.
3. Because of these communications an infection in the face can spread to the cavernous sinus leading to cavernous sinus thrombosis (see below).
4. It has been observed that such spread of infection is most likely to take place if the infection is over the upper lip or the lower part of the nose. That is why this region is called the ***dangerous area of the face***.

***Venous Pressure***

1. Clinicians examining the cardiovascular system use the level of blood in the external jugular vein as an indication of venous pressure.
   a. When the patient lies flat the vein is at the same level as the right atrium and the entire vein is full of blood.
   b. When the head rests on a pillow the level of blood in the vein lies at junction of the lower and middle-thirds of the neck.
   c. When the patient sits up the vein becomes empty.
2. Venous pressure can be raised if there is right heart failure, raised intrathoracic pressure from any cause, or obstruction to the superior vena cava.
3. Increased venous pressure leads to dilatation of veins in the neck. The internal jugular vein can be markedly dilated.

*Involvement in Malignancy*

1. Lymph nodes from all parts of the head and neck ultimately drain into the deep cervical lymph nodes that are therefore frequently involved in malignancy and in infections such as tuberculosis.
2. In the treatment of malignancy, the surgeon often has to remove these nodes.
3. Enlarged nodes become adherent to the internal jugular vein and it is sometimes necessary for the surgeon to remove a segment of the vein along with the lymph nodes.

*Intracranial Venous Sinuses*

1. Intracranial venous sinuses are of importance because they receive blood from the brain.
   a. Infection in these sinuses can spread into brain tissue with serious consequences.
   b. Infections in the scalp can spread into the venous sinuses through emissary veins that pass through foramina in the skull. Emissary veins traverse the layer of loose areolar tissue of the scalp that is therefore called the ***dangerous area of the scalp***.
   c. We have seen above that infection can reach the cavernous sinus from the face.

*Pulsating Exophthalmos*

1. Because of the peculiar relationship of the cavernous sinus to the internal carotid artery a communication between the two may occur as a result of injury.
2. When this happens the arterial pressure is communicated through the sinus to veins of the orbit (which open into the sinus). As a result, the eyeball becomes prominent and pulsates with each heart beat (***pulsating exophthalmos***).

*Thrombosis in the Cavernous Sinus*

1. The cavernous sinus can be infected by spread of infection from the dangerous area of the face (see above). Infection can also reach it from the nose and paranasal sinuses.
2. Symptoms can be produced by:
   a. Blockage to blood flow
   b. Involvement of cranial nerves.
3. As veins of the orbit drain into the cavernous sinus they become congested. Accumulation of fluid in the orbit pushes the eyeball forwards (exophthalmos).
4. The eyelids and the root of the nose show swelling.
5. Involvement of the ophthalmic nerve leads to severe pain in the region of distribution of the nerve (eye and over the forehead).
6. Involvement of the oculomotor, trochlear and abducent nerves can lead to paralysis of extraocular muscles.

*Thrombosis in the Superior Sagittal Sinus*

1. Infection can spread to this sinus from the scalp or from the nasal cavities. It can also reach it from an infected sigmoid or transverse sinus.
2. The arachnoid granulations (made up of arachnoid villi) in the superior sagittal sinus are the main site at which CSF is absorbed into the blood stream.
   a. When the sinus is thrombosed this absorption is interfered with leading to increased pressure in the CSF.
   b. This leads to various signs of increased intracranial tension. In a child it can lead to hydrocephalus.
3. Venous blood from the cerebral hemisphere is drained predominantly by superior cerebral veins that open into the superior sagittal sinus. Infection from the sinus can extend along these veins to the cerebral hemisphere.

*Thrombosis in the Sigmoid Sinus*

1. The middle ear and the mastoid air cells are very frequent sites of infection.
   a. The close relationship of the sigmoid sinus to the middle ear (lying in the petrous temporal bone) and the mastoid process often leads to spread of infection to this sinus.
   b. Thrombosis in the sinus can extend downwards into the internal jugular vein. It can spread upwards along the transverse sinus into the superior sagittal sinus.

# 43 CHAPTER

# Nerves of the Head and Neck

## CERVICAL NERVES

1. In the thoracic, lumbar and sacral regions the number of spinal nerves corresponds to that of vertebrae, each nerve lying ***below*** the numerically corresponding vertebra.
2. However, in the neck we have seven cervical vertebrae, and eight cervical nerves.
   a. The reason for this will be clear from 43.1.
   b. Note that the ***upper seven cervical nerves lie above the numerically corresponding vertebrae***.
   c. The eighth cervical nerve lies below vertebra C7.

### The Dorsal Rami of Cervical Nerves

1. The dorsal ramus of a typical spinal nerve is smaller than the ventral ramus.
2. It passes backwards and divides into medial and lateral branches that supply the deep muscles and skin of the back (43.2).
   This is all that needs to be known about the dorsal rami of most spinal nerves. The dorsal rami of the upper three cervical nerves, however, have some atypical features and are briefly described below.

#### *Dorsal Ramus of the First Cervical Nerve*

1. The dorsal ramus of the first cervical nerve is larger than the ventral ramus.
2. It is seen the suboccipital triangle which it reaches by passing above the posterior arch of the atlas (43.3). Here the nerve lies between the arch and the vertebral artery.
3. The dorsal ramus divides into branches that supply the rectus capitis posterior major and minor, the superior and inferior oblique muscles and the semispinalis capitis (43.4).
4. Some branches may reach the skin of the scalp.

#### *Dorsal Ramus of the Second Cervical Nerve*

1. The dorsal ramus of the second cervical nerve is large.
2. It reaches the suboccipital region by passing below the posterior arch of the atlas, and below the inferior oblique muscle.
3. It divides into medial and lateral branches.
4. The medial branch that is much more prominent and is called the ***greater occipital nerve*** (43.5).
   a. Winding around the lower border of the inferior oblique muscle, this nerve passes upwards and medially across the suboccipital triangle, lying deep to the semispinalis capitis.
   b. It becomes superficial by piercing first the semispinalis capitis and then the trapezius.
   c. Finally, it divides into branches that ramify in the scalp supplying its posterior part.
   d. It also gives a branch to the semispinalis capitis muscle.

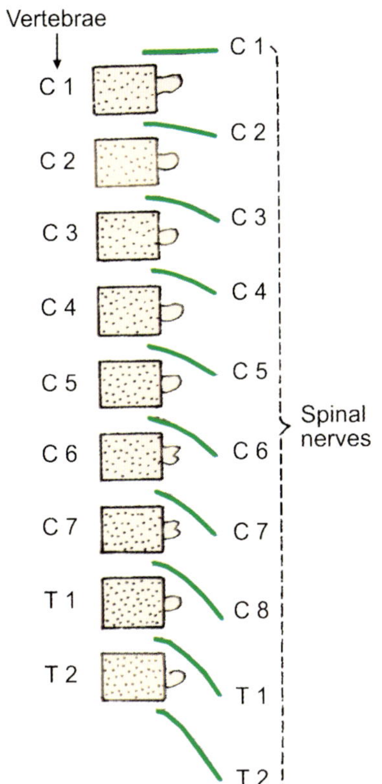


**43.1:** Scheme to show the relationship of cervical and upper thoracic nerves to vertebrae

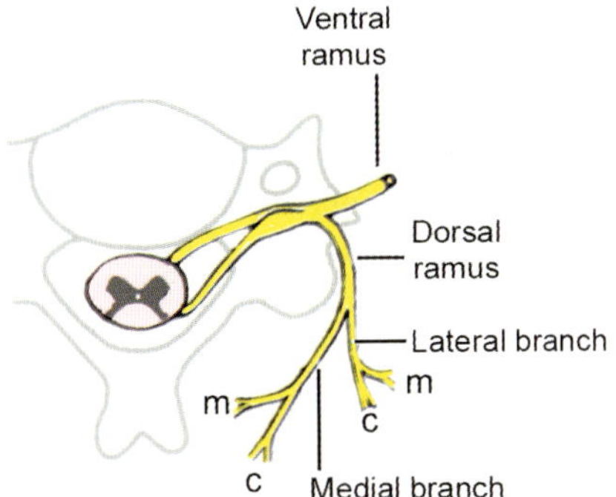


**43.2:** Dorsal ramus of a typical spinal nerve

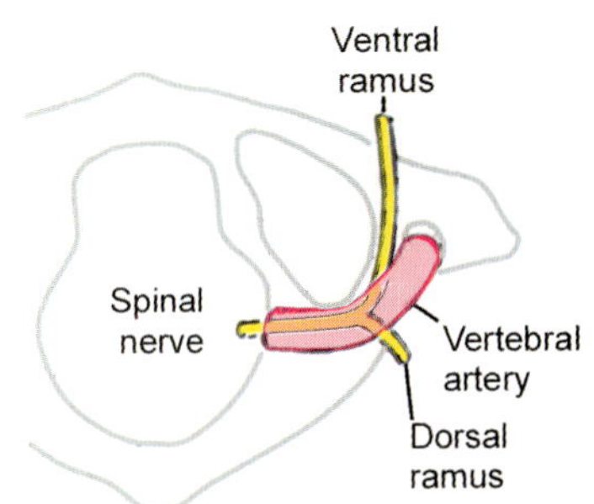


**43.3:** Dorsal ramus of the first cervical nerve

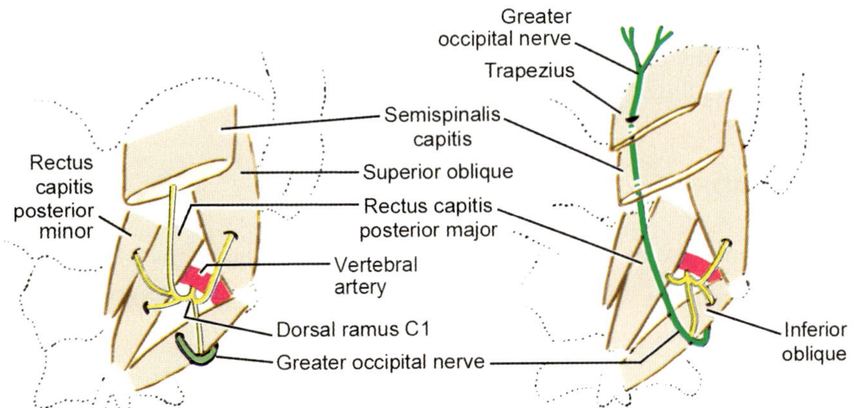


**43.4:** Distribution of the dorsal ramus of the first cervical nerve

**43.5:** Course of the greater occipital nerve

### Dorsal Ramus of the Third Cervical Nerve

1. The dorsal ramus of the third cervical nerve behaves like a typical dorsal ramus.
2. The only special feature about it is that it also gives a small branch to the skin of the occipital region. This branch is called the ***third occipital nerve.***

### The Ventral Rami of Cervical Nerves

1. The ventral rami of the first, second, third and fourth cervical nerves unite with each other to form the ***cervical plexus.***
2. The ventral rami of the fifth, sixth, seventh and eighth cervical nerves, and the greater part of the ventral ramus of the first thoracic nerve, join one another to form the brachial plexus.
3. The brachial plexus has been considered with the upper extremity (chapter 3). The cervical plexus is described below.

## THE CERVICAL PLEXUS AND ITS BRANCHES

1. The cervical plexus is formed by the ventral rami of the first, second, third and fourth cervical nerves as given below (43.6).
2. With the exception of the ramus of the first cervical nerve, each of them divides into ascending (***'a'*** in 43.6) and descending (***'d'*** in 43.6) branches.
3. The ascending branch of the second nerve joins the first nerve; and its descending branch joins the ascending branch of the third nerve.
4. Similarly, the descending branch of the third nerve joins the ascending branch of the fourth nerve.
5. The descending branch of the fourth nerve is small and joins the fifth cervical nerve.
6. The cervical plexus gives off a large number of branches. The ***cutaneous branches*** are shown in 43.7 and are as follows:
   a. The ***lesser occipital*** nerve arises from the second cervical nerve.
   b. The ***greater auricular*** nerve and the ***transverse cutaneous nerve of the neck*** arise from the second and third nerves.
   c. The ***supraclavicular*** nerves arise from the third and fourth nerves. These nerves are considered in detail on pages that follow.
7. The ***muscular branches*** of the cervical plexus are numerous. For ease of visualisation they may be subdivided as follows (43.8).

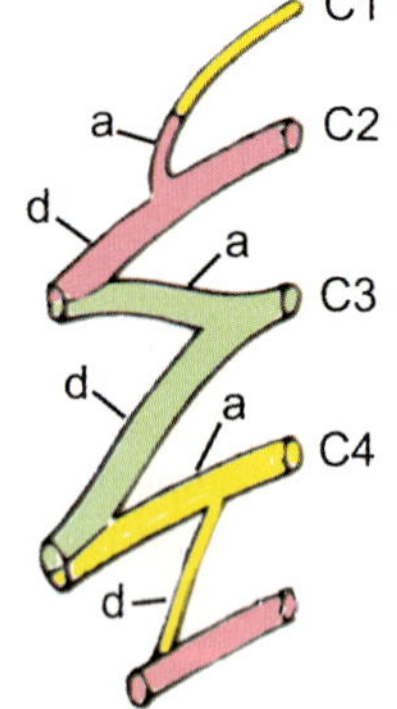


**43.6:** Plan of cervical plexus

### WANT TO KNOW MORE?

a. *Branches to prevertebral muscles:* The rectus capitis lateralis and the rectus capitis anterior receive branches from C1. The longus capitis receives branches C1, C2 and C3. The longus colli receives branches from C2, C3 and C4.

b. *Branches to muscles forming boundaries of the posterior triangle:* The sternocleidomastoid receives a branch from C2 (and sometimes from C3). The levator scapulae, the scalenus medius and the trapezius receive branches from C3 and C4.
c. The *phrenic nerve* (which supplies the diaphragm) arises by separate roots from C3, C4 and C5.
d. Branches *to infrahyoid muscles* reach them through the hypoglossal nerve and through the ansa cervicalis.

We will now consider some of these branches one by one.

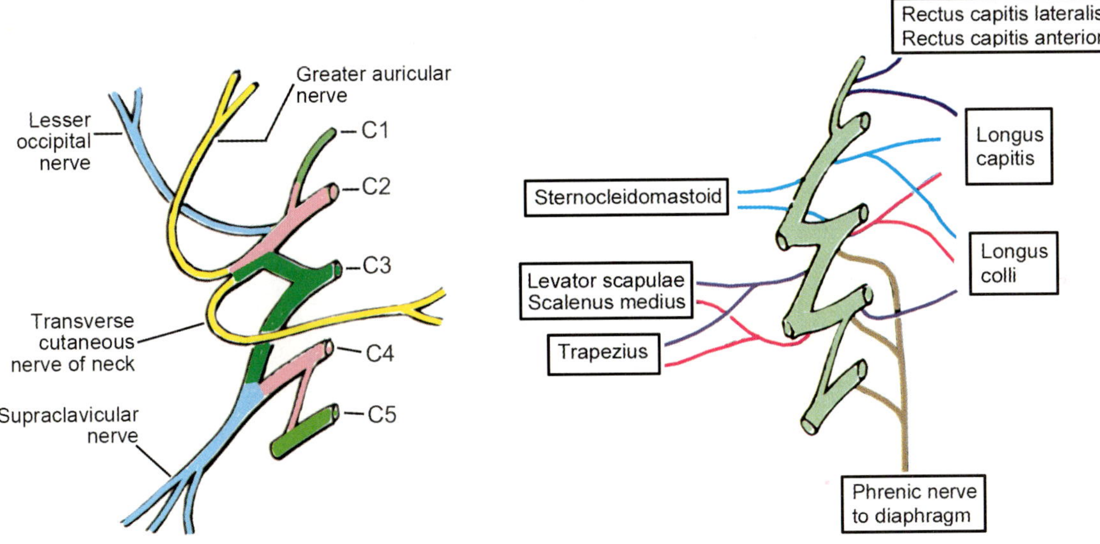


**43.7:** Cervical plexus and its cutaneous branches

**43.8:** Scheme to show the muscular branches of the cervical plexus

## Lesser Occipital Nerve

1. The lesser occipital nerve arises from the descending branch of the ventral ramus of the second cervical nerve. The origin lies deep to the sternocleidomastoid muscle (43.9).
2. The nerve forms a loop round the accessory nerve.
3. It then runs upwards and backwards for some distance along the posterior border of the sternocleidomastoid. Higher up it lies superficial to the muscle between it and the deep fascia.
4. It becomes subcutaneous behind the auricle and divides into branches that supply the skin of this region.
5. It also gives off an ***auricular branch*** that supplies the upper part of the cranial surface of the auricle (43.7).

## Greater Auricle Nerve

1. The greater auricular nerve arises from the ventral rami of the second and third cervical nerve. Its origin lies deep to the sternocleidomastoid (43.10).
2. Winding around the posterior border of the sternocleidomastoid muscle it reaches its superficial surface.
3. It pierces the deep fascia and runs upwards and somewhat forwards over the surface of the sternocleidomastoid muscle. Here it is accompanied by the external jugular vein.
4. A little below the auricle it divides into anterior and posterior branches.
5. The anterior branch supplies the skin over the parotid gland.
6. The posterior branch supplies:
   a. Most of the cranial surface of the auricle (except the part supplied by the lesser occipital)
   b. The posteroinferior part of the lateral surface of the auricle including the lobule and concha and
   c. The skin over the mastoid process (43.7 and 43.10 to 43.12).

## Transverse Cutaneous Nerve of Neck

1. The transverse cutaneous nerve of the neck is also called the anterior cutaneous nerve. It arises from the ventral rami of the second and third cervical nerves.
2. It first runs laterally deep to the sternocleidomastoid.
3. Reaching the posterior border of this muscle it curves around it and then runs forwards across the muscle.
4. The nerve becomes superficial and divides into ascending and descending branches that supply the skin on the front of the neck (43.7 and 43.10).

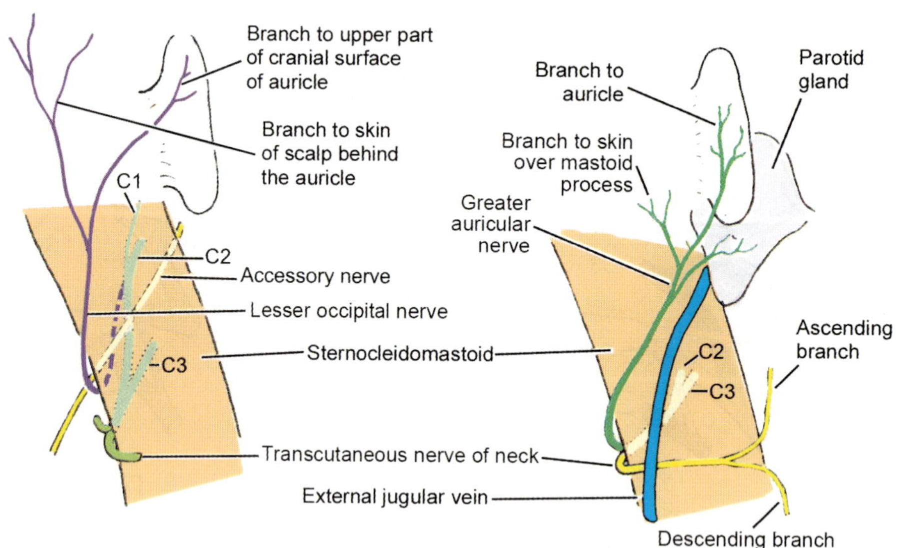


43.9: Course and distribution of lesser occipital nerve

43.10: Course and distribution of greater auricular and transverse cutaneous nerves

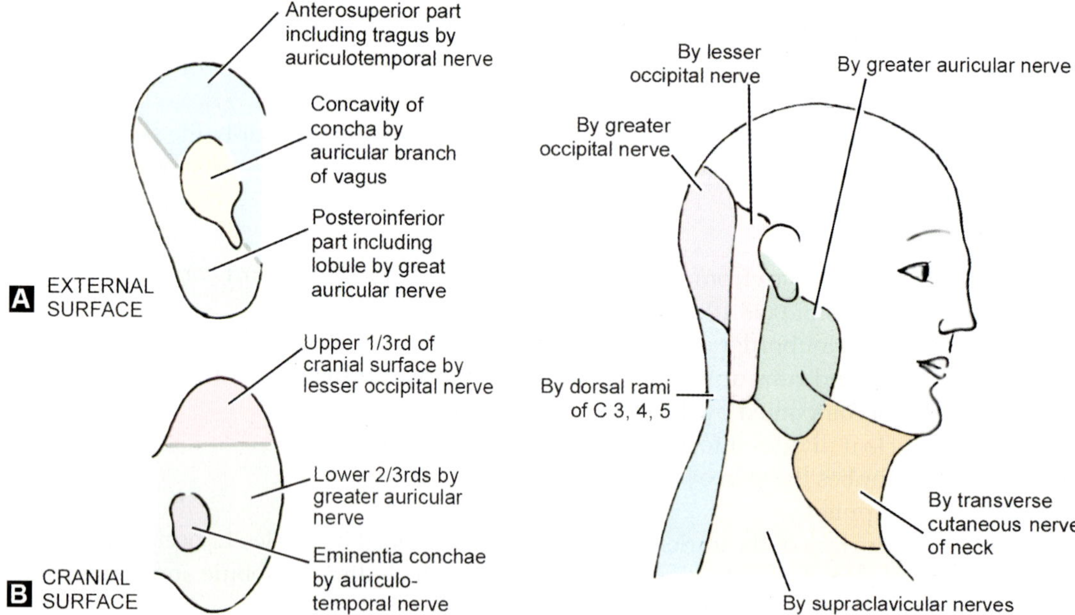


43.11A and B: Nerve supply of the auricle. (A) External surface; (B) Cranial surface

43.12: Areas of skin of neck supplied by various cutaneous nerves

## The Supraclavicular Nerves

1. The supraclavicular nerves arise (as a single ramus) from the third and fourth cervical nerves (43.7). The origin lies deep to the sternocleidomastoid.

2. The nerve trunk runs downwards and backwards deep to the muscle and appears at its posterior border.
3. Here the trunk divides into three branches called the ***medial, intermediate*** and ***lateral*** supraclavicular nerves.
4. These branches descend over the posterior triangle of the neck giving some branches to the skin here.
5. They pierce the deep fascia a little above the clavicle and then run downwards across this bone to reach the pectoral region.

## The Ansa Cervicalis

1. The ansa cervicalis is also called the ***ansa hypoglossi***. It is a nerve loop lying in front of the common carotid artery (ansa = loop) (43.13).
2. Branches arising from the ansa cervicalis innervate the sternohyoid, the sternothyroid and the omohyoid muscles (viz., all infrahyoid muscles other than the thyrohyoid).

### WANT TO KNOW MORE?

3. The ansa cervicalis is formed by union of two roots (43.13).
   a. The superior root appears to arise from the hypoglossal nerve (hence the term ansa hypoglossi given to the loop).
   b. However, the root is really made up of fibres derived from the first cervical nerve.
   c. These fibres reach the hypoglossal nerve through a communicating branch from the first cervical nerve.
   d. Apart from forming the superior root of the ansa cervicalis, these fibres from the first cervical nerve (travelling along the hypoglossal nerve) innervate the thyrohyoid and geniohyoid muscles (Also see 43.70).
4. The inferior root of the ansa cervicalis arises from the second and third cervical nerves. It descends at first lateral to the internal jugular vein and then superficial to it to join the superior root superficial to the common carotid artery.

## The Phrenic Nerve

1. The phrenic nerve is one of the most important nerves in the body as it is the only motor supply to the diaphragm.
2. This nerve arises from the (ventral rami of) spinal nerves C3, C4 and C5 the contribution from C4 being the greatest.
3. The nerve descends vertically through the lower part of the neck, and then through the thorax to reach the diaphragm.
4. Some terminal branches enter the abdomen.
5. The relations of the nerve in the neck are given below.The course and relations of the phrenic nerve in the thorax are described on page 451.

### WANT TO KNOW MORE?

*Relations in the Neck*

1. The phrenic nerve descends vertically over the scalenus anterior muscle (43.14).
2. Crossing the medial (or lower) border of the muscle it crosses in front of the first part of the subclavian artery (42.25). On the right side, however, the nerve is usually separated from the artery by a part of the scalenus anterior.
3. Throughout its course in the neck the nerve lies deep to the sternocleidomastoid muscle. It can be viewed by lifting up the lateral border of this muscle.

4. Additional relations of the phrenic nerve in the neck are as follows:
   a. While over the scalenus anterior the nerve lies deep to the prevertebral fascia. It is crossed superficially by the superior belly of the omohyoid, the transverse cervical artery and the suprascapular artery. On the left side it is also crossed by the thoracic duct (43.14).
   b. Lower down the nerve lies behind the lower end of the internal jugular vein. Still lower down the nerve passes behind the medial end of the subclavian vein.

*Accessory Phrenic Nerve*

1. The root of the phrenic nerve from C5 may sometimes follow a complicated course.
2. Instead of arising from C5 itself it may arise from the nerve to the subclavius.
3. From here the root descends through the neck lateral to the main phrenic nerve and joins it in the upper part of the thorax.
4. Such a root from C5 constitutes the accessory phrenic nerve.

## THE CRANIAL NERVES

1. There are twelve pairs of cranial nerves that emerge from the surface of the brain. They are identified by number (in cranio-caudal sequence) and also bear names as follows:
2. The ***first*** cranial nerve is called the ***olfactory*** nerve. It is the nerve of smell (Olfaction = smell).
3. The ***second*** cranial nerve is called the ***optic*** nerve. It is the nerve of sight (Optics = science of formation of images).

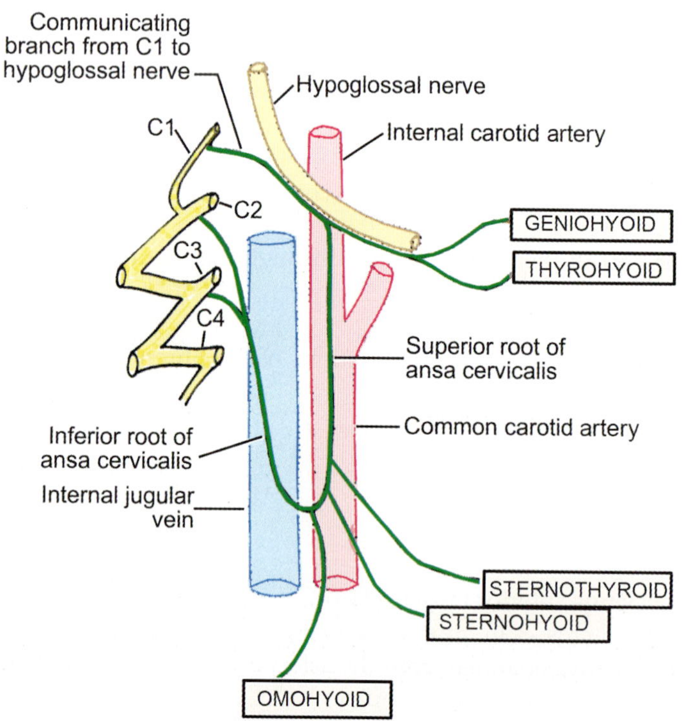


**43.13:** Scheme to show the mode of innervation of the infrahyoid muscles from the cervical plexus

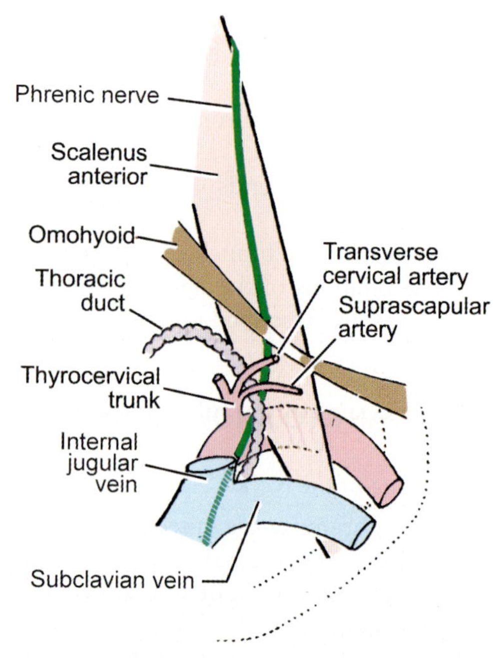


**43.14:** Some relationships of the phrenic nerve

4. The ***third*** cranial nerve is called the ***oculomotor*** nerve as it supplies several muscles that move the eyeball (Ocular = pertaining to the eye).
5. The ***fourth*** cranial nerve is called the ***trochlear*** nerve. It is so called because it supplies a muscle (superior oblique) that passes through a pulley (trochlea = pulley).
6. The ***fifth*** cranial nerve is called the ***trigeminal*** nerve because it has three major divisions. These are:
   a. The ***ophthalmic*** division to the orbit
   b. The ***maxillary*** division to the upper jaw
   c. The ***mandibular*** division to the lower jaw.
7. The ***sixth*** cranial nerve is called the ***abducent*** nerve because it supplies a muscle (lateral rectus) that 'abducts' the eyeball.
8. The ***seventh*** cranial nerve is the ***facial*** nerve because it supplies the muscles of the face.
9. The ***eighth*** cranial nerve is called the ***vestibulocochlear*** nerve because it supplies structures in the vestibular and cochlear parts of the internal ear. It is sometimes called:
   a. The auditory nerve (auditory = pertaining to hearing)
   b. The stato-acoustic nerve (stato = pertaining to equilibrium; acoustic = pertaining to sound or hearing).
10. The ***ninth*** cranial nerve is called the ***glossopharyngeal*** nerve as it is distributed to the pharynx and to part of the tongue (glossal = pertaining to the tongue).
11. The ***tenth*** cranial nerve is called the ***vagus***. It has an extensive course through the neck, the thorax and the abdomen.
12. The ***eleventh*** cranial nerve is called the ***accessory*** nerve because it appears to be a part of the vagus nerve (or 'accessory' to the vagus).
13. The ***twelfth*** cranial nerve is called the ***hypoglossal*** nerve (because it runs part of its course below the tongue before supplying the muscles in it (hypo = below; glossal = pertaining to tongue).

## TYPES OF FIBRES IN PERIPHERAL NERVES

1. Both spinal and cranial nerves contain fibres that can be classified into several types on the basis of their function.
2. It is necessary to consider this topic here as cranial nerves can contain some functional types of fibres not encountered in spinal nerves.
3. Fibres in a peripheral nerve are basically of two types.
4. Some fibres carry impulses from the spinal cord or brain to a peripheral organ like muscle.
   a. Impulses passing along such nerves cause the muscle to contract and thus result in movement. Such nerve fibres are called ***motor fibres.***
   b. They are also called ***efferent fibres*** (efferent = go away from).
   c. Some efferent fibres end in glands and their stimulation produces secretion. They are, therefore, called ***secretomotor fibres***.
5. Other nerve fibres carry impulses in the opposite direction i.e., towards the spinal cord or brain. They are called ***afferent fibres*** (afferent = come towards).
   a. Fibres bringing the sensations of touch from the skin, of sight from the eye, or of hearing from the ear are examples of afferent fibres.
   b. It is through these nerve fibres that we become conscious of such sensations. They are, therefore, also called ***sensory fibres.***
   c. Some afferent fibres carry impulses (e.g., from muscles or joints) of which we may not become conscious, but which are nevertheless very important for maintenance of posture and for proper control of movement. Such impulses are referred to as ***proprioceptive*** (as they have their origin within the body 'proper' and not from outside the body).
   d. Similar impulses arising from viscera also reach the brain. We are conscious of some of them (e.g., distension of the urinary bladder).
   e. Many of them do not reach our consciousness, but help to regulate the functions of the viscera.

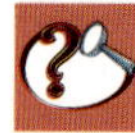

## WANT TO KNOW MORE?

6. Both afferent and efferent fibres can be further classified on the basis of the tissues supplied by them.
   a. The tissues and organs that make up the body can be broadly divided into two major parts, somatic and visceral.
   b. ***Somatic*** structures are those present in relation to the body wall (or soma); they include the tissues of the limbs (which represent a modified part of the body wall). Thus the skin, bones, joints and skeletal muscle of the limbs and body wall are classified as somatic.
   c. In contrast, the tissues that make up the internal organs like the heart, lungs or stomach are classified as ***visceral***. These include the lining epithelia of hollow viscera, and smooth muscle (including smooth muscle in the walls of blood vessels).
7. A distinction between somatic and visceral structures may also be made on embryological considerations as follows:
   a. Structures developing from specialised areas of ectoderm e.g., the retina or the membranous labyrinth, are classified as somatic.
   b. Whereas the epithelium of the tongue (and the taste buds) which is of endodermal origin is classified as visceral.
8. Skeletal muscle may be derived embryologically from three distinct sources. These are:
   a. The somites developing in the paraxial mesoderm
   b. The somatopleuric mesoderm of the body wall
   c. The mesoderm of the branchial arches.
9. The musculature of the limbs and body wall develops partly from somites and partly *in situ* from the mesoderm of the body wall. The nerves supplying this musculature are classified as somatic.
10. The muscles that move the eyeball, and the muscles of the tongue are also derived from somites and the nerves supplying them are, therefore, also classified as somatic.
11. However, skeletal muscle that develops in the mesoderm of the branchial arches is classified as visceral (or branchial).
12. Keeping in view the distinction between afferent and efferent fibres on one hand, and somatic and visceral structures on the other, we may divide fibres in peripheral nerves into four broad categories as follows:
    a. Somatic efferent
    b. Visceral efferent
    c. Somatic afferent
    d. Visceral afferent.
13. With the exception of somatic efferent fibres each of the other categories is subdivided into a ***general*** and a ***special*** group. We thus have a total of seven functional components as follows:
    a. ***Somatic efferent*** fibres supply skeletal muscle of the limbs and body wall. They also supply the extrinsic muscles of the eyeball and the muscles of the tongue.
    b. ***General visceral efferent*** fibres supply smooth muscle and glands. The nerves to glands are called secretomotor nerves.
    c. ***Special visceral efferent*** fibres supply skeletal muscle developing in branchial arch mesoderm. They are frequently called ***branchial efferent*** fibres. The muscles supplied include those of mastication, and of the face, pharynx and larynx.
    d. ***General somatic afferent*** fibres are those that carry:
       i. Sensations of touch, pain and temperature from the skin (exteroceptive sensations).
       ii. Proprioceptive impulses arising in muscles, joints and tendons. These convey information regarding movement and position of joints.
    e. ***Special somatic afferent*** fibres carry impulses of (a) vision, (b) hearing, and (c) equilibrium (from the vestibular apparatus).
    f. ***General visceral afferent*** fibres carry sensations e.g., pain from viscera (visceroceptive sensations).
    g. ***Special visceral afferent*** fibres carry the sensations of taste.

14. A typical spinal nerve contains fibres of the four general categories.
15. The special categories are present in cranial nerves only.

We will now consider the general disposition of the neurons giving rise to each of the above varieties of fibres.

## Spinal Nerve Roots

1. Each spinal nerve arises from the spinal cord by two roots, anterior (or ventral) and posterior (or dorsal).
2. Each root is formed by aggregation of rootlets that arise from one segment of the spinal cord.
3. The anterior and posterior nerve roots join each other to form a spinal nerve.
4. Just proximal to the junction of the two roots, the posterior root is marked by a swelling called the ***dorsal nerve root ganglion***.

## Neurons Supplying Typical Skeletal Muscle

1. In the spinal cord, the cell bodies of neurons supplying most skeletal muscle (derived from somites) lie in the ventral grey column. (They are, sometimes, called anterior horn cells).
2. The axons of these neurons leave the spinal cord through the ventral nerve root (43.15).
3. They then travel through the spinal nerve (and its branches) to reach a muscle and supply it.
4. The axon may divide into several branches along its course, each of which ends by supplying one muscle fibre (43.15).
5. In the case of cranial nerves the cell bodies of neurons supplying most skeletal muscle are situated in masses of grey matter present in the brainstem.

### WANT TO KNOW MORE?

6. The neurons supplying most skeletal muscle are called ***somatic efferent*** neurons.
7. In the case of cranial nerves, the neurons are located in ***somatic efferent nuclei***.
8. Some skeletal muscle is derived from branchial arches. This includes the muscles of mastication and the musculature of the face, the pharynx and the larynx.
9. Such muscle is innervated by neurons that are present in special visceral efferent nuclei of the brainstem, and are referred to as ***special visceral efferent neurons***, or ***branchial efferent neurons***.

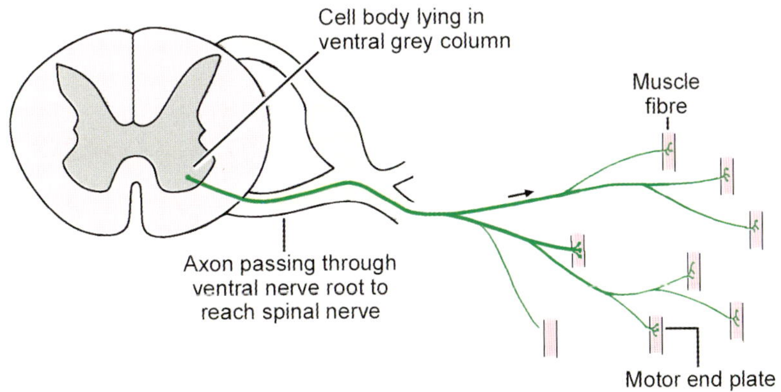


**43.15:** Scheme to show the typical arrangement of a neuron supplying skeletal muscle (somatic efferent neuron)

## Neurons Supplying Smooth Muscle and Glands

1. Nerve fibres innervating smooth muscle and glands are present in both spinal and cranial nerves.
2. The pathway for supply of smooth muscle or gland always consists of two neurons that synapse in a ganglion (43.16).
3. The first neuron carries the impulse from the brain or spinal cord to the ganglion and is, therefore, called the ***preganglionic neuron.***
4. The second neuron carries the impulse from the ganglion to smooth muscle or gland and is called the ***postganglionic neuron.***

### WANT TO KNOW MORE?

5. Neurons innervating smooth muscle or glands are ***general visceral efferent neurons***. They constitute the greater part of the autonomic nervous system.

## Afferent Neurons

1. The cell bodies of neurons that give rise to afferent fibres are located outside the central nervous system.
   a. In the case of spinal nerves, they lie in dorsal nerve root ganglia (43.17).
   b. In the case of cranial nerves, they lie in sensory ganglia (e.g., trigeminal ganglion) associated with these nerves.
2. We may illustrate the arrangement with reference to a spinal nerve (43.17).
   a. The cells of dorsal nerve root ganglia are of the unipolar type. The cell body gives off a single process that divides into a ***peripheral process*** (which is really a dendrite) and a ***central process*** (which is the axon).
   b. The peripheral process extends into the spinal nerve and courses through its branches to reach the tissue or organ supplied. It may branch repeatedly during its course. ***Such peripheral processes constitute the afferent fibres of peripheral nerves.***
   c. The sensory impulses brought by these processes from various organs of the body are conveyed to the spinal cord by the central processes. The central processes pass through the dorsal roots of spinal nerves to enter the spinal cord. In the case of cranial nerves they pass into the brainstem through the sensory roots of these nerves.

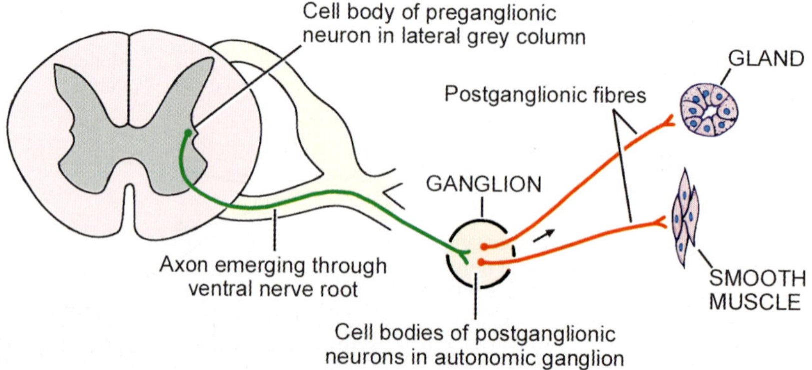


**43.16:** Scheme to show the arrangement of neurons supplying smooth muscle or gland (general visceral efferent neurons)

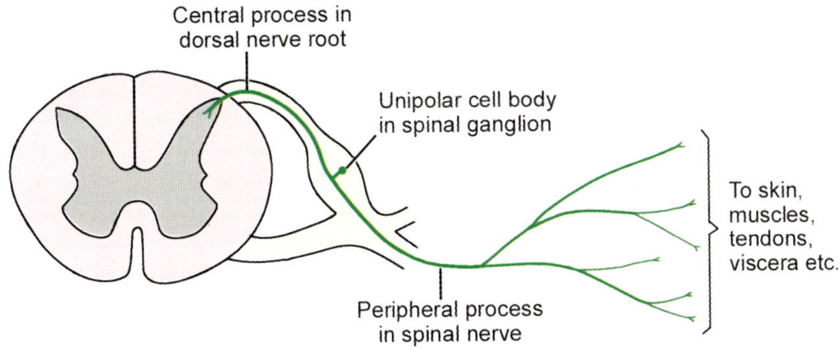


**43.17:** Scheme to show the arrangement of an afferent neuron

 **WANT TO KNOW MORE?**

3. We have seen that afferent nerve fibres can be divided into four categories viz., general somatic afferent, special somatic afferent, general visceral afferent, and special visceral afferent. The basic arrangement of neurons that give origin to all four categories of afferent fibres is similar and the description given above applies to all of them.

## CRANIAL NERVE NUCLEI

1. Cranial nerves begin or end in groups of neurons, or nuclei, present in the brain.
   a. The olfactory and optic nerves are present in relation to the cerebral hemispheres.
   b. The nuclei of remaining cranial nerves are located in the brainstem.

 **WANT TO KNOW MORE?**

2. These cranial nerve nuclei are arranged in seven groups that correspond to the seven functional types of nerve fibres described above. As a preliminary to the study of cranial nerves it is necessary to briefly consider these nuclei.
3. In the early embryo the nuclei related to the various types of fibres present in cranial nerves are arranged in vertical rows (or columns).
   a. The sequence in which the nuclei for different functional components are arranged is shown in 43.18.
   b. With further development parts of these columns disappear so that each column no longer extends through the whole length of the brainstem, but is represented by one or more discrete nuclei.
   c. These are shown schematically in 43.19. The nuclei are briefly considered below.

### Somatic Efferent Nuclei

Somatic efferent nuclei supply skeletal muscle that is derived (embryologically) from somites. They are as follows:

1. The ***oculomotor nucleus*** is situated in the midbrain (upper part, at the level of the superior colliculus). The nuclei of the two sides form a single complex that lies in the central grey matter, ventral to the aqueduct (43.20F).
2. The ***trochlear nucleus*** is situated in the midbrain (lower part, at the level of the inferior colliculus). The nucleus lies ventral to the aqueduct in the central grey matter (43.19 and 43.20E).
3. The ***abducent nucleus*** is situated in the lower part of the pons. It lies in the grey matter lining the floor of the fourth ventricle, near the midline (43.19 and 43.20C).

4. The ***hypoglossal nucleus*** lies in the medulla.
   a. It is an elongated column extending into both the open and closed parts of the medulla.
   b. Its upper part lies deep to the hypoglossal triangle in the floor of the fourth ventricle.
   c. When traced downwards it lies next to the middle line in the central grey matter ventral to the central canal (43.19 and 43.20 A and B).

**Special Visceral Efferent Nuclei**

These nuclei supply skeletal muscle derived from branchial arch mesoderm.

1. The ***motor nucleus of the trigeminal nerve*** lies in the upper part of the pons, in its dorsal part (43.19 and 43.20D).
2. The ***nucleus of the facial nerve*** lies in the lower part of the pons (43.19 and 43.20C).
3. The ***nucleus ambiguus*** lies in the medulla. It forms an elongated column that extends through both the open and closed parts of the medulla (43.19 and 43.20 A and B). It is a composite nucleus and contributes fibres to the glossopharyngeal, vagus and accessory nerves.

**General Visceral Efferent Nuclei**

1. The nuclei in this column give origin to preganglionic fibres that end in peripheral ganglia.
2. Postganglionic fibres arising in these ganglia supply smooth muscle or glands.
3. These neurons, preganglionic and postganglionic, form part of the parasympathetic nervous system.
4. The nuclei of this group are as follows. The ganglia mentioned will be studied along with the nerves concerned.
   a. The ***Edinger-Westphal nucleus*** lies in the midbrain (43.19).
      i. It is closely related to the oculomotor complex.
      ii. Fibres arising in this nucleus pass through the oculomotor nerve.
      iii. They relay in the ***ciliary ganglion*** to supply the sphincter pupillae and the ciliaris muscle.
   b. The ***salivatory nuclei*** (superior and inferior) lie in the pons (dorsal part) just above its junction with the medulla (43.19).
      i. The superior nucleus sends fibres into the facial nerve. These fibres relay in the ***submandibular ganglion*** to supply the sub-mandibular and sublingual salivary glands.
      ii. The inferior nucleus sends fibres into the glossopharyngeal nerve. These fibres relay in the ***otic ganglion*** to supply the parotid gland.
      iii. Other neurons located near the salivatory nuclei send out fibres that supply the lacrimal gland, after relaying in the ***pterygopalatine ganglion***. These fibres travel through the facial nerve.
   c. The ***dorsal (motor) nucleus of the vagus*** lies in the medulla.
      i. It is a long nucleus lying vertically.
      ii. Its upper end lies deep to the vagal triangle in the floor of the fourth ventricle.
      iii. When traced downwards it extends into the closed part of the medulla (43.19 and 43.20 A and B).
      iv. Fibres arising in this nucleus supply several thoracic and abdominal viscera.
      v. They end in ganglia closely related to these viscera.
      vi. Postganglionic fibres arising in these ganglia run a short course to supply smooth muscle and glands in these viscera.

**General and Special Visceral Afferent Nuclei**

1. Both these columns are represented by the ***nucleus of the solitary tract***, present in the medulla (43.19 and 43.20 A and B).
2. Like other cranial nerve nuclei in the medulla, the cells of this nucleus form an elongated column extending into both the open and closed parts of the medulla.
3. The nucleus of the solitary tract receives fibres carrying general visceral sensations through the vagus and glossopharyngeal nerves.

4. Fibres of taste (special visceral afferent) carried by the facial, glossopharyngeal and vagus nerves end in the upper part of the nucleus. This part is sometimes called the ***gustatory nucleus.***

**General Somatic Afferent Nuclei**

The general somatic afferent column is represented by the sensory nuclei of the trigeminal nerve. These are as follows:

1. The ***main sensory nucleus*** lies in the upper part of the pons, lateral to the motor nucleus of the nerve (43.19 and 43.20D).
2. The ***spinal nucleus*** extends from the main nucleus down into the medulla (43.19 and 43.20 A and B).
   a. It also extends into the upper two segments of the spinal cord.
   b. In addition to fibres of the trigeminal nerve, it also receives general somatic sensations carried by the facial, glossopharyngeal and vagus nerves.
3. The ***mesencephalic nucleus*** of the trigeminal nerve extends from the upper end of the main sensory nucleus into the midbrain (43.19 and 43.20 E and F).
   a. The peripheral processes of these cells are believed to carry proprioceptive impulses from muscles of mastication and possibly also from muscles of the eyeball, face and tongue.
   b. The central processes of the neurons in the nucleus probably end in the main sensory nucleus of the trigeminal nerve.

**Special Somatic Afferent Nuclei**

1. These are the cochlear and vestibular nuclei.
2. The ***cochlear nuclei*** are two in number: dorsal and ventral.
   a. They are placed dorsal and ventral to the inferior cerebellar peduncle (43.20 D and E) at the level of the junction of the pons and the medulla.
   b. These nuclei receive fibres from end organs in the cochlea that are concerned with hearing.
3. The ***vestibular nuclei*** lie in the grey matter underlying the lateral part of the floor of the fourth ventricle (43.19 and 43.20 B and C).
   a. They lie partly in the medulla and partly in the pons.
   b. They receive fibres from end organs in the vestibular part of the internal ear.
   c. They are functionally related to the maintenance of equilibrium.

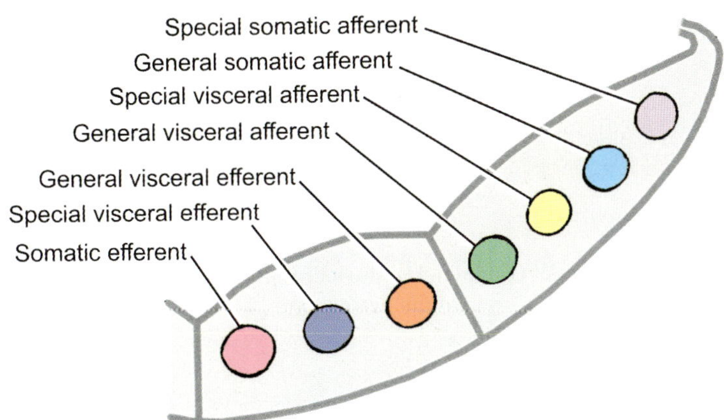


**43.18:** Arrangement of the columns of cranial nerve nuclei as seen in the embryo

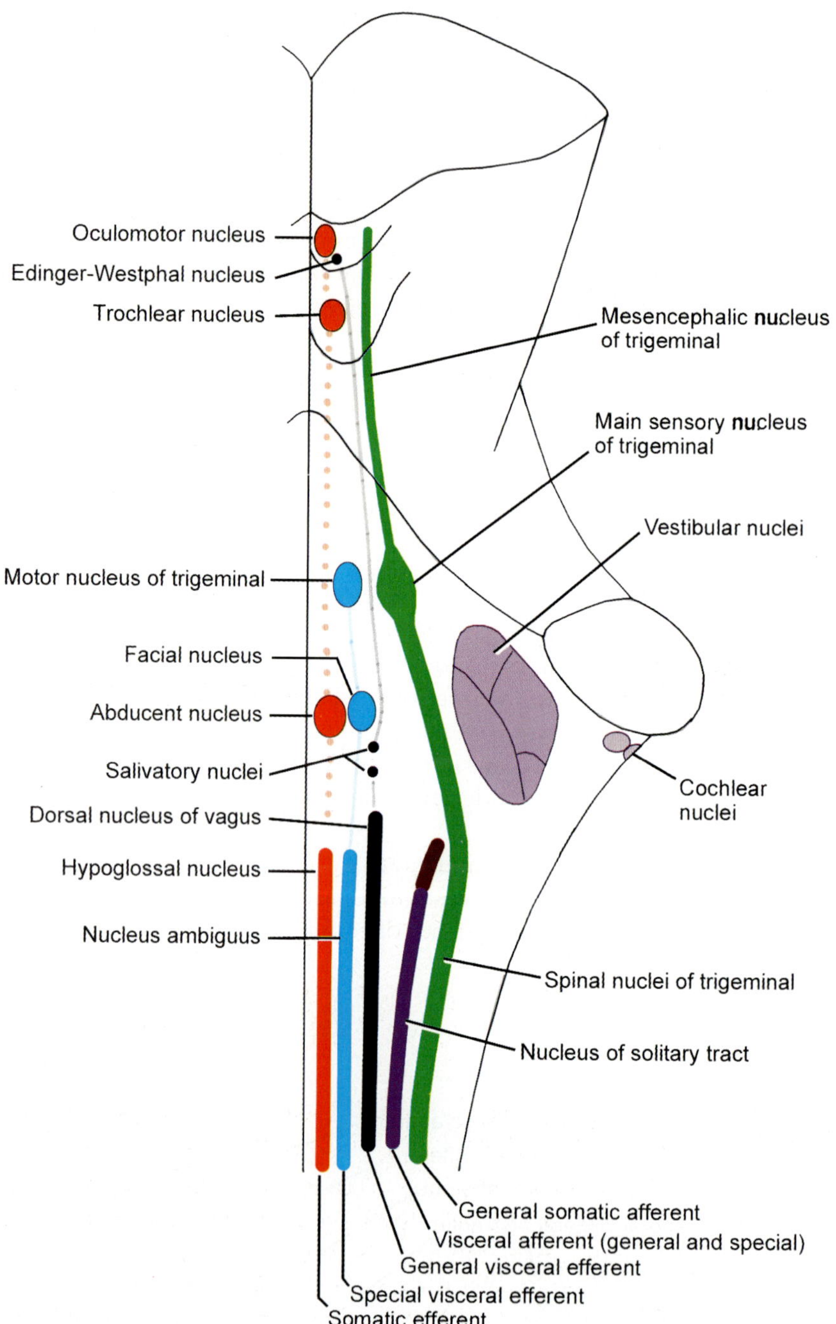


**43.19:** Schematic view of cranial nerve nuclei projected onto the posterior aspect of the brainstem

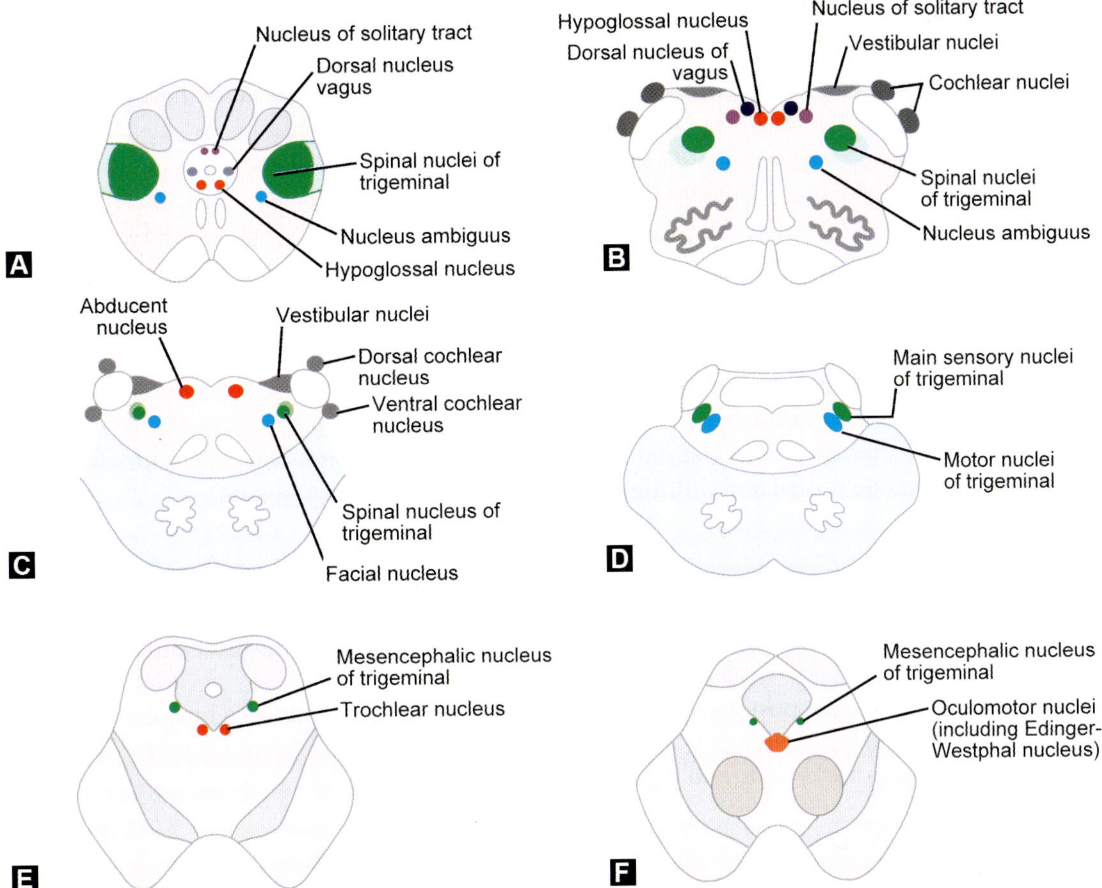


**43.20A to F:** Transverse sections through the brainstem to show the position of cranial nerve nuclei. (A and B) Upper and lower parts of midbrain; (C and D) Upper and lower parts of pons; (E and F) Upper and lower parts of medulla oblongata

## THE OLFACTORY NERVES

1. The olfactory (first cranial) nerves are purely sensory and are concerned with smell.
2. The peripheral end organ for smell is the olfactory mucosa that lines the upper and posterior part of the nasal cavity (both on the lateral wall and on the septum).
3. Nerve fibres arising in this mucosa collect to form about twenty bundles that together constitute an olfactory nerve.
4. The fibres of the olfactory nerves are processes of olfactory receptor cells located in the olfactory epithelium.
5. Each cell gives off a short peripheral process directed towards the lumen of the nasal cavity, and a larger central process that passes into the mucosa forming one fibre of the olfactory nerve.
6. These fibres collect to form about twenty bundles that collectively constitute one olfactory nerve.
   a. The bundles pass through foramina in the cribriform plate of the ethmoid bone to enter the cranial cavity (anterior cranial fossa) where they terminate in the ***olfactory bulb*** (43.21).
   b. Olfactory impulses carried by these fibres pass to other neurons located in the olfactory bulb.
   c. From the bulb they pass into the olfactory tract and ultimately end in several small areas located on the inferior surface of the cerebral hemisphere.

## WANT TO KNOW MORE?

7. The most important of these is the ***entorhinal area*** made up of the ***uncus*** and the anterior part of the ***parahippocampal gyrus*** (43.22). Smell is perceived in this region of the brain.
8. a. As the olfactory mucosa is derived from ectoderm, the olfactory nerves are classified as special somatic afferent (along with fibres for vision and hearing).
   b. However, smell is often regarded as a visceral sensation because of its close association to eating. Some authorities, therefore, classify the fibres of the olfactory nerves as special visceral afferent (like those of taste).

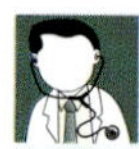

## CLINICAL CORRELATION

The olfactory nerve is tested by asking the patient to recognise various odours. The right and left nerves can be tested separately by closing one nostril and putting the substance near the open nostril.

## THE OPTIC NERVE

1. The optic nerve forms an important part of the visual pathway. It lies partly in the orbit and partly in the cranial cavity.
2. Its anterior end is attached to the posterior pole of the eyeball. The attachment lies a little medial to the antero-posterior axis of the eyeball.
3. From here the nerve passes backwards and medially:
   a. First through the orbit
   b. Next through the optic canal
   c. Finally through part of the cranial cavity.
4. The nerve ends by joining the nerve of the opposite side to form the ***optic chiasma*** (43.23).
5. The total length of the nerve is about 40 mm. Of this 25 mm is in the orbit, 5 mm in the optic canal and 10 mm in the cranial cavity.

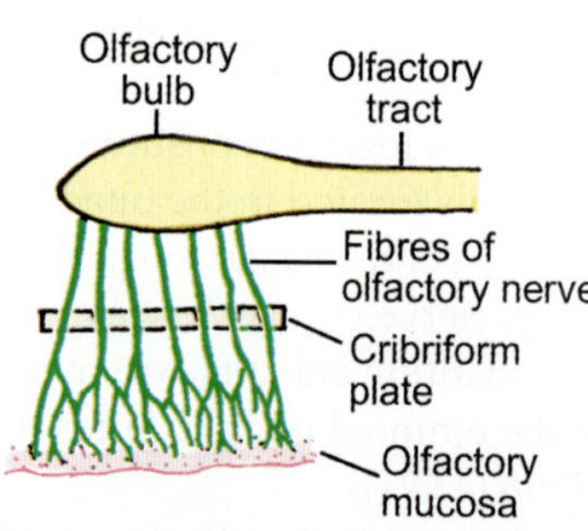


**43.21:** Scheme to show the course of the olfactory nerve

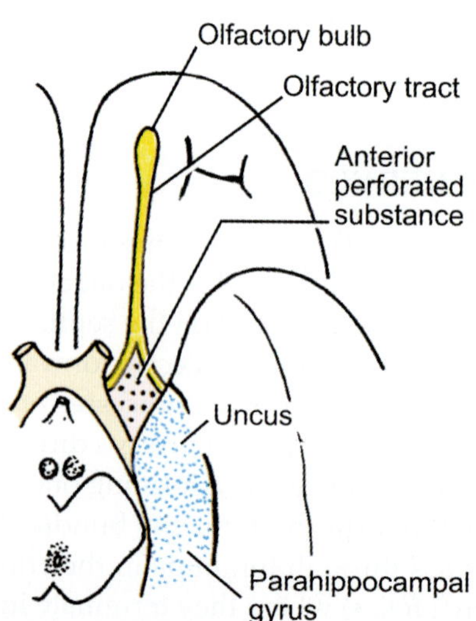


**43.22:** Diagram showing the entorhinal area made up of the uncus and the anterior part of the hippocampal gyrus

6. a. The intraorbital part of the nerve is surrounded by the superior, inferior, medial and lateral rectus muscles.
   b. The ciliary ganglion is placed between the optic nerve and the lateral rectus muscle.
   c. The ophthalmic artery is inferolateral to the nerve in the optic canal and in the posterior most part of the orbit. The artery then crosses above the nerve from lateral to medial side.
   d. Apart from the ophthalmic artery the optic nerve is crossed from medial to lateral side by:
      i. The nasociliary nerve which crosses above the optic nerve
      ii. The branch from the oculomotor nerve to the medial rectus muscle, which crosses below the nerve.
7. The central artery of the retina first lies below the optic nerve.
   a. Piercing the dural sheath of the nerve it runs forwards for a short distance between these two.
   b. About 12 mm behind the eyeball the artery enters the substance of the nerve and runs forwards in its substance to reach the eyeball.
8. The part of the optic nerve within the optic canal is related to the ophthalmic artery that lies below and lateral to it.
9. On the medial side the nerve is separated only by a thin plate of bone from the sphenoidal air sinus.
10. The intracranial part of the optic nerve is related to the internal carotid artery that is on its lateral side; and to the anterior cerebral artery that crosses above it (43.24).

**WANT TO KNOW MORE?**

11. The fibres of the optic nerve are classified as special somatic afferent (because the retina is derived from ectoderm).

## The Visual Pathway

1. The peripheral receptors for light are situated in the retina.
2. Nerve fibres arising in the retina constitute the optic nerves.
3. The two optic nerves join to form the optic chiasma in which many of their fibres cross to the opposite side.

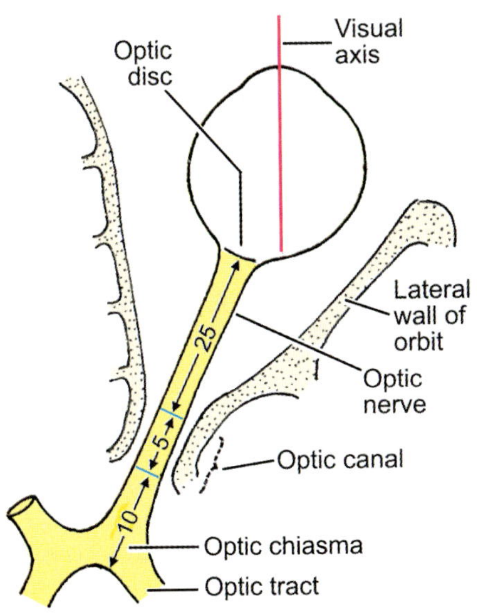


**43.23:** Scheme to show course of the optic nerve

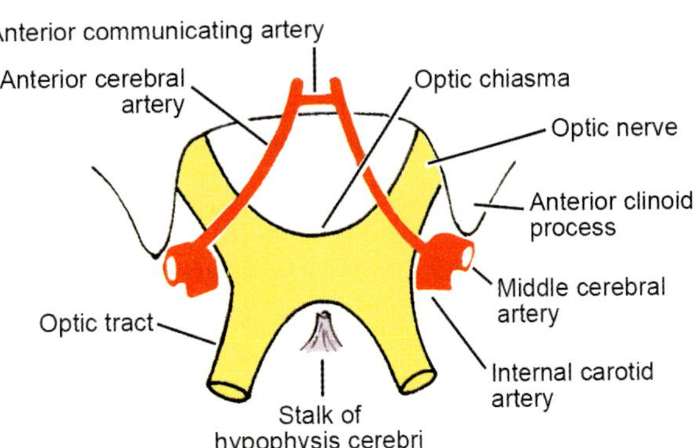


**43.24:** Some relations of the optic nerve in its intracranial part

4. The uncrossed fibres of the optic nerve, along with the fibres that have crossed over from the opposite side form the ***optic tract.***
5. The optic tract terminates predominantly in the ***lateral geniculate body***.
6. Fresh fibres arising in the lateral geniculate body form the ***geniculocalcarine tract*** (or optic radiation) that ends in the ***visual areas*** of the cerebral cortex.
7. Vision is actually perceived in the cerebral cortex.
8. Nerve fibres arising in the retina converge upon an area on the posteromedial part of the eyeball called the optic disc.
9. Here the fibres pass through the thickness of the retina, the choroid and the sclera. In this situation the sclera has numerous perforations and is, therefore, called the ***lamina cribrosa*** (crib = sieve).
10. The optic nerve is formed by the aggregation of fibres passing out through the lamina cribrosa.

## WANT TO KNOW MORE?

11. The optic nerve contains about 1,200,000 fibres.
12. The optic nerves are surrounded by sheaths formed by prolongation onto them of the dura mater, the arachnoid mater and the pia mater.
13. Fibres responsible for sharp vision arise from an area of the retina called the ***macula***. The fibres arising from the macula form the ***papillomacular bundle.***
14. Close to the eyeball the macular fibres occupy the lateral part of the optic nerve, but by the time they reach the chiasma they lie in the central part of the nerve.

15. The fibres of the optic nerve arising in the medial (or nasal) half of each retina enter the optic tract of the opposite side after crossing in the optic chiasma.
16. Fibres of the lateral (or temporal) half of each retina enter the optic tract of the same side.
17. Thus the right optic tract comes to contain fibres from the right halves of both retinae; and the left tract from the left halves.
18. The optic tract carries these fibres to the lateral geniculate body of the corresponding side.
19. From here they are relayed to the corresponding cerebral hemisphere. (For details of the visual pathway see chapter 54). The effects of damage are given later in this chapter.

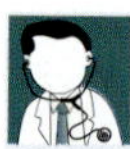

## CLINICAL CORRELATION

*Testing the Optic Nerve*

1. To test the optic nerve first ask the patient if his vision is normal.
2. Acuity (sharpness) of vision can be tested by making the patient read letters of various sizes printed on a chart from a fixed distance. It must be remembered that loss of acuity of vision can be caused by errors of refraction, or by the presence of opacities in the cornea or the lens (cataract).
3. As part of a normal clinical examination the field of vision can be tested as follows:
    a. Ask the patient to sit opposite you (about half a meter away) and look straight forwards at you.
    b. As one eye to be tested at a time, ask the patient to place a hand on one eye so that he can see only with the other eye.
    c. Stretch out one of your arms laterally so that your hand is about equal distance from your face and that of the patient.
    d. Keep moving your index finger and gradually bring the hand towards yourself until you can just see the movements of the finger. This gives you an idea of the extent of your own visual field in that direction.

e. By asking the patient to tell you as soon as he can see the moving finger (making sure that he does not turn his head) you can get an idea of the patients' field of vision in the direction of your hand.
f. By repeating the test placing your hand in different directions a good idea of the field of vision of the patient can be obtained.
g. If an abnormality is suspected, detailed testing can be done using a procedure called ***perimetry***.

4. If there is any doubt about the integrity of optic nerve, the retina is examined using an ophthalmoscope. With this instrument we can see the interior of the eye through the pupil of the eye. The optic disc and blood vessels radiating from it can be seen.

*Effects of Injury to Visual Pathway*

1. Injuries to different parts of the visual pathway can produce various kinds of defects.
2. Loss of vision in one half (right or left) of the visual field is called ***hemianopia***.
3. If the same half of the visual field is lost in both eyes the defect is said to be ***homonymous*** and if different halves are lost the defect is said to be ***heteronymous***.
4. Note that the hemianopia is named in relation to the visual field and not to the retina.
5. Injury to the optic nerve will produce total blindness in the eye concerned.
6. Damage to the central part of the optic chiasma (e.g., by pressure from an enlarged hypophysis) interrupts the crossing fibres derived from the nasal halves of the two retinae resulting in ***bitemporal heteronymous hemianopia***.
7. It has been claimed that macular fibres are more susceptible to damage by pressure than peripheral fibres and are affected first.
8. When the lateral part of the chiasma is affected a ***nasal hemianopia*** results. This may be unilateral or bilateral.
9. Complete destruction of the optic tract, the lateral geniculate body, the optic radiation or the visual cortex of one side, results in loss of the opposite half of the field of vision.
10. A lesion on the right side leads to ***left homonymous hemianopia***. Lesions anterior to the lateral geniculate body also interrupt fibres responsible for the pupillary light reflex.

## THE OCULOMOTOR NERVE

1. The oculomotor is the third cranial nerve. The distribution of this nerve is shown in 43.25.
2. Most of the fibres of this nerve arise from the oculomotor nuclear complex that is situated in the upper part of the midbrain (ventral to the aqueduct, 43.19 and 43.20F).
   a. The right and left nuclei are fused to form a midline complex.
   b. Fibres arising in the complex supply all extrinsic muscles of the eyeball except the lateral rectus and the superior oblique. These fibres also supply the levator palpebrae superioris.
3. Some fibres of the oculomotor nerve arise from the **Edinger-Westphal** nucleus that forms part of the oculomotor complex.

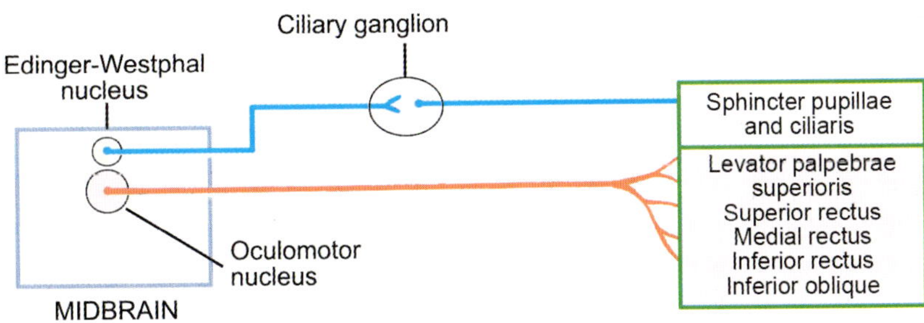


**43.25:** Scheme to show the distribution of the oculomotor nerve

a. Fibres arising in this nucleus relay in the ciliary ganglion.
b. Postganglionic fibres arising in this ganglion supply the sphincter pupillae and the ciliaris muscle.

4. Arising from these nuclei the fibres of the oculomotor nerve pass forwards through the substance of the midbrain and emerge from the cerebral peduncle (43.26 and 43.27).
   a. Just in front of the midbrain the nerve passes between the superior cerebellar artery (which lies below it) and the posterior cerebral artery (which lies above it).
   b. Here the nerve lies in the subarachnoid space.
   c. Passing forwards and laterally the nerve pierces the arachnoid. It then pierces the inner layer of dura mater in the triangular interval bounded by the free and attached margins of the tentorium cerebelli (43.26).
   d. The nerve now comes to lie in the lateral wall of the cavernous sinus (43.28). In the anterior part of this wall the nerve divides into superior and inferior rami.
5. The superior and inferior rami of the oculomotor nerve enter the orbit by passing through the superior orbital fissure (43.30). They pass through the part of the fissure that lies within the tendinous ring that gives origin to the four recti of the eyeball.
6. Within the orbit, the superior ramus supplies:
   a. The superior rectus
   b. The levator palpebrae superioris.
7. The inferior division supplies:
   a. The medial rectus
   b. The inferior rectus and
   c. The inferior oblique (43.29).

## WANT TO KNOW MORE?

8. Preganglionic fibres arising from the Edinger-Westphal nucleus travel through the trunk of the nerve, and then through its inferior division.
   a. They then pass into the nerve for the inferior oblique muscle.
   b. A short branch arising from this nerve conveys the fibres to the ciliary ganglion. This branch to the ciliary ganglion from the nerve to the inferior oblique constitutes the ***motor root*** of the ganglion.
   c. The cells of the ganglion give origin to postganglionic fibres that pass through the short ciliary nerves to reach the sphincter pupillae and the ciliaris muscles.
9. Scheme to show the connections of the ciliary ganglion is given in 43.31.
   a. The ciliary ganglion lies lateral to the optic nerve (between it and the lateral rectus).
   b. Posteriorly, it receives three roots: motor or parasympathetic, sympathetic, and sensory.
   c. The motor or parasympathetic root has been described above.
   d. The ***sympathetic root*** arises from the sympathetic plexus on the internal carotid artery. It carries postganglionic sympathetic fibres that begin in the superior cervical sympathetic ganglion.
   e. Sympathetic fibres pass through the ciliary ganglion, without relay, and enter the short ciliary nerves through which they reach the blood vessels of the eyeball.
   f. The fibres for the dilator pupillae normally follow a separate route, as described below, but sometimes they may pass through the ciliary ganglion.
   g. The sensory root of the ciliary ganglion is a branch of the nasociliary nerve. It carries sensory fibres that begin in the cornea, the iris and the choroid; pass through the short ciliary nerves and then through the ciliary ganglion; and finally enter the sensory root through which they reach the nasociliary nerve.
   h. The fibres of the oculomotor nerve that supply skeletal muscle are classified as somatic efferent, while those that supply smooth muscle (sphincter pupillae, ciliaris) are general visceral efferent.

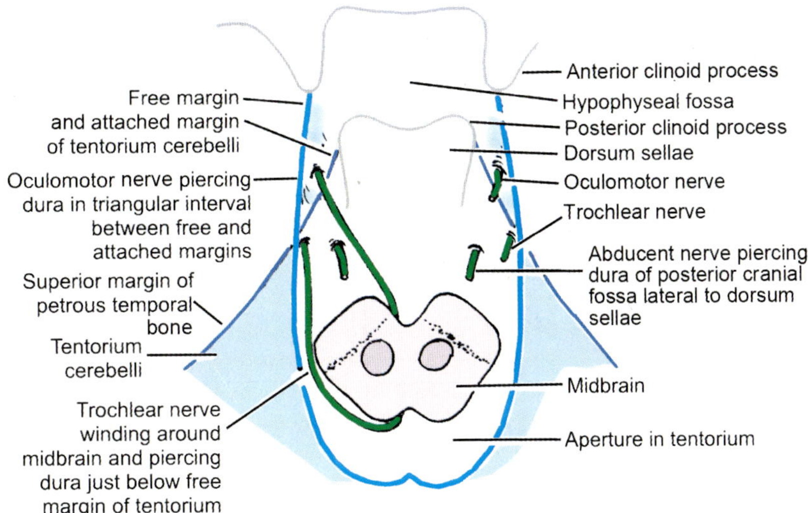


**43.26:** Diagram to show the sites of penetration of dura mater by the oculomotor, trochlear and abducent nerves

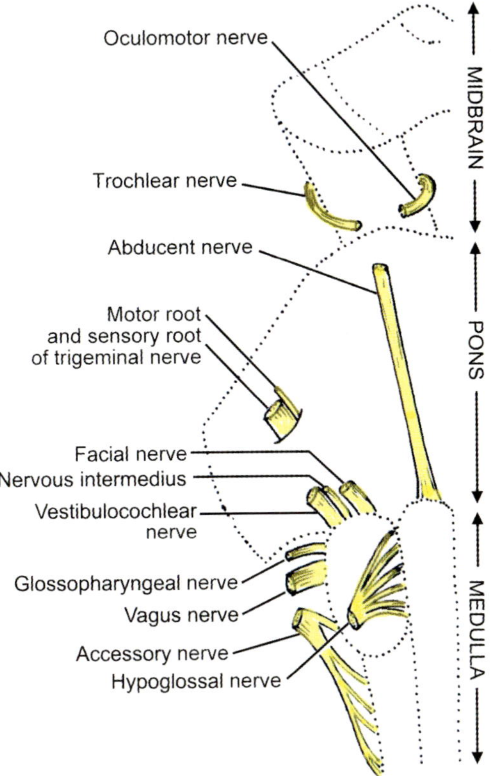


**43.27:** Attachment of cranial nerves to the surface of the brainstem

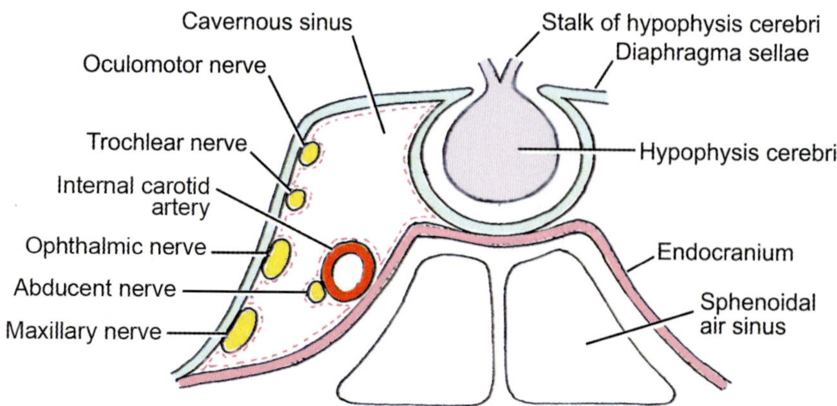


**43.28:** Relationship of cranial nerves to the cavernous sinus

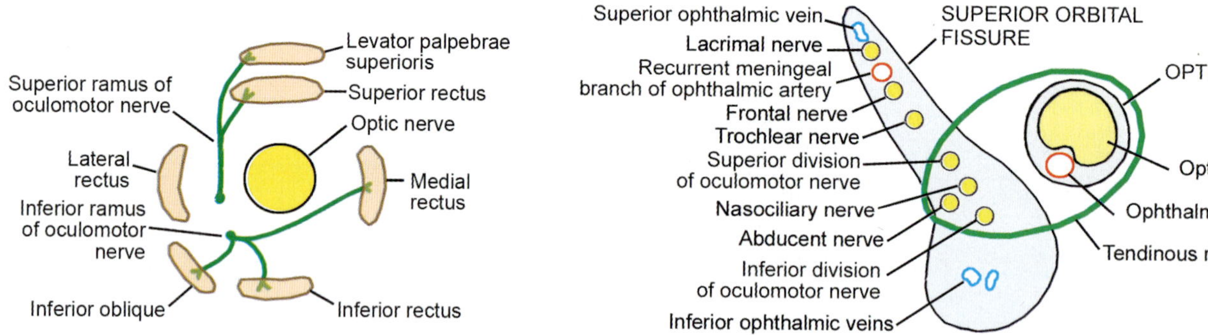


**43.29:** Distribution of oculomotor nerve

**43.30:** Position of cranial nerves in the superior orbital fissure

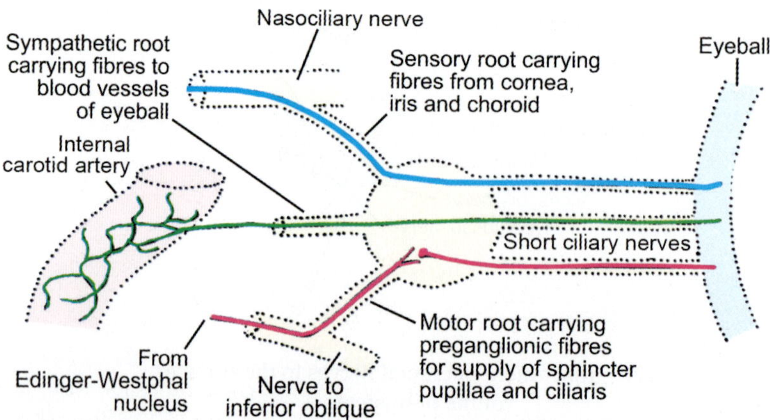


**43.31:** Scheme to show the connections of the ciliary ganglion

## THE TROCHLEAR NERVE

1. The trochlear nerve is the fourth cranial nerve.
2. It is made up of fibres that arise in the trochlear nucleus located in the lower part of the midbrain (ventral to the aqueduct, 43.19 and 43.20E).
3. Fibres arising in this nucleus pass ***backwards*** winding round the central grey matter of the midbrain to reach the upper part of the anterior (or superior) medullary velum (43.32).
   a. Here the fibres of the right and left sides ***cross.***
   b. After this decussation the fibres emerge on the posterior surface of the brainstem just below the inferior colliculus.
4. Having emerged from the midbrain the nerve winds round the cerebral peduncle to reach the front of the brain stem (43.27). While winding round the cerebral peduncle the nerve lies between the posterior cerebral artery (above it) and the superior cerebellar artery (below it).

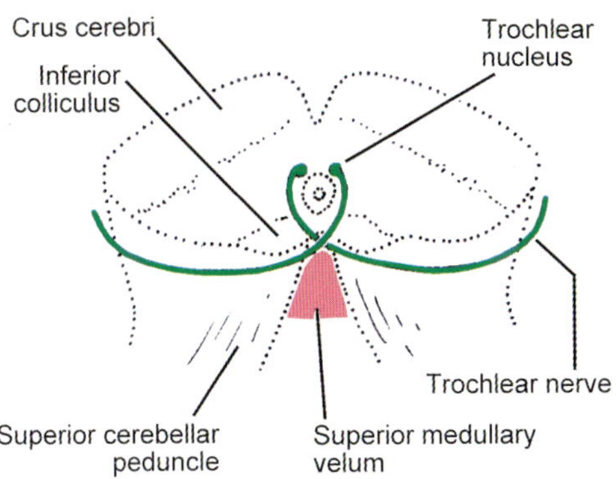


**43.32:** Schematic posterior view of the course of the trochlear nerve

5. The nerve now runs forwards and pierces the dura mater just below the free margin of the tentorium cerebelli (43.26). The point of penetration of the dura mater lies a little behind the posterior clinoid process.
6. Having pierced the dura the nerve comes to lie in the lateral wall of the cavernous sinus, below the oculomotor nerve, but above the ophthalmic division of the trigeminal nerve (43.28).
7. Continuing forwards it crosses lateral to the oculomotor nerve to enter the upper part of the superior orbital fissure (43.30). In the fissure it lies above the tendinous ring for origin of the recti of the eyeball (43.30).
8. Having entered the orbit the nerve runs forwards, above the orbital muscles, and ends in the superior oblique muscle.

### WANT TO KNOW MORE?

9. a. The trochlear nerve is the only cranial nerve that emerges on the posterior (or dorsal) aspect of the brainstem.
   b. It is also the only nerve that undergoes decussation.
   c. As a result of the decussation the left trochlear nerve is formed by fibres arising from the right trochlear nucleus and vice versa.
10. The fibres of the trochlear nerve are classified as somatic efferent.

The next cranial nerve, in order of numerical sequence, is the fifth or trigeminal. However, the abducent nerve (sixth) is considered first as its course and distribution are similar to those of the oculomotor and trochlear nerves.

## THE ABDUCENT NERVE

1. This is the sixth cranial nerve. It is made up of fibres that arise in the abducent nucleus and supply the lateral rectus muscle of the eyeball.
2. The abducent nucleus (43.19 and 43.20C) is located in the lower part of the pons, in relation to the upper part of the floor of the fourth ventricle. The position of the nucleus in relation to the floor of the fourth ventricles is indicated by an elevation called the ***facial colliculus.***

3. Arising from this nucleus the fibres of the nerve pass through the substance of the pons and emerge on the surface of the brainstem at the lower border of the pons cranial to the pyramid (43.27).
4. The nerve then runs upwards, forwards and laterally.
   a. It pierces the dura lateral to the dorsum sellae of the sphenoid bone (43.26).
   b. It then runs upwards to reach the upper border of the petrous temporal bone and bends round it to enter the middle cranial fossa.
   c. The nerve now comes to lie within the cavernous sinus, where it is closely related to the internal carotid artery. The nerve is first lateral to the artery and then inferolateral to it.
5. At the anterior end of the cavernous sinus the nerve passes through the superior orbital fissure to enter the orbit. Its position in the fissure is shown in 43.30.
6. The nerve ends by supplying the lateral rectus muscle.
7. The fibres of the abducent nerve are classified as somatic efferent (like all nerve fibres supplying extrinsic muscles of the eyeballs).

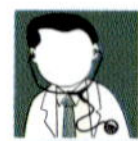

## CLINICAL CORRELATION

**Oculomotor, Trochlear and Abducent Nerves**

1. These three nerves are responsible for movements of the eyeball.
2. In a routine clinical examination, the movements are tested by asking the patient to keep his head fixed and to move his eyes in various directions i.e., upwards, downwards, inwards and outwards.
   a. An easy way is to ask the patient to keep his head fixed, and to follow the movements of your finger with his eyes.
   b. Such an examination can detect a gross abnormality in movement of the eyes.
3. Sometimes, one of the ocular muscles may not be completely paralysed but may be weak. Two indications of such weakness are given below.

***Diplopia***

1. This term means that objects are seen double.
   a. To understand this phenomenon remember that objects lying in different parts of the visual field produce images over different spots on the retina.
   b. The brain judges the position of an object by the position at which its image is formed on the retina.
2. Normally the movements of the right and left eyes are in perfect alignment, and an object casts an image on corresponding spots on the two retinae so that only one image is perceived by the brain.
3. When a muscle of the eyeball is weak, and a movement involving that muscle is performed, the movement of the defective eye is slightly less than that of the normal eye.
   a. As a result images of the object on the two retinae are not formed at corresponding points but over two points near each other.
   b. The brain therefore 'sees' two images, one from each retina.

***Squint (or Strabismus)***

1. This is a condition in which the two eyes do not look in the same direction.
2. The squint becomes obvious when the eye movement involves a muscle that is paralysed or weak, because the weak muscle cannot keep up with the muscle of the normal side.
3. As explained above squint will be accompanied by diplopia.
4. However, the patient compensates for lack of movement of the eyeball by turning the head in the direction of the object and on doing so the diplopia disappears.
5. If the normal eye is closed, the patient is unable to judge the position of objects in the field of vision correctly (because the image of the object does not fall on the part of the retina that corresponds to the true position of the object).

6. All the features described above are those of ***paralytic squint***.
7. There is another type of squint called ***concomitant squint***.
   a. This condition is congenital, and manifests itself in early childhood.
   b. Squint is present in all positions of the eyeball.
   c. There is no muscular weakness and movements are normal in all directions.
   d. There is no diplopia.

**Paralysis of Oculomotor Nerve**

1. All movements of the eyeball are lost in the affected eye.
2. When the patient is asked to look directly forwards the affected eye is directed laterally (by the lateral rectus) and downwards (by the superior oblique). There is lateral quint (***external strabismus***) and diplopia.
3. As the levator palpebrae superioris is paralysed there is drooping of the upper eyelid (***ptosis***).
4. As parasympathetic fibres to the sphincter pupillae pass through the oculomotor nerve, the sphincter pupillae is paralysed. Unopposed action of sympathetic nerves produces a fixed and dilated pupil.
5. a. Normally the pupil contracts when exposed to light (light reflex).
   b. It also contracts when the relaxed eye is made to concentrate on a near object (accommodation reflex).
   c. Both these reflexes are lost. The power of accommodation is lost because of paralysis of the ciliaris muscle.

**Paralysis of Trochlear Nerve**

1. a. The superior oblique muscle (supplied by the trochlear nerve) moves the eyeball downwards and laterally.
   b. The inferior rectus (supplied by the oculomotor nerve) moves it downwards and medially.
2. For direct downward movement synchronised action of both muscles is required.
3. When the superior oblique muscle is paralysed the eyeball deviates medially on trying to look downwards.

**Paralysis of Abducent Nerve**

1. This nerve supplies the lateral rectus muscle that moves the eyeball laterally.
2. In looking forwards the lateral pull of the lateral rectus is counteracted by the medial pull of the medial rectus and so the eye is maintained in the centre.
3. When the lateral rectus is paralysed the affected eye deviates medially (medial squint, or ***internal strabismus***).

## THE TRIGEMINAL NERVE

### Introductory Remarks

1. The trigeminal nerve is so called because it consists of three main divisions. These are:
   a. The ophthalmic nerve
   b. The maxillary nerve
   c. The mandibular nerve.
2. These nerves arise from a large trigeminal ganglion.
   a. The ganglion is connected to the brainstem (pons) by a thick sensory root.
   b. The trigeminal nerve also has a motor root (43.27) which emerges from the pons medial to the sensory root. (Note: M for motor and M for medial).
   c. The motor root passes deep to the trigeminal ganglion and joins the mandibular nerve (see 43.33).
3. The trigeminal nerve contains both afferent and efferent fibres.
4. Afferent fibres are peripheral processes of unipolar neurons located in the trigeminal ganglion.
   a. They are distributed through all three divisions of the nerve.
   b. They carry exteroceptive sensations from the skin of the face, the mucous membrane of the mouth, and the mucous membrane of the nose.

5. The central processes of the neurons in the trigeminal ganglion form the sensory root.
   a. After entering the pons these processes terminate in relation to neurons in the main sensory nucleus, and in the spinal nucleus of the trigeminal nerve (43.34).
   b. These nuclei are shown in 43.19 and 43.20 A to D.
6. Another group of afferent fibres carry proprioceptive impulses from the muscles of mastication (and possibly from the ocular, facial and lingual muscles).
   a. These fibres are believed to be peripheral processes of unipolar neurons present in the mesencephalic nucleus of the trigeminal nerve.
   b. The central processes of these neurons end in relation to the main sensory nucleus.
7. The muscles of mastication (and some other muscles) are supplied through the mandibular division of the trigeminal nerve.
   a. The cell bodies of the neurons giving origin to these fibres are located in the motor nucleus of the trigeminal nerve.
   b. Axons arising from these neurons collect to form the motor root of the nerve.
   c. The motor root joins the mandibular nerve and is distributed through it.

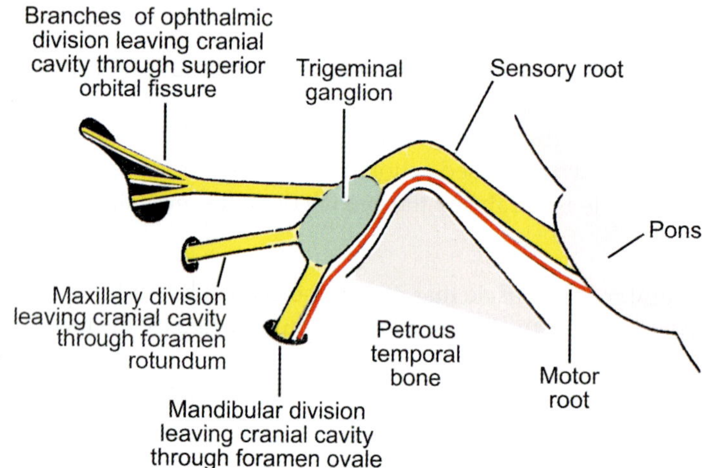


**43.33:** Roots and divisions of the trigeminal nerve

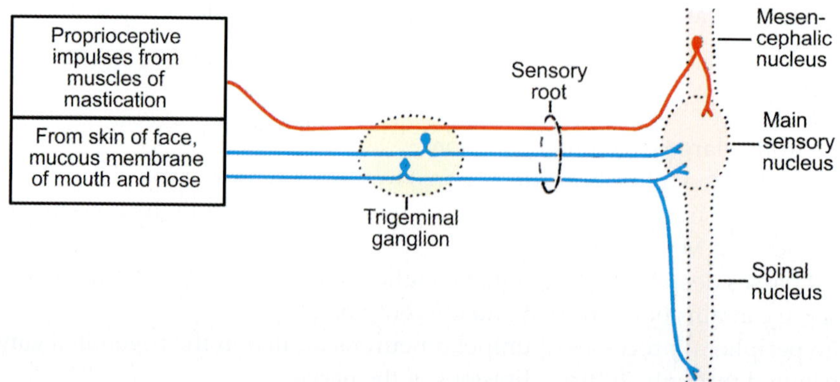


**43.34:** Scheme to show the arrangement of afferent neurons of the trigeminal nerve. The fibres that descend along the spinal nucleus constitute the spinal tract of the nerve

8. The muscles supplied by the motor fibres are as follows:
   a. ***Muscles of mastication***: Masseter, temporalis, medial and lateral pterygoids.
   b. ***Other muscles***: Mylohyoid, anterior belly of digastric, tensor palati, tensor tympani.

**WANT TO KNOW MORE?**

Functional components of trigeminal nerve:

1. The afferent fibres of the nerve (from skin and mucosa and proprioceptive from muscle) are classified as general somatic afferent.
2. The efferent fibres are classified as special visceral efferent as the muscles supplied are derived (during development) from the mesoderm of the first branchial arch.

## The Trigeminal Ganglion

1. This ganglion is shaped like a crescent (43.35). It has a convex border facing anterolaterally and a concave border facing posteromedially.
2. The convex border is continuous with the ophthalmic, maxillary and mandibular nerves; while the concave posterior border is continuous with the sensory root.
3. The ganglion is placed in a depression (called the ***trigeminal impression***) on the anterior aspect of the petrous temporal bone (near its apex).
4. The ganglion is enclosed within a pouch-like recess of dura mater. This recess is called the ***trigeminal cave***.

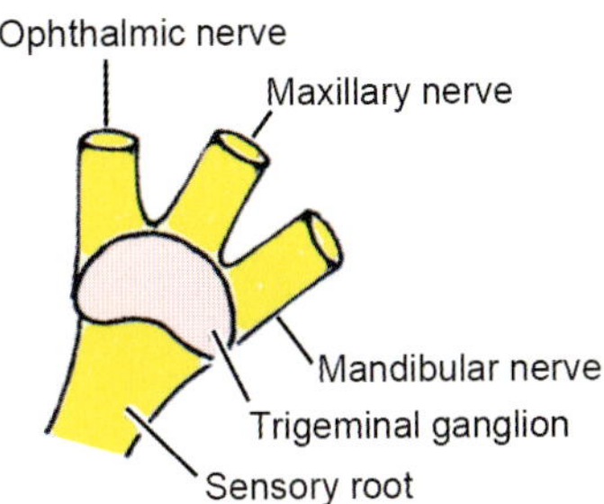


**43.35:** Trigeminal ganglion seen from above

## THE OPHTHALMIC NERVE

1. The fibres of the ophthalmic nerve are purely sensory. However, some sympathetic fibres for the eyeball travel for part of their course through the nerve and some of its branches.
2. The ophthalmic nerve arises from the trigeminal ganglion (43.36). It pierces the dura of the trigeminal cave and comes to lie in the lateral wall of the cavernous sinus, below the trochlear nerve (43.28).
3. Passing forwards it divides into three branches. These are:
   a. The lacrimal nerve
   b. The frontal nerve
   c. The nasociliary nerve.
4. These branches enter the orbit by passing through the superior orbital fissure.
   a. Their positions in the fissure are shown in 43.30.
   b. From this figure it will be obvious that on entering the orbit the lacrimal and frontal branches will lie above the orbital muscles; while the nasociliary nerve will lie between them, lateral to the optic nerve.
   c. The further course of each of these branches is as follows (43.36).
5. The ***lacrimal nerve*** runs along the lateral wall of the orbit (along the upper border of the lateral rectus).
   a. It ends in the lacrimal gland (and hence its name).
   b. Some branches pass through the gland to supply the conjunctiva and the skin of the upper eyelid.
   c. The lacrimal nerve is joined by a twig from the zygomaticotemporal branch of the maxillary nerve.
6. The ***frontal nerve*** runs forwards between the levator palpebrae superioris and the periosteum lining the roof of the orbit. It ends by dividing into supraorbital and supratrochlear branches.
7. The ***supraorbital nerve*** continues in the line of the frontal nerve (43.36), lying between the levator palpebrae superioris and the roof of the orbit.
   a. Reaching the orbital margin it passes through the supraorbital notch (on the medial part of the upper margin of the orbit) and curves upwards into the forehead.
   b. Here it divides into medial and lateral branches that supply the scalp as far back as the lambdoid suture.

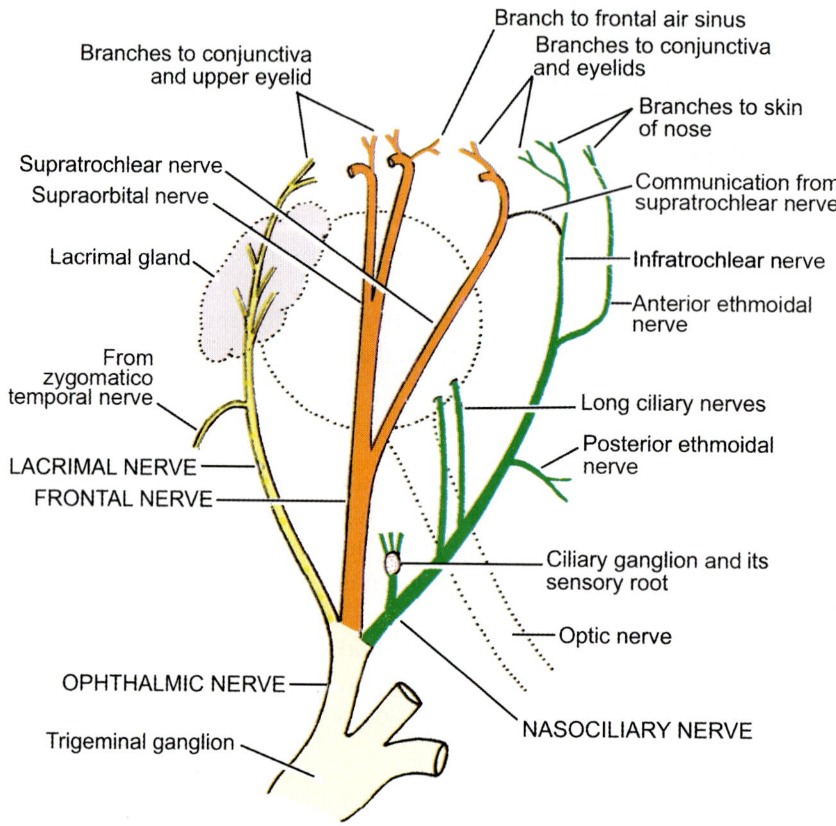


**43.36:** Scheme to show the distribution of the ophthalmic nerve

## WANT TO KNOW MORE?

Other branches given off by the supraorbital nerve are:

c. Branches to the conjunctiva and the skin of the upper eyelid.
d. Branches to the mucous membrane of the frontal air sinus.
e. Some branches to the deeper tissues of the scalp.

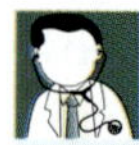

## CLINICAL CORRELATION

The nerve supply to the frontal sinus is of clinical importance. In frontal sinusitis pain is referred to the area of the scalp supplied by the supraorbital nerve (***frontal headache***).

8. The ***supratrochlear nerve*** runs forwards and medially above the orbital muscles, and medial to the supraorbital nerve.
   a. It passes above the trochlea (for the tendon of the superior oblique muscle).
   b. Reaching the upper margin of the orbital aperture, near its medial end, the nerve turns upwards into the forehead giving branches to the skin over its lower and medial part.

   Other branches given off by the supratrochlear nerve are:

   c. A descending branch which joins the infratrochlear branch of the nasociliary nerve (43.36).
   d. Branches to the conjunctiva and skin of the upper eyelid.

9. On entering the orbit the ***nasociliary nerve*** lies between the optic nerve and the lateral rectus.
   a. The nerve then runs medially crossing above the optic nerve (43.36).
   b. As it does so it lies below the superior rectus muscle.
   c. Reaching the medial wall of the orbit the nerve ends by dividing into the ***anterior ethmoidal*** and ***infratrochlear*** nerves.
10. The branches of the nasociliary nerve are as follows (43.36):
   a. Just after entering the orbit the nasociliary nerve receives the ***sensory root of the ciliary ganglion.***
   b. The ***long ciliary nerves*** (two or three) arise from the nasociliary nerve as it crosses the optic nerve.
      i. They run forwards to the eyeball where they pierce the sclera; and then run between the sclera and the choroid.
      ii. They supply sensory fibres to the ciliary body, the iris and the cornea.
      iii. They also carry postganglionic sympathetic fibres meant for the dilator pupillae.
   c. The ***posterior ethmoidal branch*** enters the posterior ethmoidal foramen (on the medial wall of the orbit) and supplies the ethmoidal and sphenoidal air sinuses.

## WANT TO KNOW MORE?

iv. These sympathetic fibres begin in the superior cervical sympathetic ganglion (43.37) and travel through a plexus surrounding the internal carotid artery. They pass to the nasociliary nerve while the latter lies in the wall of the cavernous sinus.

   d. The ***anterior ethmoidal nerve*** has a complicated course through the orbit, the anterior cranial fossa, and the nasal cavity. We will not go into details of the course. Its terminal part is seen on the face as the external nasal nerve.
      i. It gives ***internal nasal branches*** to the nasal septum and to the lateral wall of the nasal cavity.
      ii. At the lower border of the nasal bone the nerve leaves the nasal cavity, becomes superficial and supplies the skin over the lower part of the nose. This part of the nerve is called the ***external nasal nerve***.
   e. The ***infratrochlear nerve*** (43.36) runs forwards on the medial wall of the orbit and ends by supplying part of the skin of the upper and lower eyelids and over the upper part of the nose.

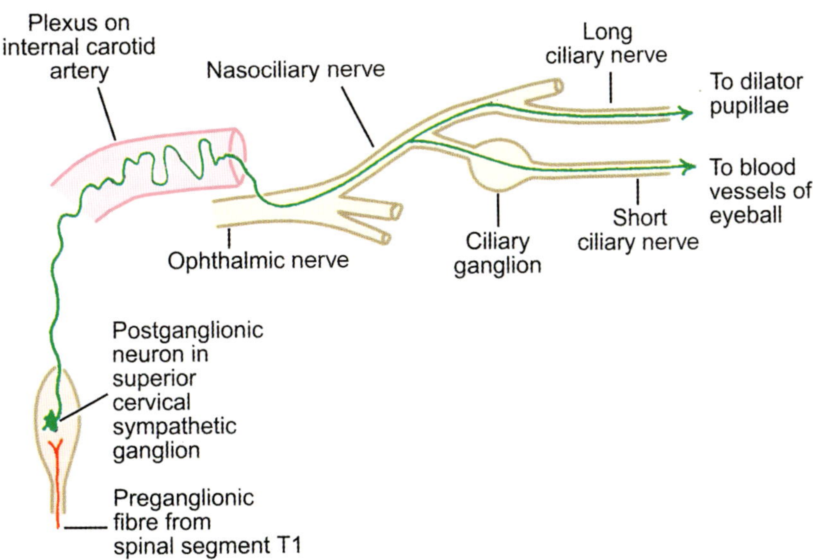


**43.37:** Two pathways followed by sympathetic fibres for the eyeball. Occasionally, the fibres for the dilator pupillae may pass through the ciliary ganglion

The nerve also gives branches to:
i. The conjunctiva
ii. The lacrimal sac
iii. The lacrimal caruncle.

11. The infratrochlear and supratrochlear nerves are joined to each other by a communicating twig.
12. The areas of skin of the face and scalp supplied by the branches of the ophthalmic nerve are shown in 37.15.

## THE MAXILLARY NERVE

1. The maxillary nerve is purely sensory. It arises from the middle of the distal edge of the trigeminal ganglion (43.33).
2. Piercing the dura forming the distal edge of the trigeminal cave it comes to lie in the lower part of the lateral wall of the cavernous sinus: its position here is shown in 43.28.
3. The nerve leaves the middle cranial fossa through the foramen rotundum to reach the pterygopalatine fossa.

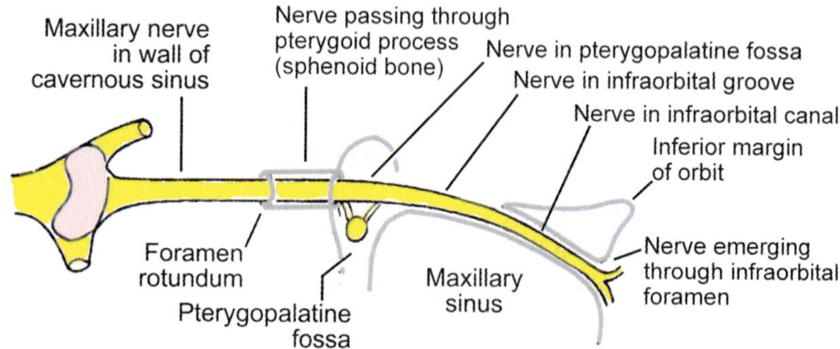


**43.38:** Scheme to show the course of the maxillary nerve

4. The nerve crosses the short distance between the anterior and posterior walls of the fossa and leaves it by passing into the orbit through the inferior orbital fissure.
5. The part of the maxillary nerve (43.38) distal to the inferior orbital fissure is called the ***infraorbital nerve.***
   a. This nerve lies first in the infraorbital groove
   b. Thereafter in the infraorbital canal.
6. It appears on the face through the infraorbital foramen and ends here by dividing into a number of terminal branches. Several branches are also given off by the maxillary and infraorbital nerves along their course as follows.

### WANT TO KNOW MORE?

**Branch in Middle Cranial Fossa**

1. Before entering the foramen rotundum the maxillary nerve gives off a ***meningeal branch*** to the dura mater of the middle cranial fossa (43.40).

**Branches Arising in Pterygopalatine Fossa**

2. In the pterygopalatine fossa the maxillary nerve is connected to the pterygopalatine ganglion by two ***ganglionic branches*** (43.24 and 43.25).
   a. Many fibres of the maxillary nerve pass through these ganglionic branches to the ganglion.
   b. They, however, have no functional relationship to the ganglion and leave it through a number of branches which are as follows (43.39).

***Branches to the Palate***

3. Two palatine nerves: greater and lesser, arise from the lower part of the ganglion.
   a. They enter the greater palatine canal that opens superiorly into the pterygopalatine fossa; and inferiorly at the posterolateral corner of the hard palate through the greater and lesser palatine foramina.
   b. The ***greater palatine nerve*** emerges through the greater palatine foramen and then runs forwards on the inferior surface of the hard palate (43.39) supplying mucous membrane and glands. (The most anterior part of the hard palate is supplied by the nasopalatine nerve described below).

c. The ***lesser palatine nerves*** (usually two) emerge through the lesser palatine foramina and run backwards into the soft palate. They also supply the tonsil.

*Branches to the Nose*

4. Some ***posterior inferior nasal branches*** arise from the greater palatine nerve and pass through minute apertures in the medial wall of the canal to enter the nasal cavity. They supply the posterior and inferior part of the lateral wall of the nasal cavity (inferior concha, middle meatus, inferior meatus).
5. Several nasal branches arise from the pterygopalatine ganglion and pass through the sphenopalatine foramen (in the medial wall of the pterygopalatine fossa) to enter the nasal cavity.
   a. These are the ***posterior superior nasal nerves***, which are in two sets, ***medial*** and ***lateral***.
   b. The lateral nerves supply the posterosuperior part of the lateral wall of the nasal cavity (superior and middle conchae).
   c. The medial nerves supply the posterior parts of the roof of the nasal cavity and of the septum.
   d. One nerve of this group is large and is called the ***nasopalatine nerve*** (43.39). It runs downwards and forwards on the nasal septum. Reaching the floor of the nasal cavity it passes through the incisive foramen to reach the anterior part of the hard palate that it supplies.

*Other Branches from Pterygopalatine Ganglion*

6. A few delicate ***orbital branches*** enter the orbit through the inferior orbital fissure. They supply the periosteum and the orbitalis muscle. (The fibres to the orbitalis are sympathetic fibres that pass through the pterygopalatine ganglion.
7. The ***pharyngeal nerve*** passes into the palatinovaginal canal (which opens on the posterior wall of the pterygopalatine fossa) and passes through it to the nasopharynx.

Apart from branches arising from the pterygopalatine ganglion the following branches arise directly from the maxillary nerve while the latter is in the pterygopalatine fossa (43.40).

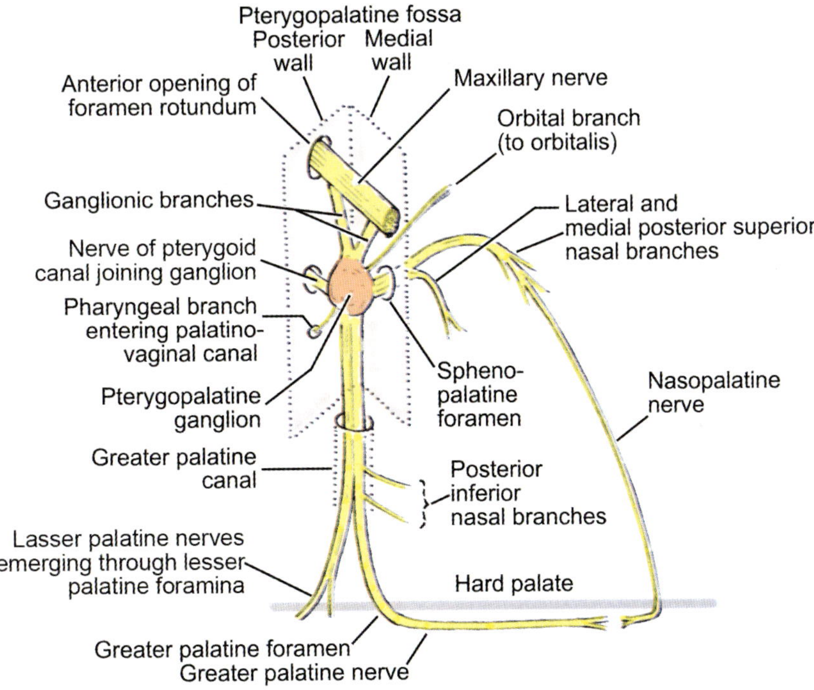


**43.39:** Scheme to show branches of the pterygopalatine ganglion

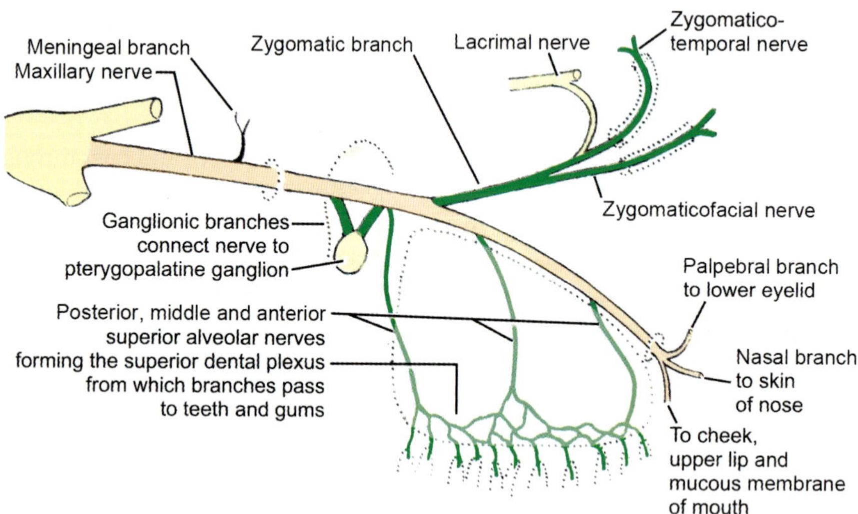


**43.40:** Scheme to show direct branches arising from the maxillary nerve (including its infraorbital continuation)

8. The ***zygomatic nerve*** enters the orbit through the inferior orbital fissure and runs forwards along its lateral wall.
   a. It divides into two branches, the zygomaticotemporal and the zygomaticofacial nerves.
   b. Both these branches enter foramina present on the orbital surface of the zygomatic bone.
   c. Travelling through the zygomatic bone the ***zygomaticotemporal nerve*** emerges from the temporal surface of the bone. The nerve ends by supplying the skin over the temple.
   d. The ***zygomaticofacial nerve*** also passes through the substance of the zygomatic bone. It emerges from the bone through the zygomaticofacial foramen present on the lateral surface of the bone and supplies the skin of the cheek.

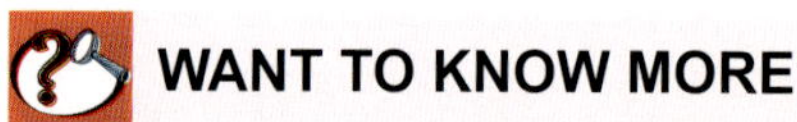

## WANT TO KNOW MORE?

9. The ***posterior superior alveolar nerve*** arises from the maxillary nerve in the pterygopalatine fossa.
   a. It runs down on the posterior surface of the maxilla (which forms the anterior wall of the pterygopalatine fossa) and then pierces it.
   b. The nerve now comes to lie in the wall of the maxillary sinus that it supplies.
   c. It then divides into branches that form a plexus over the roots of the molar teeth. Branches from the plexus supply these teeth and the related gums.

***Branches Arising in the Infraorbital Groove and Canal***

10. The ***middle superior alveolar nerve*** arises from the infraorbital nerve as the latter lies in the infraorbital groove.
    a. Entering a foramen in the floor of the groove it reaches the maxillary sinus and joins the posterior superior alveolar nerve in forming a plexus above the roots of the upper teeth.
    b. The fibres of this nerve supply the premolar teeth through the plexus.
11. The ***anterior superior alveolar nerve*** arises from the infraorbital nerve as the latter lies in the infraorbital canal.
    a. It then enters a bony canal that follows a complicated course through the maxillary bone (hence called the canalis sinuosus) to reach the incisor and canine teeth which it supplies.

b. Branches from the posterior, middle and anterior superior alveolar nerves form a continuous plexus (*superior dental plexus*) in relation to the roots of the teeth borne on the maxilla.
c. The anterior superior alveolar nerve also gives minute branches to the nasal cavity.

***Branches of Infraorbital Nerve in the Face***

12. The infraorbital nerve divides into the following branches after emerging from the infraorbital foramen:
    a. The ***palpebral branches*** supply the lower eyelid.
    b. ***Nasal branches*** supply the skin on the lateral side of the nose.
    c. ***Superior labial*** branches supply the skin of the upper lip and part of the cheek. Some branches reach the mucous membrane of the mouth.
13. The area of the skin of the face supplied by the maxillary nerve is shown in 37.15. The pterygopalatine ganglion is functionally related to the facial nerve.

## The Mandibular Nerve

1. The mandibular nerve is formed by union of two roots.
    a. The ***sensory root*** arises from the lateral part of the trigeminal ganglion, and leaves the skull through the foramen ovale.
    b. The ***motor root*** also passes through the foramen ovale and unites with the sensory root just below the foramen (43.33).
2. Emerging from the foramen ovale, the nerve enters the infratemporal fossa.
    a. After a short downward course, the trunk of the mandibular nerve divides into a smaller ***anterior division*** and a large ***posterior division*** (43.41).
3. The trunk and both divisions give off a number of branches that are given below.

### *Branches from the Trunk (or Main Stem)*

1. A ***meningeal branch*** is given off from the nerve just after the union of the motor and sensory roots.

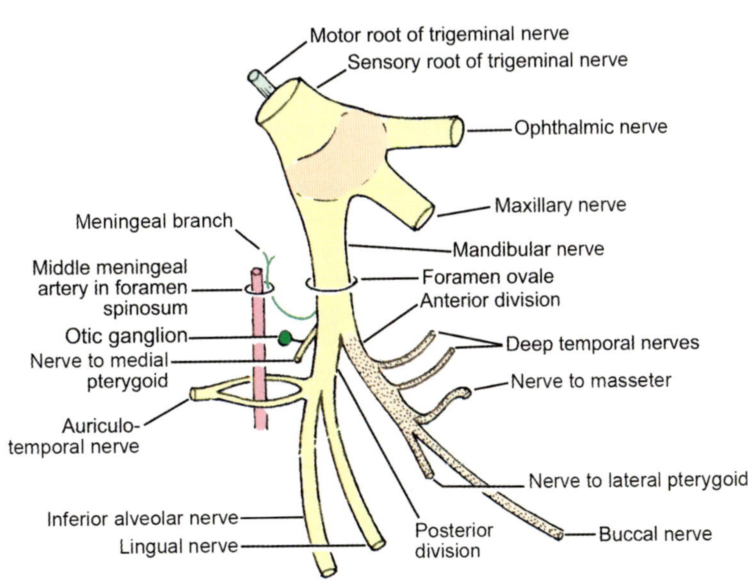


**43.41:** Scheme to show the branches of the mandibular nerve

**WANT TO KNOW MORE?**

a. The branch enters the foramen spinosum.
b. It accompanies the middle meningeal artery and its branches and is distributed to the dura mater (mainly) of the middle cranial fossa.

2. The ***nerve to the medial pterygoid*** supplies this muscle.
   a. It gives a branch to the otic ganglion.
   b. The fibres in this branch pass through the ganglion without relay and supply the tensor tympani and the tensor palati muscles (43.42).

### *Branches from the Anterior Division*

1. The ***buccal nerve*** is sensory.
   a. It runs downwards and forwards through the muscles of the infratemporal fossa to reach the surface of the buccinator muscle. Here it supplies the skin superficial to the muscle and the mucous membrane lining its deep surface.
   b. (Note: Take care not to confuse the buccal nerve with the buccal branch of the facial nerve).

   The remaining branches of the anterior division of the mandibular nerve are motor. They supply the masseter, the lateral pterygoid and the temporalis as follows (43.42).
2. The ***nerve to the masseter*** passes laterally in front of the neck of the mandible (i.e., in the posterior part of the mandibular notch) to reach the masseter.
3. The ***nerve to the lateral pterygoid*** may be independent or may arise from the buccal nerve.
4. The temporalis is supplied through the ***anterior, middle and posterior deep temporal nerves***.
   a. These nerves pass upwards (above the lateral pterygoid) to reach the deep surface of the temporalis (43.42).
   b. The anterior branch sometimes arises from the buccal nerve.
   c. The posterior branch may arise from the nerve to the masseter.

### *Branches from the Posterior Division*

The posterior division of the mandibular nerve gives rise to three important nerves. These are the auriculotemporal, the lingual and the inferior alveolar nerves.

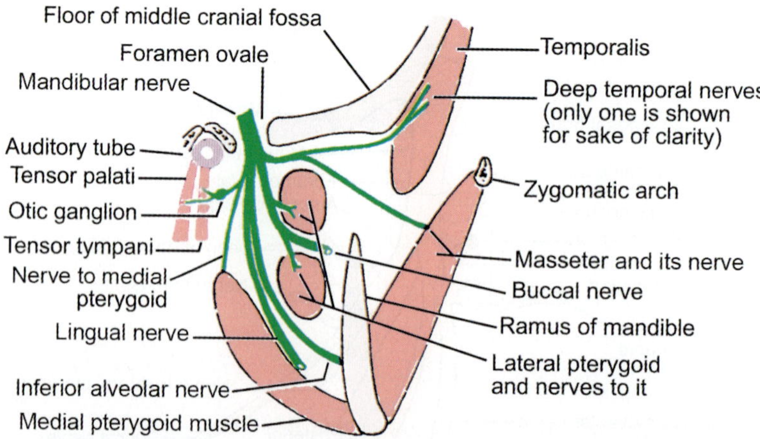


**43.42:** Schematic coronal section through the infratemporal fossa to show the relationship of some branches of the mandibular nerve to the muscles of mastication

## The Auriculotemporal Nerve

1. The auriculotemporal nerve arises by two roots that form a ring through which the middle meningeal artery passes upwards (43.41 and 43.43).
2. The nerve runs backwards deep in the infratemporal fossa; and crosses deep to the neck of the mandible.
3. It then turns laterally behind the temporomandibular joint. In this part of its course it is closely related to the upper part of the parotid gland.
4. The nerve finally turns upwards into the scalp and ends by dividing into branches that supply the skin over the temple. The other branches of the nerve are shown in 43.43.
5. The auriculotemporal nerve serves as a pathway for secretomotor fibres to the parotid gland.
   a. Preganglionic fibres travelling through the lesser petrosal nerve relay in the otic ganglion.
   b. Postganglionic fibres starting in this ganglion reach the roots of the auriculo-temporal nerve through communicating twigs.
   c. They travel through this nerve and through its branches to the parotid gland (43.43).

### WANT TO KNOW MORE?

6. Note that the auriculotemporal nerve supplies:
   ('a' in 43.43) ***Skin*** (of the temple); ('b' in 43.43) A ***gland*** (parotid); ('c' in 43.43) A ***joint*** (temporomandibular); ('d' in 43.43) A ***tube*** (external acoustic meatus); and ('e' in 43.43) A ***membrane*** (tympanic).

## The Lingual Nerve

1. The lingual nerve arises from the posterior division of the mandibular nerve (43.44).
2. Its upper part runs downward deep to the lateral pterygoid muscle (43.42).
3. It is joined here by the ***chorda tympani*** nerve (a branch of the facial nerve).
4. Lower down the lingual nerve runs downwards and forwards between the medial pterygoid (deep to it) and the ramus of the mandible (superficial to it).
5. It then enters the mouth (by passing deep to the mandibular attachment of the superior constrictor of the pharynx).
6. Within the mouth, the nerve lies deep to the mucous membrane overlying the medial surface of the mandible just below the third molar tooth. It can be felt here.
7. Leaving the gum the nerve enters the side of the tongue. The further course of the lingual nerve is shown in 43.44.
   a. The nerve crosses the styloglossus and runs forwards across the lateral surface of the hyoglossus (i.e., between the hyoglossus and the mylohyoid).

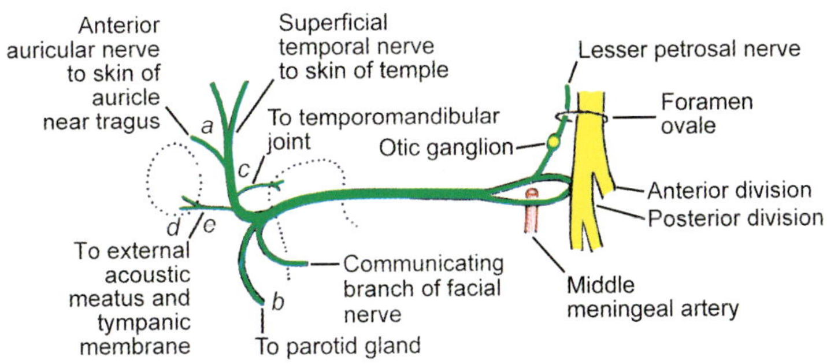


**43.43:** Branches of the auriculotemporal nerve

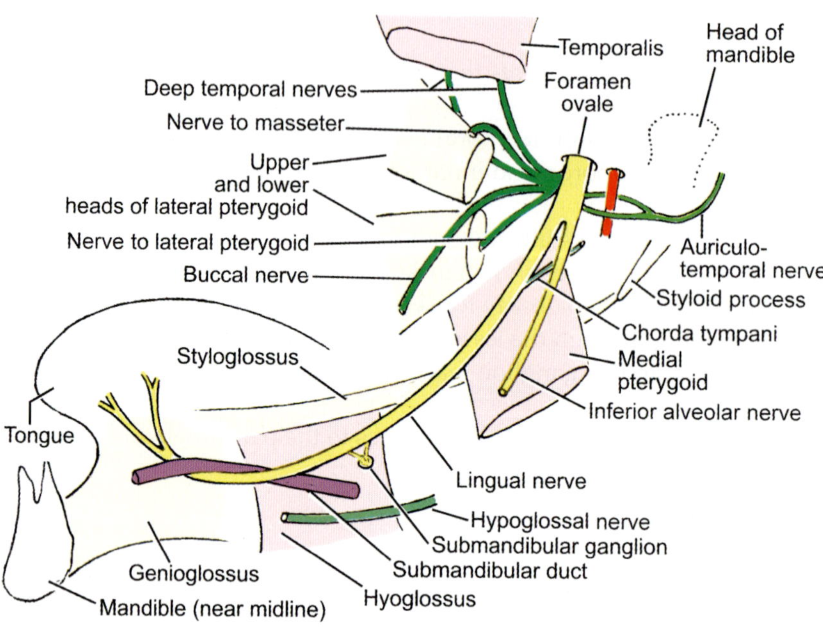


**43.44:** Course and some relations of the lingual nerve and of some other branches of the mandibular nerve

b. At the anterior margin of the hyoglossus the nerve passes onto the genioglossus and divides into a number of branches that are distributed as described below.

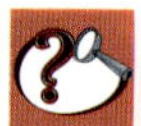

**WANT TO KNOW MORE?**

8. The following additional relations of the nerve are worth noting.
   a. While running across the hyoglossus the lingual nerve lies above the submandibular duct.
   b. Continuing forwards the nerve crosses superficial to the duct and then hooks round it to reach its medial side (43.44).
   c. Lying on the hyoglossus, a little below the lingual nerve, there is the submandibular ganglion. The lingual nerve is connected to the ganglion by two or three branches.
   d. Still lower down the hypoglossal nerve runs across the hyoglossus.

9. The lingual nerve carries three types of fibres that are distributed as follows:
   a. Most of the fibres of the lingual nerve are those of ordinary sensation. They carry the sensations of touch, pain and temperature from the anterior two-thirds of the tongue. They also supply the mucous membrane of the floor of the mouth and the gums related to the lower teeth.
   b. The part of the lingual nerve distal to the attachment of the chorda tympani carries the ***fibres for taste*** from the part of the tongue in front of the sulcus terminalis, but excluding the vallate papillae (43.45).
      i. These fibres pass from the lingual nerve into the chorda tympani (43.46).

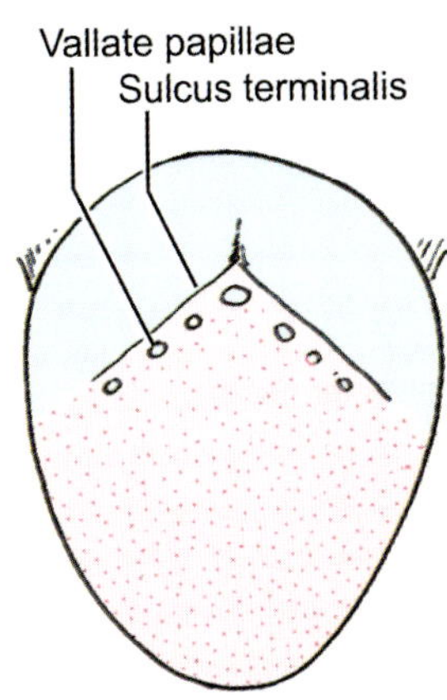

**43.45:** Area of tongue supplied by the lingual nerve (shaded pink)

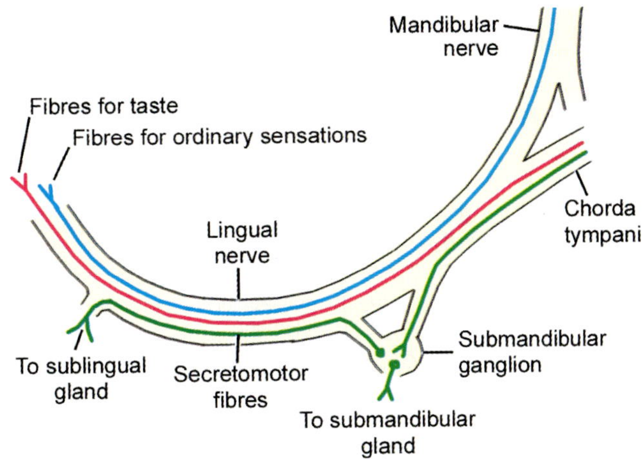

**43.46:** Course of three types of fibres carried by the lingual nerve

   ii. For further course of these fibres, see earlier chapters.
c. ***Secretomotor fibres*** for the submandibular and sublingual glands reach the lingual nerve through the chorda tympani.
   i. They end in the submandibular ganglion.
   ii. Postganglionic fibres reach the submandibular gland through branches to it from the ganglion.
   iii. The fibres for the sublingual gland re-enter the lingual nerve and pass through its distal part to reach the gland (43.46).

## The Inferior Alveolar Nerve

1. The ***inferior alveolar nerve*** is a branch of the posterior division of the mandibular nerve.
2. At its upper end the nerve lies deep to the lateral pterygoid (43.42).
   a. Emerging at the lower border of this muscle the nerve runs downwards and forwards deep to the ramus of the mandible (43.44).
   b. Here it is separated from the medial pterygoid by the sphenomandibular ligament.
3. Reaching the mandibular foramen, it passes through it into the mandibular canal. It runs forwards in this canal just below the teeth, and ends at the mental foramen by dividing into incisive and mental branches (43.48). The nerve is distributed as follows:
   a. Within the mandibular canal the nerve gives branches that supply the molar and premolar teeth.
   b. The ***incisive branch*** continues in the part of the mandibular canal anterior to the mental foramen. It supplies the canine and incisor teeth.
   c. The ***mental branch*** emerges from the mental foramen. It divides into branches that supply the skin over the chin, and that over the lower lip.
   d. The ***mylohyoid nerve*** arises from the inferior alveolar nerve just before the latter enters the mandibular foramen (43.47).
      i. It runs in a groove on the medial side of the mandible, below the mylohyoid muscle.
      ii. It supplies the mylohyoid, and the anterior belly of the digastric muscle.

The areas of skin supplied through the mandibular nerve are shown in 37.15.

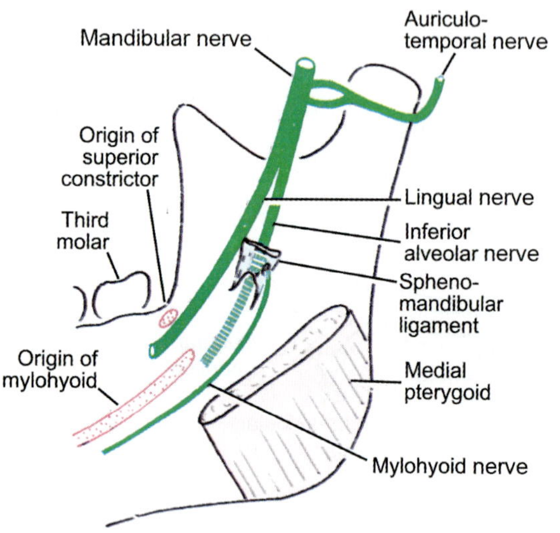


**43.47:** Lingual, inferior alveolar and auriculotemporal nerves viewed from the medial side

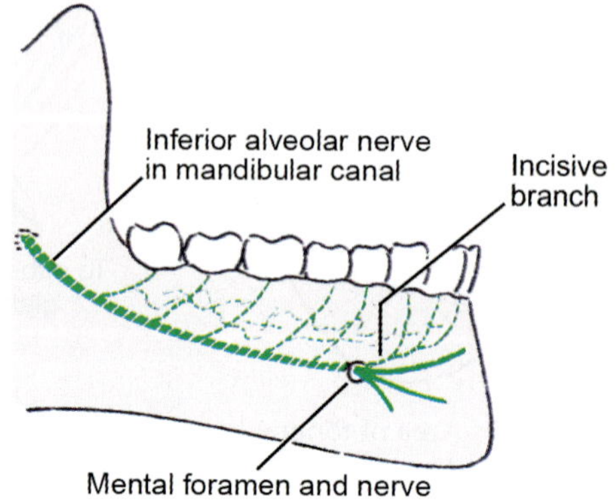


**43.48:** Course of inferior alveolar nerve through the mandibular canal as projected on to the lateral surface of the bone

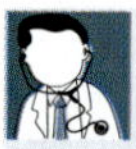

## CLINICAL CORRELATION

### *Testing of Trigeminal Nerve*

1. The trigeminal nerve has a wide sensory distribution. It also supplies the muscles of mastication.
2. The sensation of touch in the area of distribution of the nerve can be tested by touching different areas of skin with a wisp of cotton wool. The sensation of pain can be tested by gentle pressure with a pin.
3. Motor function is tested by asking the patient to clench his teeth firmly. Contraction of the masseter can be felt by palpation when the teeth are clenched.

### *Effects of Injury or Disease*

Injury to the trigeminal nerve causes paralysis of the muscles supplied and loss of sensations in the area of supply. Some features of special importance are as follows:

1. Apart from their role in opening and closing the mouth, the muscles of mastication are responsible for side to side movements of the mandible.
   a. Contraction of these muscles on one side moves the chin to the opposite side.
   b. Normally the chin is maintained in the midline by the balanced tone of the muscles of the right and left sides.
   c. In paralysis of the pterygoid muscles of one side the chin is ***pushed to the paralysed side*** by muscles of the opposite side.
2. Loss of sensation in the ophthalmic division (specially the nasociliary nerve) is of great importance.
   a. Normally the eyelids close as soon as the cornea is touched (corneal reflex).
   b. Loss of sensation in the cornea abolishes this reflex leaving the cornea unprotected.
   c. This can lead to the formation of ulcers on the cornea that can in turn lead to blindness.
3. Pain arising in a structure supplied by one branch of the nerve may be felt in an area of skin supplied by another branch: this is called referred pain. Some examples are as follows:
   a. Caries of a tooth in the lower jaw (supplied by the inferior alveolar nerve) may cause pain in the ear (auriculotemporal).

   b. If there is an ulcer or cancer on the tongue (lingual nerve), the pain may again be felt over the ear and temple (auriculotemporal).
   c. In frontal sinusitis (sinus supplied by a branch from the supraorbital nerve) the pain is referred to the forehead (skin supplied by supraorbital nerve).
   d. In fact headache is a common symptom when any structure supplied by the trigeminal nerve is involved (e.g., eyes, ears, teeth).
4. A source of irritation in the distribution of the nerve may cause severe persistent pain (***trigeminal neuralgia***). Removal of the cause can cure the pain.
   a. However, in some cases no cause can be found. In such cases pain can be relieved by injection of alcohol into the trigeminal ganglion, into one of the divisions of the nerve, or into its sensory root.
   b. In some cases it may be necessary to cut fibres of the sensory root.
   c. In this connection it is important to know that the fibres for the maxillary and mandibular divisions can be cut without destroying those for the ophthalmic division.
   d. This is possible as the fibres for the ophthalmic division lie separately in the upper medial part of the sensory root.
   e. Finally, it may be noted that trigeminal pain can also be relieved by cutting the spinal tract of the trigeminal nerve: this procedure is useful especially for relieving pain in the distribution of the ophthalmic division as pain can be abolished without loss of the sense of touch and, therefore, without the abolition of the corneal reflex.
5. ***Mandibular nerve block***
   a. This is used for anaesthesia of the lower jaw (for extraction of teeth).
   b. Palpate the anterior margin of the ramus of the mandible. Just medial to it you will feel the pterygomandibular raphe (ligament).
   c. The needle is inserted in the interval between the ramus and the raphe. The tip of the needle is now very near the inferior alveolar nerve, just before it enters the mandibular canal. Anaesthetic injected here blocks the nerve.
6. The lingual nerve lies very close to the medial side of the third molar tooth, just deep to the mucosa.
   a. The nerve can be injured in careless extraction of a third molar.
   b. In cases of cancer of the tongue, having intractable pain, the lingual nerve can be cut at this site to relieve pain.

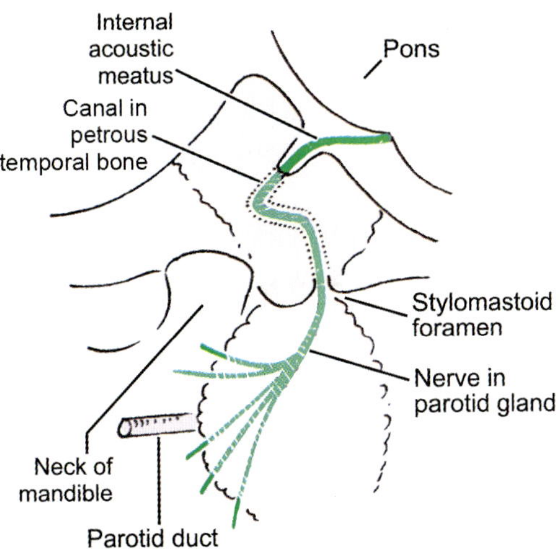


**43.49:** Scheme to show the course of the facial nerve. Structures through which the nerve passes are shown as if transparent

## THE FACIAL NERVE

### Preliminary Remarks

1. The facial nerve is the seventh cranial nerve.
   a. It is attached to the brainstem by two roots: A large ***motor root***, and a smaller ***sensory root.***
   b. These roots are attached in the lateral part of the groove between the lower border of the pons and the upper border of the medulla (43.27).
   c. The motor root is medial to the sensory root. (Note: As in the case of the trigeminal nerve, M for motor and M for medial).
   d. The sensory root is attached midway between the motor root (medially) and the vestibulocochlear nerve (laterally). It is, therefore, called the ***nervus intermedius.***
2. From this attachment the motor and sensory roots pass forwards and laterally and leave the posterior cranial fossa by entering the internal acoustic meatus (on the posterior aspect of the petrous temporal bone).
3. The nerve has a complicated course through the substance of the petrous temporal bone. This part of the nerve bears the ***genicular ganglion*** (so called because it is situated on a sharp bend of the nerve).
4. The nerve emerges on the base of the skull through the stylomastoid foramen.
5. It immediately enters the substance of the parotid gland and runs forwards within it and ends behind the neck of the mandible by dividing into several branches.

Some details of the course of the nerve are considered below. Scheme to show the course of the facial nerve is shown in 43.49.

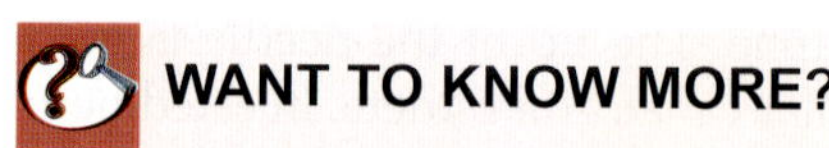


**Intrapontine Course**

(Note: The course of the facial nerve within the pons can be fully understood only after the internal structure of the pons has been studied).

1. The ***facial nucleus*** lies deep in the reticular formation of the pons, medial to the spinal nucleus of the trigeminal nerve (43.19 and 43.20C).
2. The fibres arising in the nucleus follow an unusual course.
   a. They first run backwards and medially to reach the lower pole of the abducent nucleus.
   b. They then ascend on the medial side of that nucleus.
   c. Finally, the fibres turn forwards and laterally passing above the upper pole of the abducent nucleus.
3. The abducent nucleus and the facial nerve fibres looping round it together form a surface elevation, the ***facial colliculus***, in the floor of the fourth ventricle.

**Course through the Petrous Temporal Bone**

1. The facial nerve enters the petrous temporal bone through the internal acoustic meatus.
2. The nerve then enters a bony canal.
3. Within this canal the nerve first passes laterally above the vestibule ('1' in 43.50) to reach the anterosuperior angle of the medial wall of the middle ear. At this point ('2' in 43.50) the nerve bends sharply backwards. This bend is thickened by the presence of the ***genicular ganglion.***
4. The nerve then runs horizontally backwards in a canal projecting into the medial wall of the middle ear ('3' in 43.50).
5. Reaching the junction of the medial and posterior walls of the middle ear ('4' in 43.50) the nerve turns downward.
6. Continuing downwards along the junction of the medial and posterior wall of the middle ear ('5' in 43.50) the nerve reaches the stylomastoid foramen through which it leaves the skull.

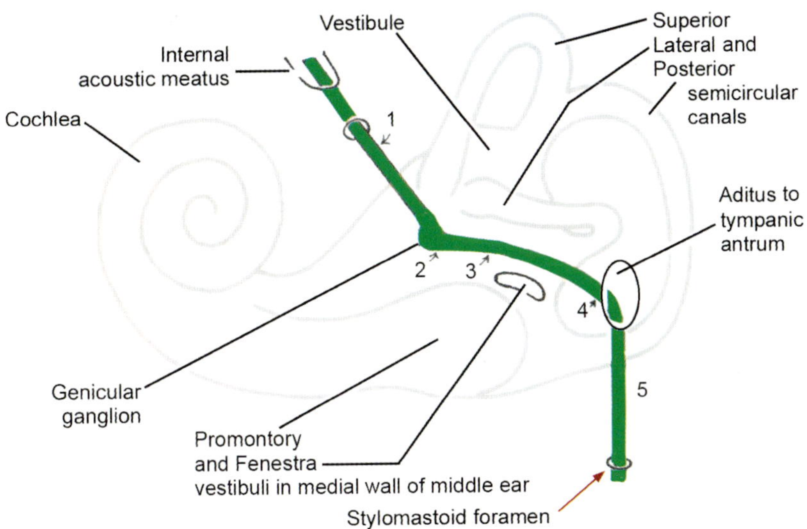


**43.50:** Scheme to show the course of the facial nerve within the petrous temporal bone

### *Course through Parotid Gland*

1. As the facial nerve runs forward through the parotid gland it crosses the styloid process, the retromandibular vein and the external carotid artery (43.52).
2. It divides into several branches while still within the gland. These branches emerge from the anteromedial surface of the gland and come into view along the anterior margin of the gland (43.51 and 43.52).

## Branches of the Facial Nerve

The branches of the facial nerve are shown in 43.53. They are as follows:

1. The ***greater petrosal nerve*** arises from the genicular ganglion. It is described in detail below.
2. The ***nerve to the stapedius*** arises from the facial as the latter turns downwards along the junction of the medial and posterior walls of the middle ear. It runs forwards through a short canal in the petrous temporal bone to reach the stapedius.
3. The ***chorda tympani*** arises from the intrapetrous part of the facial nerve about 6 mm above the stylomastoid foramen. It is considered below.
4. The ***posterior auricular nerve*** is given off just after the facial nerve emerges from the stylomastoid foramen.
   a. It runs upwards into the scalp passing behind the external acoustic meatus.
   b. It divides into an ***auricular branch***, which supplies some muscles of the auricle
   c. An ***occipital branch*** which supplies the occipital belly of the occipitofrontalis.
5. The ***nerve to the posterior belly of the digastric muscle*** and the ***nerve to the stylohyoid*** arise near the stylomastoid foramen. They end by supplying the muscles concerned.
   The remaining branches of the facial nerve arise within the parotid gland.
6. The ***temporal branches*** enter the scalp in the temporal region.
   a. They supply the frontal belly of the occipitofrontalis, the corrugator supercilii, and some muscles of the auricle.
   b. Some twigs are also given to the orbicularis oculi.
7. The ***zygomatic branches*** supply the orbicularis oculi.
8. The ***buccal branches*** are in two sets upper and lower.
   a. The upper branches (sometimes called the lower zygomatic branches) supply:
      i. The zygomaticus major and minor

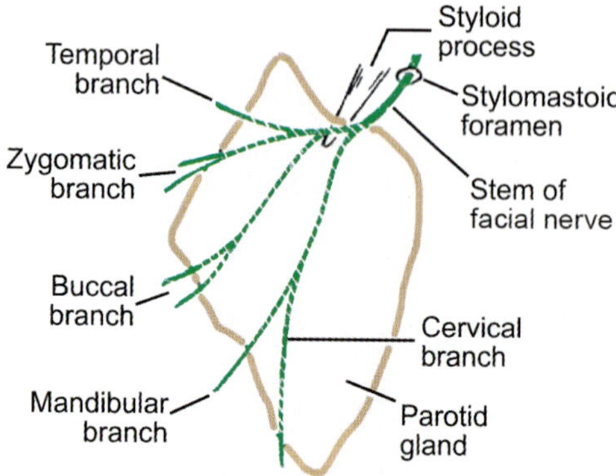


**43.51:** Course of facial nerve through parotid gland

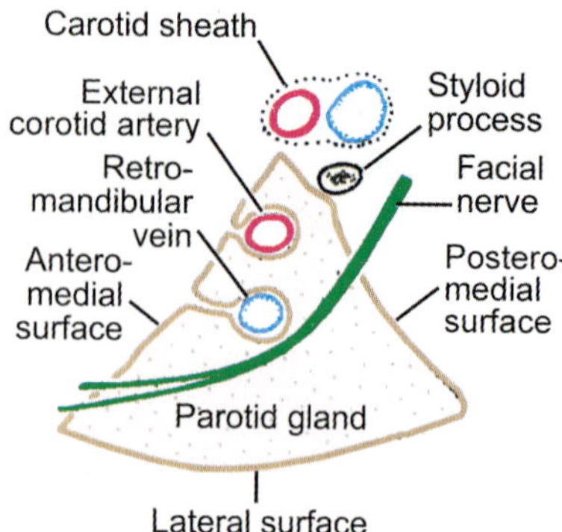


**43.52:** Transverse section through the parotid gland to show relationship to the facial nerve

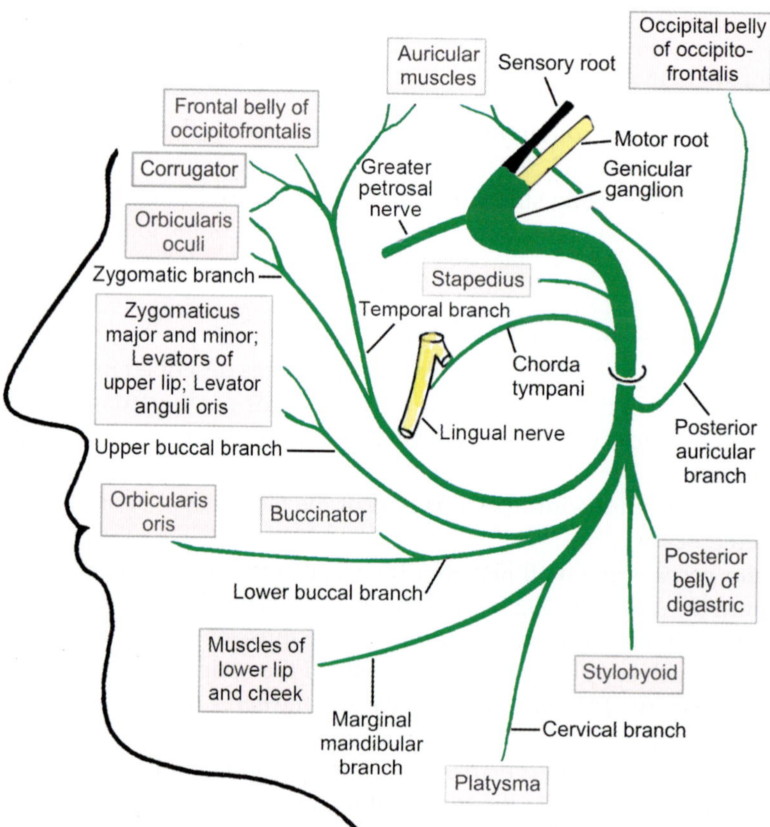


**43.53:** Scheme to show the branches of the facial nerve

ii. The levator labii superioris
iii. The levator anguli oris
iv. The levator labii superioris alaeque nasi
v. Some small muscles related to the nose.

b. The lower buccal branches supply the buccinator and the orbicularis oris.

9. The ***marginal mandibular branch*** is related to the lower border of the mandible. It supplies the muscles of the lower lip and chin.
10. The ***cervical branch*** emerges from the parotid gland near its lower end. It enters the neck and supplies the platysma.

The various branches of the facial nerve have been enumerated above. The greater petrosal nerve and the chorda tympani are considered in detail below.

**WANT TO KNOW MORE?**

**Greater Petrosal Nerve**

1. The ***greater petrosal nerve*** arises from the genicular ganglion.
2. It passes through a canal in the petrous temporal bone and reaches its anterior surface by passing through an aperture called the hiatus for the greater petrosal nerve.
3. The nerve then runs forwards and medially in a groove on the anterior surface of the bone, passing deep to the trigeminal ganglion.
4. Reaching the foramen lacerum the greater petrosal nerve ends by joining the deep petrosal nerve to form the nerve of the pterygoid canal.
5. The ***deep petrosal nerve*** consists of sympathetic fibres derived from the plexus around the internal carotid artery.
6. The ***nerve of the pterygoid canal*** passes forwards in the pterygoid canal to enter the pterygopalatine fossa.
   a. The nerve ends by joining the pterygopalatine ganglion.
   b. The greater petrosal nerve and the nerve of the pterygoid canal serve as pathways for secretomotor fibres to the lacrimal gland and to the glands of the nasal and palatine mucosa.

## Chorda Tympani

1. The chorda tympani is so called because it has an intimate relationship to the middle ear (tympanum).
2. It arises from the facial nerve as the latter descends towards the stylomastoid foramen.
3. The chorda tympani is of considerable importance as it carries fibres of taste from the anterior two thirds of the tongue and secretomotor fibres to the submandibular and sublingual glands as described below.

**WANT TO KNOW MORE?**

4. The origin of the nerve is about 6 mm above the foramen.
5. The nerve enters the middle ear through the posterior canaliculus for the chorda tympani, which opens on the posterior wall of the middle ear, close to the posterior part of the margin of the tympanic membrane (43.54).
6. The nerve now passes forwards through the substance of the tympanic membrane (lying between its fibrous basis and the mucous membrane lining its internal surface).
7. As it does so it crosses the handle of the malleus (which is embedded in the membrane).
8. Reaching the anterior margin of the tympanic membrane the chorda tympani enters the anterior canaliculus (in the anterior wall of the middle ear). It passes through this canaliculus and emerges on the base of the skull through the medial end of the petrotympanic fissure.

9. Passing medially, forwards and downwards the nerve crosses medial to the spine of the sphenoid. (Note: the auriculotemporal nerve passes lateral to the spine, See 43.54).
10. The chorda tympani ends by joining the lingual nerve from behind.
    a. To do so it has to pass deep to the inferior alveolar nerve.
    b. The junction of the chorda tympani with the lingual nerve lies deep to the lateral pterygoid muscle.

**Functional Components of the Facial Nerve**

***Special Visceral Efferent Fibres***

1. Most of the branches of the facial nerve are motor. Many of them supply the muscles of facial expression. Motor fibres also supply the occipitofrontalis, the muscles of the auricle, the stapedius, the platysma, the stylohyoid and the posterior belly of the digastric.
2. All these muscles are derived from the mesoderm of the second branchial arch.
3. The nerve fibres concerned in their innervation arise in the facial nucleus that lies in the lower part of the pons, and belongs to the ***special visceral efferent*** column (43.19 and 43.20D).
4. The axons of neurons located in this nucleus collect to form the motor root of the facial nerve.

***General Visceral Efferent Fibres***

These are as follows:

1. Preganglionic secretomotor fibres for the submandibular and sublingual glands (43.55) arise from neurons located in the ***superior salivatory nucleus***. (This nucleus lies in the lower part of the pons).
    a. The fibres leave the pons through the nervus intermedius and run for some distance in the intrapetrous part of the facial nerve.
    b. They then enter the chorda tympani to reach the lingual nerve.
    c. They leave the lingual nerve through branches to the submandibular ganglion.
    d. Postganglionic neurons are located in this ganglion.
    e. Some of the nerve fibres arising from them supply the submandibular gland.
    f. Others re-enter the lingual nerve and pass through its distal part to reach the sublingual gland.
2. Preganglionic secretomotor fibres for the lacrimal gland (43.56) arise in the lacrimatory nucleus, which is believed to lie near the salivatory nuclei.
    a. They leave the pons through the nervus intermedius, pass into the greater petrosal nerve and through it into the nerve of the pterygoid canal to end in the pterygopalatine ganglion.
    b. Postganglionic neurons are located in this ganglion.
    c. Fibres arising from them pass successively through.
        i. A ganglionic branch connecting the pterygopalatine ganglion to the maxillary nerve
        ii. The maxillary nerve itself
        iii. Its zygomatic branch
        iv. The zygomaticotemporal branch of the zygomatic nerve
        v. The loop of communication between the zygomaticotemporal and lacrimal nerves
        vi. Finally through the lacrimal nerve to reach the lacrimal gland.
3. Preganglionic secretomotor fibres for glands in the nasal and palatine mucosa arise in neurons the location of which is uncertain. They probably lie near the salivatory nuclei.
    a. The preganglionic fibres follow the same path as for the lacrimal gland.
    b. Postganglionic fibres arising in the pterygopalatine ganglion pass through its greater and lesser palatine branches to reach glands in the palate; and through its nasal branches to reach glands in the nasal mucosa.

**Special Visceral Efferent Fibres**

The facial nerve contains ***special visceral efferent*** fibres that carry the sensations of taste from the part of the tongue in front of the sulcus terminalis; and from the soft palate.

1. These fibres are processes of unipolar neurons located in the genicular ganglion.

2. Peripheral processes reach the tongue by passing successively through:
   a. Part of the intrapetrous segment of the facial nerve
   b. The chorda tympani and the lingual nerve (43.55).
3. Fibres for the soft palate pass through:
   a. The greater petrosal nerve
   b. The nerve of the pterygoid canal
   c. The pterygopalatine ganglion (without relay)
   d. The lesser palatine nerves (43.56).
4. The central processes leaving the genicular ganglion pass through the nervus intermedius to reach the brainstem. Here they terminate in relation to the upper part of the nucleus of the solitary tract (43.19 and 43.20B).

**General Somatic Afferent Fibres**

1. These fibres supply skin. Although the facial nerve gives no direct branches to skin there is evidence that some of its fibres reach part of the skin of the auricle.
2. They probably pass through communications between the facial nerve and the auricular branch of the vagus.
3. These fibres are ***general somatic afferent*** and are peripheral processes of unipolar cells located in the genicular ganglion.
4. Central processes arising in these neurons pass through the nervus intermedius and end in the nucleus of the spinal tract of the trigeminal nerve.
5. When the genicular ganglion is affected by an infection called ***herpes zoster*** vesicles appear on the skin over part of the auricle.

**The Pterygopalatine Ganglion**

1. This ganglion is located in the pterygopalatine fossa and is suspended from the maxillary nerve by two ganglionic branches (43.39). The fibres passing through the ganglion are as follows:
2. Functionally, the ganglion is autonomic and is a peripheral ganglion of the cranial parasympathetic outflow.
   a. Its motor (or parasympathetic) root is formed by the nerve of the pterygoid canal that conveys pre-ganglionic secretomotor fibres for the supply of the lacrimal gland, and for the glands of the nasal and palatine mucosa.
   b. Neurons located in this ganglion give off postganglionic fibres that innervate these glands. The pathways concerned have already been described (43.56).
3. The ganglion also receives some sympathetic fibres.
   a. These fibres, which are postganglionic, arise in the superior cervical sympathetic ganglion, run along the internal carotid plexus, pass into the deep petrosal nerve and then into the nerve of the pterygoid canal to reach the ganglion.
   b. They pass through the ganglion, without relay, and enter its orbital branches to supply the orbitalis muscle.
4. Numerous sensory fibres from the palate (greater and lesser palatine nerves), the nose (nasal branches) and the pharynx (pharyngeal branch) reach the ganglion, and pass through it without relay to enter the maxillary nerve through its ganglionic branches.
5. Fibres of taste from the soft palate reach the ganglion through the lesser palatine nerves (43.56). They pass through the nerve of the pterygoid canal and the greater petrosal nerve to reach the genicular ganglion.

**The Submandibular Ganglion**

1. This ganglion lies over the hyoglossus muscle, suspended from the lingual nerve by two or more roots (43.44).
2. It is an autonomic ganglion connected with the cranial parasympathetic outflow. The fibres passing through it are as follows:
   a. Functionally the ganglion is concerned with the secretomotor innervation of the submandibular and sublingual salivary glands. These fibres are parasympathetic. The pathway concerned is shown in 43.55 and has already been described.

b. The ganglion receives sympathetic fibres from the plexus on the facial artery. These are postganglionic fibres arising in the superior cervical sympathetic ganglion. They pass through the ganglion without relay and supply the blood vessels of the submandibular and sublingual glands.

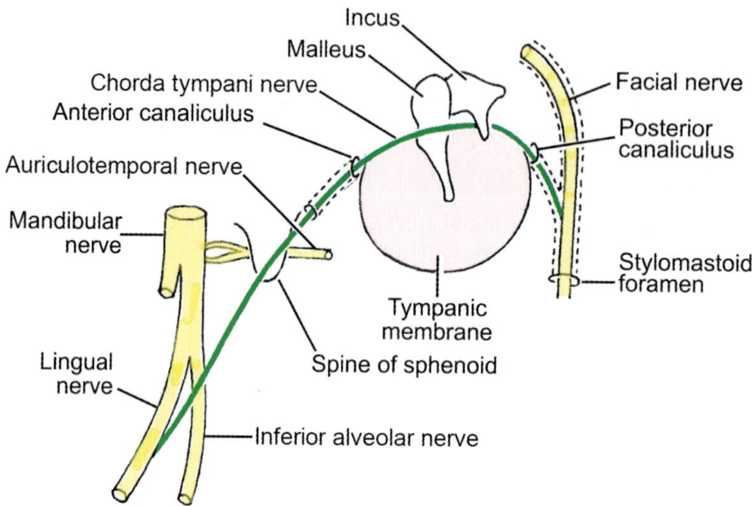


**43.54:** Course of the chorda tympani as seen from the medial side

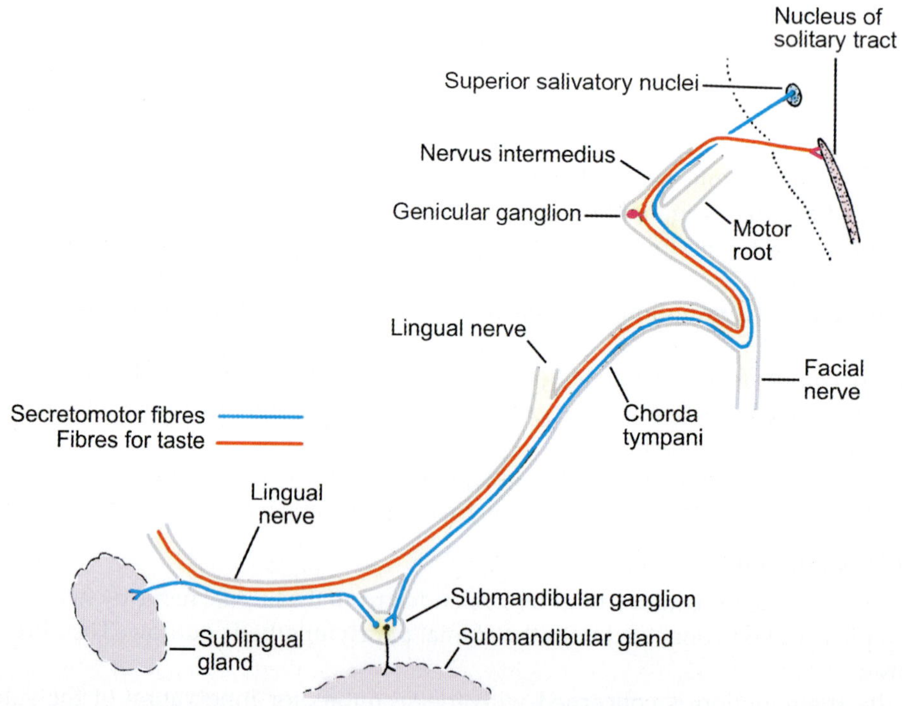


**43.55:** Scheme to show the secretomotor pathway for the submandibular and sublingual glands. The pathway for taste from the anterior two-thirds of the tongue is also shown

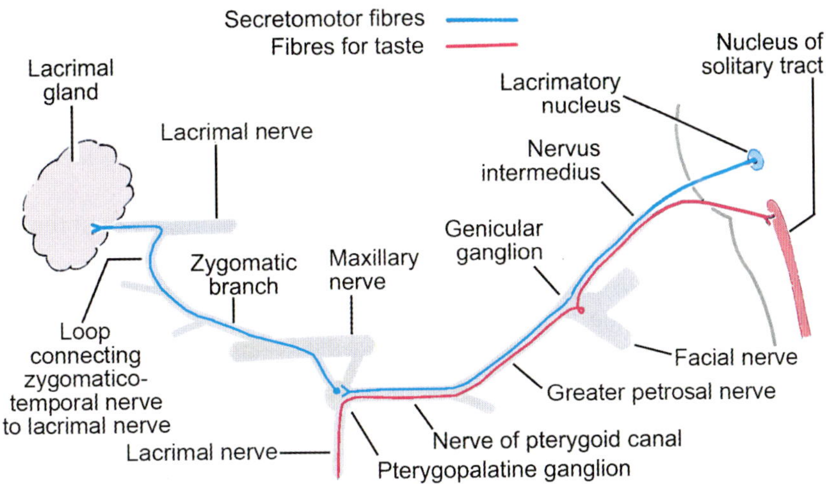


**43.56:** Scheme to show the secretomotor pathway for the lacrimal gland; and the pathway for fibres of taste from the soft palate

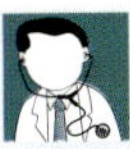

## CLINICAL CORRELATION

### Testing the Facial nerve

1. Ask the patient to close his eyes firmly. In complete paralysis of the facial nerve the patient will not be able to close the eye on the affected side. In partial paralysis the closure is weak and the examiner can easily open the closed eye with his fingers (which is very difficult in a normal person).
2. Ask the person to smile. In smiling the normal mouth is more or less symmetrical, the two angles moving upwards and outwards. In facial paralysis the angle fails to move on the paralysed side.
3. Ask the patient to fill his mouth with air. Press the cheek with your finger and compare the resistance (by the buccinator muscle) on the two sides. The resistance is less on the paralysed side. On pressing the cheek air may leak out of the mouth because the muscles closing the mouth are weak.
4. The sensation of taste should be tested on the anterior two-thirds of the tongue (as described under glossopharyngeal nerve).

### Paralysis of Facial Nerve

1. Paralysis of the facial nerve is fairly common.
2. It can occur due to injury or disease of the facial nucleus (nuclear paralysis) or of the nerve anywhere along its course (infranuclear paralysis).
3. In the most common type of infranuclear paralysis called ***Bell's palsy*** the nerve is affected near the stylomastoid foramen.
4. Facial muscles can also be paralysed by interruption of corticonuclear fibres running from the motor cortex to the facial nucleus: this is referred to as ***supranuclear paralysis***.
5. The effects of paralysis are due to the failure of the muscles concerned to perform their normal actions. Some effects are as follows:
   a. The normal face is more or less symmetrical. When the facial nerve is paralysed on one side the most noticeable feature is the loss of symmetry. (Also see para 4 in this regard).
   b. Normal furrows on the forehead are lost because of paralysis of the occipitofrontalis.
   c. There is drooping of the eyelid and the palpebral fissure is wider on the paralysed side because of paralysis of the orbicularis oculi.

   d. The conjunctival reflex is lost for the same reason.
   e. There is marked asymmetry of the mouth because of paralysis of the orbicularis oris and of muscles inserted into the angle of the mouth. This is most obvious when a smile is attempted.
   f. As a result of asymmetry the protruded tongue appears to deviate to one side, but is in fact in the midline.
   g. During mastication food tends to accumulate between the cheek and the teeth. (This is normally prevented by the buccinator).
6. Additional effects are observed in injuries to the facial nerve at levels higher than the stylomastoid foramen, as follows:
   a. If the injury is proximal to the origin of the chorda tympani there is loss of the sensation of taste on the anterior two-thirds of the tongue.
   b. The intensity of loud sounds reaching the internal ear is normally decreased by contraction of the stapedius muscle. When a lesion of the facial nerve is located proximal to the origin of the branch to the stapedius this muscle is paralysed. As a result even normal sounds appear too loud (***hyperacusis***).
   c. In fractures of the temporal bone, or in lesions near the exit of the nerve from the brain the vestibulocochlear nerve may also be affected (leading to deafness).
   d. In nuclear lesions (within the brainstem) other neighbouring nuclei may be affected leading to lesions of the abducent or trigeminal nerves.
7. Supranuclear lesions can be distinguished from nuclear or infranuclear lesions because these are usually accompanied by hemiplegia.
   a. Movements of the lower part of the face are more affected than those of the upper part.
   b. The explanation for this is that the corticonuclear fibres concerned with movements of the upper part of the face are bilateral, whereas those for movements of the lower part of the face are unilateral.
   c. Another difference is that while voluntary movements are affected, emotional expressions appear to be normal. It has been suggested that there are separate pathways from the cerebral cortex to the facial nucleus for voluntary and emotional movements, and that usually only the former are involved.

## THE VESTIBULOCOCHLEAR NERVE

1. The vestibulocochlear nerve is eighth cranial nerve. It consists of two distinct parts—vestibular and cochlear. Both of them are purely sensory.
2. The vestibular nerve carries impulses necessary for the maintenance of equilibrium from the vestibular part of the internal ear.
3. The cochlear nerve carries impulses of hearing from the cochlear part of the internal ear.
4. The vestibulocochlear nerve is attached to the surface of the brainstem at the lower border of the pons, posterolateral to the attachment of the facial nerve (43.27).
5. From here the nerve passes forwards and enters the internal acoustic meatus along with the motor and sensory roots of the facial nerve. Here the nerve divides into vestibular and cochlear parts.

### WANT TO KNOW MORE?

**The Vestibular Nerve**

1. A plan of the vestibular nerve is shown in 43.57.
2. The fibres of the nerve are processes of cells in the vestibular ganglion that is located within the internal acoustic meatus. The cells of this ganglion are bipolar (not unipolar as in typical sensory ganglia). Peripheral processes arising from neurons in the ganglion supply end organs in the vestibular part of the membranous labyrinth.
3. The central processes of neurons in the vestibular ganglion form the vestibular nerve.
4. Entering the brainstem they end in relation to the vestibular nuclei (43.19 and 43.20 B and C).

5. Fibres arising in the vestibular nuclei carry impulses for equilibrium to the cerebellum. Some fibres from the vestibular ganglion pass directly to the cerebellum.

## The Cochlear Nerve

1. A plan of the cochlear nerve is shown in 43.58.
2. The cochlear nerve is made up of the central processes of neurons located in the spiral ganglion.
3. Peripheral processes of the neurons of the spiral ganglion reach the organ of corti, which is the peripheral receptor for sound.
4. Sound is ultimately perceived in the auditory area of the cerebral cortex. A simplified scheme of the pathway for hearing from the cochlear nuclei to the cerebral cortex is given in 43.59.

### WANT TO KNOW MORE?

5. The spiral ganglion is so called because it has a spiral configuration parallel to the turns of the cochlea.
   a. The neurons in this ganglion are bipolar (like those of the vestibular ganglion).
   b. The fibres of the cochlear nerve enter the internal acoustic meatus. On reaching the brainstem they terminate in the dorsal and ventral cochlear nuclei located respectively on the dorsal and ventral sides of the inferior cerebellar peduncle.
6. The fibres in both the vestibular and cochlear nerves are classified as special somatic afferent, as the epithelium of the membranous labyrinth is of ectodermal origin.

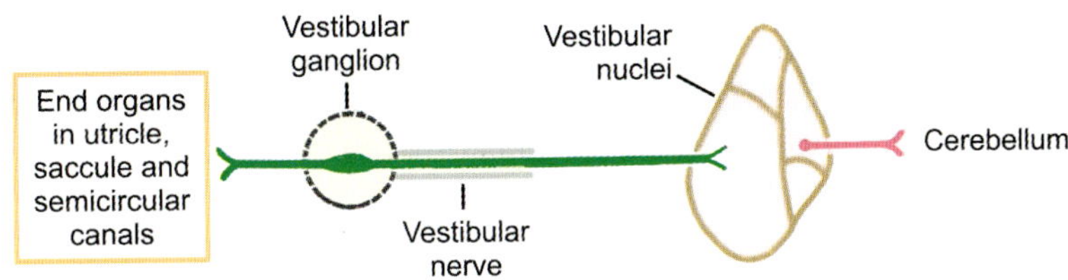


**43.57:** Basic plan of the vestibular nerve

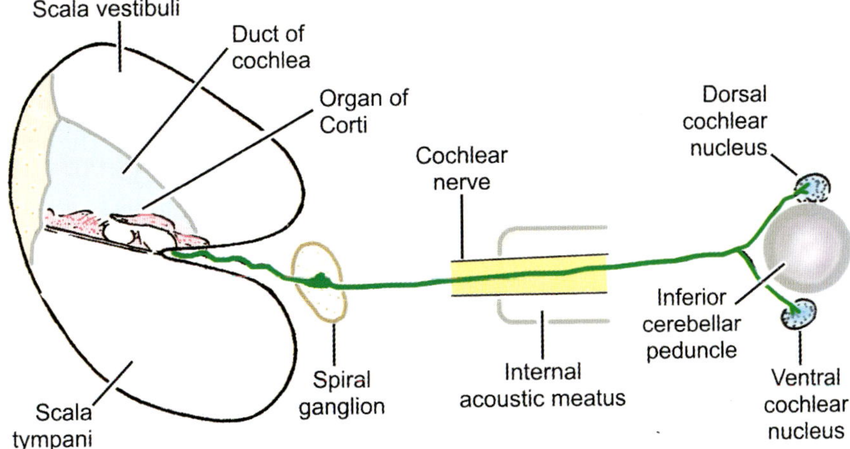


**43.58:** Simplified scheme to show the course of the cochlear nerve

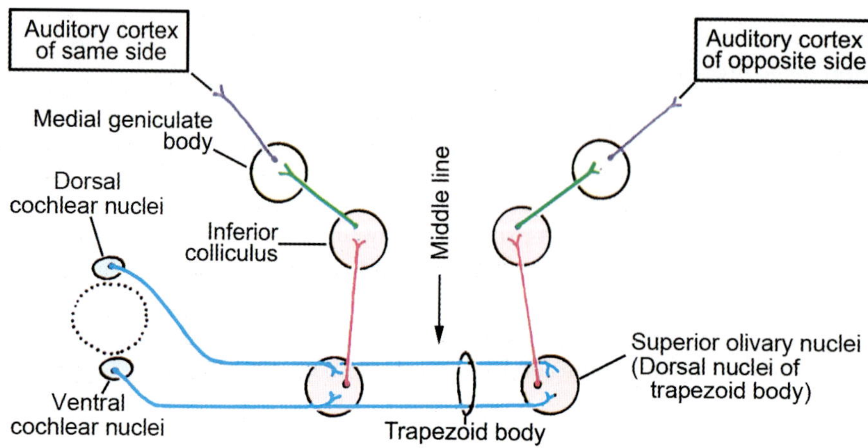


**43.59:** Scheme to show the pathway from cochlear nuclei to the auditory cortex

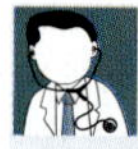

## CLINICAL CORRELATION

**Testing the Vestibulocochlear Nerve**

This nerve is responsible for hearing (cochlear part) and for equilibrium (vestibular part). Normally we test only the cochlear part.

1. The hearing of the patient can be tested by using a watch.
   a. First place the watch near one ear so that the patient knows what he is expected to hear.
   b. Next ask him to close his eyes and say so when he hears the ticking of the watch.
   c. The watch should be held away from the ear and then gradually brought towards it.
   d. The distance at which the sounds are first heard should be compared with the other ear.
2. In doing this test, it must be remembered that loss of hearing can occur from various causes such as the presence of wax in the ear, or middle ear disease.
3. Nerve deafness can be distinguished from deafness due to a conduction defect (as in middle ear disease) by noting the following:
   a. Sounds can be transmitted to the internal ear through air (normal way), and can also be transmitted through bone. Normally conduction through air is better than that through bone, but in defects of conduction the sound is better heard through bone.
   b. Air conduction and bone conduction can be compared by using a tuning fork.
   c. Strike the tuning fork against an object so that it begins to vibrate producing sound.
   d. Place the tuning fork near the patient's ear and then immediately put the base of the tuning fork on the mastoid process. Ask the patient where he hears the sound better. (This is called ***Rinne's test***).
   e. In another test the base of a vibrating tuning fork is placed on the forehead. The sound is heard in both ears but is clearer in the ear with a conduction defect. (This is ***Weber's test***).
4. Defects in the vestibular apparatus or in the vestibular nerve are difficult to test and such cases need to be examined by a specialist.

## THE GLOSSOPHARYNGEAL NERVE

1. This is the ninth cranial nerve. It is attached to the lateral side of the upper part of the medulla (between the olive and the inferior cerebellar peduncle) by three or four roots (43.27).

2. It runs forwards and laterally and leaves the cranial cavity by passing through the jugular foramen. Its position in the foramen is shown in 43.60.
3. Emerging at the base of the skull the nerve passes forwards and laterally between the internal jugular vein and the internal carotid artery.
4. It then descends in front of the internal carotid artery, passing deep to the styloid process and the structures attached to it.
5. Reaching the posterior border of the stylopharyngeus muscle it curves forwards passing lateral to the muscle (43.61).
6. The nerve then enters the pharynx by passing through the interval between the lower border of the superior constrictor of the pharynx and the upper border of the middle constrictor.
7. Passing forwards the nerve reaches the side of the tongue. Here it passes deep to the hyoglossus muscle, superficial to the genioglossus and terminates by dividing into branches to the tongue.
8. The proximal part of the glossopharyngeal nerve bears two ganglia, superior and inferior. The ***superior ganglion*** is small and lies within the jugular foramen. The ***inferior ganglion*** is larger and lies just below the foramen (43.62).

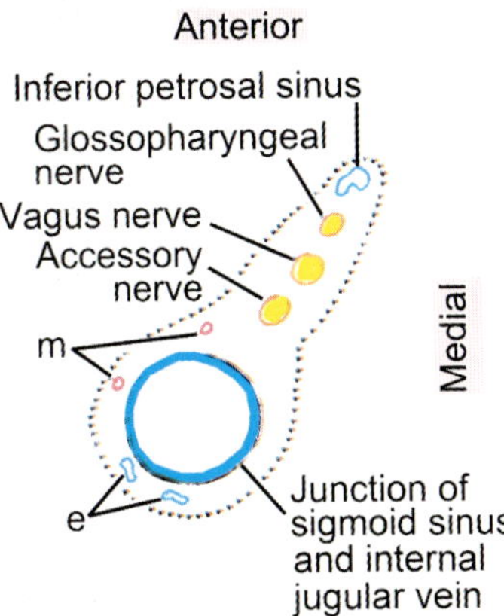


**43.60:** Relative position of structures passing through the jugular foramen. m: meningeal arteries. e: emissary veins

## Branches of Glossopharyngeal Nerve

The branches of the glossopharyngeal nerve are shown in 43.62 and are considered below:

### WANT TO KNOW MORE?

1. The ***tympanic branch*** arises from the inferior ganglion.
   a. It enters a canal (called the inferior tympanic canaliculus) within the petrous temporal bone.
   b. Passing through the canaliculus the nerve reaches the tympanic cavity and forms a plexus (***tympanic plexus***) over the promontory.
   c. Branches arising from this plexus supply the mucous membrane of the tympanic cavity, the auditory tube, and the mastoid air cells.
   d. The plexus also gives rise to the lesser petrosal nerve described below.
2. The ***lesser petrosal nerve*** leaves the tympanic cavity through a canal that opens on the anterior surface of the petrous temporal bone (lateral to the greater petrosal nerve).
   a. It leaves the cranial cavity by passing through the foramen ovale (or through a small foramen, the canaliculus innominatus present lateral to the foramen ovale).
   b. The nerve ends by joining the otic ganglion. Its importance is considered below.
3. The ***carotid branch*** arises soon after the glossopharyngeal nerve emerges on the base of the skull. It supplies the carotid sinus and carotid body (forming a plexus with sympathetic fibres from the superior cervical ganglion, and from the vagus).

4. ***Pharyngeal branches*** are given off to the mucous membrane of the pharynx. Their fibres pass through the pharyngeal plexus (which is also joined by sympathetic fibres and by fibres from the vagus).
5. As the glossopharyngeal nerve winds round the ***stylopharyngeus*** it supplies this muscle. (Note: This is the only motor branch of the nerve).
6. Some ***tonsilar branches*** supply the palatine tonsil and the soft palate.
7. The ***lingual branches*** supply the part of the tongue (mucous membrane) behind the sulcus terminalis.
   a. They also supply the vallate papillae (43.65).
   b. As described below these branches carry fibres for both general sensation and taste.

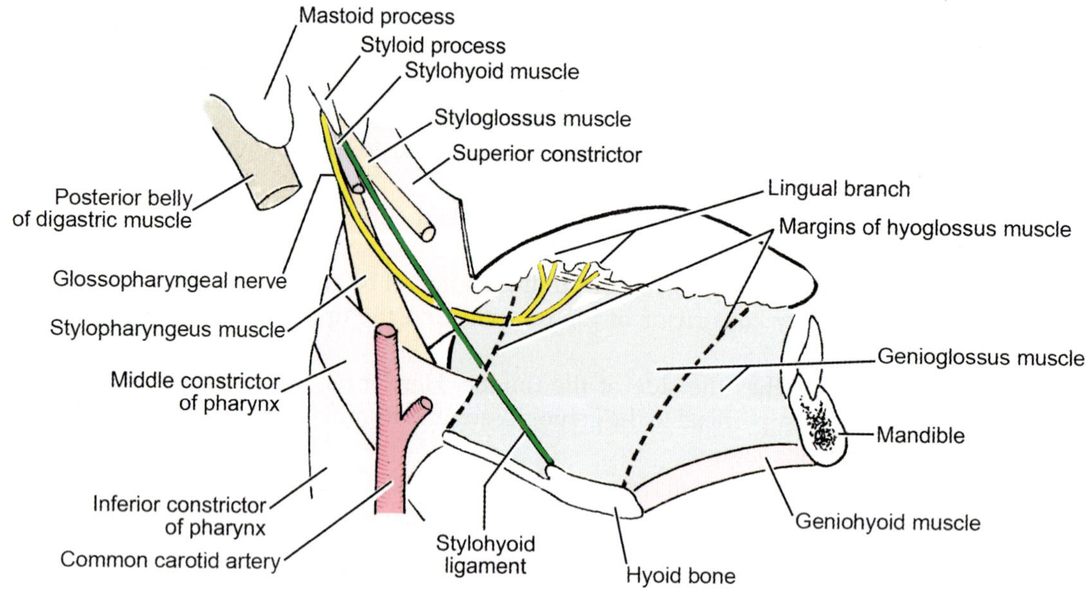


**43.61:** Some relations of the glossopharyngeal nerve. Structures deep to the hyoglossus are shown as if the muscle was transparent

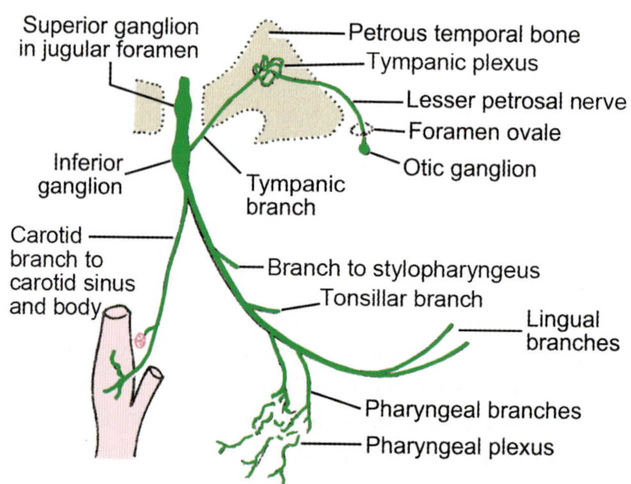


**43.62:** Branches of the glossopharyngeal nerve

## WANT TO KNOW MORE?

### Functional Components of the Glossopharyngeal Nerve

1. ***Special visceral efferent*** fibres arising in the nucleus ambiguus (43.19 and 43.20 A and B) supply the stylopharyngeus muscle.

  a. This muscle develops from the mesoderm of the third branchial arch.
  b. The glossopharyngeal is the nerve of this arch.
2. *General visceral efferent* fibres supply the parotid gland.
  a. The pathway is shown in 43.63
  b. The preganglionic neurons concerned are located in the inferior salivatory nucleus (43.19) which lies at the junction of the pons and medulla just below the superior salivatory nucleus
  c. Preganglionic fibres pass successively through:
    i. The proximal part of the glossopharyngeal nerve
    ii. Its tympanic branch
    iii. The tympanic plexus
    iv. The lesser petrosal nerve to end in the otic ganglion.
  d. Postganglionic fibres arising from neurons located in the otic ganglion (43.64) pass through a nerve connecting the otic ganglion to the auriculotemporal nerve, and then through the auriculotemporal nerve itself. They leave the latter through its parotid branch to reach the parotid gland.
3. *General visceral afferent* fibres carry general visceral sensations.
  a. They are peripheral processes of unipolar cells in the inferior ganglion of the nerve.
  b. They pass through the pharyngeal, tonsilar and lingual branches to supply the mucous membrane of the pharynx, the posterior part of the tongue, the tonsil and the soft palate.
  c. Central processes of the neurons concerned pass through the proximal part of the glossopharyngeal nerve into the brainstem.
  d. Here they end in the nucleus of the solitary tract (43.19 and 43.20 A and B).
4. *Special visceral afferent* fibres carry the sensation of taste from the part of the tongue behind the sulcus terminalis, and from the vallate papillae.
  a. The fibres are peripheral processes of unipolar cells in the inferior ganglion of the glossopharyngeal nerve.
  b. They pass through the glossopharyngeal nerve and its lingual branches to reach the tongue.
  c. Central processes of the neurons concerned pass through the proximal part of the glossopharyngeal nerve and enter the medulla where they end in the upper part of the nucleus of the solitary tract.
5. According to some authorities the glossopharyngeal nerve also contains some general somatic afferent fibres.
  a. These include some fibres from the skin of the auricle
  b. Proprioceptive fibres from the stylopharyngeus
  c. They are described as ending in the spinal nucleus of the trigeminal nerve.

### The Otic Ganglion

1. The otic ganglion is situated just below the foramen ovale medial to the trunk of the mandibular nerve (43.41).
2. It is connected to the nerve to the medial pterygoid muscle.
3. The middle meningeal artery and the roots of the auriculotemporal nerve lie close to it (see 43.63).
4. The fibres passing through the otic ganglion are as follows:
  a. Functionally the ganglion is autonomic and is a peripheral ganglion of the cranial parasympathetic outflow.
  b. It is the relay station for secretomotor fibres to the parotid gland (see above).
  c. Sympathetic fibres reach the ganglion from the plexus on the middle meningeal artery. They pass through the ganglion, without relay, and travel to the parotid gland through the auriculotemporal nerve.
  d. Motor fibres reach the ganglion through the nerve to the medial pterygoid. These fibres are derived from the motor root of the mandibular nerve. They pass through the ganglion (without relay) and enter branches of the ganglion that supply the tensor tympani and the tensor palati muscles.

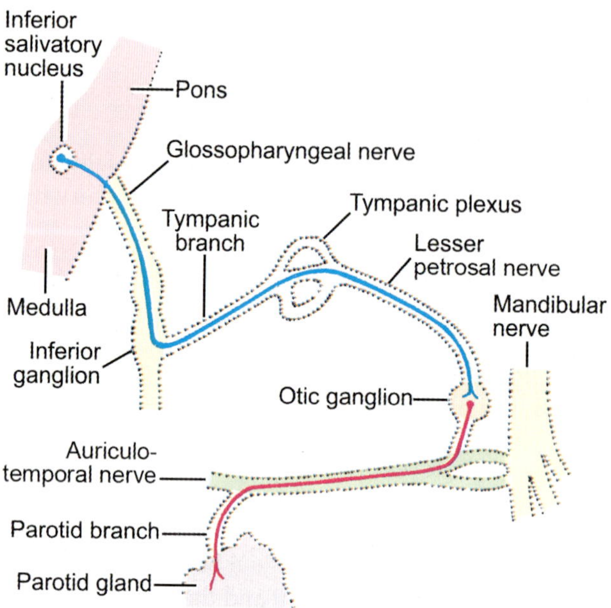


**43.63:** Secretomotor pathway for the parotid gland

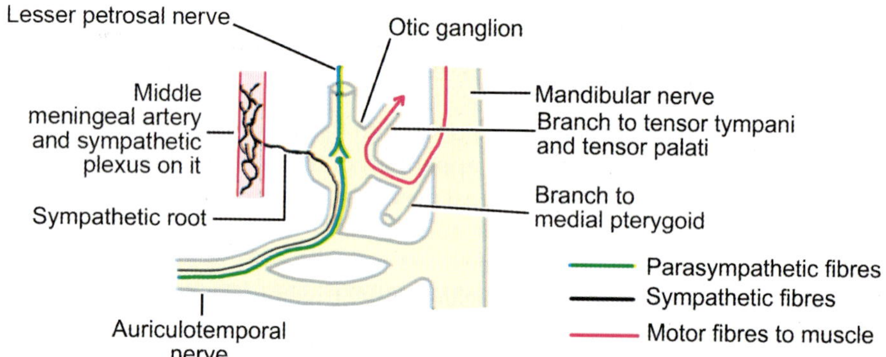


**63.64:** Connections of the otic ganglion

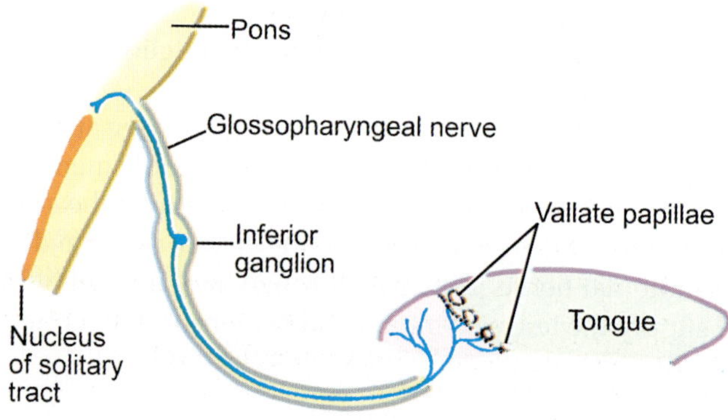


**43.65:** Pathway for taste from the posterior one-third of the tongue

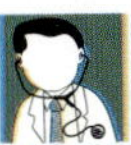

## CLINICAL CORRELATION

*Testing the Glossopharyngeal Nerve*

Testing of this nerve is based on the fact that:

1. The nerve carries fibres of taste from the posterior one-third of the tongue.
2. That it provides sensory innervation to the pharynx.
   a. Sensations of taste can be tested by applying substances that are salty (salt), sweet (sugar), sour (lemon), or bitter (quinine) to the posterior one-third of the tongue. The mouth should be rinsed and the tongue dried before the substance is applied.
   b. Touching the pharyngeal mucosa causes reflex constriction of pharyngeal muscles. The glossopharyngeal nerve provides the afferent part of the pathway for this reflex.

## THE VAGUS NERVE

1. The vagus nerve arises from the lateral side of the medulla, by about ten rootlets that are attached to the groove between the olive and the inferior cerebellar peduncle, below the rootlets of the glossopharyngeal nerve (43.27).
2. Thus formed the nerve leaves the skull through the jugular foramen. Its position relative to other structures in the foramen is shown in 43.60.
3. The part of the nerve within the jugular foramen shows an enlargement called the ***superior ganglion***. Just below the foramen the nerve has a much larger enlargement called the ***inferior ganglion***.
4. The vagus nerve descends vertically in the neck. It is enclosed within the carotid sheath. Here it lies in the interval between the posterior part of the internal or common carotid artery and the internal jugular vein. Some relations of this part of the nerve are shown in 42.3 and 42.4.
5. In the lower part of the neck the nerve crosses anterior to the first part of the subclavian artery (42.25A), and enters the thorax. Passing through the thorax the vagus enters the abdomen where it has a wide distribution.

### Branches of the Vagus Nerve in the Neck

The vagus nerve gives off numerous branches in the neck, in the thorax and in the abdomen. Branches arising in the thorax and the abdomen are considered in the appropriate sections. Here we will consider the branches that arise from the nerve in the neck.

## WANT TO KNOW MORE?

1. A ***meningeal branch*** arises near the upper end of the nerve and supplies the dura mater in the region.
2. The ***auricular branch*** arises from the superior ganglion. It is distributed to the skin of the auricle, the external acoustic meatus and the tympanic membrane.
   a. Soon after its origin the nerve enters the mastoid canaliculus (which opens on the lateral wall of the jugular fossa) and passes laterally through it within the temporal bone.
   b. The nerve emerges from the bone through the tympanomastoid fissure and divides into two branches.
   c. One of these supplies part of the skin of the auricle: the part supplied is shown in 43.11.
   d. The other branch supplies the skin lining the posterior wall and floor of the external acoustic meatus, and the posteroinferior part of the outer layer of the tympanic membrane. (The remaining parts of the meatus and of the membrane are supplied by the auriculotemporal nerve).

3. The ***pharyngeal branch*** arises from the inferior ganglion.
   a. It passes forwards on the side-wall of the pharynx crossing superficial to the internal carotid artery and deep to the external carotid artery.
   b. It divides into numerous branches that form the ***pharyngeal plexus***.
   c. Fibres continuing through the plexus supply the muscles of the pharynx and of the soft palate (except the tensor palati that is supplied by the mandibular nerve through the otic ganglion).
   d. The pharyngeal plexus is joined by branches from the glossopharyngeal nerve (sensory fibres) and by branches from the sympathetic trunk.

## WANT TO KNOW MORE?

4. One or more branches are given off to the carotid body. They may arise from the inferior ganglion or from the pharyngeal branch.

5. The ***superior laryngeal nerve*** arises from the inferior ganglion.
   a. It descends on the side-wall of the pharynx posterior to the internal carotid artery.
   b. It then curves forwards passing deep to the artery and ends by dividing into the internal and external laryngeal nerves.
6. The ***internal laryngeal nerve*** is sensory. It enters the larynx by piercing the thyrohyoid membrane. It divides into branches that supply:
   a. The mucous membrane of the upper half of the larynx (up to the vocal folds); and
   b. The mucous membrane of part of the pharynx, the epiglottis, the vallecula, and the posteriormost part of the tongue.
7. The ***external laryngeal nerve*** descends over the inferior constrictor muscle. It ends by supplying the cricothyroid muscle.
8. The course of the ***recurrent laryngeal nerve*** is different on the right and left sides. The course on the right side is as follows:
   a. The ***right recurrent laryngeal nerve*** arises from the right vagus as the latter passes in front of the subclavian artery.
   b. It passes backwards below the artery and then upwards behind the artery forming a loop.
   c. The nerve then runs upwards and medially deep to the common carotid artery to reach the side of the trachea.
9. The course of the ***left recurrent laryngeal nerve*** is as follows:
   a. The left recurrent laryngeal nerve arises from the left vagus in the thorax, as the latter crosses lateral to the arch of the aorta.
   b. The nerve winds below the arch, immediately behind the ligamentum arteriosum and then passes upwards and medially to reach the side of the trachea.

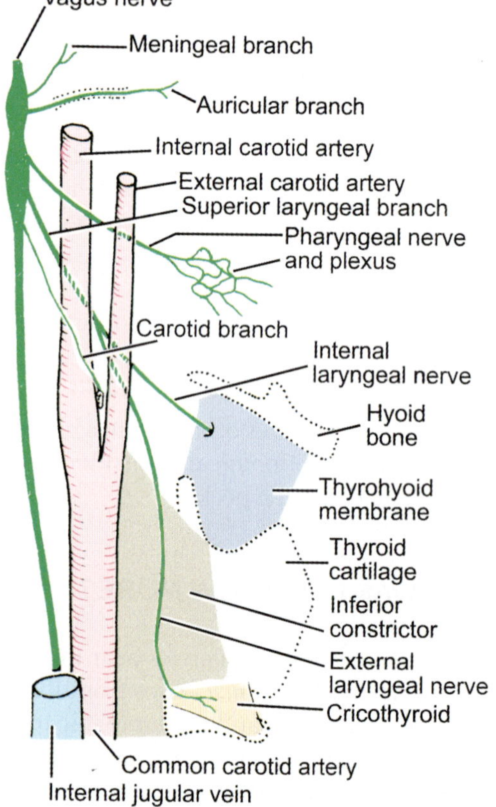


**43.66:** Scheme to show some branches of the vagus nerve in the neck

10. Having reached the trachea ***both the right and left nerves*** ascend in the groove between it and the oesophagus, deep to the medial surface of the thyroid gland. At the upper end of the trachea and oesophagus the nerve passes deep to the lower border of the inferior constrictor muscle and enters the larynx. It is distributed as follows:
    a. The nerve provides the motor supply to all intrinsic muscles of the larynx (except the cricothyroid supplied by the external laryngeal nerve).

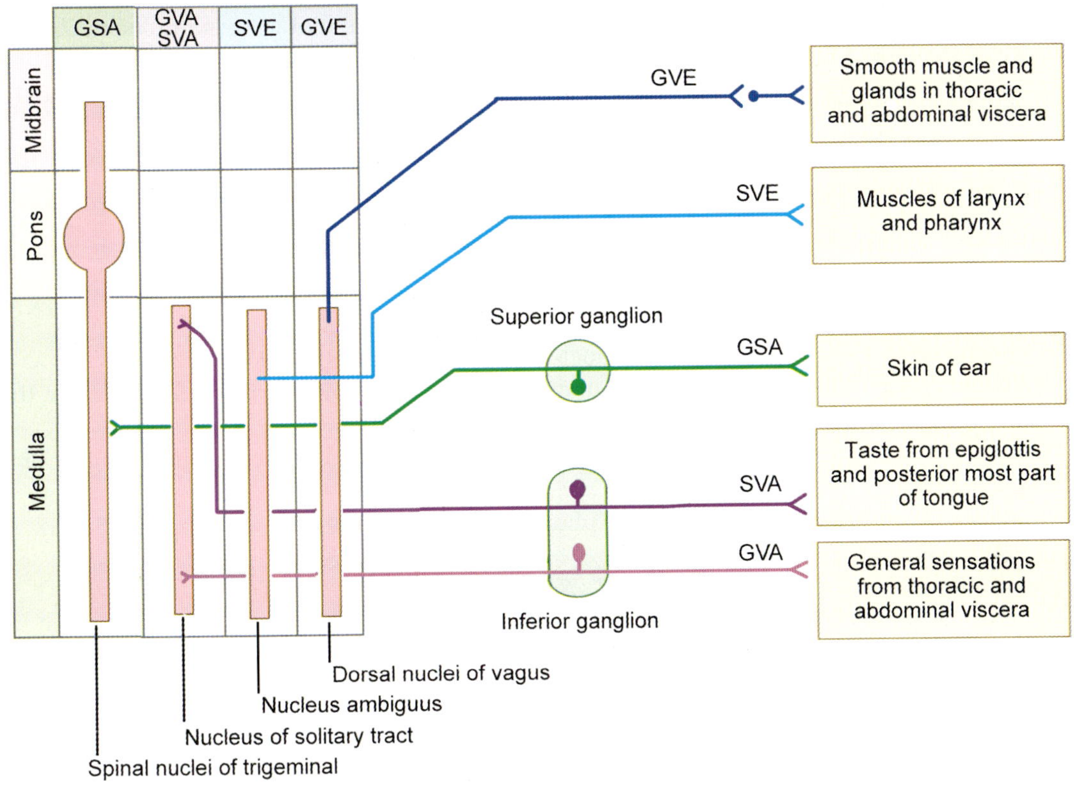


**43.67:** Scheme to show the functional components of the vagus nerve

b. The nerve provides the sensory supply to the mucous membrane of the lower half of the larynx i.e., the part below the level of the vocal folds.
c. It gives sensory branches to the trachea, the oesophagus and to the inferior constrictor muscle. It also gives branches to the cardiac plexus (see below).

At the lower pole of thyroid gland the recurrent laryngeal nerve is intimately related to the terminal branches of the inferior thyroid artery. Variations in the relationship are of surgical importance.

## WANT TO KNOW MORE?

11. **Cardiac Branches**
    a. Each vagus nerve gives one (or more) superior cervical cardiac branch in the upper part of the neck.
    b. An inferior cervical cardiac branch in its lower part.
    c. Additional cardiac branches arise from the nerve in the superior mediastinum.
    d. Also from the recurrent laryngeal branches.
    e. These branches end in the superficial and deep cardiac plexuses.

### Functional Components of the Vagus Nerve

1. The vagus nerve is composed predominantly of parasympathetic fibres.
    a. We have seen that these are classified as ***general visceral efferent.***
    b. These fibres are very widely distributed.

c. The vagi are responsible for parasympathetic innervation of the thoracic viscera including the heart and bronchi and of the greater part of the gastrointestinal tract.

d. Because of this fact the term 'vagal' is synonymous with parasympathetic while referring to these organs.

2. The fibres in the vagus nerves are preganglionic.
   a. They arise from the dorsal nucleus of the vagus (43.19 and 43.20 E and F) and pass through the nerve and its ramifications to reach the viscera supplied.
   b. As a rule postganglionic neurons are located in plexuses situated close to the viscera, or in the walls of the viscera themselves. They innervate:
      i. Smooth muscle
      ii. Glands present in the walls of the viscera.
3. ***Special visceral efferent*** fibres arise from the nucleus ambiguus (43.19 and 43.20 E and F).
   a. They pass through branches of vagus to innervate some of the musculature derived from the branchial arches.
   b. The superior laryngeal branch is the nerve of the fourth arch, and the recurrent laryngeal branch that of the sixth arch.
   c. Through these branches (and through the pharyngeal branches) the vagus supplies muscles of the pharynx, soft palate and larynx.
4. The vagus contains numerous ***general visceral afferent*** fibres.
   a. The neurons concerned are unipolar and are located in the inferior ganglion.
   b. The peripheral processes pass through the vagus and its branches to reach the pharynx, larynx, trachea, and oesophagus; and the thoracic and abdominal viscera.
   c. Central processes of these neurons end in the nucleus of the solitary tract.
   d. According to some authorities some of these fibres terminate in the dorsal nucleus of the vagus.
5. The vagus carries the sensation of taste from the posterior-most part of the tongue and from the epiglottis. These fibres are ***special visceral afferent.***
   a. The neurons concerned lie in the inferior ganglion of the nerve.
   b. Their peripheral processes pass through the superior laryngeal nerve to reach the tongue and epiglottis.
   c. The central processes end in the nucleus of the solitary tract (43.19 and 43.20 E and F).
6. Finally the vagus also contains ***general somatic afferent*** fibres that supply skin.
   a. The neurons concerned lie in the superior ganglion of the nerve.
   b. Peripheral processes pass through the auricular branch to reach the skin of the auricle. The area supplied is shown in 43.11.

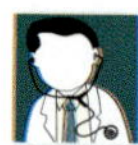

## CLINICAL CORRELATION

**Vagus Nerve (and Cranial Part of Accessory Nerve)**

This nerve has an extensive distribution but testing is based on its motor supply to the soft palate and to the larynx.

1. Ask the patient to open the mouth wide and say 'aah'. Observe the movement of the soft palate.
   a. In a normal person the soft palate is elevated.
   b. When one vagus nerve is paralysed the palate is pulled towards the normal side.
   c. When the nerve is paralysed on both sides the soft palate does not move at all.
2. In injury to the superior laryngeal nerve the voice is weak due to paralysis of the cricothyroid muscle. At first there is hoarseness but after some time the opposite cricothyroid muscle compensates for the deficit and hoarseness disappears.
3. Injury to the recurrent laryngeal nerve also leads to hoarseness, but this hoarseness is permanent.
   a. On examining the larynx through a laryngoscope it is seen that on the affected side the vocal fold does not move. It is fixed in a position midway between adduction and abduction.

b. In cases where the recurrent laryngeal nerve is pressed upon by a tumour it is observed that nerve fibres that supply abductors are lost first.

4. In paralysis of both recurrent laryngeal nerves voice is lost as both vocal folds are immobile.
5. It may be remembered that the left recurrent laryngeal nerve runs part of its course in the thorax. It can be involved in bronchial or oesophageal carcinoma, or in secondary growths in mediastinal lymph nodes.

## THE ACCESSORY NERVE

This is the eleventh cranial nerve. It consists of two distinct parts, cranial and spinal. Both parts consist predominantly of efferent fibres as follows:

1. The fibres of the ***cranial part*** arise from the nucleus ambiguus. These fibres join the vagus nerve and are distributed through its pharyngeal and laryngeal branches to muscles of the pharynx, soft palate and larynx.
2. The fibres of the spinal part arise from the lateral part of the ventral grey column of the upper five or six cervical segments of the spinal cord. They supply the sternocleidomastoid and trapezius muscles.

### WANT TO KNOW MORE?

**Cranial Part of Accessory Nerve**

1. The cranial part of the nerve is attached, by four or five rootlets, to the side of the medulla in the groove between the olive and the inferior cerebellar peduncle.
2. The rootlets are attached in line with, but below, those of the vagus nerve (43.27 and 43.68).
3. From here the nerve runs laterally to reach the jugular foramen where it is joined by the spinal root (see below).
4. Its position in the jugular foramen is shown in 43.60.
5. After passing through the jugular foramen the cranial root again separates from the spinal root and merges with the inferior ganglion of the vagus.
6. The fibres of the cranial root of the accessory nerve pass into the pharyngeal and recurrent laryngeal branches of the vagus.
7. They contribute to the innervation of the muscles of the pharynx and larynx.
8. It is believed that fibres of the accessory nerve supply all the muscles of the soft palate (except the tensor palati).

**Spinal Part of Accessory Nerve**

1. The spinal part of the accessory nerve is formed by union of a number of rootlets that emerge from the upper five or six cervical segments of the spinal cord.
2. The rootlets emerge along a vertical line midway between the line of attachment of the ventral and dorsal roots of the spinal nerves.
3. Thus formed the spinal root ascends lateral to the spinal cord.
4. It enters the skull through the foramen magnum. Here it lies behind the vertebral artery.
5. The spinal root then runs upwards and laterally to reach the jugular foramen. The spinal root joins the cranial root within the foramen, but leaves it again on emerging from the foramen.

### Course in the Neck

1. In the neck the spinal accessory nerve first runs backwards and laterally to reach the transverse process of the atlas.
2. It then downwards and backwards across the lateral side of the neck (43.69).

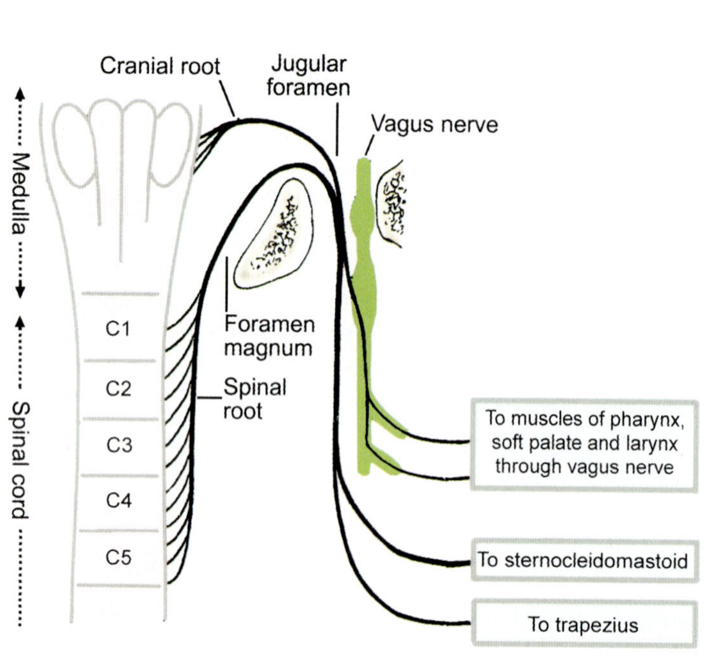


**43.68:** Scheme to show the formation and distribution of the accessory nerve

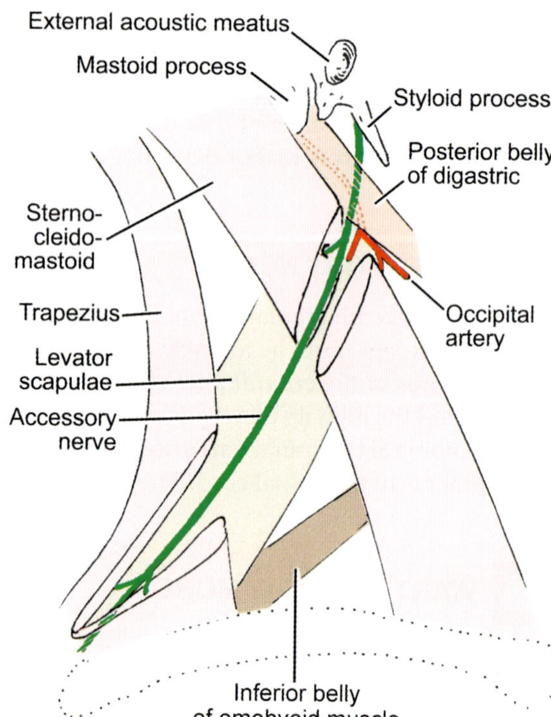


**43.69:** Course and some relations of the accessory nerve

3. In this part of its course the nerve passes through the sternocleidomastoid. It enters the deep surface of the muscle and passing through it emerges at its posterior border (near the middle).
4. The nerve now runs downwards and backwards across the posterior triangle to reach the anterior margin of the trapezius about 5 cm above the clavicle.
5. The terminal part of the nerve runs down the back deep to the trapezius.
6. The spinal part of the accessory nerve supplies the sternocleidomastoid (as it passes through it) and the trapezius (by its terminal branches). Note that these muscles also receive branches from the cervical plexus, but these branches are generally regarded as having only proprioceptive fibres.
7. Some important relations of the accessory nerve as it runs through the neck are as follows:

## WANT TO KNOW MORE?

a. Between the jugular foramen and the transverse process of the atlas the nerve usually passes posterior to the internal jugular vein. In this part of its course the nerve lies deep to the styloid process and the posterior belly of the digastric muscle.
b. Over the transverse process of the atlas the nerve is crossed by the occipital artery (43.69).
c. While crossing the posterior triangle of the neck the nerve lies on the levator scapulae (43.69).

The fibres of the accessory nerve are regarded as special visceral efferent as the muscles supplied are derived from branchial arches.

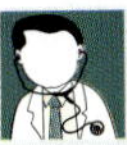

### CLINICAL CORRELATION

This nerve is tested as follows:

1. Put your hands on the right and left shoulders of the patient and ask him to elevate (shrug) his shoulders. In paralysis, the movement will be weak on one side (due to paralysis of the trapezius).
2. Ask the patient to turn his face to the opposite side (against resistance offered by your hand). In paralysis the movement is weak on the affected side (due to paralysis of the sternocleidomastoid muscle).

## THE HYPOGLOSSAL NERVE

1. This is the twelfth cranial nerve. Its fibres are purely motor. They supply the muscles of the tongue.
2. The neurons that give origin to these fibres are located in the hypoglossal nucleus that is shown in 43.19 and 43.20 E and F.
3. The hypoglossal nerve emerges from the medulla by ten to fifteen rootlets that are attached in the vertical groove separating the pyramid from the olive (43.27). (The rootlets are in line with those of the ventral root of the first cervical nerve).
4. The hypoglossal nerve leaves the cranial cavity through the hypoglossal canal (or anterior condylar) canal.
5. On emerging at the base of the skull the nerve lies deep (medial) to the internal jugular vein and internal carotid artery.
   a. It passes downwards to reach the interval between these vessels, and then runs vertically between them, up to the level of the angle of the mandible (43.71).
   b. Here the nerve passes forwards crossing the internal and external carotid arteries, and enters the submandibular region.
6. In the submandibular region the hypoglossal nerve at first lies superficial to the hyoglossus muscle and then to the genioglossus.
   a. It ends by dividing into its terminal branches.
   b. These supply all the intrinsic and extrinsic muscles of the tongue (except the palatoglossus that is supplied, along with other muscles of the palate, by the cranial accessory nerve) (also see below).

### WANT TO KNOW MORE?

7. Some relations of the hypoglossal nerve are as follows:
   a. In the initial part of its course the nerve passes laterally behind the internal carotid artery, the glossopharyngeal nerve and the vagus. The nerve then winds round the lateral side of the inferior ganglion of the vagus to reach the front of the nerve.
   b. Just before the nerve turns forwards (near the angle of the mandible) it lies deep to the posterior belly of the digastric muscle.
   c. Emerging from under this muscle the nerve loops round the inferior sterno-cleidomastoid branch of the occipital artery (43.71).
   d. As the nerve runs forwards in the neck it crosses the internal carotid artery, the external carotid artery and the loop formed by the lingual artery. The loop of the lingual artery is crossed just above the tip of the greater cornu of the hyoid bone.
   e. As the nerve runs forwards above the greater cornu of the hyoid bone it is crossed by the digastric tendon and the stylohyoid.
   f. As the hypoglossal nerve crosses the hyoglossus the lingual nerve, the submandibular duct and the deep part of the submandibular gland lie above it (43.71). This part of the nerve is deep to the mylohyoid muscle.

## Branches of the Hypoglossal Nerve

The branches of the hypoglossal nerve may be divided:

1. Branches of the nerve proper
2. Branches that represent fibres which reach it from the first cervical nerve.

## Branches of the Hypoglossal Nerve Proper

1. The hypoglossal nerve itself supplies the muscles of the tongue (styloglossus, hyoglossus, genioglossus, and intrinsic muscles).

### WANT TO KNOW MORE?

**Branches Carrying Fibres of Cervical Nerves**

2. A ***meningeal branch*** arises from the nerve as it passes through the hypoglossal canal. It supplies the dura mater of the posterior cranial fossa. The fibres of this branch are probably derived from the upper cervical nerves and from the superior cervical sympathetic ganglion.
3. The nerve gives a ***descending branch*** that forms the superior root of the ansa cervicalis. Its fibres are derived from the first cervical nerve (43.13 and 43.70).

4. Branches from the hypoglossal nerve also supply the thyrohyoid and geniohyoid muscles (43.70). Like the fibres of the descending branch the fibres of these branches are also derived from the first cervical nerve.

### WANT TO KNOW MORE?

**Functional Component**

The fibres of the hypoglossal nerve are classified as somatic efferent because the muscles of the tongue develop from somites (occipital somites).

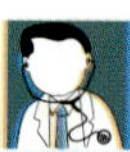

### CLINICAL CORRELATION

1. This nerve supplies muscles of the tongue. To test the nerve, ask the patient to protrude the tongue.
   a. In a normal person the protruded tongue lies in the midline.
   b. If the hypoglossal nerve is paralysed the tongue deviates to the paralysed side.
2. The explanation for this is as follows:
   a. Protrusion of the tongue is produced by the pull of the right and left genioglossus muscles.
   b. The origin of the right and left genioglossus muscles lies anteriorly (on the hyoid bone), and the insertion lies posteriorly (onto the posterior part of the tongue).
   c. Each muscle draws the posterior part of the tongue forwards and medially.
   d. Normally, the medial pull of the two muscles cancels out, but when one muscle is paralysed it is this medial pull of the intact muscle that causes the tongue to deviate to the opposite side.
3. Deviation of the tongue should be assessed with reference to the incisor teeth, and not to the lips. Remember that in facial paralysis the tongue may protrude normally, but may appear to deviate to one side because of asymmetry of the mouth.

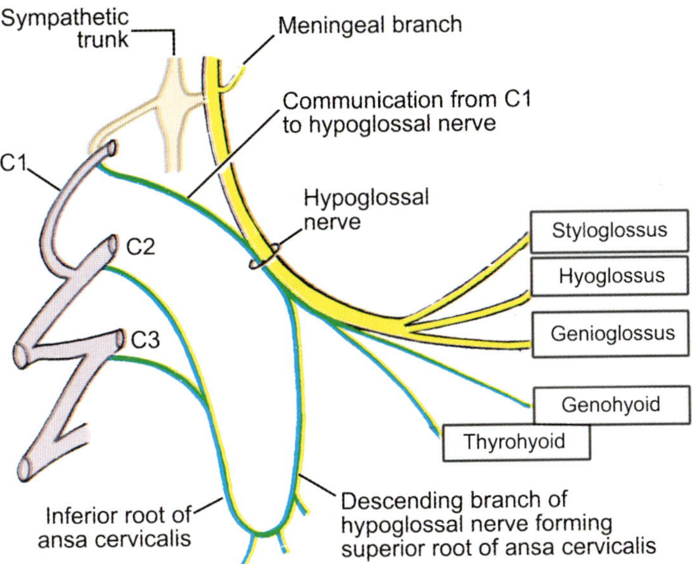


43.70: Scheme to show the distribution of the hypoglossal nerve

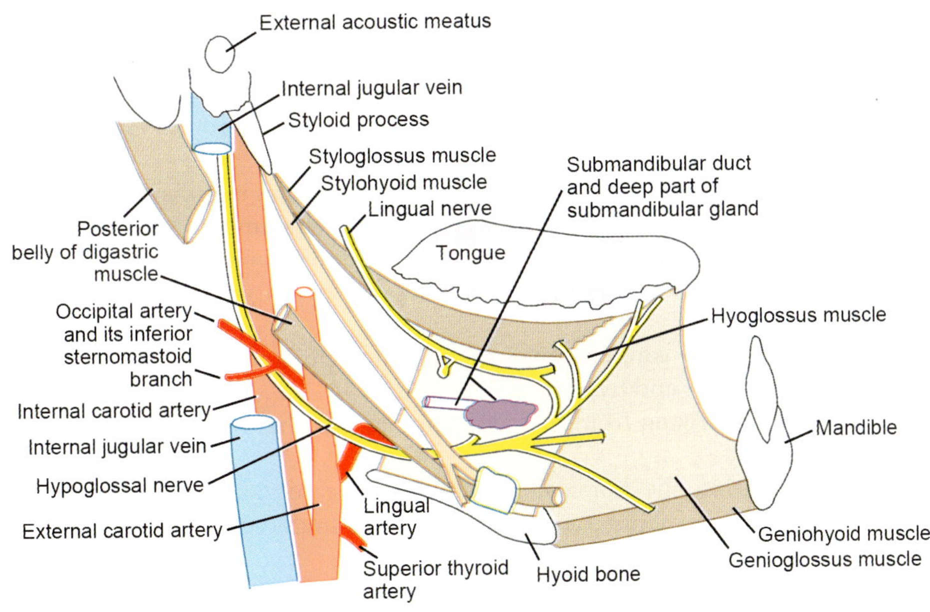


43.71: Some relations of the hypoglossal nerve

## CERVICAL PART OF SYMPATHETIC TRUNK

1. The cervical part of the sympathetic trunk bears three ganglia: Superior, middle and cervicothoracic.
   a. The ***superior ganglion*** represents fused ganglia C1 to C4.
   b. The ***middle ganglion*** represents ganglia C5 and C6.
   c. The ***cervicothoracic ganglion*** represents ganglia C7, C8 and T1. This ganglion has numerous branches that give it a star-like appearance and so it is also called the ***stellate ganglion***.

2. a. The superior cervical ganglion lies in front of the transverse processes of vertebrae C2 and C3.
   b. The middle ganglion in front of C6.
   c. The cervicothoracic ganglion between the transverse process of C7 and the neck of the first rib.

## WANT TO KNOW MORE?

### Branches of Superior Cervical Ganglion

The branches of the superior cervical sympathetic ganglion are as follows (43.73):

1. The ***internal carotid nerve*** arises from the upper pole of the ganglion.
   a. It is composed mainly of postganglionic fibres arising in the superior cervical ganglion.
   b. The nerve ascends along the internal carotid artery and divides into branches that form a plexus over it.
   c. This plexus has numerous connections the more important of which are as follows (43.72).
2. While in the carotid canal the plexus gives off the ***caroticotympanic nerves*** which enter the middle ear and join the tympanic plexus.
3. In the foramen lacerum the internal carotid plexus gives off the ***deep petrosal nerve***.
   a. This branch joins the greater petrosal nerve to form the nerve of the pterygoid canal through which the fibres reach the pterygopalatine ganglion.
   b. They pass through this ganglion, without relay, and travel through its orbital branches to supply the orbitalis muscle.
4. While the internal carotid nerve lies in the cavernous sinus it communicates with the ophthalmic division of the trigeminal nerve.
   a. These fibres pass into its nasociliary branch, and then into the long ciliary nerves to reach the eyeball where they supply the dilator pupillae muscle, and the blood vessels of the eyeball.
   b. Some fibres pass from the nasociliary nerve, or direct from the plexus round the internal carotid artery, to the ciliary ganglion.
   c. These fibres pass through this ganglion without relay and then pass into the short ciliary nerves to supply blood vessels of the eyeball. The fibres to the dilator pupillae sometimes follow the second route.
   d. It may be noted here that preganglionic sympathetic fibres for the eyeball begin in segment T1 of the spinal cord and ascend in the sympathetic trunk to the superior cervical ganglion in which the postganglionic neurons lie.
5. The superior cervical sympathetic ganglion gives grey rami to spinal nerves C1 to C4. It also communicates with the glossopharyngeal, vagus and hypoglossal nerves.
6. ***Laryngopharyngeal branches*** arising from the ganglion join the pharyngeal plexus. They also supply the carotid body.
7. The ***cardiac branch*** descends into the thorax along the common carotid artery.
   a. On the left side the nerve runs across the lateral side of the arch of the aorta and ends in the superficial cardiac plexus.
   b. On the right side it joins the deep cardiac plexus.
8. Branches are also given off from the ganglion to the common carotid and external carotid arteries and form plexuses over them.
   a. Branches of the plexus on the external carotid artery extend along its branches.
   b. The plexus on the middle meningeal artery gives a branch to the otic ganglion.
   c. And that on the facial artery to the submandibular ganglion.
   d. Fibres running along the facial artery supply the sweat glands of the face.

### Branches of Middle Cervical Ganglion

The branches of the middle cervical ganglion and its connections are as follows (43.74):

1. The ganglion is connected superiorly to the superior cervical ganglion.

2. It is connected inferiorly to the cervicothoracic ganglion by an anterior and two posterior cords.
   a. The posterior cords enclose the vertebral artery.
   b. The anterior cord passes down across the subclavian artery, forms a loop below it and then passes up behind the artery to join the cervicothoracic ganglion. The loop formed is called the ***ansa subclavia***.
3. The middle cervical ganglion gives grey rami to nerves C5 and C6.
4. A cardiac branch descends into the thorax and ends in the deep cardiac plexus.
5. Branches are also given off to the thyroid and parathyroid glands. They pass along the inferior thyroid artery.

**Branches of Cervicothoracic Ganglion**

The branches of the cervicothoracic ganglion (or stellate ganglion) are as follows (43.74):

1. The connections of the ganglion to the middle cervical ganglion, including that through the ansa subclavia have been described above.
2. The ganglion gives grey rami to nerves C7, C8 and T1.
3. A cardiac branch arising from this ganglion ends in the deep cardiac plexus.
4. The cervicothoracic ganglion gives branches that form a plexus on the subclavian artery. This plexus extends onto:
   a. The axillary artery
   b. Branches of the subclavian artery including the vertebral and inferior thyroid arteries.
5. The plexus on the vertebral artery extends along the artery into the cranial cavity and communicates with the internal carotid plexus.
6. Branches from the vertebral plexus also pass to the cervical nerves.

**Sympathetic Innervation of Upper Limb**

1. The cervicothoracic ganglion is intimately concerned with the sympathetic innervation of the upper limb.
2. The preganglionic neurons concerned lie in spinal segments T2 to T6 and emerge through the corresponding spinal nerves.
3. These fibres ascend in the sympathetic trunk to reach the cervicothoracic ganglion in which they relay.
4. Postganglionic fibres starting in the ganglion reach the blood vessels and sweat glands of the upper limb through the brachial plexus and its branches (mainly through nerves C8 and T1).
5. The plexus on the subclavian artery was at one time considered to be the main pathway for sympathetic innervation of the upper limb, but it is now known that the fibres in the plexus do not extend much beyond the first part of the axillary artery.

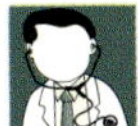

## CLINICAL CORRELATION

**Horner's Syndrome**

Interruption of sympathetic supply to the head and neck results in ***Horner's syndrome.*** The features of this syndrome are as follows:

1. There is ***constriction of the pupil*** because of paralysis of the dilator pupillae. Unopposed action of the sphincter pupillae leads to ***constriction of the pupil***.
2. There is drooping of the upper eyelid (***ptosis***) because of paralysis of smooth muscle fibres present in the levator palpebrae superioris.
3. The eyeball is less prominent than normal (***enophthalmos***).
4. There is ***absence of sweating*** on the affected side of the face. (Remember that secretomotor supply to sweat glands is through sympathetic nerves).

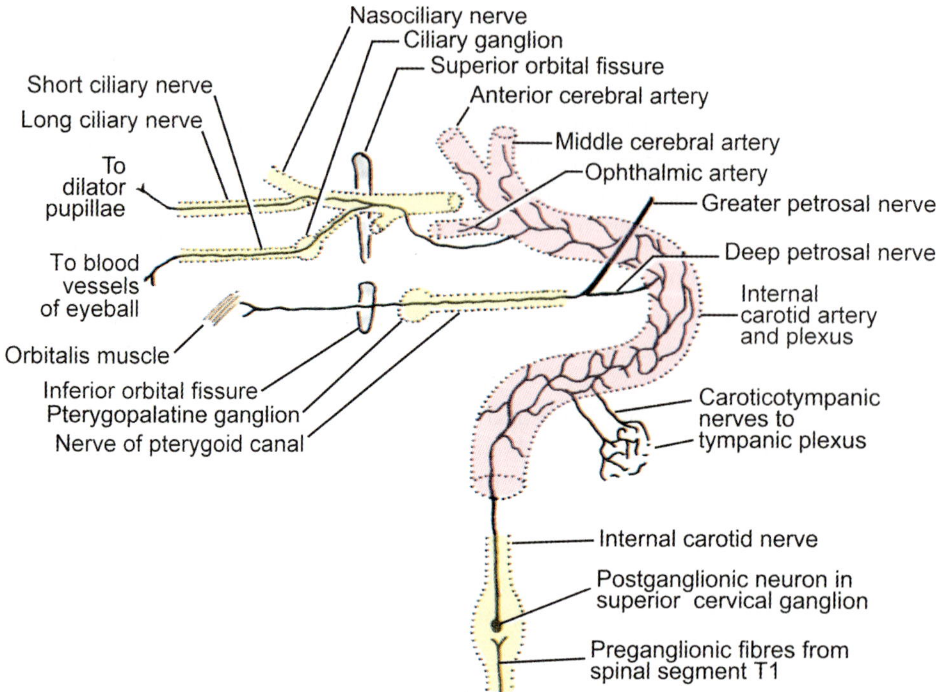


**43.72:** Distribution of internal carotid nerve

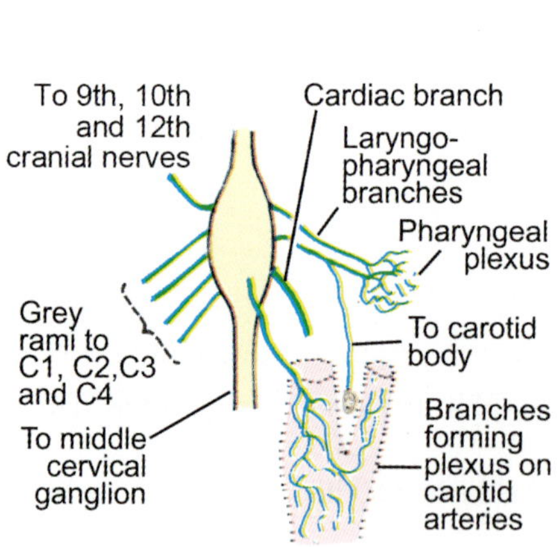


**43.73:** Branches of superior cervical sympathetic ganglion

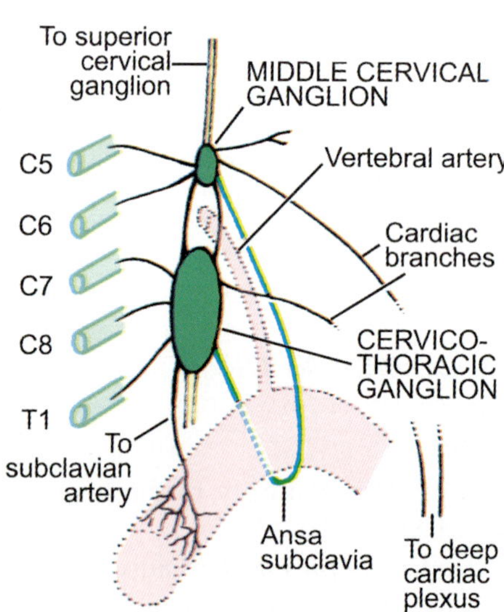


**43.74:** Branches of the middle cervical sympathetic and cervicothoracic ganglia

# 44 CHAPTER

# Orbit, Eye and Ear

## THE ORBIT

### CONTENTS OF THE ORBIT

These are as follows:

1. The eyeball
2. Extraocular muscles
3. Nerves of the orbit (all described in Chapter 43)
   a. Optic nerve
   b. Oculomotor nerve
   c. Trochlear nerve
   d. Abducent nerve
   e. Ophthalmic division of trigeminal nerve and its branches
   f. Part of maxillary division of trigeminal nerve.
4. Arteries: ophthalmic branch of internal carotid (Chapter 42)
5. Ophthalmic veins (Chapter 42).
6. Lacrimal gland.

### MUSCLES OF THE ORBIT

1. The muscles of the orbit include the ***extraocular muscles*** that are:
   a. The four recti (superior, inferior, medial and lateral)
   b. Two oblique muscles (superior and inferior)
   c. The levator palpebrae superioris.
2. In addition, we have some muscles made up of smooth muscle fibres and supplied by autonomic nerves. These are the ***superior tarsal, inferior tarsal*** and ***orbitalis*** muscles. Some muscles that lie within the eyeball (***sphincter and dilator pupillae, ciliaris***) will be considered when we study that organ.
3. The extraocular muscles are described in 44.1 and shown in 44.2 to 44.6.

#### Actions of Rectus and Oblique Muscles: Movements of the Eyeball

Actions of individual muscles are given in 44.1. Here, we consider important points about movements of the eyeball. As a convention movements of the eyeball are described with reference to its anterior end (or more simply, the cornea).

1. The cornea can move upwards or downwards, the movement occurring on an imaginary axis passing transversely through the equator of the eyeball.
2. Upward movement can be produced by:
   a. Pulling the anterior part of the eyeball upwards (superior rectus)
   b. Pulling the posterior part downwards (inferior oblique).

**44.1: Extraocular muscles**

| *Muscle* | *Origin* | *Insertion* | *Action* | *Nerve supply* |
|---|---|---|---|---|
| Superior rectus | All recti arise from posterior part of orbit through a common tendinous ring which surrounds the optic canal, and encloses part of the superior orbital fissure. The superior, inferior, medial and lateral recti arise from the corresponding parts of the ring. | The recti run forwards to reach the corresponding side of the sclera about 6 mm behind the junction of the sclera and cornea. Insertions are in front of the equator of the eyeball. | 1. Upward movement of eyeball.<br>2. Inward movement of eyeball.<br>3. Intorsion of eyeball. | Oculomotor nerve |
| Inferior rectus | | | 1. Downward movement of eyeball.<br>2. Inward movement of eyeball.<br>3. Extorsion of eyeball. | Oculomotor nerve |
| Medial rectus | | | Inward movement of eyeball. | Oculomotor nerve |
| Lateral rectus | | | Outward movement of eyeball. | Abducent nerve |
| Superior oblique | Body of sphenoid bone just above and medial to optic canal. | 1. Runs forward in upper part of orbit.<br>2. Near orbital margin the muscle ends in a tendon the passes through a tendinous pulley.<br>3. Tendon then runs backwards and laterally to be inserted into the upper lateral quadrant of eyeball behind the equator. | 1. Outward movement of eyeball.<br>2. Intorsion of eyeball. | Trochlear nerve |
| Inferior oblique | Anterior and medial part of floor of orbit (maxilla) | Muscle winds round eyeball to reach the lateral part of the sclera behind equator of eyeball. | 1. Outward movement of eyeball.<br>2. Extorsion of eyeball. | Oculomotor nerve |
| Levator palpebrae superioris | Posterior part of orbit (lesser wing of sphenoid above optic canal. | Upper eyelid (tarsus and superior conjunctival fornix) | Elevates eyelid and keeps palpebral fissure open. | Oculomotor nerve |

3. Similarly, downward movement can be produced by:
    a. Pulling the anterior part downwards (inferior rectus)
    b. Pulling the posterior part upwards (superior oblique).
4. The cornea can move medially or laterally on an axis passing vertically through the equator of the eyeball.
    a. Medial movement can be produced by pulling the anterior part of the eyeball medially. This action is performed by the medial rectus.
    b. The superior and inferior recti can also move the cornea medially as they pass forwards and laterally from origin to insertion.
5. Lateral movement can be produced by:
    a. Pulling the anterior part of the eyeball laterally (lateral rectus)
    b. Pulling the posterior part medially (superior and inferior oblique).
6. The cornea can move obliquely by combination of the movements described above e.g., upwards and medially, downwards and laterally and so on.

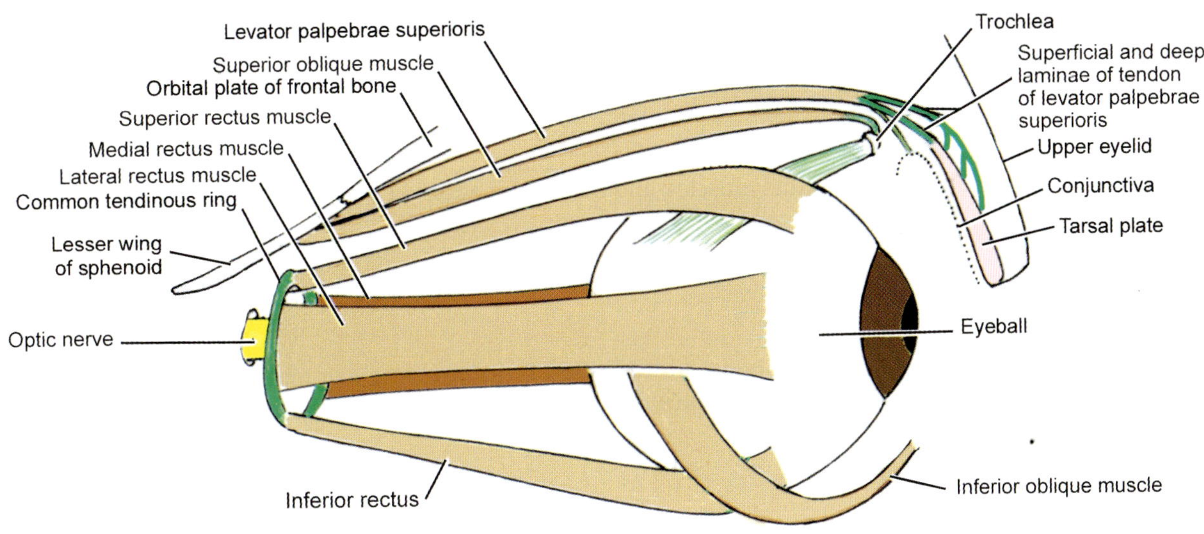


**44.2:** Scheme to show extraocular muscles as seen from the lateral side

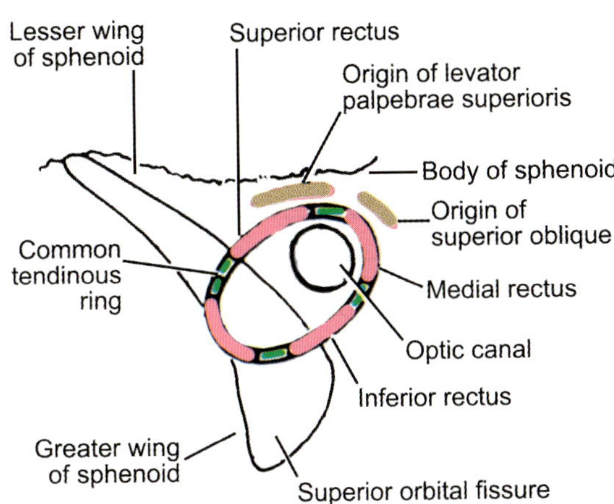


**44.3:** Diagram showing the common tendinous ring for origin of the rectus muscles of the orbit. Note its relationship to the optic canal and to the superior orbital fissure

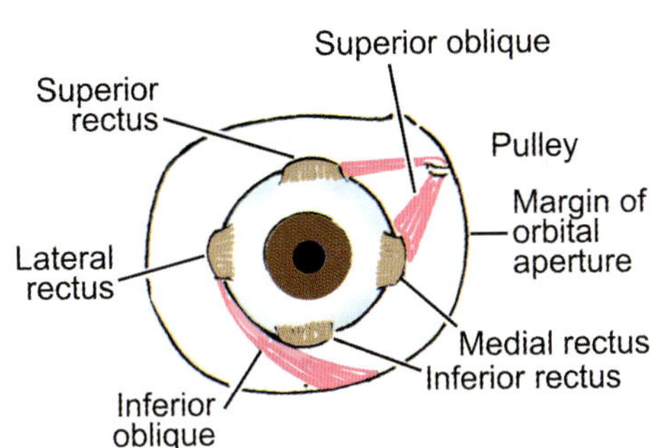


**44.4:** Schematic anterior view of the orbit to show the attachment of extraocular muscles to the eyeball. In particular note the arrangement of the superior and inferior oblique muscles

## WANT TO KNOW MORE?

7. The eyeball undergoes torsional movements on an anteroposterior axis.
   a. To understand these movements imagine a vertical line drawn through the middle of the cornea dividing it into medial and lateral halves (44.5A).
   b. Torsion is described with reference to the ***upper*** end of this line (arrow).
   c. When the eyeball rotates so that the upper end of the line moves medially the movement is described as ***intorsion***
   d. When it moves laterally the movement is called ***extorsion.***

8. From 44.5B, it will be obvious that intorsion will be produced mainly by the superior oblique and partly by the superior rectus; while extorsion will be produced (44.5C) mainly by the inferior oblique, and partly by the inferior rectus.

9. The movements produced by individual muscles, and the combinations of muscles producing a given movement, are summarised in 44.6.

## Arrangement of Fascia in the Orbit

### *Periorbita (Orbital Fascia)*

1. The periosteum lining the inside of the bony orbit is called the orbital fascia or periorbita.
2. At the anterior aperture of the orbit, it becomes continuous with periosteum covering the bones around the aperture.

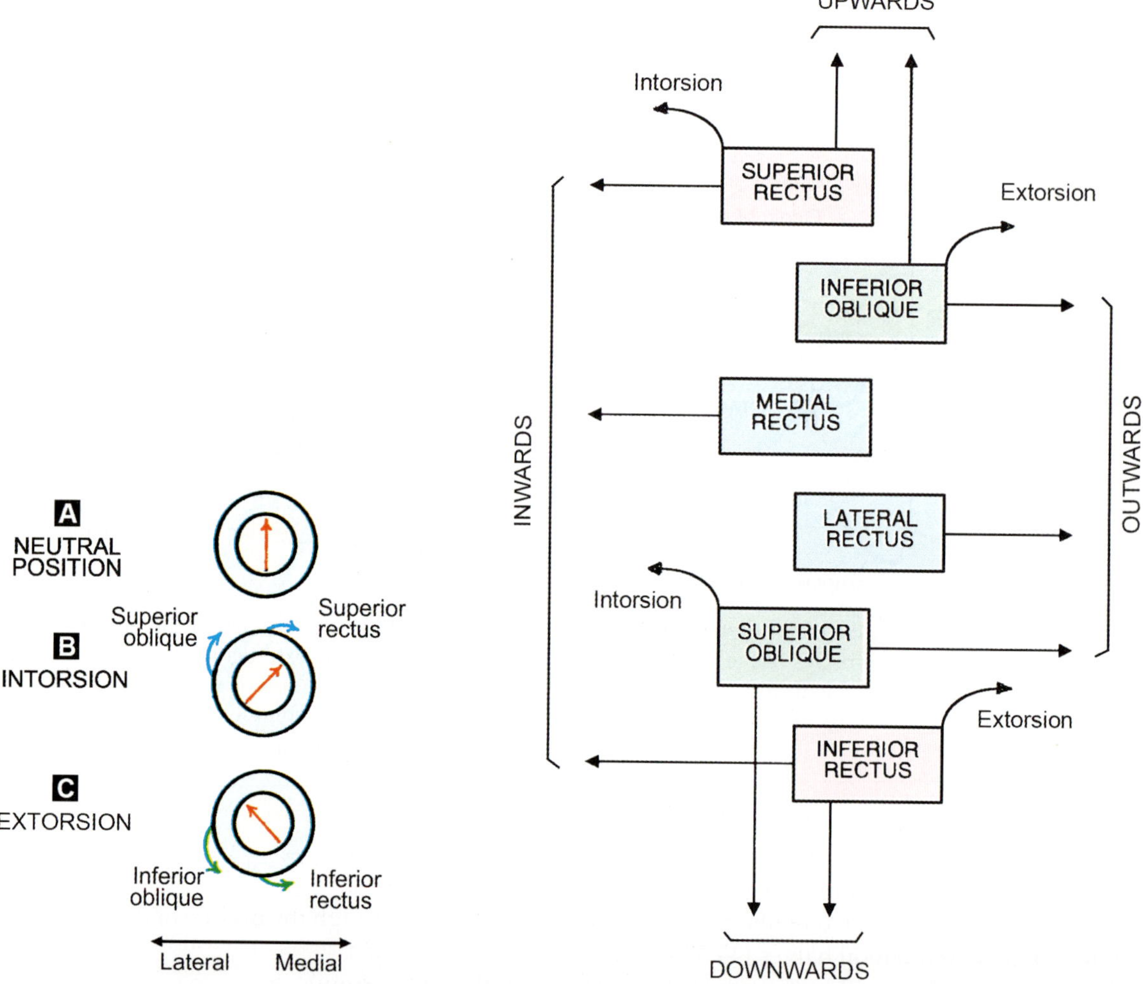


**44.5:** Schematic diagram of the eye to explain the movements of intorsion and extorsion. The inner circle represents the cornea, and the outer circle represents the sclera

**44.6:** Scheme showing the movements of the eyeball produced by individual extraocular muscles, and the muscles responsible for each movement

3. At the superior orbital fissures, and at the optic canal, it becomes continuous with the endocranium of the middle cranial fossa.
4. At the inferior orbital fissure, it becomes continuous with periosteum lining the pterygopalatine fossa.
5. The periorbita sends expansions into the eyelids. These extensions form the ***orbital septum***.
6. The lacrimal fascia (37.8), and the trochlea for the superior oblique tendon can be regarded as special regions of the periorbita.

### *Fascial Sheath of the Eyeball*

1. The eyeball is surrounded by a fascial sheath that extends posteriorly up to the attachment of the optic nerve, where the fascial sheath fuses with the sheath of the nerve.
2. Anteriorly, it extends up to the sclerocorneal junction.
3. It is separated from the eyeball by the ***episcleral space*** .
4. The sheath is closely related to the ocular muscles that perforate it, and receive extensions from it. These extensions form tubular sheaths round the muscles: fibrous bands pass from them to the orbital wall.
5. The most important bands are the ***medial and lateral check ligaments***.
   a. The medial check ligament passes from the sheath around the medial rectus to the medial wall of the orbit.
   b. The lateral check ligament passes from the sheath over the lateral rectus to the lateral wall of the orbit.
   c. They are called check ligaments on the assumption that they limit the contraction of these muscles.
6. The space between the fascial sheath of the eyeball and the orbital periosteum is filled mostly by fat. The sheath and the fat keep the eyeball in place.
7. The sheath provides a smooth surface over which the surface of the eyeball can move freely. In this connection, it is interesting to note that the fascial sheath has been compared to a hammock supporting the eyeball (44.7).

## THE LACRIMAL GLAND

1. The lacrimal gland lies in relation to the upper lateral part of the wall of the orbit (formed here by the zygomatic process of the frontal bone) (37.7).
2. The gland is related inferiorly to the levator palpebrae superioris and to the lateral rectus muscle.
3. An extension of the gland, that enters the upper eyelid, is called its ***palpebral part*** (37.7).
   a. The palpebral part is continuous with the ***main (or orbital) part*** around the lateral side of the aponeurosis of the levator palpebrae superioris.

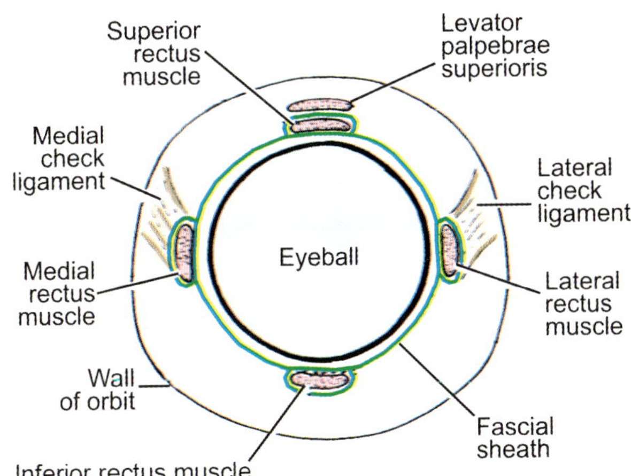


**44.7:** Scheme to show some parts of the fascial sheath of the eyeball. Note the 'hammock' formed by the lower part of the sheath and the check ligaments

   b. In other words, the palpebral part of the gland lies deep to the aponeurosis of the levator palpebrae superioris (37.5).
4. The lacrimal gland drains into the superior conjunctival fornix through about twelve ducts. All ducts pass through the palpebral part of the gland.
5. Accessory lacrimal glands may be present in relation to the superior conjunctival fornix, or less commonly in relation to the inferior fornix.
6. The lacrimal gland is supplied by twigs from the lacrimal branch of the ophthalmic artery.
7. The secretomotor fibres to the gland follow a complicated course that is shown in 43.56.

## NERVES AND VESSELS OF ORBIT

These have been described in detail in Chapters 42 and 43. The parts pertaining to the orbit are repeated here for convenience. For further details, illustrations and clinical correlations see the chapters cited.

### The Ophthalmic Artery

1. The ophthalmic artery passes forwards to enter the cavity of the orbit through the optic canal.
2. In this canal, it lies inferolateral to the optic nerve.
   a. Having entered the orbit the artery is at first lateral to the optic nerve (42.9).
   b. It then crosses above the nerve to reach the medial wall of the orbit and runs forwards along this wall.

#### *Branches of the Ophthalmic Artery*

The branches of the ophthalmic artery are shown in 42.9.

1. The ***central artery of the retina*** is the first branch of the ophthalmic artery.
   a. It arises from the ophthalmic artery when the latter is still within the optic canal.
   b. It first lies below the optic nerve.
   c. It pierces the dural sheath of the nerve and runs forwards for a short distance between these two.
   d. It then enters the substance of the nerve and runs forwards in its centre to reach the optic disc.
   e. Here, it divides into branches that supply the retina (42.10).
2. The largest branch of the ophthalmic artery is the ***lacrimal artery*** that runs forwards along the lateral wall of the orbit. The further branches given off by the lacrimal artery are as follows:
   a. Just near its origin from the ophthalmic artery, the lacrimal artery gives off a ***recurrent meningeal*** branch that runs backwards to enter the middle cranial fossa through the superior orbital fissure.
   b. The lacrimal artery gives off two ***zygomatic*** branches that enter canals in the zygomatic bone. One branch appears on the face through the zygomaticofacial foramen. The other appears on the temporal surface of the bone through the zygomaticotemporal foramen.
   c. Terminal ramifications of the lacrimal artery supply the lacrimal gland.
   d. The lateral palpebral branches supply the eyelids.

   The other branches of the ophthalmic artery arise from the main stem of the artery (42.9).
3. The ***posterior ciliary arteries*** arise as the ophthalmic artery crosses the optic nerve. They run forwards around the optic nerve and supply the eyeball.
4. The ***supraorbital*** branch supplies the skin of the forehead.
5. The ***anterior*** and ***posterior ethmoidal*** branches:
   a. Enter foramina in the medial wall of the orbit to supply the ethmoidal air sinuses.
   b. They then enter the anterior cranial fossa.
   c. Their terminal branches (specially of the anterior artery) enter the nose and supply part of it.
6. The ***anterior ciliary arteries*** arise from the ophthalmic artery near the anterior part of the eyeball and supply it.
7. The ***medial palpebral*** branches supply the eyelids.
8. The ***supratrochlear artery*** is one of the terminal branches of the ophthalmic artery. It supplies the skin of the forehead (along with the supraorbital artery).

9. The ***dorsal nasal branch*** supplies the upper part of the nose.
   In addition to the branches shown in 42.9, the ophthalmic artery and its branches give off several ***muscular*** branches to muscles of the orbit.
   **Veins of orbit**: See previous chapters.

## The Optic Nerve

1. The optic nerve forms an important part of the visual pathway. It lies partly in the orbit and partly in the cranial cavity.
2. Its anterior end is attached to the posterior pole of the eyeball. The attachment lies a little medial to the anteroposterior axis of the eyeball.
3. From here, the nerve passes backwards and medially:
   a. First through the orbit
   b. Next through the optic canal
   c. Finally through part of the cranial cavity.
4. The nerve ends by joining the nerve of the opposite side to form the ***optic chiasma*** (43.23).
5. The total length of the nerve is about 40 mm. Of this 25 mm is in the orbit, 5 mm in the optic canal and 10 mm in the cranial cavity.
6. a. The intraorbital part of the nerve is surrounded by the superior, inferior, medial and lateral rectus muscles.
   b. The ciliary ganglion is placed between the optic nerve and the lateral rectus muscle.
   c. The ophthalmic artery is inferolateral to the nerve in the optic canal and in the posteriormost part of the orbit. The artery then crosses above the nerve from lateral to medial side.
   d. Apart from the ophthalmic artery, the optic nerve is crossed from lateral to medial side by:
      i. The nasociliary nerve which crosses above the optic nerve.
      ii. The branch from the oculomotor nerve to the medial rectus muscle, which crosses below the nerve.
7. The central artery of the retina first lies below the optic nerve.
   a. Piercing the dural sheath of the nerve it runs forwards for a short distance between these two.
   b. About 12 mm behind the eyeball the artery enters the substance of the nerve and runs forwards in its substance to reach the eyeball.

## The Oculomotor Nerve

1. The oculomotor is the third cranial nerve.
2. The nerve arises from the midbrain.
3. It runs part of its course in the cavernous sinus. Here, it divides into superior and inferior rami.
4. The superior and inferior rami of the oculomotor nerve enter the orbit by passing through the superior orbital fissure (43.30). They pass through the part of the fissure that lies within the tendinous ring that gives origin to the four recti of the eyeball.
5. Within the orbit the superior ramus supplies:
   a. The superior rectus
   b. The levator palpebrae superioris.
6. The inferior division supplies:
   a. The medial rectus
   b. The inferior rectus
   c. The inferior oblique (43.29).
7. The oculomotor nerve also carries secremotor fibres. Preganglionic fibres arising from the Edinger Westphal nucleus travel through the trunk of the nerve, and then through its inferior division.
   a. They then pass into the nerve for the inferior oblique muscle.
   b. A short branch arising from this nerve conveys the fibres to the ciliary ganglion. This branch to the ciliary ganglion from the nerve to the inferior oblique constitutes the ***motor root*** of the ganglion.
   c. The cells of the ganglion give origin to postganglionic fibres that pass through the short ciliary nerves to reach the sphincter pupillae and the ciliaris muscles.

8. ***The ciliary ganglion***
   a. The ciliary ganglion lies lateral to the optic nerve (between it and the lateral rectus).
   b. Posteriorly, it receives three roots: motor or parasympathetic, sympathetic, and sensory.
   c. The motor or parasympathetic root carries fibres for the sphincter pupillae and ciliaris (see above).
   d. The ***sympathetic root*** arises from the sympathetic plexus on the internal carotid artery. It carries postganglionic sympathetic fibres that begin in the superior cervical sympathetic ganglion.
   e. Sympathetic fibres pass through the ciliary ganglion, without relay, and enter the short ciliary nerves through which they reach the blood vessels of the eyeball.
   f. The fibres for the dilator pupillae normally follow a separate route, as described below, but sometimes they may pass through the ciliary ganglion.
   g. The sensory root of the ciliary ganglion is a branch of the nasociliary nerve. It carries sensory fibres that begin in the cornea, the iris and the choroid; pass through the short ciliary nerves and then through the ciliary ganglion; and finally enter the sensory root through which they reach the nasociliary nerve.

## The Trochlear Nerve

1. The trochlear nerve is the fourth cranial nerve.
2. It enters the orbit through the upper part of the superior orbital fissure (43.30). In the fissure, it lies above the tendinous ring for origin of the recti of the eyeball (43.30).
3. Having entered the orbit the nerve runs forwards, above the orbital muscles, and ends in the superior oblique muscle.

## The Abducent Nerve

1. This is the sixth cranial nerve.
2. The nerve passes through the superior orbital fissure to enter the orbit.
3. The nerve ends by supplying the lateral rectus muscle.

## The Ophthalmic Nerve

1. The fibres of the ophthalmic nerve are purely sensory. However, some sympathetic fibres for the eyeball travel for part of their course through the nerve and some of its branches.
2. Passing forwards it divides into three branches. These are:
   a. The lacrimal nerve
   b. The frontal nerve
   c. The nasociliary nerve.
3. These branches enter the orbit by passing through the superior orbital fissure.
4. The ***lacrimal nerve*** runs along the lateral wall of the orbit (along the upper border of the lateral rectus).
   a. It ends in the lacrimal gland (and hence its name).
   b. Some branches pass through the gland to supply the conjunctiva and the skin of the upper eyelid.
   c. The lacrimal nerve is joined by a twig from the zygomaticotemporal branch of the maxillary nerve.
5. The ***frontal nerve*** runs forwards between the levator palpebrae superioris and the periosteum lining the roof of the orbit. It ends by dividing into supraorbital and supratrochlear branches.
6. The ***supraorbital nerve*** continues in the line of the frontal nerve (43.36), lying between the levator palpebrae superioris and the roof of the orbit.
   a. Reaching the orbital margin it passes through the supraorbital notch (on the medial part of the upper margin of the orbit) and curves upwards into the forehead.
7. The ***supratrochlear nerve*** runs forwards and medially above the orbital muscles, and medial to the supraorbital nerve.
   a. It passes above the trochlea (for the tendon of the superior oblique muscle).
   b. Reaching the upper margin of the orbital aperture, near its medial end, the nerve turns upwards into the forehead giving branches to the skin over its lower and medial part.
   Other branches given off by the supratrochlear nerve are:

c. A descending branch which joins the infratrochlear branch of the nasociliary nerve (43.36).
d. Branches to the conjunctiva and skin of the upper eyelid.

8. On entering the orbit, the ***nasociliary nerve*** lies between the optic nerve and the lateral rectus.
   a. The nerve then runs medially crossing above the optic nerve (43.36).
   b. As it does so it lies below the superior rectus muscle.
   c. Reaching the medial wall of the orbit, the nerve ends by dividing into the ***anterior ethmoidal*** and ***infratrochlear*** nerves.

   The branches of the nasociliary nerve are as follows (43.36):
   i. Just after entering the orbit, the nasociliary nerve receives the ***sensory root of the ciliary ganglion***.
   ii. The ***long ciliary nerves*** (two or three) arise from the nasociliary nerve as it crosses the optic nerve.
      - They run forwards to the eyeball where they pierce the sclera; and then run between the sclera and the choroid.
      - They supply sensory fibres to the ciliary body, the iris and the cornea.
      - They also carry postganglionic sympathetic fibres meant for the dilator pupillae.
      - These sympathetic fibres begin in the superior cervical sympathetic ganglion (43.37) and travel through a plexus surrounding the internal carotid artery. They pass to the nasociliary nerve while the latter lies in the wall of the cavernous sinus.
   iii. The ***posterior ethmoidal branch*** enters the posterior ethmoidal foramen (on the medial wall of the orbit) and supplies the ethmoidal and sphenoidal air sinuses.
   iv. The ***anterior ethmoidal nerve*** has a complicated course through the orbit, the anterior cranial fossa, and the nasal cavity. We will not go into details of the course.
   v. The ***infratrochlear nerve*** (43.36) runs forwards on the medial wall of the orbit and ends by supplying part of the skin of the upper and lower eyelids and over the upper part of the nose.

9. The nerve also gives branches to:
   a. The conjunctiva
   b. The lacrimal sac
   c. The lacrimal caruncle.

## THE EYEBALL

### Preliminary Remarks

1. The greater part of the eyeball (posterior five-sixths) is shaped like a sphere and has a diameter of about 24 mm.
2. The anterior one sixth is much more convex than the posterior part. It represents part of a sphere having a diameter of about 15 mm.
3. The posterior five-sixths of the eyeball, are covered by a thick white opaque membrane called the *sclera*.
4. The wall of the anterior one-sixth of the eyeball is transparent and is called the *cornea*.
5. When the 'eye' is viewed in the living person we see only a small part of the eyeball that appears in the interval between the upper and lower eyelids (i.e., in the palpebral fissure).
   a. The 'white' of the eye is formed by the sclera.
   b. The dark central part is formed by the cornea. The cornea itself is transparent. The dark appearance is because of the presence of a pigmented diaphragm, the ***iris***, deep to the cornea.
6. In the centre of the iris, there is an aperture called the ***pupil***. The pupil appears black in colour as the interior of the eye is dark.
7. A horizontal section across an eyeball is shown in 44.8. Note the following features:
   a. The wall of the eyeball is made up of three main layers.
   b. The outermost layer is called the ***fibrous coat***. It is formed posteriorly by the sclera and anteriorly by the cornea.
   c. The next layer is the ***vascular coat***. It has the following subdivisions:
      i. The part lining the inner surface of most of the sclera is thin and is called the ***choroid***.
      ii. Near the junction of the sclera with the cornea the vascular coat is thick and forms the ***ciliary body***.
      iii. The ciliary body is continuous with the ***iris*** that lies a short distance behind the cornea.

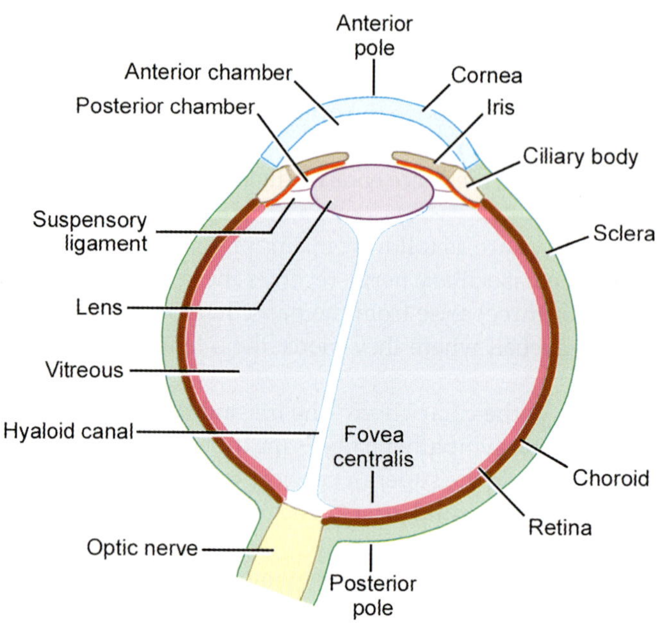


**44.8:** Horizontal section across the eyeball to show the main features of its structure

8. The space between the iris and the cornea is called the ***anterior chamber***. The space between the iris and the front of the lens is called the ***posterior chamber***.
9. The innermost layer of the wall of the eyeball is called the ***retina.***
10. Light falling on the retina has to pass through a number of ***refracting media*** before reaching the retina and forming an image on it. These are:
    a. The cornea
    b. A fluid, the ***aqueous humour***, which fills the anterior and posterior chambers
    c. The lens
    d. A jelly like ***vitreous body*** which fills the eyeball posterior to the lens.
11. The centre of the cornea is called the ***anterior pole*** of the eyeball.
12. The opposite end of the eyeball is called the ***posterior pole***.
13. The ***visual axis*** of the eye passes from the anterior pole to the posterior pole.
14. In 44.8 note that the optic nerve is attached to the back of the eyeball a short distance medial to the posterior pole.
15. An imaginary line passing round the eyeball midway between the anterior and posterior poles is called the ***equator*** of the eyeball.
16. Any line passing through both the poles (i.e., at right angles to the equator) is called a ***meridian***.

 **WANT TO KNOW MORE?**

**THE SCLERA**

1. The sclera is made up mainly of fibrous tissue. Its external surface gives attachment to the extrinsic muscles of the eyeball.
2. Posteriorly, in the region of the attachment of the optic nerve the sclera is perforated like a sieve. This area is called the ***lamina cribrosa*** (44.9). Bundles of nerve fibres arising in the retina pass through these perforations to form the optic nerve.

3. At the centre of the lamina cribrosa, there is a larger aperture (44.9) for passage of the central artery and vein of the retina.
4. Just around the lamina cribrosa, the sclera becomes continuous with the dural sheath of the optic nerve.
5. A short distance from the lamina cribrosa the sclera is perforated by the short ciliary nerves and arteries, and further away by the long ciliary nerves and arteries.
6. A little behind the equator of the eyeball, the sclera has four or five apertures for veins called the ***venae vorticosae*** (44.9).
7. Anteriorly, the sclera becomes continuous with the cornea at the ***sclerocorneal junction***. As this junction is circular it is also called the ***limbus***.
8. A circular channel called the ***sinus venosus sclerae*** (or ***canal of Schlemm***) is located in the sclera just behind the sclerocorneal junction (44.13).
9. A triangular mass of scleral tissue projects into the cornea just medial to the sinus. This projection is called the ***scleral spur*** (44.13).
10. The sclera over the anterior part of the eyeball is covered by the ocular conjunctiva.
11. The rest of the sclera is in contact with a ***fascial sheath*** that surrounds the eyeball.
12. The deep surface of the sclera is separated from the choroid by the ***perichoroidal space***.
13. Delicate connective tissue present in this space constitutes the ***suprachoroid lamina*** (or ***lamina fusca***).
14. The contents of the eyeball are under positive pressure. This pressure is resisted by the sclera, which is not extensible. These two factors together maintain the shape of the eyeball.
15. The sclera provides a smooth external surface that facilitates movements of the eyeball. This surface also provides attachment to the extrinsic muscles of the eyeball.

## THE CORNEA

1. The cornea is not exactly circular.
   a. Its horizontal diameter is somewhat greater than 11 mm.
   b. But its vertical diameter is slightly less.
2. As the cornea is more convex than the sclera the junction of the two is marked, on the exterior of the eyeball, by a groove called the ***sulcus sclerae***.
3. The cornea is made up of five layers that are shown in 44.10. For details of these layers consult the author's HUMAN HISTOLOGY.

## THE CHOROID

1. The choroid consists of a network of blood vessels supported by connective tissue containing many pigmented cells that give it a dark brown colour.
   a. It is the dark colour of the choroid that darkens the interior of the eyeball.
   b. It also prevents reflection of light within the eyeball.
   c. Both these factors are necessary for formation of sharp images on the retina.
2. Within the choroid, there is an outer ***vascular layer*** made up of small arteries and veins, and an inner ***capillary layer***.
   a. The short ciliary arteries that pierce the posterior part of the sclera (44.9) run forwards in the vascular lamina.
   b. However, most of the vascular lamina is filled by veins that converge on four or five ***venae vorticosae***. We have seen that these veins pierce the sclera a short distance behind the equator of the eyeball.
3. The choroid is separated from the sclera by a layer of delicate connective tissue called the ***suprachoroid lamina*** (or lamina fusca).
4. The choroid is separated from the retina by a thin membrane called the ***basal lamina*** (or membrane of Bruch). Nutrients diffusing through this membrane, from capillaries in the choroid, provide nutrition to the outer part of the retina.

## THE CILIARY BODY

1. The ciliary body represents an anterior continuation of the choroid.
2. Anteromedially, it becomes continuous with the iris. It is made up of vascular tissue, muscle and connective tissue.
3. When the eyeball is cut coronally, some distance behind the lens, and is viewed from behind we see the appearance shown in 44.11. Identify, the following in this figure.
   a. The retina proper ends anteriorly (a short distance behind the sclerocorneal junction) in a wavy line called the ***ora serrata***. This line also represents the junction of the choroid with the ciliary body.
   b. The ciliary body extends forwards (and medially) from the ora serrata to end near the periphery of the lens.
   c. Anterior to the ora serrata, the retina is continued forwards as a double layer of simple epithelium that lines the inner surface of the ciliary body and the posterior surface of the iris.
4. The ciliary body can be divided into a posterior part called the ***ciliary ring***, and an anterior part made of the ciliary processes.
   a. The ***ciliary ring*** is about 3.5 mm wide. It has a relatively flat surface on which there are shallow radial grooves (Fig. 44.11).
   b. The ***ciliary processes*** lie between the ciliary ring and the base of the iris (44.11). The ciliary processes secrete the aqueous humour. They may also produce some components of the vitreous body.
   c. There are about 70 processes arranged radially (meriodonally).
   d. Each process may be regarded as an infolding of the surface of the ciliary body, and having a very irregular surface because of the presence of secondary folds.
   e. The substance of each process is made up of a plexus of blood vessels covered by the double layer of retinal epithelium mentioned above.
5. The ciliary processes and the furrows between them give attachment to numerous delicate fibres that pass to them from the periphery of the lens. Many of these fibres can run into the ciliary ring.
6. A meridional section (i.e., a section along a line joining the anterior and posterior poles of the eyeball) is shown in 44.12. In such a section, the ciliary body appears to be triangular. Lateral to the ciliary processes (and medial to the anterior part of the sclera), there is a triangular mass of the ***ciliary muscle***. The fibres of the ciliary muscle are arranged in two main groups.
   a. The ***circular fibres*** lie in the anterior and inner part of the ciliary body. They form a ring of muscle, contraction of which relaxes the fibres of the suspensory ligament. Release of tension on the lens makes it more convex.
   b. The ***meriodonal fibres*** take origin from the scleral spur (44.12 and 44.13). They pass backwards and get attached to the ciliary processes and the ciliary ring. Some fibres extend into the choroid. When these fibres contract the ciliary ring is drawn forwards (i.e., towards the lens). As a result, the suspensory ligament is again relaxed. In this way, the circular and meriodonal fibres act together to make the lens more convex; and enable it to focus images of near objects on the retina. This is called ***accommodation***.
7. The ciliary muscle (or ciliaris) is supplied by parasympathetic nerve fibres that travel to it via the oculomotor nerve and the ciliary ganglion.

## THE IRIS

1. The iris is the most anterior part of the vascular coat of the eyeball.
2. It forms a diaphragm placed immediately in front of the lens. At its periphery it is continuous with the ciliary body. In its centre there is an aperture, the ***pupil***.
3. The iris is composed of a stroma of connective tissue containing numerous pigment cells, and in which are embedded blood vessels and smooth muscle (see below).
4. The pupil regulates the amount of light passing into the eye.
   a. In bright light the pupil contracts, and in dim light it dilates.
   b. In this way, the optimum amount of light required for proper vision reaches the retina, within a considerable range in intensity of illumination.

5. Changes in the size of the pupil are produced by the smooth muscle of the iris that consists of two parts.
   a. The ***sphincter pupillae*** is a ring of circularly arranged muscle situated just around the pupil. Its contraction narrows the pupil.
   b. The ***dilator pupillae*** is in the form of muscle fibres that are arranged radially in the iris (44.13). These fibres are intimately related to the anterior of the two layers of epithelium lining the posterior surface of the iris. Near the pupil, these radial fibres merge with the sphincter pupillae.

*Nerve Supply of the Sphincter and Dilator Pupillae*

1. The sphincter pupillae has a parasympathetic nerve supply (similar to that of the ciliary muscle).
   a. Preganglionic neurons that are located in the Edinger Westphal nucleus (in the upper part of the midbrain) give off axons that pass through the oculomotor nerve and its branches to reach the ciliary ganglion.
   b. Postganglionic nerve fibres pass through the short ciliary nerves to reach the muscle.
2. The dilator pupillae is supplied by sympathetic nerves.
   a. The preganglionic neurons concerned are located in segment TI of the spinal cord.
   b. The postganglionic neurons lie in the superior cervical sympathetic ganglion.

## THE IRIDIOCORNEAL ANGLE

1. The angle between the peripheral margins of the iris and of the cornea is a region of importance.
   a. From 44.12 and 44.13, it will be seen that the most anterior part of the ciliary body appears in this angle.
   b. Laterally, the angle is related to the sinus venosus sclerae.
   c. The lateral wall of this sinus is formed by a groove in the sclera. Medially, it is related to the scleral spur. It is also intimately related to the pectinate ligament described below.
2. The ***pectinate ligament*** is formed by numerous interlacing filaments that represent continuations of the posterior limiting lamina of the cornea (44.10), into the iris.
   a. These filaments are separated by spaces called the ***spaces of the iridocorneal angle***, or ***trabecular spaces***.
   b. These spaces communicate medially with the anterior chamber, and laterally with the sinus venosus sclerae.
   c. Aqueous humour secreted by the ciliary processes passes into the posterior chamber of the eye (i.e., the space between the posterior surface of the iris and the lens).
   d. It passes through the pupil into the anterior chamber.
   e. From here, it filters through the spaces of the iridocorneal angle to enter the sinus venosus sclerae through which it is drained into the veins of the region.
   f. The clinician often refers to the iridocorneal angle as the ***angle of filtration***. With advancing age, these spaces may get blocked resulting in increased tension within the eyeball. This disease, called ***glaucoma,*** may have serious consequences.

## THE RETINA

1. To understand the structure of the retina brief reference to its development is necessary.
   a. The retina develops as an outgrowth from the brain (diencephalon).
   b. The proximal part of the diverticulum remains narrow and is called the ***optic stalk***. It later becomes the optic nerve.
   c. The distal part of the diverticulum forms a rounded hollow structure called the ***optic vesicle***.
   d. This vesicle is invaginated by the developing lens (and other surrounding tissues) so that it gets converted into the two-layered ***optic cup***.
   e. At first each layer of the cup is made up of a single layer of cells. The outer layer persists as a single layered epithelium that becomes pigmented and forms the ***pigment cell layer*** of the retina (44.14).
   f. Over the greater part of the optic cup, the cells of the inner layer multiply to form several layers of cells that become the ***nervous layer*** of the retina.
   g. The anterior limit of the region where this transformation takes place is later marked by the ora serrata.

   h. The part of the retina behind the ora serrata now consists of an outer, pigmented layer, and an inner nervous layer. The two are separated by a cleft representing the original cavity of the optic cup. It is only this part of the retina that is light sensitive and is referred to as the ***optical part*** of the retina, or the retina proper.
   i. Anterior to the ora serrata, both layers of the optic cup remain single layered. These two layers of epithelium line the inner surface of the ciliary body forming the ***ciliary part*** of the retina, and the posterior surface of the iris forming the ***iridial part*** of the retina.
2. The layer of pigment cells has greater adherence to the choroid than to the nervous layer of the retina. In some cases, part of the retina may get detached from its normal position. In such ***detachment of the retina***, it is only the nervous layer that gets detached, the pigment cells remaining attached to the choroid.
3. The essential features of the structure of the retina are shown in 44.15.
4. It contains photoreceptors that convert the stimulus of light into nervous impulses. These receptors are of two kinds, ***rods*** and ***cones***.
   a. There are about seven million cones in each retina. The rods are far more numerous: they number more than 100 million.
   b. The cones respond best to bright light. They are responsible for sharp vision and for discrimination of colour.
5. Opposite the posterior pole of the eyeball, the retina shows a ***central region*** about 6 mm in diameter. This region is responsible for sharp vision.
6. In the centre of this region, an area about 2 mm in diameter has a yellow colour and is called the ***macula lutea.***
7. The ***fovea centralis***, that is a depression in the centre of the macula is only 0.4 mm in diameter. Cones are most numerous in the central region. The fovea centralis is believed to contain cones only.
8. Rods can respond to poor light and specially to movement across the field of vision. They predominate in peripheral parts of the retina.
9. Each rod or cone can be regarded as a modified neuron.
   a. It consists of a cell body, a peripheral process and a central process. The cell body contains the nucleus.
   b. The peripheral process is rod-shaped in the case or rods, and cone-shaped in the case of cones (hence the names rods and cones).
   c. The ends of the peripheral processes are separated from one another by processes of pigment cells (44.15).
   d. The central processes of rods and cones are like those of neurons: they end by synapsing with other neurons within the retina.
10. The basic neuronal arrangement within the retina is shown in 44.15.
   a. The central processes of rods and cones synapse with the peripheral processes of ***bipolar cells***.
   b. The central processes of bipolar cells synapse with dendrites of ***ganglion cells***.
   c. Axons arising from ganglion cells form the ***fibres of the optic nerve.***
11. The various elements mentioned above form a series of layers within the retina. The outermost layer (towards the choroid) is formed by the pigment cells, followed in sequence by:
   a. The rods and cones
   b. The bipolar cells
   c. The ganglion cells
   d. A layer of optic nerve fibres.
12. The layer of nerve fibres is apposed to the vitreous.
13. Light has to pass through several layers of the retina to reach the rods and cones. At the fovea centralis, the other layers are 'swept aside' to allow direct access of light to the cones here.
14. The optic nerve is attached to the eyeball a short distance medial to the posterior pole. The nerve fibres arising from the ganglion cells all over the retina converge to this region, where they pass through the lamina cribrosa to form the optic nerve.
15. When viewed from the retinal side this region is seen as a circular area called the ***optic disc*** (44.16). There are no photoreceptors here. The optic disc is, therefore, insensitive to light and is called the ***blind spot***.
16. The optic disc is pierced, near its centre, by the central artery and vein of retina (see below).

## THE LENS

1. The lens lies in front of the vitreous body and behind the iris. It is enclosed by a capsule.
2. It has convex anterior and posterior surfaces, and a peripheral margin (or equator) to which the suspensory ligament is attached.
3. The anterior surface is less convex than the posterior surface. It comes into contact with the iris near the margin of the pupil.
4. The posterior surface of the lens lies in a depression in the vitreous body called the ***hyaloid fossa***.

### *The Suspensory Ligament*

1. The suspensory ligament of the lens is also called the ***zonule*** (44.12). It is made up of fibres passing from the equator of the lens to the ciliary processes, and to the recesses between them.
2. Changes in the tension on the suspensory ligament, produced by contraction of the ciliary muscle, produce alterations in the convexity of the lens and enable it to focus objects at varying distances from the eye.

## BLOOD VESSELS AND NERVES OF THE EYEBALL

1. The arteries supplying the retina are all branches of the ophthalmic artery.
2. The ***short ciliary arteries*** are several in number.
   a. They pierce the sclera near the lamina cribrosa (44.9).
   b. They end in numerous branches that form a plexus in the choroid and supply it (44.17).
   c. The capillary plexus in the choroid is also responsible for providing nutrition (by diffusion) to the outer part of the retina (i.e., the part nearer the choroid).
3. The ***long ciliary arteries*** are two in number (one medial and one lateral).
   a. They pierce the sclera a short distance to the corresponding side of the lamina cribrosa (44.9).
   b. These arteries then run forward between the sclera and the choroid to reach the region of the ciliary body. Here, each artery divides into one upper and one lower branch (44.18).
   c. The upper branches of the medial and lateral sides anastomose with each other. Similarly, the lower branches of the two sides anastomose to form the ***greater arterial circle*** at the periphery of the iris.
   d. This circle is joined by small anterior ciliary arteries that reach the region through the attachments of the rectus muscles to the eyeball. Branches pass radially into the iris from the greater circle, and join each other just round the pupil to form the ***lesser arterial circle***.
4. The veins draining the iris, the ciliary body and the choroid form a dense plexus deep to the sclera. The veins of this plexus converge on four or five ***venae vorticosae***. These veins pierce the sclera a little behind the equator of the eyeball (44.9) to end in the ophthalmic veins.
5. The main blood supply to the retina reaches it through the central artery of the retina.
   a. This artery runs forwards through the distal part of the optic nerve to enter the retina through the optic disc.
   b. It divides into upper and lower branches, each of which divides into medial (or nasal) and lateral (or temporal) branches. Further ramifications supply the entire retina.
   c. These arteries can be seen in the living subject by looking into the eye through the pupil using an instrument called an ophthalmoscope (44.16).
6. Branches of the central artery of the retina are end arteries i.e., they do not anastomose with each other. Blockage of any branch results in death of the part of the retina supplied by it, and to consequent loss of the part of the field of vision concerned. No large vessels are to be seen in the central region of the retina.
7. The blood from the retina is drained by tributaries that correspond to the branches of the central artery, but do not accompany them closely. These tributaries end in two veins superior and inferior that pierce the lamina cribrosa and join each other to form the ***central vein of the retina***.
8. The nerves (other than the optic nerve) that supply the eyeball are the ***long and short ciliary nerves***.
   a. The long ciliary nerves are branches of the nasociliary nerve, while the short ciliary nerves arise from the ciliary ganglion.

b. They enter the eyeball along with the corresponding arteries (44.9).
c. The short ciliary nerves carry parasympathetic postganglionic fibres from the ciliary ganglion to the ciliary muscle and to the sphincter pupillae. They also carry sympathetic postganglionic fibres to blood vessels of the eyeball.
d. Sympathetic postganglionic fibres meant for the dilator pupillae normally travel through the long ciliary nerves. Occasionally, they may pass through the short ciliary nerves.
e. In addition to autonomic efferents, the long and short ciliary nerves carry sensory fibres from various structures in the eyeball including the ciliary body, the iris and the cornea.

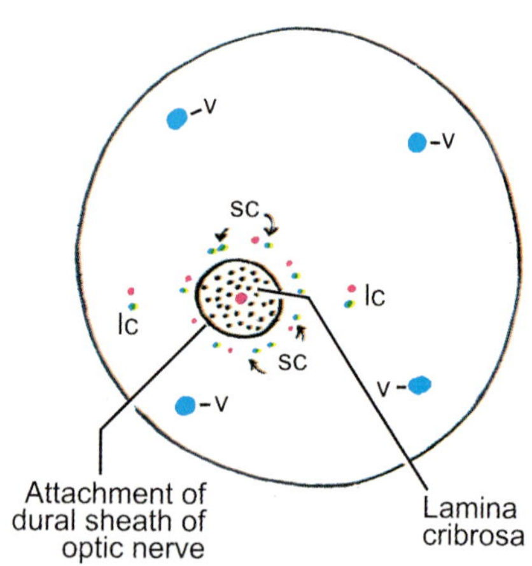


**44.9:** Eyeball seen from behind to show the openings in the sclera. sc: foramina for short ciliary nerves and arteries; lc: foramina for long ciliary nerves and arteries; v: foramina for venae vorticosae

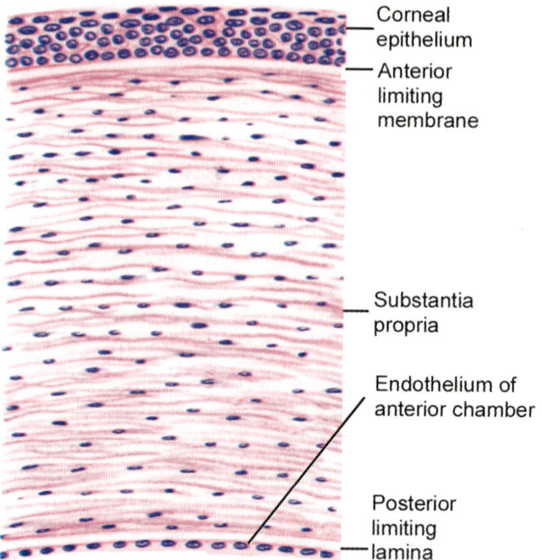


**44.10:** Diagram of a section through the cornea to show its layers

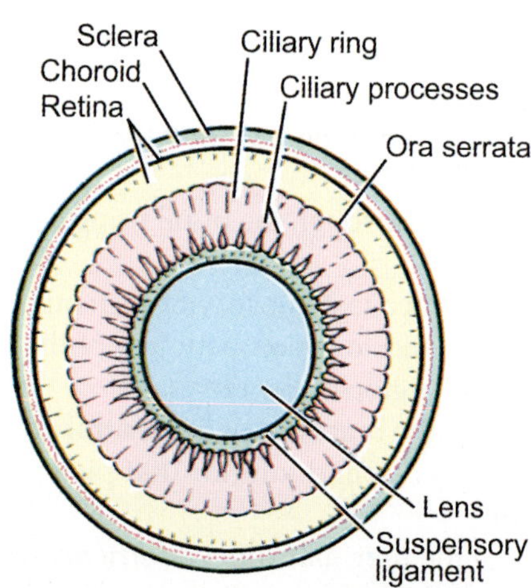


**44.11:** Anterior part of the eyeball viewed from behind after cutting the eyeball in the coronal plane

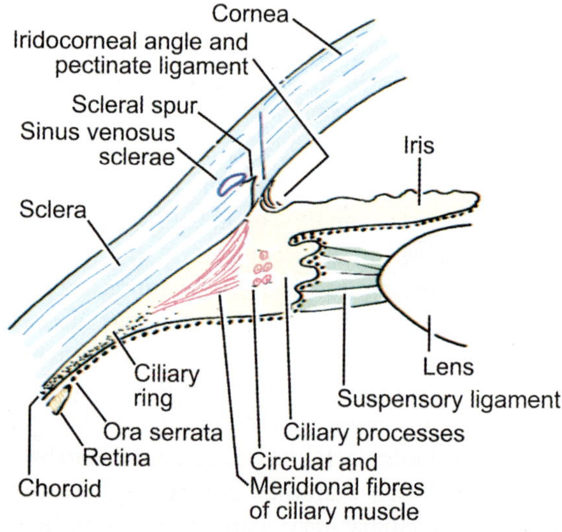


**44.12:** Meriodonal section through the ciliary body and iris

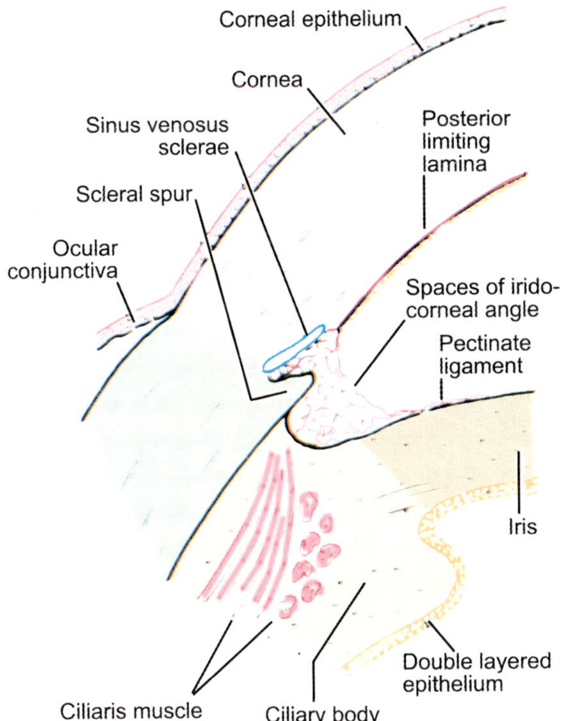


**44.13:** Some features of the iridocorneal angle. Blood vessels in the ciliary body and iris are omitted

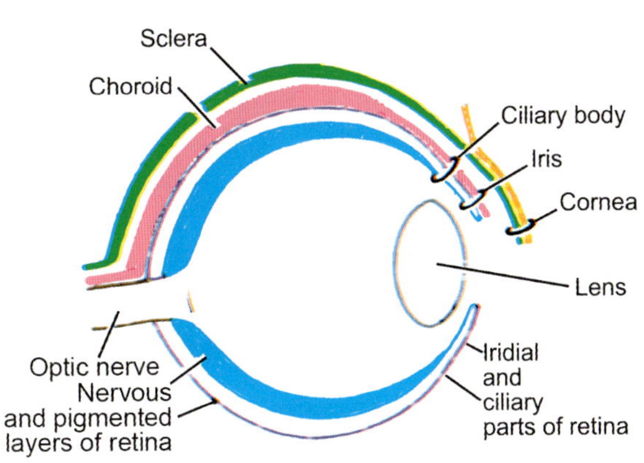


**44.14:** Scheme to show some features of the developing eye

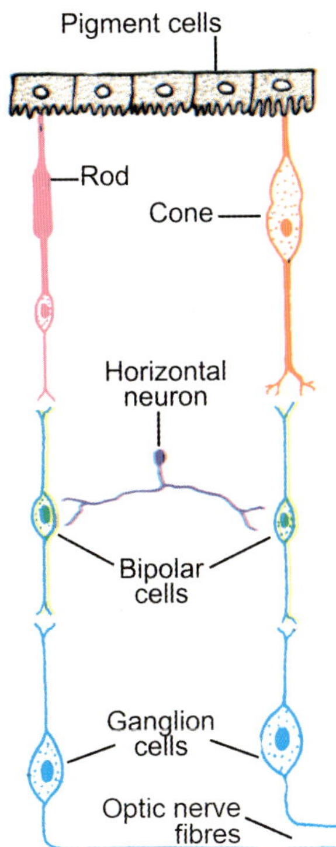


**44.15:** Simplified scheme to show the main elements of the retina

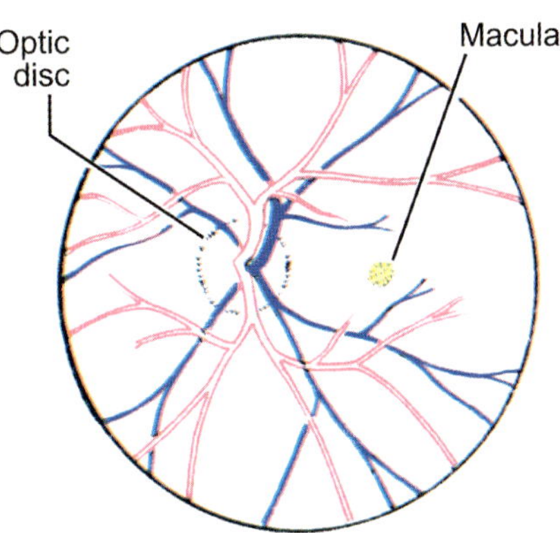


**44.16:** Blood vessels of the retina as seen through an ophthalmoscope

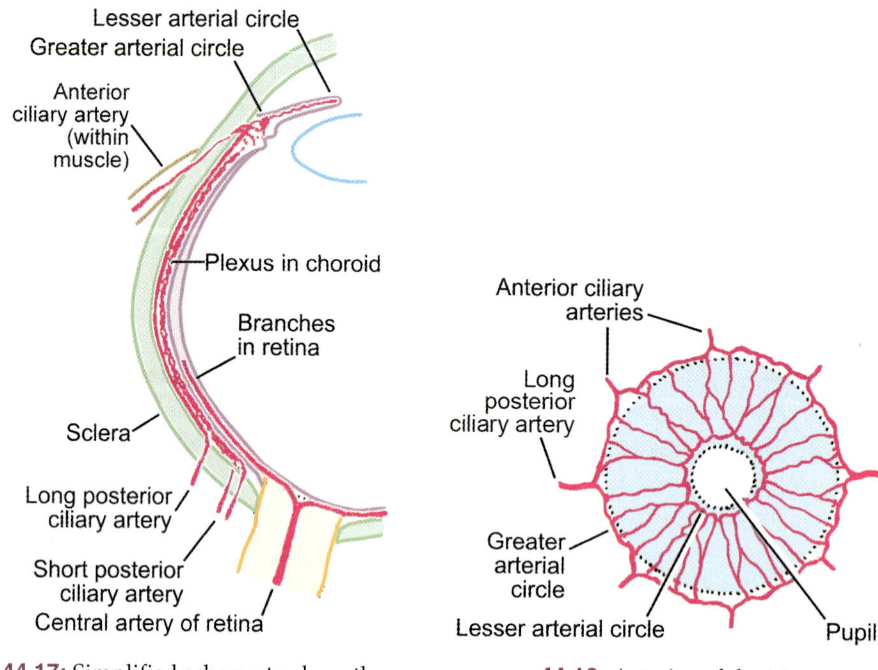


**44.17:** Simplified scheme to show the arteries supplying the eyeball

**44.18:** Arteries of the iris

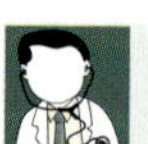

## CLINICAL CORRELATION

### Eyes and Related Structures

*Infections*

1. Infections are common in the eyelids (***blepharitis***).
2. A pus-filled swelling near the edge of the eyelid is a ***stye***. It is caused by infection in large sebaceous glands present here.
3. Inflammation of a tarsal gland results in a localised swelling called ***chalazion***.
4. Inflammation of the conjunctiva is called ***conjunctivitis***.
5. Other structures in the eye that may be infected are the iris (***iritis***), the ciliary body (***cyclitis***), and a combination of both these (***iridocyclitis***).
6. Infection in the cornea is called ***keratitis***. It can lead to formation of a corneal ulcer. Corneal ulcers can also be caused by injury or by foreign bodies that enter the eye.
7. A superficial infection of the sclera is ***episcleritis***, and a deeper infection is ***scleritis***.
8. Inflammation of the retina is ***retinitis***.
9. Inflammation of the optic nerve is ***optic neuritis***.

*Cornea*

1. Injuries to the cornea can result in ***corneal opacities*** that can lead to blindness. Blindness due to corneal opacity can be cured by corneal grafting.
2. The so-called eye transplantations that are advertised so much in the lay press are really corneal transplants. A whole eye cannot be transplanted.
3. Alterations in the curvature of the cornea can lead to an error of refraction called ***astigmatism*** (see below).

*Lens*

1. Opacity in the lens of the eyeball is called ***cataract***. It occurs in many old persons and is a common cause of blindness.

2. Vision can be restored by removing the lens, and this is one the most common operations done on the eyeball.
3. Focussing power is restored by use of appropriate spectacles, or by implanting an artificial lens into the eye (***intraocular lens transplantation***).

*Errors of Refraction*

Defects in the shape of the eyeball, or in refractive media, lead to errors of refraction in which images are not focussed on the retina. Common errors are as follows:

1. In ***myopia*** (near sightedness), the image comes into focus in front of the plane of the retina. Objects can be seen clearly only when placed close to the eyes. Myopia is corrected with convex (plus) lenses.
2. ***Hypermetropia*** is a condition in which the image comes to a focus behind the plane of the retina. Only distant objects can be seen. It is corrected with concave (minus) lenses.
3. ***Presbyopia*** is a condition caused by decreased elasticity of the lens in persons over 40 years old. Presbyopia can be corrected by convex lenses.
4. In ***astigmatism,*** the image is correctly focussed in some planes but not in others. This is due to abnormalities in curvature of the cornea or of the lens. Correction requires the use of cylindrical lenses.
5. The degree of refractive error is determined by a procedure called ***retinoscopy***.

*Fundus Examination*

1. The retina can be examined through an ***ophthalmoscope***. The procedure is commonly referred to as fundus examination.
2. Apart from diagnosis of diseases of the retina itself, such examination also helps in assessing the status of patients in diseases like hypertension and diabetes.

*Tumours*

1. Tumours may occur in the eye.
2. A ***melanoma*** may arise from the iris or the choroid.
3. Another tumour seen in the eye is a ***retinoblastoma***.

*Retinal Detachment*

1. The retina consists of a nervous layer (the retina proper) and an outer layer of pigment cells.
2. In the embryo, the two layers are separated by a cavity.
3. Sometimes, the nervous layer gets detached from the pigment layer (detachment of the retina). It causes serious impairment of vision.

*Other Conditions*

See optic nerve (page 884), visual pathway (page 885), squint (page 892), and corneal reflex (page 906).

## THE EAR AND SOME RELATED STRUCTURES

### Preliminary Remarks About The Ear

1. Anatomically speaking, the ear is made up of three main parts called:
   a. The external ear
   b. The middle ear
   c. The internal ear.
2. The external ear and the middle ear are concerned exclusively with hearing. The internal ear has:
   a. A ***cochlear part*** concerned with hearing
   b. A ***vestibular part*** which provides information to the brain regarding the position and movements of the head.
3. The main parts of the ear are shown in 44.19.

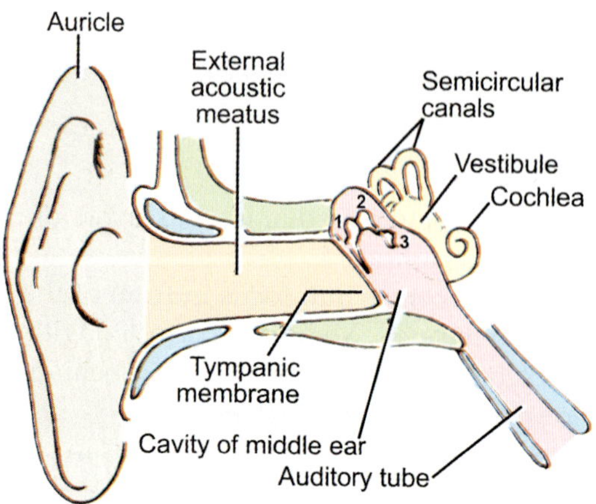


**44.19:** Scheme to show the main parts of the ear. 1: Malleus; 2: Incus; 3: Stapes

4. The part of the ear that is seen on the surface of the body (i.e., the part that the lay person calls the ear) is anatomically speaking the ***auricle*** or ***pinna***.
5. Leading inwards from the auricle there is a tube called the ***external acoustic meatus***. The auricle and external acoustic meatus together form the ***external ear***.
6. The inner end of the external acoustic meatus is closed by a thin membranous diaphragm called the ***tympanic membrane***. This membrane separates the external acoustic meatus from the middle ear.
7. The ***middle ear*** is a small space placed deep within the petrous part of the temporal bone. It is also called the ***tympanum*** (from which we get the adjective tympanic applied to structures connected with the middle ear).
8. Medially, the middle ear is closely related to parts of the internal ear. The cavity of the middle ear is continuous with that of the nasopharynx through a passage called the ***auditory tube***.
9. Within the cavity of the middle ear, there are three small bones that are collectively called the ***ossicles*** of the ear. The ossicles are called:
   a. The ***malleus*** (= like a hammer)
   b. The ***incus*** (= like an anvil, used by blacksmiths)
   c. The ***stapes*** (= like a stirrup in which the foot of a horse rider fits).
10. The three ossicles form a chain that is attached on one side to the tympanic membrane and at the other to a part of the internal ear.
11. The ***internal ear*** is in the form of a cavity within the petrous temporal bone having a very complex shape.
    a. This bony cavity (or ***bony labyrinth***) has a central part called the ***vestibule***.
    b. Continuous with the front of the vestibule, there is a spiral shaped cavity, the bony ***cochlea***.
    c. Posteriorly, the vestibule is continuous with three ***semicircular canals***.
12. Sound waves travelling through air reach the ears.
    a. Waves striking the tympanic membrane produce vibrations in it.
    b. These vibrations are transmitted through the chain of ossicles present in the middle ear to reach the internal ear.
    c. Specialised end organs in the cochlea act as transducers that convert the mechanical vibrations into nervous impulses.
    d. These impulses travel through the cochlear part of the vestibulocochlear nerve to reach the brain.
    e. Actual perception of sound takes place in the auditory (or acoustic) areas in the cerebral cortex.

We will now consider the different parts of the ear one by one. However, the descriptions that follow will be confined only to those facts that undergraduate students need to know.

## THE AURICLE

1. The auricle is made up of a skeleton of elastic cartilage and fibrous tissue, which is covered on both sides by a layer of thin skin.
2. The cartilage of the auricle is continuous with that of the external acoustic meatus.
3. The auricle has an external surface facing laterally, and an inner or cranial surface that lies against the side of the head.
   a. The skin over the external surface is continuous with the skin lining the external acoustic meatus. Part of it passes forwards to become continuous with the skin over the parotid gland.
   b. The skin over the cranial surface passes backwards to become continuous with the skin lining the head behind the auricle. [These facts help in understanding why the nerves and blood vessels that supply the cranial surface of the auricle reach it (mainly) from the back, and those supplying the external surface reach it from the front].

### WANT TO KNOW MORE?

4. The cartilage of the auricle is curved on it self in a complicated manner so that a number of elevations and depressions are produced.
   a. Elevations on the external surface correspond to depressions on the cranial surface and vice versa. These elevations and depressions are given names that are shown in 44.20A.
   b. In particular note that the lowest part of the auricle is soft. It does not contain cartilage and is composed only of a fold of skin with enclosed connective tissue. This part is called the ***lobule***.
   c. At the centre of the external surface of the auricle, there is a large depression called the ***concha***. Its anterior part is continued into the external acoustic meatus.
   d. On the cranial surface, the position of the concha is marked by an elevation called the ***eminentia conchae***.

#### *Auricular Muscles*

A number of extrinsic auricular muscles pass from the skull to the auricle. Some intrinsic muscles that are confined to the auricle are also present. In man, the auricular muscles are to be regarded as vestigial structures of no importance. They, however, receive a nerve supply through branches of the facial nerve.

*Blood vessels, lymphatics and nerves of the auricle*

1. The auricle is supplied by:
   a. The posterior auricular branch of the external carotid artery
   b. The anterior auricular branch of the superficial temporal artery
   c. Branches from the occipital artery
   d. The veins accompany the arteries.

   The ***lymphatic drainage*** of the auricle is shown in 44.20B.
2. The ***sensory nerves*** supplying the auricle are:
   a. The auriculotemporal branch of the mandibular nerve
   b. The great auricular nerve
   c. The auricular branch of the vagus nerve.

   The area supplied by each of these nerves is shown in 43.11.

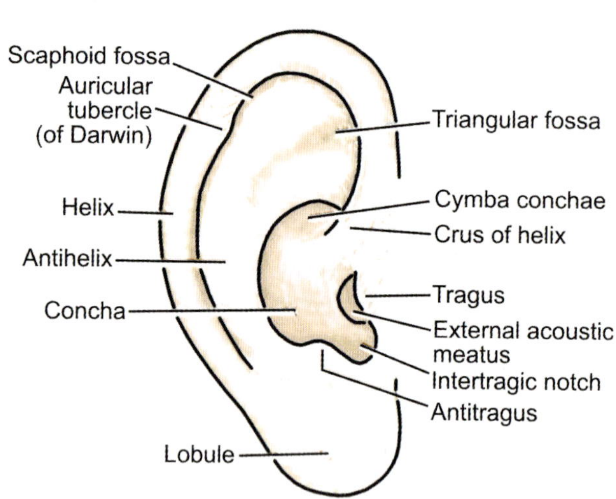


**44.20A:** Scheme to show elevations on the external surface corresponding to depressions on the cranial surface of the ear and vice versa

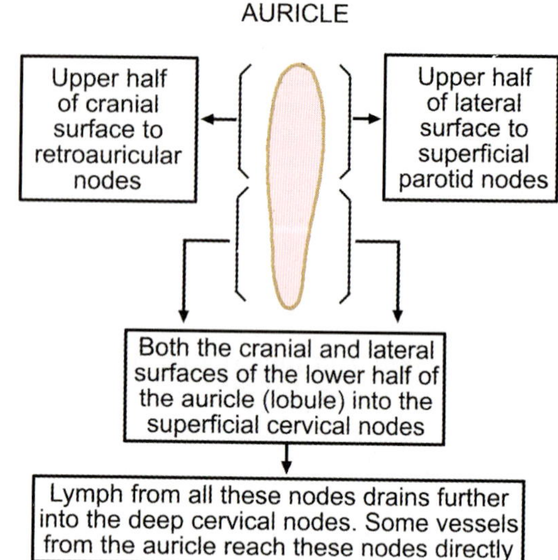


**44.20B:** Scheme to show the lymphatic drainage of the auricle

## EXTERNAL ACOUSTIC MEATUS

1. The external acoustic meatus is a tube passing medially from the bottom of the concha of the auricle.
   a. It is closed medially by the tympanic membrane.
   b. The total length of the tube is approximately 24 mm. Of this the wall of the outer 8 mm is cartilaginous, while that of the inner 16 mm is bony (44.19).
2. The cartilage or bone forming the wall of the meatus is lined by a layer of thin skin that is continuous with that over the concha.
   a. The cartilage forming the wall of the outer part of the meatus is continuous with the cartilage of the auricle.
   b. The cartilage does not form a complete tube, but is deficient in its posterosuperior part.
   c. Medially, the cartilage is firmly attached to the rough edge of the bony part of the tube.
3. The wall of the bony part of the meatus is formed mainly by the tympanic plate of the temporal bone. The posterosuperior region of the wall is formed by the squamous part of the temporal bone.
4. The medial end of the meatus is closed by the tympanic membrane. Here, the bony wall is marked by a groove called the ***tympanic sulcus***.
5. The tympanic membrane is placed obliquely both in the anteroposterior and vertical planes (44.19 and 44.25). As a result, the floor and anterior wall are longer than the roof and posterior wall. Further details of the tympanic membrane are considered with the middle ear.
6. The external acoustic meatus is not straight, but follows an S-shaped course. This is so because the cartilaginous part is not in line with the bony part, and is also bent on itself.
   a. The cartilaginous part first passes medially: forwards and upwards.
   b. It then passes medially: backwards and upwards.
   c. The bony part runs medially: forwards and downwards.
7. In clinical examination of the meatus, and through it of the tympanic membrane, the auricle is pulled upwards, backwards and somewhat laterally. This renders the meatus straight. It then has a uniform medial, forward and downward direction.
8. The meatus shows a narrowing at the junction of the cartilaginous and bony parts.
   a. It shows another narrowing called the ***isthmus*** about 4 mm from the tympanic membrane (i.e., 20 mm from the floor of the concha).

b. The floor of the meatus shows a depression immediately lateral to the tympanic membrane. Foreign bodies entering the meatus can get stuck here.

9. The skin lining the external acoustic meatus contains numerous ***ceruminous glands***. These are modified sweat glands that produce the wax of the ear, or ***cerumen***.

## WANT TO KNOW MORE?

*Relations of external acoustic meatus*

1. The meatus is related in front to the temporomandibular joint.
2. Behind to the mastoid process in the substance of which there are the mastoid air cells.
3. Inferiorly, it is related to the parotid gland.
4. Superiorly (in its deeper part), it is related to the middle cranial fossa.

*Blood vessels, lymphatics and nerves*

1. The external acoustic meatus is supplied by:
   a. The posterior auricular branch of the external carotid artery
   b. The auricular branches of the superficial temporal artery
   c. By the deep auricular branch of the maxillary artery.
2. The veins of the meatus drain into the external jugular vein, the maxillary vein and veins of the pterygoid plexus.

   The lymphatic drainage of the meatus is shown in 44.20C.
3. The sensory nerve supply to:
   a. The anterior wall and roof of the meatus is derived from the auriculotemporal nerve
   b. The posterior wall and floor from the auricular branch of the vagus nerve.

## THE MIDDLE EAR

1. The middle ear is also called the ***tympanic cavity*** or ***tympanum*** (44.19).
2. It is a space lying in the petrous temporal bone.
3. The middle ear is separated from the external acoustic meatus by the tympanic membrane.

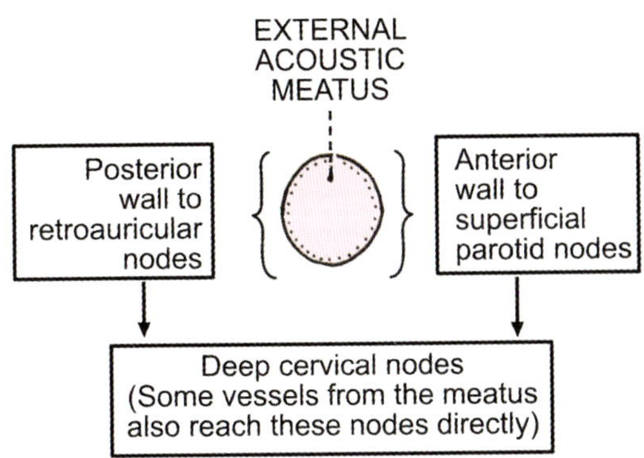


**44.20C:** Scheme to show the lymphatic drainage of the external acoustic meatus

4. From 44.19, it will be seen that part of the tympanic cavity lies above the level of the tympanic membrane: this part is called the ***epitympanic recess.***
5. Three ossicles, the malleus, the incus and the stapes lie within the middle ear.
6. The tympanic cavity communicates with the cavity of the nasopharynx through the ***auditory tube***.
7. It also communicates with a large space in the petrous part of the temporal bone called the ***mastoid antrum,*** and with smaller spaces within the mastoid process called the ***mastoid air cells.***
8. These spaces, the tympanic cavity itself, and the auditory tube are all lined by mucous membrane. Because of their communication with the nasopharynx these spaces are filled with air.
9. The tympanic cavity is shaped like a box (44.21).
   a. It has six sides: a roof, a floor, anterior, posterior, medial and lateral walls.
   b. The approximate dimensions of these walls are shown in 44.21.
   c. The anteroposterior and vertical diameters are each about 15 mm.
   d. The cavity is narrow from side to side. The distance between the medial and lateral wall is about 6 mm near the roof; about 4 mm near the floor; and only about 2 mm in the middle of the cavity.

## Ossicles of Middle Ear

### The Malleus

1. The malleus is so called because it resembles a hammer (mallet = hammer) (44.22).
2. It has an upper rounded part called the ***head*** to which is attached a relatively long ***handle*** (or ***manubrium***).
3. At the junction of the head with the handle, there is a slight constriction called the ***neck***.
4. Just below the neck, the bone gives off two ***processes: anterior and lateral.***

### The Incus

1. The incus (= anvil) has a main part or ***body*** and two ***processes***: ***long and short.***
2. The long process is directed downwards parallel to the handle of the malleus.
3. The short process is directed backwards (44.22).

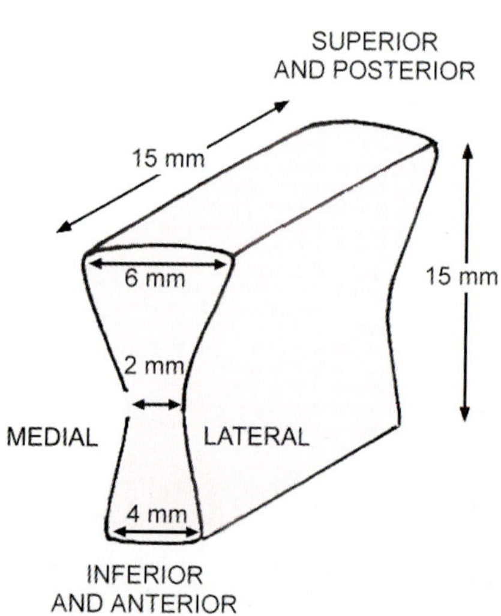


**44.21:** Dimensions of the tympanic cavity

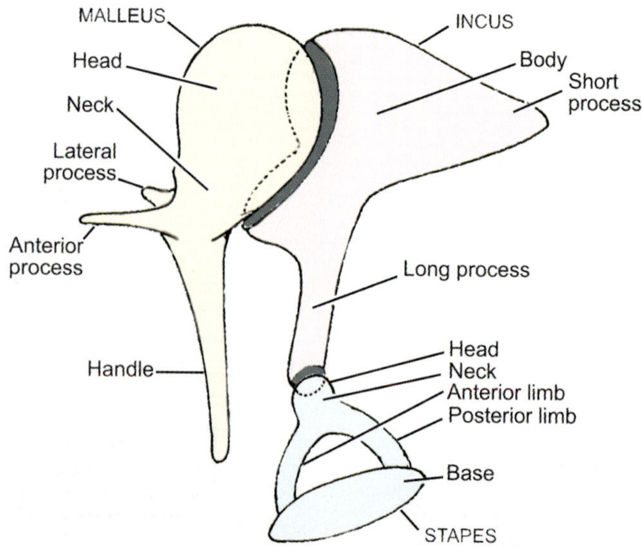


**44.22:** Ossicles of the ear as seen from the medial side

### *The Stapes*

1. The stapes is shaped like a stirrup (44.22).
2. It has a ***head***, that is connected by two ***limbs*** or ***crura*** (anterior and posterior), to an oval plate called the ***base***.
3. The constricted part adjoining the head is called the ***neck***.

## Roof of Middle Ear

1. The roof of middle ear cavity is formed by a plate of bone called the ***tegmen tympani***. (This plate forms the intracranial surface of the petrous temporal bone that is seen in the floor of the middle cranial fossa).
2. The same plate of bone extends forwards to form the roof of the canal for the tensor tympani (see below), and backwards to form the roof of the mastoid antrum.

## Floor of Middle Ear

The floor of middle ear is formed by a thin plate of bone, that separates it from the bulb of the internal jugular vein (44.23).

## Lateral Wall of Middle Ear

1. The greater part of the lateral wall of the middle ear is formed by the tympanic membrane.
2. The part of the middle ear cavity lying above the level of the tympanic membrane is the ***epitympanic recess***.
3. The lateral wall of the epitympanic recess is formed by part of the temporal bone (44.23).

### *The Tympanic Membrane*

1. This is an oval membrane about 9 mm in long diameter, and about 8 mm in its short diameter (44.24). The long diameter passes downwards and forwards.
2. The membrane is placed obliquely both in the vertical and anteroposterior planes. In the vertical plane its upper end is distinctly lateral to its lower end (44.19), and the membrane forms an acute angle of about 55° with the floor of the external acoustic meatus (44.25).

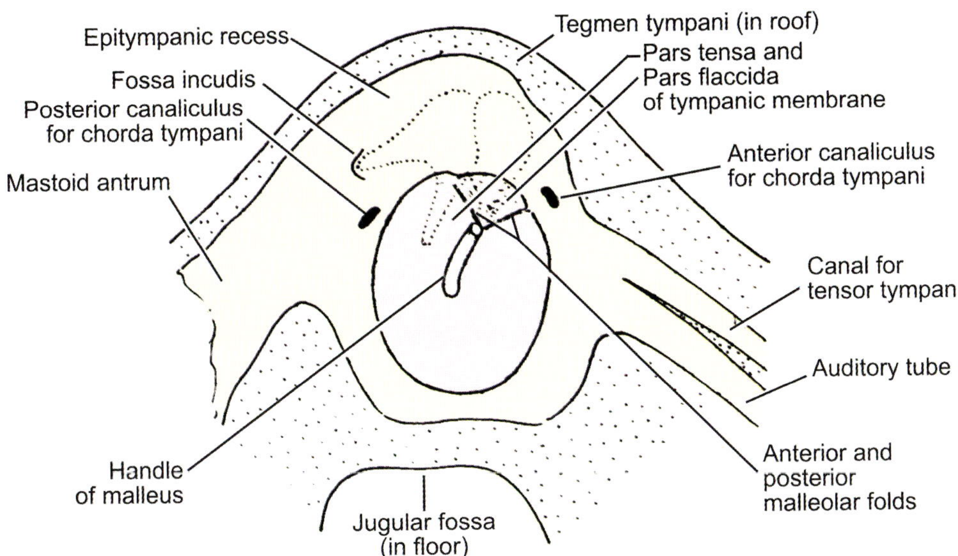


44.23: Lateral wall of tympanic cavity. Parts of the roof, floor, anterior and posterior walls (adjoining the lateral wall) are also seen. The position of the upper part of the malleus, and of the incus is shown in dotted line

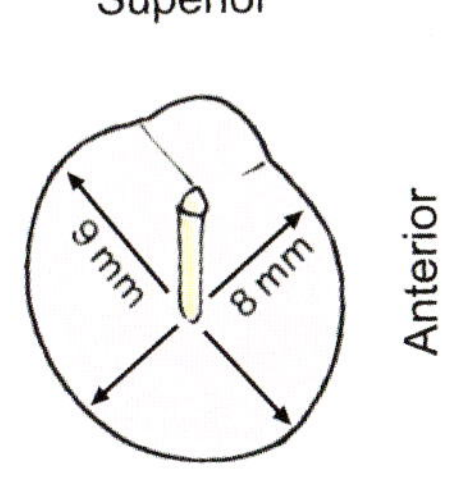


44.24: Dimensions of the tympanic membrane

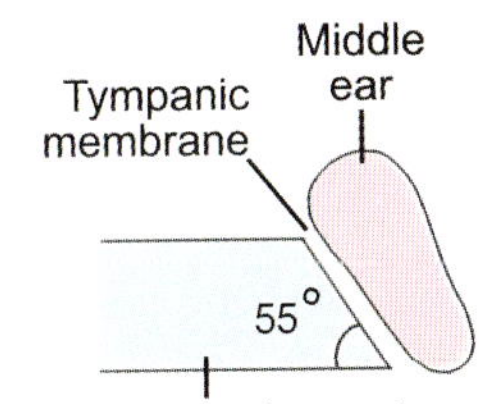


44.25: Angle between the tympanic membrane and the floor of the external acoustic meatus

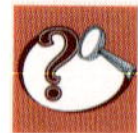

## WANT TO KNOW MORE?

3. Structurally, the tympanic membrane has three layers.
   a. The outer layer is continuous with the skin lining the external acoustic meatus.
   b. The inner layer is formed by the mucous membrane of the tympanic cavity.
   c. Between these two there is a layer of fibrous tissue. Some of the fibres in this tissue are arranged radially and some circularly.
4. With the exception of a small area in its anterosuperior part, the circumference of the tympanic membrane is thickened because of the presence here of fibrocartilage. This ring of fibrocartilage fits into a groove, the ***tympanic sulcus***, present at the medial end of the external acoustic meatus.
5. From 44.23, it will be seen that the handle of the malleus is closely attached to the medial side of the tympanic membrane.
   a. Its lower end lies approximately at the centre of the membrane.
   b. From here the handle passes upwards and forwards ending a little short of the circumference of the membrane.
   c. The lateral process of the malleus projects towards the membrane at this point.
6. From 44.23, it will also be seen that a small area of the tympanic membrane, located in its anterosuperior region, is separated from the rest of the membrane by two small folds.
   a. This part of the membrane is not stretched like the rest of it; and is therefore called the ***pars flaccida***.
   b. In contrast, the rest of the membrane is called the ***pars tensa***.
   c. The folds separating the pars flaccida from the pars tensa are called the ***anterior and posterior malleolar folds***. They pass from the lateral process of the malleus to the circumference of the tympanic membrane.
7. The part of the circumference of the tympanic membrane, formed by the pars flaccida is not thickened by fibrocartilage. Here, the tympanic sulcus is replaced by a notch.
8. On the whole, the tympanic membrane is convex medially.
   a. The point of greatest convexity corresponds to the lower end of the handle of the malleus and is called the ***umbo***.
   b. However, in passing from the umbo to the tympanic sulcus the layers of the membrane show a slight convexity outwards.

***Relationship of Chorda Tympani to Lateral Wall of Middle Ear***

1. The chorda tympani nerve has an intimate relationship to the tympanic membrane. To understand the relationship, note the following points:
   a. Just posterior to the upper part of the tympanic membrane, there is a small aperture in the angle between the lateral and posterior walls of the middle ear. This aperture is called the ***posterior canaliculus*** for the chorda tympani (44.23).
   b. Just anterior to the upper part of the tympanic membrane, there is a transverse slit (in the angle between the anterior and lateral walls of the middle ear). This slit is called the ***petrotympanic fissure*** (44.26). At the medial end of this fissure, there is an opening called the ***anterior canaliculus*** for the chorda tympani. In 44.26 note that the anterior ligament of the malleus passes into the petrotympanic fissure.
   c. The handle of the malleus is actually embedded within the tympanic membrane and lies between the fibrous and mucosal layers.
2. The chorda tympani, that is a branch of the facial nerve arising within the substance of the temporal bone, enters the middle ear through the posterior canaliculus (44.26).
   a. It passes forwards through the substance of the upper part of the tympanic membrane, lying between the fibrous and mucosal layers.
   b. As it does so it crosses medial to the handle of the malleus, near the upper end of the latter.
   c. The chorda tympani leaves the middle ear by passing through the anterior canaliculus to reach the infratemporal fossa.

*Tympanic Membrane as seen through the External Acoustic Meatus*

1. Many of the features of the tympanic membrane described in the preceding paragraphs can be seen in the living through the external acoustic meatus (44.27).
2. The pars flaccida can be seen in the anterosuperior corner of the membrane, and the anterior and posterior malleolar folds can also be distinguished.
3. The lateral process of the malleus can be seen as a white dot where these folds meet.
4. Running downwards and backwards from this dot to the centre of the membrane there is the handle of the malleus.
5. A little behind and parallel to the upper part of the handle of the malleus the long process of the incus may be visible as a faint white streak.
6. The anteroinferior part of the membrane (between the lower end of the handle of the malleus and the circumference of the membrane) reflects light more than the rest of the membrane and is referred to as the *cone of light*.

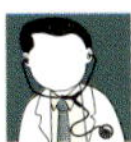

## CLINICAL CORRELATION

It is sometimes necessary to incise the tympanic membrane to let out pus from the middle ear. Such an incision is always made in the lower part to avoid damage to the chorda tympani. Another advantage of such an incision is that the lower part of the membrane is less vascular.

## WANT TO KNOW MORE?

*Blood Vessels and Nerves of Tympanic Membrane*

1. a. The blood vessels and nerves to the external surface of the tympanic membrane are derived from those supplying the external acoustic meatus.
   b. Those to its internal surface are derived from vessels and nerves that supply the middle ear.
2. a. The external surface is supplied by the deep auricular branch of the maxillary artery, and drains into the external jugular vein.
   b. It is supplied by the auriculotemporal nerve, and the auricular branch of the vagus (Compare with external acoustic meatus).
3. The internal surface of the tympanic membrane is supplied by:
   a. The tympanic branches of the maxillary artery
   b. The stylomastoid branch which arises either from the posterior auricular artery or from the occipital artery.
   c. The nerves to the internal surface are derived from the tympanic branch of the glossopharyngeal nerve.

### *Anterior Wall of Middle Ear*

1. The medial and lateral walls of the middle ear are fairly close to each other. It follows that the anterior and posterior walls are narrow.
2. The various structures to be seen on the anterior wall are shown in 44.23.
   a. In the upper part of the wall, there are two openings.
   b. The upper opening leads into a canal in which the tensor tympani muscle lies.
   c. The lower opening is that of the auditory tube.
   d. The two openings are separated by a thin bony septum. This septum extends onto the medial wall of the middle ear where it curves on itself to form a pulley *(processus trochleariformis)*.

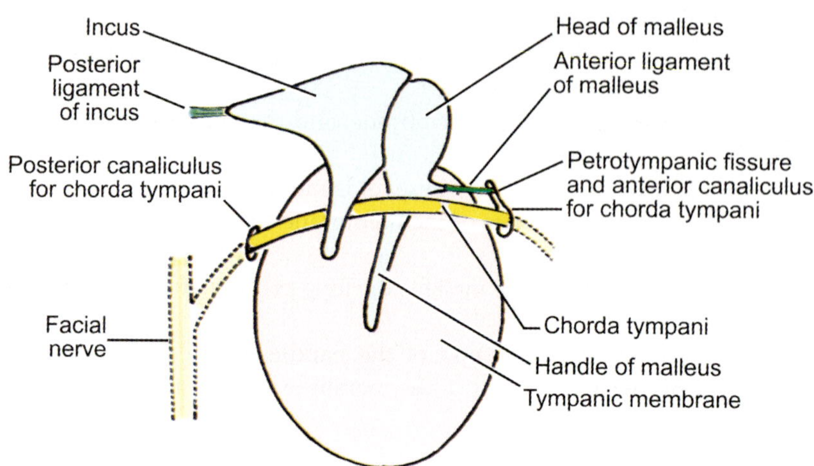


**44.26:** Relationship of the chorda tympani to the lateral wall of the middle ear

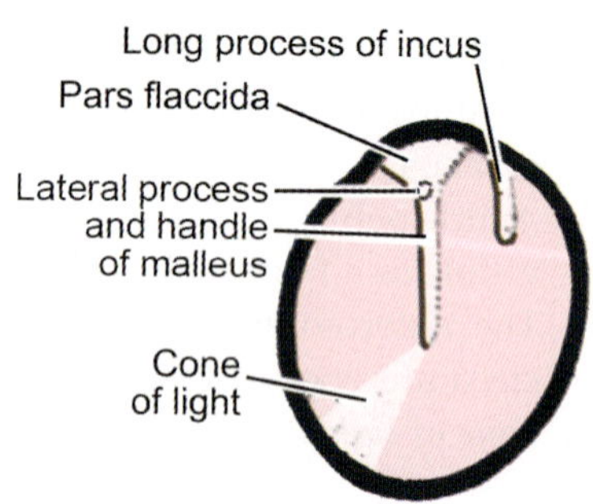


**44.27:** Tympanic membrane as seen through the external acoustic meatus

**WANT TO KNOW MORE?**

e. The tendon of the tensor tympani winds around this pulley (to change from a backward direction to a lateral one) (44.29 and 44.30).

3. The part of the anterior wall of the middle ear lying below the opening for the auditory tube, is formed by a plate of bone that separates the middle ear from the carotid canal (through which the internal carotid artery passes).
4. Minute apertures in this plate give passage to branches from the internal carotid artery to the middle ear, and also to ***caroticotympanic nerves*** that arise from the sympathetic plexus surrounding the artery to reach the middle ear.

### *Posterior Wall of Middle Ear*

1. The features to be seen on the posterior wall of the middle ear are shown in 44.28.
2. The upper part of the wall is relatively broad. It shows a large round aperture through which the middle ear communicates with the mastoid antrum. This aperture is called the ***aditus to the mastoid antrum***.
3. On the medial wall of the aditus, there is a bulging produced by the lateral semicircular canal.

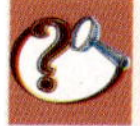

**WANT TO KNOW MORE?**

4. Anterior to the aditus there is the posterior wall of the epitympanic recess.
   a. On it we see a depression, the ***fossa incudis***.
   b. The tip of the short process of the incus extends into this depression, and is attached to the fossa by fibres of the posterior ligament of the incus. The aditus to the mastoid antrum and the fossa incudis are also seen in 44.23.

5. Inferior to the aditus, the medial end of the posterior wall of the middle ear bears a conical elevation called the ***pyramid***.
   a. The tip of the pyramid projects forwards, and has an opening that leads into a canal in which the stapedius muscle is lodged.

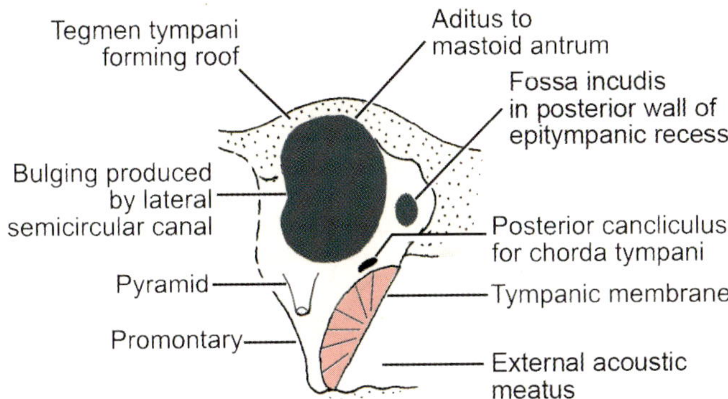


**44.28:** Features to be seen on the posterior wall of the middle ear

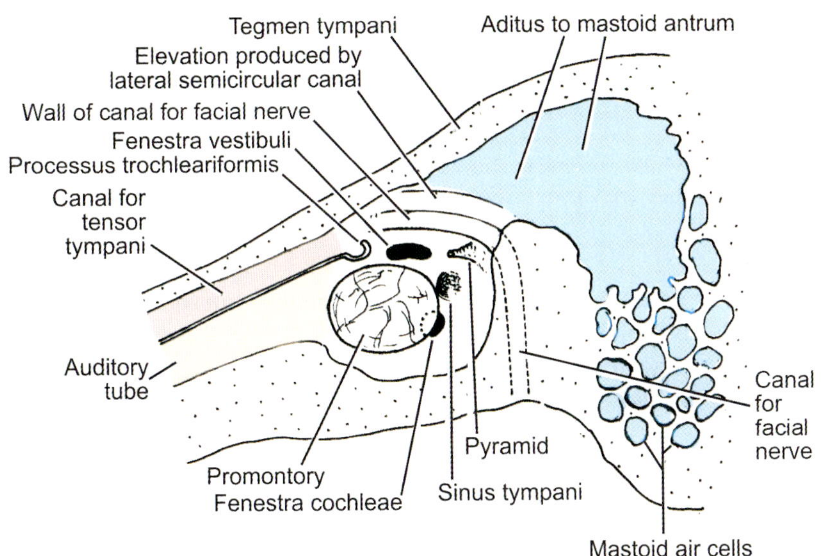


**44.29:** Medial wall of middle ear. Parts of the anterior and posterior walls, and of the mastoid antrum and mastoid air cells, are also seen. Compare with Fig. 44.28

   b. The tendon of the stapedius emerges from the opening at the tip of the pyramid and runs forwards to be inserted into the posterior surface of the neck of the stapes (44.30).
6. The facial nerve is closely related to the internal ear and to the medial and posterior walls of the middle ear. Part of it runs vertically downwards in a bony canal placed along the junction of the medial and posterior walls (See 43.50).

### *Medial Wall of Middle Ear*

1. The medial wall of the middle ear is also the lateral wall of the internal ear. It can be properly understood only after examining some features of the internal ear as follows:
   a. The bony internal ear consists of a central part called the vestibule, which is connected anteriorly to the cochlea, and posteriorly to three semicircular canals.

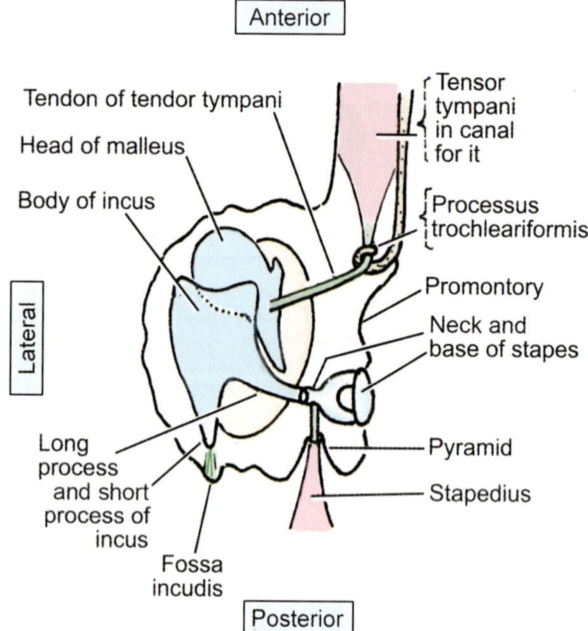


**44.30:** Scheme to show the muscles of the middle ear. They are viewed from above after removing the roof of the middle ear

b. Further details should be noted by examining 44.34 in which the internal ear is seen from the lateral side.
   i. Note that the cochlea is in the form of a spiral and that its 'turns' are narrow in the centre and become wider as we proceed outwards.
   ii. The lowest (or basal) turn of the cochlea is large and is continuous posteriorly with the vestibule.
   iii. If we look into the interior of the basal turn of the cochlea (44.36) we find that its cavity consists of two parts, upper and lower.

c. The upper part, which is called the ***scala vestibuli***, becomes continuous with the cavity of the vestibule.
   i. The vestibule communicates with the middle ear through a large oval aperture called the ***fenestra vestibuli***.
   ii. Thus, the scala vestibuli is in indirect communication with the middle ear.
   iii. The lower part of the cavity of the cochlea (or ***scala tympani***) opens independently into the middle ear through a round opening called the ***fenestra cochleae***. This fenestra is situated inferior to the vestibule.
   iv. In 44.34 observe that the three semicircular canals are named anterior, posterior and lateral. Note further that the lateral canal bulges in a lateral direction and is, therefore, closest to the middle ear.

2. With this brief introduction, we can now proceed to study the features to be seen on the medial wall of the middle ear as shown in 44.29. In the anterior and posterior parts of this figure, we see some features of the anterior and posterior walls of the middle ear already described.
3. Anteriorly, identify the canal for the tensor tympani, and below it the auditory tube. In particular note that the septum between these tubes reaches the medial wall and curves on itself to form the processus trochleariformis (or cochleariformis).
4. Posteriorly, note the aditus to the tympanic antrum and below it the pyramid. Also note that superiorly the medial wall meets the roof, formed by the tegmen tympani; and inferiorly it meets the floor.
5. The most prominent feature to be seen on the medial wall is the ***promontory***.
   a. This is a large circular bulging produced by the basal turn of the cochlea.
   b. Its surface bears a number of grooves.

   c. The apex of the cochlea comes in contact with the medial wall of the middle ear just in front of the promontory.
6. Posterosuperior to the promontory, we see the ***fenestra vestibuli*** that is also called the ***oval window***.
   a. Note its shape in 44.29.
   b. The base of the stapes fits into this opening and is attached to its margins by the annular ligament.
7. Posteroinferior to the promontory there is a round aperture called the ***fenestra cochleae*** (also called the ***round window***).
   a. This aperture is only partially seen (or not seen at all) because it is overlapped by the lower edge of the promontory which overhangs it.
   b. This opening is continuous with part of the cavity of the cochlea.
   c. It is closed by the ***secondary tympanic membrane***.
8. Posterior to the promontory, there is a depression called the ***sinus tympani***, which lies between the fenestra vestibuli and the fenestra cochleae. A part of the posterior semicircular canal (ampulla) lies deep to the sinus tympani.
9. The part of the medial wall above the promontory and the fenestra vestibuli, is marked by two rounded ridges that run anteroposteriorly.
   a. The upper of these is produced by the lateral semicircular canal.
   b. The lower ridge is the wall of a canal through which the facial nerve runs backwards.
10. Only a thin layer of bone separates the nerve from the cavity of the middle ear. Occasionally, this bone may be missing and the nerve may lie just under the mucosa.
11. Running backwards across the medial wall of the middle ear, the facial canal reaches the aditus to the mastoid antrum. Here, it bends downwards and runs through bone just behind the angle between the medial and posterior walls of the middle ear to reach the stylomastoid foramen (See 43.50).

## WANT TO KNOW MORE?

*Muscles of the Middle Ear*

These are the stapedius and the tensor tympani.

1. The ***stapedius*** is a small muscle lying in a bony canal that is related to the posterior wall of the middle ear.
   a. Posteriorly and below, this canal is continuous with the vertical part of the canal for the facial nerve. Anteriorly, the canal opens into the middle ear at the apex of the pyramid.
   b. The fibres of the stapedius arise from the walls of this canal.
   c. They end in a tendon that enters the middle ear through the pyramid and runs forwards to be inserted into the posterior surface of the neck of the stapes.
   d. The stapedius muscle is supplied by a branch from the facial nerve (44.30).
2. The ***tensor tympani*** lies in a canal that opens into the anterior wall of the middle ear.
   a. At its other end, this canal opens on the base of the skull.
   b. Muscle fibres arise from the wall of this canal. Some fibres arise from the cartilaginous part of the auditory tube and some from the base of the skull formed here by the greater wing of the sphenoid.
   c. The muscle ends in a tendon that reaches the middle ear cavity near its medial wall.
   d. Here, it bends sharply to the lateral side by passing around the processus trochleariformis.
   e. It is inserted into the upper end of the handle of the malleus.
3. Both the tensor tympani and the stapedius protect the ear against very loud sounds by restricting the vibrations of the tympanic membrane and the ossicles.
4. Paralysis of the muscles (specially of the stapedius) gives rise to a condition called ***hyperacusis*** in which even normal sounds appear too loud.

### *The Mastoid Antrum*

1. The mastoid antrum is of considerable importance as it is a frequent site of infection, which may be difficult to eradicate. Furthermore, infection may spread from it to neighbouring structures with serious consequences.
2. Although, it is called the 'mastoid' antrum this space lies in the ***petrous*** part of the temporal bone.
3. Anteriorly the antrum opens, through its aditus, into the epitympanic recess. The medial side of the aditus is related to the lateral semicircular canal (44.28 and 44.29).

**WANT TO KNOW MORE?**

4. The following additional relationships are seen in 44.29.
   a. Superiorly, the roof of the antrum is formed by the tegmen tympani that separates it from the middle cranial fossa; and from the temporal lobe of the cerebral hemisphere.
   b. Inferiorly, the mastoid antrum is continuous with the mastoid air cells (see below).
   c. Anteriorly, below the aditus, the antrum is related to the facial nerve as it descends within its bony canal.
   d. Posteriorly, the antrum is close to the posterior surface of the temporal bone (i.e., to the posterior cranial fossa) and here, it may be separated only by a thin plate of bone from the sigmoid sinus.
   e. Medially, behind the aditus, the antrum is related to the posterior semicircular canal.
5. The lateral wall of the mastoid antrum is related to the ***suprameatal triangle*** (44.31). This triangle is bounded:
   a. Above by the supramastoid crest.
   b. Anteroinferiorly by the posterosuperior margin of the (bony) external acoustic meatus.
   c. Posteriorly by a vertical line drawn as a tangent to the posterior margin of the meatus.
6. The thickness of bone separating the mastoid antrum from the surface of the skull is only about 2 mm at birth, but it increases by about 1 mm for every year of age until it is about 13 to 14 mm thick. (In other words, it attains its full thickness by puberty).

### *The Mastoid Air Cells*

1. These are a series of intercommunicating spaces of variable size present within the mastoid process. They communicate above with the mastoid antrum.
2. Their number varies considerably. Sometimes there are just a few, and are confined to the upper part of the mastoid process. In other case, they may extend throughout the process. Occasionally, they may extend beyond the mastoid process into the squamous or petrous parts of the temporal bone.

**WANT TO KNOW MORE?**

3. Some of the cells may occasionally lie:
   a. Very close to the sigmoid sinus
   b. In the roof of the external acoustic meatus
   c. In the floor of the tympanic cavity close to the jugular bulb
   d. In the medial part of the petrous temporal bone in relation to the internal ear, the carotid canal, the auditory tube, and the abducent nerve.

4. Infection can reach the mastoid air cells though the tympanic cavity and the mastoid antrum, and can spread to any of the structures related to them.

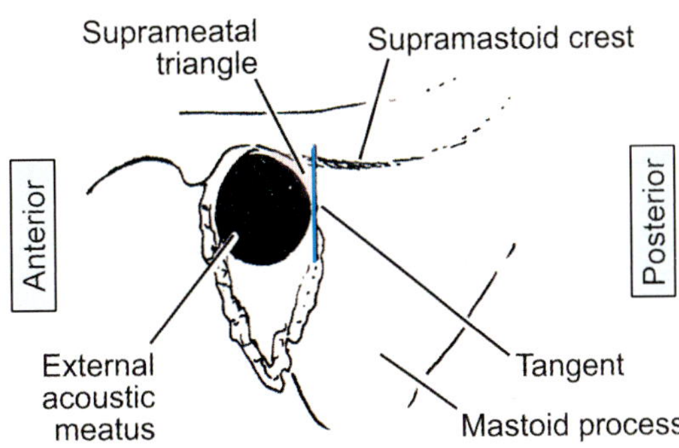


**44.31:** Boundaries of the suprameatal triangle

## *The Auditory Tube*

### *Importance of tube*

1. The auditory tube is also called the ***pharyngotympanic tube***, or the ***Eustachian tube***.
2. It provides a communication between the nasopharynx and the middle ear (44.19).
3. Because of this communication air passes into the tympanic cavity (and into the mastoid antrum and air cells).
4. As a result, air pressure on both sides of the tympanic membrane is the same. This is important for proper vibration of the tympanic membrane.
5. However, the auditory tube is not patent all the time. It opens during deglutition, or even during the swallowing of saliva.
6. When we suddenly ascend to a higher altitude (as in going up a hill in a car) the air pressure on the outside of the tympanic membrane falls, but that on its inner side remains the same as before.
   a. This inequality in pressure gives rise to a change in the quality of sound perceived.
   b. However, on swallowing of saliva, and the consequent equalisation of pressure, the sound suddenly returns to normal.
7. The same phenomenon takes place much more acutely during the take off of an aircraft, and can give rise to distress in the ear; more so in persons who have a mild infection. [The sweets handed out by air-hostesses just before take off are meant to keep passengers swallowing so that discomfort is avoided or lessened].

## CLINICAL CORRELATION

8. The communication between the pharynx and the middle ear is a path along which infection frequently reaches the middle ear. This occurs more commonly in children, in whom the auditory tube is shorter and wider than in the adult.
9. In the presence of infection, the tube is easily blocked. When this happens air within the tympanic cavity is gradually absorbed and pressure on the outside of the tympanic membrane becomes greater than on the inside. This can give rise to discomfort that can be relieved by introducing air into the auditory tube through a catheter.
10. If obstruction to the auditory tube is prolonged pus can accumulate in middle ear resulting in severe pain. The pus may burst through the tympanic membrane leading to discharge from the ear, and to the formation of a perforation in the membrane. It is for these reasons that the anatomy of the auditory tube is of much practical importance.

## WANT TO KNOW MORE?

*Anatomical Features*

1. The auditory tube is about 36 mm long.
   a. It consists of an outer bony part, which is about 12 mm long.
   b. An inner cartilaginous part which is about 24 mm long.
2. Both these parts are directed downwards, forwards and medially.
3. The lateral end of the bony part opens on the anterior wall of the middle ear (44.23 and 44.29).
4. The medial end of the bony part opens on the base of the skull (at the lateral end of the groove between the anterior margin of the petrous temporal bone and the posterior margin of the greater wing of the sphenoid bone).
5. The cartilaginous part extends from the medial end of the bony part to the lateral wall of the nasopharynx.
6. The auditory tube is narrowest at the junction of the bony and cartilaginous parts: this part is called the ***isthmus***.
7. The cartilage forming the wall of the auditory tube is not tubular, but consists of a triangular plate that is bent on itself.
   a. Its lateral end (that joins the bony part) is narrow.
   b. Its medial end is broad and lies just under the mucous membrane of the lateral wall of the nasopharynx where it forms the tubal elevation.
   c. The cartilage consists of a larger medial lamina (facing backwards and medially) and of a smaller lateral lamina (facing forwards and laterally).
   d. There is a gap in the cartilage in the inferolateral wall of the tube. This gap is filled by fibrous tissue.
8. The cartilaginous part of the auditory tube lies in close relation to the base of the skull in the groove between the anterior margin of the petrous temporal bone and the posterior margin of the greater wing of the sphenoid bone.
9. The interior of the auditory tube is lined by mucous membrane continuous with that of the nasopharynx and of the middle ear.
10. The cartilaginous part of the auditory tube lies in close relationship to the roof of the infratemporal fossa (44.32A).
    a. The tensor palati muscle lies immediately to its lateral side, and the levator palati lies immediately medial to it.
    b. Both the muscles partially arise from the wall of the tube.
    c. The part of the tensor palati arising from the tube is believed to be responsible for opening the auditory tube during swallowing. It is, therefore, called the ***dilator tubae***.
    d. The salpingopharyngeus (44.32A) takes origin from the lower part of the tube near its medial end.
11. The tensor palati separates the tube from several structures in the infratemporal fossa including the mandibular nerve, the chorda tympani, the middle meningeal artery and the otic ganglion.

*Blood Vessels, Lymphatics and Nerves of Middle Ear*

1. The middle ear receives several small branches that arise from arteries that lie in its neighbourhood. Branches are received from:
   a. Anterior tympanic branch of maxillary artery
   b. Middle meningeal artery
   c. Artery of pterygoid canal
   d. Stylomastoid branch of posterior auricular artery (or of occipital artery)
   e. Ascending pharyngeal artery
   f. Directly from internal carotid artery.

2. The veins of the middle ear drain downward (along the auditory tube) towards the infratemporal fossa where they end in the pterygoid plexus. Some veins drain through apertures in the petrous temporal bone to end in the superior petrosal sinus.
3. The lymphatics from the middle ear and the mastoid air cells end in the parotid lymph nodes while those from the auditory tube reach the deep cervical nodes (44.32B).
4. The nerves supplying the mucous membrane of the middle ear, the mastoid antrum and air cells and the auditory tube are derived from the tympanic plexus that lies over the promontory.
   a. The tympanic plexus is formed mainly by branches from the tympanic branch of the glossopharyngeal nerve.
   b. It also receives some fibres from the sympathetic plexus around the internal carotid artery (caroticotympanic nerves).
   c. The tympanic plexus gives off the lesser petrosal nerve, which ends in the otic ganglion.

## THE INTERNAL EAR

### Preliminary Remarks

1. The internal ear is in the form of a complex system of cavities within the petrous temporal bone. Because of the complex shape of these intercommunicating cavities the internal ear is referred to as the ***labyrinth***.
2. The basic arrangement of the labyrinth is best understood by looking at a transverse section through a relatively simple part of it like a semicircular canal (44.33).
   a. The wall of the ***bony labyrinth*** is made up of dense bone. Its inner surface is lined by periosteum.
   b. Lying within the bony labyrinth, there is a system of ducts which constitute the ***membranous labyrinth***.
   c. The spaces within the membranous labyrinth are filled by a fluid called the ***endolymph***.
   d. The space between the membranous labyrinth and the bony labyrinth is filled by another fluid called the ***perilymph***.
3. The ***parts of the bony labyrinth*** are shown in 44.34. These are as follows:
   a. In the central part of the bony labyrinth, there is a cavity called the ***vestibule***.
   b. Anterior to the vestibule, we see the ***bony cochlea***. The cavity of the bony cochlea is divided into two parts:
      i. One part, called the ***scala vestibuli*** (44.36), is continuous posteriorly with the cavity of the vestibule.
      ii. The second part is called the ***scala tympani***. The scala tympani opens into the middle ear at the fenestra cochleae (44.36).

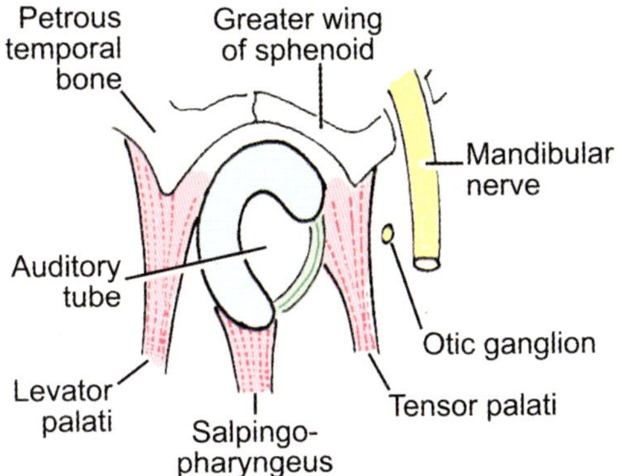


**44.32A:** Some relations of the cartilaginous part of the auditory tube

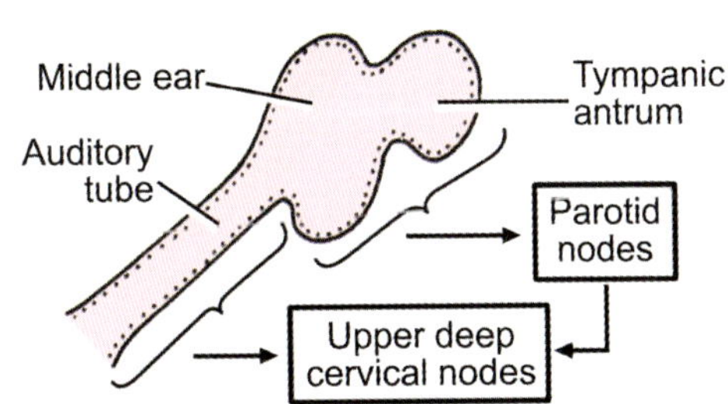


**44.32B:** Scheme to show the lymphatic drainage of the middle ear

4. Posteriorly, the cavity of the vestibule is continuous with the three ***semicircular canals*** (44.34).
5. The ***parts of the membranous labyrinth*** are shown in 44.35.
6. The part of the membranous labyrinth within each semicircular canal is called a ***semicircular duct*** [It is important to distinguish carefully between the terms semicircular canal, and semicircular duct].
7. The part of the membranous labyrinth in the cochlea is called the ***duct of the cochlea.***
8. The part of the membranous labyrinth lying in the vestibule is represented by two distinct membranous sacs called the ***saccule*** and the ***utricle.***

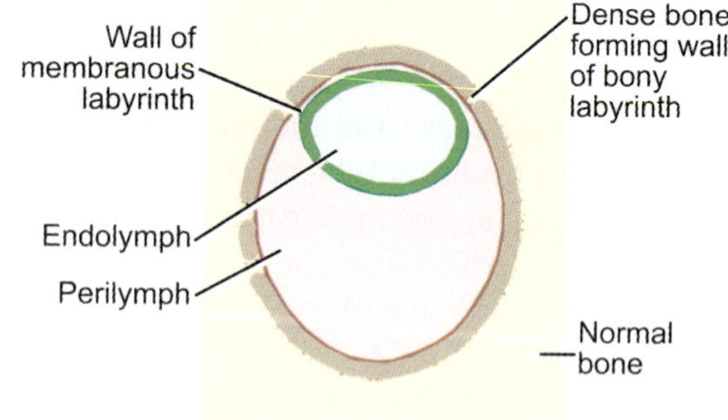


**44.33:** Basic structure of the internal ear as seen in a section through a semicircular canal

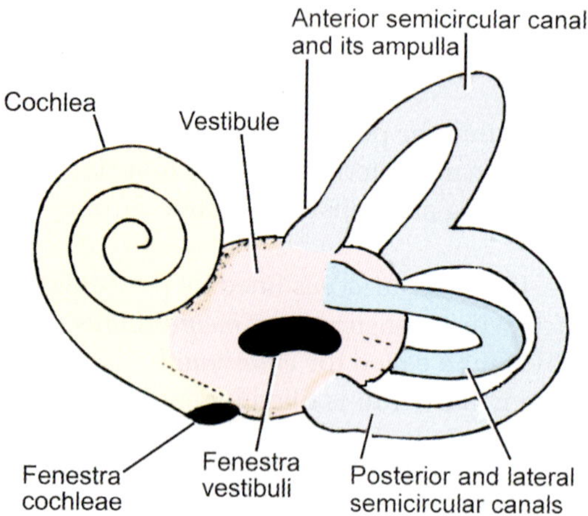


**44.34:** Bony labyrinth seen from the lateral side

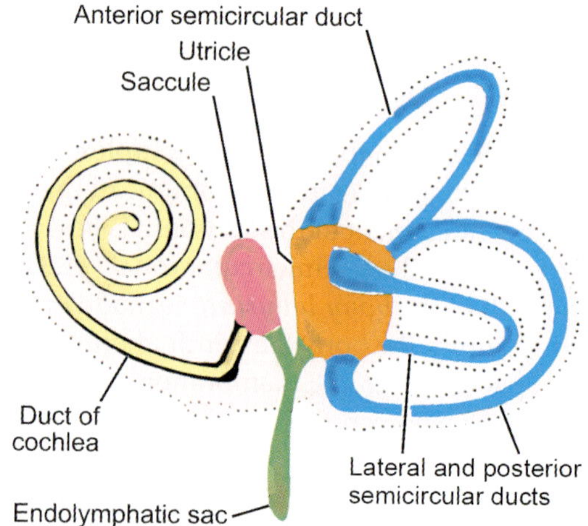


**44.35:** Scheme to show the parts of the membranous labyrinth. Note the ampullated ends of the semicircular ducts

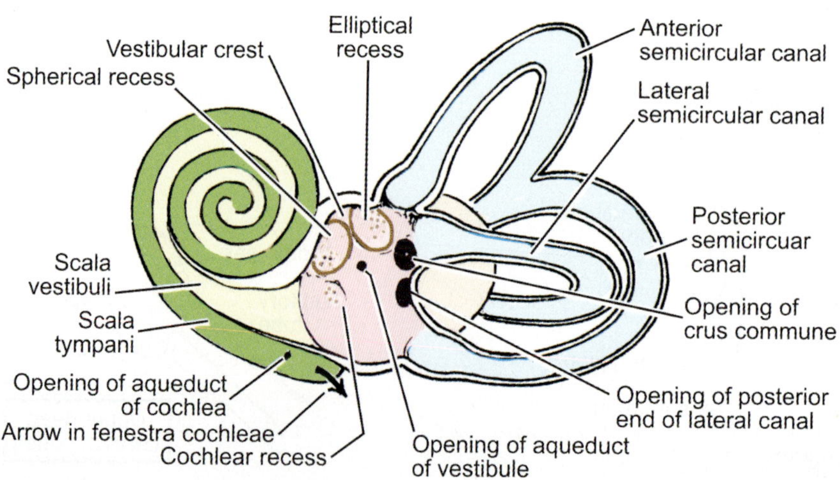


**44.36:** Interior of the bony labyrinth as seen from the lateral side

**WANT TO KNOW MORE?**

1. The saccule communicates with the duct of the cochlea through a narrow duct called the ***ductus reunions***.
2. The semicircular ducts open into the utricle.
3. The utricle and the saccule communicate with each other through the ***utriculosaccular duct***.
4. The utriculosaccular duct is also connected to a diverticulum called the ***saccus endolymphaticus***.

We will now consider the parts of the bony and membranous labyrinth one by one.

**WANT TO KNOW MORE?**

**The Vestibule**

1. The vestibule is an oval space about 5 mm in diameter.
2. Anteriorly, it is continuous with the scala vestibuli of the cochlea.
3. Posterosuperiorly, the vestibule has five openings for the semicircular canals.
4. Its lateral wall is formed by the part of the same plate of bone that forms the medial wall of the middle ear.
5. In this wall, there is an aperture, the fenestra vestibuli, through which the vestibule and middle ear communicate. This aperture is closed by the base of the stapes and by the annular ligament.
6. The plate of bone that forms the medial wall of the vestibule closes the inner end of the internal acoustic meatus.

## The Semicircular Canals

1. There are three semicircular canals, ***anterior*** (or superior), ***posterior***, and ***lateral*** (44.34).
2. One end of each canal is dilated, and the dilatation is called an ***ampulla***.
3. The non-ampullated ends of the anterior and posterior canals join to form a common channel, the ***crus commune***. As a result, the semicircular canals open into the vestibule through five (not six) openings.
4. The most important facts about the semicircular canals concern their orientation.
   a. The three canals lie in planes at right angles to one another (44.37).
   b. The anterior and posterior canals are both vertical, while the lateral canal is horizontal.
   c. The plane of the posterior canal is parallel to the long axis of the petrous temporal bone.
   d. The plane of the anterior canal is at right angles to this axis.
   e. The plane of the lateral canal is transverse.
5. From 44.37, it will be clear that the right and left lateral semicircular canals lie in the same plane. The anterior canal of one side lies in the same plane as the posterior canal of the opposite side.

## The Bony Cochlea

1. The cochlea is continuous with the anterior part of the vestibule. From 44.34, it is seen that the cochlea is basically a tube that is coiled on itself for two and three quarter turns.
2. The diameter of the tube is greatest at its junction with the vestibule, and this part is called the ***basal turn*** of the cochlea.
3. The tube becomes progressively narrower towards the centre or ***apex*** of the cochlea.
4. The basal turn of the cochlea produces an elevation, the promontory, on the medial wall of the middle ear. The apex of the cochlea is related to this wall of the middle ear just in front of the promontory.
5. If we examine the basal turn of the cochlea shown in 44.36 we find that it is made up of an upper channel the scala vestibuli that is continuous with the vestibule; and of a lower channel, the scala tympani, that opens into the middle ear through the fenestra cochleae.

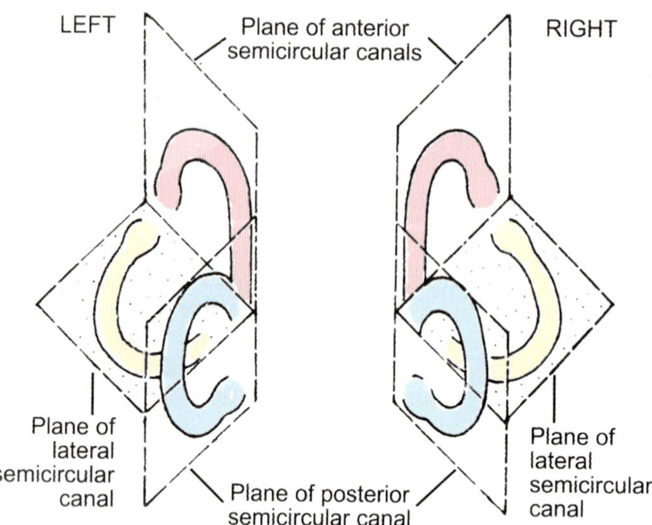


**44.37:** Planes in which the semicircular canals lie as seen from behind

6. The fenestra cochleae is closed by the ***secondary tympanic membrane.***
7. The scala vestibuli and the scala tympani are partially separated from each other by a shelf of bone. The shelf follows the coiling of the cochlea and is, therefore, called the ***spiral lamina***. The spiral lamina is a projection from the modiolus.
8. Further details of the cochlea can be appreciated if we study a transverse section through one turn of the cochlea (44.38).
   a. In this figure, we see that the spiral lamina extends only partially into the canal of the cochlea.
   b. The division of the canal into the scala vestibuli and the scala tympani is completed by the ***basilar membrane*** that stretches from the 'free' edge of the spiral lamina to the outer wall of the cochlear canal.
9. The spiral lamina ends just short of the apex of the cochlea so that the scala vestibuli becomes continuous with the scala tympani at the apex (44.36). This communication is called the ***helicotrema***.
10. The part of the membranous labyrinth in the cochlea is called the ***duct of the cochlea***. This duct lies just above the basilar membrane. It is separated from the scala vestibuli by a thin ***vestibular membrane.***
11. Near the attached margin of the spiral lamina there is a canal. This canal is also shaped like a spiral and is called the ***spiral canal***. This canal contains a collection of neurons that constitute the ***spiral ganglion***. Fibres arising from the ganglion pass through the spiral lamina to supply the spiral organ (See below).

**WANT TO KNOW MORE?**

**The Membranous Labyrinth**

The parts of the membranous labyrinth are shown in 44.35.

1. The membranous labyrinth lying within each semicircular canal forms a ***semicircular duct*** [It is important to distinguish carefully between the terms semicircular canal, and semicircular duct].
2. The part of the membranous labyrinth in the cochlea is called the ***duct of the cochlea***.
3. The part of the membranous labyrinth lying within the vestibule is represented by two distinct membranous sacs called the ***saccule*** and the ***utricle.***
4. The duct of the cochlea opens into the saccule. The semicircular ducts open into the utricle.

5. The saccule and the utricle are indirectly interconnected by a Y-shaped tube. The stem of the 'Y' is blind, and slightly expanded. It is called the ***endolymphatic sac***.
6. This sac lies outside the bony labyrinth on the posterior surface of the petrous temporal bone.

## Specialised End Organs in the Membranous Labyrinth

### *The Spiral Organ of Corti*

1. The end organ for hearing is the ***spiral organ (of Corti)***. It lies in the duct of the cochlea, just above the basilar membrane (44.38).
2. Sound waves travelling through air produce vibrations in the tympanic membrane.
   a. These are transmitted through the malleus and incus to the stapes.
   b. The base of the stapes (that fits into the fenestra vestibuli) transmits these vibrations to the perilymph of the vestibule.
   c. From there, the vibrations pass into the scala vestibuli.
3. Each time the base of the stapes moves inwards into the vestibule it creates a pressure wave that extends along the perilymph filling the entire length of the scala vestibuli.
   a. Reaching the helicotrema, the pressure wave passes into the perilymph filling the scala tympani.
   b. Traversing the entire length of the scala tympani, it reaches the secondary tympanic membrane (which closes the fenestra cochleae) causing it to bulge into the middle ear.

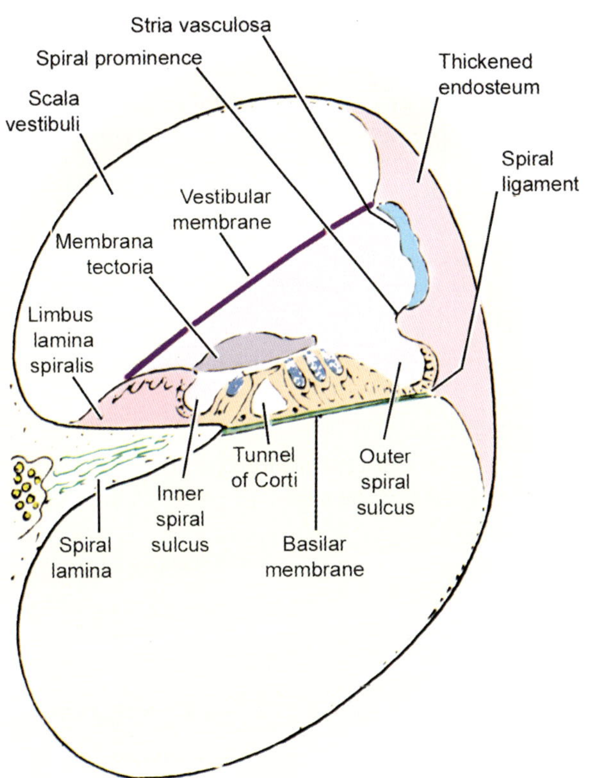


**44.38:** Transverse section through one turn of the cochlea

4. The process is reversed when the base of the stapes moves outwards. These changes take place almost instantaneously.
   a. In this way, vibrations are set up in the perilymph.
   b. These in turn produce vibrations of the basilar membrane and of the spiral organ.
   c. The spiral organ contains highly specialised ***hair cells***. Distortions produced in these cells as a result of vibrations generate nervous impulses.
5. These impulses travel along nerve fibres that are peripheral processes of neurons located in the spiral ganglia. These processes reach the hair cells through canals in the spiral lamina.
6. Central processes arising from neurons of the spiral ganglion constitute the cochlear nerve.

### *Maculae*

1. Information about changes in the position of the head is provided by end organs called ***maculae*** (singular = macula) present in the utricle and saccule.
2. Each macula consists essentially of hair cells, surrounded by supporting cells.
   a. The 'hair' of the hair cells are covered by a membrane which contains crystals of calcium carbonate (***otoliths***).
   b. With changes in the position of the head, the otoliths are displaced leading to distortion of hair cells.
   c. Nervous impulses are generated as a result of this distortion.

### *Cristae Ampullae*

1. Information about angular movements (acceleration) of the head is provided by end organs called the ***ampullary crests*** (or ***cristae ampullae***) one of which is present in the ampulla of each semicircular duct.
   a. Each crista consists of hair cells (and supporting cells) that are surmounted by a gelatinous covering that forms a partition (***cupola***) within the ampulla.
   b. Movements of the head produce currents in the endolymph within the semicircular ducts. These cause the cupolae to move resulting in deformation of hair cells and production of nerve impulses.
   c. The nerve fibres innervating the cristae of the semicircular ducts and the maculae of the utricle and saccule are peripheral processes of neurons located in the vestibular ganglion.
   d. This ganglion lies in the internal acoustic meatus. The central processes of cells of the ganglion form the vestibular nerve.

## WANT TO KNOW MORE?

***Blood Vessels of the Internal Ear***

1. The internal ear is supplied by the labyrinthine artery which usually arises from the anterior inferior cerebellar artery.
2. It sometimes arises from the basilar artery.
3. The internal ear also receives some twigs from the stylomastoid artery that supplies the middle ear.
4. The internal ear drains into veins that end in the superior petrosal sinus or in the transverse sinus.

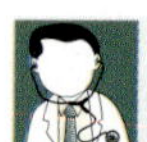

## CLINICAL CORRELATION

**The Ear**

1. The anatomy of the external acoustic meatus, of the middle ear, and of the mastoid antrum is of great clinical importance as these are frequent sites of infection.
2. Middle ear infection is referred to as ***otitis media***.
   a. It is usually caused by extension of infection from the pharynx through the auditory tube.
   b. Such infections are more frequent in children as the tube is relatively wide in them.

c. Infection in the middle ear can spread to the mastoid antrum and the mastoid air cells. This makes eradication of the infection much more difficult.

d. Middle ear infection can also lead to perforation of the tympanic membrane. The pus then flows out of the external acoustic meatus.

e. As the middle ear is closely related to the sigmoid sinus and the bulb of the internal jugular vein infection can spread to them. Through the sigmoid sinus infection can reach the temporal lobe of the brain.

3. Disease of the middle ear, of the ossicles, of the internal ear, and of the vestibulocochlear nerve can lead to deafness.
4. Viral infection of the labyrinth can lead ***labyrinthitis***. There is giddiness and difficulty in maintaining the balance of the body. Similar symptoms can be produced by degeneration in old age but they are much milder.

# 45 CHAPTER

# Oral Cavity, Nasal Cavity, Pharynx, Larynx, Trachea and Oesophagus

## THE ORAL CAVITY AND SOME RELATED STRUCTURES

In this section we will consider:

1. The oral cavity
2. The palate
3. The teeth.

The tongue and salivary glands which are closely related to the oral cavity have been described in chapters 37 and 39.

## THE ORAL CAVITY

1. The lay person uses the word 'mouth' loosely both for the external opening and for the cavity it leads to.
2. Strictly speaking, the term mouth should be applied only to the external opening which is also called the ***oral fissure.***
3. The cavity (containing the tongue and teeth) is the mouth cavity or ***oral cavity***.
4. A basic idea of the boundaries of the oral cavity can be had from 45.1 which is a coronal section through it.
   a. Laterally the oral cavity is bounded by the cheeks.
   b. Above by the palate (which separates it from the nasal cavity).
   c. Below, it has a floor to which the tongue is attached.
5. Projecting into the cavity from above and below, just medial to the each cheek, there are the alveolar processes of the upper and lower jaws which bear the teeth.
6. When the mouth is closed bringing the upper and lower teeth into apposition, the oral cavity is seen to consist of:
   a. A part between the teeth of the two sides (the ***oral cavity proper***)
   b. A part between the alveolar processes and the cheeks. The latter is called the ***vestibule***.
7. In 45.1 the vestibule is seen in two halves right and left.
   a. When traced anteriorly, the two halves become continuous in the middle line in front of the teeth.
   b. Here, the vestibule communicates with the exterior; and its external walls are formed by the upper and lower lips.
   c. When the teeth are in apposition, the vestibule communicates with the oral cavity proper through a space behind the last tooth. (This is a point of practical importance. It means that any liquid put into the vestibule will find its way into the mouth even if the jaws are kept closed).
8. With the exception of the teeth all structures in the oral cavity are covered by mucous membrane. The mucous membrane over the alveolar processes of the jaws is firmly attached to underlying bone and is referred to as the ***gum***.
9. The oral cavity proper communicates posteriorly with the oral part of the pharynx. The communication between the two is called the ***oropharyngeal isthmus*** (45.2).

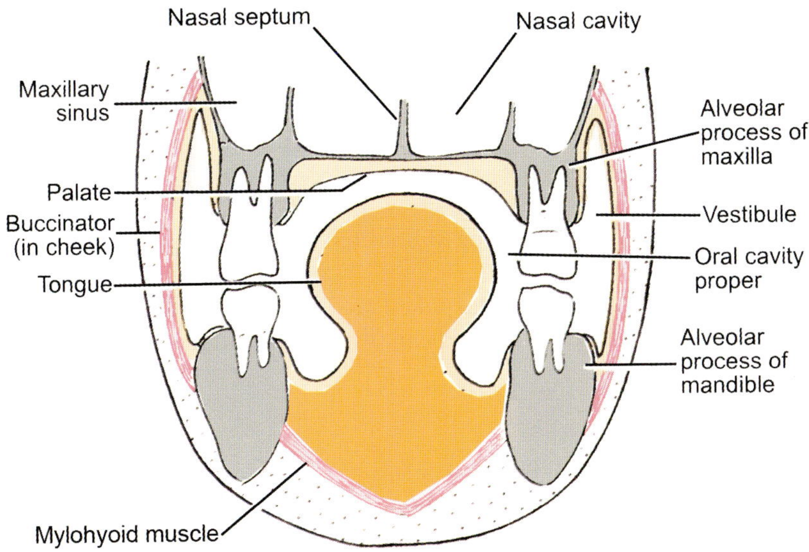


**45.1:** Schematic coronal section through the oral cavity

10. The roof of the cavity is formed by the palate (described below).
11. The chief structure in the floor is the tongue. The rest of the floor is formed by mucous membrane passing from the sides of the tongue to the gum.
    a. The anterior part of the tongue is not attached to the floor and that is why it can be protruded out of the mouth.
    b. This part of the tongue is attached to the floor by a median fold of mucosa called the ***frenulum linguae***.
12. Three pairs of salivary glands are present near the oral cavity and pour their secretions into it. These are:
    a. The parotid glands
    b. The submandibular glands
    c. The sublingual glands.

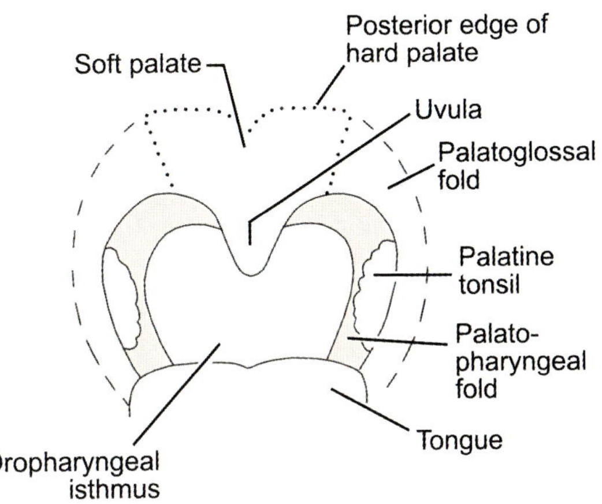


**45.2:** Soft palate as seen through the mouth. The dotted line indicates its upper and lateral limits

13. The secretions of the parotid glands are poured into the mouth through the right and left parotid ducts which open into the corresponding half of the vestibule, on the inner side of the cheek, opposite the crown of the second upper molar tooth.
14. The duct for each submandibular gland opens on the ***sublingual papilla*** located just lateral to the frenulum linguae (39.11).
15. The sublingual glands lie just below the mucosa on the floor of the mouth. Each gland raises a ridge of mucosa which starts at the sublingual papilla and runs laterally and backwards. This ridge is called the ***sublingual fold*** (39.11).
16. ***Lymphatics*** from the floor of the mouth, gums and teeth drain to submandibular nodes and submental nodes and from them to deep cervical lymph nodes.

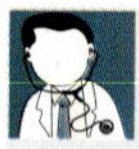

## CLINICAL CORRELATION

### Mouth

1. The mouth is always examined as part of a general physical examination. Hence, a doctor must be aware of common conditions affecting the region.
2. The lips are blue in cyanosis.
3. Inflammation at the angles of the mouth (angular stomatitis) occurs in some vitamin deficiencies.
4. See harelip page 760 (chapter 37).
5. Conditions affecting the teeth and gums, and the palate are considered later in this chapter.
6. Conditions affecting the tongue and salivary glands are given in chapter 37 and 39.

## THE PALATE

1. The palate separates the oral cavity from the nasal cavity.
2. It is divisible into an anterior, larger, part the ***hard palate***, and a posterior part the ***soft palate***.
3. The hard palate has a skeletal basis formed by the palatal processes of the right and left maxillae, and the horizontal plates of the palatine bones. This bony basis is covered by periosteum.
4. The lower surface of the palate is lined by mucous membrane of the mouth and its upper surface by mucous membrane of the nasal cavity.
5. The soft palate is shown as seen from the front (i.e., through the mouth) in 45.2. It is shown in median section in 45.7.
   a. The soft palate is attached to the posterior margin of the hard palate. In its normal relaxed position it has one surface directed upwards and backwards, and another surface directed forwards and downwards (45.7).
   b. Its median part is prolonged downwards as a conical projection called the ***uvula*** (45.2).
   c. The lateral margins of the palate are continuous with two folds of mucous membrane.
   d. The anterior of these connects the palate to the lateral margin of the posterior part of the tongue and is called the ***palatoglossal fold.***
   e. The posterior fold connects the palate to the wall of the pharynx and is called the ***palatopharyngeal fold***. (Also see 39.10).
6. The soft palate consists of two layers of mucous membrane (continuous with those lining the upper and lower surfaces of the hard palate). Between these layers of mucosa there is a fibrous basis called the ***palatine aponeurosis*** (see below). Several muscles are present in the soft palate.

## MUSCLES OF THE SOFT PALATE

These are:

1. The tensor palati
2. The levator palati
3. The musculus uvulae
4. The palatoglossus
5. The palatopharyngeus (45.3).

The attachments and layout of these muscles is complicated and details will not be described. Note the following.

## WANT TO KNOW MORE?

1. The ***tensor palati*** arises from the base of the skull (45.3). It descends and ends in a tendon which winds round the pterygoid hamulus and expands into a wide fibrous band called the ***palatine aponeurosis***. The palatine aponeurosis forms the fibrous basis of the soft palate and gives attachment to other muscles of the palate.

2. The ***levator palati*** also arises in relation to the base of the skull (45.3). It is inserted into the upper surface of the palatine aponeurosis near the uvula.
3. The ***musculus uvulae*** is attached to the posterior edge of the hard palate near the middle line. Its fibres run backwards (on either side of the middle line) through the palatine aponeurosis (45.3). They gain insertion into the mucous membrane of the uvula.
4. The ***palatopharyngeus*** arises from the palatine aponeurosis and descends to the wall of the pharynx.
5. The ***palatoglossus*** arises from the palatine aponeurosis. It passes downwards to reach the side of the tongue (45.3). The muscle lies within the palatoglossal fold (39.10 and 45.2).

### Nerve Supply of Muscles of the Palate

1. All muscles of the palate, except the tensor palati, are supplied by the cranial part of the accessory nerve through the pharyngeal branch of the vagus.
2. The tensor palati is supplied by the mandibular nerve.

### Actions of Palatine Muscle

1. The palatine muscles are responsible for movements of the palate associated with deglutition and with speech.
2. The levator palati helps to close the pharyngeal isthmus (communication between nasopharynx and oropharynx) by elevating the palate and bringing it into contact with the posterior wall of the pharynx.
3. In this action it is helped by the ***palatopharyngeal sphincter*** that produces a ridge on the pharyngeal wall that comes in contact with the palate.
4. The tensor palati helps in deglutition by pressing the bolus between the palate and the tongue.
5. The palatopharyngeus helps in deglutition by pulling the pharynx up thus shortening its length. The palatoglossus closes the oropharyngeal isthmus.

### Nerve Supply, Blood Supply and Lymphatics of the Palate

1. The palate is supplied by the greater palatine branch of the maxillary artery, the ascending palatine branch of the facial artery, and by the palatine branch of the ascending pharyngeal artery.
2. The veins from the palate end in the pterygoid and tonsilar plexuses.
3. The lymph vessels drain into the deep cervical lymph nodes.
4. The nerves supplying the palate are the greater and lesser palatine nerves and the nasopalatine nerves.
5. ***Lymphatics*** from the palate drain into retropharyngeal and deep cervical nodes.

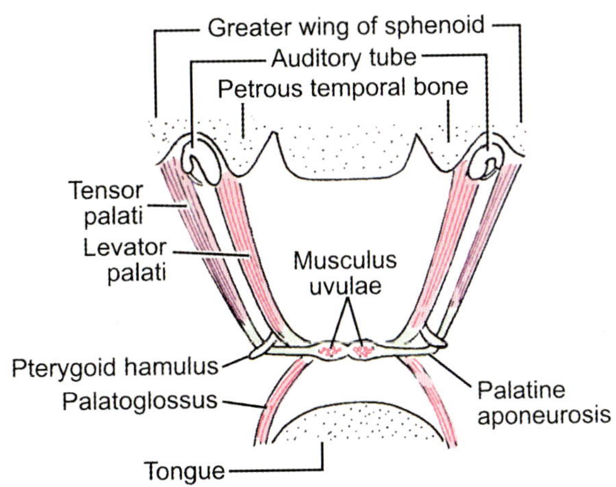


**45.3:** Schematic coronal section through palate to show arrangement of muscles

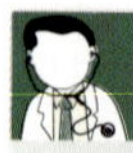

**CLINICAL CORRELATION**

**Harelip and Cleft Palate**

1. Embryologically, both the upper lip and the palate are derived from three elements. These are:
   a. The right and left maxillary processes
   b. The frontonasal process which is a median structure.

***Harelip***

Harelip is not an anomaly of the palate but of the lip. It is given here because both harelip and cleft palate have a common basis.

1. The frontonasal process forms the median part of the upper lip. This part is called the ***philtrum***.
2. On each side the frontonasal process fuses with the corresponding maxillary process.
   a. Abnormalities in fusion of these processes lead to clefts in the upper lip (called hare lip because the hare normally has an upper lip with a cleft).
   b. The defect may be unilateral or bilateral.
   c. When defect in fusion is minimal only a small indentation may be seen in the margin of the lip.
   d. When non-union is complete the defect extends into the nostril, and is continuous with a defect in the palate as described below.

***Cleft Palate***

1. As stated above the palate is derived from the frontonasal process and the right and left maxillary processes.
2. The frontonasal process forms the part of the palate that bears the incisor teeth. This part of the palate is also called the ***premaxilla***.
3. The rest of the palate is formed by shelf-like projections of the right and left maxillary process.
   a. These processes grow towards the midline.
   b. Anteriorly, each maxillary process fuses with the corresponding edge of the premaxilla.
   c. Behind the level of the premaxilla the two maxillary processes fuse with each other.
   d. From the manner of fusion it will be clear that the line of union of the three elements forming the palate is Y-shaped.
4. Defects in the process of union lead to the formation of different varieties of cleft palate as follows. Remember that fusion of components of the palate starts anteriorly and proceeds posteriorly.
   a. Complete non-union gives rise to a Y-shaped cleft. Anteriorly the limbs of the 'Y' become continuous with clefts in the upper lip (i.e., bilateral harelip is also present).
   b. The premaxilla may fuse with the maxillary process on one side, but not on the other side. At the same time the two maxillary processes do not fuse with each other. This results in a defect that is oblique anteriorly and median posteriorly. It will be associated with a unilateral harelip.
   c. Both the maxillary processes fuse with the premaxilla but their fusion to each other is deficient. This can give rise to median defects of varying extent. The cleft may involve both the hard palate and the soft palate, may be confined to the soft palate, or may be represented only by a cleft in the uvula.
5. It has been said above that fusion of the elements forming the palate begins anteriorly and progresses backwards. This statement does not apply to the upper lip. A harelip can exist without there being any cleft in the palate.

## THE TEETH

1. As the teeth can be seen and felt some facts about them are commonly known.
   a. We know that the newborn have no teeth
   b. That the first tooth appears when the infant is about six months old
   c. That the teeth in young children gradually fall off and are replaced by new ones that can last throughout life.

2. The teeth that appear in children and fall off with time are called ***deciduous*** (or milk) teeth.
3. The teeth of the second set that gradually replace the deciduous teeth constitute the ***permanent*** teeth.
4. The teeth, both deciduous and permanent, have varying shapes.
   a. Some have sharp cutting edges and are, therefore, called ***incisors***.
   b. Others are sharp and pointed: These are called ***canines*** as they form the most prominent teeth in canine species (e.g., dogs).
   c. Still others have edges suitable for a grinding function: These are called ***molars***.
   d. In the permanent set we also have grinding teeth that are somewhat smaller than the molars and are called the ***premolars*** (as they lie in front of the molars).
5. A set of deciduous teeth consists of the following. Beginning from the middle line (in front) there is:
   a. A central incisor
   b. A lateral incisor (i.e., two incisors)
   c. One canine
   d. Two molars (distinguished from each other by being called the first and second molars).

   There are, thus, five teeth in each half of each jaw i.e., twenty in all.
6. A set of permanent teeth consists of the following. Beginning from the middle line there is:
   a. A central incisor
   b. A lateral incisor
   c. A canine
   d. Two premolars (first and second, that replace the deciduous molars)
   e. Three molars (first, second and third).

   Thus, in each half of each jaw there are eight teeth, or thirty two in all.

## WANT TO KNOW MORE?

7. There is considerable variation in the ages at which the various teeth erupt. The following scheme gives the approximate ages of appearance in a form easy to remember.

   *Deciduous teeth*

   | | | |
   |---|---|---|
   | Central incisor | = | 6 months |
   | Lateral incisor | = (+ 2) | 8 months |
   | First molar | = (+ 4) | 12 months |
   | Canine | = (+ 4) | 16 months |
   | Second molar | = (+ 4) | 20 months |

   Note that the first deciduous molar appears before the canine.

   *Permanent teeth*

   | | | |
   |---|---|---|
   | First molar | = | 6 years |
   | Central incisor | = (+ 1) | 7 years |
   | Lateral incisor | = (+ 1) | 8 years |
   | Canine | = (+ 1) | 9 years |
   | Premolars | = (+ 1) | 10 years |
   | Second molar | = (+ 1) | 11 years |
   | Third molar | = | 17 years + |

   a. Note that the first permanent tooth to appear is the first molar. Approximately, one tooth appears every year from the 6th to 11th years.
   b. The third molar teeth appear at the age of 17 years or later and are, therefore, called the ***wisdom teeth***. Not infrequently one or more third molars may fail to erupt.

## Structure of a Typical Tooth

1. A tooth consists of an upper part, the ***crown***, which is seen in the mouth; and of one or more ***roots*** which are embedded in sockets in the jaw bone (mandible or maxilla). Vertical section through a typical tooth is shown in 45.4.
2. The greater part of the tooth is formed by a bone-like material called ***dentine***.
3. In the region of the crown the dentine is covered by a much harder white material called the ***enamel***.
4. Over the root the dentine is covered by a thin layer of ***cement***.
5. The cement is united to the wall of the bony socket in the jaw through a layer of fibrous tissue called the ***periodontal ligament***.
6. The external surface of the alveolar process is covered by the gum which normally overlaps the lower edge of the crown.
7. Within the dentine there is a ***pulp canal*** which contains a mass of cells, blood vessels and nerves which constitute the pulp.
8. The blood vessels and nerves enter the pulp canal at the apex of the root through an ***apical foramen***.

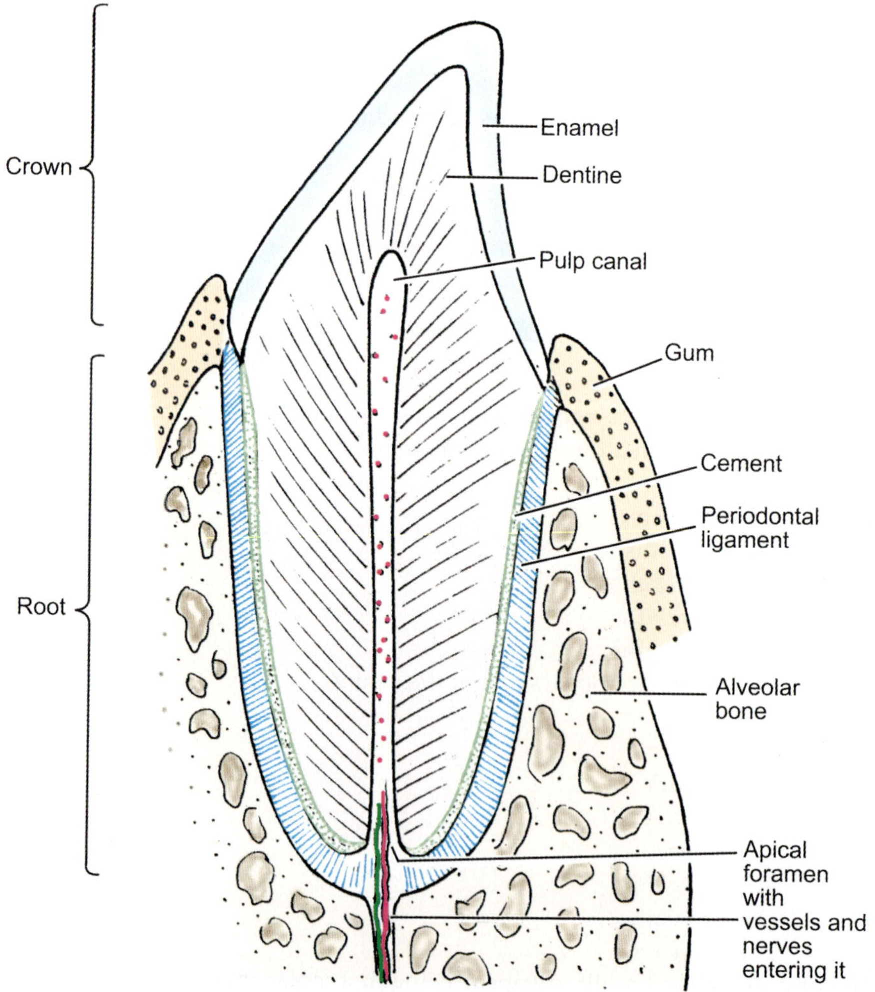


**45.4:** Vertical section through a typical tooth

## WANT TO KNOW MORE?

### Differences in Structure of Different Teeth

Details of the anatomy of individual teeth are beyond the scope of this book. The following information is, however, sufficient for medical students.

1. In describing teeth, the dentist uses certain terms that the medical student should be familiar with.
   a. As the teeth are arranged in an arch, terms like anterior, posterior, medial or lateral are confusing.
   b. The surface of the tooth facing the lip or cheek is the ***buccal*** (or ***labial***) surface
   c. The surface towards the tongue is the ***lingual*** (or ***palatal***) surface.
   d. The surface nearest to the middle line is the ***mesial*** surface: This term corresponds to 'medial' in case of the anterior teeth, and to 'anterior' for the posterior teeth.
   e. The surface opposite to the mesial surface is called the ***distal*** surface.
   f. The upper surfaces of the lower teeth, and the lower surfaces of the upper teeth are referred to as the ***occlusal*** surfaces.
2. In the case of the incisors the occlusal surface forms a sharp cutting edge. In the canines it is pointed. In the molars and premolars the occlusal surface bears rounded elevations or ***cusps***. Typically there are two cusps on each premolar and four or five in each molar.
3. The incisors and canines have one root each. The premolars may have one or two roots. The molars have two or three roots, but the last molar may have only one.
4. The meeting of the upper and lower teeth is called ***occlusion***.
   a. In the relaxed mouth the upper and lower teeth are a short distance apart.
   b. In proper occlusion there is minimal space between the upper and lower teeth, the cusps of one set fitting into the depressions on the occlusal surface of the other set.
   c. The upper incisors lie slightly in front of the lower.

### Blood Supply and Nerve Supply of Teeth

1. The lower teeth are supplied by:
   a. Branches from the inferior alveolar artery (branch of maxillary artery)
   b. The inferior alveolar nerve (branch of mandibular nerve, 43.48).
2. The upper teeth are supplied by:
   a. The anterior and posterior superior alveolar branches of the maxillary artery
   b. The anterior, middle and posterior superior alveolar nerves (branches of the maxillary nerve and its infraorbital continuation).

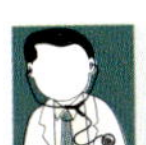

## CLINICAL CORRELATION

### Teeth and Gums

1. The number of teeth present should be compared with the age of the patient.
2. The ages at which various teeth erupt have been described above. Delayed eruption may be a sign of malnutrition or some other growth disorder.
3. In older people who have lost some teeth the absence of sufficient teeth for mastication may result in digestive disorders.
4. Peg shaped upper central incisors (***Hutchinson's teeth***) may be an indication of syphilis. In this condition the teeth may show notches.
5. Notching may also be present in rickets.
6. In acromegaly the lower jaw becomes relatively larger than the upper jaw so that the teeth go out of alignment.
7. Gums are often the site of chronic inflammation specially in persons with poor oral hygiene.

8. Inflammation of gums is called ***gingivitis***.
   a. The gums may be inflamed and bleed easily.
   b. Pockets may form and pus may be present in them (***pyorrhea***). Infection in the gums can lead to digestive and respiratory problems.
9. A blue line running along the edge of the gum may be a sign of lead poisoning.
10. The gums are swollen and spongy and bleed easily in scurvy which is caused by a deficiency of vitamin C.
11. ***Dental caries*** is a very common disease of the teeth.
   a. Microorganisms produce small cavities that gradually enlarge.
   b. The patient is usually unaware of them until the cavity invades the dentine when the teeth become sensitive to hot and cold, or to sugar.
   c. If untreated the cavity ultimately reaches the pulp of the tooth resulting in severe pain.
   d. Dental caries can be prevented by teaching children to brush their teeth after meals.
   e. Prevention can also be ensured by regular check up by a dentist. If cavities are discovered early they can be filled up and the tooth can be saved.
   f. Caries is common in milk teeth and is ignored on the assumption that these teeth are going to be replaced. However, caries can result in too early loss of milk teeth and this can result in abnormal eruption of permanent teeth.

**Medicolegal Importance of Teeth**

Being very hard, teeth are preserved for a very long time after death. They can be very useful in identifying a dead person specially if a dentist's record of the state of the teeth is available.

## THE NASAL CAVITIES AND PARANASAL SINUSES

### Preliminary Remarks

1. The nasal cavity is divided by a median septum into right and left halves.
2. Each half of the nasal cavity opens to the exterior through the ***external*** (or anterior) ***nares***, and posteriorly it opens into the nasopharynx.
3. A schematic coronal section through the nasal cavity is shown in 45.6. It is seen that each half of the cavity is triangular.
   a. It has a vertical medial wall formed by the nasal septum
   b. A sloping lateral wall
   c. A relatively broad floor formed by the palate (which separates it from the oral cavity)
   d. A narrow roof which lies at the junction of the medial and lateral walls.
4. These walls have a skeletal basis that is made up predominantly of bone, but is cartilaginous at some places.
5. The skeletal basis is covered (over most of the nasal cavity) by mucous membrane.
   a. Typically the mucosa is moist and highly vascular. It serves to warm inspired air and also helps to remove dust (which sticks to the moist wall). For these reasons the mucosa is referred to as ***respiratory***.
   b. The mucosa lining the uppermost part of the septum, and the adjoining part of the lateral wall, differs from that present elsewhere in the nasal cavity. It is characterised by the presence of receptor cells that are sensitive to smell: The mucosa in this region is, therefore, called the ***olfactory mucosa.***
   c. Olfactory nerves arise from olfactory mucosa.
6. A small area of the nasal cavity (near the anterior nares) is lined not by mucous membrane, but by skin. This skin bears hair that serve to trap dust present in inspired air.

### Medial Wall of Nasal Cavity: Nasal Septum

1. The skeletal basis of the medial wall of the nasal cavity (formed by the nasal septum) is shown in 45.5. It is formed mainly by:

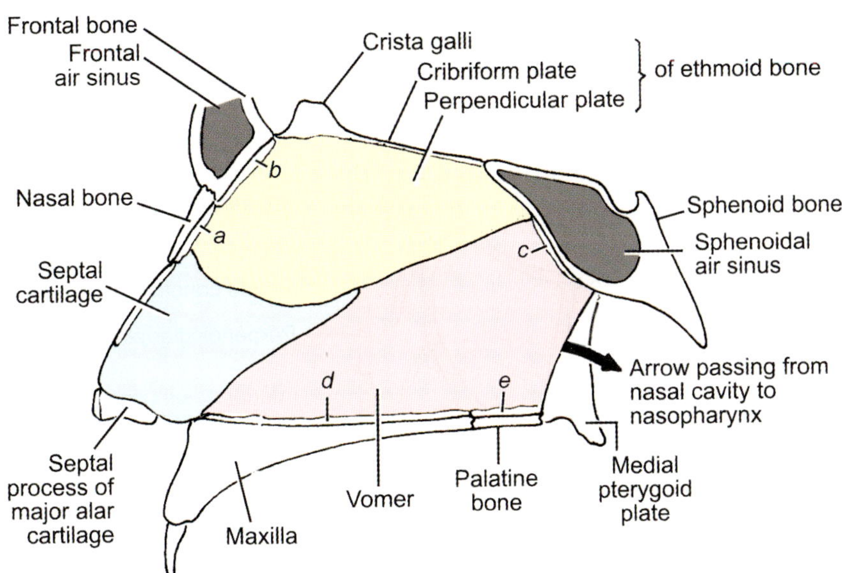


**45.5:** Skeletal basis of the nasal septum

   a. The perpendicular plate of the ethmoid bone (posterosuperior part)
   b. The vomer (posteroinferior part)
   c. The septal cartilage (anterior part).
2. Around the edges of the septum there are small contributions from the nasal, frontal, sphenoid, maxillary and palatine bones ('a' to 'e' in 45.5).
3. As a point of practical importance it may be remembered that the septum is fairly often deflected to one side so that one-half of the nasal cavity may be larger than the other.

## Lateral Wall of Nasal Cavity

1. The bones taking part are (45.6):
   a. The maxilla (medial surface)
   b. The ethmoid bone
   c. The palatine bone
   d. The inferior nasal concha
   e. The lacrimal bone.
2. Note that the lateral wall of the external nose also forms the anterior part of the lateral wall of the nasal cavity. Some cartilages appear in this part of the lateral wall of the nasal cavity.
3. The lateral wall of the nasal cavity as seen with the mucous membrane intact is shown in 45.7. The following points may be noted.
4. There are three anteroposterior elevations on the lateral wall. These are the superior, middle and inferior nasal *conchae.*
   a. Each concha has a core of bone covered by mucous membrane.
   b. The bony core of the superior and middle conchae is formed by parts of the ethmoid bone, while that of the inferior concha is independent (45.6).
   c. Each concha has an upper border attached to the rest of the lateral wall and a free lower margin.
5. The spaces deep to the superior, middle and inferior conchae are called the superior, middle and inferior *meatuses* respectively ('2', '3', '4' in 45.6).

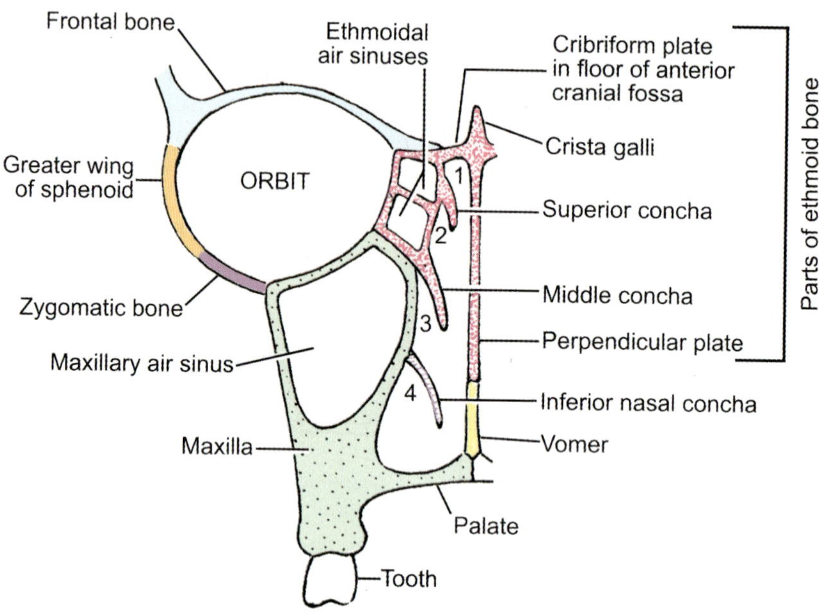


**45.6:** Lateral wall of the nasal cavity with the mucous membrane intact

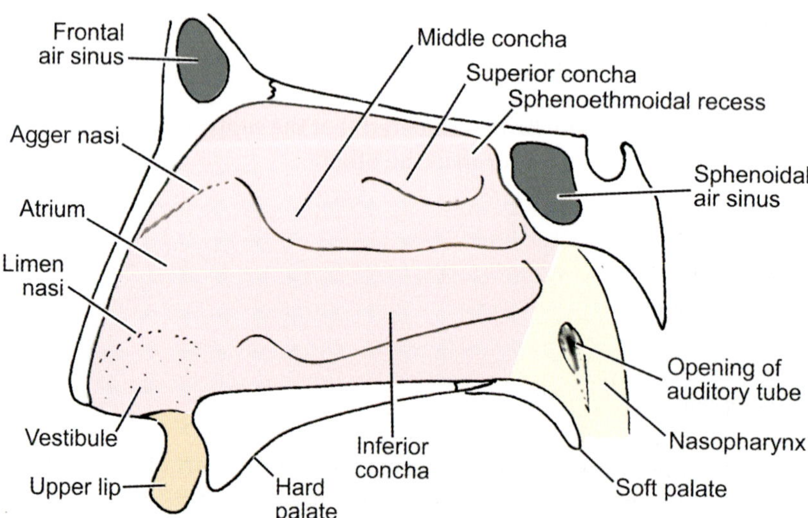


**45.7:** Schematic coronal section through the nasal cavity to show some bones forming its walls. The orbit is also shown

6. There is a triangular space above the superior concha ('1' in 45.6). This is the ***sphenoethmoidal recess*** (also see 45.7).
7. Occasionally, an additional concha (called the highest nasal concha) may be present on the lateral wall of the sphenoethmoidal recess.

8. The part of the nasal cavity just above the anterior nares is called the ***vestibule.***
   a. The vestibule is lined by skin.
   b. At the upper limit of the vestibule (where skin meets mucous membrane) there is a curved elevation called the ***limen nasi*** (45.7).
   c. Above the limen nasi there is a depression called the ***atrium.***
   d. The upper limit of the atrium is marked by another curved ridge called the ***aggar nasi.***
9. Some structures in the lateral wall of the nose can be seen only when the conchae are cut away (45.8).
   a. In the middle meatus we see a rounded elevation called the ***bulla ethmoidalis.***
   b. Below and in front of the bulla there is a curved groove called the ***hiatus semilunaris***. The lower curved margin of the hiatus is sharp: it is produced by a process of the ethmoid bone called the uncinate process.
   c. The anterior end of the hiatus is continuous with a depression called the ***ethmoidal infundibulum.***
   d. The upper end of the infundibulum is usually continuous with the ***frontonasal duct*** which connects the frontal sinus to the nasal cavity.
10. There are a number of openings in the meatuses of the nose (45.8A and B). They are described in connection with paranasal sinuses below.
11. The presence of conchae in the lateral wall of the nasal cavity greatly increases the surface area of the nasal mucosa. This factor combined with the presence of a highly vascular and moist mucous membrane enables the nose to effectively warm inspired air and to make it moist.

## Roof of Nasal Cavity

1. We have already seen that the roof of the nasal cavity lies at the junction of the medial and lateral walls (45.6).
2. From 45.5, it will be seen that when traced anteroposteriorly, the roof is divisible into three parts:
   a. The middle part is formed by the mucous membrane covering the ethmoid bone and is almost horizontal.
   b. The anterior part slopes downwards and forwards. It is formed by the mucous membrane covering the frontal bone above, and the nasal bone below.
   c. The posterior part slopes downwards and backwards. It is formed by the mucous membrane covering the sphenoid bone.

## Floor of Nasal Cavity

1. The floor of the nasal cavity is formed by the mucous membrane covering the upper surface of the hard palate.
2. Each half of the hard palate is formed (45.5):
   a. In its anterior three-fourths by the maxilla (palatine process)
   b. In its posterior one-fourth by the palatine bone (horizontal plate).

## WANT TO KNOW MORE?

### Blood Supply of the Nasal Cavity

1. The chief artery to the mucous membrane of the nose is the sphenopalatine branch of the maxillary artery.
   a. It gives off posterolateral nasal branches to the lateral wall of the nose
   b. Posterior septal branches to the septum.
2. Smaller arteries helping in the supply are:
   a. The anterior and posterior ethmoidal branches (of the ophthalmic artery)
   b. The terminal part of the greater palatine artery
   c. Twigs from the superior labial branch of the facial artery.
3. The veins accompany the arteries.
4. For *lymphatic drainage* of the nasal cavity see 45.8B.

### Nerve Supply of the Nasal Cavity

The nerves innervating the nasal mucosal are as follows:

1. The olfactory mucosa is innervated by the olfactory nerves.
2. The posterior three-fourths of the cavity (including lateral wall, septum, roof and floor) are supplied by:
   a. The lateral and medial posterior superior nasal branches (including the nasopalatine nerve) that arise directly from the pterygopalatine ganglion.
   b. The posterior inferior nasal branches of the greater palatine nerves (see 43.39).
3. The upper and anterior part of the cavity is innervated by the anterior ethmoidal branch of the nasociliary nerve.
4. The lower and anterior part of the cavity is supplied by twigs from the anterior superior alveolar nerve (43.40).

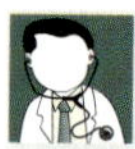

## CLINICAL CORRELATION

### Nasal Cavity

1. Infection of the nasal cavity is called ***rhinitis***.
2. Infection from the nasal cavity can spread to paranasal sinuses, to the middle ear, to the pharynx and larynx, and even to the anterior cranial fossa (through the roof of the cavity).
3. Rhinitis may be caused by viruses (as in common cold), by bacteria, and by allergy (allergic rhinitis). In allergic rhinitis the nasal mucosa can undergo hypertrophy resulting in chronic blockage.
4. Children often insert foreign bodies into the nose and they can get impacted there.
5. Bleeding from the nose is called ***epistaxis***. In most cases it is caused by rupture of blood vessels on the anterior inferior part of the nasal septum (***Little's area***).
6. The nasal septum is commonly deflected (i.e., it comes to lie to one side of the middle line). This can cause blocking of the nasal cavity on one side and may require surgical correction.
7. In cleft palate, the nasal cavity is in communication with the mouth. Because of leakage of air into the nose during speech the person has a nasal twang.

## THE PARANASAL SINUSES

These are spaces present in the substance of bones related to the nasal cavities. Each sinus opens into the nasal cavity, and is lined by mucous membrane continuous with that of the latter. Because of this communication each sinus is normally filled with air.

### Frontal Sinuses

1. The right and left frontal sinuses are present in the part of the frontal bone deep to the superciliary arches. Each sinus lies deep to a triangular area the angles of which lie:
   a. At the nasion
   b. At a point about 3 cm above the nasion
   c. At a point on the supraorbital margin at the junction of the medial one-third with the lateral two-thirds.
2. The cavity of the frontal sinus extends for some distance into the orbital plate of the frontal bone between the roof of the orbit and the floor of the anterior cranial fossa.
3. Each frontal sinus usually opens into the middle meatus through the frontonasal duct. This duct is usually continuous, below, with a funnel-like space the ethmoidal infundibulum (45.8A) that is continuous with the upper end of the hiatus semilunaris.

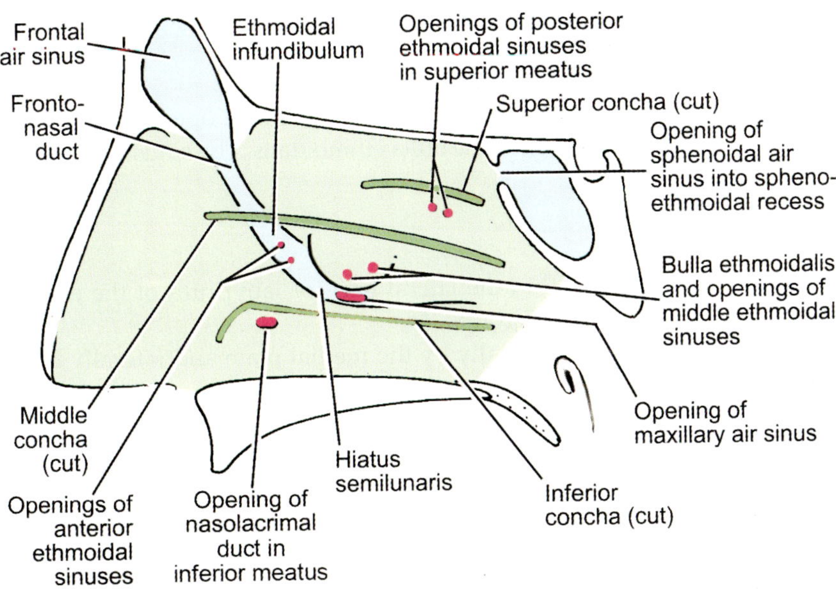


**45.8A:** Lateral wall of the nasal cavity after removing the conchae to reveal structures deep to them

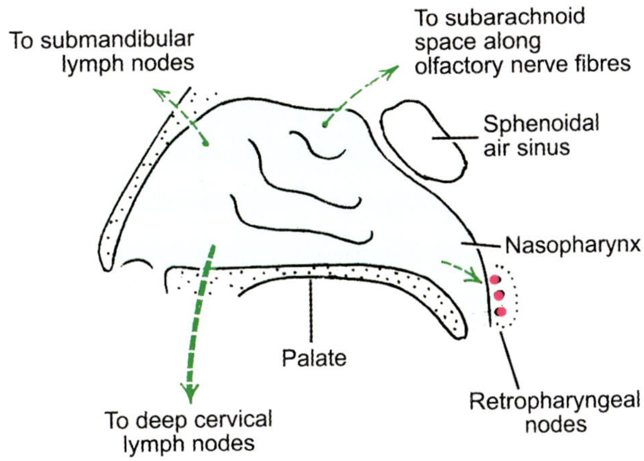


**45.8B:** Scheme to show the lymphatic drainage of the nasal cavity

## Sphenoidal Sinuses

1. The right and left sphenoidal sinuses are present in the body of the sphenoid bone.
2. Each sinus opens into the corresponding half of the nasal cavity through an aperture on the anterior aspect of the body of the sphenoid.
3. The part of the nasal cavity into which the sinus opens lies above the superior nasal concha and is called ***sphenoethmoidal recess*** (45.8B).

### Maxillary Sinuses

1. Each maxillary sinus lies within the maxilla.
2. On the medial aspect of this bone there is a large maxillary hiatus.
3. The sinus usually opens into middle meatus of the nasal cavity by an opening in the lower part of the hiatus semilunaris (45.8A). The opening lies just below the bulla ethmoidalis. The sinus may have an additional opening behind the main one.

### Ethmoidal Air Sinuses

1. The ethmoidal air sinuses are located within the lateral part (or labyrinth) of the ethmoid bone. They can be divided into anterior, middle and posterior groups.
2. Each labyrinth (right or left) is bounded medially by the medial plate and laterally by the orbital plate of the ethmoid bone. The ethmoidal air sinuses lie between these plates. They are seen in coronal section in 45.6 in which their close relationship to the orbit can be appreciated.
3. The walls of some of the ethmoidal sinuses are incomplete. In the intact skull they are completed by parts of the frontal, maxillary, lacrimal, sphenoidal and palatine bones.
4. The anterior ethmoidal sinuses open into the ethmoidal infundibulum, or into the upper part of the hiatus semilunaris.
5. The middle ethmoidal sinuses open on or near the bulla ethmoidalis.
6. The posterior ethmoidal sinuses open into the superior meatus.

### Other Openings in the Nasal Cavity

1. In addition to the openings of the paranasal sinuses, the lateral wall of the nose shows the opening of the ***nasolacrimal duct.***
2. This duct conveys lacrimal fluid from the conjunctival sac, via the lacrimal sac.
3. It opens into the anterior part of the inferior meatus (45.8A). The nasolacrimal duct is described in chapter 37.

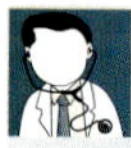

### CLINICAL CORRELATION

**Paranasal Sinuses**

***Sinusitis***

1. Paranasal sinuses are frequently sites of infection (sinusitis). The infection usually reaches them from the nasal cavity.
2. As the sinuses open into the nasal cavity through narrow openings, slight swelling of the mucosa, or presence of thick secretions at the orifice, can block outflow of secretions that accumulate within the sinus.
3. This is one reason why sinusitis so often becomes chronic.
4. This is specially true in the case of the maxillary sinus because the level of the opening of the maxillary air sinus into the nose is placed at a higher level than the floor of the sinus, so that natural drainage is difficult.
5. To facilitate drainage it is sometimes necessary to make an artificial opening into the sinus through the inferior meatus of the nose. The sinus can also be drained through the vestibule of the mouth near the canine tooth.
6. A study of the anatomy of the lateral wall of the nose shows that secretions draining out of the frontal air sinus flow towards the opening into the maxillary sinus. For this reason frontal sinusitis often leads to maxillary sinusitis.
7. Infection in the maxillary sinus can spread to the orbit. (Remember that the plate of bone that forms the roof of the maxillary sinus also forms the floor of the orbit).

***Diagnosis of Sinusitis***

1. Infection in paranasal sinus leads to headache. In addition tenderness can often be elicited by pressure over the sinus.

2. In frontal sinusitis tenderness is felt by upward pressure over the medial part of the superior orbital margin.
3. In maxillary sinusitis there may be tenderness over the cheek below the inferior orbital margin.
4. In ethmoidal sinusitis there can be tenderness over the medial wall of the orbit.
5. Pain originating in the paranasal sinuses may be referred to other sites.
   a. The frontal sinus is supplied by the supraorbital nerve which also supplies the skin of the forehead and anterior part of the scalp. Therefore, frontal headache is almost always present in frontal sinusitis.
   b. In maxillary sinusitis pain may be felt in the upper jaw and teeth.
6. Diagnosis of maxillary sinusitis can be confirmed by transillumination. In a darkened room light (from a torch) is directed towards the wall of the sinus through the mouth or through the cheek. The presence of fluid, rather than air, reduces transmission of light.
7. Radiography is also useful in confirming presence of sinusitis.

## THE PHARYNX

### Preliminary Remarks

1. The pharynx is a median passage that is common to the alimentary and respiratory systems (45.9).
2. It is divisible (from above downwards) into:
   a. A ***nasal part*** (or ***nasopharynx***) into which the nasal cavities open
   b. An ***oral part*** (or ***oropharynx***) which is continuous with the posterior end of the oral cavity
   c. A ***laryngeal part*** (or ***laryngopharynx***) which is continuous in front with the larynx, and below with oesophagus.
3. The communication between the nasopharynx and the oropharynx is called the ***pharyngeal isthmus***.
   a. This isthmus can be closed (e.g., during swallowing) by elevation of the soft palate.

**WANT TO KNOW MORE?**

   b. Closure is helped by contraction of muscle fibres in the pharyngeal wall that constitute the ***palatopharyngeal sphincter***. Contraction of this sphincter produces a ridge (of Passavant) on the posterior pharyngeal wall with which the soft palate comes in contact.

4. The communication between the oral cavity and the pharynx is called the ***oropharyngeal isthmus*** (45.2). It is bounded:
   a. Above by the soft palate
   b. Below by the posterior part of the tongue
   c. On either side by the palatoglossal arches.
5. The oropharyngeal isthmus can be closed by contraction of the palatoglossus muscles. This closure plays an important part in deglutition.
6. The laryngopharynx lies just behind the inlet of the larynx, and behind the posterior wall of the larynx.

**WANT TO KNOW MORE?**

**The Nasal Part of the Pharynx**

1. On each lateral wall of the nasopharynx there is an opening which leads into the auditory tube (45.9).
2. This tube connects the nasopharynx to the middle ear.

3. Above and behind the opening of the auditory tube the wall of the nasopharynx shows a bulging called the ***tubal elevation***. This elevation is produced by the projecting end of a cartilage which forms part of the wall of the auditory tube.
4. A fold of mucous membrane starting at the tubal elevation passes down the pharyngeal wall. This is the ***salpingopharyngeal fold*** and is produced by a muscle called the salpingopharyngeus.
5. Another mucosal fold passes from the tubal elevation to the soft palate. This is the ***salpingopalatine fold***.
6. Behind the tubal elevation the wall of the nasopharynx shows a depression called the ***pharyngeal recess***.
7. The nasopharynx has a roof continuous with the posterior end of the roof of the nasal cavity. The roof and posterior wall of the nasopharynx form a continuous curve that rests on the posterior part of the body of the sphenoid, the basilar part of the occipital bone, and the anterior arch of the atlas.

8. The mucosa of the median part of the roof shows a bulging produced by a mass of lymphoid tissue. This lymphoid tissue constitutes the ***pharyngeal tonsil***. (When enlarged, the pharyngeal tonsils are referred to as ***adenoids***).
9. Some lymphoid tissue is also present behind the opening of the auditory tube. This collection of lymphoid tissue is called the ***tubal tonsil***.

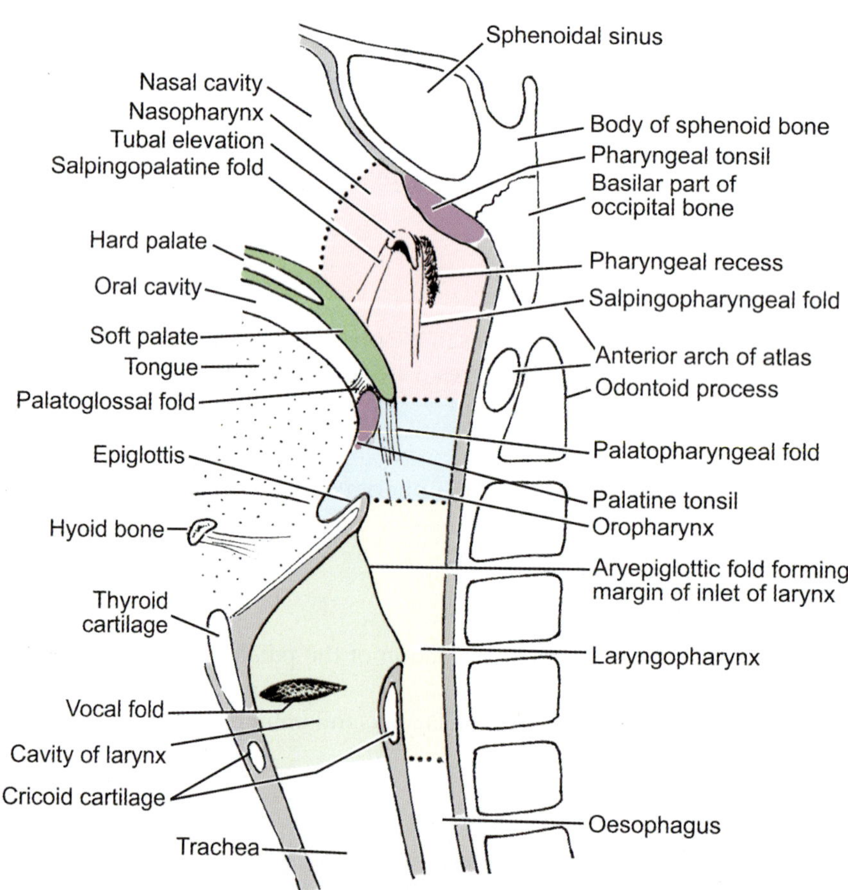


**45.9:** Schematic median section through the pharynx (and neighbouring structures) to show its lateral wall. The limits of the subdivisions of the pharynx are indicated in dotted lines

## The Oral Part of the Pharynx

1. The oropharynx lies in front of the second cervical vertebra and the upper part of the third.
2. The only features to be noted on its lateral walls are the ***palatopharyngeal folds*** (or arches). These stretch from the uvula to the lateral wall of the pharynx and enclose the palatopharyngeus muscle.
3. The palatine tonsil lies between the palatoglossal and palatopharyngeal folds. The depression in which the palatine tonsil lies is called the ***tonsilar sinus***. The palatine tonsil is considered later in this Chapter.

## Laryngeal Part of Pharynx

1. The laryngeal part of the pharynx lies in front of the third to sixth cervical vertebrae. (Its relationships can be properly appreciated after the larynx has been studied. They are given here for sake of completeness).
2. In terms of laryngeal cartilages the upper end of the laryngeal part of the pharynx corresponds to the upper end of the epiglottis; and its lower end lies at the caudal border of the cricoid cartilage. In other words it is coextensive with the larynx.
3. The upper part of the anterior wall is formed by the inlet of the larynx; and below by the posterior surfaces of the arytenoid and cricoid cartilages. Lateral to the inlet of the larynx the mucosa shows a depression called the ***piriform recess*** or fossa.

## Walls of the Pharynx

1. The walls of the pharynx are constituted mainly by muscles. The muscles of the pharynx are considered below.
2. The layer of muscle is covered on the outside by a layer of fascia called the ***buccopharyngeal fascia***. This fascia extends forwards onto the buccinator (and hence its name).
3. Between the mucous membrane and the layer of muscle there is a thicker fascia called the ***pharyngobasilar*** fascia. This fascia is so called because it is thickest in its upper part where it bridges across a gap between the muscle layer of the pharynx and the base of the skull (45.10).

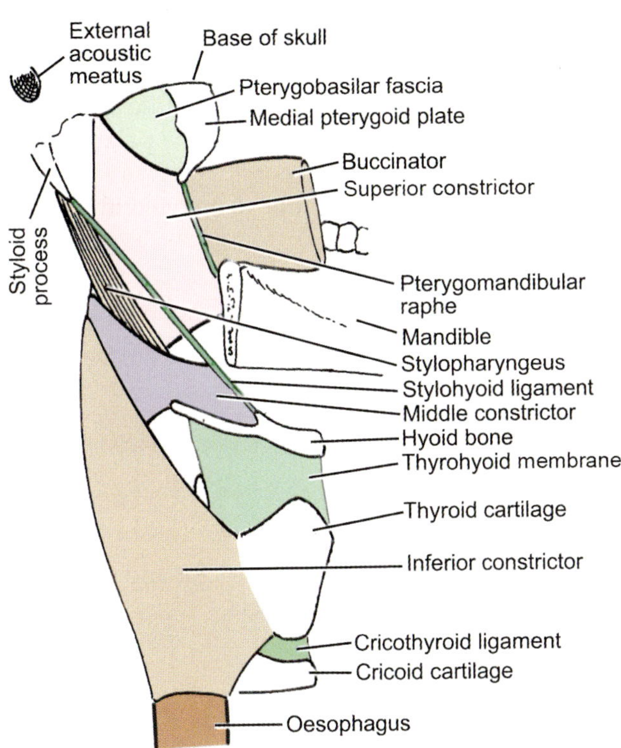


**45.10:** Muscles of the pharynx seen from the lateral side

## MUSCLES OF THE PHARYNX

The muscular basis of the wall of the pharynx is formed by the following muscles:

### Constrictors of the Pharynx

There are three pairs of constrictors:

1. Superior constrictor
2. Middle constrictor
3. Inferior constrictor.
   a. The origins of the constrictors are situated anteriorly in relation to the posterior openings of the nose, mouth and larynx (from above downwards).
   b. From here their fibres pass into the lateral and posterior walls of the pharynx, the fibres of the two sides meeting posteriorly, in the middle line in a fibrous raphe.
   c. The three constrictors are so arranged that the inferior overlaps the middle, which in turn, overlaps the superior.
   d. The fibres of the superior constrictor reach the base of the skull posteriorly, in the middle line.
   e. On the sides, however, there is a gap between the base of the skull and the upper edge of the superior constrictor. This gap is filled by the upper part of the pharyngobasilar fascia that is thickened in this situation.
   f. The lower edge of the inferior constrictor becomes continuous with the circular muscle of the oesophagus.

   The attachments of individual constrictors are complex and will not be considered. Some details can be seen in 45.10.

### Longitudinal Muscles

1. In addition to the constrictors, the pharynx has three muscles the fibres of which run longitudinally. These are:
   a. The stylopharyngeus
   b. The palatopharyngeus
   c. The salpingopharyngeus.
2. The ***stylopharyngeus*** arises from the styloid process. It passes through the gap between the superior and middle constrictors to run downwards on the inner surface of the middle and inferior constrictors.
3. The fibres of the ***palatopharyngeus*** descend from the sides of the palate and run longitudinally on the inner aspect of the constrictors.
4. The ***salpingopharyngeus*** descends from the auditory tube to merge with the palatopharyngeus.

### Insertion of Constrictors of Pharynx

1. All the constrictors of the pharynx are inserted into a median raphe on the posterior wall of the pharynx. The upper end of the raphe reaches the base of the skull where it is attached to the pharyngeal tubercle on the basilar part of the occipital bone.

**WANT TO KNOW MORE?**

2. There is a gap between the upper edge of the superior constrictor and the base of the skull. It gives passage to the auditory tube and is closed by the pharyngobasilar fascia.

### Actions of Muscles of the Pharynx

1. The muscles of the pharynx play an important part in deglutition.

## WANT TO KNOW MORE?

2. Food entering the oropharynx is carried downwards by successive contraction of the superior, middle and inferior constrictors.
3. The stylopharyngeus, salpingopharyngeus and the palatopharyngeus help by pulling the pharynx upwards and by shortening it.
4. The inferior constrictor is divided into two parts:
   a. The cricopharyngeal part
   b. Thyropharyngeal part.
5. It is often held that the cricopharyngeal part is 'sphincteric' in contrast to the thyropharyngeal part which is 'propulsive'. Incoordination in the action of the two parts may result in the formation of a diverticulum on the posterior wall of the pharynx at the junction of the two parts (see further below).
6. The inner surface of the superior constrictor is lined by a band of muscle fibres arising from the sides of the palate. These fibres form the ***palatopharyngeal sphincter*** which produces a ridge (of Passavant) on the pharyngeal wall at the junction of nasopharynx with the oropharynx. Acting along with the soft palate the palatopharyngeal sphincter closes the pharyngeal isthmus preventing food from entering the nasopharynx.

### Nerve Supply of Muscles of Pharynx

1. The constrictors of the pharynx, and the salpingopharyngeus are supplied by the pharyngeal branch of the vagus, through the pharyngeal plexus (also see below).
2. The stylopharyngeus is supplied by the glossopharyngeal nerve.
3. The palatopharyngeus is supplied by the cranial part of the accessory nerve.

### Blood Vessels, Lymphatics and Nerves of Pharynx

1. The pharynx receives numerous small branches which arise from the ascending pharyngeal, lingual, facial and maxillary arteries.
2. The veins drain into a plexus which surrounds the pharynx and drains into the internal jugular and facial veins.
3. The ***lymph vessels*** of the pharynx drain into the deep cervical lymph nodes. Some of the lymph passes through the retropharyngeal nodes.
4. The nerve supply of the pharynx is through the ***pharyngeal plexus*** which is formed by branches from the glossopharyngeal, vagus and cranial accessory nerves; and from the sympathetic trunk.
   a. The fibres of the cranial accessory nerve run through the vagus and constitute the main supply of the muscles of the pharynx, including that of the soft palate.
   b. Sensory fibres travel through the glossopharyngeal and vagus nerves. Some sensory fibres also travel through the lesser palatine branch of the pterygopalatine ganglion.

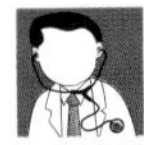

## CLINICAL CORRELATION

### Pharynx

1. The division of the inferior constrictor of the pharynx into a cricopharyngeal part and a thyropharyngeal part has been noted above.
2. The cricopharyngeus is believed to act as a sphincter at the junction of the pharynx and oesophagus, and to prevent passage of air into the latter.
3. The thyropharyngeus (along with other constrictors) helps to push the bolus of food down the pharynx.
4. The posterior wall of the pharynx is weakest just above the cricopharyngeus.
5. There may be a gap here between the thyropharyngeal and cricopharyngeal fibres. This gap is referred to as ***Killian's dehiscence***.

6. Pressure of food over this area can lead to the formation of a pouch (diverticulum). This is more likely to occur if there is incoordination of muscles (the crico-pharyngeus failing to relax when the thyropharyngeus is contracting.
7. The pharyngeal pouch thus formed cannot expand posteriorly (because of the presence of the vertebral column). It, therefore, grows downwards and can press on the oesophagus resulting in dysphagia (difficulty in swallowing).

## THE PALATINE TONSILS

1. The palatine tonsils are masses of lymphoid tissue.
2. Each palatine tonsil (right or left) lies in the tonsilar sinus on the lateral wall of the oropharynx (45.2 and 45.9).
3. This sinus is bounded by the palatoglossal fold in front and the palatopharyngeal fold behind. Relative to the surface of the body the palatine tonsil lies just in front of and above the angle of the mandible.
4. The medial surface of the palatine tonsil is covered by mucous membrane which is continuous with that of the palatoglossal folds; and below with the mucous membrane on the tongue.
5. Deep to the mucosa the lymphoid tissue of the tonsil extends upwards into the soft palate and downwards into the tongue.
6. The mucosa over the upper part of the tonsil dips into the substance of the tonsil forming a deep ***intratonsillar cleft*** (45.11). A number of smaller recesses called the ***tonsilar crypts*** are also present.
7. The lateral surface of the tonsil is covered by fascia which forms a ***capsule*** for it and separates it from the superior constrictor of the pharynx.
8. The right and left palatine tonsils form the most conspicuous parts of a ring of lymphoid tissue ***(Waldeyer's ring)*** present near the oropharyngeal isthmus (45.12). The ring is completed below by the lingual tonsil and above by the pharyngeal and tubal tonsils.

### WANT TO KNOW MORE?

9. The tonsil receives branches from several arteries in the region. The chief supply is through the tonsilar branch of the facial artery. One other branch of the facial artery, the ascending palatine branch, also supplies it.
   a. The tonsillar branch of the facial artery reaches the tonsil by piercing the superior constrictor of the pharynx (See below for clinical significance).
   b. Note that the ascending palatine branch of the facial artery (and sometimes the facial artery itself) is separated from the tonsil only by the superior constrictor muscle. It can be injured in operations for removal of the tonsil ***(tonsillectomy)***.
10. Veins from the tonsil may join a vein descending from the soft palate across its lateral side (between the capsule and the superior constrictor).
    a. This is the external palatine or paratonsilar vein (45.11).
    b. It can be injured during tonsillectomy and can cause troublesome bleeding.
    c. Some veins from the tonsil may pierce the superior constrictor muscle to end in the facial vein or in the pharyngeal plexus of veins.
11. The sensory nerves supplying the tonsil are derived from the glossopharyngeal and lesser palatine nerves. As the glossopharyngeal nerve also supplies the middle ear, pain caused by tonsillitis may be referred to the ear.

12. Palatine tonsils are best developed in children. Like other lymphoid tissue they undergo retrogression after puberty
13. *Lymphatics* from the tonsil pass through the superior constrictor to reach the jugulodigastric nodes and other nodes of the deep cervical group.

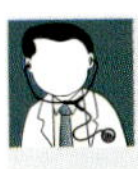

## CLINICAL CORRELATION

**Palatine Tonsils**

1. When we talk of tonsils we are really referring to palatine tonsils.
2. Infection of the tonsils is common and is referred to as ***tonsillitis***.
3. Infection can spread from them to peritonsillar tissues leading to a ***peritonsillar abscess*** (also called ***quinsy***).
4. Infected tonsils can be responsible for spread of infection to the nasal cavities, the ears, and the respiratory passages.
5. An operation for surgical removal of the tonsils is called ***tonsillectomy***.
   a. The main danger during the operation is bleeding from the external palatine (paratonsillar) vein.
   b. The ascending branch of the facial artery (and sometimes the facial artery itself) is separated from the tonsil only by the superior constrictor muscle, and can in injured in a crudely performed tonsillectomy.

## The Pharyngeal Tonsil

1. This is a collection of lymphoid tissue present in relation to the roof of the nasopharynx (45.9).
2. Hence, it is also called the nasopharyngeal tonsil.

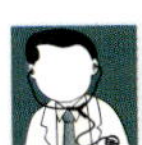

## CLINICAL CORRELATION

1. When enlarged (because of chronic infection) the pharyngeal tonsil is referred to as ***adenoids***.
2. Adenoids lead to obstruction in the nasopharynx forcing the child to breathe through the mouth.
3. A constantly open mouth can lead to deformities of the teeth and palate (as normal pressure of the tongue on the palate is not present).
4. Infection frequently spreads to the middle ear (through the auditory tube).
5. Removal of adenoids is called ***adenoidectomy***.

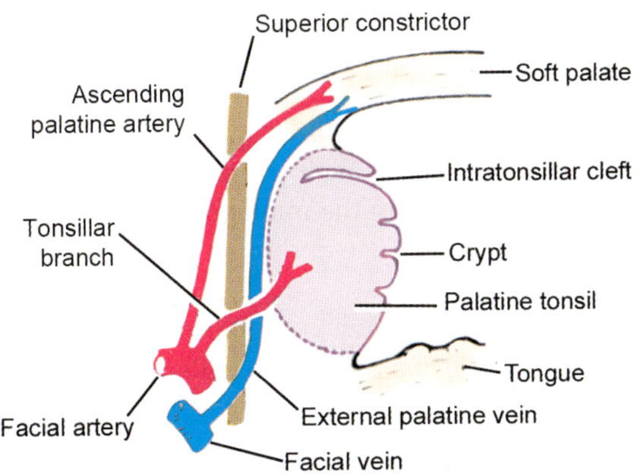


**45.11:** Coronal section through the palatine tonsil

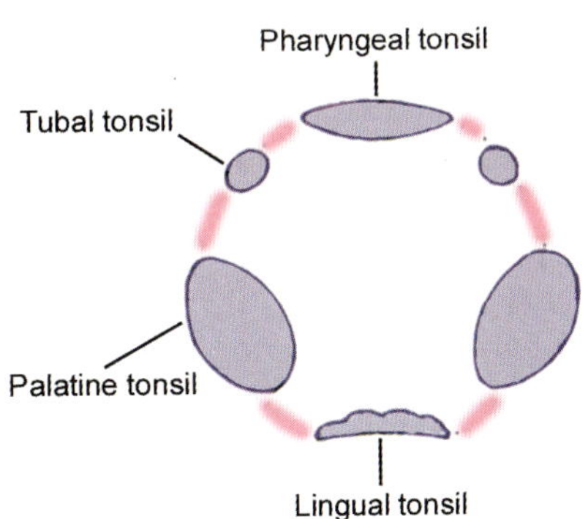


**45.12:** Waldeyer's ring of lymphoid tissue

# THE LARYNX

## Introductory Remarks about the Larynx

1. The larynx is a space that communicates above with the laryngeal part of the pharynx, and below with the trachea.
2. Apart from being a respiratory passage the larynx is the organ where voice is produced.
3. Near the middle of the larynx there are ***vocal folds*** (one right and one left) that project into the laryngeal cavity. Between these folds there is an interval called the ***rima glottidis.***
4. The rima is fairly wide in ordinary breathing.
   a. When we wish to speak the two vocal folds come close together narrowing the rima glottidis.
   b. Expired air passing through the narrow gap causes the vocal folds to vibrate resulting in the production of sound.
   c. Variation in the loudness of sound is produced by the force with which air is expelled through the rima glottidis.
   d. Variation in pitch is achieved by stretching of the vocal folds to different degrees.
   e. The difference in the voice of a man and that of a woman (or of a child) is due to the fact that the vocal folds are considerably longer in the male adult. The structure of the larynx has to be studied keeping these facts in view.
5. The larynx has a rigid framework made up of cartilages.
   a. The cartilages are joined to one another by ligaments.
   b. A number of muscles are attached to the cartilages. They produce movements of the vocal folds that are necessary for speech.
   c. The cartilages, ligaments and muscles are covered on the inside by mucous membrane that is continuous above with that of the laryngeal part of the pharynx and below with that of the trachea.

## Cartilages of the Larynx

1. These are seen from the front in 45.13; from the lateral side in 45.14; from above in 45.15 and from behind in 45.16A.
2. There are three unpaired cartilages. These are:
   a. The thyroid cartilage
   b. The cricoid cartilage
   c. The cartilage of the epiglottis.
3. The paired cartilages are:
   a. The right and left arytenoid cartilages
   b. Corniculate and cuneiform cartilages which are small nodules (of little importance).

## Thyroid Cartilage

1. The thyroid cartilage consists of right and left ***laminae.*** Each lamina is roughly quadrilateral (45.14).
2. As seen in 45.15, the laminae are placed obliquely relative to the midline: their posterior borders are far apart but the anterior borders approach each other at an angle that is about 90° in the male and about 120° in the female.
3. The lower parts of the anterior borders of the right and left laminae fuse and form a median projection called the ***laryngeal prominence*** (45.13).
4. The upper parts of the anterior borders (of the laminae) do not meet: they are separated by a ***notch.***
5. The posterior margin of each laminae is prolonged upwards to form a projection called the ***superior cornu***; and downwards to form a smaller projection called the ***inferior cornu***.
6. The medial side of each inferior cornu articulates with the corresponding lateral aspect of the cricoid cartilage.
7. The lateral surface of each lamina is marked by an ***oblique line*** that runs downwards and forwards. At its upper and lower ends the oblique line ends in projections called the ***superior*** and ***inferior tubercles***, respectively (45.13 and 45.14).

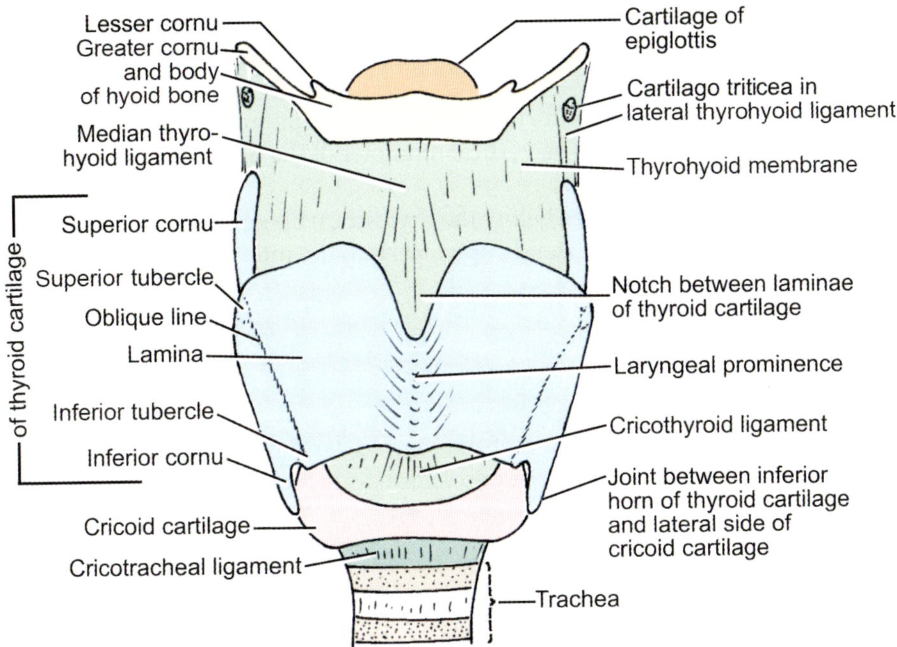


**45.13:** Cartilages of the larynx as seen from the front

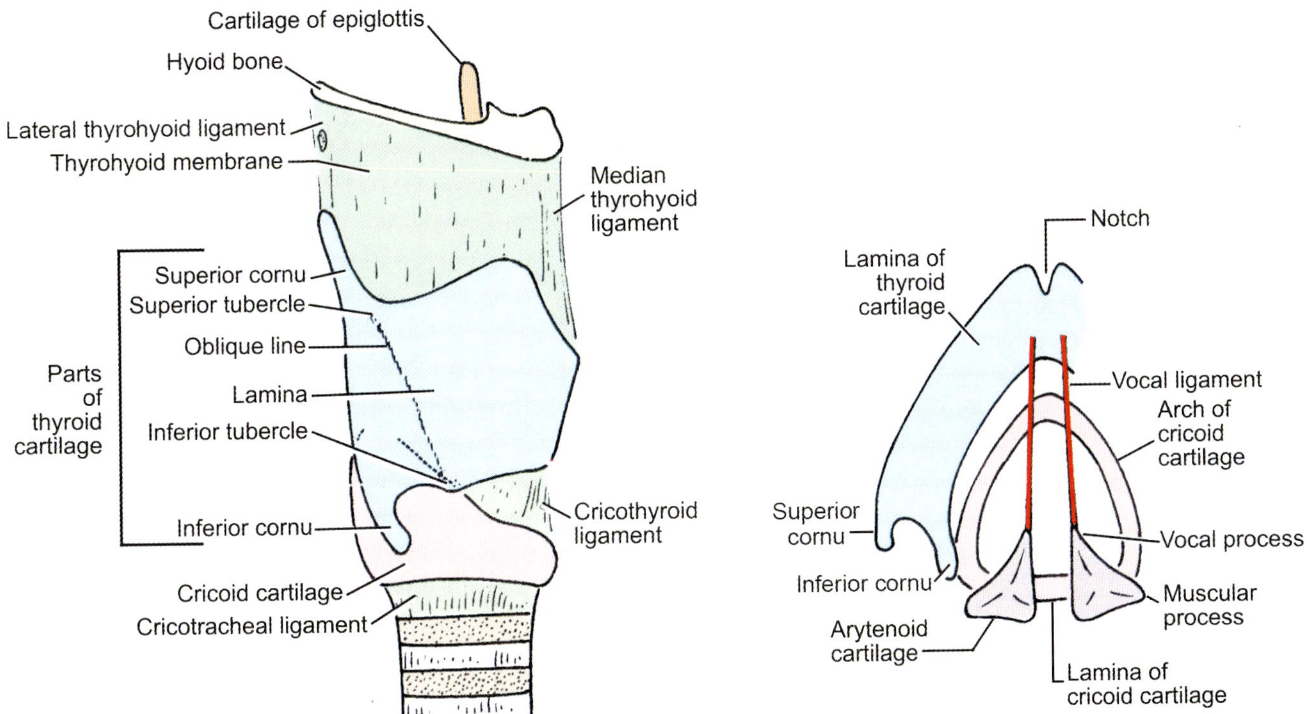


**45.14:** Cartilages of the larynx seen from the lateral side

**45.15:** Cartilages of the larynx seen from above

### Cricoid Cartilage

1. The cricoid cartilage is shaped like a ring. This fact is best appreciated when the cartilage is viewed from above (45.15).
2. The posterior part of the ring is enlarged to form a roughly quadrilateral ***lamina*** (45.16A).
3. The rest of the cartilage is called the ***arch.*** The vertical diameter of the arch is greatest where it joins the lamina, and least near the midline, in front (45.14).
4. The anterior part of the cricoid cartilage lies below the thyroid cartilage (45.13).
5. The posterior part of the cricoid cartilage extends upwards into the interval between the laminae of the thyroid cartilage (45.14 and 45.16A).

#### WANT TO KNOW MORE?

6. We have already seen that the inferior cornua of the thyroid cartilage articulate with the lateral sides of the arch of the cricoid cartilage. On each side the superolateral aspect of the lamina of the cricoid cartilage bears a facet for articulation with the arytenoid cartilage.

**Cartilage of Epiglottis**

1. The cartilage of the epiglottis is tongue-shaped, having a broad upper part, and a narrow lower end.
2. The upper broad part lies just behind the tongue. The lower end is attached to the angle formed by the anterior margins of the laminae of the thyroid cartilage, just below the notch.
3. The lower part of the epiglottis shows a backward projection in the midline. This projection is called the ***tubercle*** of the epiglottis.

**Arytenoid Cartilage**

1. Each arytenoid cartilage (right or left) is pyramidal (45.16B).
2. It has:
   a. A ***base*** (below) which articulates with the cricoid cartilage.
   b. An ***apex*** which is directed upwards and to which the corniculate cartilage is attached.
   c. Three ***surfaces-medial, posterior*** and ***anterolateral.***
3. The anteroinferior angle of the cartilage is prolonged forwards to form the ***vocal process.*** The inferolateral angle is enlarged to form the ***muscular process.***

## INTERIOR OF THE LARYNX

1. Almost midway between the upper and lower ends of the larynx, two pairs of mucosal folds project into its cavity.
2. The upper folds are the right and left ***vestibular folds.***
3. The lower folds are the right and left ***vocal folds.***
4. The part of the laryngeal cavity lying above the vestibular folds is called the ***vestibule.***
5. The narrow recess between the levels of the vestibular and vocal folds (on either side) is called the ***sinus*** or ***ventricle*** of the larynx.
6. The upper aperture of the larynx is called its ***inlet***, or ***aditus.***
   a. The aperture is directed backwards and a little upwards (so that its anterior margin lies distinctly higher than the posterior margin).
   b. It is bounded on either side by the ***aryepiglottic folds***. These folds are made of mucous membrane that extend from the sides of the epiglottis (in front) to the arytenoid cartilages.
7. Each vestibular fold encloses a bundle of fibres that constitute the ***vestibular ligament*** .

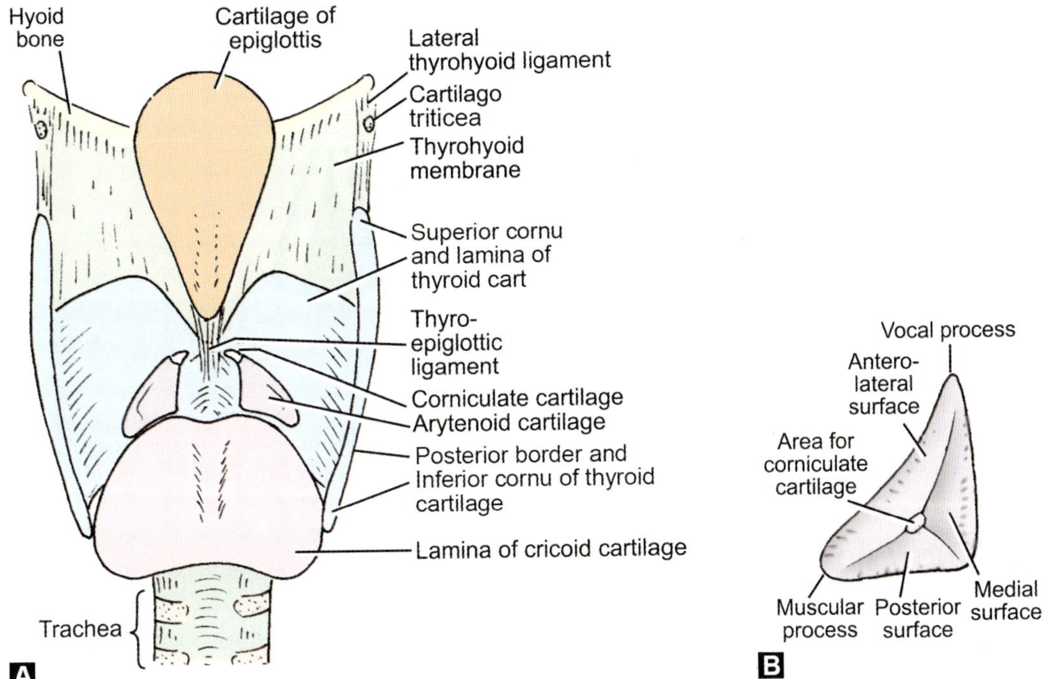


**45.16A and B:** (A) Cartilages of the larynx seen from behind. (B) Arytenoid cartilage of the left side seen from above

## WANT TO KNOW MORE?

8. The ligament is attached, in front, to the angle of the thyroid cartilage; and, behind, to the anterolateral surface of the arytenoid cartilage.
9. The fissure separating the right and left vestibular folds is called the ***rima vestibuli*** (shown but not labelled in 45.18).

10. Each vocal fold contains a bundle of elastic fibres that constitute the ***vocal ligament***.
    a. The ligament is attached in front to the angle of the thyroid cartilage (below the attachment of the vestibular ligament)
    b. Behind to the vocal process of the arytenoid cartilage (45.15).
11. The function of voice production (by vibration) demands that the vocal folds be firm and of uniform thickness.
    a. This aim is achieved by close adherence of the lining epithelium to the vocal ligaments, and by the absence of blood vessels.
    b. As a result the vocal folds withstand the stress of repeated and intense vibration.
12. The right and left vocal folds are separated by the anterior or ***intermembranous*** part of a fissure called the ***rima glottidis***. The posterior part of the fissure lies between the two arytenoid cartilages and is, therefore, called the ***intercartilaginous*** part (45.17).
13. The shape of the rima varies in different phases of respiration and of phonation.

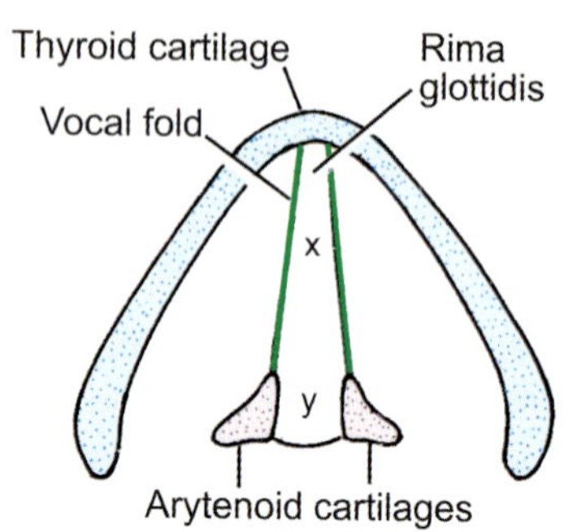


**45.17:** Scheme to show the intermembranous (x) and intercartilaginous (y) parts of the rima glottidis

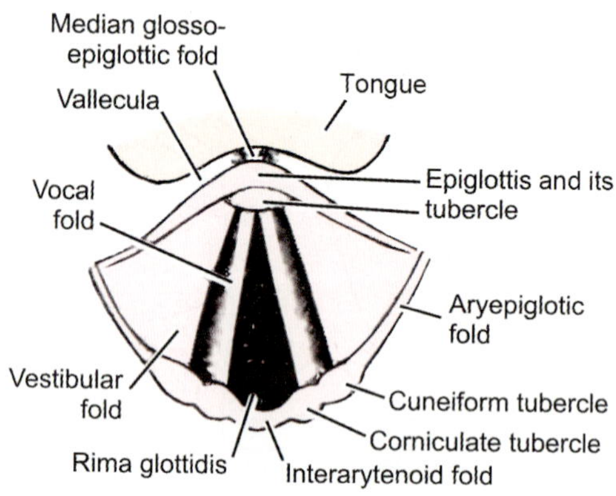


**45.18:** Some features of the larynx as seen through a laryngoscope (i.e., from above). The gap between the two vestibular folds is the rima vestibuli

### WANT TO KNOW MORE?

14. We have seen that the part of the cavity of the larynx lying between the vocal and vestibular folds of each side is called the sinus or ventricle of the larynx.
    a. A pouch like diverticulum arises from the anterior part of each sinus.
    b. This pouch is called the ***saccule*** of the larynx.

## MUSCLES OF THE LARYNX

1. The muscles of the larynx are extrinsic and intrinsic.
2. The ***extrinsic muscles*** are those in which one end of the muscle is attached to a cartilage of the larynx whereas the other end is attached elsewhere.
   a. These muscles raise or lower the larynx as a whole during deglutition.
   b. The extrinsic muscles include the sternothyroid and thyrohyoid muscles and the inferior constrictor of the pharynx. Some muscles attached to the hyoid bone can raise the larynx indirectly.
3. The ***intrinsic muscles*** are confined to the larynx. They may be classified in accordance with their actions as follows.
   a. ***Muscles that increase or decrease tension of the vocal folds.***
   These are:
      i. The cricothyroid
      ii. The thyroarytenoid
      iii. The vocalis.
   b. ***Muscles that open or close the glottis.***
   These are:
      i. The posterior cricoarytenoid
      ii. The lateral cricoarytenoid
      iii. The transverse arytenoid.
   c. ***Muscles that open or close the inlet of the larynx.***
   These are:
      i. The oblique arytenoids
      ii. The aryepiglottic
      iii. Thyroepiglottic muscles.

## WANT TO KNOW MORE?

The attachments of the intrinsic muscles of the larynx are complicated and will not be described. However, note the following:

1. The cricothyroid is the only intrinsic muscle of the larynx that is seen on its outer aspect. It passes from the cricoid cartilage to the thyroid cartilage.
2. The cricothyroid lengthens the vocal folds and makes them tense.
3. The thyroarytenoid passes from the thyroid cartilage to the arytenoid cartilage. It relaxes the vocal fold.
4. The deeper fibres of the thyroarytenoid muscle form a band that runs along the vocal ligament, just lateral to it.
   a. This band is called the ***vocalis***.
   b. The fibres of this muscle are attached at different distances along the vocal ligament.
   c. Contraction of this muscle can cause different lengths of the vocal ligament to become tense, thus varying the pitch of the voice. The muscle is therefore called the tuning fork of the larynx.
5. The posterior cricoarytenoid muscle arises from the posterior aspect of the lamina of the cricoid cartilage. Its fibres pass upwards and laterally to be inserted on the back of the muscular process of the arytenoid cartilage of that side. The muscle abducts the vocal folds.
6. The lateral cricoarytenoid muscle arises from the arch of the cricoid cartilage. Its fibres are inserted on the front of the muscular process of the arytenoid cartilage. This muscle adducts the vocal folds.
7. The oblique arytenoids and the aryepiglottic muscle close the inlet of the larynx.
8. The thyroepiglottic muscles open the inlet of the larynx.

## Alterations in Shape of Rima Glottides

These are shown in 45.19A to D.

1. The glottis has an anterior (membranous) part placed between the two vocal folds, and a posterior (cartilaginous) part placed between the medial surfaces of the two arytenoid cartilages (45.19A).
2. The size and shape of the glottis undergoes changes during different phases of respiration and of speech.
3. During quiet respiration (and after death) the glottis is moderately wide, the anterior part being triangular and the posterior part rectangular (45.19A). In this position the laryngeal muscles are relaxed.
4. The glottis is narrowest during speech (45.19B), both the vocal folds and the arytenoid cartilages being close together. This position is produced mainly by contraction of the transverse arytenoid which pulls the cartilages towards each other.
5. In whispering (45.19C) the glottis is closed in its anterior part, but the posterior part is wide open.
6. The glottis is widely opened in forced respiration, both the anterior and posterior parts becoming triangular (45.19D).

## Vessels and Nerves of Larynx

1. The ***arteries*** supplying the larynx are branches from the superior and inferior thyroid arteries.
2. The ***veins*** accompany the arteries.
3. The ***lymphatic drainage*** of the larynx is shown in 45.20.
4. The sensory ***innervation*** of the part of the larynx above the vocal folds is by the internal laryngeal nerve.
5. Sensations of taste from the epiglottis also travel through this nerve.
6. The part of the larynx below the vocal folds receives its sensory innervation through branches of the recurrent laryngeal nerve.
7. Most of the intrinsic muscles of the larynx are supplied by the recurrent laryngeal nerve. The only exception is the cricothyroid that is supplied by the external laryngeal nerve.

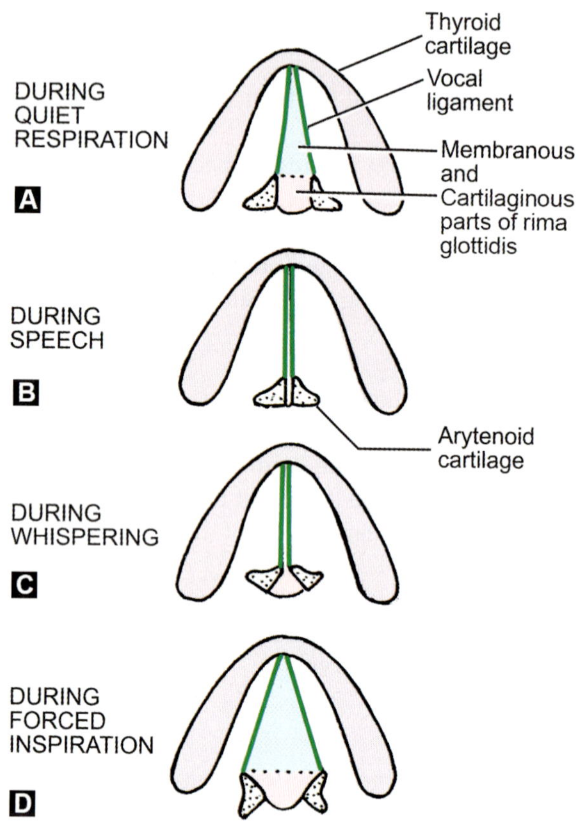


**45.19A to D:** Alterations in shape of the rima glottidis during respiration and during speech

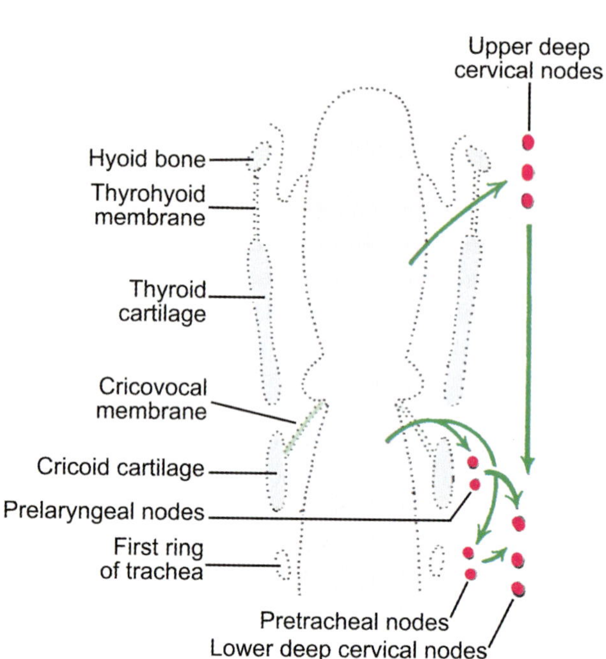


**45.20:** Scheme to show the lymphatic drainage of the larynx

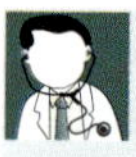

## CLINICAL CORRELATION

**Larynx**

1. Entry of any foreign matter (including water or food) into the larynx can result in suffocation and death. The intense cough that is set up on the entry of even a small particle is a protective mechanism against suffocation.
2. Inflammation of the mucous membrane of the larynx (***laryngitis***) can cause hoarseness of voice, or even complete loss of voice, because of oedema above the level of the vocal folds.
   a. Note that laryngeal mucous membrane is firmly adherent to the vocal folds and that is why fluid accumulates above this level.
   b. In the presence of severe inflammation or irritation the oedema may be of such a degree as to lead to suffocation. In such cases it may become necessary to create an artificial opening in the trachea (***tracheostomy***) to save the life of the person.
3. Paralysis of one or more muscles of the larynx also leads to hoarseness of voice.
   a. The hoarseness is temporary in case of injury to the external laryngeal nerve (as the function of the paralysed cricothyroid is gradually taken up by the muscle of the normal side).
   b. When the recurrent laryngeal nerve is injured, hoarseness is permanent.
4. In this connection it may be noted that in some cases only some groups of muscles may be affected.
   a. When all intrinsic laryngeal muscles are paralysed, the vocal folds are immobile and lie midway between abduction and adduction. This is the position occupied by the vocal folds after death.

b. Paralysis of abductors alone leads to adduction of the vocal folds (by unopposed action of the adductors): this leads to closure of the glottis with consequent suffocation. Hence, paralysis of abductors alone is much more dangerous than paralysis of both abductors and adductors of the vocal folds.

5. The interior of the larynx can be examined in a living person using an instrument called a ***laryngoscope***. The procedure is called ***laryngoscopy***.

## THE TRACHEA

1. The trachea is a wide tube lying on the front of the neck more or less in the middle line.
2. The upper end of the trachea is continuous with the lower end of the larynx.
3. The junction lies opposite the lower part of the body of the sixth cervical vertebra.
4. At the root of the neck the trachea passes into the superior mediastinum of the thorax. Here, we will consider the relations of the trachea in the neck.

### Relations of the Trachea in the Neck

The trachea is related to a large number of structures in the neck as follows:

1. Posteriorly the trachea is related to the oesophagus which runs vertically behind it, and separates it from the bodies of vertebrae C6 and C7 (45.21).
2. Anteriorly, over its entire length, the trachea is covered by skin, superficial and deep fascia.
   a. The deep fascia is represented by a superficial part, the investing layer.
   b. A deeper part, the pretracheal fascia.
3. The right and left sternohyoid and sternothyroid muscles overlap the part of the trachea near the inlet of the thorax.
4. Near its upper end (over the 2nd, 3rd and 4th rings) the trachea is covered anteriorly by the isthmus of the thyroid gland.
5. The right and left lobes of the gland overlap the corresponding sides of the trachea (45.16).
6. The right and left common carotid arteries ascend along the corresponding side of the cervical part of the trachea.

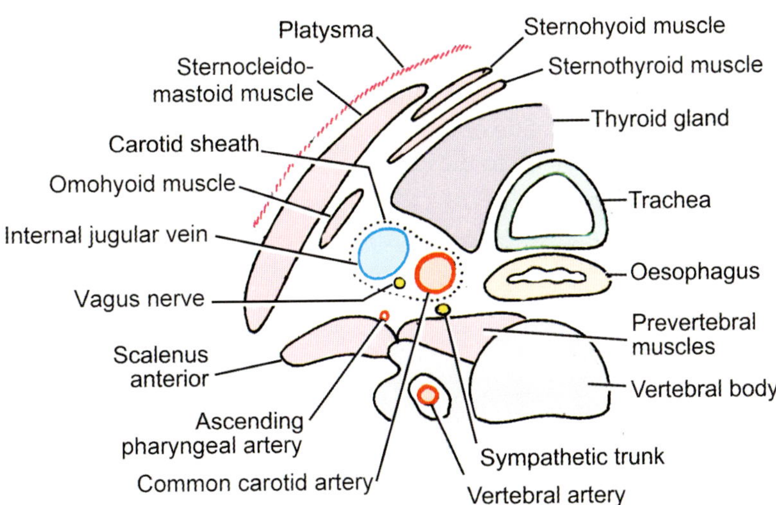


**45.21:** Transverse section through the upper part of the trachea to show some of its relations in the neck

7. On either side the inferior thyroid artery is closely related to the trachea (42.1).
8. On either side, the recurrent laryngeal nerve lies in the groove between the trachea and the oesophagus. (On the left side the nerve is related to both the thoracic and cervical parts of trachea, but on the right side it is related to the cervical part only).
9. Small structures lying in front of the trachea are as follows:
   a. An anastomosis between branches of the right and left superior thyroid arteries lies along the upper margin of the isthmus of the thyroid gland.
   b. The inferior thyroid veins pass from the lower border of the isthmus of the thyroid gland to their termination in the left brachiocephalic vein.
   c. A small artery, the thyroidea ima, is sometimes present. It arises from the brachiocephalic trunk or from the arch of the aorta and runs upwards in front of the trachea to reach the isthmus of the thyroid gland.
   d. The jugular arch connecting the right and left anterior jugular veins runs across the trachea just above the manubrium sterni.
10. Lymphatic vessels of the trachea drain into pretracheal and paratracheal nodes and through them (or directly) to the deep cervical nodes

## THE OESOPHAGUS

1. The oesophagus is a tubular structure which starts at the lower end of the oropharynx (i.e., in front of the sixth cervical vertebra: 45.9).
2. It descends through the lower part of the neck, and enters the thorax through its inlet.
3. After passing through the thorax the oesophagus enters the abdomen and ends by joining the cardiac end of the stomach.
4. The cervical part of the oesophagus receives branches from the inferior thyroid artery. Veins drain into the inferior thyroid vein.
5. Lymphatics from the cervical part of the oesophagus drain to the deep cervical nodes. Some lymph passes through paratracheal nodes.

### Relations of Oesophagus in the Neck

These are shown in 45.21.

a. Posteriorly, the oesophagus is related to the sixth and seventh cervical vertebrae (covered by prevertebral muscles and fascia).
b. Anteriorly it is related to the trachea.
c. Laterally the oesophagus is related to the corresponding common carotid artery.
d. The upper part of the oesophagus is overlapped, laterally, by the corresponding lobe of the thyroid gland.
e. The thoracic duct ascends along the left side of the oesophagus in the lower part of the neck. The right and left recurrent laryngeal nerves lie anterolateral to the oesophagus in the corresponding grooves between it and the trachea.

### Clinical Correlations of Oesophagus

See chapter 22, pp. 440-41.

46

CHAPTER

# Endocrine Glands of the Head and Neck, Carotid Sinus and Carotid Body

The endocrine glands that lie in the head and neck are:

1. The hypophysis cerebri
2. The pineal gland
3. The thyroid gland
4. The parathyroid glands.

Some endocrine functions are also ascribed to the carotid body. The carotid body, and the carotid sinus, will also be considered.

## THE HYPOPHYSIS CEREBRI

1. The hypophysis cerebri is also called the pituitary gland.
2. It is placed in the cranial cavity, in the floor of the middle cranial fossa. It lies in a depression on the superior surface of the body of the sphenoid bone called the ***hypophyseal fossa*** or ***sella turcica***.
3. The hypophysis is suspended from the floor of the third ventricle of the brain by a narrow funnel shaped stalk called the ***infundibulum.***
4. The hypophysis cerebri is a small ovoid structure measuring about 13 mm from side to side, about 10 mm front to back, and about 8 mm in vertical diameter.
5. The relations of the hypophysis cerebri are shown in 46.1, that is a coronal section; and in 46.2 which is a sagittal section.

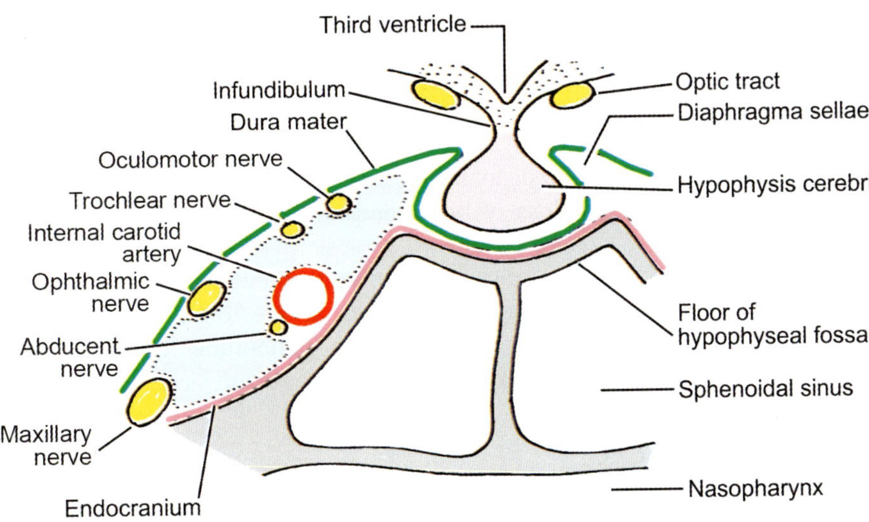


**46.1:** Coronal section through hypophysis cerebri to show some of its relations

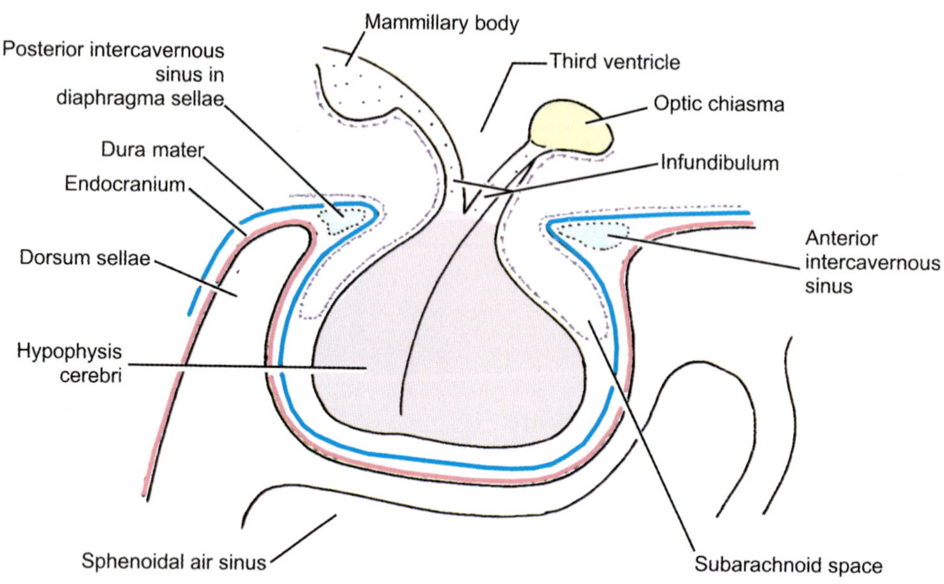


**46.2:** Sagittal section through the hypophysis cerebri to show its relations

6. The hypophyseal fossa is lined by dura mater.
   a. Superior to the hypophysis, the dura mater is folded on itself to form the ***diaphragma sellae***.
   b. The infundibulum passes through an aperture in the diaphragma to join the inferior wall of the third ventricle.
   c. The optic chiasma lies antero-superior to the hypophysis cerebri being separated from it by the anterior part of the diaphragma. It lies anterior to the infundibulum.
   d. Inferiorly, the hypophysis cerebri is related to the sphenoidal air sinuses and beyond them to the nasopharynx.
   e. On the right and left sides, the hypophysis cerebri is related to the corresponding cavernous sinus (and to structures in its wall).
   f. The cavernous sinuses are connected across the midline by anterior and posterior intercavernous sinuses that are located within the layers of the diaphragma sellae.

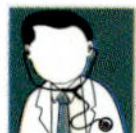

**CLINICAL CORRELATION**

1. The relations of the hypophysis cerebri help us to understand the effects of pressure by a tumour of the organ.
2. Pressure on the optic chiasma leads to loss of both temporal halves of the fields of vision (bitemporal hemianopia).
3. Lateral pressure may lead to paralysis of muscles supplied by the oculomotor nerve.
4. The trochlear and abducent nerves are rarely affected (as they are too low down).
5. Downward pressure of an enlarging hypophysis leads to 'ballooning' of the hypophyseal fossa; and backward pressure can cause erosion of the dorsum sellae. These features can be recognised on a skiagram.

## Subdivisions of the Hypophysis Cerebri

1. The hypophysis cerebri has, in the past, been usually divided into an anterior part, the ***pars anterior***; an intermediate part, the ***pars intermedia***; and a posterior part, the ***pars posterior*** (or ***pars nervosa***) (46.3).

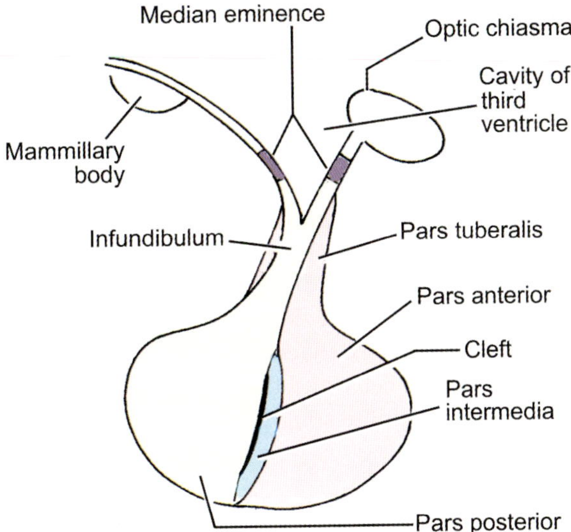


**46.3:** Sagittal section to show the subdivisions of the hypophysis cerebri

2. The pars posterior contains numerous nerve fibres. It is directly continuous with the central core of the infundibulum, which is made up of nervous tissue. These two parts are together referred to as the ***neurohypophysis***.
3. The area of the floor of the third ventricle (tuber cinerium) immediately adjoining the attachment to it of the infundibulum is referred to as the ***median eminence***. Some authorities include the median eminence in the neurohypophysis.
4. The pars anterior (which is also called the ***pars distalis***) and the pars intermedia are both made up of cells having a direct secretory function and are collectively referred to as the ***adenohypophysis***.
5. An extension of the pars anterior surrounds the central nervous core of the infundibulum. Because of the tubular shape of this extension (46.3) it is called the ***pars tubularis***. The pars tubularis is part of the adenohypophysis.

### WANT TO KNOW MORE?

6. A distinction between the adenohypophysis and the neurohypophysis can also be made on the basis of their development.
   a. The neurohypophysis is formed as a down growth from the floor of the third ventricle.
   b. In contrast, the adenohypophysis is derived from ***Rathke's pouch*** that arises from the ectoderm lining the roof of the primitive mouth (stomodaeum). This pouch has a cavity.
   c. The pars anterior is formed in the anterior wall of the pouch and the pars intermedia in its posterior wall.
   d. The original cavity of Rathke's pouch may persist as a cleft separating the pars anterior and intermedia.

## Structure and Hormones of Hypophysis Cerebri

Students interested in detailed study of the histology of the hypophysis cerebri should consult the author's HUMAN HISTOLOGY. A brief summary is given below.

### Pars Anterior

1. The pars anterior is made up of cords of cells separated by sinusoids.
2. Several types of cells can be recognised on the basis of their staining characters. More recently, the cells responsible for production of individual hormones have been distinguished by a technique called immunofluorescence.
3. Using routine staining procedures the cells of the adenohypophysis can be divided into:
   a. ***Chromophil*** cells that have brightly staining granules in their cytoplasm.
   b. ***Chromophobe*** cells in which the granules are not present.
4. Chromophil cells are further classified as:
   a. ***Acidophil*** when they stain with acid dyes (like eosin or orange G).
   b. ***Basophil*** when they stain with basic dyes (like haematoxylin).
   c. The acidophil cells are often called alpha cells, and the basophils are called beta cells.
5. Both acidophils and basophils can be divided into subtypes on the basis of structural details and on the basis of the hormones produced by them. The following types of cells are described.

### Types of Acidophil Cells

1. ***Somatotrophs (or somatotropes)*** produce the somatotropic hormone (also called ***somatotropin, STH*** or ***growth hormone***). This hormone controls body growth, specially before puberty.
2. ***Mammotrophs*** (or ***mammotropes***) produce the ***mammotropic hormone*** (also called ***mammotropin, prolactin, lactogenic hormone***, or ***LTH***) which stimulates the growth and activity of the female mammary gland, during pregnancy and lactation.

### Types of Basophil Cells

1. ***Corticotrophs*** (or ***corticotropes***) produce the ***corticotropic hormone*** (also called ***adrenocorticotropin*** or ***ACTH***). This hormone stimulates the secretion of some hormones of the adrenal cortex. [Note: The staining characters of these cells are intermediate between acidophils and basophils; and they are sometimes classified amongst acidophils].
2. ***Thyrotrophs*** (or ***thyrotropes***) produce the ***thyrotropic hormone*** (***thyrotropin*** or ***TSH***)) which stimulates the activity of the thyroid gland.
3. ***Gonadotrophs*** (***gonadotropes*** or delta basophils) produce two types of hormones each type having a separate action in the male and female.
   a. In the female, the first of these hormones stimulates the growth of ovarian follicles. It is, therefore, called the ***follicle stimulating hormone (FSH)***. It also stimulates the secretion of oestrogens by the ovaries. In the male, the same hormone stimulates spermatogenesis.
   b. In the female, the second hormone stimulates the maturation of the corpus luteum and the secretion by it of progesterone. It is called the ***luteinising hormone (LH)***.
   c. In the male, the same hormone stimulates the production of androgens by interstitial cells of the testes, and is called the ***interstitial cell stimulating hormone (ICSH)***.

   The secretion of hormones by the cells of the adenohypophysis is under the control of the hypothalamus.

### Chromophobe Cells

The chromophobe cells probably represent alpha or beta cells that have been depleted of their granules. Some of them are stem cells that give rise to new chromophil cells.

### Pars Tubularis and Pars Intermedia

See a book on histology.

### *The Pars Posterior*

1. The pars posterior consists of numerous unmyelinated nerve fibres, and of cells called pituicytes.
2. The nerve fibres are the axons of neurons located in the hypothalamus. Situated between these axons there are pituicytes. These cells have long dendritic processes many of which lie parallel to the nerve fibres. The axons descending into the pars posterior from the hypothalamus end in terminals closely related to capillaries.
3. The pars posterior of the hypophysis is associated with the release into the blood of two hormones.
   a. One of these is ***vasopressin*** (also called the ***antidiuretic hormone*** or *ADH*): This hormone controls the reabsorption of water by kidney tubules.
   b. The second hormone is ***oxytocin***: This hormone controls the contraction of smooth muscle of the uterus and also of the mammary gland.
4. It is now known that these two hormones are not produced in the hypophysis at all.
   a. They are synthesised in neurons located mainly in the supraoptic and paraventricular nuclei of the hypothalamus.
   b. Vasopressin is produced mainly in the supraoptic nucleus; and oxytocin in the paraventricular nucleus.
   c. These secretions (which are bound with other proteins) pass down the axons of the neurons concerned, through the infundibulum into the pars posterior. Here they are released into the capillaries of the region and enter the general circulation (46.4).

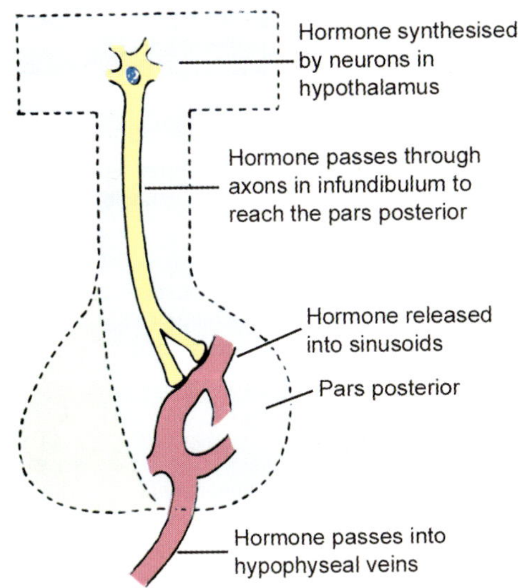


**46.4:** Scheme to show the relationship of the hypothalamus and the pars posterior of the hypophysis cerebri

## WANT TO KNOW MORE?

### *Blood Supply of the Hypophysis Cerebri*

1. The hypophysis cerebri is supplied by superior and inferior branches arising from the internal carotid arteries. Some branches also arise from the anterior and posterior cerebral arteries.
2. The inferior hypophyseal arteries are distributed mainly to the pars posterior.
3. Branches from the superior set of arteries supply the median eminence and infundibulum.
   a. Here they end in capillary plexuses from which ***portal*** vessels arise (46.5).
   b. These portal vessels descend through the infundibulum and end in the sinusoids of the pars anterior.
   c. The sinusoids are drained by veins that end in neighbouring venous sinuses.
4. It will be noticed that the above arrangement is unusual in that two sets of capillaries intervene between the arteries and veins.
   a. One of these is in the median eminence and the upper infundibulum.
   b. The second set of capillaries is represented by the sinusoids of the pars anterior.
5. This arrangement is referred to as the ***hypothalamo-hypophyseal portal system***. (Compare with ***the*** portal system). The functional significance of this system is described below.

### *Control of Secretion of Hormones of Adenohypophysis*

1. The secretion of hormones by the adenohypophysis takes place under higher control of neurons in the hypothalamus, notably those in the median eminence and in the infundibular nucleus.
2. The axons of these neurons end in relation to capillaries in the median eminence and in the upper part of the infundibulum.

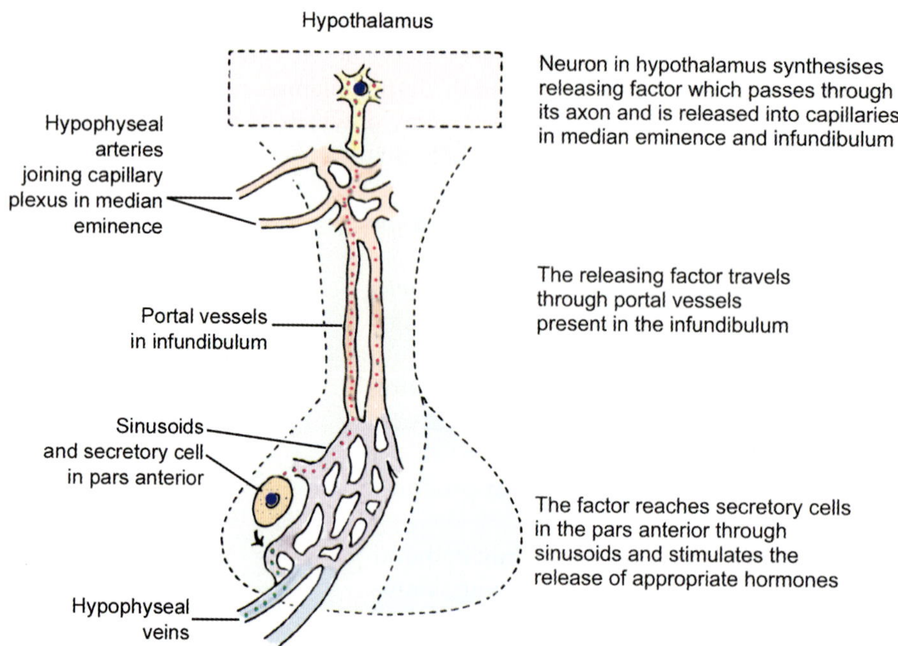


**46.5:** Scheme to show the hypothalamo-hypophyseal portal circulation and the control of secretions of the adenohypophysis by the hypothalamus

3. Different neurons produce specific ***releasing factors*** (or releasing hormones) for each hormone of the adenohypophysis.
4. These factors are released into the capillaries mentioned above.
5. Portal vessels arising from the capillaries carry these factors to the pars anterior of the hypophysis.
6. Here, they stimulate the release of appropriate hormones. Some factors inhibit the release of hormones.

*FURTHER CLINICAL CORRELATIONS OF HYPOPHYSIS CEREBRI*

1. Various types of tumours may arise in the hypophysis cerebri. The effects of the tumour (adenoma) may be caused by pressure on surrounding structures, or by increased or decreased production of hormones.
2. An adenoma arising from chromophobe cells can become quite large and can produce pressure effects as follows.
   a. Pressure on the walls of the hypophyseal fossa (sella turcica) leads to its enlargement, and this enlargement can be seen in a skiagram.
   b. The enlarging tumour presses on and destroys other cells (acidophils, basophils) of the pars anterior, and gives rise to deficiency of the hormones produced by them. Pressure on the pars posterior can lead to diabetes insipidus (see below).
   c. Pressure on the optic chiasma can lead to loss of vision in the temporal halves of vision in both eyes (bitemporal hemianopia). Stretching of the optic nerves can lead to optic atrophy.
   d. Pressure on the hypothalamus can interfere with various visceral functions. It can lead to ***Frohlich's syndrome*** that is characterised by obesity, poor development of sex organs including the gonads, and altered secondary sex characters.
   e. Pressure on the third ventricle, can result in obstruction to flow of CSF, and raised intracranial tension.
3. An adenoma can be removed surgically.
   a. The approach can be through the roof of the pharynx, through the sphenoidal sinuses.
   b. In extensive tumours, the cranial cavity has to be opened so that the tumour can be seen directly.
4. In an eosinophil adenoma, pressure effects are negligible. The main effects arise from excessive production of growth hormone.

a. In a young individual (before the epiphyses have fused), the condition results in excessive growth (***gigantism***).
b. If the adenoma is formed after the epiphyses have fused, overgrowth mainly affects the head, the hands and the feet (***acromegaly***).
c. The scalp, lips, tongue and face become thick because of increased amount of subcutaneous tissue, and the same happens to the hands and feet.
d. The paranasal sinuses enlarge making the facial region prominent.
e. There is overgrowth of hair, and the man's appearance tends to resemble that of an ape.

5. a. In the case of a basophil adenoma, there is excessive secretion of adrenotropic hormones. It leads to ***Cushings's syndrome*** that can also be caused by a tumour of the adrenal cortex.
   b. The syndrome is seen mostly in females. Abnormal deposition of fat takes place over the face, neck and trunk. The limbs remain thin and weak.
6. The posterior lobe of the hypophysis cerebri produces antidiuretic hormone (ADH) that is responsible for reabsorption of water from renal tubules.
   a. Destruction of the posterior lobe (e.g., by pressure from an adenoma), can result in ***diabetes insipidus***.
   b. In this condition, large amounts of urine are passed (polyuria). The urine is of very low specific gravity and contains no sugar or albumin. The resultant dehydration leads to excessive thirst (polydipsia) and to dryness of skin.
   c. Apart from pressure by a tumour diabetes insipidus can be caused by trauma to the region. In many cases, there is no obvious cause for the condition.

## THE PINEAL BODY

1. The pineal body is a small piriform structure present in relation to the posterior wall of the third ventricle of the brain. It is also called the ***epiphysis cerebri***.
2. It is about 8 mm in length, and about 4 cm in width and in thickness.
3. It is situated in the median plane just below the splenium of the corpus callosum, and just above the superior colliculi of the midbrain (46.6).
4. The pineal body is made up mainly of cells called ***pinealocytes***. In the adult, sections of the pineal gland show aggregations of salts containing calcium. These are referred to as ***corpora arenacea***, or 'brain sand'. They are by products of secretory activity.
5. The pineal body has for long been regarded as a vestigial organ of no functional importance.
   a. Recent investigations have shown that the pineal body is an endocrine gland of great importance.
   b. It produces hormones that may have an important regulatory influence on many other endocrine organs (including the adenohypophysis, the neurohypophysis, the thyroid, the parathyroids, the adrenal cortex and medulla, and the gonads).
6. The hormones of the pineal body reach the hypophysis both through the CSF and through blood.
7. The best known hormone of the pineal body is the amino acid ***melatonin*** (so called because it causes changes in skin colour in amphibia).
8. The pineal body may act as a kind of biological clock that may produce circadian rhythms (variations following a 24 hour cycle) in various parameters.

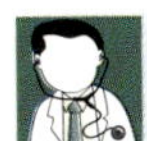

### CLINICAL CORRELATION

1. Tumours of the pineal gland can press on the tectum of the midbrain.
2. This can damage the oculomotor nucleus and can thus lead to paralysis of the oculomotor nerve.
3. Pressure of the tumour may obstruct the aqueduct and cause hydrocephalus.

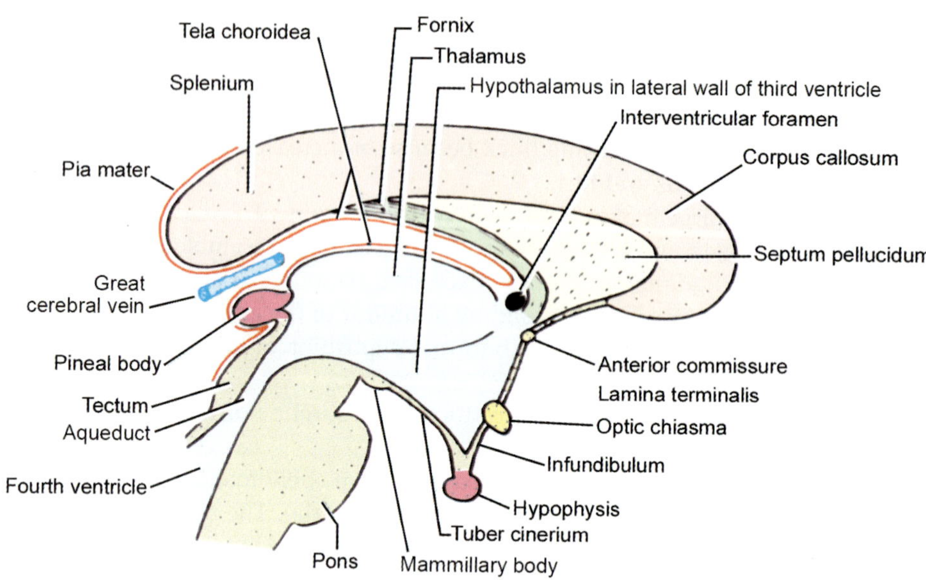


**46.6:** Diagram to show the position of the hypophysis cerebri and of the pineal body relative to the third ventricle of the brain

## THE THYROID GLAND

1. The thyroid gland lies in the front of the neck, in front of the lower part of the larynx and the upper part of the trachea (46.7).
2. It consists of right and left ***lobes*** that are joined, across the midline, by an ***isthmus*** (46.7).
3. The vertical diameter of each lobe is about 5 cm (2 inches) and that of the isthmus is about 1 cm (half inch).
   a. The anteroposterior diameter of each lobe is about 2 cm.
   b. The transverse diameter of the entire thyroid is about 8 cm.
4. When seen in cross section each lobe of the thyroid is seen to have three surfaces, lateral (or superficial), medial and posterior.
5. The ***lateral surface*** is directed forwards and laterally (46.8). It is covered by:
   a. Skin and fascia
   b. The sternothyroid and sternohyoid muscles
   c. The superior belly of the omohyoid muscle
   d. The anterior part of the sternocleidomastoid muscle.
6. The ***medial surface*** lies over:
   a. The thyroid and cricoid cartilages of the larynx.
   b. The uppermost parts of the trachea and oesophagus.
7. Other structures deep to it are:
   a. Parts of two muscles: The inferior constrictor of the pharynx, and the cricothyroid.
   b. Two important nerves: The recurrent laryngeal nerve and the external laryngeal nerve.
8. The recurrent laryngeal nerve is deep to the thyroid as it ascends in the groove between the trachea and oesophagus; while the external laryngeal nerve lies deep to the thyroid as it descends to reach the cricothyroid (46.9A).
9. The ***posterior surface*** of the lobe is directed posterolaterally. It is in contact with the carotid sheath and its contents.
10. The lateral and medial surfaces of the lobe are separated by a sharp ***anterior border.*** A branch of the superior thyroid artery descends along this border.

11. The posterior and medial surfaces of the lobe are separated by the ***posterior border*** which is rounded. It is related to:
    a. Inferior thyroid artery
    b. Parathyroid glands
    c. On the left side, the posterior border is related to the thoracic duct (46.10).
12. The ***upper end*** of each lobe extends up to the oblique line of the thyroid cartilage (46.7). [It is prevented from extending further upwards by the insertion of the sternothyroid muscle to the oblique line]. The upper end lies opposite vertebra C5.

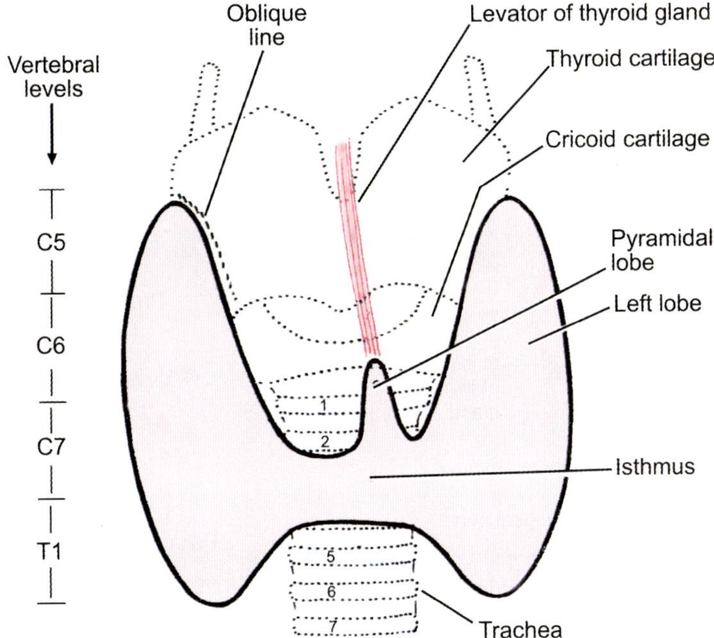


**46.7:** Outline of the thyroid gland as seen from the front, and its relationship to the larynx and trachea

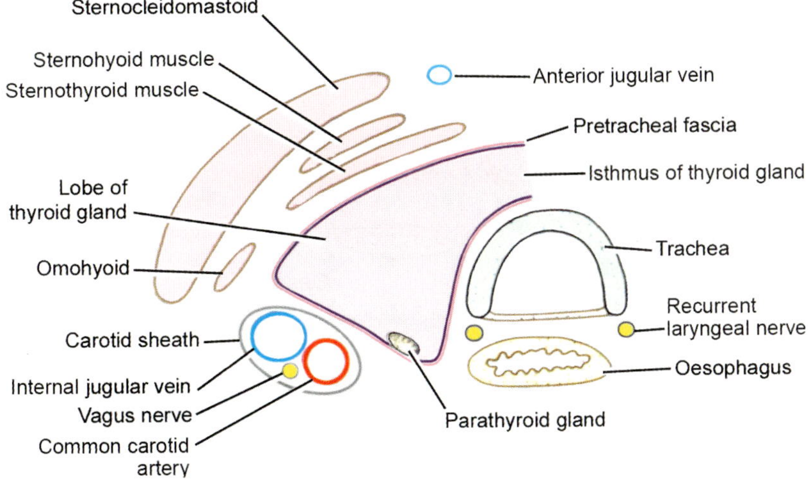


**46.8:** Transverse section across the thyroid gland and related structures

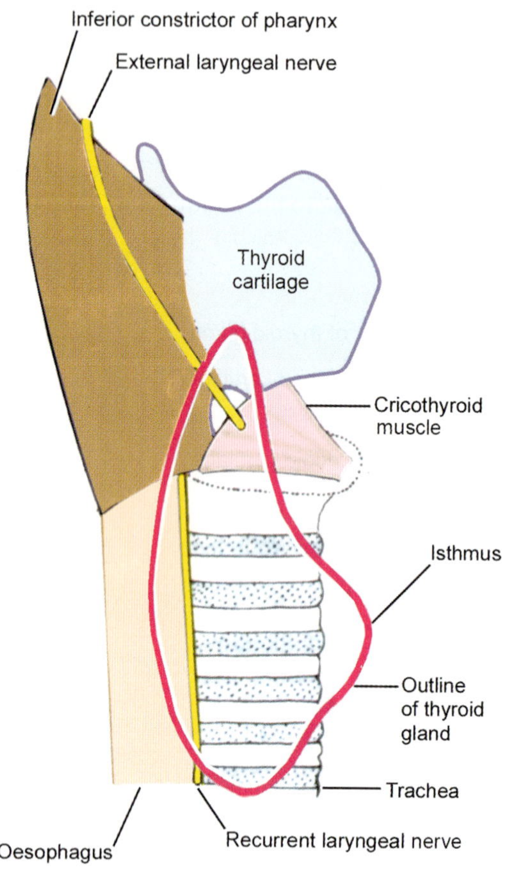


**46.9A:** Medial relations of the thyroid gland. The outline of the gland is shown in pink line

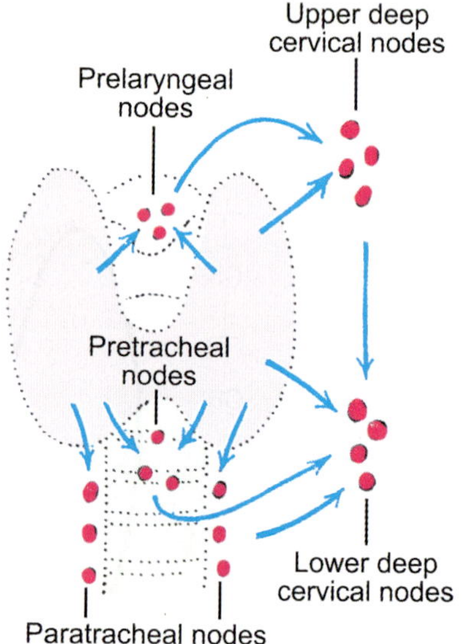


**46.9B:** Scheme to show the lymphatic drainage of the thyroid gland

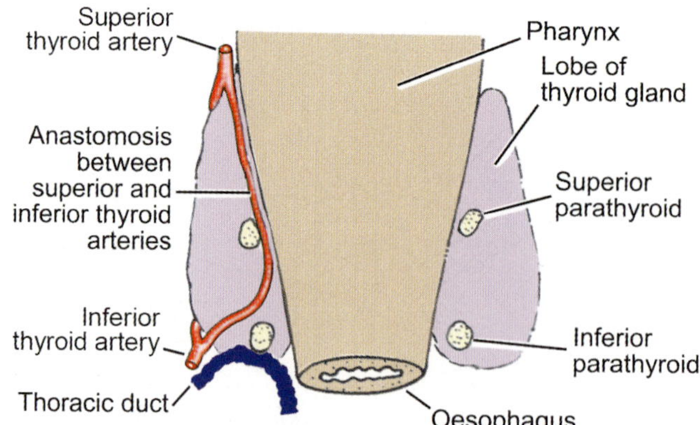


**46.10:** Thyroid and parathyroid glands seen from behind

13. The ***lower end*** of the lobe lies at the level of the fifth or sixth tracheal ring (corresponding to vertebra T1).
    a. The level of the lower end is variable.
    b. An enlarging thyroid usually extends downwards.
14. The isthmus of the thyroid gland lies in front of the second, third and fourth rings of the trachea. It is covered in front by:

a. Skin and fascia
b. Sternothyroid and sternohyoid muscles
c. Anterior jugular veins.

15. A finger like projection of thyroid tissue frequently arises from the upper border of the isthmus. This is called the ***pyramidal lobe*** (46.7).
16. Its upper end is attached to the hyoid bone by fibrous tissue or muscle (***levator of the thyroid gland***).
17. The thyroid gland is surrounded by a ***capsule*** made up of connective tissue.
18. Outside this capsule, the thyroid has another sheath (or ***false capsule***) formed by the pretracheal fascia.
    a. On each side, this fascia is thickened posteromedially to form a band connecting the lobe of the thyroid gland to the side of the cricoid cartilage.
    b. This band is called the ***lateral ligament*** or the ligament of Berry.
19. The thyroid has a rich blood supply. The arteries supplying it are:
    a. The superior thyroid branch of the external carotid artery.
    b. The inferior thyroid branch of the thyrocervical trunk.
    c. A small artery the thyroidea ima arising from the brachiocephalic trunk.
    d. Accessory thyroid arteries derived from those supplying the trachea and oesophagus.
20. The superior thyroid artery gives an anterior branch that runs down along the anterior border of the lobe, and along the upper border of the isthmus, to anastomose with the corresponding artery of the opposite side.
21. An anastomotic branch joining the superior and inferior thyroid arteries runs along the posterior border of the lobe.
22. It is important to note that:
    a. The superior thyroid artery is relatively superficial, whereas the inferior artery is very deep.
    b. The superior artery is closely related to the external laryngeal nerve. In operations for removal of the thyroid gland, the surgeon has to carefully separate the nerve from the artery before ligating the latter to avoid injury to the nerve.
23. The thyroid gland is drained by three veins—superior, middle and inferior.
    a. The veins form a plexus deep to the capsule of the gland.
    b. In order to avoid injury to them the surgeon removes the thyroid along with its true capsule.
24. The lymphatic drainage of the thyroid gland is shown in 46.9B.

## A Brief Note on Structure and Function of the Thyroid Gland

1. We have seen that the thyroid gland is covered by a fibrous ***capsule***. Septa extending into the gland from the capsule divide it into ***lobules***.
2. Each lobule is made up of an aggregation of ***follicles***.
3. Each follicle is lined by a layer of ***follicular cells***. Typical follicular cells are cubical. The follicle has a cavity that is filled by a homogeneous material called ***colloid*** (which appears pink in haematoxylin and eosin stained preparations). The follicular cells rest on a basement membrane.
4. At some places, cells of a different type intervene between the follicular cells and the basement membrane. These are called the ***parafollicular cells***.
5. The follicular cells secrete hormones that influence the rate of metabolism.
    a. Iodine is an essential constituent of these hormones.
    b. One hormone containing three atoms of iodine in each molecule is called ***triiodothyronine*** or T3.
    c. Another hormone containing four atoms of iodine is called ***tetraiodothyronine*** or T4.
6. Colloid present in the follicles is an intermediate product (iodinated thyroglobulin).
7. a. During moderate activity of the thyroid gland, the follicular cells are cubical, and a moderate amount of colloid is present in the follicles.
    b. When the gland is inactive, the follicles get distended with stored colloid and the cells are flattened.
    c. In highly active states, there is little colloid in the follicles and the cells become columnar.
8. The parafollicular cells are completely different in function from the follicular cells. They produce a hormone called ***calcitonin***, the significance of which is considered below, along with that of the parathyroid hormone.

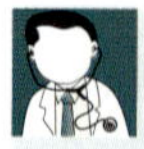

## CLINICAL CORRELATION

### Thyroid Gland

*Congenital Anomalies*

1. Parts of the thyroid (isthmus, or one lobe) may be absent.
2. A pyrimidal lobe may pass upwards from the isthmus or from one of the lobes. It may be just a short stump or may reach right up to the hyoid bone.
3. Thyroid tissue is derived from a median diverticulum arising from the floor of the primitive pharynx.
   a. In later life, the site of origin of the diverticulum lies over the posterior part of the tongue (foramen caecum).
   b. As the diverticulum elongates, it grows downwards as the thyroglossal duct. This duct lies in the midline of the neck.
   c. The tip of the diverticulum divides into two parts each of which forms one lobe of the thyroid gland.
   d. Abnormal thyroid tissue may develop anywhere along the course of the thyroglossal duct.
4. Thyroid tissue present under the mucosa of the dorsum of the tongue is called a ***lingual thyroid***.
   a. Thyroid tissue may be embedded within the lingual musculature.
   b. May lie in the midline of the neck above or below the hyoid bone.
   c. May even be found in the thorax.
5. A fact of considerable surgical importance is that before removing an abnormally situated mass of thyroid tissue the surgeon must make sure that a thyroid gland is present at the normal site. Sometimes, it may not be present.
6. Apart from these masses of thyroid tissue present along the path of the thyroglossal duct ectopic thyroid tissue may be present in other locations. These include:
   a. Larynx
   b. Trachea
   c. Oesophagus
   d. Pleura or pericardium
   e. Ovaries.
7. Remnants of the thyroglossal duct may persist and may form ***thyroglossal cysts*** that may be seen anywhere along the course of the duct.
   a. When a cyst opens on to the surface of the neck a fistula is created.
   b. In treating these conditions, the surgeon has to remove the entire track of the thyroglossal duct.
   c. The duct forms a loop deep to the hyoid bone, and part of this bone may have to be excised for complete removal of the duct.
   d. Finally note that remnants of the thyroglossal duct may give rise to a carcinoma.

*Other correlations*

1. In examining a patient in whom an enlargement of the thyroid is suspected, it is useful to remember that the thyroid moves up and down during swallowing.
2. Deficient intake of iodine (common in areas where drinking water does not contain iodine) can lead to benign enlargement of the thyroid gland. The enlarged thyroid is referred to as ***goitre***. The symptoms are those of hypothyroidism.
3. Hypothyroidism in infants leads to ***cretinism***. A child with cretinism has a puffed face with a protruding tongue, a bulky belly, and sometimes an umbilical hernia.
4. Hypothyroidism in adults is manifested by symptoms including:
   a. A slow pulse
   b. Cold intolerance
   c. Mental and physical lethargy
   d. A hoarse voice.

5. In advanced cases, the condition is called ***myxoedema***.
   a. There is deposition of mucopolysaccharides in subcutaneous tissue at various sites resulting in a non-pitting oedema.
   b. The face is bloated, the lips are thick and protuberant and the expression is dull.
6. Hypothyroidism can be caused by underdevelopment of the thyroid gland and this can be caused by maternal and fetal iodine deficiency.
7. It can also take place as a result of destruction of thyroid tissue because of carcinoma, thyroiditis, surgical removal of the thyroid gland, or prolonged use of antithyroid drugs.
8. Hyperthyroidism is also referred to as ***thyrotoxicosis***, or ***toxic goitre***.
   a. The condition is much more common in women than in men.
   b. The condition is marked by nervousness, loss of weight, tachycardia and palpitation, excitability, tremors of the outstretched hands, and exophthalmos.
   c. The most important causes are ***Graves' disease*** (or ***diffuse toxic goitre***, in which no nodules are felt on palpation of the thyroid); ***multinodular goitre***, and a ***toxic adenoma***.
9. Tumours of the thyroid may be benign or malignant.
   a. A tumour can press upon or involve the trachea, or carotid sheath. Involvement of the recurrent laryngeal nerve may occur.
   b. Upward expansion of a tumour of the thyroid is limited by the fact that the sternothyroid muscles, which cover the thyroid gland in front, are attached above to the thyroid cartilage. The tumours therefore tend to grow downwards and can even enter the thorax (retrosternal goitre).
10. An operation for removal of the thyroid gland is called ***thyroidectomy***.
   a. This may be required in some cases of hyperthyroidism.
   b. Normally, the posterior parts of the gland (and the parathyroids) are left behind.
   c. It is of interest to note that the part left behind receives an adequate blood supply through branches from the tracheal and oesophageal arteries (even after the main thyroid arteries have been ligated).
11. In thyroidectomy, the main arteries have to be cut and tied.
   a. The superior thyroid artery is intimately related to the external laryngeal artery at a high level, but they separate near the upper pole of the gland. The surgeon, therefore, always cuts this artery as near the gland as possible so that the nerve is not cut.
   b. In contrast, the inferior thyroid artery is closely related to the recurrent laryngeal nerve near the gland and has to be ligated as far away as possible from the gland.
12. Inflammation of the thyroid gland is called ***thyroiditis***. It can be caused by infection or by various other causes. The most important form of thyroiditis is caused by an autoimmune process (***autoimmune or lymphatic thyroiditis***). It is also called ***Hashimoto's disease***. The thyroid gland is enlarged and is infiltrated with lymphocytes.
13. The thyroid gland can be imaged using radioactive iodine. Different patterns of take up of iodine help in diagnosis of disorders. The parathyroid glands can also be seen.
14. Ultrasound examination of the thyroid is also a useful diagnostic technique.

## THE PARATHYROID GLANDS

1. The parathyroid glands are so called because they lie in close relationship to the thyroid gland.
2. Normally, there are two glands, one superior and one inferior, on either side, there being four glands in all. However, the number can be more or less.
3. Each gland is roughly oval and weighs about 50 mg.
4. On each side, the ***superior parathyroid gland*** lies near the middle of the posterior border of the thyroid gland. It is relatively constant in position.

5. The ***inferior parathyroid gland*** lies near the lower end of the posterior border of the thyroid gland.
   a. Its position is variable. It may lie above or below the inferior thyroid artery.
   b. It may lie outside the false capsule of the thyroid, between the false and true capsules; or deep to the true capsule within the substance of the thyroid.
   c. Occasionally, the inferior parathyroid gland may lie below the level of the thyroid gland, and may even descend into the superior or posterior mediastinum.
6. The superior parathyroid gland receives a branch from the anastomotic channel connecting the superior and inferior thyroid arteries. The inferior gland receives a branch from the inferior thyroid artery.

### A Brief Note on Parathyroid Structure and Function

1. The parathyroid glands consist essentially of columns of cells separated by sinusoids.
2. The cells are of two types:
   a. The large majority of cells are called ***chief cells*** or ***principal cells.***
   b. Cells of the second type are called ***oxyphil or eosinophil cells*** as they contain granular structures that stain with eosin.
3. The parathyroid glands produce a hormone called the ***parathyroid hormone*** (PTH) or ***parathormone***.
   a. This hormone helps to maintain a suitable level of calcium ions in blood.
   b. When there is a tendency for serum calcium levels to fall calcium is removed from stores in bone bringing serum levels back to normal.
   c. Simultaneously, the excretion of calcium by the kidney is decreased, and calcium absorption by the intestines is increased.
4. Calcitonin secreted by the parafollicular cells of the thyroid gland has effects opposite to those of the parathyroid hormone. A decrease in serum calcium levels stimulates the secretion of parathyroid hormone, while an increase stimulates the secretion of calcitonin.

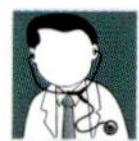

### CLINICAL CORRELATION

#### Parathyroid Glands

1. The variations in position of parathyroid glands described above are of considerable importance to a surgeon trying to locate the glands.
2. The parathyroid glands can be seen when the thyroid is imaged using radioactive iodine. The areas where radioactive materials are located can be recorded on a gamma camera. Computer separation of images reveals the location of the parathyroids.

*Hyperparathyroidism*

3. Excessive amounts of circulating parathormone can be present in tumours of the parathyroid gland (***parathyroid adenoma***).
   a. As a result calcium is depleted from bones that become weak (and can fracture).
   b. Increased urinary excretion of calcium may lead to formation of urinary calculi.

*Hypoparathyroidism*

4. Calcium levels in blood fall leading to muscular irritability and convulsions. The condition may be spontaneous or may occur following accidental removal of parathyroid glands during thyroidectomy.

## THE CAROTID SINUS

1. The term carotid sinus is applied to a dilated segment of the common carotid body located at its bifurcation. The dilatation usually extends on to the initial part of the internal carotid artery, and may be confined to it.

### WANT TO KNOW MORE?

2. In the region of the dilatation, the tunica media in the arterial wall is thin, but the adventitia is thick.
3. Numerous nerve endings are seen in the adventitia.
4. The region of the carotid sinus is surrounded by a nerve plexus.
   a. The main contribution to this plexus is by the carotid branch of the glossopharyngeal nerve.
   b. The plexus also receives fibres from the superior cervical sympathetic ganglion, and from the vagus nerve.
5. The afferent nerve terminals present over the carotid sinus are stimulated by alterations in blood pressure. Afferent impulses arising from the sinus play an important role in reflex control of blood pressure.

## THE CAROTID BODIES AND PARAGANGLIA

1. These are small oval structures, present one on each side of the neck, at the bifurcation of the common carotid artery (i.e., near the carotid sinus).
2. The main function of the carotid bodies is that they act as chemoreceptors that monitor the oxygen and carbon dioxide levels in blood.
   a. They exercise reflex control on the rate and depth of respiration through respiratory centres located in the brainstem.
   b. In addition to this function the carotid bodies are also believed to have an endocrine function.
3. The most conspicuous cells of the carotid body are called ***glomus cells*** (or type I cells). These are large cells that have several similarities to neurons.
4. Apart from the glomus cells various other cells present in the carotid bodies. They include a few sympathetic and parasympathetic postganglionic neurons.
5. The carotid bodies are included under the general heading of ***paraganglia***. This term is used to describe small collections of neuroendocrine cells present in association with autonomic nerves.
   a. Structures similar to the carotid bodies, present in relation to the inferior aspect of the arch of the aorta are also included in paraganglia.
   b. They are called the ***aortic bodies***, or ***aortico-pulmonary paraganglia***.

# 47 CHAPTER

# Surface Marking and Radiological Anatomy of Head and Neck

## SURFACE MARKING

The study of the surface projections of various structures is best undertaken while studying their gross anatomy. For sake of convenience in revision the descriptions are grouped together in this chapter.

## SURFACE MARKING OF SOME VISCERA

### Parotid Gland

The parotid gland has been described on page 760. Its projection on the surface can be marked as follows:

1. To mark the ***anterior border***, begin at the upper border of the head of the mandible.
   a. Draw a line downwards and forwards to reach the centre of the masseter muscle.
   b. Now carry the line downwards and backwards to reach a point just posteroinferior to the angle of the mandible.
2. To mark the ***posterior border*** begin at the lower end of the anterior border. Draw a line upwards to reach the anterior border of the mastoid process, near its upper end.
3. To mark the ***superior border*** join the upper ends of the posterior and anterior borders by a line that is convex downwards.
   a. This line corresponds to the lower part of the margin of the external acoustic meatus.
   b. It can be marked on the lobule of the ear, but it is more useful to mark it by lifting the lobule upwards.

#### *Parotid Duct*

1. Draw a line running forwards from the lower border of the tragus to a point midway between the ala of the nose and the upper lip.
2. Divide this line into three parts.
3. The position of the parotid duct corresponds to the middle one-third of this line.

### Thyroid Gland

The thyroid gland has been described in chapter 45. Before marking the gland you must have an idea of its shape and of its division into the isthmus and the right and left lobes.

1. To mark the isthmus of the gland, begin by feeling the lower border of the arch of the cricoid cartilage.
   a. Take one point half an inch below the border of the cricoid cartilage, and another point half inch lower down (Remember that one-inch is equal to 2.5 cm approximately).
   b. At each of these levels draw transverse lines, half an inch long. These lines represent the upper and lower borders of the isthmus.
2. Each lobe of the thyroid gland is marked as follows:
   a. To mark the anterior border start at the lateral end of the upper border of the isthmus (marked above).
   b. Carry the line upwards and slightly backwards to reach the anterior border of the sternocleidomastoid muscle, at the level of the middle of the thyroid cartilage.

c. To mark the posterior border, begin at the upper end of the anterior border.
d. Draw a line running downwards (with a slight backward convexity) to reach the clavicle.
e. To complete the marking of the lobe, join the lower end of the posterior border to the lateral end of the lower border of the isthmus by a broad line convex downwards.

### Submandibular Gland

The submandibular gland has been described on page 779.

1. The outline of this gland is oval. To mark it feel the angle of the mandible.
2. To draw the upper margin of the gland, draw a line convex upwards, starting at the angle and reaching the middle of the base of the mandible.
3. To mark the lower margin of the gland join the two ends of the upper margin (drawn as described above) by a line convex downwards.
4. The curve should extend below to the level of the greater cornu of the hyoid bone.

#### *Palatine Tonsil*

The palatine tonsil is described on page 996.

1. To mark it draw a small oval just in front of, and above, the angle of the mandible.
2. The marking will lie over the masseter muscle.

## PARANASAL SINUSES

The paranasal sinuses have been described on page 988. We will consider the surface marking only of the frontal and maxillary sinuses (as these are large and lie near the surface).

### Frontal Air Sinus

1. The projection of this sinus lies above the medial part of the orbit. It is triangular.
2. To mark the medial border of the sinus draw a vertical line one inch (2.5 cm) long over the lower part of the forehead, in the middle line.
   a. The lower end of the line should be just above the depression between the forehead and the upper end of the nose.
   b. (The point corresponds to the ***nasion*** that is the point at which the internasal and frontonasal sutures meet).
3. To mark the lower border of the sinus draw a line starting at the lower end of the medial border, and passing laterally and slightly upwards to reach the upper margin of the orbit. The line should lie just above the medial one-third of the superior orbital margin.
4. The third border (above and laterally) is drawn by joining the upper end of the medial border with the lateral end of the lower border.

### Maxillary Sinus

1. The outline of this sinus is irregular. It can be marked on the face following the outline of the maxilla.
2. Above, the line is just below the orbit.
3. Below, the line lies just above the alveolar process of the maxilla.
4. Medially it reaches the lateral wall of the nose.
5. Laterally it reaches the zygomatic process of the maxilla.

## ARTERIES

### Common Carotid Artery

1. The common carotid artery has been described on page 833.
2. The left artery runs part of its course in the thorax where its surface marking has been studied in an earlier chapter.
3. In the neck the position of the artery is similar on both sides.

4. To mark the artery draw a broad line:
   a. Starting over the sternoclavicular joint.
   b. Passing upwards along the anterior border of the sternocleidomastoid muscle.
   c. Ending at the level of the upper border of the thyroid cartilage.

### Internal Carotid Artery

The internal carotid artery has been described on page 834.

1. The lower end of this artery corresponds to the termination of the common carotid artery.
2. It lies over the anterior border of the sternocleidomastoid muscle at the level of the upper border of the thyroid cartilage.
3. From this level draw a broad line running upwards and ending just behind the condyle of the mandible.

### External Carotid Artery

The external carotid artery has been described on page 838.

1. The lower end of this artery corresponds to the termination of the common carotid artery.
2. It lies over the anterior border of the sternocleidomastoid muscle at the level of the thyroid cartilage.
3. From here draw a line upwards to end just behind the neck of the mandible.
4. The line should be slightly convex forwards in its lower half, and slightly convex backwards in its upper half.

### Subclavian Artery

The subclavian artery has been described on page 847.

1. The left subclavian artery runs part of its course in the thorax where its surface marking has been described earlier. The course of the right and left arteries is similar in the neck.
2. The artery can be marked by drawing a broad line:
   a. Beginning over the sternoclavicular joint.
   b. Passing laterally with an upward convexity to a point over the middle of the clavicle.
   c. The highest point of the upward convexity rises 2 cm above the clavicle.

### Facial Artery

The facial artery has been described on page 841.

1. We have seen that the artery runs part of its course in the neck, and passes through the submandibular region before entering the face. Its course in the face can be marked as follows.
2. Ask the subject to clench his teeth. This makes the masseter prominent and its anterior border can be felt.
3. The facial artery enters the face where the anterior border of the masseter cuts the lower border of the mandible. The pulsations of the artery can be felt here.
4. From here the artery runs upwards and forwards to reach a point half an inch (1.2 cm) lateral to the angle of the mouth.
5. It then bends more sharply upwards to reach the medial angle of the eye.

### Middle Meningeal Artery

This artery has been described in chapter 42. Its relationship to the surface of the skull is shown in 42.21. The artery can be marked as follows:

1. Feel the zygomatic arch (zygoma) and take its midpoint. This is the level at which the artery enters the skull.
2. Draw a line vertically upwards from this point for 2 cm. This line represents the stem of the artery. The artery divides into frontal and parietal branches at the upper end of this line.
3. The frontal branch is marked as follows.
   a. Draw a line starting at the upper end of the main stem (see above) and running upwards with a forwards convexity (42.21).

   b. The upper end of the line ends over the centre of pterion which lies 3.5 cm behind and 1.5 cm above the frontozygomatic suture.
   c. From here the frontal branch runs upwards and backwards to end approximately midway between the root of the nose and the external occipital protuberance.
4. The parietal branch begins at the upper end of the main stem of the middle meningeal artery (see above). It runs backwards to a point about 6 cm above the external occipital protuberance.

## VEINS

### Internal Jugular Vein

The internal jugular vein has been described on page 854.

1. The upper end of the vein lies on the neck just deep to the lobule of the ear.
2. Its lower end lies deep to the medial end of the clavicle.
3. The vein can be marked by drawing a broad line joining these points.

### Subclavian Vein

The subclavian vein has been described on page 855.

1. Its lateral end lies behind the clavicle a little medial to its midpoint.
2. Its medial end lies behind the medial end of the clavicle.
3. The vein can be marked as a broad line over the clavicle joining these points.
4. Note that the vein lies at a lower level than the subclavian artery.

### External Jugular Vein

This vein has been described on page 863.

1. Its upper end lies a little behind and below the angle of the mandible.
2. The vein runs downwards across the sternocleidomastoid and ends deep to the clavicle immediately behind the sternocleidomastoid muscle.
3. The vein can be marked by drawing a line joining these points.
4. The vein can often be seen in the living subject.

## INTRACRANIAL VENOUS SINUSES

The intracranial venous sinuses have been described on page 855.

### Superior Sagittal Sinus

1. The relationship of this sinus to the surface of the body is simple.
2. It lies in the midline of the vault of the skull.
3. Its anterior end reaches the raised area between the right and left eyebrows (glabella).
4. Its posterior end reaches the external occipital protuberance.
5. The sinus is narrow at its anterior end. At the posterior end it is about 1 cm broad.

### Transverse Sinus

1. The sinus is about 1 cm broad.
2. Its posterior end (beginning) lies deep to the external occipital protuberance.
3. Its anterior end lies deep to the mastoid process.
4. The sinus is marked by a line joining these points.
5. The line should be drawn with an upward convexity.

### Sigmoid Sinus

1. This sinus is also about 1 cm broad.
2. It begins where the transverse sinus ends i.e., deep to the upper part of the mastoid process.
3. Its lower end lies about 1 cm above the tip of the mastoid process.
4. The line joining the two points is short because of foreshortening of the projection.

## NERVES

Of the many nerves to be seen in the head and neck the surface projection of only a few is considered below. The nerves considered are those than can be approached surgically from the surface (It is always useful to read the course of the nerve before trying to understand surface marking).

### Some Branches of Trigeminal Nerve

1. The ***mandibular nerve*** is described on page 901.
2. The *main stem* of the mandibular nerve can be marked on the surface as a short vertical line just in front of the head of the mandible.
3. The ***auriculotemporal nerve*** is described on page 903.
4. It can be marked by a line that runs backwards from the main stem of the mandibular nerve, across the neck of the mandible.
5. The nerve then turns upwards passing immediately in front of the tragus (preauricular point).
6. The ***lingual nerve*** is described on page 903.
7. To mark it draw a line continuous with the main stem of the mandibular nerve (see above).
8. It is represented by a line that runs downwards and forwards to reach opposite the lower third molar tooth.
9. It then runs forwards in relation to the mandible up to the level of the first molar tooth.

#### *Facial Nerve*

The facial nerve is described on page 908.

1. It is useful only to mark the extracranial part of the nerve, before it divides into several branches.
2. Remember that the nerve emerges from the skull through the stylomastoid foramen.
3. This foramen lies deep to the middle of the anterior border of the mastoid process (In the adult, the nerve lies at a depth of 2 cm, but the depth is much less in children).
4. From here draw a horizontal line that runs forwards to end just behind the neck of the mandible.

#### *Glossopharyngeal Nerve*

The glossopharyngeal nerve is described on page 918-19.

1. This nerve is marked by a line that runs downwards and forwards with a downward convexity.
2. The line begins over the tragus and runs to the angle of the mandible.
3. It then runs for a short distance along the lower border of the mandible.

#### *Vagus Nerve*

The vagus nerve is described on page 923.

1. It can be represented by a straight line running down the entire length of the neck.
2. The upper end of the line should lie over the anterior part of the tragus.
3. The lower end should lie over the medial end of the clavicle.

#### *Spinal Accessory Nerve*

This nerve is described on page 927.

1. Its upper end lies over the same point as for the vagus (i.e., over the anterior part of the tragus).

2. From here draw a line downwards and backwards to reach a point midway between the mastoid process and the angle of the mandible.
3. (Deep pressure here will show that the point lies over the transverse process of the atlas).
4. From this point carry the line further downwards and backwards to reach the middle of the posterior border of the sternocleidomastoid muscle.
5. The nerve then runs across the posterior triangle to reach the anterior border of the trapezius about two inches above the clavicle.

### *Phrenic Nerve*

This nerve is described on page 873.

1. To mark this nerve first feel for the upper border of the thyroid cartilage.
2. At this level take a point 3.5 cm from the anterior midline of the neck. This is the upper end of the nerve.
3. From here draw a line downwards and medially to reach the medial end of the clavicle.

### *Sympathetic Chain in the Neck*

This is described in chapter 43.

1. To mark this chain remember that it runs vertically immediately behind the carotid sheath.
2. Its upper end lies just behind the condyle of the mandible.
3. Its lower end lies over the sternoclavicular joint.

## RADIOLOGICAL ANATOMY

Some radiographs of the head and neck are shown in 47.1 to 47.4.

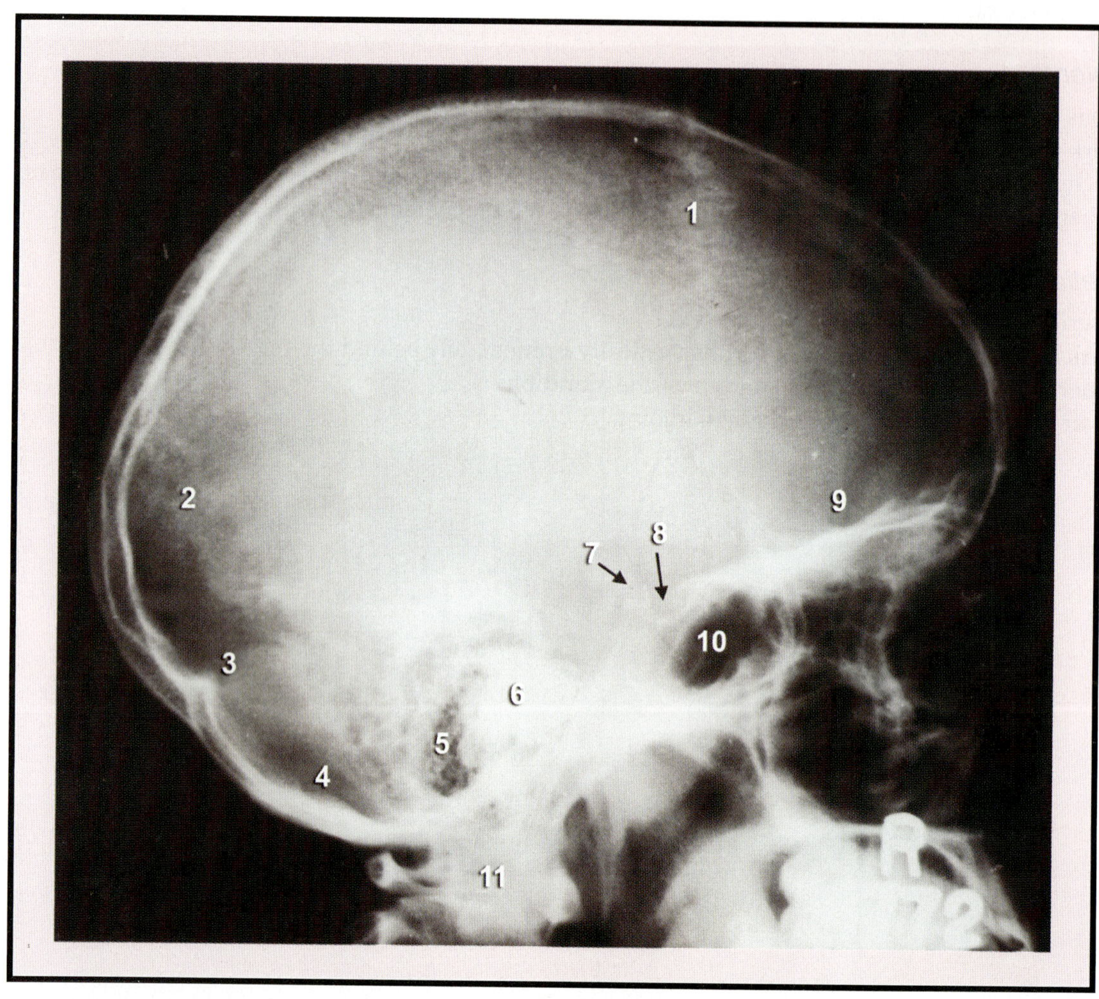


**47.1:** Radiograph of the skull, lateral view. 1: Coronal suture; 2: Lambdoid suture; 3: Internal occipital protuberance; 4: Floor of posterior cranial fossa; 5: Mastoid air cells; 6: Petrous temporal bone; 7: Dorsum sellae; 8: Hypophyseal fossa; 9: Floor of anterior cranial fossa; 10: Sphenoidal sinus; 11: Cervical vertebrae

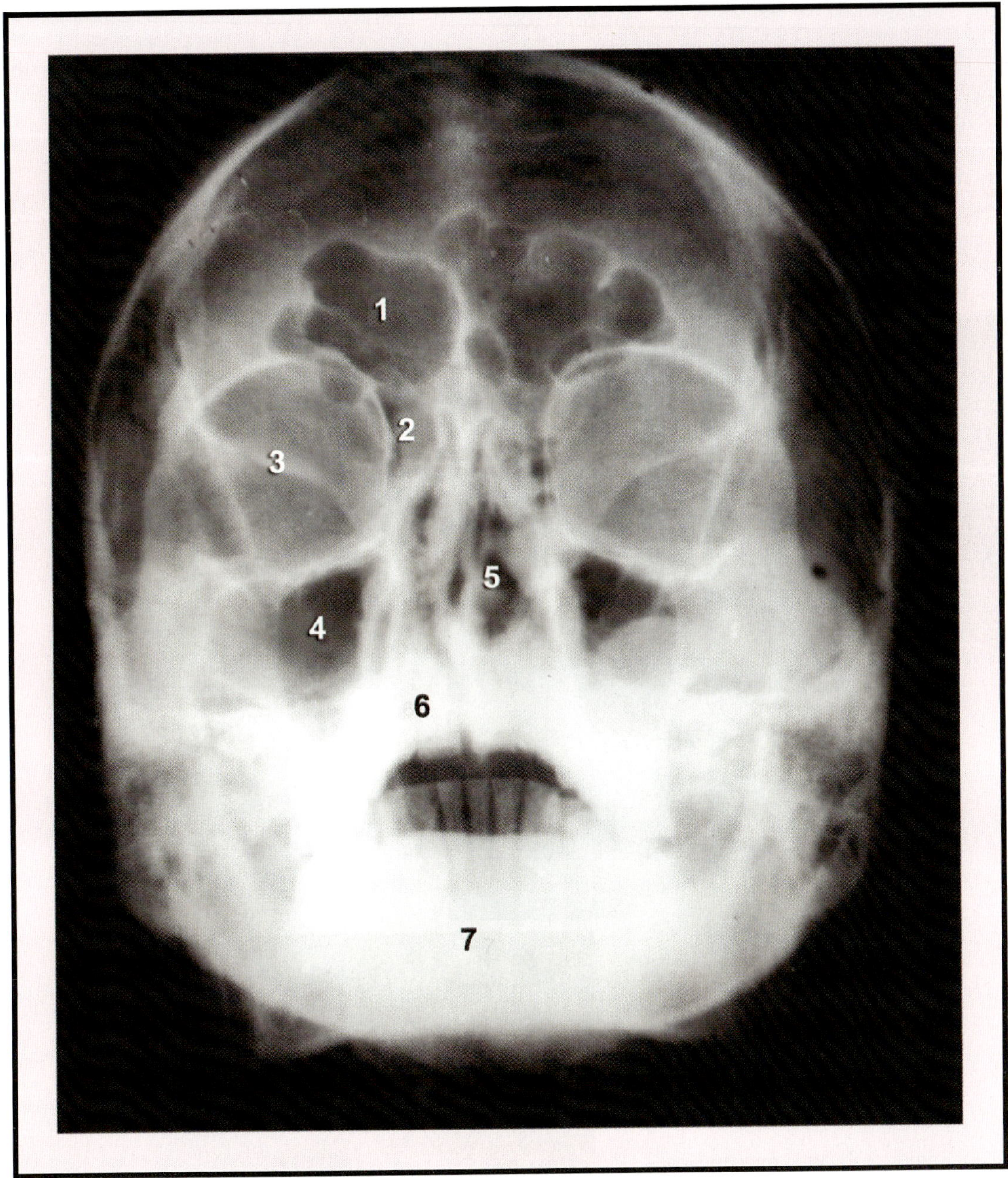


**47.2:** Radiograph of the skull to show paranasal sinuses (PNS view).
1: Frontal sinus; 2: Ethmoidal sinuses; 3: Orbit; 4: Maxillary sinus;
5: Nasal cavity; 6: Maxilla; 7: Mandible

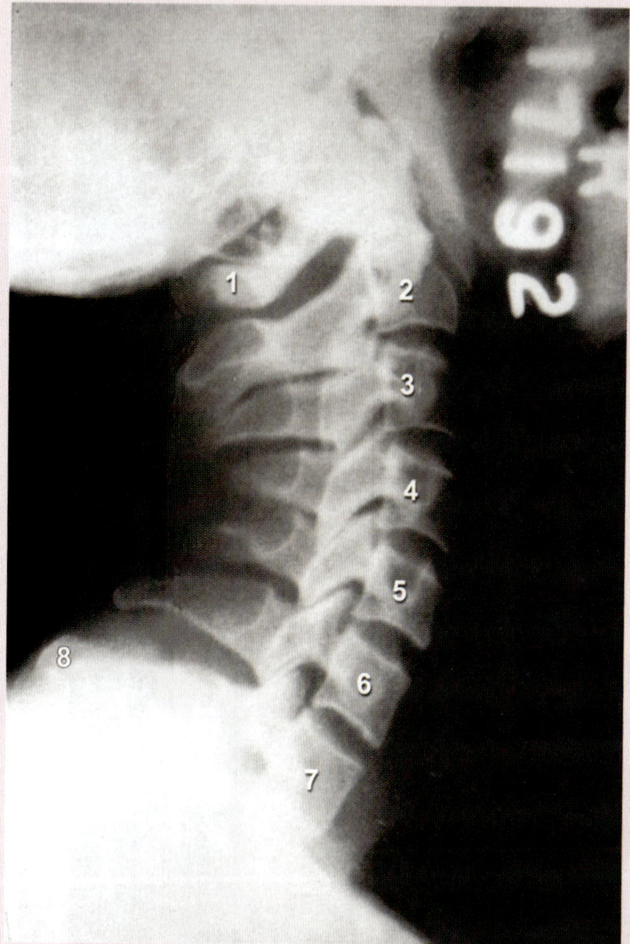


**47.3:** Radiograph to show the cervical spine (lateral view).

1: Posterior arch of atlas;
2 to 7: Bodies of second to seventh cervical vertebrae;
8: Tip of spine of C7

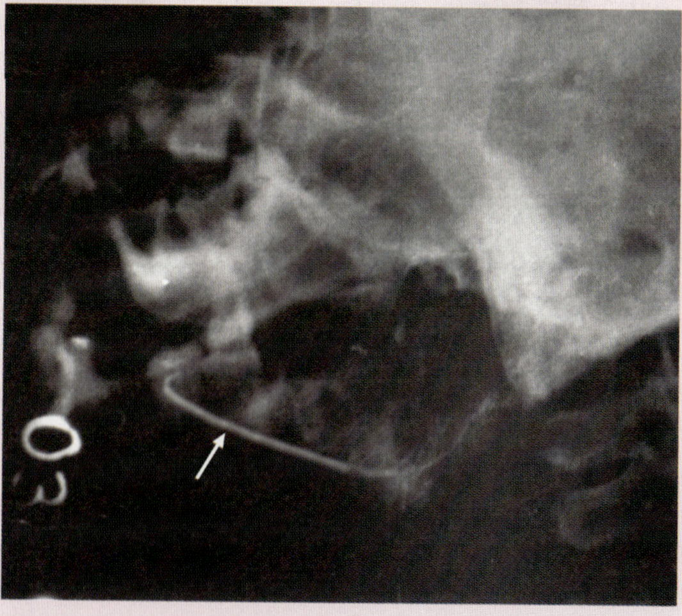

**47.4:** Radiograph after injecting contrast medium into the submandibular duct (Sialography). The arrow points to the duct

# PART 6

# Central Nervous System

# 48 CHAPTER

# Introduction to Central Nervous System and Internal Structure of Spinal Cord

## INTRODUCTION TO THE CENTRAL NERVOUS SYSTEM

1. The *central nervous system* is made up of the brain and spinal cord. In contrast, the *peripheral nervous system* consists of the cranial nerves and the spinal nerves.
2. The brain consists of:
   a. The cerebrum, made up of two large cerebral hemispheres
   b. The cerebellum
   c. The brainstem.
3. The brainstem is made up of:
   a. The midbrain
   b. The pons
   c. The medulla oblongata. The medulla oblongata is continuous with the spinal cord.

### Some Elementary Facts About Neurons

1. The nervous system is made up, predominantly, of tissue that has the special property of being able to conduct impulses rapidly from one part of the body to another.
2. The specialised cells that constitute the functional units of the nervous system are called ***neurons***.
3. Within the brain and spinal cord, neurons are supported by a special kind of connective tissue that is called ***neuroglia.***
4. Nervous tissue, composed of neurons and neuroglia, is richly supplied with blood, but lymph vessels are not present.

### The Neuron

1. A neuron consists of a ***cell body*** that gives off a variable number of ***processes***.
2. The cell body is also called the ***soma*** or ***perikaryon***.
3. The processes arising from the cell body of a neuron are called ***neurites.*** These are of two kinds:
   a. Most neurons give off a number of short branching processes called ***dendrites*** and one longer process called an ***axon.***
   b. There are various structural differences between dendrites and axons.
   c. However, the most important difference is functional. In a dendrite, the nerve impulse travels ***towards the cell body*** whereas in an axon the impulse travels ***away from the cell body.***
4. Peripheral nerves are made up of aggregations of axons (and in some cases of dendrites).
5. During its formation, each axon (and some dendrites) comes to be associated with certain cells that provide a sheath for it.
   a. The cells providing this sheath for axons lying outside the central nervous system are called ***Schwann cells***.
   b. Axons lying within the central nervous system are provided a similar covering by a kind of neuroglial cell called an ***oligodendrocyte***.

6. All nerve fibres in peripheral nerves have an outer sheath called the ***neurilemma***. This forms the outer covering of the nerve fibre.
7. Deep to the neurilemma, most nerve fibres also have a second sheath that is rich in lipids. This is the ***myelin sheath***.
8. Axons having a myelin sheath are called ***myelinated axons***. Those without this sheath are ***unmyelinated axons***.
9. An axon (or its branches) can terminate in two ways:
   a. Within the central nervous system, it always terminates by coming in intimate relationship with another neuron, the junction between the two neurons being called a ***synapse***.
   b. Outside the central nervous system, the axon may end in relation to an effector organ (e.g., muscle or gland), or may end by synapsing with neurons in a peripheral ganglion.
10. Neurons vary considerably in the size and shape of their cell bodies (somata) and in the length and manner of branching of their processes.
    a. The shape of the cell body is dependent on the number of processes arising from it.
    b. The most common type of neuron gives off several processes and the cell body is, therefore, ***multipolar***.
    c. Some neurons have only one axon and one dendrite and are ***bipolar.***
    d. Another type of neuron has a single process and is therefore described as ***unipolar***. However, this process almost immediately divides into two. One of the divisions represents the axon; the other is functionally a dendrite, but its structure is indistinguishable from that of an axon.
    e. Depending on the shapes of their cell bodies some neurons are referred to as ***stellate*** (star shaped) or ***pyramidal.***
11. Apart from structural differences neurons can also be classified on the basis of their functions.
    a. A classification of types of nerve fibres to be seen in peripheral nerves; and the arrangement of neurons giving origin to various functional types of nerve fibres has been discussed in chapter 43.
    b. These descriptions will be essential in understanding some aspects of the structure of the brain.

### *Grey and White Matter*

1. Sections through the spinal cord or through any part of the brain show certain regions that appear whitish, and others that have a darker greyish colour. These constitute the ***white*** and ***grey matter*** respectively.
2. Microscopic examination shows that the grey matter contains:
   a. Cell bodies of neurons
   b. Dendrites and axons starting from or ending on the cell bodies.
3. Most of the fibres within the grey matter are unmyelinated.
4. On the other hand, the white matter consists predominantly of myelinated fibres. It is the reflection of light by myelin that gives this region its whitish appearance.
5. Neuroglia and blood vessels are present in both grey and white matter.
6. The arrangement of the grey and white matter differs at different situations in the brain and spinal cord.
   a. In the spinal cord and brainstem the white matter is on the outside whereas the grey matter forms one or more masses embedded within the white matter.
   b. In the cerebrum and cerebellum there is an extensive, but thin, layer of grey matter on the surface. This layer is called the ***cortex***.
   c. Deep to the cortex there is white matter, but within the latter several isolated masses of grey matter are present. Such isolated masses of grey matter, present anywhere in the central nervous system, are referred to as ***nuclei.***
   d. As grey matter is made of cell bodies of neurons (and the processes arising from or terminating on them) nuclei can be defined as groups of cell bodies of neurons.
7. Aggregations of the cell bodies of neurons may also be found outside the central nervous system. Such aggregations are referred to as ***ganglia.***
8. Ganglia are of two distinct functional types.
9. ***Sensory ganglia*** contain neurons that give off processes that form the afferent fibres of peripheral nerves. Examples of sensory ganglia are the dorsal nerve root ganglia of spinal nerves, and the trigeminal ganglion.

10. ***Autonomic ganglia*** include ***sympathetic ganglia*** located on the sympathetic chain, and ***parasympathetic ganglia***. Examples of the latter are the ciliary ganglion and the submandibular ganglion.
11. Some autonomic neurons are located in ***nerve plexuses*** (often called ganglia) present in close relationship to some viscera.
12. The axons arising in one mass of grey matter terminate very frequently by synapsing with neurons in other masses of grey matter.
    a. The axons connecting two (or more) masses of grey matter are frequently numerous enough to form recognisable bundles.
    b. Such aggregations of fibres are called ***tracts***.
    c. Larger collections of fibres are also referred to as ***funiculi, fasciculi*** or ***lemnisci***.
    d. Large bundles of fibres connecting the cerebral or cerebellar hemispheres to the brainstem are called ***peduncles.***

## Arrangement of Neurons within the Central Nervous System

The various functional categories of nerve fibres present in peripheral nerves, and the arrangement of neurons associated with these fibres, has been described in chapter 43.

1. We have seen that neurons giving rise to fibres of peripheral nerves are basically of two types as follows:
    a. Neurons having cell bodies that lie within the brain and spinal cord, send out efferent processes that leave the CNS to form the motor fibres of peripheral nerves.
    b. Neurons having cell bodies located in ganglia outside the CNS, give origin to peripheral processes that form afferent nerve fibres of peripheral nerves. Their central processes form the sensory roots of the nerves in question. They enter the brain or spinal cord and synapse with neurons within them.
2. The bulk of the CNS is, however, made up of neurons that lie entirely within it.
    a. As explained earlier, the cell bodies of these neurons are invariably located in masses of grey matter.
    b. The axons may be short, ending in close relation to the cell body, or may be long and may travel to other masses of grey matter lying at considerable distances from the grey matter of origin.
3. The neurons within the CNS are interconnected in an extremely intricate manner. The description that follows illustrates some of the basic arrangements encountered.
4. The simplest pathways are those concerned with reflex activities, such as the contraction of a muscle in response to an external stimulus. For example, if the skin of the sole of a sleeping person is scratched, the leg is reflexly drawn up. Let us see how this happens.
5. The simplest possible arrangement is shown in 48.1.
    a. The stimulus applied to skin gives rise to a nerve impulse that is carried by the peripheral process of a unipolar neuron to the dorsal nerve root ganglion.
    b. From here the impulse passes into the central process that terminates by directly synapsing with an anterior grey column cell supplying the muscle which draws the leg up.
    c. The complete pathway constitutes a ***reflex arc*** and in the above example it consists of two neurons — one afferent and the other efferent.
6. In actual practice, however, the reflex arc is generally made up of three neurons as shown in 48.2.
    a. The central process of the dorsal nerve root ganglion cell ends by synapsing with a neuron lying in the posterior grey column.
    b. This neuron has a short axon that ends by synapsing with a neuron in the anterior grey column, thus completing the reflex arc.
    c. The third neuron interposed between the afferent and efferent neurons is called an ***internuncial neuron,*** or simply an ***interneuron.***
7. The purpose served by an interneuron may be basically of three types:
    a. Firstly, the axon arising from an interneuron may divide into a number of branches and may synapse with a number of different efferent neurons. As a result an impulse coming along a single afferent neuron may result in an effector response by a large number of efferent neurons.

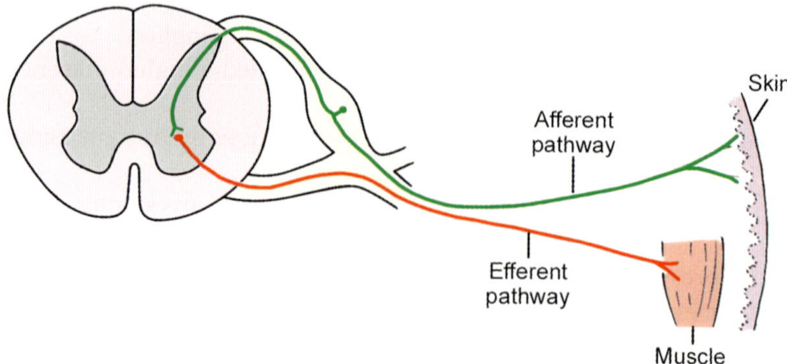


**48.1:** A spinal reflex arc composed of two neurons

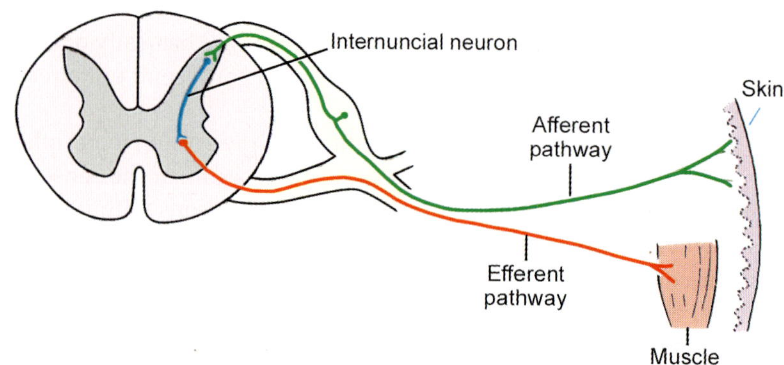


**48.2:** A spinal reflex arc composed of three neurons

   b. Secondly, afferent impulses brought by a number of afferent neurons may converge on a single efferent neuron through the agency of interneurons.

8. Some of these impulses tend to induce activity in the efferent neuron (i.e., they are ***facilitatory)*** while others tend to suppress activity (i.e., they are ***inhibitory).***
9. Thirdly, through interneurons an afferent neuron may establish contact with efferent neurons in the opposite half of the spinal cord, or in a higher or lower segment of the cord.
10. Every time a stimulus reaches a neuron it does not mean that it must become active and must produce an impulse.
    a. A neuron receives inputs from many neurons (in some cases from hundreds of them).
    b. Some of these inputs are facilitatory and others are inhibitory.
    c. Activity in the neuron (in the form of initiation of an impulse) depends on the sum total of these inputs.
11. Thus, each neuron may be regarded as a decision-making centre.
    a. The greater the number of neurons involved in any pathway, the greater the possibility of such interactions.
    b. Viewed in this light it will become clear that interneurons interposed in a pathway increase the number of levels at which 'decisions' can be taken.
    c. It will also be appreciated that most of the neurons within the nervous system are, in this sense, interneurons that are involved in numerous highly complex interactions on which the working of the nervous system depends.
12. From what has been said above it will be seen that some activities occur due to reflex action, and may involve only neurons within the spinal cord.

   a. However, most activities of the spinal cord are subjected to influence from higher centres.
   b. In the more complicated types of activity, several higher centres may be involved and the pathways may be extremely complicated.
13. Afferent impulses reaching these higher centres (e.g., the cerebral cortex) would appear to be somehow stored and this stored information (of which we may or may not be conscious) is used to guide responses to similar stimuli received in future. This accounts for memory and for learning processes.
14. From the above it will be appreciated that in a study of the nervous system we must first of all have some knowledge of the various masses of grey matter in the CNS and of their interconnections.
15. To this end we will begin by studying the internal structure of the spinal cord below.

### Projection, Association and Commissural Fibres

1. When a considerable number of fibres pass from a mass of grey matter in one part of the brain to another mass of grey matter in another part of the brain or spinal cord, these are referred to as ***projection fibres.***
2. Fibres interconnecting different areas of the cerebral cortex or of the cerebellar cortex are called ***association fibres.***
3. Fibres connecting identical areas of the two halves of the brain are called ***commissural fibres.***
4. When fibres originating in a mass of grey matter in one-half of the CNS end in some other mass of grey matter in the opposite half they are referred to as ***decussating fibres,*** and the sites where such crossings take place are referred to as ***decussations.***

## INTERNAL STRUCTURE OF SPINAL CORD

1. The gross anatomy of the spinal cord, and some elementary facts about its internal structure, have been described in Chapter 40. The concept of spinal segments, and the relationship of the spinal cord to spinal nerves has also been examined therein.
2. We have seen that the grey matter of the spinal cord is divided into ventral, dorsal and lateral columns, and that the white matter is divided into anterior, posterior, and lateral funiculi.
3. The relative amount of grey and white matter, and the shape and size of the grey columns, vary at different levels of the spinal cord (48.3).
   a. The amount of grey matter to be seen at a particular level can be correlated with the mass of tissue to be supplied.
   b. It is, therefore, greatest in the region of the cervical and lumbar enlargements that supply the limbs.
   c. The amount of white matter undergoes progressive increase as we proceed up the spinal cord. This is a result of the fact that:
      (i) Progressively more and more ascending fibres are added as we pass up the cord.
      (ii) The number of descending fibres decreases as we go down the cord as some of them terminate in each segment.

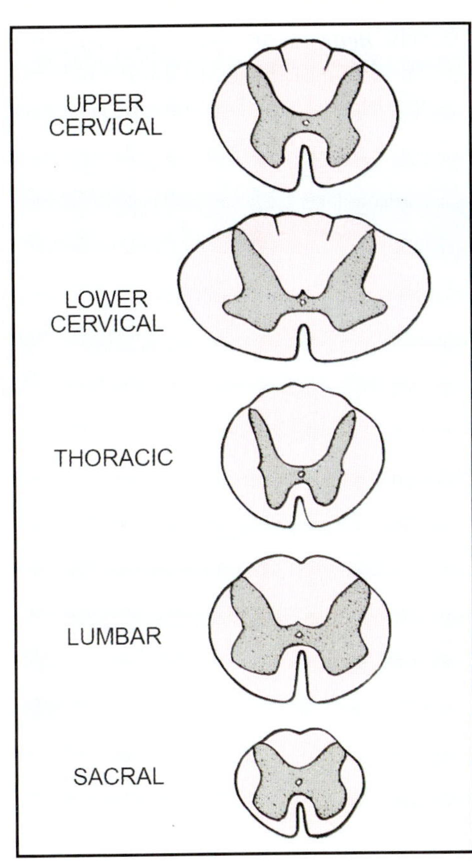


**48.3:** Diagrams to show differences in appearance of transverse sections through various levels of the spinal cord

### Subdivisions of Grey Matter

The grey matter of the spinal cord may be subdivided in more than one manner.

1. Traditionally, the ventral grey column has been divided into a ventral part, the ***head***, and a dorsal part, the ***base.***
2. Similarly, the dorsal grey column has been subdivided (from anterior to posterior side) into a ***base***, a ***neck***, and a ***head***. These subdivisions have, however, been found to have little importance.

3. An attempt has been made to recognise discrete collections of neurons (or nuclei) in various regions of the spinal grey matter. These are illustrated in the left half of 48.4 and will not be described in detail. However, identify the following:
   a. ***Substantia gelatinosa*** near the apex of the dorsal column.
   b. ***Dorsal nucleus*** (also called the thoracic nucleus or Clark's column) lying on the medial side of the base.
   c. Between the ventral and dorsal grey columns an intermediate zone is sometimes described. This contains the ***intermediolateral*** and ***intermediomedial*** nuclei.
4. Recent studies have shown that from the point of view of neuronal connections the grey matter of the spinal cord may be divided into ten areas or laminae. These are illustrated in the right half of 48.4.

## Significance of Neurons in Grey Matter of Spinal Cord

1. The ***ventral column neurons*** of the spinal cord may be functionally divided into three major categories as follows:
   a. The most prominent neurons with large cell bodies and prominent Nissl substance are designated ***alpha neurons***. These are somatic efferent neurons. Their axons (***alpha efferents***) leave the spinal cord through the ventral nerve roots of spinal nerves and innervate striated muscle.
   b. Some smaller neurons designated as ***gamma neurons*** are also located in lamina IX. They supply intrafusal fibres of muscle spindles.
   c. A considerable number of smaller neurons in the ventral grey column are internuncial neurons.
2. Another variety of neuron that is believed (on physiological grounds) to exist in the ventral grey column is the so-called ***Renshaw cell***.
3. The ***neurons of the dorsal grey column*** may be subdivided as follows:
   a. Some of these are internuncial neurons.
   b. Many dorsal column neurons receive afferent impulses through the central processes of neurons in dorsal nerve root ganglia.

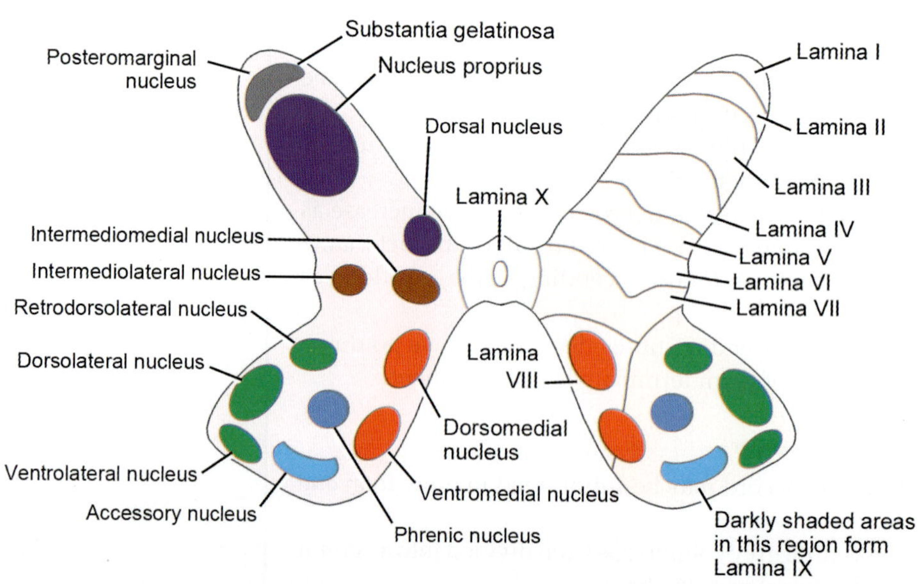


**48.4:** Subdivisions of grey matter of the spinal cord. The left half of the figure shows the cell groups as usually described. The right half shows the concept of laminae

4. These dorsal column neurons give off axons that enter the white matter of the spinal cord either on the same or opposite side. These axons may behave in one of the following ways:
   a. They may ascend or descend for some segments before terminating in relation to neurons at other levels of the spinal cord. Such axons constitute ***intersegmental tracts.***
   b. A considerable number of axons arising from dorsal column neurons run upwards in the spinal cord and constitute ***ascending tracts*** that terminate in various masses of grey matter in the brain. These tracts form a considerable part of the white matter of the spinal cord.
5. The ***neurons of the intermediolateral group*** (lateral grey column) are visceral efferent neurons. They are present at two levels of the spinal cord.
6. One group is present in the thoracic and upper two or three lumbar segments.
   a. These are preganglionic neurons of the sympathetic nervous system.
   b. Their axons terminate in relation to postganglionic neurons in sympathetic ganglia (and occasionally in some other situations).
   c. Axons of these postganglionic neurons are distributed to various organs, and to blood vessels.
7. The second group of visceral efferent neurons is found in the second, third and fourth sacral segments of the spinal cord.
   a. These are preganglionic neurons of the parasympathetic nervous system.
   b. Their axons leave the spinal cord through the ventral nerve roots to reach spinal nerves.
   c. They leave the spinal nerves as the ***pelvic splanchnic nerves*** that are distributed to some viscera in the pelvis and abdomen.
   d. They end by synapsing with ganglion cells located in intimate relationship to the viscera concerned.
   e. The postganglionic fibres arising in these ganglia are short and supply smooth muscle and glands in these viscera.

## White Matter of the Spinal Cord

The anterior, lateral and posterior funiculi of the spinal cord are made up of nerve fibres running up or down the cord. These constitute the ascending and descending tracts that are described in chapter 51.

# 49 CHAPTER

# Gross Anatomy of Brain

## GROSS ANATOMY OF THE BRAINSTEM

1. The brainstem consists (from above downwards) of the midbrain, the pons and the medulla (49.1 and 49.2).
2. The midbrain is continuous, above, with the cerebral hemispheres.
3. The medulla is continuous, below, with the spinal cord.
4. Posteriorly, the pons and medulla are separated from the cerebellum by the fourth ventricle (49.3).
5. The ventricle is continuous, below, with the central canal, which traverses the lower part of the medulla, and becomes continuous with the central canal of the spinal cord.
6. Cranially, the fourth ventricle is continuous with the aqueduct, which passes through the midbrain.
7. The midbrain, pons and medulla are connected to the cerebellum by the superior, middle and inferior cerebellar peduncles, respectively.
8. A number of cranial nerves are attached to the brainstem.
   a. The third and fourth nerves emerge from the surface of the midbrain.
   b. The fifth from the pons.

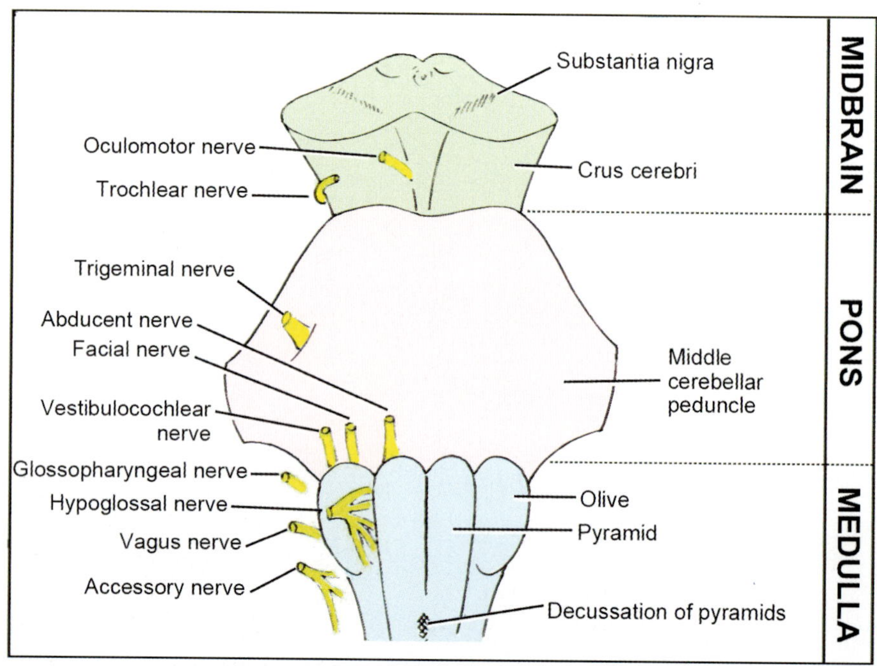


**49.1:** Ventral aspect of the brainstem

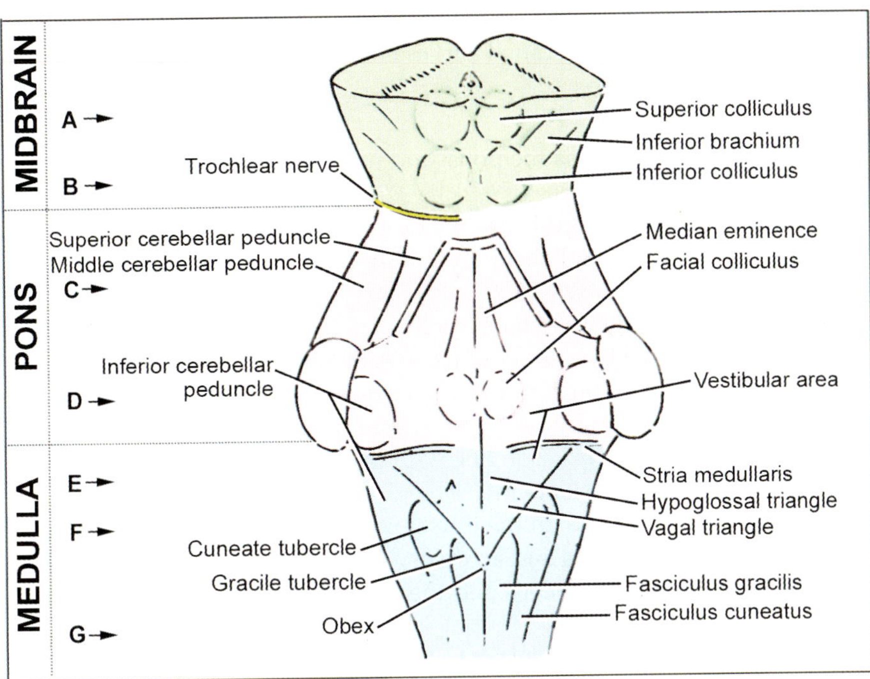


**49.2:** Dorsal aspect of the brainstem. Letters G to A represent levels at which transverse sections are shown in 49.4 to 49.10

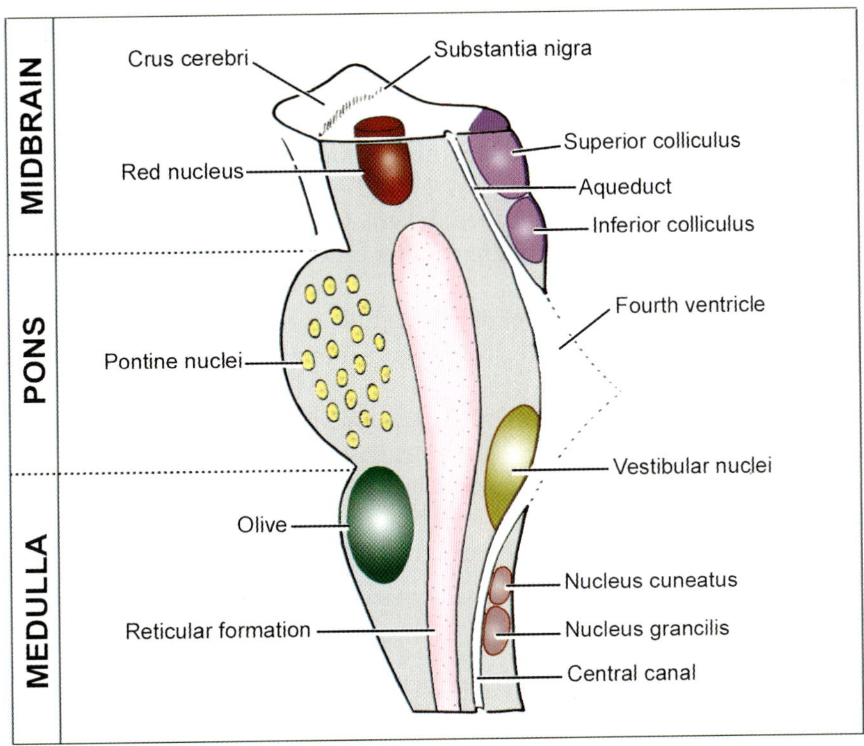


**49.3:** Median section through the brainstem. Some important masses of grey matter are shown projected onto the median plane

  c. The sixth, seventh and eighth nerves emerge at the junction of the pons and medulla.
  d. The ninth, tenth, eleventh and twelfth cranial nerves emerge from the surface of the medulla.

## Gross Anatomy of the Medulla

1. The medulla is broad above, where it joins the pons; and narrows down below, where it becomes continuous with the spinal cord.
2. The junction of the medulla and spinal cord is usually described as lying at the level of the upper border of the atlas vertebra. The transition is, in fact, not abrupt but occurs over a certain distance.
3. The medulla is divided into a lower ***closed part***, which surrounds the central canal; and an upper ***open part***, which is related to the lower part of the fourth ventricle.
4. The surface of the medulla is marked by a series of fissures or sulci that divide it into a number of regions.
   a. The ***anterior median fissure*** and the ***posterior median sulcus*** are upward continuations of the corresponding features seen on the spinal cord.
   b. On each side, the ***anterolateral sulcus*** lies in line with the ventral roots of spinal nerves. The rootlets of the hypoglossal nerve emerge from this sulcus.
   c. The ***posterolateral sulcus*** lies in line with the dorsal nerve roots of spinal nerves, and gives attachment to rootlets of the glossopharyngeal, vagus and accessory nerves.
5. The region between the anterior median sulcus and the anterolateral sulcus is occupied (on either side of the midline) by an elevation called the ***pyramid.***
   a. The elevation is caused by a large bundle of fibres that descend from the cerebral cortex to the spinal cord.
   b. Some of these fibres cross from one side to the other in the lower part of the medulla, obliterating the anterior median fissure. These crossing fibres constitute the ***decussation of the pyramids***.
   c. Some other fibres emerge from the anterior median fissure, above the decussation, and wind laterally over the surface of the medulla. These are the ***anterior external arcuate fibres.***
6. In the upper part of the medulla, the region between the anterolateral and posterolateral sulci shows a prominent, elongated, oval swelling named the ***olive.*** It is produced by a large mass of grey matter called the ***inferior olivary nucleus.***
7. The posterior part of the medulla, between the posterior median sulcus and the posterolateral sulcus, contains tracts that enter the medulla from the posterior funiculus of the spinal cord.
   a. These are the ***fasciculus gracilis*** lying medially, next to the middle line, and the ***fasciculus cuneatus*** lying laterally.
   b. These fasciculi end in rounded elevations called the ***gracile*** and ***cuneate tubercles.***
   c. These tubercles are produced by masses of grey matter called the ***nucleus gracilis*** and the ***nucleus cuneatus*** respectively.
8. Just above these tubercles, the posterior aspect of the medulla is occupied by a triangular fossa that forms the lower part of the floor of the fourth ventricle. This fossa is bounded on either side by the inferior cerebellar peduncle.
9. The lower part of the medulla, immediately lateral to the fasciculus cuneatus, is marked by another longitudinal elevation called the ***tuberculum cinereum.***
   a. This elevation is produced by an underlying collection of grey matter called the ***spinal nucleus of the trigeminal nerve.***
   b. The grey matter of this nucleus is covered by a layer of nerve fibres that form the ***spinal tract of the trigeminal nerve.***

## Gross Anatomy of the Pons

1. The pons shows a convex ***anterior surface***, marked by prominent transversely running fibres.
2. Laterally, these fibres collect to form a bundle, the ***middle cerebellar peduncle.***
3. The trigeminal nerve emerges from the anterior surface, and the point of its emergence is taken as a landmark to define the plane of junction between the pons and the middle cerebellar peduncle.

4. The anterior surface of the pons is marked, in the midline, by a shallow groove, the ***sulcus basilaris,*** which lodges the basilar artery.
5. The line of junction between the pons and the medulla is marked by a groove through which a number of cranial nerves emerge.
   a. The abducent nerve emerges just above the pyramid and runs upwards in close relation to the anterior surface of the pons.
   b. The facial and vestibulo-cochlear nerves emerge in the interval between the olive and the pons.
6. The posterior aspect of the pons forms the upper part of the floor of the fourth ventricle.

### Gross Anatomy of the Midbrain

1. When the midbrain is viewed from the anterior aspect, we see two large bundles of fibres, one on each side of the middle line.
   a. These are the ***crura*** of the midbrain.
   b. The right and left crura are separated by a deep fissure. Near the pons the fissure is narrow, but broadens as the crura diverge to enter the corresponding cerebral hemispheres.
   c. The parts of the crura just below the cerebrum form the posterior boundary of a space called the ***interpeduncular fossa*** (49.21). The oculomotor nerve emerges from the medial aspect of the crus (singular of crura) of the same side.
2. The posterior aspect of the midbrain is marked by four rounded swellings.
   a. These are the ***colliculi,*** one ***superior*** and one ***inferior*** on each side.
   b. Each colliculus is related laterally to a ridge called the ***brachium.*** The ***superior brachium*** connects the superior colliculus to the lateral geniculate body, while the ***inferior brachium*** connects the inferior colliculus to the medial geniculate body.
3. Just below the colliculi, there is the uppermost part of a membrane, the ***superior medullary velum,*** which stretches between the two superior cerebellar peduncles, and helps to form the roof of the fourth ventricle.
4. The trochlear nerve emerges from the velum, and then winds round the side of the midbrain to reach its ventral aspect.

## PRELIMINARY REVIEW OF THE INTERNAL STRUCTURE OF THE BRAINSTEM

1. The following description is confined to those features of internal structure that can be seen with the naked eye. A detailed consideration of the internal structure of the brainstem will be taken up in Chapter 51.
2. The main features of the internal structure of the brainstem are most easily reviewed by examining transverse sections at various levels. These are illustrated in 49.4 to 49.8. The levels represented in these figures are indicated in 49.2.

### Internal Structure of the Medulla

#### *At Level of Pyramidal Decussation*

1. A section at the level of the pyramidal decussation (49.4) shows some similarity to sections through the spinal cord.
2. The central canal is surrounded by central grey matter.
3. The ventral grey columns are present, but are separated from the central grey matter by decussating pyramidal fibres.
4. The region behind the central grey matter is occupied by the fasciculus gracilis, medially; and by the fasciculus cuneatus laterally.
5. Closely related to these fasciculi, there are two tongue-shaped extensions of the central grey matter. The medial of these extensions is the ***nucleus gracilis,*** and the lateral is the ***nucleus cuneatus.***
6. More laterally, there is the ***spinal nucleus of the trigeminal nerve.***
   a. When traced inferiorly, this nucleus reaches the second cervical segment of the spinal cord, where it becomes continuous with the substantia gelatinosa.

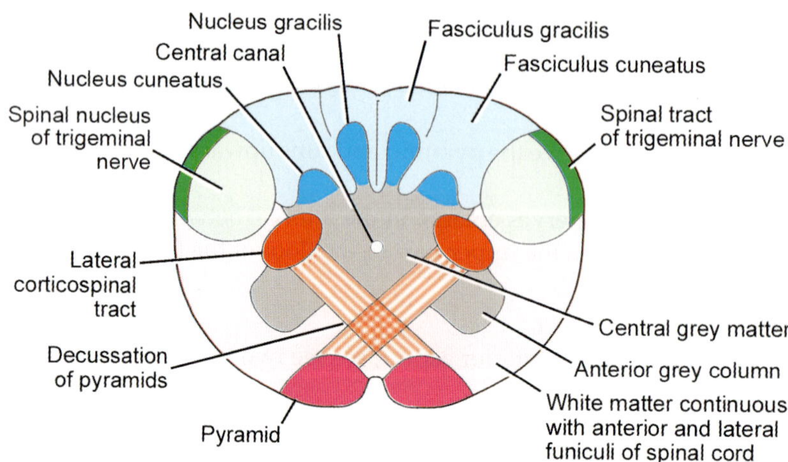


**49.4:** Main features to be seen in a transverse section through the medulla at the level of the pyramidal decussation

   b. Above, the nucleus extends as far as the upper part of the pons. The spinal nucleus of the trigeminal nerve is related superficially to the ***spinal tract*** of the nerve.
7. The ventral part of the medulla is occupied, on either side of the middle line, by a prominent bundle of fibres: these fibres form the ***pyramid***.
   a. The fibres of the pyramids are ***corticospinal fibres*** on their way from the cerebral cortex to the spinal cord.
   b. At this level in the medulla, many of these fibres run backwards and medially to cross in the middle line. These crossing fibres constitute the ***decussation of the pyramids***.
   c. Having crossed the middle line, the corticospinal fibres turn downwards to enter the lateral white column of the spinal cord.
8. The anterolateral region of the medulla is continuous with the anterior and lateral funiculi of the spinal cord.

### At Level of Sensory Decussation

1. A section thorough the medulla at a somewhat higher level is shown in 49.5. The central canal surrounded by central grey matter, the nucleus gracilis, the nucleus cuneatus, the spinal nucleus of the trigeminal nerve, and the pyramids occupy the same positions as at lower levels.
2. The nucleus gracilis and the nucleus cuneatus are, however, much larger and are no longer continuous with the central grey matter.
3. The fasciculus gracilis and the fasciculus cuneatus are less prominent.
4. The region just behind the pyramids is occupied by a prominent bundle of fibres, the ***medial lemniscus***, on either side of the middle line.
   a. The medial lemniscus is formed by fibres arising in the nucleus gracilis and the nucleus cuneatus.
   b. These fibres cross the middle line and turn upwards in the lemniscus of the opposite side.
   c. Crossing fibres of the two sides constitute the ***sensory decussation***.
5. The region lateral to the medial lemniscus contains scattered neurons mixed with nerve fibres. This region is the ***reticular formation***.
6. More laterally, there is a mass of white matter containing various tracts.

### At Level of Olive

1. A section through the medulla at the level of the olive is shown in 49.6. The pyramids, the medial lemniscus, the spinal nucleus and tract of the trigeminal nerve, and the reticular formation are present in the same relative position as at lower levels.

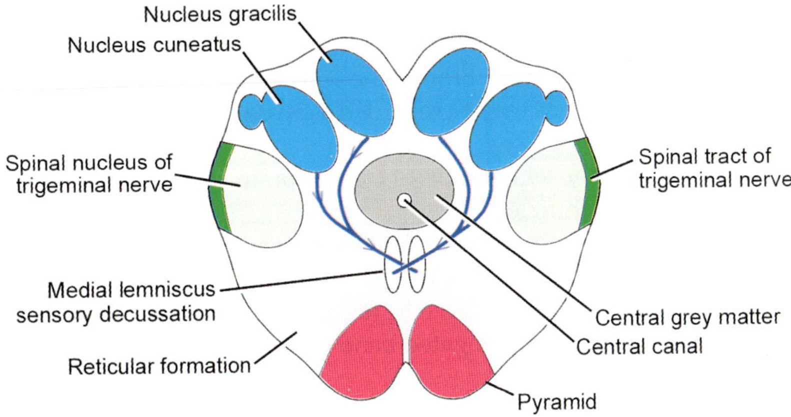


**49.5:** Transverse section through the medulla to show the main features seen at the level of the sensory decussation

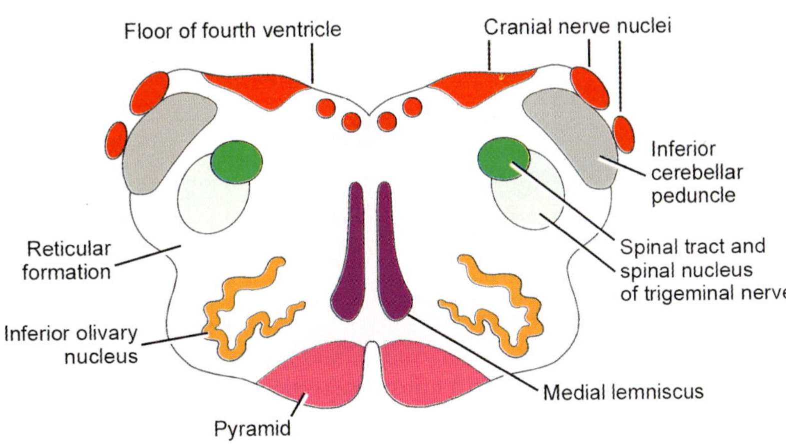


**49.6:** Main features to be seen in a transverse section through the medulla at the level of the olive

2. The medial lemniscus is, however, much more prominent and is somewhat expanded anteriorly.
3. Lateral to the spinal nucleus (and tract) of the trigeminal nerve, we see a large compact bundle of fibres. This is the ***inferior cerebellar peduncle*** that connects the medulla to the cerebellum.
4. Posteriorly, the medulla forms the floor of the fourth ventricle. Here, it is lined by a layer of grey matter in which are located several important cranial nerve nuclei.
5. The ***inferior olivary nucleus*** forms a prominent feature in the anterolateral part of the medulla at this level. It is made-up of a thin lamina of grey matter that is folded on itself like a crumpled purse. The nucleus has a hilum that is directed medially.

## Internal Structure of the Pons

1. The pons is divisible into a ventral part and a dorsal part (49.7).
2. The ***ventral (or basilar) part*** consists of transverse and vertical fibres.
3. Amongst the fibres are groups of cells that constitute the ***pontine nuclei***.
4. When traced laterally the transverse fibres form the ***middle cerebellar peduncle***.

5. The vertical fibres are of two types.
   a. Some of them descend from the cerebral cortex to end in the pontine nuclei.
   b. Others are corticospinal fibres that descend through the pons into the medulla where they form the pyramids.
6. The ***dorsal part (or tegmentum)*** of the pons may be regarded as an upward continuation of the part of the medulla behind the pyramids.
   a. Superiorly, it is continuous with the tegmentum of the midbrain.
   b. Posterior to it we see the fourth ventricle.
   c. Laterally, it is related to the ***superior cerebellar peduncles*** in its upper part (49.7); and to the inferior cerebellar peduncles in its lower part (49.8).
7. The spinal nucleus and tract of the trigeminal nerve lie just medial to these peduncles.
8. The medial lemniscus forms a transversely elongated band of fibres just behind the ventral part of the pons.

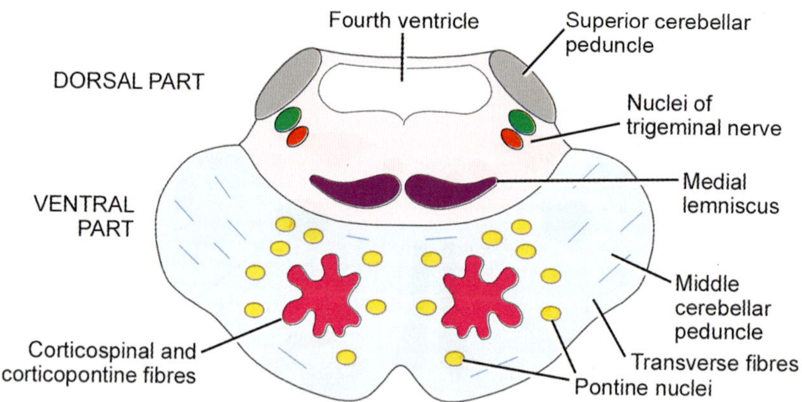


**49.7:** Main features to be seen in a transverse section through the upper part of the pons

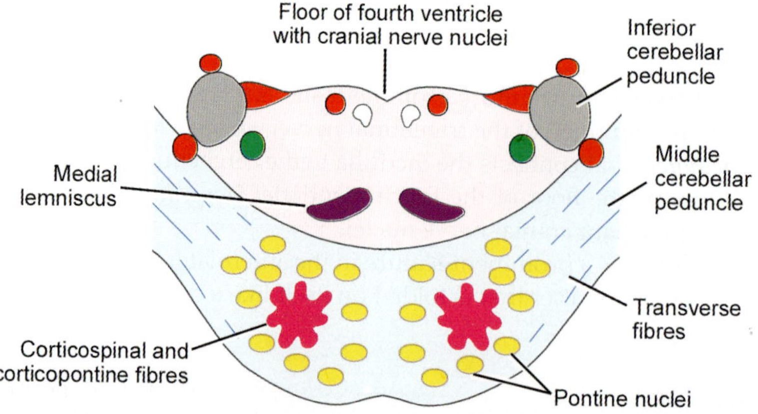


**49.8:** Main features to be seen in a transverse section through the lower part of the pons

## Internal Structure of the Midbrain

1. For convenience of description, the midbrain may be divided as follows (49.9):
   a. The part lying behind a transverse line drawn through the cerebral aqueduct is called the ***tectum.*** It consists of the superior and inferior colliculi of the two sides.
   b. The part lying in front of the transverse line is made up of right and left halves called the ***cerebral peduncles.***
2. Each peduncle consists of three parts. From anterior to posterior side these are:
   a. The crus cerebri (or basis pedunculi)
   b. The substantia nigra
   c. The tegmentum.
3. The ***crus cerebri*** consists of a large mass of vertically running fibres.
   a. These fibres descend from the cerebral cortex.
   b. Some of these pass through the midbrain to reach the pons, while others reach the spinal cord. The two crura are separated by a notch seen on the anterior aspect of the midbrain.
4. The ***substantia nigra*** is made up of pigmented grey matter and, therefore, appears dark in colour.
5. The ***tegmentum*** of the two sides is continuous across the middle line. It contains important masses of grey matter as well as fibre bundles.
6. The largest of the nuclei is the ***red nucleus*** (49.10) present in the upper half of the midbrain.
7. The tegmentum also contains the ***reticular formation*** that is continuous below with that of the pons and medulla.
8. The fibre bundles of the tegmentum include the medial lemniscus that lies just behind the substantia nigra, lateral to the red nucleus.
   a. The lower part of the tegmentum is traversed by a large number of fibres that cross the middle line from one side to the other.
   b. These are the fibres of the superior cerebellar peduncles that have their origin in the cerebellum and decussate before ending in the red nucleus (and in some other centres).
9. It may be noted that some authorities describe the corresponding half of the tectum as part of the cerebral peduncle.

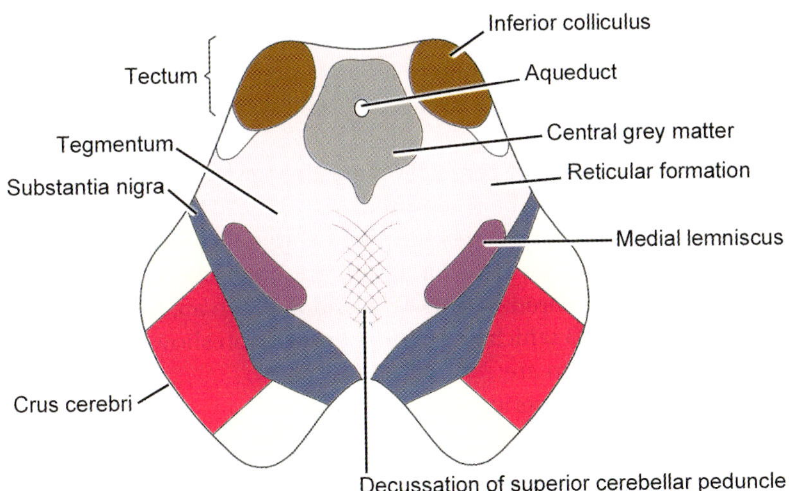


**49.9:** Main features to be seen in a transverse section through the lower part of the midbrain

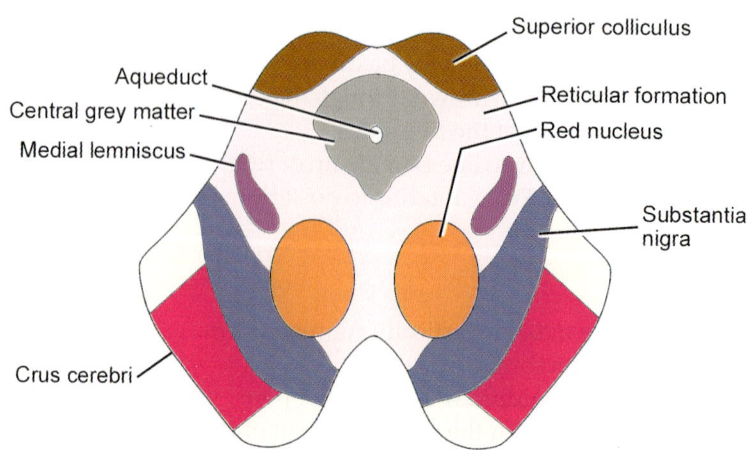


**49.10:** Main features to be seen in a transverse section through the upper part of the midbrain

## GROSS ANATOMY OF THE CEREBELLUM

### Subdivisions of the Cerebellum

1. The cerebellum lies in the posterior cranial fossa, behind the pons and the medulla.
2. It is separated from the cerebrum by a fold of dura mater called the ***tentorium cerebelli.***
3. The cerebellum consists of a part lying near the middle line called the ***vermis,*** and of two lateral ***hemispheres.*** It has two surfaces, ***superior*** and ***inferior.***
4. On the superior aspect, there is no line of distinction between vermis and hemispheres.
5. On the inferior aspect, the two hemispheres are separated by a deep depression called the ***vallecula.*** The vermis lies in the depth of this depression.
6. Anteriorly and posteriorly, the hemispheres extend beyond the vermis and are separated by anterior and posterior ***cerebellar notches.***
7. The surface of the cerebellum is marked by a series of fissures that run more or less parallel to one another.
   a. The fissures subdivide the surface of the cerebellum into narrow leaf like bands or ***folia***.
   b. The long axis of the majority of folia is more or less transverse.
8. Sections of the cerebellum cut at right angles to this axis have a characteristic tree-like appearance to which the term ***arbor-vitae*** (tree of life) is applied.
9. Some of the fissures on the surface of the cerebellum are deeper than others. They divide the cerebellum into ***lobes*** within which smaller ***lobules*** may be recognised.
10. To show the various subdivisions of the cerebellum in a single illustration, it is usual to represent the organ as if it has been 'opened out' so that the superior and inferior aspects can both be seen. Such an illustration is shown in 49.11. This should be compared with 49.12 A and B which are more realistic drawings of the superior and inferior surfaces, and with 49.13 which is a middle line section showing the subdivisions of the vermis.
11. The deepest fissures in the cerebellum are:
    a. The ***primary fissure*** seen on the superior surface
    b. The ***posterolateral fissure*** seen on the inferior aspect.
12. These fissures divide the cerebellum into three lobes:
    a. The part anterior to the primary fissure is the ***anterior lobe.***
    b. The part between the two fissures is the ***middle lobe*** (sometimes called the ***posterior lobe***).
    c. The remaining part is the ***flocculonodular lobe.***
13. The anterior and middle lobes together form the ***corpus cerebelli.***

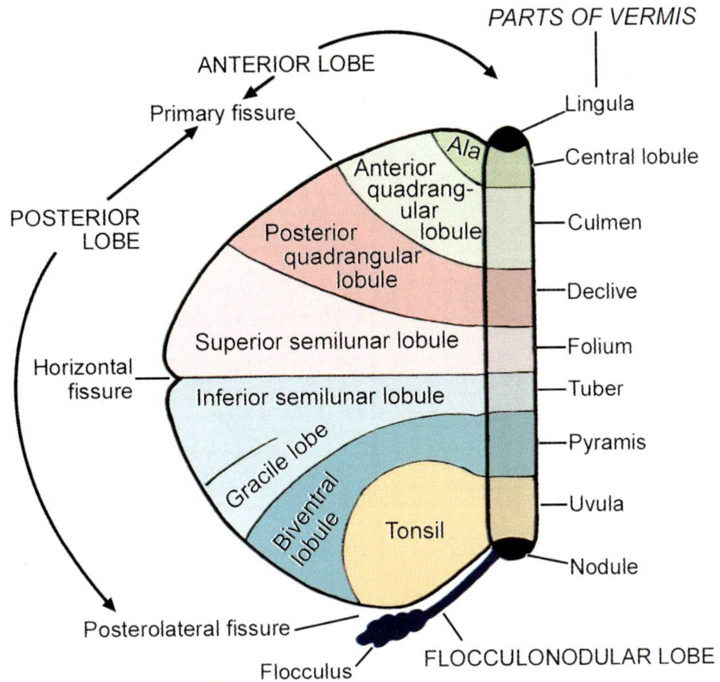


**49.11:** Scheme to show the subdivisions of the cerebellum

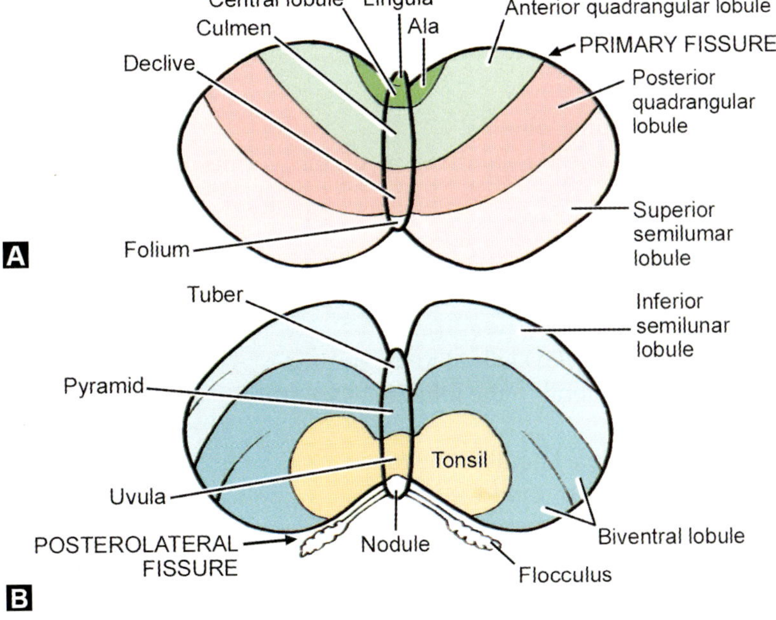


**49.12A and B:** Subdivisions of the cerebellum. (A) As seen on the superior aspect; (B) As seen on the inferior aspect

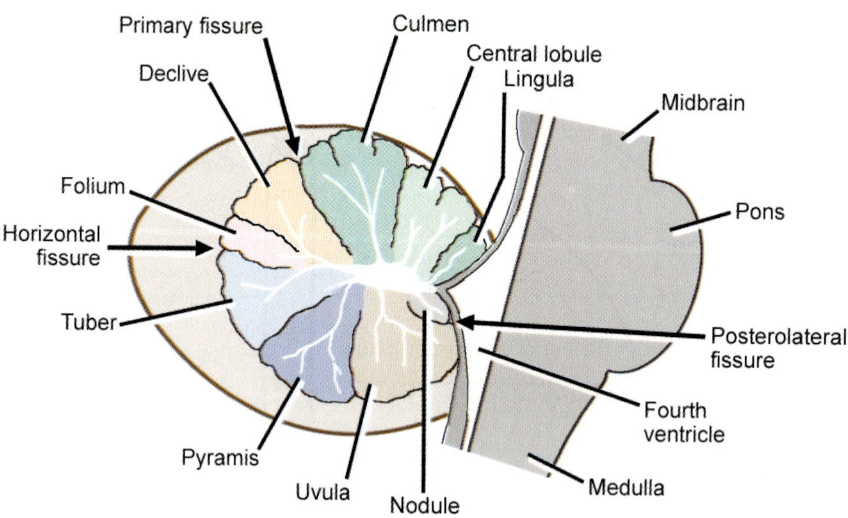


49.13: Subdivisions of the vermis of the cerebellum as seen in a median section

## WANT TO KNOW MORE?

14. The vermis is so called because it resembles a worm. Proceeding from above downwards in 49.11 it is seen to consist of 49.13
    a. The lingula
    b. Central lobule
    c. Culmen (in the anterior lobe)
    d. The declive
    e. Folium (or folium vermis)
    f. Tuber (or tuber vermis)
    g. Pyramid
    h. Uvula (in the middle lobe)
    i. The nodule (in the flocculonodular lobe).
15. With the exception of the lingula, each subdivision of the vermis is related laterally to a part of the hemisphere.
16. In the anterior lobe, we have:
    a. The ***ala*** lateral to the central lobule
    b. The ***quadrangular lobule*** lateral to the culmen.
17. In the middle lobe, we have:
    a. The ***simple lobule*** (or ***lobulus simplex)*** lateral to the declive
    b. The ***superior semilunar lobule*** lateral to the folium
    c. The ***inferior semilunar lobule***
    d. The ***gracile*** (or ***paramedian) lobule*** lateral to the tuber
    e. The ***biventral lobule*** lateral to the pyramid
    f. The ***tonsil*** lateral to the uvula.
18. The ***nodule*** is continuous laterally with the flocculus through the inferior medullary velum.
19. The fissures separating the subdivisions of the cerebellum are shown in 49.11.
    a. In particular note the ***horizontal fissure.*** This fissure divides the cerebellum into upper and lower halves.
    b. The parts shown above this fissure in 49.11 are seen on the superior surface of the cerebellum (49.12A), and those below it on the inferior surface (49.12B).

## Cerebellar Peduncles

1. The fibres entering or leaving the cerebellum pass through three thick bundles called the cerebellar peduncles.
   a. The ***inferior cerebellar peduncle*** connects the posterolateral part of the medulla with the cerebellum.
   b. The ***middle cerebellar peduncle*** looks like a lateral continuation of the ventral part of the pons. It connects the pons to the cerebellum.
   c. The ***superior cerebellar peduncle*** is the main connection between the midbrain and the cerebellum.
2. The fibres passing through each peduncle are enumerated in chapter 50.

### *White Matter of the Cerebellum*

1. The central core of each cerebellar hemisphere is formed by white matter. The peduncles are continued into this white matter.
2. The white matter of the two sides is connected by a thin lamina of fibres that are closely related to the fourth ventricle.
   a. The upper part of this lamina forms the superior medullary velum.
   b. Its inferior part forms the inferior medullary velum.
   c. Both these take part in forming the roof of the fourth ventricle.

### *Grey Matter of the Cerebellum*

1. Most of the grey matter of the cerebellum is arranged as a thin layer covering the central core of white matter. This layer is the ***cerebellar cortex***.
2. The subdivisions of the cerebellar cortex correspond to the subdivisions of the cerebellum described above.
3. Embedded within the central core of white matter there are masses of grey matter that constitute the ***cerebellar nuclei***. These are as follows (49.14):
   a. The ***dentate nucleus*** lies in the centre of each cerebellar hemisphere. Cross-sections through the nucleus have a striking resemblance to those through the inferior olivary nucleus. Like the latter, it is made up of a thin lamina of grey matter that is folded upon itself so that it resembles a crumpled purse. Both the nuclei have a hilum directed medially.
   b. The ***emboliform nucleus*** lies on the medial side of the dentate nucleus.
   c. The ***globose nucleus*** lies medial to the emboliform nucleus.
   d. The ***fastigial nucleus*** lies close to the middle line in the anterior part of the superior vermis.

# GROSS ANATOMY OF THE CEREBRAL HEMISPHERES

## Exterior of the Cerebral Hemispheres

### *Poles, Surfaces, and Borders*

1. The cerebrum consists of two cerebral hemispheres that are partially connected with each other.
2. When viewed from the lateral aspect, each cerebral hemisphere has the appearance shown in 49.15.
3. Three somewhat pointed ends or ***poles*** can be recognised:
   a. These are the ***frontal pole*** anteriorly
   b. The ***occipital pole*** posteriorly
   c. The ***temporal pole*** that lies between the frontal and occipital poles, and points forwards and somewhat downwards.
4. A coronal section through the cerebral hemispheres (49.16) shows that each hemisphere has three borders, ***superomedial, inferolateral*** and ***inferomedial.***
5. These borders divide the surface of the hemisphere into three large surfaces, ***superolateral, medial*** and ***inferior.***
6. The inferior surface is further subdivided into an anterior ***orbital*** part and a posterior ***tentorial*** part. (49.16).
7. Corresponding to these subdivisions, the inferomedial border is divided into
   a. An anterior part called the ***medial orbital border***
   b. A posterior part called the ***medial occipital border.***

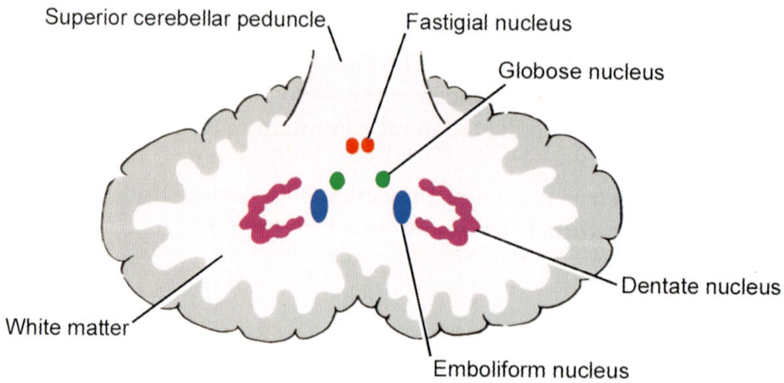


**49.14:** Scheme to show the cerebellar nuclei

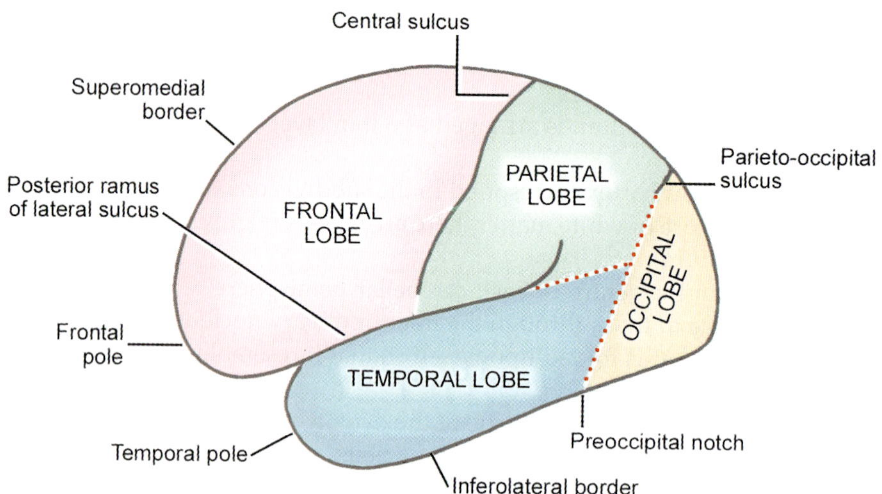


**49.15:** Lateral aspect of the cerebral hemisphere to show borders, poles and lobes

8. The orbital part of the inferolateral border is called the ***superciliary border*** (as it lies just above the level of the eyebrows).
9. The surfaces of the cerebral hemisphere are not smooth. They show a series of grooves or ***sulci*** that are separated by intervening areas that are called ***gyri.***

### *Lobes*

1. For convenience of description, each cerebral hemisphere is divided into four major subdivisions or ***lobes.*** To consider, the boundaries of these lobes reference has to be made to some sulci and other features to be seen on each hemisphere (49.15).
2. On the superolateral surface of the hemisphere, there are two prominent sulci:
   a. One of these is the ***posterior ramus of the lateral sulcus*** that begins near the temporal pole and runs backwards and slightly upwards. Its posterior-most part curves sharply upwards.
   b. The second sulcus that is used to delimit the lobes is the ***central sulcus.*** It begins on the superomedial margin a little behind the midpoint between the frontal and occipital poles, and runs downwards and forwards to end a little above the posterior ramus of the lateral sulcus.

3. On the medial surface of the hemisphere, near the occipital pole, there is a sulcus called the ***parieto-occipital sulcus*** (49.19). The upper end of this sulcus reaches the superomedial border and a small part of it can be seen on the superolateral surface (49.15).
4. A little anterior to the occipital pole the inferolateral border shows a slight indentation called the ***preoccipital notch*** (or ***preoccipital incisure***).
5. To complete the subdivision of the hemisphere into lobes we now have to draw two imaginary lines.
   a. The first imaginary line connects the upper end of the parieto-occipital sulcus to the preoccipital notch.
   b. The second imaginary line is a backward continuation of the posterior ramus of the lateral sulcus (excluding the posterior upturned part) to meet the first line.
6. We are now in a position to define the limits of the various lobes as follows:
   a. The ***frontal lobe*** lies anterior to the central sulcus, and above the posterior ramus of the lateral sulcus.
   b. The ***parietal lobe*** lies behind the central sulcus. It is bounded below by the posterior ramus of the lateral sulcus and by the second imaginary line, and behind by the upper part of the first imaginary line.
   c. The ***occipital lobe*** is the area lying behind the first imaginary line.
   d. The ***temporal lobe*** lies below the posterior ramus of the lateral sulcus and the second imaginary line. It is separated from the occipital lobe by the lower part of the first imaginary line.
7. Before going onto consider further subdivisions of each of the lobes named above, attention has to be directed to details of some structures already mentioned.
   a. The upper end of the central sulcus winds round the superomedial border to reach the medial surface. Here, its end is surrounded by a gyrus called the ***paracentral lobule*** (49.19). The lower end of the central sulcus is always separated by a small interval from the posterior ramus of the lateral sulcus (49.15).
   b. The lateral sulcus begins on the inferior aspect of the cerebral hemisphere where it lies between the orbital surface and the anterior part of the temporal lobe (49.21). It runs laterally to reach the superolateral surface.
   c. On reaching this surface, it divides into three rami (branches).
   d. These rami are ***anterior*** (or ***anterior horizontal***), ***ascending*** (or ***anterior ascending***) and ***posterior*** (49.18).
   e. The anterior and ascending rami are short and run into the frontal lobe in the directions indicated by their names.
   f. The posterior ramus of the lateral sulcus has already been considered.
8. Unlike most other sulci, the lateral sulcus is very deep. Its walls cover a fairly large area of the surface of the hemisphere called the ***insula*** (49.17).

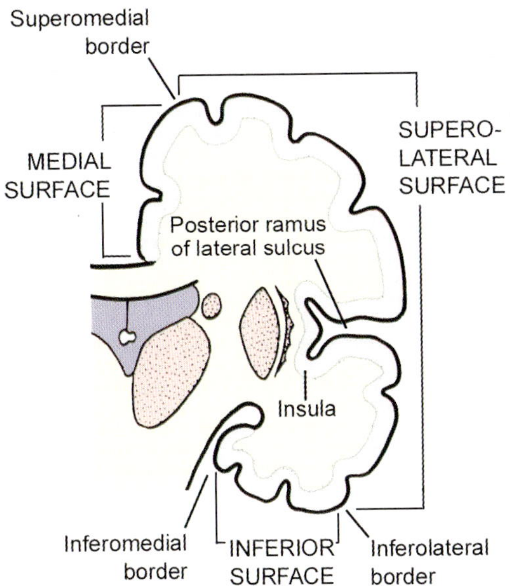


**49.16:** Coronal section through a cerebral hemisphere to show its borders and surfaces

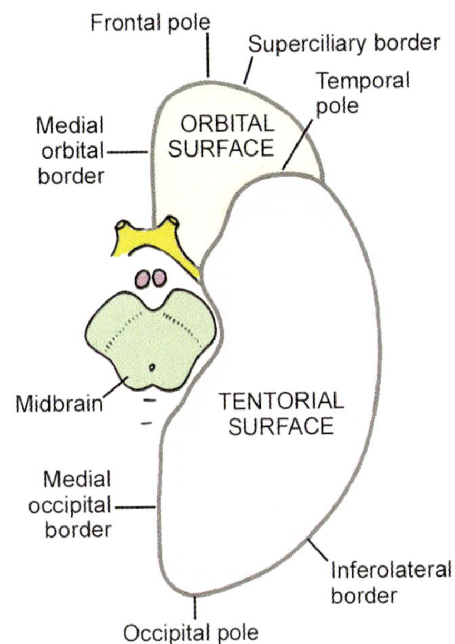


**49.17:** Inferior aspect of a cerebral hemisphere to show its borders, poles and surfaces

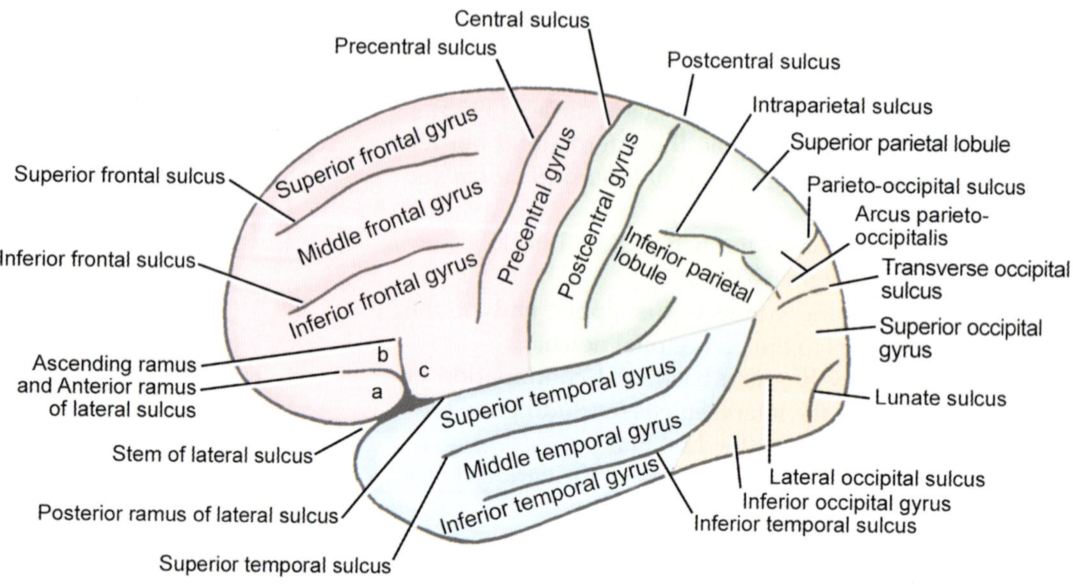


**49.18:** Simplified presentation of sulci and gyri on the superolateral surface of the cerebral hemisphere. a: pars orbitalis; b: pars triangularis; c: pars opercularis

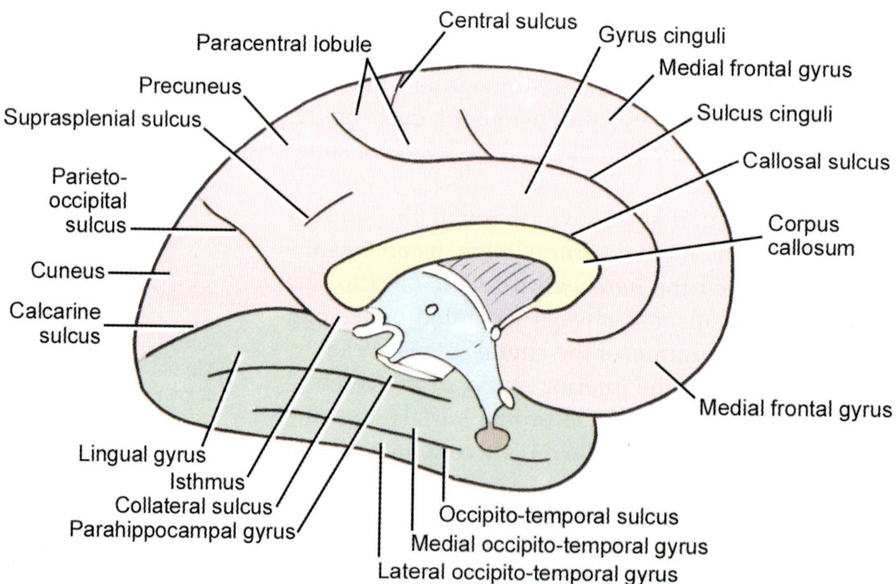


**49.19:** Simplified presentation of sulci and gyri on the cerebral hemisphere as seen from the medial aspect. The medial surface and the tentorial surface (shaded green) are seen. The corpus callosum and some other median structures have been cut across

## Further Subdivisions of the Superolateral Surface

### Frontal Lobe

The frontal lobe is further subdivided as follows (49.18):

1. The ***precentral sulcus*** runs downwards and forwards parallel to and a little anterior to the central sulcus.
2. The area between it and the central sulcus is the ***precentral gyrus.***
3. In the region anterior to the precentral gyrus, there are two sulci that run in an anteroposterior direction. These are the ***superior*** and ***inferior frontal sulci.***
4. They divide this region into ***superior, middle*** and ***inferior frontal gyri.***
5. The anterior and ascending rami of the lateral sulcus extend into the inferior frontal gyrus dividing it into three parts:
   a. The part below the anterior ramus is the ***pars orbitalis***.
   b. The part between the anterior and ascending rami is the ***pars triangularis***.
   c. The part posterior to the ascending ramus is the ***pars opercularis.***

### Temporal Lobe

1. The temporal lobe has two sulci that run parallel to the posterior ramus of the lateral sulcus. They are termed the ***superior*** and ***inferior temporal sulci.***
2. They divide the superolateral surface of this lobe into ***superior, middle*** and ***inferior temporal gyri.***

### Parietal Lobe

1. The parietal lobe shows the following subdivisions.
2. The ***postcentral sulcus*** runs downwards and forwards parallel to and a little behind the central sulcus. The area between these two sulci is the ***postcentral gyrus.***
3. The rest of the parietal lobe is divided into a ***superior parietal lobule*** and an ***inferior parietal lobule*** by the ***intraparietal sulcus.***
4. The upturned posterior end of the posterior ramus of the lateral sulcus extends into the inferior parietal lobule. The posterior ends of the superior and inferior temporal sulci also turn upwards to enter this lobule.
5. The upturned ends of these three sulci divide the inferior parietal lobule into three parts:
   a. The part that arches over the upturned posterior end of the posterior ramus of the lateral sulcus is called the ***supramarginal gyrus.***
   b. The part that arches over the superior temporal sulcus is called the ***angular gyrus.***
   c. The part that arches over the posterior end of the inferior temporal sulcus is called the ***arcus temporo-occipitalis.***

### Occipital Lobe

1. The occipital lobe shows three rather short sulci.
2. One of these, the ***lateral occipital sulcus*** lies horizontally and divides the lobe into ***superior and inferior occipital gyri.***
3. The ***lunate sulcus*** runs downwards and slightly forwards just in front of the occipital pole. The vertical strip just in front of it is the ***gyrus descendens.***
4. The ***transverse occipital sulcus*** is located in the uppermost part of the occipital lobe.
5. The upper end of the parieto-occipital sulcus (which just reaches the superolateral surface from the medial surface) is surrounded by the ***arcus parieto-occipitalis.*** As its name suggests, it belongs partly to the parietal lobe and partly to the occipital lobe.

### Insula

1. In the depth of the stem and posterior ramus of the lateral sulcus, there is a part of the cerebral hemisphere called the ***insula*** (insula = insulated or hidden). It is surrounded by a ***circular sulcus.***

2. During development of the cerebral hemisphere, this area grows less than surrounding areas that, therefore, come to overlap it and occlude it from surface view. These surrounding areas are called ***opercula*** (= lids).
   a. The ***frontal operculum*** lies between the anterior and ascending rami of the lateral sulcus.
   b. The ***frontoparietal operculum*** lies above the posterior ramus of the lateral sulcus.
   c. The ***temporal operculum*** lies below this sulcus.
3. The temporal operculum has a superior surface hidden in the depth of the lateral sulcus (49.17). On this surface, we see two gyri called the ***anterior and posterior transverse temporal gyri.***

## Medial Surface of Cerebral Hemisphere

1. When the two cerebral hemispheres are separated from each other by a cut in the middle line the appearances seen are shown in 49.19 and 49.20. The structures seen are as follows.
2. The ***corpus callosum*** is a prominent arched structure consisting of commissural fibres passing from one hemisphere to the other (49.20).
   a. It consists of a central part called the ***trunk.***
   b. A posterior end or ***splenium.***
   c. An anterior end or ***genu.***
3. A little below the corpus callosum we see the third ventricle of the brain. A number of structures can be identified in relation to this ventricle.
   a. The ***interventricular foramen*** through which the third ventricle communicates with the lateral ventricle can be seen in the upper and anterior part.
   b. Posteroinferiorly, the ventricle is continuous with the ***cerebral aqueduct.***
   c. The lateral wall of the ventricle is formed in greater part by a large mass of grey matter called the ***thalamus.*** The right and left thalami are usually interconnected (across the middle line) by a strip of grey matter called the ***interthalamic connexus.***
   d. The anteroinferior part of the lateral wall of the third ventricle is formed by a collection of grey matter that constitutes the ***hypothalamus.***
4. Above the thalamus, there is a bundle of fibres called the ***fornix.***
   a. Posteriorly, the fornix is attached to the undersurface of the corpus callosum.
   b. But anteriorly, it disappears from view just in front of the interventricular foramen.

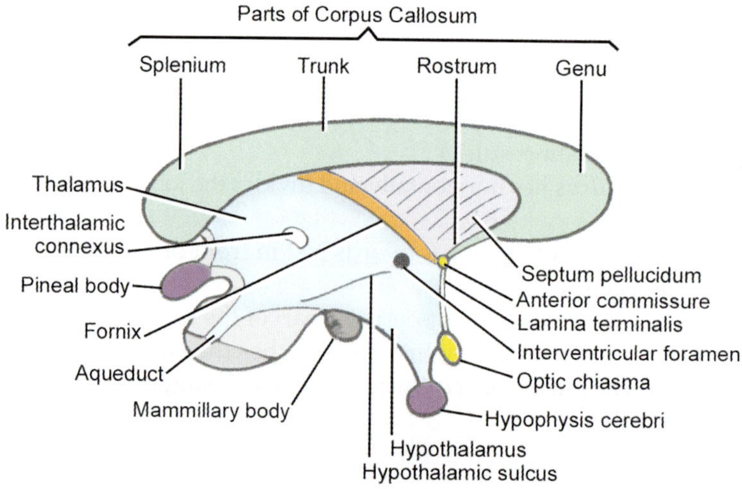


**49.20:** Enlarged view of part of 49.19 to show some structures to be seen on the medial aspect of the cerebral hemisphere

5. Extending between the fornix and the corpus callosum, there is a thin lamina called the ***septum pellucidum*** (or ***septum lucidum***), which separates the right and left lateral ventricles from each other. Removal of the septum pellucidum brings the interior of the lateral ventricle into view.
6. In the anterior wall of the third ventricle, there are the ***anterior commissure*** and the ***lamina terminalis.***
7. The anterior commissure is attached to the genu of the corpus callosum through a thin lamina of fibres that constitutes the ***rostrum*** of the corpus callosum.
8. Below, the anterior commissure is continuous with the lamina terminalis that is a thin lamina of nervous tissue. The lower end of the lamina terminalis is attached to the optic chiasma.
9. Posteriorly, the third ventricle is related to the ***pineal gland*** and inferiorly to the ***hypophysis cerebri.***
10. Above the corpus callosum (and also in front of and behind it), we see the sulci and gyri of the medial surface of the hemisphere (49.19).
    a. The most prominent of the sulci is the ***cingulate sulcus*** that follows a curved course parallel to the upper convex margin of the corpus callosum.
    b. Anteriorly, it ends below the rostrum of the corpus callosum. Posteriorly, it turns upwards to reach the superomedial border a little behind the upper end of the central sulcus.
    c. The area between the cingulate sulcus and the corpus callosum is called the ***gyrus cinguli.*** It is separated from the corpus callosum by the ***callosal sulcus.***
    d. The part of the medial surface of the hemisphere between the cingulate sulcus and the superomedial border consists of two parts.
    e. The smaller posterior part that is wound around the end of the central sulcus is called the ***paracentral lobule.***
    f. The large anterior part is called the ***medial frontal gyrus.*** These two parts are separated by a short sulcus continuous with the cingulate sulcus.
11. The part of the medial surface behind the paracentral lobule and the gyrus cinguli shows two major sulci that cut off a triangular area called the ***cuneus.***
    a. The triangle is bounded anteriorly and above by the ***parieto-occipital sulcus.***
    b. Inferiorly by the ***calcarine sulcus.***
    c. Posteriorly by the superomedial border of the hemisphere.
12. The calcarine sulcus extends forwards beyond its junction with the parieto-occipital sulcus and ends a little below the splenium of the corpus callosum.
13. The small area separating the splenium from the calcarine sulcus is called the ***isthmus.***
14. Between the parieto-occipital sulcus and the paracentral lobule there is a quadrilateral area called the ***precuneus.*** Anteroinferiorly, the precuneus is separated from the posterior part of the gyrus cinguli by the ***suprasplenial (or subparietal) sulcus.***

### Inferior Surface of Cerebrum

1. When the cerebrum is separated from the hindbrain by cutting across the midbrain, and is viewed from below, the appearances seen are shown in 49.21.
2. Posterior to the midbrain, we see the undersurface of the splenium of the corpus callosum.
3. Anterior to the midbrain, there is a depressed area called the ***interpeduncular fossa.*** The fossa is bounded in front by the ***optic chiasma*** and on the sides by the right and left ***optic tracts.***
4. The optic tracts wind round the sides of the midbrain to terminate on its posterolateral aspect. In this region two swellings, the ***medial and lateral geniculate bodies***, can be seen.
5. Certain structures are seen within the interpeduncular fossa. These are closely related to the floor of the third ventricle (see also 49.20).
    a. Anterior and medial to the crura of the midbrain, there are two rounded swellings called the ***mammillary bodies.***
    b. Anterior to these bodies, there is a median elevation called the ***tuber cinereum,*** to which the infundibulum of the hypophysis cerebri is attached.

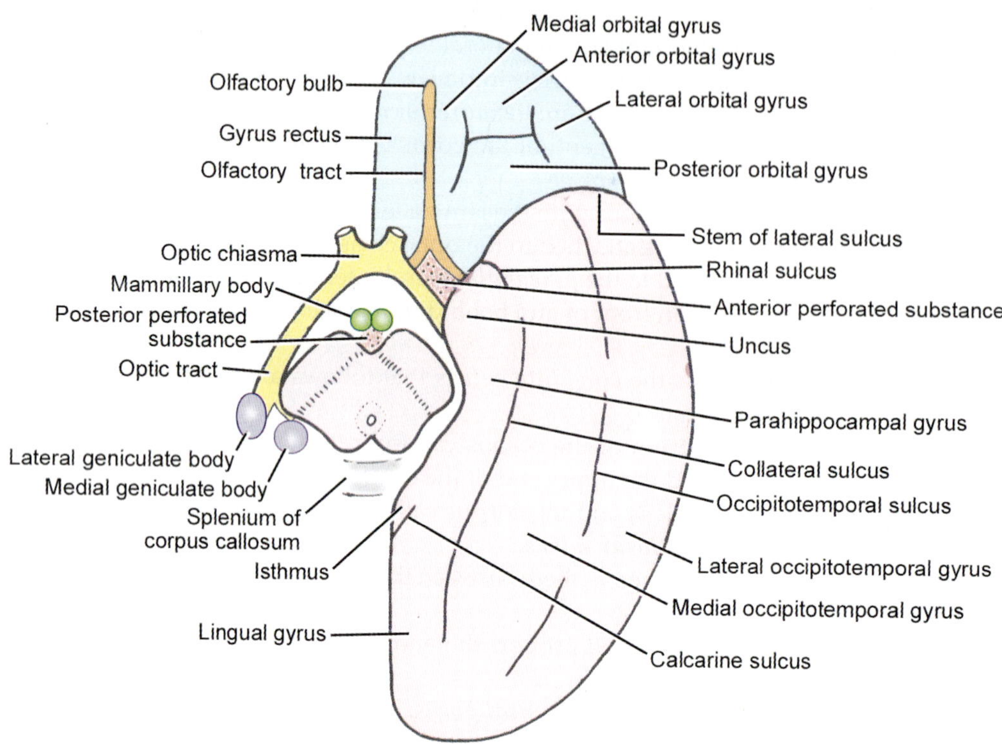


**49.21:** Structures to be seen on the inferior aspect of the cerebral hemisphere

c. The triangular interval between the mammillary bodies and the midbrain is pierced by numerous small blood vessels and is called the ***posterior perforated substance.***
d. A similar area lying on each side of the optic chiasma is called the ***anterior perforated substance.***
e. The anterior perforated substance is connected to the insula by a band of grey matter called the ***limen insulae*** that lies in the depth of the stem of the lateral sulcus.

6. In addition to these structures, we see the sulci and gyri on the orbital and tentorial parts of the inferior surface of the each cerebral hemisphere (described below). The orbital and tentorial parts of the inferior surface are separated from each other by the stem of the lateral sulcus.

## Orbital Surface

1. Close to the medial border of the orbital surface, there is an anteroposterior sulcus: it is called the ***olfactory sulcus*** because the olfactory bulb and tract lie superficial to it.
2. The area medial to this sulcus is called the ***gyrus rectus.***
3. The rest of the orbital surface is divided by an H-shaped ***orbital sulcus*** into ***anterior, posterior, medial*** and ***lateral orbital gyri.***

## Tentorial Surface

1. The tentorial surface is marked by two major sulci that run in an anteroposterior direction.
   a. These are the ***collateral sulcus*** medially.
   b. The ***occipitotemporal sulcus*** laterally.
2. The posterior part of the collateral sulcus runs parallel to the calcarine sulcus: the area between them is the ***lingual gyrus.***

3. Anteriorly, the lingual gyrus becomes continuous with the ***parahippocampal gyrus***. This is related medially to the midbrain and to the interpeduncular fossa.
4. The anterior end of the parahippocampal gyrus is cut off from the curved temporal pole of the hemisphere by a curved ***rhinal sulcus.***
5. This part of the parahippocampal gyrus forms a hook-like structure called the ***uncus.***
6. Posteriorly, the parahippocampal gyrus becomes continuous with the gyrus cinguli through the isthmus (49.19).
7. The area between the collateral sulcus and the rhinal sulcus medially, and the occipitotemporal sulcus laterally, is the ***medial occipitotemporal gyrus.***
8. The area lateral to the occipitotemporal sulcus is called the ***lateral occipitotemporal gyrus.*** This gyrus is continuous (around the inferolateral margin of the cerebral hemisphere) with the inferior temporal gyrus.

## AN INTRODUCTION TO SOME STRUCTURES WITHIN THE CEREBRAL HEMISPHERES

### Early Development of the Brain

1. For a proper understanding of the structure of the cerebrum, brief reference to the development of the brain is necessary.
2. At an early stage of development, the brain is made up of three hollow vesicles. These are the ***prosencephalon,*** the ***mesencephalon*** and the ***rhombencephalon*** (in craniocaudal sequence) (49.22).
3. The mesencephalon gives rise to the midbrain, while the rhombencephalon forms the hindbrain (i.e., the pons, the medulla, and the cerebellum).
4. The cerebrum develops from the prosencephalon that soon shows a subdivision into a median part, the ***diencephalon,*** and two lateral evaginations (the ***telencephalic vesicles***). These together constitute the ***telencephalon.***
5. In subsequent development, the telencephalic vesicles grow much faster than the diencephalon.
   a. As they enlarge, they eventually overlap the diencephalon and fuse with its lateral aspect.
   b. One telencephalic vesicle, along with the corresponding half of the diencephalon constitutes one cerebral hemisphere.
   c. From what has been said above, it will be clear that the diencephalic part of the hemisphere lies medially and inferiorly relative to the part derived from the telencephalon.
6. The developing brain has a series of cavities within it.
   a. The cavity of each telencephalic vesicle becomes one ***lateral ventricle.***
   b. The ***third ventricle*** may be regarded as the cavity of the diencephalon.

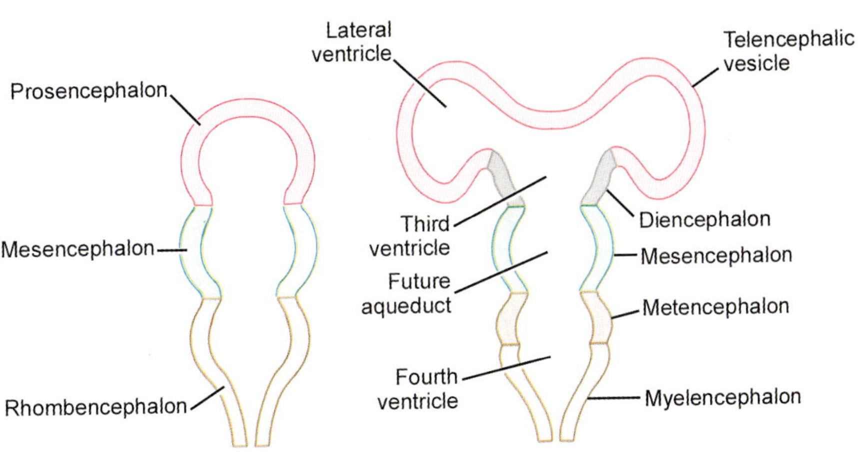


**49.22:** Two stages in the development of the brain

c. The interventricular foramina connecting the lateral ventricles to the third ventricle represent the sites of the original telencephalic evaginations.

## Basic Structure of Cerebral Hemisphere

Keeping these facts in mind, we may now examine the basic structure of the cerebral hemispheres as seen in a coronal section (49.23).

1. The surface of the cerebral hemisphere is covered by a thin layer of grey matter called the ***cerebral cortex***.
   a. The cortex follows the irregular contour of the sulci and gyri of the hemisphere and extends into the depths of the sulci.
   b. As a result of this folding of the cerebral surface, the cerebral cortex acquires a much larger surface area than the size of the hemispheres would otherwise allow.
2. The greater part of the cerebral hemisphere deep to the cortex is occupied by white matter within which are embedded certain important masses of grey matter.
3. Immediately lateral to the third ventricle, there are the ***thalamus*** and ***hypothalamus*** (and certain smaller masses) derived from the diencephalon.
4. More laterally, there is the ***corpus striatum*** that is derived from the telencephalon.
   a. It consists of two masses of grey matter, the ***caudate nucleus*** and the ***lentiform nucleus***.
   b. A little lateral to the lentiform nucleus we see the cerebral cortex in the region of the insula.
   c. Between the lentiform nucleus and the insula there is a thin layer of grey matter called the ***claustrum.***
5. The caudate nucleus, the lentiform nucleus, the claustrum and some other masses of grey matter (all of telencephalic origin) are referred to as ***basal ganglia.***
6. The white matter that occupies the interval between the thalamus and caudate nucleus medially, and the lentiform nucleus laterally, is called the ***internal capsule.*** It is a region of considerable importance as major ascending and descending tracts pass through it.
7. The white matter that radiates from the upper end of the internal capsule to the cortex is called the ***corona radiata.***

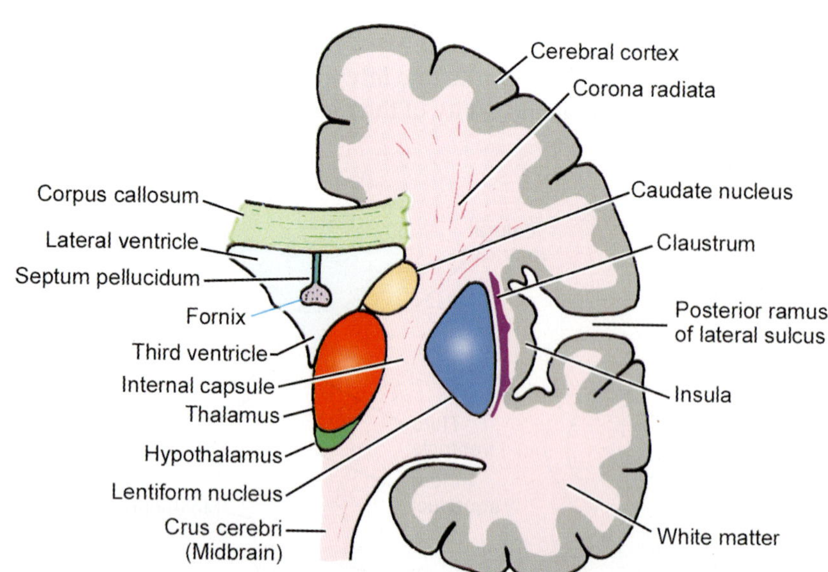


**49.23:** Coronal section through a cerebral hemisphere to show some important masses of grey matter, and some other structures, within it

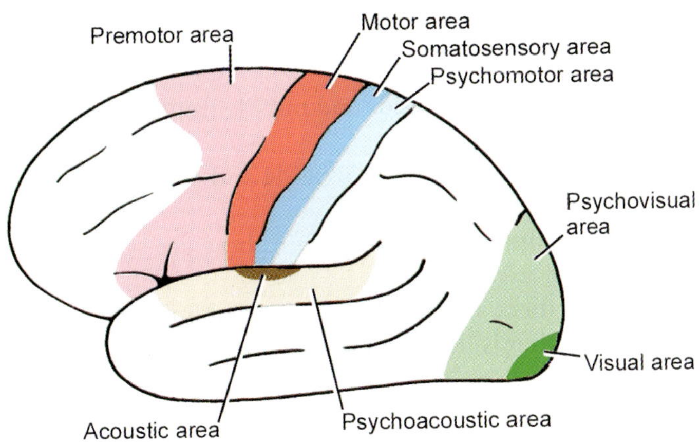


49.24: Functional areas on the superolateral aspect of the cerebral hemisphere

8. The two cerebral hemispheres are interconnected by fibres passing from one to the other. These fibres constitute the ***commissures*** of the cerebrum. The largest of these is the ***corpus callosum*** that is seen just above the lateral ventricles in 49.23.

## IMPORTANT FUNCTIONAL AREAS OF THE CEREBRAL CORTEX

Some areas of the cerebral cortex can be assigned specific functions. These areas can be defined in terms of sulci and gyri described in preceding pages. The subdivisions, as classically described, are as follows 49.24:

### Motor Area

The motor area of classical description is located in the precentral gyrus on the superolateral surface of the hemisphere, and in the anterior part of the paracentral lobule on the medial surface.

#### WANT TO KNOW MORE?

1. Specific regions within the area are responsible for movements in specific parts of the body.
   a. Stimulation of the paracentral lobule produces movement in the lower limbs.
   b. The trunk and upper limb are represented in the upper part of the precentral gyrus.
   c. The face and head are represented in the lower part of the gyrus.
2. Another feature of interest is that the area of cortex representing a part of the body is not proportional to the size of the part, but rather to intricacy of movements in the region. Thus, relatively large areas of cortex are responsible for movements in the hands or in the lips.

### Premotor Area

1. The premotor area is located just anterior to the motor area. It occupies the posterior parts of the superior, middle and inferior frontal gyri.

**WANT TO KNOW MORE?**

2. The part of the premotor area located in the superior and middle frontal gyri corresponds to areas 6 and 8 of Brodmann.
3. The part in the inferior frontal gyrus (corresponds to areas 44 and 45) and constitutes the ***motor speech area (of Broca).***
4. Stimulation of the premotor area results in movements, but these are somewhat more intricate than those produced by stimulation of the motor area.
5. Closely related to the premotor area, there are two specific areas of importance. One is the motor speech area of Broca, mentioned above; and the other is the frontal eye field.

**Motor Speech Area**

1. The motor speech area of Broca lies in the inferior frontal gyrus (areas 44 and 45).
2. Injury to this region results in inability to speak (***aphasia)*** even though the muscles concerned are not paralysed.
3. These effects occur only if damage occurs in the left hemisphere in right handed persons; and in the right hemisphere in left handed persons.
4. In other words, motor control of speech is confined to one hemisphere: that which controls the dominant upper limb.

**Frontal Eye Field**

1. The frontal eye field lies in the middle frontal gyrus just anterior to the precentral gyrus. It includes parts of areas 6, 8, and 9.
2. Stimulation of this area causes both eyes to move to the opposite side. These are called ***conjugate movements.***
3. Movements of the head and dilatation of the pupil may also occur.
4. This, area is connected to the cortex of the occipital lobe that is concerned with vision.

## Sensory Area

1. The sensory area of classical description is located in the postcentral gyrus. It corresponds to areas 1, 2, and 3 of Brodmann.
2. It also extends onto the medial surface of the hemisphere where it lies in the posterior part of the paracentral lobule.
3. Responses can be recorded from the sensory area when individual parts of the body are stimulated.
4. A definite representation of various parts of the body can be mapped out in the sensory area.
5. It corresponds to that in the motor area in that the body is represented upside down.
6. The area of cortex that receives sensations from a particular part of the body is not proportional to the size of that part, but rather to the complexity of sensations received from it.
7. Thus, the digits, the lips and the tongue have a disproportionately large representation.

## Visual Areas

1. The areas concerned with vision are located in the occipital lobe, mainly on the medial surface, both above and below the calcarine sulcus (area 17).
2. Area 17 extends into the cuneus, and into the lingual gyrus. Posteriorly, it may extend onto the superolateral surface where it is limited (anteriorly) by the lunate sulcus.
3. Area 17 is continuous, both above and below, with area 18 and beyond this with area 19.
4. Areas 18 and 19 are responsible mainly for interpretation of visual impulses reaching area 17: They are often described as ***psychovisual areas.***

### Acoustic Area

1. The acoustic area, or the area for hearing, is situated in the temporal lobe.
2. It lies in that part of the superior temporal gyrus that forms the inferior wall of the posterior ramus of the lateral sulcus.
3. In this situation, there are two short oblique gyri called the anterior and posterior ***transverse temporal gyri*** (areas 41, 42 and 52).
4. The acoustic area lies in the anterior transverse temporal gyrus (area 41) and extends to a small extent onto the surface of the hemisphere in the superior temporal gyrus.

## WHITE MATTER OF CEREBRAL HEMISPHERES

Deep to the cerebral cortex, the greater part of each cerebral hemisphere is occupied by nerve fibres that constitute the white matter.

These fibres may be:

1. ***Association fibres*** that interconnect different regions of the cerebral cortex.
2. ***Projection fibres*** that connect the cerebral cortex with other masses of grey matter; and ***vice versa.***
3. ***Commissural fibres*** that interconnect identical areas in the two hemispheres.

### Association Fibres

1. These may be short and may connect adjoining gyri.
2. Alternatively, they may be long and may connect distant parts of the cerebral cortex.
3. Many of the association fibres form bundles that can be seen by gross dissection.
4. Some association fibres pass through commissures to connect ***dissimilar*** areas in the two cerebral hemispheres.

### Projection Fibres

1. These fibres connect the cerebral cortex to centres in the brainstem and spinal cord, in both directions.
2. Fibres to the cortex are often referred to as ***corticopetal fibres***, while those going away from the cortex are referred to as ***corticofugal fibres.***
3. Fibres connecting the cortex with the thalamus, the hypothalamus and the basal ganglia, are also projection fibres.
4. Many of the major projection fibres pass through the internal capsule, which is considered below.

### The Internal Capsule

1. A large number of nerve fibres interconnect the cerebral cortex with centres in the brainstem and spinal cord, and with the thalamus.
2. Most of these fibres pass through the interval between the thalamus and caudate nucleus medially, and the lentiform nucleus laterally. This region is called the ***internal capsule.***
3. Superiorly, the internal capsule is continuous with the corona radiata; and, below, with the crus cerebri (of the midbrain). The internal capsule may be divided into the following parts (49.25).
4. The ***anterior limb*** lies between the caudate nucleus medially, and the anterior part of the lentiform nucleus laterally.
5. The ***posterior limb*** lies between the thalamus medially, and the posterior part of the lentiform nucleus on the lateral side.
6. In transverse sections through the cerebral hemisphere, the anterior and posterior limbs of the internal capsule are seen to meet at an angle open outwards. This angle is called the ***genu*** (genu = bend).
7. Some fibres of the internal capsule lie behind the posterior end of the lentiform nucleus. They constitute its ***retrolentiform part.***
8. Some other fibres pass below the lentiform nucleus (and not medial to it). These fibres constitute the ***sublentiform part*** of the internal capsule.

   Details of the fibres passing through the internal capsule are considered in chapter 53.

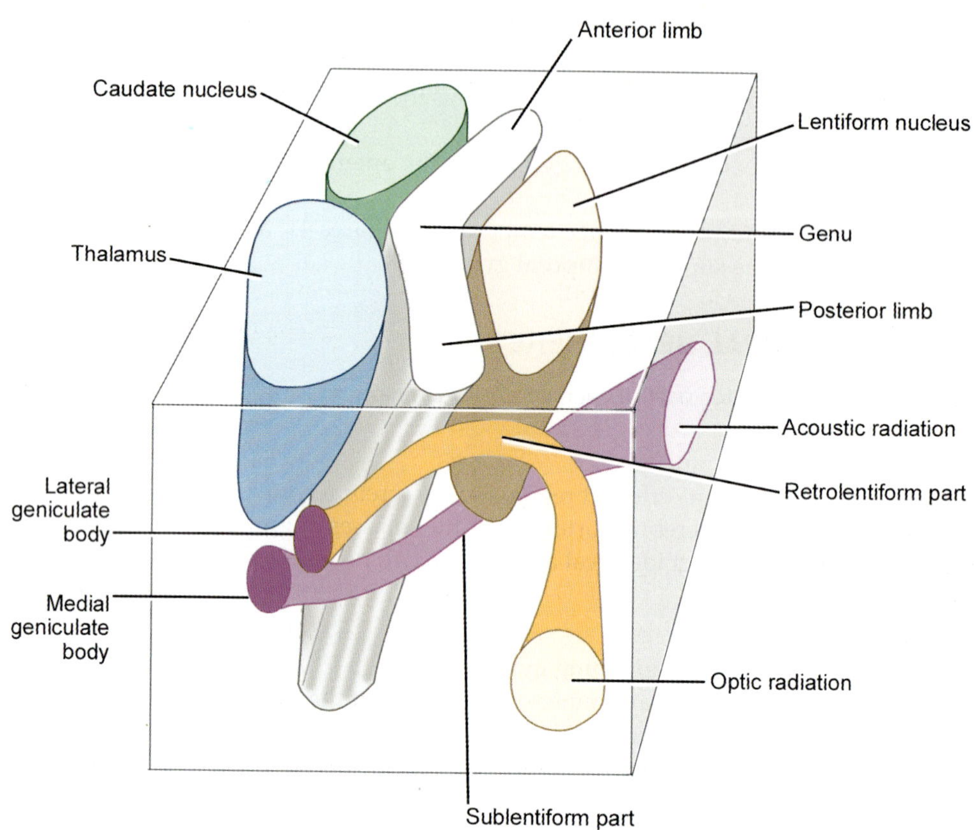


**49.25:** Scheme to show the subdivisions of the internal capsule

## Corpus Callosum

1. The corpus callosum is made up of a large mass of nerve fibres that connect the two cerebral hemispheres (49.20). It is subdivided into:
   a. A central part or ***trunk***
   b. An anterior end that is bent on itself to form the ***genu***
   c. An enlarged posterior end called the ***splenium***
   d. A thin lamina of nerve fibres connects the genu to the upper end of the lamina terminalis. These fibres form the ***rostrum*** of the corpus callosum.
2. The corpus callosum is intimately related to the lateral ventricles. Its undersurface gives attachment to the septum pellucidum (49.20).
3. The fibres of the corpus callosum interconnect the corresponding regions of almost all parts of the cerebral cortex of the two hemispheres.
4. The fibres of the genu run forwards into the frontal lobes, the fibres of the two sides forming a fork-like structure called the ***forceps minor***.
5. Many fibres of the splenium run backwards into the occipital lobe to form a similar structure called the ***forceps major.***
6. Each half of the forceps major bulges into the posterior horn of the corresponding lateral ventricle, forming the ***bulb of the posterior horn***.
7. The fibres of the trunk of the corpus callosum (and some from the splenium) run laterally and as they do so they intersect the fibres of the corona radiata.

8. Some fibres of the trunk and of the splenium, of the corpus callosum form a flattened band called the ***tapetum***. The tapetum is closely related to the posterior and inferior horns of the lateral ventricle.
9. All fibres passing through the corpus callosum are not strictly commissural. Some fibres that interconnect dissimilar areas in the two hemispheres are really association fibres.

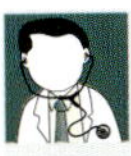

## CLINICAL CORRELATION

**Injuries to the Brain following Injury to the Skull**

1. Fractures of the skull often lead to injury to the brain. An impact on the head can damage the brain even in the absence of a fracture.
2. In this connection, it is to be remembered that the brain is a very delicate tissue. However, it is not damaged by normal bodily movements because
   a. It is surrounded by a cushion of CSF.
   b. Its displacement is prevented by folds of dura mater (falx cerebri, tentorium cerebelli, falx cerebelli).
   c. Veins passing from the brain to the dural venous sinuses (specially the superior cerebral veins passing to the superior sagittal sinus) also help to keep the brain in position.
3. A strong impact on the head can shake up the brain. When this shaking up leaves no apparent physical damage the condition is called ***cerebral concussion***. It is usually followed by a variable period of unconsciousness. On regaining consciousness, the patient may suffer from headaches and loss of memory.
4. An injury in which there is superficial injury to brain tissue (but without any break on its surface) is called ***cerebral contusion***; and when there is tearing of brain tissue it is a ***cerebral laceration***.
5. Severe damage to the brain, specially the brain stem, can lead to prolonged periods of deep unconsciousness (*coma*) and to death. Patients who come out of coma may show various neurological symptoms depending on the part of the brain injured.
6. Apart from direct injury to the brain, injury to the skull can affect the brain by causing haemorrhage. Such bleeding can be of various types.
   a. ***Extradural haemorrhage***: Injury to meningeal vessels can cause bleeding into the potential space between the inner (meningeal) layer of dura mater and the skull. The haematoma can press upon the brain surface and produce symptoms. Extradural haemorrhage is often caused by injury to the anterior division of the middle meningeal artery, resulting in pressure over the motor area of the brain.
   b. ***Subdural haemorrhage***: Blood accumulates in the space between the dura and arachnoid. It is often caused by rupture of superior cerebral veins at their entry into the superior sagittal sinus. Such injury is most likely to be caused by a blow on the front or back of the head (as such injury causes anteroposterior displacement of the brain stretching the veins).
   c. ***Subarachnoid haemorrhage***: Blood flows into the subarachnoid space and mixes with CSF. Such haemorrhage can be caused by rupture of aneurysms that are not uncommon on arteries forming the circulus arteriosus.

# 50 CHAPTER Tracts of Spinal Cord and Brainstem; and Cerebellar Connections

## TRACTS OF SPINAL CORD AND BRAINSTEM

1. A collection of nerve fibres within the central nervous system, that connects two masses of grey matter, is called a tract.
2. A tract may be defined as a collection of nerve fibres having the same origin, course, and termination.
3. Tracts may be ascending or descending.
4. They are usually named after the masses of grey matter connected by them.
   a. Thus, a tract beginning in the cerebral cortex and descending to the spinal cord is called the corticospinal tract.
   b. A tract ascending from the spinal cord to the thalamus is called the spinothalamic tract.
5. Tracts are sometimes referred to as fasciculi or lemnisci.
6. The major tracts passing through the spinal cord and brainstem are shown schematically in 50.1. The tracts seen in a transverse section through the spinal cord are shown in 50.2. They are seen in transverse sections through various levels of the brainstem in 51.1 to 51.7 (in chapter 51).

## DESCENDING TRACTS ENDING IN THE SPINAL CORD

### Corticospinal Tract

1. A scheme showing the main features of this tract is given in 50.3. The corticospinal tract is made up, predominantly, of axons of cells lying in the motor area of the cerebral cortex (area 4).
2. Some fibres also arise from the premotor area (area 6) and some from the somatosensory area (areas 3, 2, 1).
3. From this origin fibres pass through the corona radiata to enter the internal capsule where they lie in the posterior limb (50.3).
4. After passing through the internal capsule the fibres enter the crus cerebri (of the midbrain): they occupy the middle two-thirds of the crus.
5. The fibres then descend through the ventral part of the pons to enter the pyramids in the upper part of the medulla.
6. Near the lower end of the medulla about 80 percent of the fibres cross to the opposite side. (The crossing fibres of the two sides constitute the decussation of the pyramids.)
7. The fibres that have crossed in the medulla enter the lateral funiculus of the spinal cord and descend as the ***lateral corticospinal tract*** (50.2).
   a. The fibres of this tract terminate in grey matter at various levels of the spinal cord.
   b. The internuncial neurons carry the impulses brought by fibres of the tract to ventral column neurons.
8. The corticospinal fibres that do not cross in the pyramidal decussation enter the anterior funiculus of the spinal cord to form the ***anterior corticospinal tract.***
   a. On reaching the appropriate level of the spinal cord the fibres of this tract cross the middle line to reach grey matter on the opposite side of the cord.
   b. In this way the corticospinal fibres of both the lateral and anterior tracts ultimately connect the cerebral cortex of one side with ventral column neurons in the opposite half of the spinal cord.

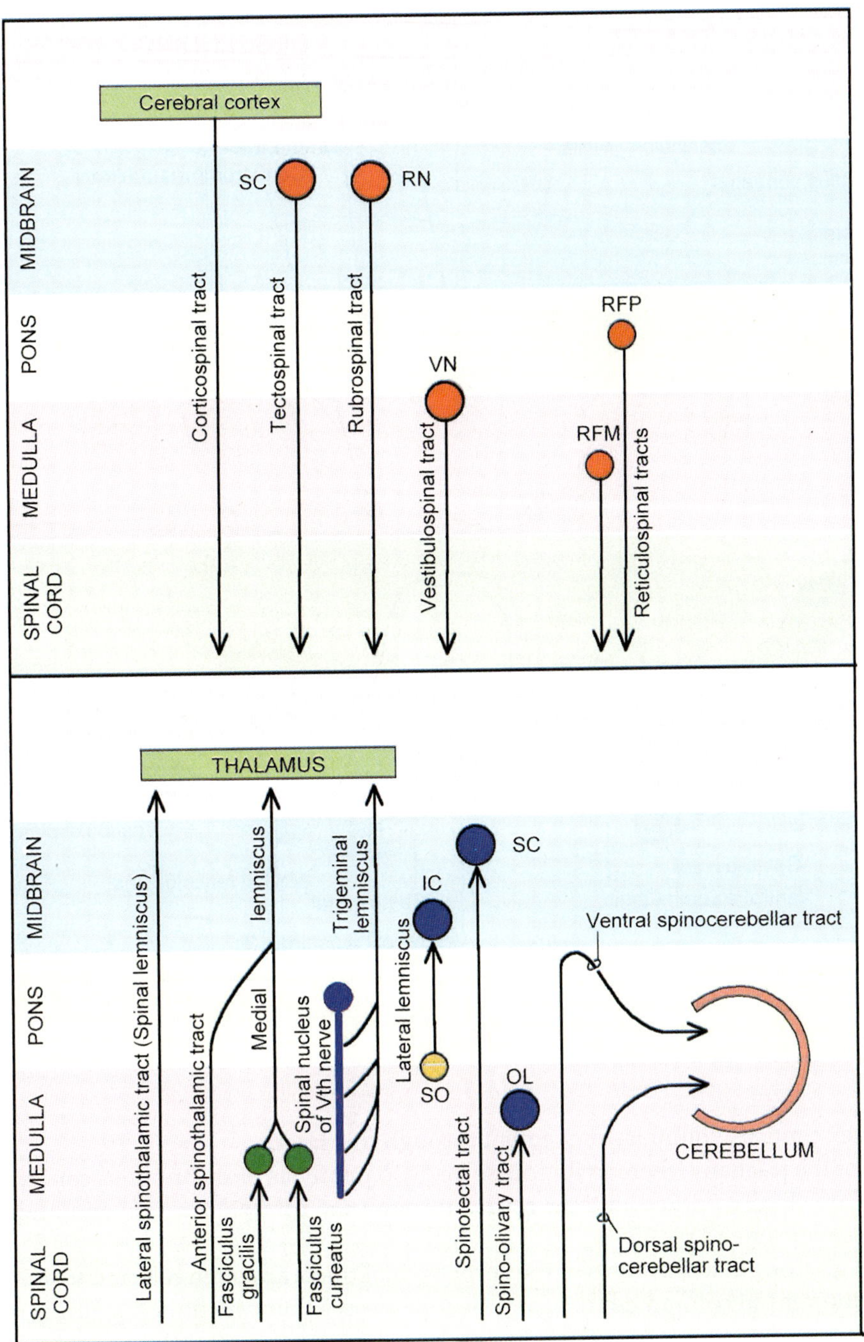


**50.1:** Scheme to show the various tracts passing through the brainstem. SC: superior colliculus; RN: red nucleus; VN: vestibular nuclei; OL: inferior olivary nucleus; RFP: reticular formation of pons; RFM: reticular formation of medulla; IC: inferior collicus; SO: superior olivary nucleus

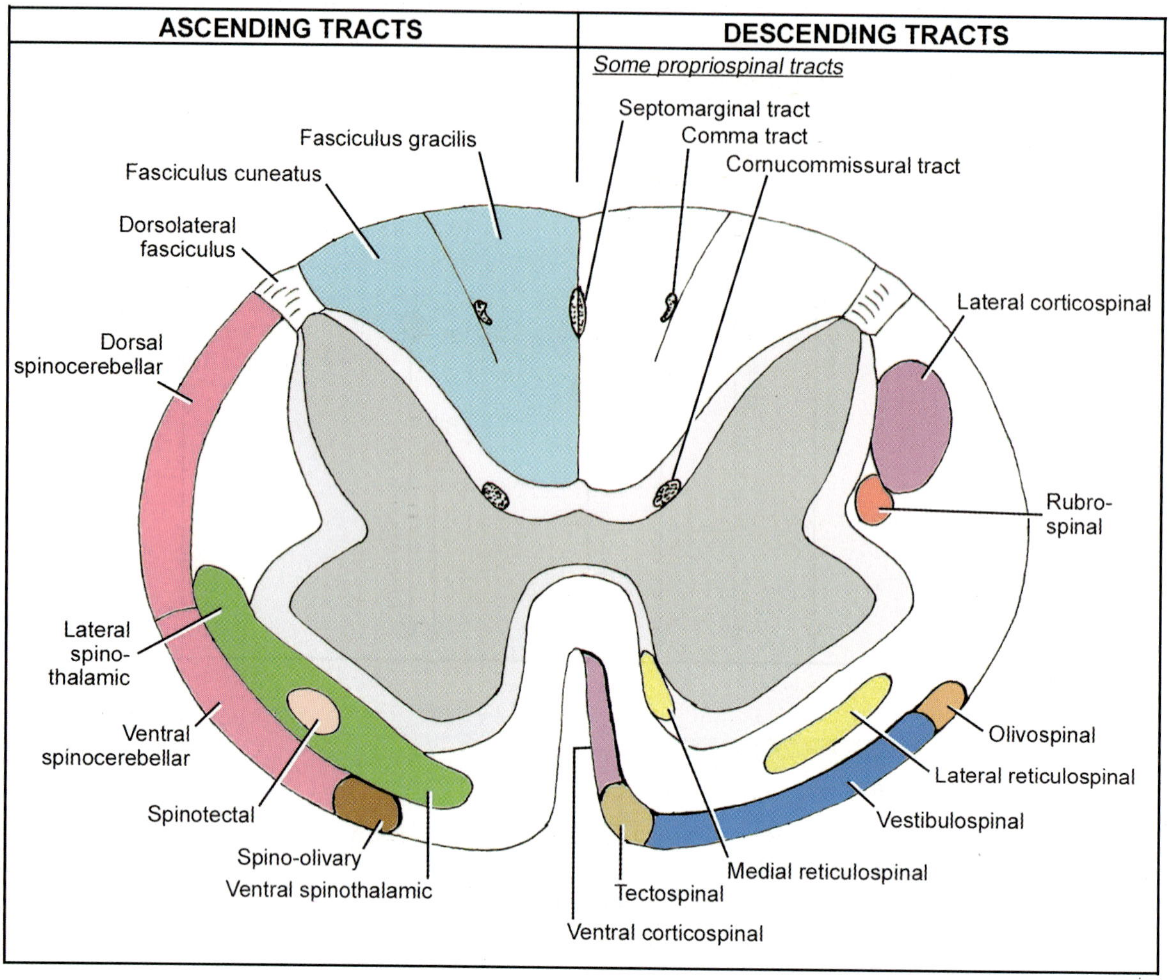

**50.2:** Simplified scheme to show the positions of the main ascending and descending tracts present in the spinal cord

9. The cerebral cortex controls voluntary movement through this tract.
   a. Interruption of the tract anywhere in its course leads to paralysis of the muscles concerned.
   b. As the fibres are closely packed in their course through the internal capsule and brainstem small lesions here can cause widespread paralysis.
10. The neurons that give origin to the fibres of the corticospinal tracts are often referred to as ***upper motor neurons*** in distinction to the ventral column neurons and their processes that constitute the ***lower motor neurons.***
11. Interruption of either of these neurons leads to paralysis, but the nature of the paralysis is distinctive in each case.

## WANT TO KNOW MORE?

***Rubrospinal Tract***

1. This tract is made up of axons of neurons lying in the red nucleus (which lies in the upper part of the midbrain).

2. The fibres of the tract cross to the opposite side in the lower part of the tegmentum of the midbrain. The crossing fibres constitute the ***ventral tegmental decussation*** (51.7).
3. The tract descends through the pons and medulla to enter the lateral funiculus of the spinal cord.
4. The fibres of the tract end by synapsing with ventral column neurons through internuncial neurons located in spinal grey matter.

*Tectospinal Tract*

1. The fibres of this tract arise from neurons in the superior colliculus (midbrain).
2. The fibres cross to the opposite side in the upper part of the tegmentum of the midbrain. The crossing fibres form the ***dorsal tegmental decussation*** (51.7).
3. The tract descends through the pons and medulla into the anterior funiculus of the spinal cord.
4. The fibres terminate by synapsing with ventral column neurons in cervical segments of the cord, through internuncial neurons located in spinal grey matter.

*Vestibulospinal Tract*

1. The neurons of origin of the vestibulospinal tract lie in the lateral vestibular nucleus.
2. This tract is uncrossed and lies in the anterior funiculus of the spinal cord (50.2).
3. Its fibres end in relation to neurons in the ventral grey column.
4. This tract is an important efferent path for equilibrium.

*Olivospinal Tract*

1. This tract is generally described as arising from the inferior olivary nucleus (medulla) and terminating in relation to ventral column neurons of the spinal cord.
2. Its exact connections are, however, unknown.

*Reticulospinal Tracts*

1. Fibres arising in the reticular formation of the brainstem descend to end in relation to internuncial neurons in the spinal cord.
2. Reticulospinal fibres are widely scattered in the anterior and lateral funiculi.
3. Usually, two tracts medial and lateral are recognised.
4. The ***medial reticulospinal tract*** begins in the reticular formation of the pons. Most of its fibres are uncrossed.
5. The ***lateral reticulospinal tract*** begins in the reticular formation of the medulla. It contains both crossed and uncrossed fibres.
6. The fibres of the reticulospinal tracts influence the alpha and gamma motor neurons.

## Significance of Descending Tracts

1. The various descending tracts described above, that end in relation to ventral column neurons, influence their activity, and thereby have an effect on contraction and tone of skeletal muscle.
2. Although, a small number of the fibres of these tracts may synapse directly with ventral column neurons, most of them influence these cells through intervening internuncial neurons.
3. This influence is exerted both on alpha neurons and gamma neurons. Gamma neurons indirectly influence the activity of alpha neurons via muscle spindles. Hence all these influences ultimately reach the alpha neurons. Such influences may be either facilitatory or inhibitory.

### WANT TO KNOW MORE?

4. The corticospinal and rubrospinal tracts are described as being facilitatory to flexors and inhibitory to extensors, while the vestibulospinal tract is said to have the opposite effect. The medial reticulospinal tract is generally regarded as facilitatory and the lateral tract as inhibitory.

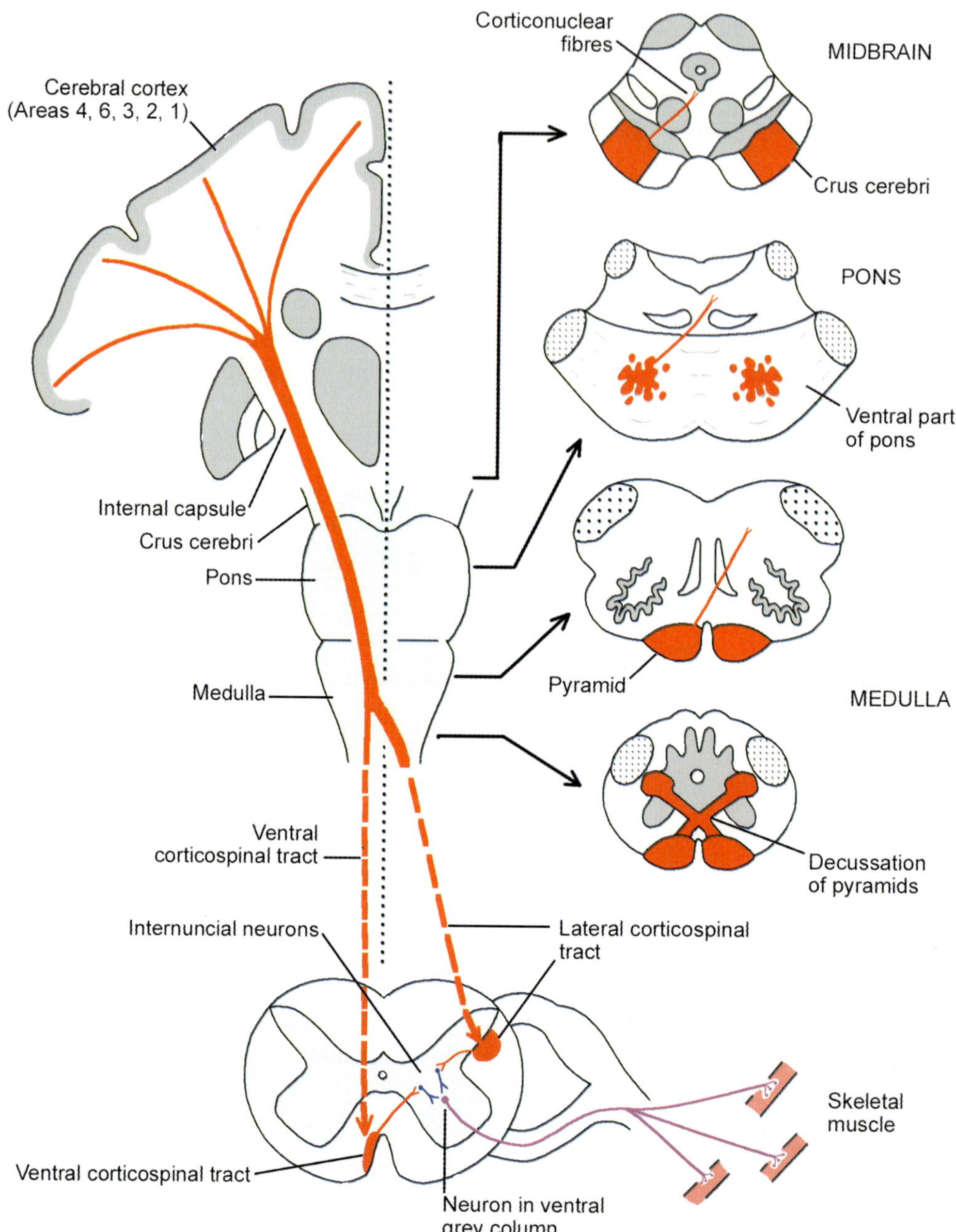


**50.3:** Scheme to show the course of the corticospinal tracts

5. The corticospinal tracts are often referred to as ***pyramidal tracts***.
6. Traditionally all other descending tracts have been collectively referred to as ***extrapyramidal tracts***.
7. It has often been presumed that the pyramidal and extrapyramidal tracts act in opposition to each other. It has also been said that the pyramidal fibres end in relation to alpha neurons, and extrapyramidal fibres in relation to gamma neurons.
8. However, it is now recognised that such a distinction is artificial and of little significance either physiological or clinical.

9. In addition to their influence on motor activity, it has been relatively recently recognised that descending tracts may influence the transmission of afferent impulses through ascending tracts.

## DESCENDING TRACTS ENDING IN THE BRAINSTEM

### Corticonuclear Tracts

1. The nuclei of cranial nerves that supply skeletal muscle (i.e., somatic efferent and special visceral efferent nuclei) are functionally equivalent to ventral column neurons of the spinal cord.
2. They are under cortical control through fibres that are closely related in their origin and course to corticospinal fibres.
3. At various levels of the brainstem these fibres cross to the opposite side to end by synapsing with cells in cranial nerve nuclei, either directly or through interneurons (50.3).

### Cortico-ponto-cerebellar Pathway

1. Fibres arising in the cerebral cortex of the frontal, temporal, parietal and occipital lobes descend through the corona radiata and internal capsule to reach the crus cerebri.
2. The frontopontine fibres occupy the medial one-sixth of the crus; and the temporopontine fibres (along with occipitopontine and parieto-pontine fibres) occupy the lateral one-sixth of the crus (51.6).
3. These fibres enter the ventral part of the pons to end in pontine nuclei of the same side.
4. Axons of neurons in the pontine nuclei form the transverse fibres of the pons. These fibres cross the middle line and pass into the middle cerebellar peduncle of the opposite side. The fibres of this peduncle reach the cerebellar cortex.
5. The cortico-ponto-cerebellar pathway forms the anatomical basis for control of cerebellar activity by the cerebral cortex.

## WANT TO KNOW MORE?

**Disorders of Motor Function**

1. Inability to move a part of the body is referred to as ***paralysis***. This can be produced by interruption of motor pathways anywhere between the motor area of the cerebral cortex and the muscles themselves.
2. We have seen that the pathway from cortex to muscle involves at least two neurons. The first of these is located in the cerebral cortex. Its axon terminates in the spinal cord or in motor cranial nerve nuclei in the brainstem. From a physiological and clinical point of view this neuron is referred to as the upper motor neuron.
3. The second neuron is located in the anterior grey column of the spinal cord (or in motor nuclei of the brainstem) and sends out an axon that travels through a peripheral nerve to innervate muscle. This neuron is referred to as the lower motor neuron.
4. When lower motor neurons are destroyed, or their continuity interrupted, the effects are as follows:
   a. Muscles supplied by them lose their tone (i.e., they become flaccid).
   b. In course of time the muscles undergo atrophy.
   c. Changes in electrical responses of the muscles also take place.
   d. These alterations constitute the ***reaction of degeneration***.
   e. In addition, because of interruption of the efferent part of reflex pathways tendon reflexes are abolished.
5. Destruction or interruption of the upper motor neuron is not followed by any of these changes.
   a. On the other hand it is usually accompanied by an increase in muscle tone.
   b. By exaggeration of tendon reflexes.
6. It is, therefore, possible to distinguish between an ***upper motor neuron paralysis*** (often called ***spastic paralysis***) and a ***lower motor neuron*** (or ***flaccid***) ***paralysis***.
7. Paralysis may be confined to one limb (***monoplegia***) or to both limbs on one side of the body (***hemiplegia***).

8. Paralysis of both lower limbs is called ***paraplegia***, and that of all four limbs is called ***quadriplegia***.
9. Paralysis of muscles supplied by one or more cranial nerves may occur in isolation, or in combination with hemiplegia.
10. Destruction of a particular region often destroys lower motor neurons situated at that level resulting in a localised flaccid paralysis of muscles supplied from that level. This lesion may at the same time interrupt descending tracts (representing upper motor neurons) resulting in a spastic paralysis below the level of the lesion. The presence of a localised flaccid paralysis can thus serve as a pointer to the level of lesion.
11. It is also important to remember that the fibres of upper motor neurons meant for the limbs cross the midline in the lower part of the medulla (in the decussation of the pyramids); and those for the cranial nerves cross just above the level of their termination. A lesion above the level of crossing produces a paralysis in the opposite half of the body, and a lesion below this level produces a lesion on the same side.
12. Keeping the considerations discussed above in mind we may now consider the effects of lesions of the motor pathways at various levels.
    a. Because of the large extent of the motor areas of the cerebral cortex lesions here produce a relatively localised paralysis e.g., a ***monoplegia***.
    b. A lesion in the internal capsule is capable of producing widespread paralysis on the opposite half of the body (***hemiplegia***) which may also involve the lower part of the face and the tongue. A lesion in the internal capsule is most likely to result from thrombosis or rupture of one of the arteries supplying the capsule. The artery most often involved is ***Charcot's artery of cerebral haemorrhage***.
13. Lesions of corticospinal fibres at various levels in the brainstem, above the level of the pyramidal decussation, can produce contralateral hemiplegia. If the lesion crosses the midline symptoms can be bilateral. Involvement of motor cranial nerve nuclei (or of fibres arising from them) may result in various combinations.
    a. For example, a lesion in the upper part of the midbrain can produce a paralysis of muscles supplied by the oculomotor nerve on the side of lesion, along with a hemiplegia on the opposite side (***Weber's syndrome***).
    b. A similar lesion in the pons, results in a paralysis of the lateral rectus muscle (abducent nerve) on the side of lesion with hemiplegia on the opposite side (***Raymond's syndrome***).
    c. Alternatively, facial paralysis of one side can be combined with contralateral hemiplegia (***Millard Gubler syndrome***). Various such combinations may result depending on the level of lesion.
14. Lesions affecting the lateral corticospinal tract in the spinal cord produce an upper motor neuron paralysis of muscles on the same side of the body.
    a. Lesions above the fifth cervical segment result in paralysis of both upper and lower extremities.
    b. While lesions below the first thoracic segment affect only the lower limbs.
    c. As in the brainstem, lesions in the spinal cord may be bilateral.
15. Involvement of lower motor neurons at the level of lesion produces a flaccid paralysis of muscles supplied from that level, along with spastic paralysis below the level of injury. Knowledge of muscles supplied by individual spinal segments can thus help in locating the level of a lesion in the spinal cord.
16. In some diseases (e.g., ***poliomyelitis***) damage may be confined to lower motor neurons, and the resulting paralysis may be purely flaccid.

## ASCENDING TRACTS

### Introductory Remarks

1. The ascending tracts of the spinal cord and brainstem represent one stage of multi-neuron pathways by which afferent impulses arising in various parts of the body are conveyed to different parts of the brain.
2. The ***first order neurons*** of these pathways are usually located in spinal (dorsal nerve root) ganglia (43.17).
    a. The neurons in these ganglia are unipolar (pseudounipolar).
    b. Each neuron gives off a peripheral process and a central process.
    c. The peripheral processes of the neurons form the afferent fibres of peripheral nerves.

d. They end in relation to sensory end organs (receptors) situated in various tissues.
e. The central processes of these neurons enter the spinal cord through the dorsal nerve roots. Having entered the cord the central processes, as a rule, terminate by synapsing with cells in spinal grey matter.
f. Some of them may run upwards in the white matter of the cord to form ascending tracts (50.4).

3. The majority of ascending tracts are, however, formed by axons of cells in spinal grey matter. These are ***second order*** sensory neurons (50.6).
4. In the case of pathways that convey sensory information to the cerebral cortex, the second order neurons end by synapsing with neurons in the thalamus.

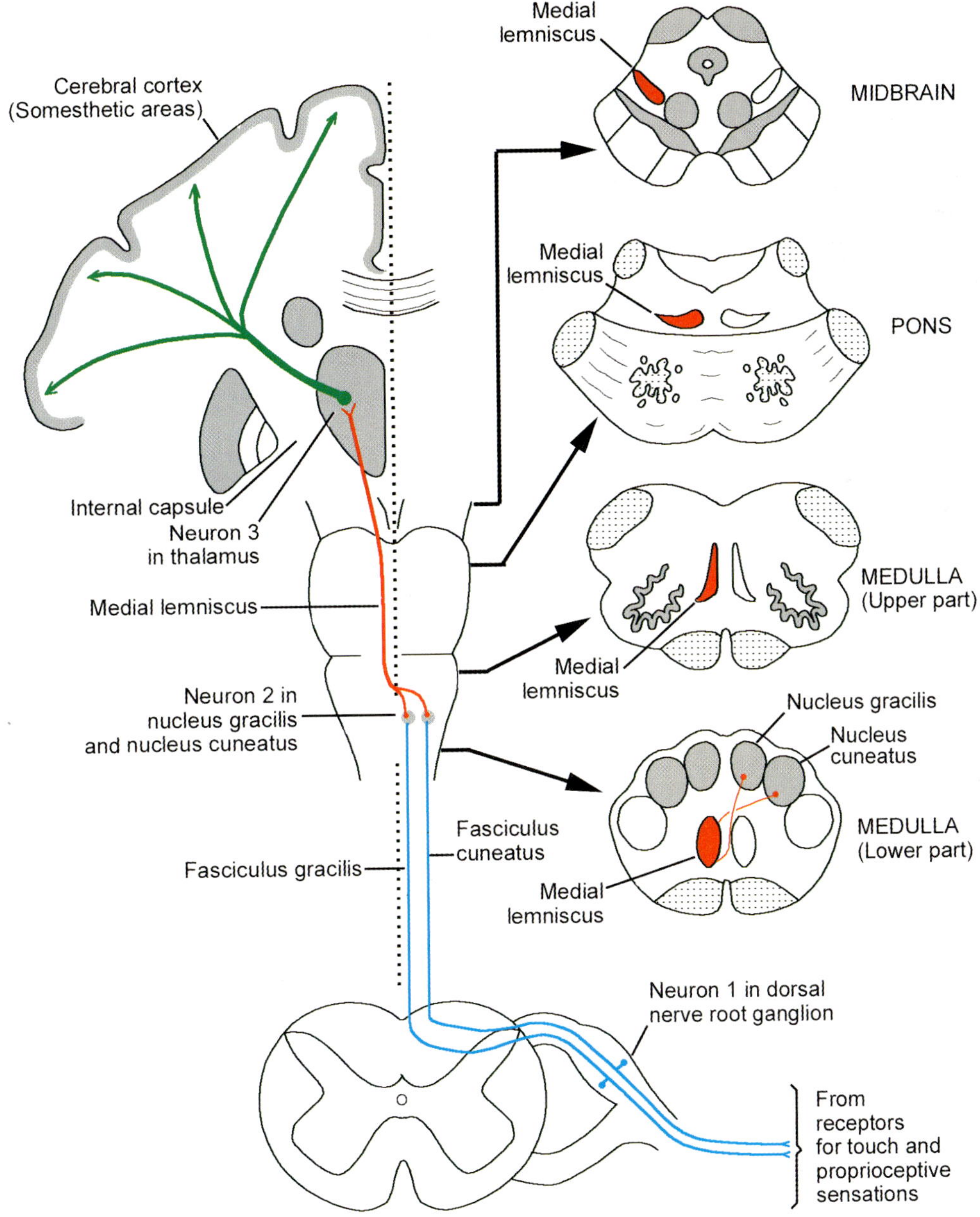


**50.4:** Scheme to show the main features of the posterior column—medial lemniscus pathway

5. ***Third order*** sensory neurons located in the thalamus carry the sensations to the cerebral cortex.
   The following additional points may now be noted:
   a. The axons of the second orders neurons may enter white matter on the same side, forming an uncrossed tract; or on the opposite side, forming a crossed tract.
   b. In the case of the head (and other parts supplied by cranial nerves) the first order neurons are located in sensory ganglia situated on the cranial nerves.
      i. The central processes of these neurons end in relation to afferent nuclei of cranial nerves.
      ii. The neurons in these nuclei constitute second order neurons.
   c. Only those afferent impulses that reach the cerebral cortex are consciously perceived.
      i. One exception to this may be perception of some degree of pain in the thalamus.
      ii. Afferent impulses ending in the cerebellum or in the brainstem influence the activities of these centres.

## Ascending Pathways Connecting the Spinal Cord to the Cerebral Cortex

### *The Posterior Column — Medial Lemniscus Pathway*

### *Fasciculus Gracilis and Fasciculus Cuneatus*

1. These tracts occupy the posterior funiculus of the spinal cord and are, therefore, often referred to as the ***posterior column tracts*** (50.2).
   a. They are unique in that they are formed predominantly by the central processes of neurons located in dorsal nerve root ganglia i.e., by first order sensory neurons (50.4).
   b. The fibres derived from the lowest ganglia are situated most medially; while those from the highest ganglia are most lateral.
   c. The fasciculus gracilis, which lies medially is, therefore, composed of fibres from the sacral, lumbar and lower thoracic ganglia; while the fasciculus cuneatus that lies laterally consists of fibres from upper thoracic and cervical ganglia.
2. The fibres of these fasciculi extend upwards as far as the lower part of the medulla. Here the fibres of the gracile and cuneate fasciculi terminate by synapsing with neurons in the nucleus gracilis and nucleus cuneatus respectively.

### *Medial Lemniscus*

1. The neurons of the gracile and cuneate nuclei are second order sensory neurons.
   a. Their axons run forwards and medially (as ***internal arcuate fibres***) to cross the middle line.
   b. The crossing fibres of the two sides constitute the ***sensory decussation.***
   c. Having crossed the middle line, the fibres turn upwards to form a prominent bundle called the ***medial lemniscus*** (50.4).
   d. The medial lemniscus runs upwards through the medulla, pons and midbrain to end in the thalamus (ventral posterolateral nucleus). Note the position of the medial lemniscus at different levels of the brainstem in 50.4.
2. Third order sensory neurons located in the thalamus give off axons that pass through the internal capsule and the corona radiata to reach the somatosensory areas of the cerebral cortex.
   The posterior column—medial lemniscus pathway described above carries:
   a. Some components of the sense of touch. These include:
      i. Deep touch and pressure.
      ii. The ability to localise exactly the part touched (tactile localisation).
      iii. The ability to recognise as separate two points on the skin that are touched simultaneously (tactile discrimination).
      iv. The ability to recognise the shape of an object held in the hand (stereognosis).

b. Proprioceptive impulses that convey the sense of position and of movement of different parts of the body.
c. The sense of vibration.

## Spinothalamic Pathway

1. The first order neurons of this pathway are located in spinal ganglia. The central processes of these neurons enter the spinal cord and terminate in relation to spinal grey matter. They may ascend in the dorsolateral tract (situated near the tip of the dorsal grey column, 50.2) for one or more segments before ending in grey matter.
2. The second order neurons of this pathway are located in the spinal grey matter.
3. The axons of these neurons constitute the anterior and lateral spinothalamic tracts.
4. They cross to the opposite side of the spinal cord in the white commissure.
   a. This crossing is oblique.
   b. The fibres for the lateral spinothalamic tract cross within the same segment of the cord, while those of the anterior spinothalamic tract may ascend for one or more segments before they cross to the opposite side.
5. The fibres for the anterior spinothalamic tract enter the anterior funiculus (50.2 and 50.5) and ascend to the medulla. This tract merges with the medial lemniscus in the medulla and travels in the lemniscus to the thalamus.
6. The fibres for the lateral spinothalamic tract enter the lateral funiculus. They ascend through the medulla, pons and midbrain (where this tract is often referred to as the ***spinal lemniscus***) to end in the thalamus (ventral posterolateral nucleus).

## Ascending Pathways Ending in the Brainstem

1. A number of tracts arising in spinal grey matter, and ending in masses of grey matter in the brainstem, are described.
2. The ***spinotectal tract*** connects the spinal grey matter to the superior colliculus. It is a crossed tract. It carries impulses that regulate reflex movements of the head and eyes in response to stimulation of some parts of the body. The tract may also carry sensations of pain and temperature.
3. The ***spino-olivary tract*** is also a crossed tract. It conveys proprioceptive impulses to the accessory olivary nuclei. The tract may also carry exteroceptive impulses.

## Spinocerebellar Pathways

1. These pathways carry proprioceptive impulses arising in muscle spindles, Golgi tendon organs, and other receptors to the cerebellum.
2. They constitute the afferent component of reflex arcs involving the cerebellum for control of posture.
3. Some exteroceptive sensations (e.g., touch) may reach the cerebellum through these pathways.
4. The first order neurons of these pathways are located in dorsal nerve root ganglia.
   a. Their peripheral processes end in relation to muscle spindles, Golgi tendon organs and other proprioceptive receptors.
   b. The central processes of the neurons concerned ascend in the posterior funiculi for varying distances before ending in spinal grey matter. Some of them ascend all the way to the medulla and end in the accessory cuneate nucleus.
5. The second order neurons of the pathway are arranged in a number of groups.
   a. Neurons located in the dorsal nucleus (situated on the medial side of the base of the dorsal grey column in segments C8 to L3 of the spinal cord: 49.4) give origin to fibres of the ***dorsal (posterior) spinocerebellar tract.*** This is an uncrossed tract lying in the lateral funiculus (50.2). It ascends to the medulla where its fibres become incorporated in the inferior cerebellar peduncle and pass through it to reach the cerebellum (50.6).
   b. The ***ventral (anterior) spinocerebellar tract*** is predominantly crossed. The fibres ascend in the lateral funiculus, anterior to the fibres of the dorsal spinocerebellar tract (50.2), and pass through the medulla and pons. At the upper end of the pons the fibres turn downwards to enter the superior cerebellar peduncle through which they reach the cerebellum (50.6).

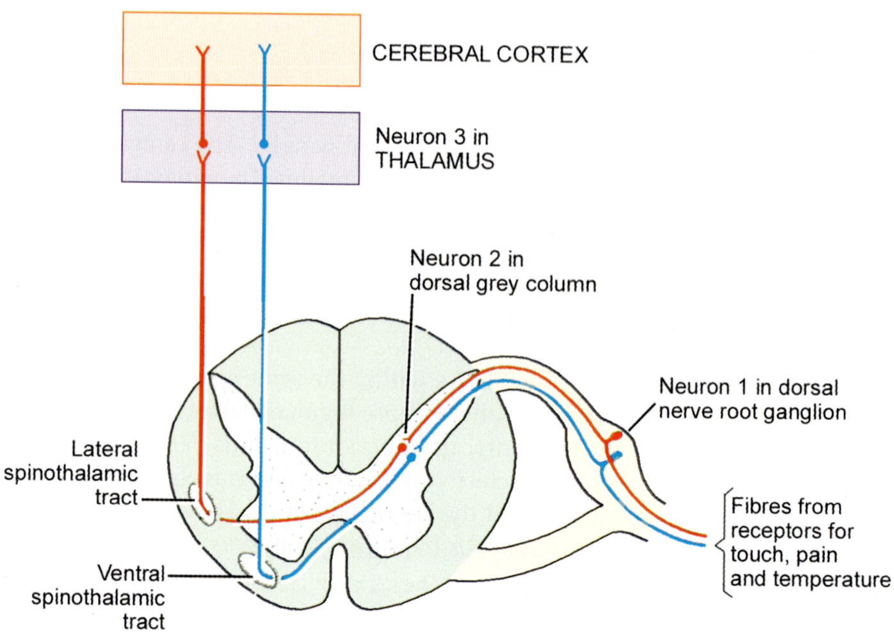


**50.5:** Scheme to illustrate the main features of the spinothalamic tracts

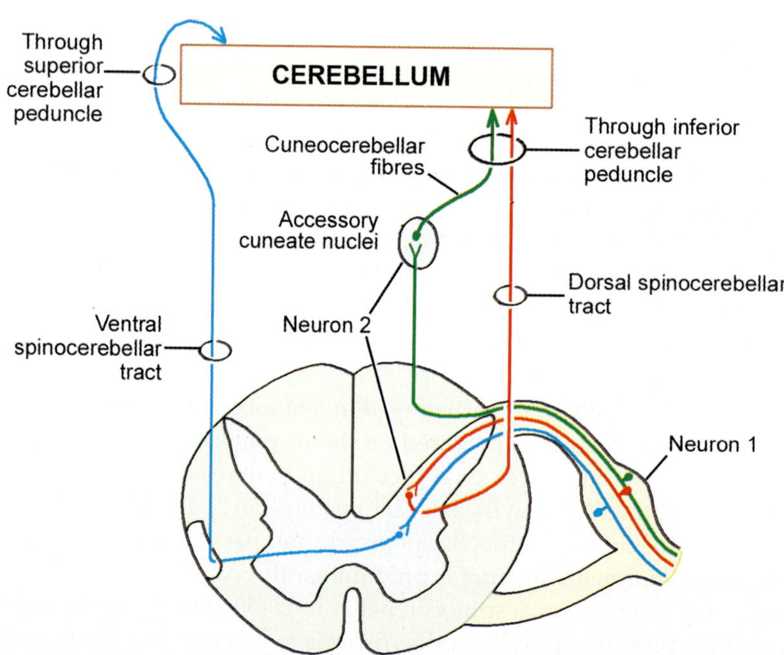


**50.6:** Scheme to illustrate the main features of spinocerebellar pathways

## WANT TO KNOW MORE?

### Sensory Disorders

1. Interruption of ascending pathways carrying various sensations results in loss of sensory perception (***anaesthesia***) over parts of the body concerned.
2. In case of peripheral nerves the area of anaesthesia following injury is often much less than the area of distribution of the nerve. This is so because of considerable overlap in the areas supplied by different nerves.
3. The area of skin supplied from one spinal segment is called a ***dermatome.*** Dermatomes for adjoining segments overlap, a given area of skin being innervated by two or more segments.
4. In the case of spinal cord lesions, the level of disease can be inferred from the level of sensory loss.
   a. In this connection it must be remembered that the finer modalities of touch are carried by the posterior column tracts which are uncrossed.
   b. Crude touch, pain and temperature are carried by the spinothalamic tracts which are crossed.
   c. Thus, a unilateral lesion in the spinal cord can result in loss of the power of tactile localisation, tactile discrimination and of stereognosis on the side of lesion with loss of crude touch, pain and temperature on the opposite side.
   d. Because of a double pathway for touch, loss of sensations of pain and temperature is often more obvious than interference with touch.
5. We have seen that, while crossing the midline, fibres of the spinothalamic tracts do not run horizontally.
   a. They ascend as they cross so that their path is oblique.
   b. The degree of obliquity is greater in the case of fibres carrying touch as compared to those carrying pain and temperature.
   c. Because of this there can be a difference of a few segments in the level at which (or below which) these sensations are lost when the crossing fibres are interrupted by a lesion.
6. In a disease called ***syringomyelia***, the region of the spinal cord near the central canal undergoes degeneration with formation of cavities.
   a. Fibres of spinothalamic tracts crossing in this region are interrupted.
   b. Sensations of pain and temperature are lost over the part of the skin from which fibres are interrupted, but touch is retained as there is an additional pathway for it through the posterior column tracts.
   c. This phenomenon is called ***dissociated anaesthesia.***
7. Sensory disturbances can also result from lesions in the brainstem because of damage to the medial lemniscus or to the spinal and trigeminal lemnisci.
8. Lesions of the thalamus can produce bizarre sensory disturbances.
9. Lesions in the internal capsule can cause sensory loss in the entire opposite half of the body as thalamocortical fibres pass through this region.
10. Pressure on sensory areas of the cerebral cortex can result in various abnormal sensations, or in anaesthesia over certain regions.
11. Damage to pathways carrying special sensations of smell, vision and hearing can result in various defects.

### *Referred Pain*

It sometimes happens that when one of the viscera is diseased pain is not felt in the region of the organ itself; but is felt in some part of the skin and body wall. This phenomenon is called ***referred pain.*** This pain is usually (but not always) referred to areas of skin supplied by the same spinal segments that innervate the viscus. Some classical examples of referred pain are as follows:

1. Pain arising in the diaphragm, or diaphragmatic pleura, is referred to the shoulder (C4).
2. Pain arising in the heart is referred to the lower cervical and upper thoracic segments. It is felt in the chest wall and along the medial side of the left arm. It may also be referred to the neck or jaw.

3. Referred pain from the stomach is felt in the epigastrium (T6 to T9); and that from the intestines is felt in the epigastrium and around the umbilicus (T7 to T10). Pain from the ileocaecal region is felt in the right iliac region. Pain from the appendix is felt in the umbilical region.
4. Pain from the gall bladder is referred to the epigastrium. It may also be referred to the back just below the inferior angle of the right scapula.
5. Pain arising in the area of distribution of one division of the trigeminal nerve may be referred along other branches of the same division, or even along branches of other divisions.

## CONNECTIONS OF THE CEREBELLUM

1. The fundamental points to be appreciated in considering the connections of the cerebellum are that, as a rule (50.7):
   a. Afferent fibres terminate in the cortex.
   b. Efferent fibres arising in the cortex end in cerebellar nuclei.
   c. Fibres arising in the nuclei project to centres outside the cerebellum.
2. There are, however, important exceptions to these rules.
   a. Some fibres (notably vestibular) project directly to the cerebellar nuclei.
   b. Some parts of the cortex give off efferents that bypass the nuclei to reach centres outside the cerebellum.

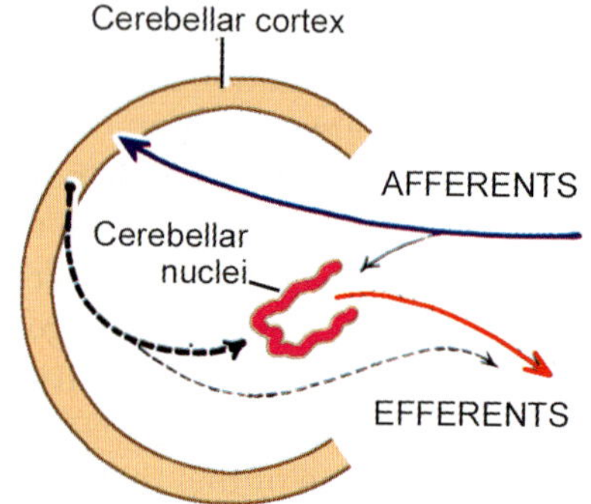


**50.7:** Scheme to show the fundamental arrangement of cerebellar afferents and efferents

### Afferent Fibres Entering the Cerebellum

The cerebellum receives direct afferents from the spinal cord and from various centres in the brainstem. The main afferents are (50.8):

1. ***Spinocerebellar*** (through the various tracts described above). These terminate predominantly in the paleocerebellum.
2. ***Pontocerebellar***. These are part of the cortico-ponto-cerebellar pathway. They end predominantly in the neocerebellum.
3. ***Olivocerebellar***. These end mainly in the neocerebellum and partly in the paleocerebellum.
4. ***Vestibulocerebellar***, from the vestibular nuclei, and also direct fibres of the vestibular nerve.
5. ***Reticulocerebellar*** fibres from the reticular formation of the pons and of the medulla.

The cerebellum also receives fibres from the tectum, the arcuate nuclei, the accessory cuneate nucleus, and from the sensory nuclei of the trigeminal nerve.

### Efferent Fibres leaving the Cerebellum

The main efferents of the cerebellum are (50.8):

1. ***Cerebello-rubral***, to the red nucleus of the opposite side.
2. ***Cerebello-thalamic***, to the thalamus of the opposite side.
3. ***Cerebello-vestibular***, to the vestibular nuclei.
4. ***Cerebello-reticular***, to the reticular formation.

Some fibres from the cerebellum are also believed to reach the inferior olivary nucleus, the nucleus of the oculomotor nerve, and the tectum.

## CEREBELLAR PEDUNCLES

The various fibres entering or leaving the cerebellum pass through the superior, middle and inferior cerebellar peduncles. These connect the cerebellum to the midbrain, the pons and the medulla respectively. The main fibres composing each peduncle are enumerated below. (For additional details see the author's HUMAN NEUROANATOMY).

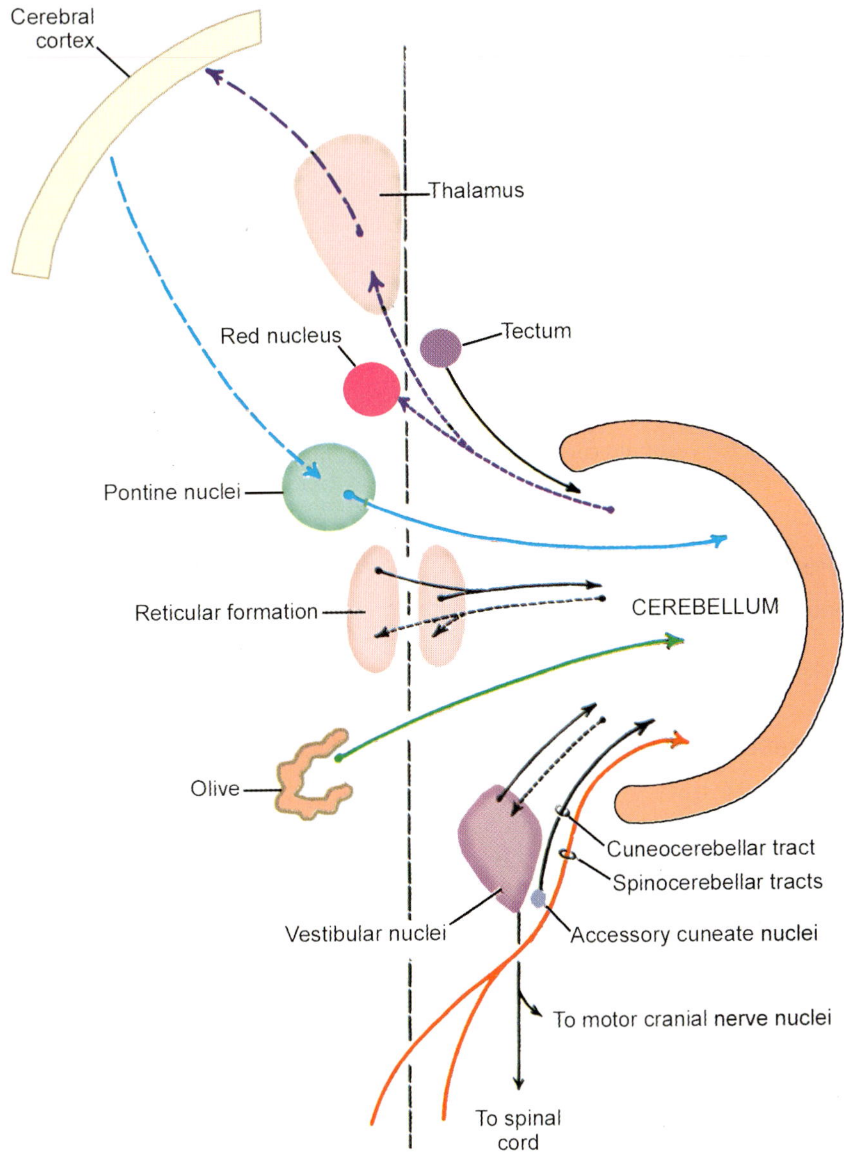


**50.8:** Scheme to show the connections of the cerebellum as a whole

## Superior Cerebellar Peduncle

### *Fibres Entering the Cerebellum*

1. Ventral spinocerebellar tract
2. Rostral (or superior) spinocerebellar tract.

### *Fibres Leaving the Cerebellum*

1. Cerebello-rubral fibres
2. Cerebello-thalamic fibres
3. Cerebello-reticular fibres (from dentate nucleus, some from the fastigial nucleus).

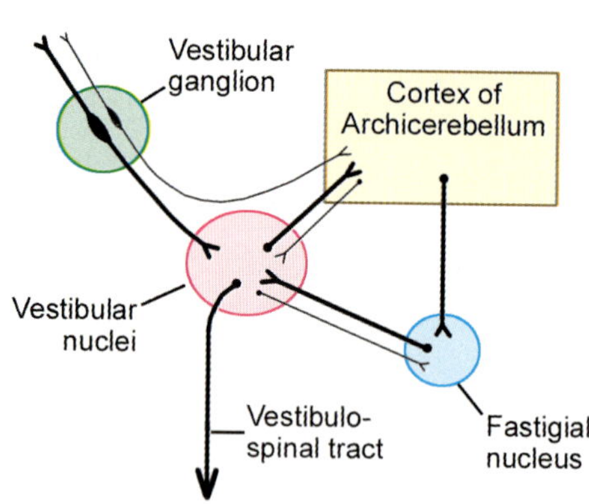


**50.9:** Scheme to show the vestibulo-cerebellar connections

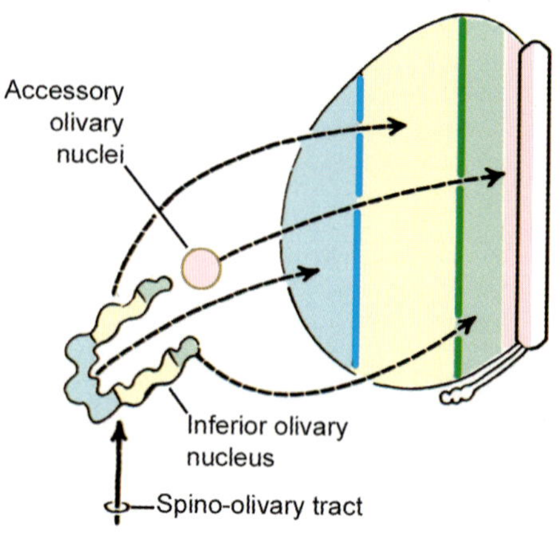


**50.10:** Scheme to show the olivocerebellar connections

## Middle Cerebellar Peduncle

This is made up of pontocerebellar fibres.

## Inferior Cerebellar Peduncle

### *Fibres Entering the Cerebellum*

1. Posterior spinocerebellar tract
2. Cuneocerebellar tract (posterior external arcuate fibres
3. Olivocerebellar fibres from inferior olivary nucleus
4. Reticulocerebellar fibres
5. Vestibulocerebellar fibres
6. Parolivocerebellar fibres from accessory olivary nuclei
7. Anterior external arcuate fibres from arcuate nuclei.

### *Fibres Leaving the Cerebellum*

1. Cerebello-olivary fibres
2. Cerebello-vestibular fibres
3. Cerebello-reticular fibres (from fastigial nucleus)
4. Some cerebello-spinal and cerebello-nuclear fibres are also present.

## WANT TO KNOW MORE?

**Further Details of Cerebellar Connections**

***Vestibulocerebellar Connections***

1. The vestibular nerves carry impulses necessary for maintaining equilibrium (from semicircular ducts, utricle and saccule) to the cerebellum (50.9).
2. The fibres of this nerve are constituted by central processes of bipolar neurons in the vestibular ganglion. They terminate in vestibular nuclei.
3. New fibres arising in the nuclei carry these impulses to the cortex of the flocculonodular lobe (and some adjoining areas).

4. Fibres arising in the flocculonodular lobe project to the fastigial nuclei.
5. Finally, fibres arising in the fastigial nuclei project to the vestibular nuclei.
6. The vestibular nuclei project to the spinal cord through the vestibulospinal tract.
7. Through these connections the cerebellum is able to influence the musculature of the limbs in response to vestibular stimuli.

*Olivocerebellar Connections*

The inferior olivary nucleus (and the accessory olivary nuclei) sends numerous fibres to the opposite half of the cerebellum (50.10).

*Reticulocerebellar Connections*

1. The cerebellum receives fibres from and sends fibres to the reticular formation.
2. Impulses passing from the cerebellum to the reticular formation are relayed to the spinal cord and to cranial nerve nuclei through reticulospinal and reticulonuclear pathways; and to the thalamus through reticulothalamic fibres.

*Cerebello-rubral Connections*

1. Fibres arising in the emboliform and globose nuclei (and some from the dentate nucleus) pass through the superior cerebellar peduncle to reach the red nucleus.
2. These enable the cerebellum to influence the spinal cord through the rubrospinal tract.
3. In this cerebello-rubro-spinal pathway, there is a double decussation.
   a. The cerebellorubral fibres cross in the decussation of the superior cerebellar peduncle while
   b. The rubrospinal fibres cross in the ventral tegmental decussation.
4. As a result the cerebellum influences the same side of the spinal cord.

*Cerebello-thalamic Connections*

Fibres arising in the dentate nucleus (and a few in the emboliform and globose nuclei) pass through the superior cerebellar peduncle, to reach the thalamus of the opposite side, either directly, or after relay in the red nucleus.

***Connections of Cerebellar Nuclei***

1. We have seen that the cerebellar nuclei receive afferents from the cerebellar cortex. As a broad generalisation it can be said that:
   a. The fastigial nuclei receive fibres from the flocculonodular lobe and other parts of the vermis (archicerebellum).
   b. The emboliform and globose nuclei from the paravermal cortex (mainly paleocerebellum).
   c. The dentate nuclei from the lateral part of the cerebellar hemispheres.
2. Efferent fibres from the dentate nucleus (accompanied by some fibres from the emboliform and globose nuclei) constitute the greater part of the superior cerebellar peduncle.
3. On reaching the lower part of the midbrain most of these fibres cross the middle line (in the decussation of the superior cerebellar peduncle) and ascend to the red nucleus and to the thalamus. For details see 50.11.
4. Fibres arising in fastigial nuclei pass through the inferior cerebellar peduncle and reach the vestibular nuclei and the reticular formation.

## Summary of Pathways Interconnecting the Cerebellum and Spinal Cord

Spinocerebellar pathways convey to the cerebellum proprioceptive information necessary for controlling muscle tone and for maintaining body posture. These pathways also carry exteroceptive impulses.

### *Direct Pathways from Spinal Cord to Cerebellum*

1. These are the ventral spinocerebellar tract, and the dorsal spinocerebellar tract that convey information from the hindlimb.

2. Information from the forelimb is probably conveyed by the rostral spinocerebellar tract and the cuneocerebellar tract. The cuneocerebellar tract begins in the medulla, but is included here as it is functionally equivalent to spinocerebellar tracts.

### *Indirect Pathways from Spinal Cord to Cerebellum*

These are:

1. Spino-olivo-cerebellar
2. Spino-reticulo-cerebellar
3. Spino-vestibulo-cerebellar
4. Spino-tecto-cerebellar pathways.

### *Cerebello-spinal Pathways*

The cerebellum can influence the spinal cord through the following pathways:

1. Cerebello-rubro-spinal
2. Cerebello-vestibulo-spinal
3. Cerebello-reticulo-spinal
4. Cerebello-tecto-spinal
5. Cerebello-thalamo-cortico-spinal.

### *Summary of Connections between the Cerebellum and the Cerebral Cortex*

The connections between the cerebellum and the cerebral cortex are all indirect.

### *Corticocerebellar Pathways*

The cerebral cortex influences the cerebellum through various centres in the brainstem (and possibly even through the spinal cord) through the following pathways.

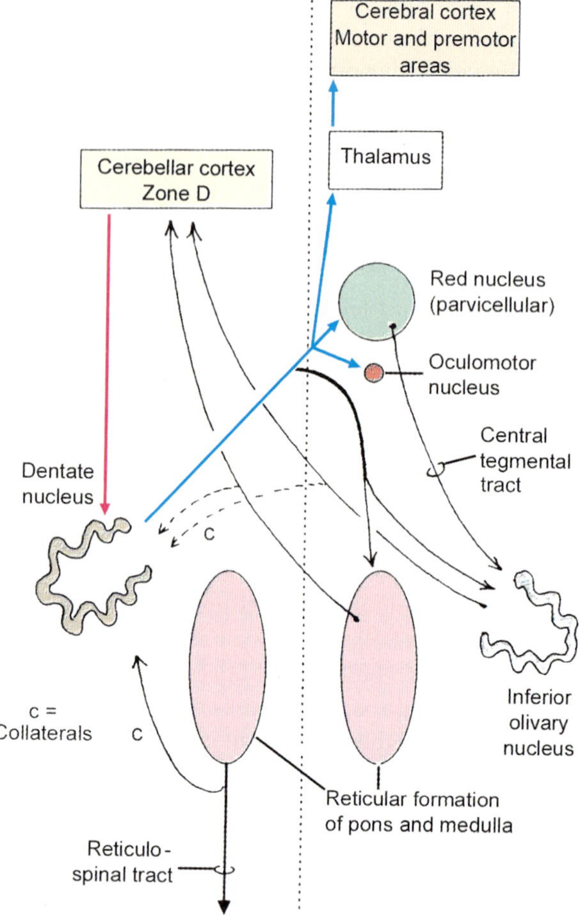


**50.11:** Scheme to show the connections of the dentate nucleus

The most important of these is the cortico-ponto-cerebellar pathway. The arcuate nuclei and the pontobulbar body represent displaced pontine nuclei. The cortico-arcuato-cerebellar, and the cortico-ponto-bulbar cerebellar pathways are, functionally, equivalent to the cortico-ponto-cerebellar pathway.

Other pathways connecting the cerebral cortex to the cerebellum are as follows:

1. Cortico-olivo-cerebellar
2. Cortico-reticulo-cerebellar
3. Cortico-rubro-cerebellar
4. Cortico-tecto-cerebellar
5. Cortico-spino-cerebellar.

Some of the impulses may reach these intermediary centres through the corpus striatum.

### *Cerebello-cortical Pathways*

We have seen that the cerebellum projects upon the cerebellar nuclei from where fresh fibres relay to the thalamus. Thalamocortical fibres carry these impulses to the cerebral cortex.

## Functions of the Cerebellum

1. The cerebellum plays an essential role in the control of movement.
2. It is responsible for ensuring that movement takes place smoothly, in the right direction, and to the right extent.

3. It is responsible for maintaining the equilibrium of the body.
4. These functions are possible because the cerebellum receives constant information regarding the state of contraction of muscles, and of the position of various joints.
5. It also receives information from the eyes, the ears, the vestibular apparatus, the reticular formation and the cerebral cortex.
6. All this information is integrated, and is used to influence movement through motor centres in the brainstem and spinal cord, and also through the cerebral cortex.

## WANT TO KNOW MORE?

**Disorders of Equilibrium**

1. The maintenance of equilibrium, and of correct posture, is dependent on reflex arcs involving various centres including the spinal cord, the cerebellum, and the vestibular nuclei.
2. Interruption of any of these pathways; or lesions in the cerebellum, the vestibular nuclei and other centres concerned; can result in various abnormalities involving maintenance of posture and coordination of movements.
3. Inability to maintain the equilibrium of the body, while standing, or while walking, is referred to as ***ataxia***.
   a. This may occur as a result of the interruption of afferent proprioceptive pathways (sensory ataxia).
   b. Disease of the cerebellum itself, or of efferent pathways, results in more severe disability.
4. Coordination of the activity of different groups of muscles is interfered with, leading to various defects.
5. The person is unable to stand with his feet close together: the body sways from side-to-side and the person may fall.
6. While walking, the patient staggers and is unable to maintain progression in the desired direction.
7. Lack of proprioceptive information can be compensated to a considerable extent by information received through the eyes. The defects mentioned are, therefore, much more pronounced with the eyes closed (***Romberg's sign***).
8. Lack of coordination of muscles also interferes with purposeful movements (***asynergia***). Movements are jerky and lack precision.
   a. For example, the patient finds it difficult to touch his nose with a finger, or to move a finger along a line.
   b. There is difficulty in performing movements involving rapid alternating action of opposing groups of muscles (e.g., tapping one hand with the other; repeated pronation and supination of the forearm). This phenomenon is called ***dysdiadokokinesis***.
   c. Incoordination of the muscles responsible for the articulation of words leads to characteristic speech defects (***dysarthria***).
   d. For the same reason, the eyes are unable to fix the gaze on an object for any length of time.
   e. Attempts to bring the gaze back to the same point result in repeated jerky movements of the eyes. This is called ***nystagmus***.
9. Apart from incoordination, cerebellar disease is characterised by diminished muscle tone (***hypotonia***).
   a. The muscles are soft, and tire easily (***asthenia***).
   b. Joints may lack stability (***flail joints***).
   c. Tendon reflexes may be diminished. Alternatively, tapping a tendon may result in oscillating movements of the part concerned, like a pendulum.

# 51 CHAPTER

# Internal Structure of Brainstem

1. A brief outline of the internal structure of the brainstem has been given in Chapter 49. (This chapter should be revised before proceeding further).
2. We have also considered the cranial nerve nuclei and their connections, and the tracts passing through the brainstem (Chapter 50).
3. With this background we will now consider the internal structure of the brainstem as seen in transverse sections at various levels.

## THE MEDULLA

### Section through the Medulla at the Level of the Pyramidal Decussation

1. A section through the medulla ***at the level of the pyramidal decussation*** is shown in 51.1.
2. Some features to be seen at this level have been reviewed on page 1044 (49.4).
   a. The pyramids and their decussation
   b. The nucleus gracilis
   c. The nucleus cuneatus

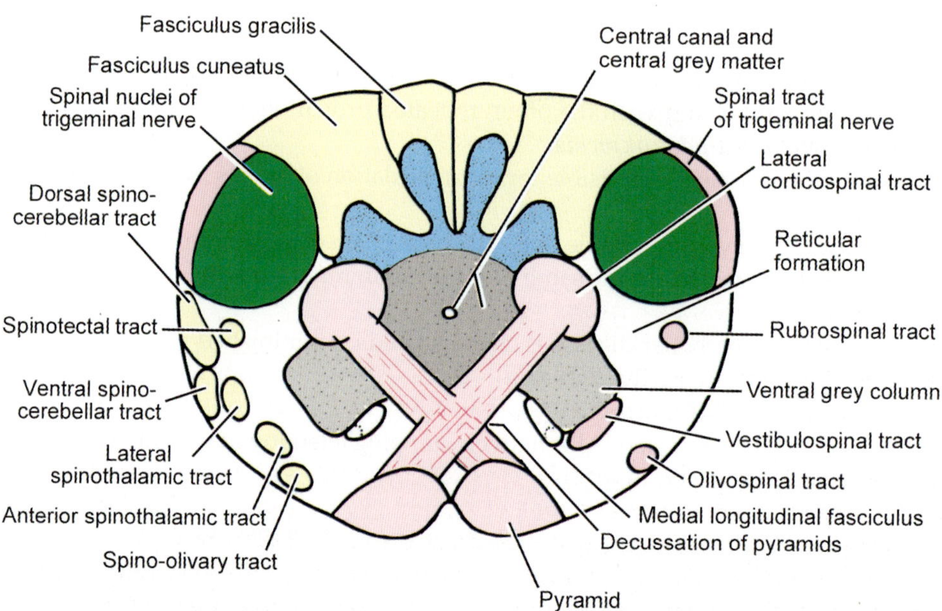


**51.1:** Transverse section through the medulla at the level of the pyramidal decussation

   d. The spinal nucleus of the trigeminal nerve
   e. The central grey matter
   f. The central canal
   g. The uppermost part of the ventral grey column have been identified.
3. The ventral grey column is separated from the central grey matter by decussating pyramidal fibres.
   a. The neurons in it give origin to the uppermost rootlets of the first cervical nerve, and to some fibres in the spinal root of the accessory nerve.
   b. The area between the ventral grey column and the spinal nucleus of the trigeminal nerve is occupied by the lower part of the reticular formation.
4. The main descending fibres to be seen at this level are:
   a. The corticospinal fibres that form the pyramids.
   b. After crossing the midline, these fibres turn downwards in the region lateral to the central grey matter to form the lateral corticospinal tract.
   c. We have already seen that those fibres of the pyramids that do not cross descend into the ventral funiculus of the spinal cord to form the ventral corticospinal tract.
5. Other descending tracts to be seen at this level (in the anterolateral part of the medulla, 51.1, right half) are:
   a. The rubrospinal tract
   b. The vestibulospinal tract
   c. The olivospinal tract
   d. The tectospinal tract. The tectospinal tract is incorporated within the medial longitudinal fasciculus.
   e. Among descending tracts we may also include the spinal tract of the trigeminal nerve, which forms a layer of fibres superficial to the spinal nucleus of this nerve.
6. The ascending tracts to be seen at this level include:
   a. The fasciculus gracilis
   b. Fasciculus cuneatus which occupy the areas behind the corresponding nuclei
   c. The spinothalamic
   d. Spinocerebellar
   e. Spinotectal
   f. Spino-olivary tracts that occupy the anterolateral region.

## Section through the Medulla at the Level of the Lemniscal Decussation

1. A section through the medulla ***at the level of the sensory decussation*** is shown in 51.2. Some features of a section at this level have already been seen (page 1045, 49.5).
   a. The central canal surrounded by central grey matter
   b. The medial lemniscus
   c. The pyramids
   d. The nucleus gracilis
   e. The nucleus cuneatus
   f. The spinal nucleus of the trigeminal nerve
   g. The reticular formation have been identified.
2. The nucleus gracilis and the nucleus cuneatus are much larger than at lower levels.
3. Internal arcuate fibres arising in these nuclei arch forwards and medially around the central grey matter to cross the middle line.
4. Having crossed the middle line these fibres turn cranially to constitute the medial lemniscus.
5. As the fibres from the nucleus gracilis and the nucleus cuneatus pass forwards they intercross so that the fibres from the nucleus gracilis come to lie ventral to those from the nucleus cuneatus.
   a. The most medial fibres (from the legs) come to lie most anteriorly in the medial lemniscus.
   b. These are followed by fibres from the trunk and from the upper limb in that order.

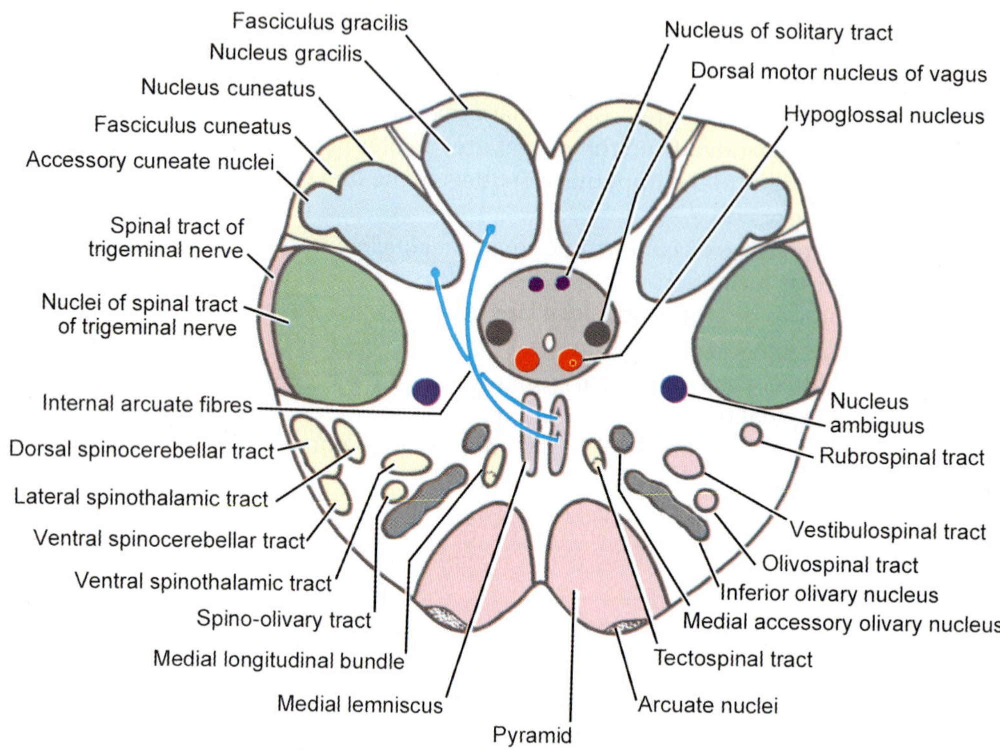


**51.2:** Transverse section through the medulla at the level of the lemniscal decussation

6. Higher up in the brainstem the medial lemniscus changes its orientation, its long axis (as seen in cross section) becoming transverse (51.5).
   a. The most anterior fibres become lateral, and the posterior fibres become medial.
   b. As it ascends through the medulla, the medial lemniscus is probably joined by the anterior spinothalamic tract.
7. A number of cranial nerve nuclei can be identified at this level. Several of these are present in relation to the central grey matter.
   a. The hypoglossal nucleus is located ventral to the central canal just lateral to the middle line.
   b. The dorsal vagal nucleus lies dorsolateral to the hypoglossal nucleus.
   c. The nucleus of the solitary tract is seen dorsal to the central canal near the middle line.
   d. The lower ends of these nuclei of the two sides become continuous with each other to form the ***commissural nucleus*** of the vagus.
   e. The nucleus ambiguus lies in the reticular formation medial to the spinal nucleus of the trigeminal nerve.
8. Other masses of grey matter that may be recognised at this level are:
   a. The lowest part of the ***inferior olivary nucleus***.
   b. The ***medial accessory olivary nucleus*** which lies dorsal to the medial part of the inferior olivary nucleus (see below).
   c. The ***lateral reticular nucleus*** lying in the lateral part of the reticular formation.
   d. ***Arcuate nuclei*** lying on the anterior aspect of the pyramids.
9. The gracile and cuneate fasciculi are much smaller than at lower levels as the fibres of these tracts progressively terminate in the gracile and cuneate nuclei.

10 Other ascending tracts to be seen at this level are:
   a. The spinothalamic
   b. Spinocerebellar

c. Spinotectal
d. Spino-olivary tracts all of which lie in the anterolateral region (51.2, left half).

11. The descending tracts present are (51.2, right half):
   a. The pyramids
   b. The rubrospinal
   c. Vestibulospinal
   d. Olivospinal tracts
   e. Medial longitudinal fasciculus which includes the tectospinal tract.

## Section through the Medulla at the Level of the Olive

1. A section through the medulla ***at the level of the olive*** is shown in 51.3.
2. Some features of a transverse section at this level have been introduced on page 1045 (49.6).
   a. The floor of the fourth ventricle lined by grey matter
   b. The reticular formation
   c. The spinal nucleus and tract of the trigeminal nerve
   d. The inferior cerebellar peduncle
   e. The inferior olivary nucleus
   f. The medial lemniscus
   g. The pyramids have been briefly considered.

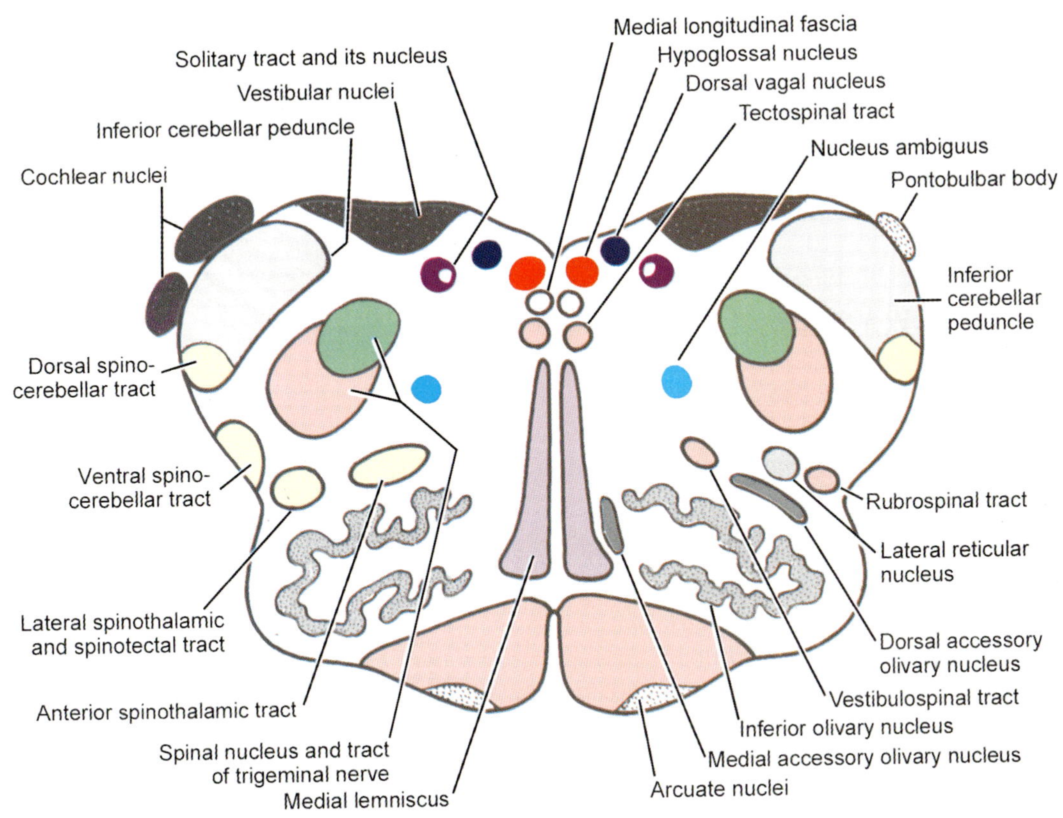


**51.3:** Transverse section through the medulla at the level of the olive

3. Several cranial nerve nuclei can be recognised in relation to the floor of the fourth ventricle. From medial to lateral side these are:
   a. The hypoglossal nucleus.
   b. The dorsal vagal nucleus.
   c. The vestibular nuclei.
   d. The solitary tract and its nucleus lie ventrolateral to the dorsal vagal nucleus.
   e. The nucleus ambiguus lies much more ventrally within the reticular formation.
4. The dorsal and ventral cochlear nuclei can be seen in relation to the inferior cerebellar peduncle. (They are shown schematically in 51.3. They are actually seen at higher levels of the medulla, near its junction with the pons).
5. Other masses of grey matter present are:
   a. The medial and dorsal accessory olivary nuclei (lying medial and dorsal, respectively, to the inferior olivary nucleus).
   b. The lateral reticular nucleus and arcuate nuclei which occupy the same relative positions as at lower levels.
   c. The pontobulbar body lies on the dorsolateral aspect of the inferior cerebellar peduncle (51.3, right).
6. The descending tracts to be seen at this level (51.3, right half) are:
   a. The pyramids
   b. The tectospinal
   c. Vestibulospinal
   d. Rubrospinal tracts
   e. The spinal tract of the trigeminal nerve.
7. The ascending tracts are:
   a. The medial lemniscus forming an anteroposterior L-shaped band lying next to the middle line
   b. The spinothalamic
   c. Spinocerebellar
   d. Spinotectal tracts.
8. At this level, the dorsal spinocerebellar tract lies within the inferior cerebellar peduncle. The ventral spinocerebellar tract lies more anteriorly near the surface of the medulla. The spinothalamic tracts lie dorsolateral to the inferior olivary nucleus.
9. The medial longitudinal fasciculus lies dorsal to the medial lemniscus.

## WANT TO KNOW MORE?

*Connections of the Inferior Olivary Nucleus*

1. The main afferents of the inferior olivary nucleus are from the cerebral cortex and from the spinal cord.
2. The main efferents are to the cerebellar cortex and to the spinal cord.

*Connections of Other Nuclei*

1. The ***accessory olivary nuclei*** are connected to the cerebellum by parolivocerebellar fibres.
2. The ***arcuate nuclei*** are generally regarded as displaced pontine nuclei.
   a. Cortical fibres reach them through the pyramids.
   b. These are relayed to the cerebellum by fibres that follow two separate pathways.
   c. Some of them wind round the anterior and lateral aspect of the medulla as anterior external arcuate fibres to reach the inferior cerebellar peduncle of the opposite side.
   d. Other fibres pass dorsally through the substance of the medulla to reach the floor of the fourth ventricle. Here they run under the ependyma to the inferior cerebellar peduncle of the opposite side as fibres of the striae medullares.
   e. Fibres from the arcuate nuclei probably end in the flocculus of the cerebellum.

3. Like the arcuate nuclei, the ***pontobulbar body*** is made up of neurons that represent displaced pontine nuclei.
   a. Fibres arising in this body form the ***circumolivary bundle***.
   b. These fibres join those from the arcuate nuclei to reach the inferior cerebellar peduncle of the opposite side.
   c. Some of them possibly pass through the striae medullares.

## THE PONS

1. Transverse sections through the upper and lower parts of the pons are illustrated in 51.5 and 51.4. Some features common to both these levels have been already considered (page 1046, 49.7).
   a. The subdivision of the pons into dorsal and ventral parts and its relationship to the superior, middle and inferior cerebellar peduncles has been noted.
   b. We have seen that the ventral part of the pons contains:
      i. The pontine nuclei
      ii. Vertically running corticospinal and corticopontine fibres
      iii. Transversely running fibres arising in the pontine nuclei and projecting to the opposite half of the cerebellum through the middle cerebellar peduncle.
2. The ***pontine nuclei*** (or ***nuclei pontis***) receive corticopontine fibres from the frontal, temporal, parietal and occipital lobes of the cerebrum.
   a. Their efferents form the transverse fibres of the pons.
   b. We have seen that most of these fibres cross to the opposite side, but some may end ipsilaterally.

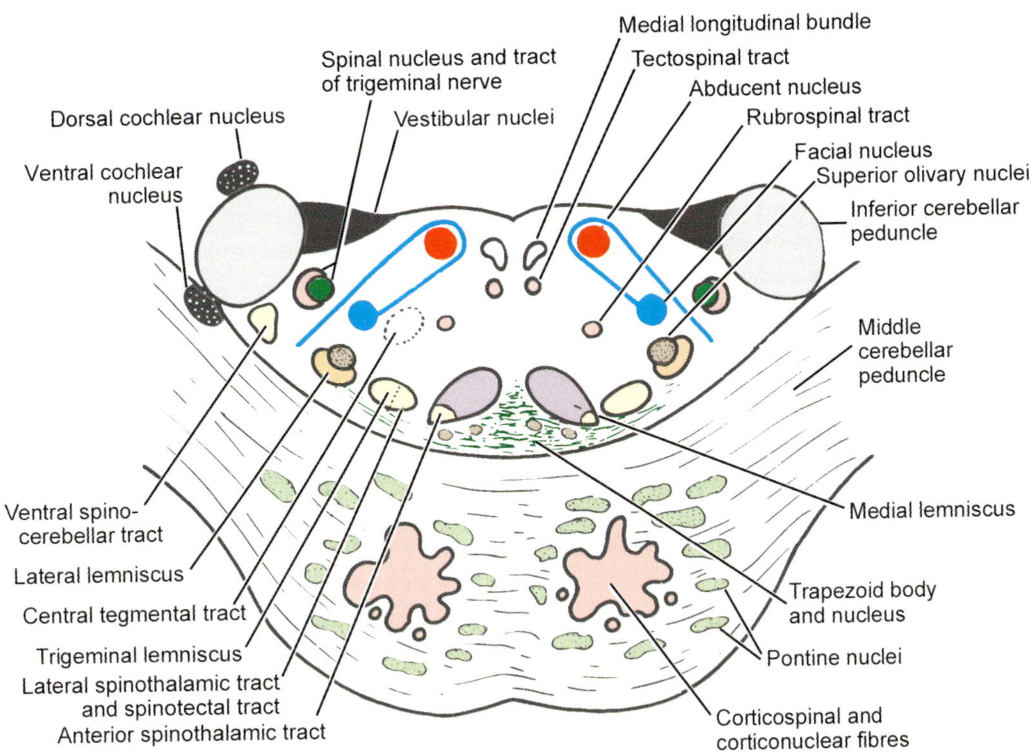


**51.4:** Transverse section through the lower part of the pons

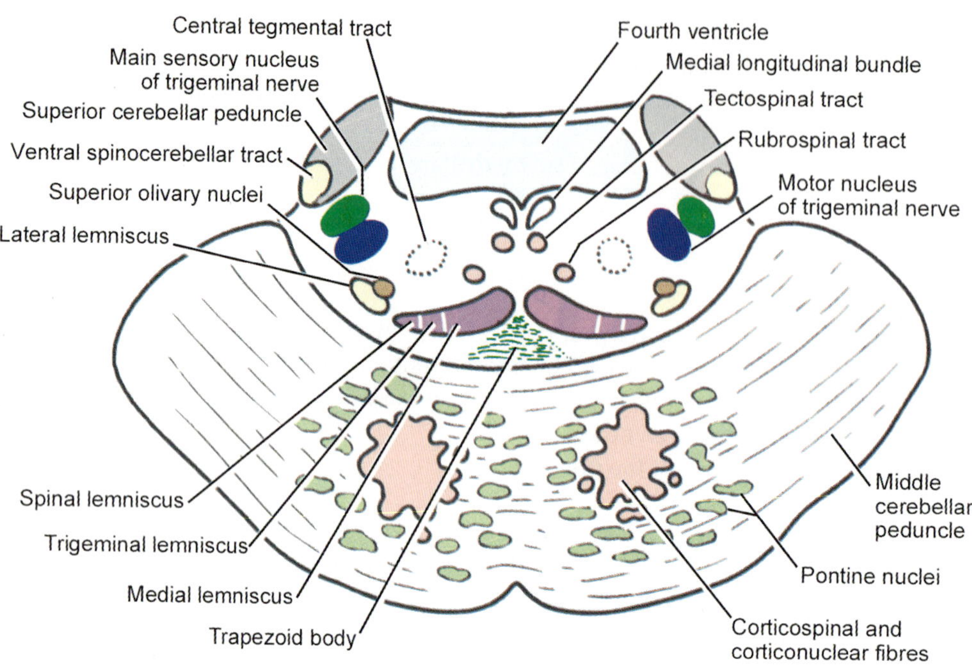


**51.5:** Transverse section through the upper part of the pons

3. The dorsal part of the pons is occupied, predominantly, by the reticular formation.
4. Its posterior surface helps to form the floor of the fourth ventricle. This surface is lined by grey matter and is related to some cranial nerve nuclei.
5. The dorsal part is bounded laterally by the inferior cerebellar peduncle in the lower part of the pons, and by the superior cerebellar peduncle in the upper part.
6. The region adjoining the ventral part is occupied by important ascending tracts.
   a. The medial lemniscus occupies a transversely elongated oval area next to the middle line.
   b. Lateral to this are the trigeminal lemniscus and the spinal lemniscus (lateral spinothalamic tract).
   c. The fibres of the spinotectal tract run along with the spinal lemniscus, while those of the ventral spinothalamic tract lie within the medial lemniscus.
   d. Still more laterally, there is the lateral lemniscus.
   e. Ventral to these lemnisci there are conspicuous transversely running fibres that form the ***trapezoid body***.
   f. The ventral spinocerebellar tract lies ventromedial to the inferior cerebellar peduncle in the lower part of the pons (51.4). In the upper part of the pons it is seen within the superior cerebellar peduncle (51.5).
7. Descending tracts passing through the dorsal part of the pons are:
   a. The tectospinal tract
   b. The rubrospinal tract.
8. The medial longitudinal fasciculus lies dorsally near the middle line.

We will now consider those features of the pons that are different in the upper and lower parts.

## Section through Lower Part of Pons

1. A section through the lower part of the pons (51.4) shows two cranial nerve nuclei that are closely related to the floor of the fourth ventricle.
   a. These are the abducent nucleus lying medially and the vestibular nuclei that lie laterally.
   b. At a deeper level in the lateral part of the reticular formation two additional nuclei are seen.

   c. These are the spinal nuclei of the trigeminal nerve (along with its tract) lying laterally.
   d. The facial nucleus lying medially.
   e. The dorsal and ventral cochlear nuclei lie dorsal and ventral, respectively, to the inferior cerebellar peduncle.
2. The fibres arising from the facial nucleus follow an unusual course that has been described earlier. We have seen that the abducent nucleus and the facial nerve fibres looping around it together form a surface elevation, the *facial colliculus,* in the floor of the fourth ventricle.
3. The vestibular nuclei occupy the vestibular area in the lateral part of the floor of the fourth ventricle. These nuclei are to be seen in the lower part of the pons and in the upper part of the medulla (51.3 and 51.4).
4. Other masses of grey matter to be seen in the lower part of the pons are:
   a. The superior olivary complex (made up of several nuclei) which lies dorsomedial to the lateral lemniscus.
   b. The nuclei of the trapezoid body which consist of scattered cells lying within this body.

### Section through Upper Part of Pons

1. A section through the upper part of the pons (51.5) shows that the dorsal part is bounded laterally by the superior cerebellar peduncles.
2. Medial to the peduncle there is the main sensory nucleus of the trigeminal nerve, and further medially there is the motor nucleus of the same nerve.
3. The superior olivary nucleus extends to this level, but is less prominent; while the lateral lemniscus forms a more conspicuous bundle.
4. Some fibres of the trapezoid body can be seen ventral to the medial lemniscus.
5. The reticular formation of the pons is described later in this chapter.

## THE MIDBRAIN

1. Some features of the internal structure of the midbrain have been considered on page 1047 (49.9).
   a. The subdivision of the midbrain into the tectum, the tegmentum, the substantia nigra, and the crus cerebri (or basis pedunculi) has been noted.
   b. The superior and inferior colliculi, the red nucleus and the reticular formation have been identified.

### Transverse Sections through the Midbrain

1. A transverse section through the midbrain at the level of the inferior colliculus is shown in 51.6 and a section at the level of the superior colliculus in 51.7. We will first consider those features that are common to both these levels.
2. The *crus cerebri* (or *basis pedunculi*) consists of fibres descending from the cerebral cortex.
   a. Its medial one-sixth is occupied by corticopontine fibres descending from the frontal lobe.
   b. The lateral one-sixth is occupied by similar fibres from the temporal, occipital and parietal lobes.
   c. The intermediate two-thirds of the crus cerebri are occupied by corticospinal and corticonuclear fibres.
   d. The fibres for the leg are most lateral and those for the head are most medial.
3. The *substantia nigra* lies immediately behind and medial to the basis pedunculi. It appears dark in unstained sections as neurons within it contain pigment (neuromelanin).
4. The midbrain is traversed by the cerebral aqueduct that is surrounded by central grey matter.
5. Ventrally, the central grey matter is related to cranial nerve nuclei (oculomotor and trochlear).
6. The region between the substantia nigra and the central grey matter is occupied by the reticular formation.

### Section through Midbrain at Level of Inferior Colliculus

1. A section through the midbrain at the level of the inferior colliculus shows the following additional features (51.6).

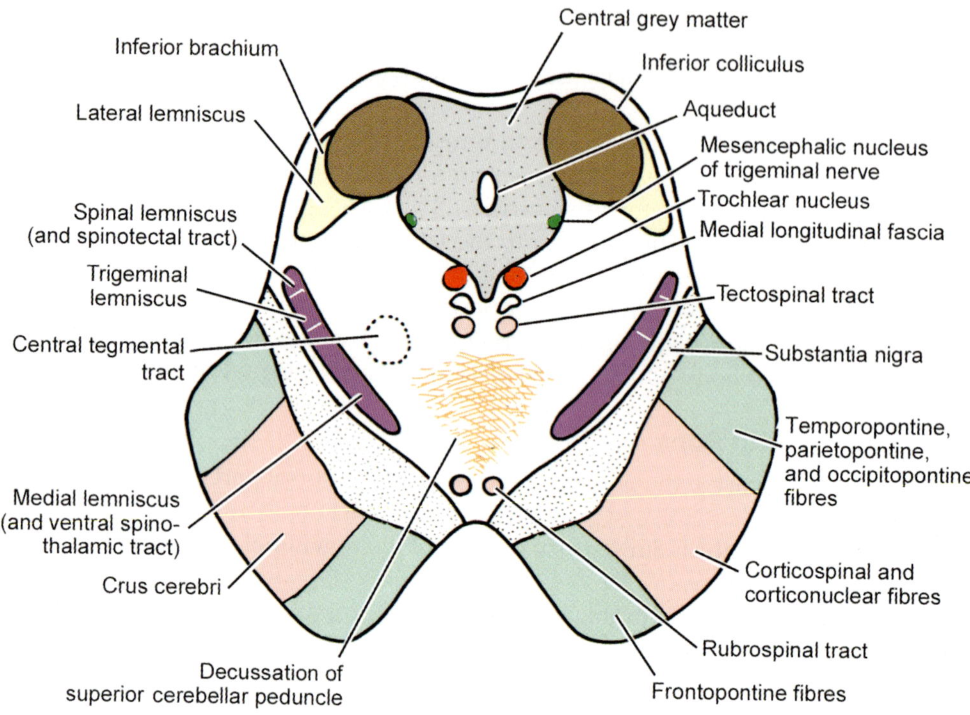


**51.6:** Transverse section through the lower part of the midbrain

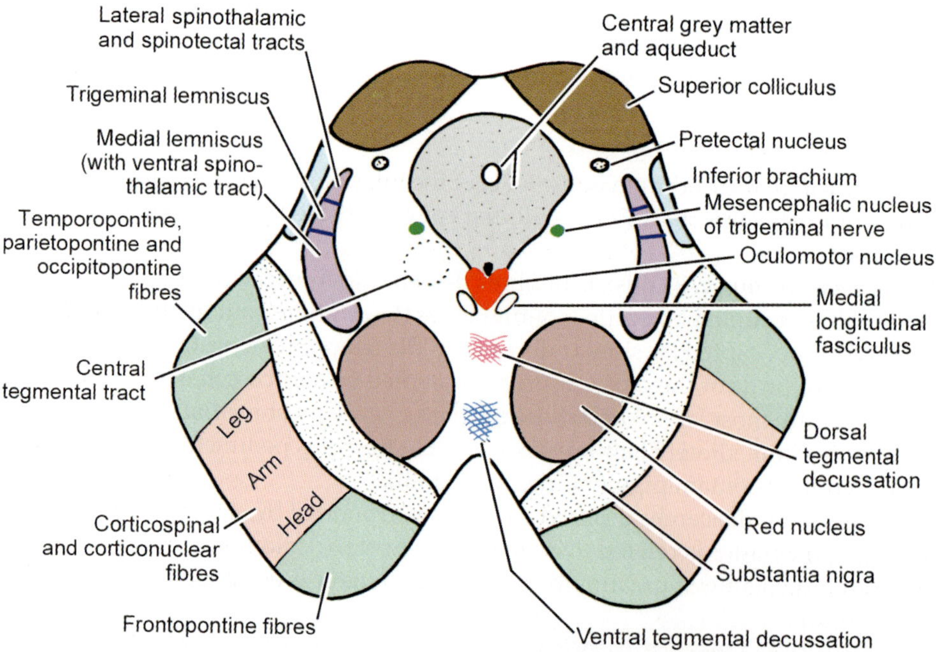


**51.7:** Transverse section through the upper part of the midbrain

2. The ***inferior colliculus*** is a large mass of grey matter lying in the tectum. It forms a cell station in the auditory pathway and is probably concerned with reflexes involving auditory stimuli.
3. The ***trochlear nucleus*** lies in the ventral part of the central grey matter.
   a. Fibres arising in this nucleus follow an unusual course.
   b. They run dorsally and decussate (in the superior medullary velum) before emerging on the dorsal aspect of the brainstem.
4. The ***mesencephalic nucleus of the trigeminal nerve*** lies in the lateral part of the central grey matter.
5. A compact bundle of fibres lies in the tegmentum dorsomedial to the substantia nigra. It consists of:
   a. The medial lemniscus
   b. The trigeminal lemniscus
   c. The spinal lemniscus in that order from medial to lateral side.
6. The medial lemniscus includes fibres of the ventral spinothalamic tract while the spinal lemniscus (made up mainly of the lateral spinothalamic tract) includes fibres of the spinotectal tract.
7. More dorsally, the lateral lemniscus forms a bundle ventrolateral to the inferior colliculus (in which most of its fibres end).
8. Important fibre bundles are also located near the middle line of the tegmentum.
   a. The medial longitudinal fasciculus lies ventral to the trochlear nucleus.
   b. Ventral to the fasciculus there is the tectospinal tract.
9. The region ventral to the tectospinal tracts is occupied by decussating fibres of the superior cerebellar peduncle.
   a. These fibres have their origin in the dentate nucleus of the cerebellum.
   b. They cross the middle line in the lower part of the tegmentum.
   c. Some of these fibres end in the red nucleus while others ascend to the thalamus.
10. The part of the tegmentum ventral to the decussation of the superior cerebellar peduncle is occupied by the rubrospinal tracts.

## Section through Midbrain at Level of Superior Colliculus

1. A section through the upper part of the midbrain (51.7) shows two large masses of grey matter not seen at lower levels. These are:
   a. The ***superior colliculus*** in the tectum
   b. The ***red nucleus*** in the tegmentum.
2. The superior colliculus is a centre concerned with visual reflexes.
3. The red nucleus (so called because of a reddish colour in fresh material) lies in the anterior part of the tegmentum dorsomedial to the substantia nigra.
4. The ***oculomotor nucleus*** lies in relation to the ventral part of the central grey matter. The nuclei of the two sides lie close together forming a single complex.
5. The ***Edinger Westphal nucleus*** (which supplies the sphincter pupillae and ciliaris muscle) forms part of the oculomotor complex.
6. The oculomotor complex is related ventrally to the medial longitudinal fasciculus.
7. Closely related to the cranial part of the superior colliculus there is a small collection of neurons that constitute the ***pretectal nucleus***. This nucleus is concerned with the pathway for the pupillary light reflex.
8. The bundle of ascending fibres consisting of the medial lemniscus, the trigeminal lemniscus and the spinal lemniscus lies more dorsally than at lower levels (because of the presence of the red nucleus).
9. The lateral lemniscus is not seen at this level as its fibres end in the inferior colliculus.
10. However, the ***inferior brachium*** that conveys auditory fibres to the medial geniculate body can be seen near the surface of the tegmentum.
11. The middle line region of the tegmentum shows two groups of decussating fibres.
    a. The ***dorsal tegmental decussation*** consists of fibres that have their origin in the superior colliculus and cross to the opposite side to descend as the tectospinal tract.
    b. The ***ventral tegmental decussation*** consists of fibres that originate in the red nucleus and decussate to form the rubrospinal tracts.

## WANT TO KNOW MORE?

*Connections of the Red Nucleus*

1. The nucleus receives its main afferents from:
   a. The cerebral cortex.
   b. The cerebellum (dentate, emboliform and globose nuclei).
2. The main efferents are to the spinal cord through the rubrospinal tract, and also to motor cranial nerve nuclei.
3. The red nucleus may, therefore, be considered as an integrating and relay centre on the following pathways:
   a. Cortico rubrospinal
   b. Cortico rubronuclear
   c. Cerebello rubrospinal.

*Connections of the Inferior Colliculus*

1. The inferior colliculus is an important relay centre in the acoustic (auditory) pathway.
2. It receives fibres of the lateral lemniscus arising in the superior olivary complex.
3. Each colliculus receives auditory impulses from both ears.
4. These impulses are relayed to the medial geniculate body and from there to the acoustic area of the cerebral cortex.

*Connections of the Superior Colliculus*

1. The superior colliculus has a complex laminar structure, being made up of six (or more) layers.
2. Its most important afferents are those that bring visual impulses from the retina.
3. The major efferents are the tectospinal tract, and tectonuclear fibres to the nuclei of cranial nerves responsible for moving the eyes and head.
4. The colliculus has, therefore, been regarded as a centre for reflex movements of the head and eyes in response to visual stimuli.

*Connections of the Substantia Nigra*

1. The main connections (both afferent and efferent) are with the striatum (i.e., caudate nucleus and putamen).
2. Dopamine produced by neurons in the substantia nigra passes along their axons to the striatum.
3. Dopamine is much reduced in patients with a disease called Parkinsonism in which there is a degeneration of the striatum.

## Reticular Formation of the Brainstem

1. The term reticular formation was originally used to designate areas of the central nervous system that were not occupied by well-defined nuclei or fibre bundles, but consisted of a network of fibres within which scattered neurons were situated.
2. Such areas are to be found at all levels in the nervous system.
   a. In the spinal cord there is an intermingling of grey and white matter on the lateral side of the neck of the dorsal grey column. This area is sometimes referred to as the reticular formation of the spinal cord.
   b. The reticular formation is, however, best defined in the brainstem where it is now recognised as an area of considerable importance.
3. Some centres in the cerebrum and cerebellum are regarded, by some authorities, to be closely related, functionally, to this region.
4. The reticular formation extends throughout the length of the brainstem.
   a. In the medulla it occupies the region dorsal to the inferior olivary nucleus.
   b. In the pons it lies in the dorsal part.
   c. In the midbrain it lies in the tegmentum.

**WANT TO KNOW MORE?**

*Connections of the Reticular Formation*

1. The reticular formation has numerous connections. Directly, or indirectly, it is connected to almost all parts of the nervous system.
2. The pathways involved are both ascending and descending; crossed and uncrossed, somatic and visceral.
3. The reticular formation receives impulses from the motor and other areas of the cerebral cortex and relays them to the spinal cord through the medial and lateral reticulospinal tracts.
4. It is also connected to the cerebellum and to the thalamus.
5. Fibres passing from the reticular formation to the thalamus constitute the ***ascending reticular activating system*** (ARAS).

## Functions of the Reticular Formation

Because of its diverse connections the reticular formation is believed to have a controlling or modifying influence on many functions. Some of them are as follows:

### *Somatomotor Control*

Through its direct connections with the spinal cord; and indirectly through the corpus striatum, the cerebral cortex and the cerebellum, the reticular formation has an influence on fine control of movements including those involved in postural adjustments, locomotion, skilled use of the hands, speech etc.

### *Somatosensory Control*

The reticular formation influences conduction through somatosensory pathways. Similar effects may also be exerted on visual and auditory pathways.

### *Visceral Control*

1. Physiological studies have shown that stimulation of certain areas in the reticular formation of the medulla has great influence on respiratory and cardiovascular function.
2. These effects are mediated through connections between the reticular formation and autonomic centres in the brainstem and spinal cord, but the pathways concerned are not well defined.

### *Neuroendocrine Control*

Through its connections with the hypothalamus, the reticular formation influences activity of the adenohypophysis and of the neurohypophysis. A similar influence is also exerted on the pineal body.

### *Alertness*

Through the ascending reticular activating system the reticular formation helps to maintain a state of alertness.

52

CHAPTER

# Diencephalon, Basal Ganglia, Olfactory Region and Limbic System

## THE DIENCEPHALON

1. The diencephalon consists of:
   a. The thalamus (or dorsal thalamus)
   b. The hypothalamus
   c. The epithalamus
   d. The subthalamus (or ventral thalamus)
   e. The metathalamus.
2. The third ventricle may be regarded as the cavity of the diencephalon.

### THE THALAMUS

1. The thalamus (or dorsal thalamus) is a large mass of grey matter that lies immediately lateral to the third ventricle. It has two ends (or poles), anterior and posterior; and four surfaces, superior, inferior, medial and lateral.
2. The ***anterior end (or pole)*** lies just behind the interventricular foramen (49.19 and 49.20).
3. The ***posterior end (or pole)*** is called the pulvinar. It lies just above and lateral to the superior colliculus.
4. The ***medial surface*** forms the greater part of the lateral wall of the third ventricle, and is lined by ependyma.
   a. The medial surfaces of the two thalami are usually interconnected by a mass of grey matter called the ***interthalamic connexus***.
   b. Inferiorly, the medial surface is separated from the hypothalamus by the ***hypothalamic sulcus***. This sulcus runs from the interventricular foramen to the aqueduct.
5. The lateral surface of the thalamus is related to the internal capsule that separates it from the lentiform nucleus (52.1).
6. The ***superior (or dorsal) surface*** of the thalamus is related laterally to the caudate nucleus from which it is separated by a bundle of fibres called the ***stria terminalis***, and by the thalamostriate vein.
7. The thalamus and the caudate nucleus together form the floor of the central part of the lateral ventricle. The medial part of the superior surface of the thalamus is, however, separated from the ventricle by the fornix, and by a fold of pia mater called the ***tela choroidea*** (52.1).
8. At the junction of the medial and superior surfaces of the thalamus the ependyma of the third ventricle is reflected from the lateral wall to the roof.
   a. The line of reflection is marked by a line called the ***taenia thalami.***
   b. Underlying it, there is a narrow bundle of fibres called the ***stria medullaris thalami*** (not to be confused with the stria medullares present in the floor of the fourth ventricle).
9. The ***inferior surface*** of the thalamus is related to the hypothalamus anteriorly (49.20), and to the subthalamus posteriorly (52.1). The subthalamus separates the thalamus from the tegmentum of the midbrain.

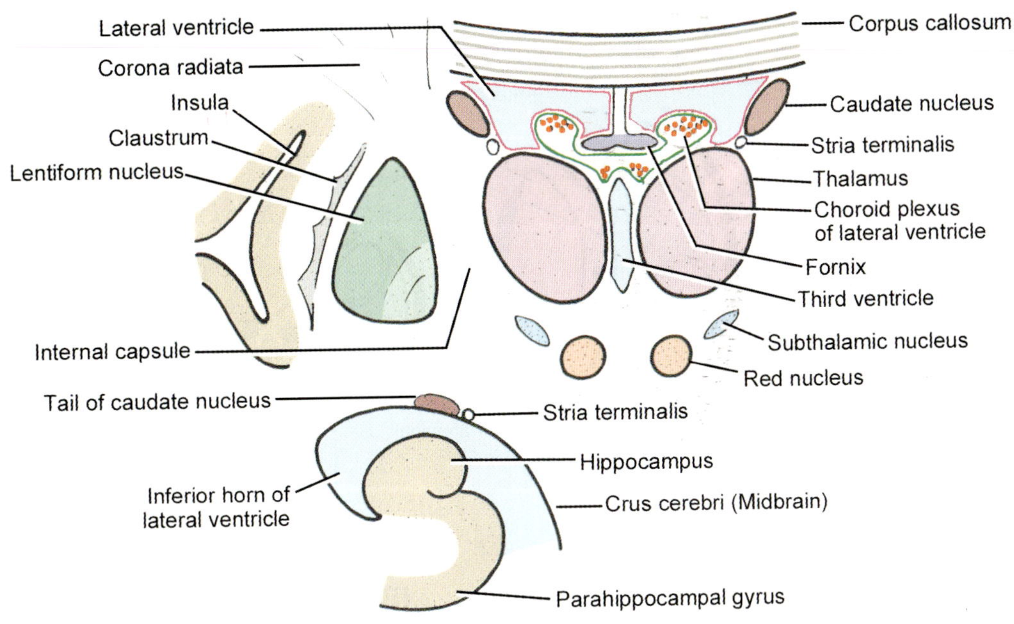


52.1: Coronal section through the cerebrum to show structures related to the thalamus

## Internal Structure of the Thalamus

1. The thalamus consists mainly of grey matter. Its superior surface is covered by a thin layer of white matter called the ***stratum zonale;*** and its lateral surface by a similar layer called the ***external medullary lamina.***
2. The grey matter of the thalamus is subdivided into three main parts by a Y-shaped sheet of white matter which is called the ***internal medullary lamina*** (52.2A).
   a. This lamina is placed vertically.
   b. It divides the thalamus into a lateral part, a medial part, and an anterior part situated between the two limbs of the 'Y'.
3. A number of nuclei can be distinguished within each of these parts. Only the more important of these are listed below.

### *Nuclei in the Anterior Part*

A number of nuclei can be distinguished, but we shall refer to them collectively as the ***anterior nucleus.***

### *Nuclei in the Medial Part*

The largest of these is the ***medial dorsal nucleus.***

### *Nuclei in the Lateral Part*

1. The nuclei in the lateral part can be subdivided into a ***ventral group*** and a ***lateral group.***
2. The ***nuclei in the ventral group*** are as follows (in anteroposterior order):
   a. ***Ventral anterior nucleus***
   b. ***Ventral intermediate nucleus*** (also called the ***ventral lateral nucleus***).
   c. ***Ventral posterior nucleus,*** which is further subdivided into:
      i. A lateral part called the ***ventral posterolateral nucleus.***
      ii. A medial part called the ***ventral posteromedial nucleus*** (52.2B).

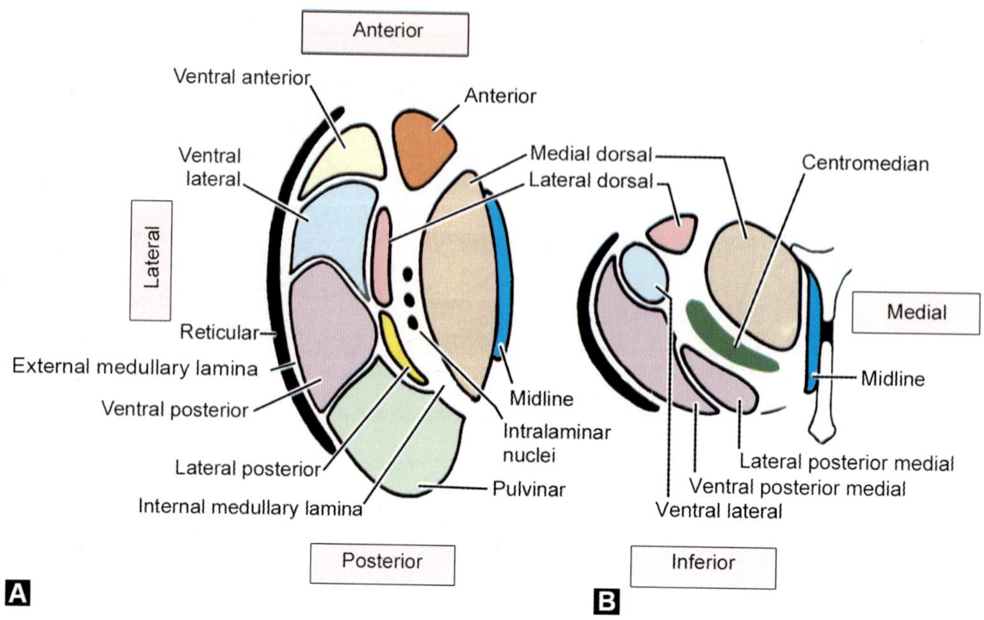


**52.2A and B:** Scheme to show the nuclei of the thalamus. (A) Superior aspect; (B) Coronal section

3. The ***nuclei of the lateral group*** are as follows (in anteroposterior order):
   a. ***Lateral dorsal nucleus***
   b. ***Lateral posterior nucleus***
   c. ***Pulvinar.***

*In addition to the above, the thalamus contains the following nuclei:*

1. The ***intralaminar nuclei*** are embedded within the internal medullary lamina. The most important of these is the ***centromedian nucleus*** (52.2B).
2. The ***midline nuclei*** consist of scattered cells that lie between the medial part of the thalamus and the ependyma of the third ventricle.
3. The ***reticular nucleus*** is made up of a thin layer of cells covering the lateral aspect of the thalamus. The cells of this nucleus are separated from the rest of the thalamus by the external medullary lamina. The reticular nucleus is related laterally to the internal capsule.
4. The ***medial and lateral geniculate bodies*** (described under metathalamus) are often included as part of the thalamus.

## Connections of the Thalamus

1. Afferent impulses from a large number of subcortical centres converge on the thalamus (52.3).
2. Exteroceptive and proprioceptive impulses ascend to it through the medial lemniscus, the spinothalamic tracts, and the trigeminothalamic tract.
3. Visual and auditory impulses reach the lateral and medial geniculate bodies respectively.
4. Sensations of taste are conveyed to the thalamus through solitario-thalamic fibres.
5. Although the thalamus does not receive direct olfactory impulses they probably reach it through the amygdaloid complex.
6. Visceral information is conveyed from the hypothalamus, and probably through the reticular formation.
7. In addition to these afferents, the thalamus receives profuse connections from all parts of the cerebral cortex, the cerebellum, and the corpus striatum.

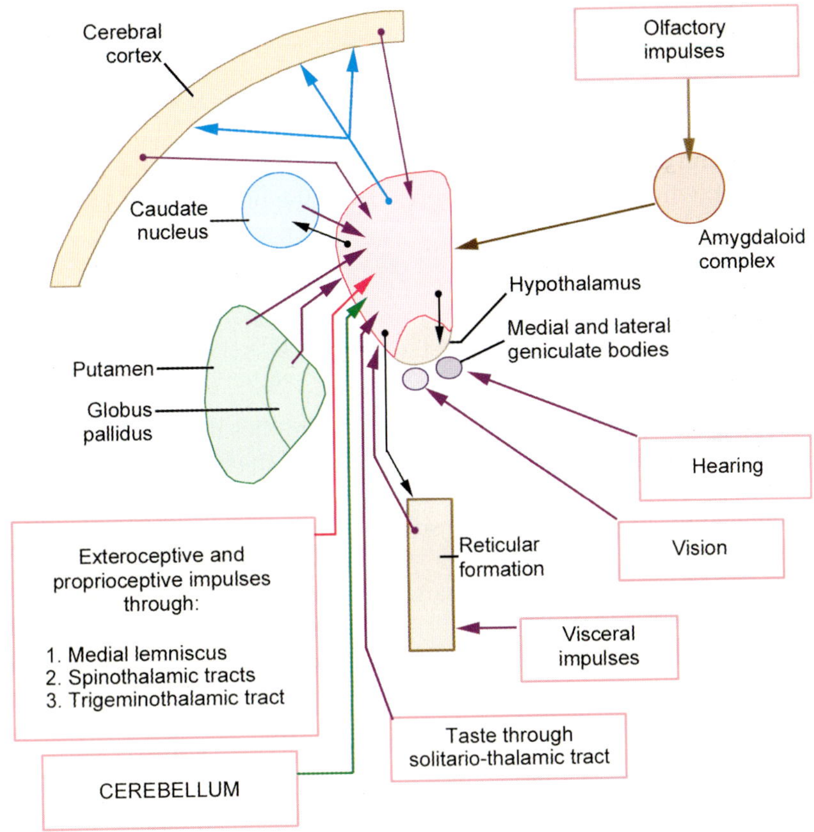


**52.3:** Scheme to show the connections of the thalamus

8. The thalamus is, therefore, regarded as a great integrating centre where information from all these sources is brought together.
9. This information is projected to almost the whole of the cerebral cortex through profuse thalamocortical projections.
10. These thalamocortical fibres form large bundles that are described as ***thalamic radiations*** or as ***thalamic peduncles***. These radiations are ***anterior*** (or ***frontal***), ***superior*** (or ***dorsal***), ***posterior*** (or ***caudal***), and ***ventral.***
11. Efferent projections from the thalamus also reach the corpus striatum, the hypothalamus, and the reticular formation.
12. Besides its integrating function, the thalamus is believed to have some degree of ability to perceive exteroceptive sensations, specially pain.
13. Some further details are as follows.
14. The most important connections of the thalamus are those of the ***ventral posterior nucleus*** that receives the terminations of the major sensory pathways ascending from the spinal cord and brainstem. These include:
    a. The medial lemniscus
    b. The spinothalamic tracts
    c. The trigeminal lemniscus
    d. The solitario-thalamic fibres carrying sensations of taste.
15. All these sensations are carried to the sensory areas of the cerebral cortex (areas 3,2,1) by fibres passing through the posterior limb of the internal capsule (superior thalamic radiation).

**WANT TO KNOW MORE?**

16. Within the ventral posterior nucleus fibres from different parts of the body terminate in a definite sequence.
    a. The fibres from the lowest parts of the body end in the most lateral part of the nucleus.
    b. The medial lemniscus and spinothalamic tracts carrying sensations from the limbs and trunk end in the ventral posterolateral part; while the trigeminal fibres (from the head) end in the ventral posteromedial part, which also receives the fibres for taste.

## THE HYPOTHALAMUS

1. The hypothalamus is a part of the diencephalon. As its name implies it lies below the thalamus.
2. On the medial side, it forms the wall of the third ventricle below the level of the hypothalamic sulcus.
3. Laterally, it is in contact with the internal capsule, and (in the posterior part) with the subthalamus.
4. Posteriorly, the hypothalamus merges with the subthalamus, and through it with the tegmentum of the midbrain.
5. Anteriorly, it extends up to the lamina terminalis, and merges with certain olfactory structures in the region of the anterior perforated substance.
6. Inferiorly, the hypothalamus is related to structures in the floor of the third ventricle. These are:
    a. The tuber cinereum
    b. The infundibulum
    c. The mammillary bodies, which are considered as parts of the hypothalamus.

### Subdivisions of the Hypothalamus

1. For convenience of description, the hypothalamus may be subdivided, roughly, into a number of regions (52.4).
2. Some authorities divide it (from medial to lateral side) into three ***zones*** that are as follows:
    a. Periventricular zone
    b. Intermediate zone
    c. Lateral zone.
3. The periventricular and intermediate zones are often described collectively as the ***medial zone***.
4. The column of the fornix lies between the medial and lateral zones. (The mammillo-thalamic tract also lies in this plane).
5. The hypothalamus is also subdivided anteroposteriorly into four ***regions***. These are as follows:
    a. The ***preoptic region*** adjoins the lamina terminalis.
    b. The ***supraoptic region*** lies above the optic chiasma.
    c. The ***tuberal (or infundibulo-tuberal) region*** includes the infundibulum, the tuber cinereum and the region above it.
    d. The ***mammillary region*** consists of the mammillary body and the region above it.
6. The preoptic region differs from the rest of the hypothalamus in being a derivative of the telencephalon. (The lamina terminalis also belongs to the telencephalon).

### Hypothalamic Nuclei

The entire hypothalamus contains scattered neurons within which some aggregations can be recognised. These aggregations, termed the hypothalamic nuclei, are as follows (52.4):

1. The ***preoptic nucleus*** extends through the periventricular, intermediate, and lateral zones of the preoptic part.
2. The ***mammillary nuclei*** lie within the mammillary body.

   The remaining nuclei of the hypothalamus lie either in the periventricular, intermediate, or lateral zones.

**52.4: Hypothalamic regions and nuclei in them**

| | *Medial zone (Periventricular and intermediate)* | *Lateral zone* |
|---|---|---|
| | | Preoptic nucleus |
| Supraoptic region | Paraventricular nucleus<br>Periventricular cell groups<br>Suprachiasmatic nucleus<br>Intermediate cell groups<br>(= anterior nucleus ?) | Supraoptic nucleus* |
| Tuberal region | Dorsimedial nucleus<br>Ventrimedial nucleus<br>Arcuate (infundibular) nucleus Premammillary nucleus | Lateral tuberal nucleus |
| Mammillary or posterior region | Posterior nucleus<br>(lies partly in tuberal region) | Tuberomammillary nucleus* |
| | | Mammillary nuclei |

* From a functional point of view the supraoptic and tuberommamillary nuclei are grouped with the nuclei of the intermediate zone

## Nuclei in the Periventricular Zone

1. The ***paraventricular nucleus***
2. The ***suprachiasmatic nucleus,*** lie in the supraoptic region
3. The ***infundibular nucleus*** lies in the tuberal region
4. The ***posterior nucleus*** extends into both the tuberal and mammillary regions.

## Nuclei in the Intermediate Zone

1. The ***anterior nucleus*** occupies the supraoptic region
2. The ***dorsimedial nucleus***
3. The ***ventromedial nucleus*** lie in the tuberal part, which also contains small aggregations of cells that constitute
4. The ***premammillary nuclei.***

## Nuclei in the Lateral Zone

1. The lateral zone contains a diffuse collection of cells that extends through the supraoptic, tuberal and mammillary regions. These cells constitute the ***lateral nucleus.*** The lateral zone also contains the following nuclei:
2. The ***supraoptic nucleus*** lies in the supraoptic region.
3. The ***tuberomammillary nucleus*** extends into the tuberal and mammillary regions.
4. Small aggregations of neurons in the tuberal region constitute the ***lateral tuberal nuclei.***

## Connections of the Hypothalamus

The hypothalamus is concerned with visceral function and is, therefore, connected to other areas having a similar function. These include:

1. The various parts of the limbic system
2. The reticular formation
3. Autonomic centres in the brainstem and spinal cord (52.5).

### *Afferent Connections*

1. The hypothalamus receives visceral afferents (including those of taste) through the spinal cord and brainstem. The exact pathways are not known. They probably pass through the reticular formation and consist of several relays.

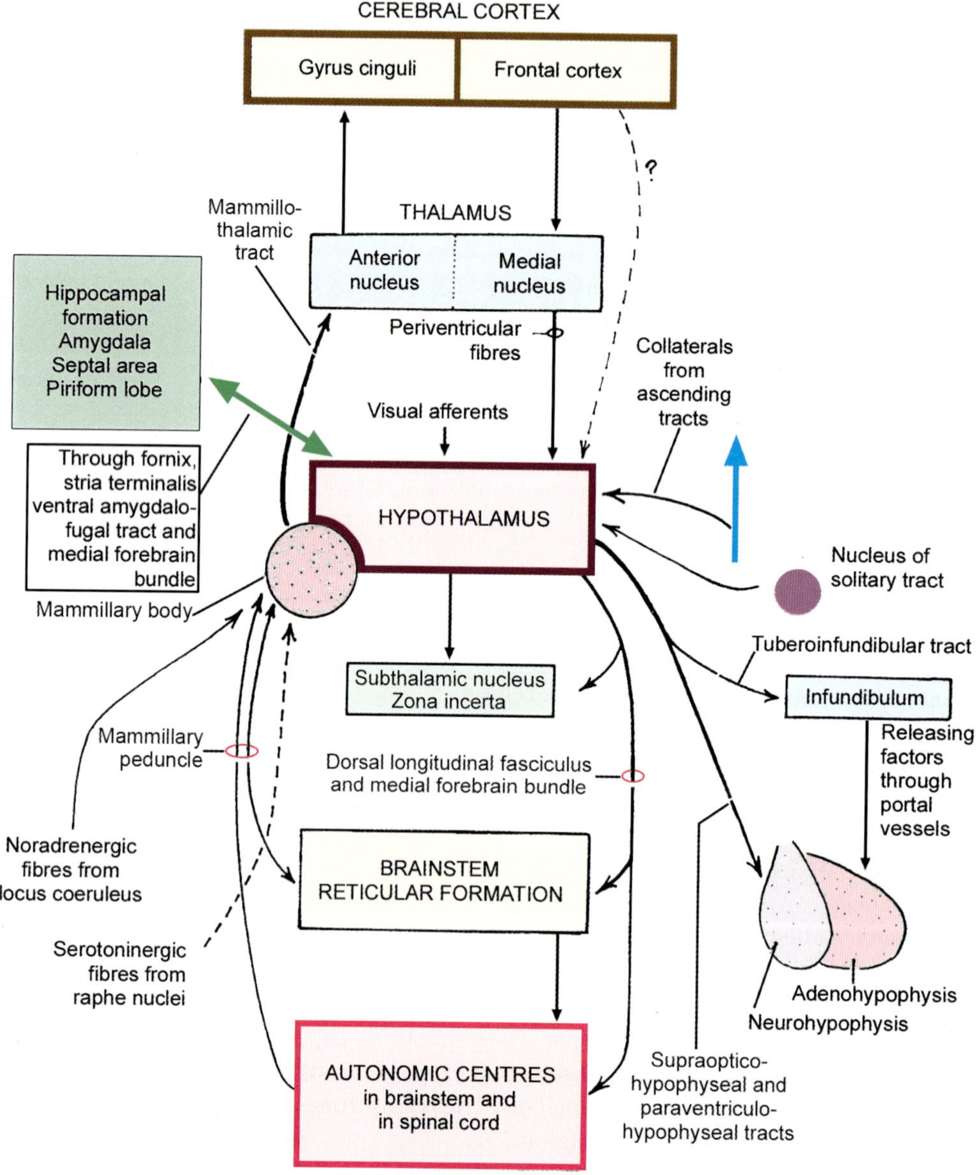


**52.5:** Simplified scheme of the main connections of the hypothalamus

### WANT TO KNOW MORE?

a. Many of these fibres pass through a bundle called the ***mammillary peduncle***.
b. Other fibres pass through a bundle called the ***dorsal longitudinal fasciculus***.
c. Fibres from the tegmentum of the midbrain also reach the hypothalamus through the ***medial forebrain bundle.***

2. The hypothalamus receives afferents from several centres connected to olfactory pathways, and to the limbic system.

### WANT TO KNOW MORE?

These are:

a. The anterior perforated substance
b. The septal nuclei
c. The amygdaloid complex
d. The hippocampus
e. The piriform cortex.

3. Many of these fibres reach the hypothalamus through the medial forebrain bundle. Fibres from the hippocampus travel through the fornix. Some fibres from the amygdaloid complex pass through the stria terminalis, and some through the medial forebrain bundle.

4. The hypothalamus receives afferents from several parts of the cerebral cortex, and some from the cerebellum.

*Efferent Connections*

1. The hypothalamus sends fibres to autonomic centres in the brainstem and spinal cord. It also sends fibres to:

### WANT TO KNOW MORE?

a. The hippocampal formation
b. The septal nuclei
c. The amygdaloid complex
d. The tegmentum of the midbrain.

These fibres pass through the same bundles that convey afferent fibres from these centres.

2. Fibres from the mammillary body pass through the mammillo-thalamic tract to reach the anterior nucleus of the thalamus. New fibres arising here project to the gyrus cinguli.

3. The supraoptic, paraventricular and infundibular nuclei exert an important influence on the hypophysis cerebri.
4. Fibres arising from the supraoptic and paraventricular nuclei reach the pars posterior (neurohypophysis) through the ***supraoptico-hypophyseal*** and ***paraventriculo-hypophyseal*** tracts.
5. The cells in these nuclei are peculiar in that they produce a secretion that travels along their axons and is released into the sinusoids of the neurohypophysis. This phenomenon is called ***neurosecretion.***

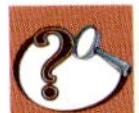

### WANT TO KNOW MORE?

6. The supraoptic nucleus is believed to mainly produce the antidiuretic hormone, and the paraventricular nucleus is believed to mainly produce oxytocin; though both nuclei produce both hormones.
7. Axons of cells in the infundibular (arcuate) nucleus end in the median eminence and infundibulum.
   a. They travel through the ***tubero-hypophyseal tract*** that also receives fibres from several other hypothalamic nuclei.
   b. The axon terminals of the fibres in these tracts are closely related to capillaries in the region.
   c. The cells of the infundibular nucleus are believed to produce ***releasing factors*** that travel along their axons and are released into the capillaries.
   d. These capillaries carry these factors into the pars anterior of the hypophysis cerebri through the ***hypothalamo-hypophyseal portal system***.

e. In the pars anterior these factors are responsible for release of appropriate hormones.
f. It may be noted, however, that in the case of some hormones their secretion is inhibited by such factors. (See chapter 46).

## Functions of the Hypothalamus

The hypothalamus plays an important role in the control of many functions that are vital for the survival of an animal. In exercising such control the hypothalamus acts in close coordination with higher centres including the limbic system and the prefrontal cortex, and with autonomic centres in the brainstem and spinal cord. The main functions attributed to the hypothalamus are as follows:

### *Regulation of Eating and Drinking Behaviour*

The hypothalamus is responsible for feelings of hunger and of satiety, and this determines whether the animal will accept or refuse food. Stimulation of the lateral zone stimulates hunger while stimulation of the medial zone produces satiety. The lateral zone is also responsible for thirst and drinking.

### *Regulation of Sexual Activity and Reproduction*

The hypothalamus controls sexual activity, both in the male and female. It also exerts an effect on gametogenesis, on ovarian and uterine cycles, and on the development of secondary sexual characters. These effects are produced by influencing the secretion of hormones by the hypophysis cerebri.

### *Control of Autonomic Activity*

The hypothalamus exerts an important influence on the activity of the autonomic nervous system, and thus has considerable effect on cardiovascular, respiratory and alimentary functions. Sympathetic activity is said to be controlled, predominantly, by caudal parts of the hypothalamus; and parasympathetic activity by cranial parts, but there is considerable overlap between the regions concerned.

### *Emotional Behaviour*

The hypothalamus has an important influence on emotions like fear, anger and pleasure. Stimulation of some areas of the hypothalamus produces sensations of pleasure, while stimulation of other regions produces pain or other unpleasant effects.

### *Control of Endocrine Activity*

The influence of the hypothalamus in the production of hormones by the pars anterior of the hypophysis cerebri, and the elaboration of oxytocin and the antidiuretic hormone by the hypothalamus itself, have been described above. Through control of the adenohypophysis the hypothalamus indirectly influences the thyroid gland, the adrenal cortex, and the gonads.

### *Temperature Regulation*

The hypothalamus acts as a thermostat to control body temperature. When body temperature rises or falls, appropriate mechanisms are brought into play to bring the temperature back to normal.

### *Biological Clock*

Several functions of the body show a cyclic variation in activity, over the twenty four hours of a day. The most conspicuous of these is the cycle of sleep and waking. Such cycles (called ***circadian rhythms***) are believed to be controlled by the hypothalamus, which is said to function as a biological clock. The suprachiasmatic nucleus is believed to play an important role in this regard. Lesions of the hypothalamus disturb the sleep-waking cycle.

## THE METATHALAMUS

1. The metathalamus is constituted by the medial and lateral geniculate bodies. These are small oval collections of grey matter situated below the posterior part of the thalamus, lateral to the colliculi of the midbrain (52.6).
2. Each mass of grey matter is bent on itself, hence the term 'geniculate'.

### The Medial Geniculate Body

1. The medial geniculate body is a relay station on the auditory pathway.
2. The medial geniculate body receives fibres of the lateral lemniscus either directly, or after relay in the inferior colliculus (52.7).
3. These fibres pass through the brachium of the inferior colliculus.
4. Fibres arising in the medial geniculate body constitute the acoustic radiation.
5. The acoustic radiation passes through the sublentiform part of the internal capsule to reach the acoustic areas of the cerebral cortex.
6. Some other connections of the medial geniculate body are shown in 52.7.
7. Each medial geniculate body receives impulses from the cochleae of both sides.

### The Lateral Geniculate Body

1. The lateral geniculate body is a relay station on the visual pathway.
2. It receives fibres from the retinae of both eyes (52.8).
3. Efferents arising in this body constitute the optic radiation that passes through the retrolentiform part of the internal capsule to reach the visual areas of the cerebral cortex.

## THE EPITHALAMUS

1. The epithalamus lies in relation to the posterior part of the roof of the third ventricle, and in the adjoining part of its lateral wall. It consists of:
   a. The pineal gland
   b. The habenular nuclei, and related structures.

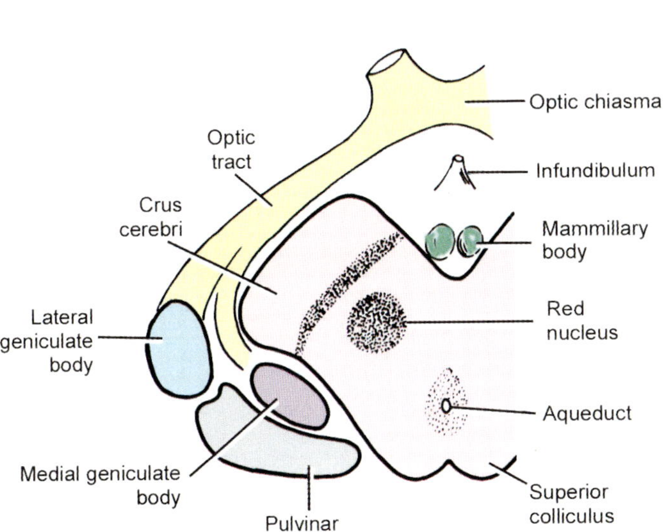


52.6: Diagram to show the location of the medial and lateral geniculate bodies

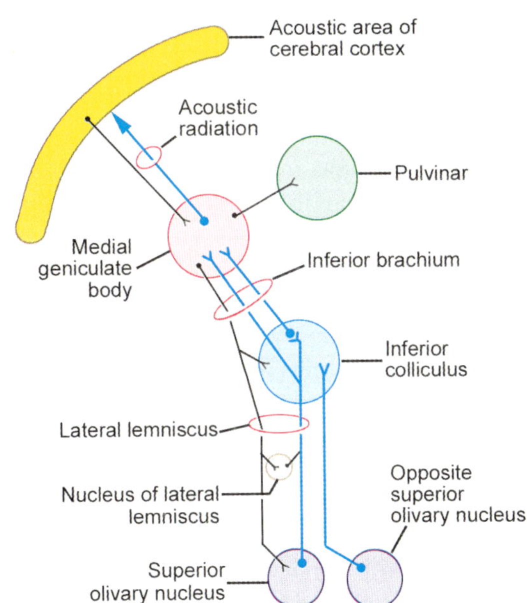


52.7: Connections of the medial geniculate body

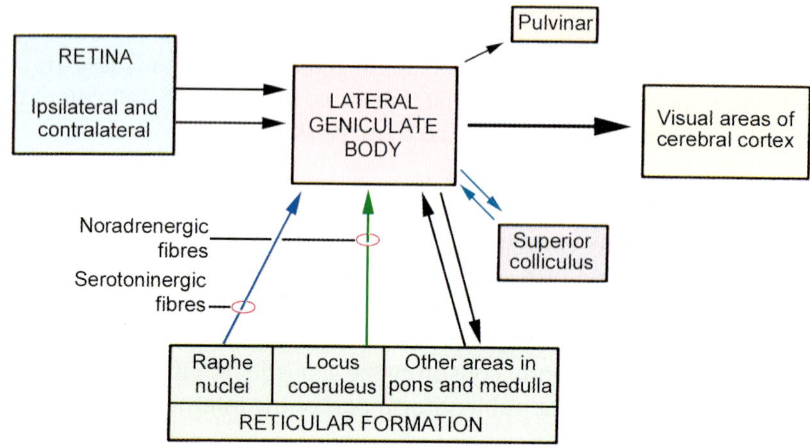


**52.8:** Connections of the lateral geniculate body

2. The pineal gland has been described on page 1013 (chapter 46). The other structures will not be described here.

## THE SUBTHALAMIC REGION

1. The part of the diencephalon that is called the subthalamus lies below the posterior part of the thalamus, behind and lateral to the hypothalamus.
2. It is also referred to as the ***ventral thalamus***.
3. Inferiorly, it is continuous with the tegmentum of the midbrain. Laterally, it is related to the lowest part of the internal capsule.
4. Apart from some small aggregations of neurons, the grey matter of the region consists of the ***subthalamic nucleus*** and the ***zona incerta***. The upper ends of the red nucleus, and the substantia nigra, project into the region.
5. Detailed studies of connections of the subthalamic nucleus show that this nucleus is closely related to the basal ganglia and some authorities include the subthalamic nucleus among these ganglia.

## THE BASAL GANGLIA

1. The basal ganglia (or basal nuclei) are large masses of grey matter situated in the cerebral hemispheres. They are derived from the telencephalon. The basal ganglia are as follows (52.9):
   a. Caudate nucleus
   b. Lentiform nucleus, which consists of two functionally distinct parts, the putamen and the globus pallidus
   c. Amygdaloid nuclear complex
   d. The claustrum is often included among the basal ganglia
   e. Some authorities include the subthalamic nucleus amongst the basal ganglia
2. Various other terms commonly used for some of the above nuclei are as follows:
   a. The caudate nucleus and the lentiform nucleus together constitute the ***corpus striatum.***
   b. This consists of two functionally distinct parts.
   c. The caudate nucleus and the putamen form one unit called the ***striatum***
   d. The globus pallidus forms the other unit, the ***pallidum.***
3. From an evolutionary point of view, the amygdaloid complex is the oldest of the basal ganglia and is, therefore, sometimes referred to as the ***archistriatum.***
4. The globus pallidus constitutes the ***paleostriatum*** while the caudate nucleus and the putamen form the ***neostriatum.***

## The Caudate Nucleus

1. The caudate nucleus is a C-shaped mass of grey matter (52.9). It consists of a large head, a body and a thin tail.
2. The caudate nucleus is intimately related to the lateral ventricle. The head of the nucleus bulges into the anterior horn of the ventricle and forms the greater part of its floor.
3. The body of the nucleus lies in the floor of the central part of the ventricle; and the tail in the roof of the inferior horn.
4. The anterior part of the head of the caudate nucleus is fused, inferiorly, with the lentiform nucleus.
5. In this situation the grey matter of these two nuclei is continuous with that of the anterior perforated substance.
6. The anterior end of the tail of the caudate nucleus ends in relation to the amygdaloid complex.
7. The body of the caudate nucleus is related medially to the thalamus, and laterally to the internal capsule which separates it from the lentiform nucleus (52.10). Some other relationships of the caudate nucleus are shown in 52.1.

## The Lentiform Nucleus

1. The lentiform nucleus lies lateral to the internal capsule.
2. Laterally, it is separated from the claustrum by fibres of the external capsule.
3. Superiorly, the lentiform nucleus is related to the corona radiata, and inferiorly to the sublentiform part of the internal capsule.
4. Some other relationships are evident in 52.1.
5. The lentiform nucleus appears triangular (or wedge-shaped) in coronal section.
6. It is divided, by a thin lamina of white matter, into a lateral part, the ***putamen;*** and a medial part, the ***globus pallidus.*** The globus pallidus is further subdivided into medial and lateral segments.
7. The corpus striatum is regarded as an important integrating centre. It plays an important role in motor activity.
   a. It receives afferents from various sources including the motor cortex and, in turn, sends out efferents to several important centres in the brainstem from which descending tracts arise.
   b. The striatum constitutes the receiving centre of the corpus striatum, as most of the afferents end in this part. It sends fibres to the pallidum, which, in turn, projects fibres to various centres.

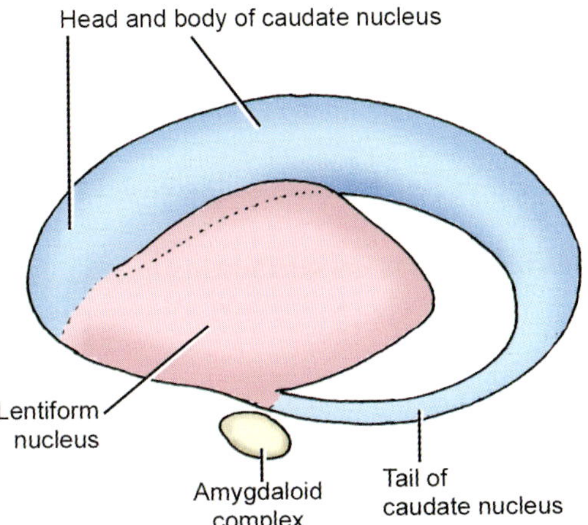


**52.9:** The corpus striatum viewed from the lateral aspect

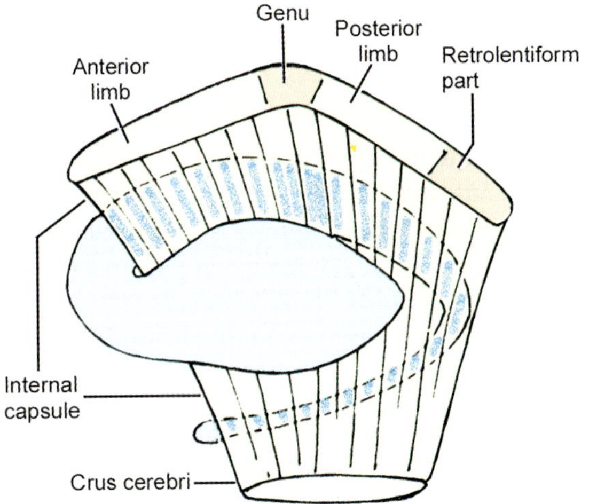


**52.10:** Relationship of the corpus striatum to the internal capsule (viewed from the lateral side)

## WANT TO KNOW MORE?

**The Claustrum**

This is a thin lamina of grey matter that lies lateral to the lentiform nucleus. It is separated from the latter by fibres of the external capsule. Laterally, it is separated by a thin layer of white matter from the cortex of the insula. Its connections are unknown.

## The Amygdaloid Complex

1. This complex (also called the amygdaloid body, amygdala) lies in the temporal lobe of the cerebral hemisphere, close to the temporal pole.
2. It lies deep to the uncus, and is related to the anterior end of the inferior horn of the lateral ventricle.

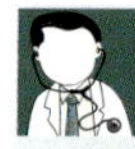

## CLINICAL CORRELATION

Clinicians often use the term basal ganglia in a wider sense than used here. The thalamus, the red nucleus, the substantia nigra and the subthalamic nuclei are included.

**Abnormal Movements**

1. Various kinds of abnormal movements are seen in neurological disorders involving the basal ganglia, the subthalamic nucleus and the cerebellum.
2. These may take the form of involuntary shaking (***tremor***) of the hands, head or other parts of the body, because of rapid alternating contraction of opposing groups of muscles.
3. In some instances, the tremor comes on when the patient tries to perform voluntary movement (***intention tremor***).
4. Another type of abnormal movement consists of a slow twisting of a limb, or of the face or neck (***athetosis***).
5. Sudden, jerky, shock-like movements involving any part of the body (***myoclonus***) may also occur. These can cause objects held in the hand to be thrown away (***hemiballism***).
6. Sometimes different, complex, involuntary movements occur in succession, particularly in the distal parts of the limbs (***chorea***).
7. It has not been possible to precisely correlate specific abnormal movements with disease in specific regions of the basal ganglia and neighbouring structures. The movements are not a result of inactivity of the diseased centres but are, on the contrary, to be regarded as release phenomena, due to abolition of inhibitory influences.
   a. Hemiballism is seen in lesions in the subthalamic nucleus.
   b. Intention tremor is seen in disorders of the cerebellum.
8. In many cases, abnormal movements are accompanied by rigidity of muscles, because of increased muscle tone. The increased tone is also a release phenomenon.
9. One common syndrome characterised by rigidity and abnormal movements is called ***Parkinsonism*** or ***paralysis agitans*** (shaking palsy).
10. It is characterised by marked rigidity that leads to:
    a. A stooped posture
    b. A slow shuffling gait
    c. Difficulty in speech
    d. A mask-like face.
11. Characteristic involuntary 'pill-rolling' movements of the hands are seen in Parkinsonism. The condition is believed to be due to degenerative changes in the striatum and the substantia nigra.

# THE OLFACTORY REGION AND LIMBIC SYSTEM

## THE OLFACTORY REGION

1. The peripheral end organ for smell is the ***olfactory mucosa*** that lines the upper and posterior parts of the nasal cavity.
2. Nerve fibres arising in this mucosa collect to form about twenty bundles that together constitute an ***olfactory nerve.***
3. The bundles pass through foramina in the cribriform plate of the ethmoid bone to enter the cranial cavity where they terminate in the ***olfactory bulb*** (52.11 and 52.13).
4. The olfactory bulb is an elongated oval structure that lies just above the cribriform plate.
5. It is continuous posteriorly with the ***olfactory tract*** through which it is connected to the base of the cerebral hemisphere.
6. When traced posteriorly, the olfactory tract divides into ***medial and lateral olfactory striae*** (52.11 and 52.13).
7. The point of bifurcation is expanded and forms the ***olfactory trigone.***
8. An ***intermediate stria*** is sometimes present.
9. The olfactory striae are intimately related to a mass of grey matter called the ***anterior perforated substance.***
   a. The medial and lateral striae form the anteromedial and anterolateral boundaries of this substance.
   b. The intermediate stria extends into the anterior perforated substance and ends in a slight elevation (in the anterior part of the substance) called the ***olfactory tubercle.***
   c. Posterolaterally, the anterior perforated substance is related to the uncus (52.11), while
   d. Posteromedially it is bounded by a bundle of fibres called the ***diagonal band*** (of Broca)(52.12).
10. The uncus is a part of the cerebral hemisphere that lies on the tentorial surface a little behind and medial to the temporal pole. It represents the anterior end of the ***parahippocampal gyrus*** and is separated from the temporal pole by the rhinal sulcus.
11. The anterior part of the parahippocampal gyrus, including the uncus, is referred to as the ***entorhinal area*** (area 28).

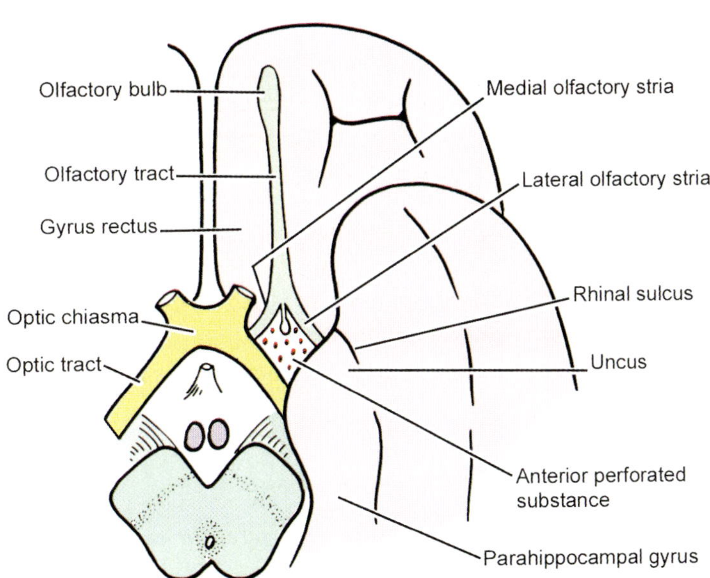


**52.11:** Relationship of the corpus striatum to the internal capsule (viewed from the lateral side)

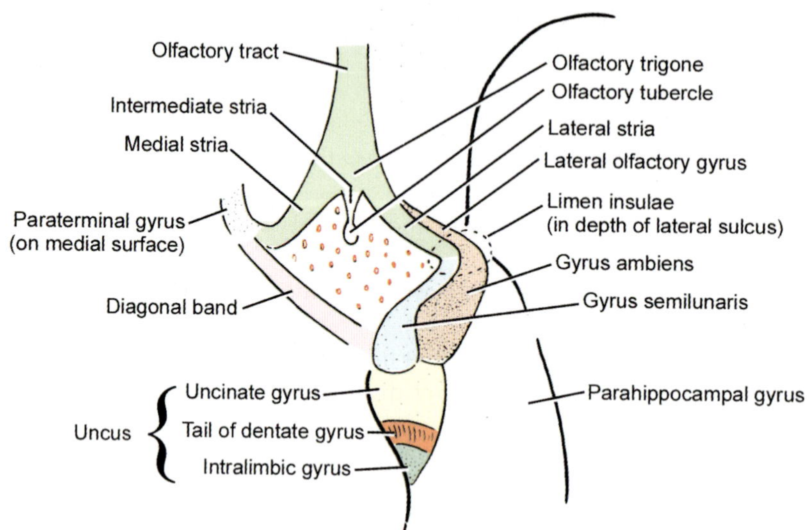


**52.12:** Details of olfactory structures present in relation to the anterior perforated substance. Note the subdivisions of the uncus

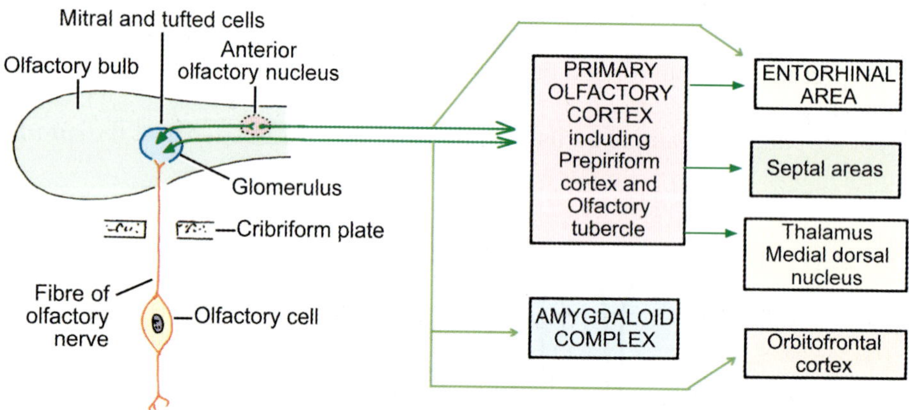


**52.13:** Scheme to show the main features of the olfactory pathway

12. Some other areas present in the region are shown in 52.12. Their names may be noted, but further description is unnecessary.

## THE OLFACTORY PATHWAY

1. The fibres of the olfactory nerves are processes of ***olfactory receptor cells*** lying in the epithelium lining the olfactory mucosa (52.13).
   a. These receptor cells are homologous to sensory neurons located in sensory ganglia.
   b. In other words, the first order sensory neurons of the olfactory pathway are located within the olfactory epithelium itself.

2. Each receptor cell consists of a cell body and of two processes i.e., it is a bipolar cell.
   a. The peripheral process (dendrite) reaches the surface of the olfactory epithelium and ends in a small swelling. A number of cilia are attached to this swelling.
   b. The central process (axon) enters the submucosa, and forms one fibre of the olfactory nerve.
3. The olfactory nerve fibres terminate in the olfactory bulb.
4. Fibres arising in the olfactory bulb form the olfactory tract.
5. The fibres of the olfactory tract pass through the lateral olfactory stria to terminate in the anterior perforated substance and in some neighbouring areas that collectively constitute the ***primary olfactory cortex.***
6. Fibres arising in the primary cortex project to the entorhinal area. The entorhinal area is, therefore, called the ***secondary olfactory cortex.***
7. The sense of smell is believed to be perceived in both the primary and secondary olfactory cortex.
8. Some fibres of the olfactory tract, which pass through the medial stria, end in the anterior perforated substance.
9. Others cross to the opposite side through the anterior commissure.
10. The primary olfactory cortex is connected to various other areas. In the past, many of these areas have been included under the term ***rhinencephalon*** or smell brain. It is now recognised, however, that although these areas might receive olfactory impulses their primary functions are not olfactory. Some of these areas and their connections are considered below as part of the limbic system.

## THE LIMBIC SYSTEM

1. The term limbic system is applied to certain regions of the brain that are believed to play an important role in the control of visceral activity. Many of these areas have, in the past, been considered to have a predominantly olfactory function; but it is now realised that this is not so.

### WANT TO KNOW MORE?

2. Some of the functions attributed to the limbic system are as follows:
   a. Integration of olfactory, visceral, and somatic impulses reaching the brain.
   b. Control of activities necessary for survival of the animal, including the procuring of food and eating behaviour.
   c. Control of activities necessary for survival of the species including sex behaviour.
   d. Emotional behaviour.
   e. Retention of recent memory.
3. The areas to be included under the heading limbic system are not completely agreed upon. The most important of these are as follows:
   a. Gyrus cinguli.
   b. Entorhinal area (area 28), consisting of the anterior part of the parahippocampal gyrus, including the uncus.
   c. Anterior perforated substance.
   d. Prepiriform area consisting of the lateral olfactory gyrus and the gyrus ambiens (See 52.12).
   e. Gyrus semilunaris (or periamygdaloid area) (52.12).
   f. Hippocampal formation including:
      i. The hippocampus, which is made up of the cornu ammonis and the dentate gyrus.
      ii. The indusium griseum and smaller related structures.
   g. Amygdaloid nuclear complex.
   h. Septal region consisting of:
      i. The septal area (cortex)
      ii. The septal nuclei (see below).

i. Olfactory nerves, bulb, tract, striae, trigone, tubercle; and the anterior olfactory nucleus.
j. Fornix, stria terminalis, stria medullaris thalami (or stria habenularis), diagonal band, and the anterior commissure.
k. The piriform lobe that includes the prepiriform area, the entorhinal area, the lateral olfactory stria and the gyrus semilunaris.
l. In addition to the above, other regions that are included in the limbic system by some authorities are the hypothalamus and the reticular formation of the midbrain.
m. The medial part of the thalamus, and the frontal cortex are closely related functionally to the limbic system.

Several of the above areas have been considered along with the olfactory pathway. The hypothalamus has already been considered. We shall now consider some other areas.

**Amygdaloid Nuclear Complex**

1. This region is also called the amygdaloid body or amygdala.
2. It is situated near the temporal pole of the cerebral hemisphere in close relation to the anterior end of the inferior horn of the lateral ventricle.
3. Superiorly, the complex is related to the anterior part of the lentiform nucleus.
4. Inferiorly, the complex is related to the gyrus semilunaris, the gyrus ambiens and the uncinate gyrus.
5. Posteriorly, it becomes continuous with the tail of the caudate nucleus and with the stria terminalis (52.9).

**Stria Terminalis**

1. This bundle of fibres is closely related to the inferior horn and central part of the lateral ventricle.
2. It begins in the amygdaloid complex and runs backwards in the roof of the inferior horn.
3. It then winds upwards and forwards to lie in the floor of the central part of the ventricle.
4. Finally, it terminates near the interventricular foramen and anterior commissure by dividing into various smaller bundles.
5. Throughout its course, it is closely related to the medial side of the caudate nucleus (52.1).
   a. In the inferior horn it is related to the tail of this nucleus.
   b. In the central part of the ventricle it lies medial to the body of the caudate nucleus. Here, the thalamus is medial to it.

**Anterior Commissure**

1. The anterior commissure is situated in the anterior wall of the third ventricle at the upper end of the lamina terminalis (52.14).
2. When traced laterally, it divides into anterior and posterior bundles.
3. Fibres passing through the commissure interconnect the regions of the two cerebral hemispheres concerned with the olfactory pathway.

**Septal Region**

1. This term is used to designate certain masses of grey matter that lie immediately anterior to the lamina terminalis and the anterior commissure (52.14).
2. The cerebral cortex of this region shows two small vertical sulci called the anterior and posterior ***parolfactory sulci.***
3. The region between the lamina terminalis and the posterior parolfactory sulcus is the ***paraterminal gyrus.***
4. The anterior part of this region that adjoins the posterior parolfactory sulcus is called the ***prehippocampal rudiment.***
5. The region between the anterior and posterior parolfactory sulci is the ***subcallosal area*** (or ***parolfactory gyrus***).
6. The cortex of this region is referred to as the ***septal area*** in distinction to the ***septal nuclei*** that lie deep to the cortex.

## Hippocampal Formation

1. In the human embryo, the hippocampal formation develops in relation to the medial surface of each cerebral hemisphere close to the choroid fissure of the lateral ventricle.
   a. It is at first approximately C-shaped in accordance with the outline of the body and inferior horn of the ventricle.
   b. The upper part of the formation is, however, separated from the ventricle because of the development of the corpus callosum between the two.
   c. For the same reason, this part of the formation remains underdeveloped and is represented by a thin layer of grey matter lining the upper surface of the corpus callosum. This layer is the ***indusium griseum.***
2. Within the indusium griseum are embedded two bundles of longitudinally running fibres called the ***medial*** and ***lateral longitudinal striae*** (on each side of the middle line).
3. Posteriorly, the indusium griseum is continuous with a thin layer of grey matter related to the inferior aspect of the splenium of the corpus callosum. This grey matter is the ***splenial gyrus*** or ***gyrus faciolaris.***
4. The splenial gyrus runs forwards to become continuous with the ***dentate gyrus*** present in relation to the inferior horn of the lateral ventricle.
5. In the region of the inferior horn of the lateral ventricle, the developing hippocampus is pushed into the cavity of the ventricle because of the great development of the neighbouring neocortex. The hippocampal formation is best developed in this region and forms the ***hippocampus***: This term includes the dentate gyrus.
6. Several subdivisions of the region are described. These are shown in 52.15 which shows a coronal section through the inferior horn of the lateral ventricle.
   a. In this figure, note that the cavity of the inferior horn is closed, on the medial side, only by apposed layers of pia mater and ependyma.
   b. A fold of pia mater (tela choroidea) projects into the ventricle and encloses a bunch of capillaries that constitute the choroid plexus.
   c. This fissure through which the tela choroidea projects into the ventricle is the ***choroid fissure.***
   d. The cerebral cortex that lies below the choroid fissure is S-shaped in cross-section.
   e. The ***hippocampal fissure*** separates the upper and middle limbs of the 'S'.
   f. The superior limb of the 'S' forms the hippocampus. The dentate gyrus lies in the lower part of the same area and is considered to be a part of the hippocampus.
7. The hippocampus forms a longitudinal projection that occupies the greater part of the floor of the inferior horn of the lateral ventricle.
   a. Its anterior end is expanded and notched and resembles a foot. It is therefore called the ***pes hippocampi.***
   b. A layer of nerve fibres that covers the ventricular surface of the hippocampus is called the ***alveus.***
   c. The fibres of the alveus pass medially and collect to form a bundle of fibres, the ***fimbria,*** which projects above the medial part of the hippocampus (52.15).
   d. The fimbria runs backwards along the medial side of the hippocampus to become continuous with the fornix (see below).
8. The dentate gyrus is a longitudinal strip of grey matter.
   a. Laterally, it is fused with the hippocampus.
   b. Its medial margin is free, and bears a series of notches that give it a dentate appearance (52.15): hence the name dentate gyrus.
   c. When traced anteriorly, the dentate gyrus runs medially across the inferior surface of the uncus. This part is called the ***tail of the dentate gyrus*** (52.12).
   d. As stated above, the posterior end of the dentate gyrus is continuous with the splenial gyrus (gyrus fasciolaris) (52.14).
9. Because of its close relationship to the dentate gyrus, the uncus is sometimes regarded as part of the hippocampal formation.

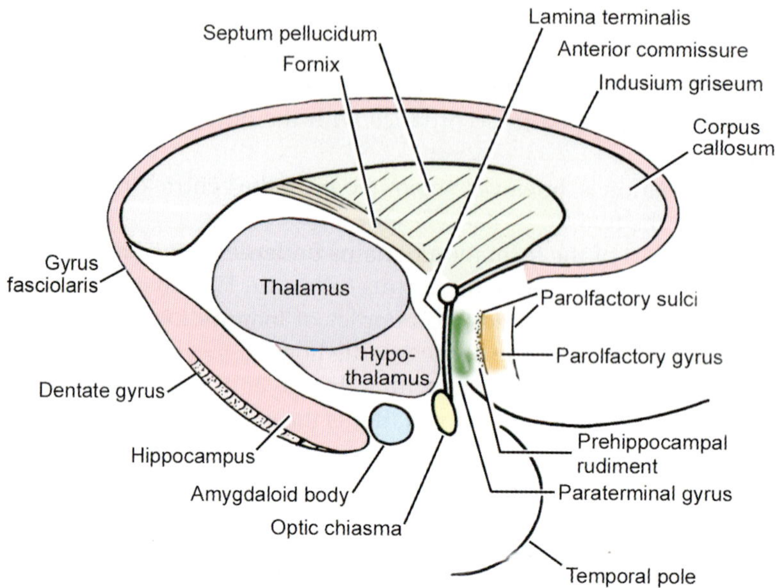


**52.14:** The hippocampal formation and related structures. Note the positions of the parolfactory sulci and gyri

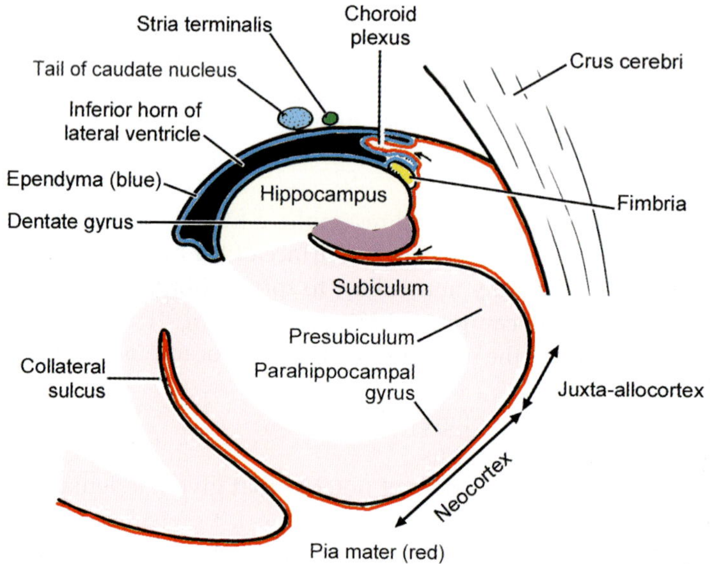


**52.15:** Coronal section through the cerebral hemisphere in the region of the inferior horn of the lateral ventricle to show the hippocampus and related structures
C: choroid fissure;
H: hippocampal fissure

## The Fornix

1. The fornix is a prominent bundle of fibres seen on the medial aspect of the cerebral hemisphere.
2. It is made up, predominantly, of fibres arising in the hippocampus.
3. The ***body*** of the fornix is suspended from the corpus callosum by the septum pellucidum (52.1) and comes into close relationship with the tela choroidea in the roof of the third ventricle.
4. When traced posteriorly, the body of the fornix divides into two parts called ***crura.*** Each crus of the fornix becomes continuous with the fimbria of the corresponding side.
5. The two crura are interconnected by fibres passing from one to the other. These crossing fibres constitute the ***hippocampal commissure*** or ***commissure of the fornix.***
6. The anterior end of the body of the fornix also divides into right and left halves called the ***columns*** of the fornix. Each column turns downward just in front of the interventricular foramen and passes through the hypothalamus to reach the mammillary body.

### WANT TO KNOW MORE?

**Review of Main Connections of the Limbic System**

Having considered some of the important components of the limbic system we are now in a position to review the major interconnections.

1. The main inputs into the limbic system are:
   a. Olfactory (from primary olfactory areas).
   b. Visceral through fibres ascending from the brainstem and terminating in the hypothalamus, the septal region and the amygdaloid complex.
   c. Probably somatic through interconnections between the thalamus and the hypothalamus.
2. The limbic system may possibly be influenced by afferents from some areas of the neocortex.
3. Impulses received from all these centres can spread to all centres within the limbic system through numerous interconnections, most of which are reciprocal.
4. The output from the limbic system is concentrated upon the midbrain reticular formation. These inputs reaching the midbrain reticular formation are relayed to autonomic centres in the brainstem and spinal cord.

# 53 Internal Capsule Commissures

CHAPTER

## THE INTERNAL CAPSULE

1. A preliminary description of the internal capsule is given in the preceding chapters. This should be read before studying the details of the fibres passing through the capsule.
2. The fibres passing through the capsule may be ascending (to the cerebral cortex) or descending (from the cortex).
3. The arrangement of fibres is easily remembered if it is realised that any group of fibres within the capsule takes ***the most direct path*** to its destination.
   a. Thus, fibres to and from the anterior part of the frontal lobe pass through the anterior limb of the internal capsule.
   b. Those to and from the posterior part of the frontal lobe, and from the greater part of the parietal lobe, occupy the genu and posterior limb of the capsule.
   c. Fibres to and from the temporal lobe occupy the sublentiform part, while those to and from the occipital lobe pass through the retrolentiform part.
   d. Some fibres from the lowest parts of the parietal lobe accompany the temporal fibres through the sublentiform part.

### Ascending Fibres

1. These are predominantly ***thalamocortical fibres*** that go from the thalamus to all parts of the cerebral cortex (53.1 and 53.2A and B).
2. Fibres to the frontal lobe constitute the ***anterior thalamic radiation*** (or ***frontal thalamic peduncle***).
   a. They pass through the anterior limb of the internal capsule.
   b. The anterior thalamic radiation also carries fibres from the hypothalamus and limbic structures to the frontal lobe.
3. Fibres travelling from the ventral posterior nuclei of the thalamus to the somatosensory area (in the postcentral gyrus) constitute the ***superior thalamic radiation*** (or the ***superior, or dorsal, thalamic peduncle***).
   a. These fibres occupy the genu and posterior limb of the capsule.
   b. It should be noted that these fibres are third order sensory neurons responsible for conveying somesthetic sensations to the cerebral cortex.
   c. The superior thalamic radiation also contains some fibres that go from the thalamus to parts of the frontal and parietal lobes adjoining the postcentral gyrus.
4. Fibres from the thalamus to the occipital lobe constitute the ***posterior thalamic radiation*** (or the ***posterior, or caudal, thalamic peduncle***).
   a. This includes the ***optic radiation*** from the lateral geniculate body to the visual cortex.
   b. This radiation lies in the retrolentiform part of the internal capsule.
   c. The retrolentiform part also contains some fibres passing from the thalamus to the posterior part of the parietal lobe.

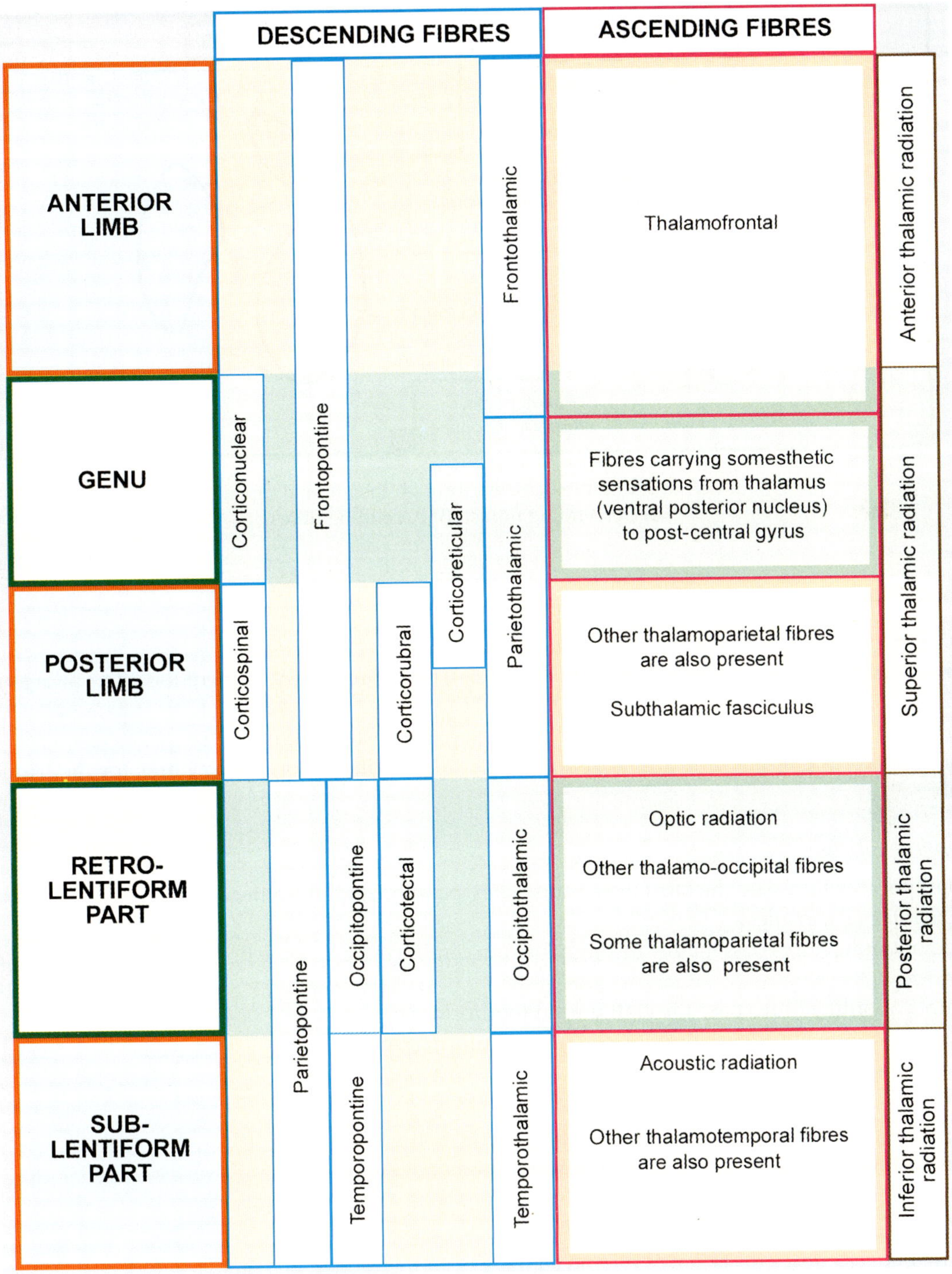

**53.1:** Scheme to show the fibres passing through the internal capsule

5. Fibres from the thalamus to the temporal lobe constitute the ***inferior thalamic radiation*** (or ***ventral thalamic peduncle***).
   a. It includes the ***acoustic radiation*** from the medial geniculate body to the acoustic area of the cerebral cortex.
   b. These fibres pass through the sublentiform part of the internal capsule.

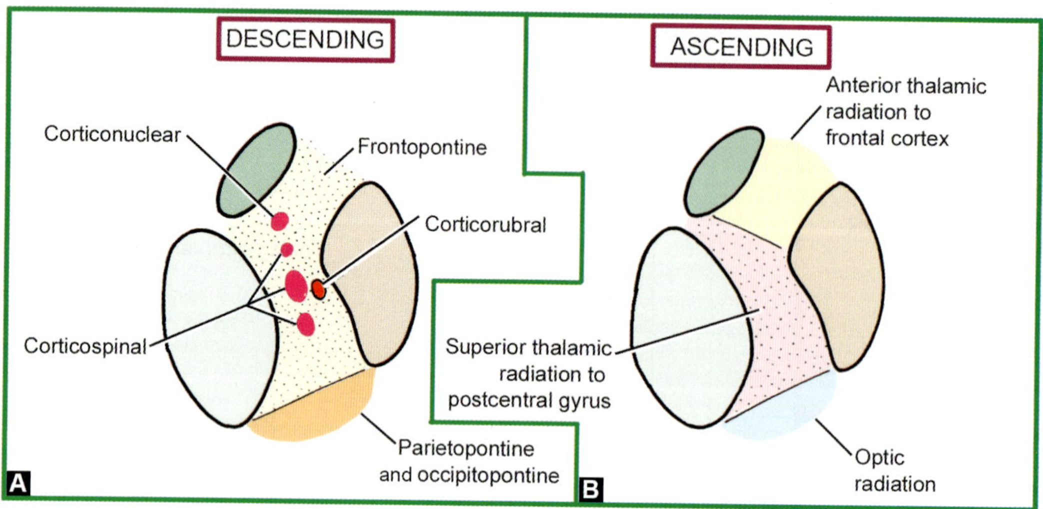


**53.2A and B:** Fibres passing through the internal capsule. (A) Descending fibres; (B) Ascending fibres

## Descending Fibres

### *Corticospinal and Corticonuclear Fibres*

1. Corticonuclear fibres (for motor cranial nerve nuclei) pass through the genu of the internal capsule (53.1 and 53.2A).
2. Corticospinal fibres form several discrete bundles in the posterior limb.
3. The fibres for the upper limb are most anterior, followed (in that order) by fibres for the trunk and lower limb.

### *Corticopontine Fibres*

1. Frontopontine fibres are the most numerous. They pass through the anterior limb, genu, and posterior limb of the internal capsule.
2. Parietopontine fibres pass mainly through the retrolentiform part. Some fibres pass through the sublentiform part.
3. Temporopontine fibres pass through the sublentiform part.
4. Occipitopontine fibres pass through the retrolentiform part.

### *Corticothalamic Fibres*

1. These pass from various parts of the cerebral cortex to the thalamus.
2. They form part of the thalamic radiations described above.

### *Fibres from Cerebral Cortex to Brainstem Nuclei*

1. ***Corticonuclear*** fibres to cranial nerve nuclei have been mentioned above.
2. ***Corticorubral fibres*** pass through the posterior limb.
3. ***Corticoreticular fibres*** pass through the genu and posterior limb.
4. ***Occipitotectal fibres*** pass through the retrolentiform part.

### *Fibres of the Subthalamic Fasciculus*

These pass transversely through the posterior limb (intersecting the vertically running fibres). The fibres of this fasciculus connect the subthalamic nucleus to the globus pallidus.

## COMMISSURES OF THE BRAIN

1. The two halves of the brain and spinal cord are interconnected by numerous fibres that cross the middle line.
2. In some situations, such fibres form recognisable bundles that are called commissures.
3. Strictly speaking, commissural fibres are those that connect corresponding regions of the two sides.
4. Many of the fibres passing through the so-called commissures do not fulfil this criterion as they connect different regions of the two sides. Such fibres are really association fibres.
5. We have seen that several tracts passing through the spinal cord and brainstem cross from one side to the other. These crossings are ***decussations***, but collections of such fibres are sometimes loosely referred to as commissures e.g., the ventral white commissure of the spinal cord.

### The Corpus Callosum

1. The corpus callosum is the largest commissure connecting the right and left cerebral hemispheres. It has been described in chapter 49.
2. The fibres passing through the corpus callosum are generally believed to interconnect corresponding regions of the entire neocortex of the right and left sides.

### Other Commissures

1. Other commissures connecting the two cerebral hemispheres are:
   a. The anterior commissure
   b. The posterior commissure
   c. The hippocampal commissure or commissure of the fornix
   d. The habenular commissure.
2. In close relationship to the optic chiasma a number of commissures carrying fibres not concerned with vision are described. These include:
   a. The ***ventral supraoptic commissure*** (of Gudden)
   b. The ***dorsal supraoptic commissure*** (of Meynert)
   c. The anterior hypothalamic commissure (of Ganser).

54

CHAPTER

# Pathways for Special Senses

In this chapter we will consider the pathways responsible for perception of the special senses of vision, smell, taste, and hearing. In considering each pathway we have to consider:

1. The peripheral organ concerned
2. Pathways through the cranial nerves
3. Centres and pathways within the central nervous system.

## VISUAL PATHWAY

1. The peripheral organ for sight is the eyeball. It has been described in chapter 44.
2. We have seen that receptors for vision are the rods and cones located in the retina.
   a. It may be repeated here that the rods and cones are modified neurons.
   b. They give off central processes that synapse with peripheral processes of bipolar cells.
   c. The central processes of bipolar cells synapse with the dendrites of ganglion cells.
   d. Axons arising from ganglion cells form the fibres of the optic nerve.
3. Opposite the posterior pole of the eyeball the retina shows a ***central region*** about 6 mm in diameter. This region is responsible for sharp vision.
4. In the centre of this region an area about 2 mm in diameter has a yellow colour and is called the ***macula lutea***.
5. The fovea centralis is a depression in the centre of the macula and is 0.4 mm in diameter.
6. Visual impulses arising in the retina are carried to the brain through the optic nerve. The anatomy of the optic nerve and the main features of the visual pathway have been described in chapter 43.
   a. We have seen that the optic nerves enter the cranial cavity through the optic canal and join each other to form the optic chiasma (54.1).
   b. Many fibres of each optic nerve cross to the opposite side through the chiasma.
   c. The uncrossed fibres, along with those that have crossed over from the opposite side, form the optic tract.
   d. The optic tract terminates predominantly in the lateral geniculate body.
   e. Fresh fibres arising in the lateral geniculate body form the geniculocalcarine tract (or optic radiation) which ends in the visual areas of the cerebral cortex.

### The Visual Field and Retinal Quadrants

1. When the head and eyes are maintained in a fixed position, and one eye is closed, the area seen by that eye constitutes the visual field for that eye.
2. Now if the other eye is also opened the area seen is more or less the same as was seen with one eye.
   a. In other words, the visual fields of the two eyes overlap to a very great extent.
   b. On either side, however, there is a small area seen only by the eye of that side.
3. Although, the two eyes view the same area, the relative position of objects within the area appears somewhat dissimilar to the two eyes as they view the object from slightly different angles.

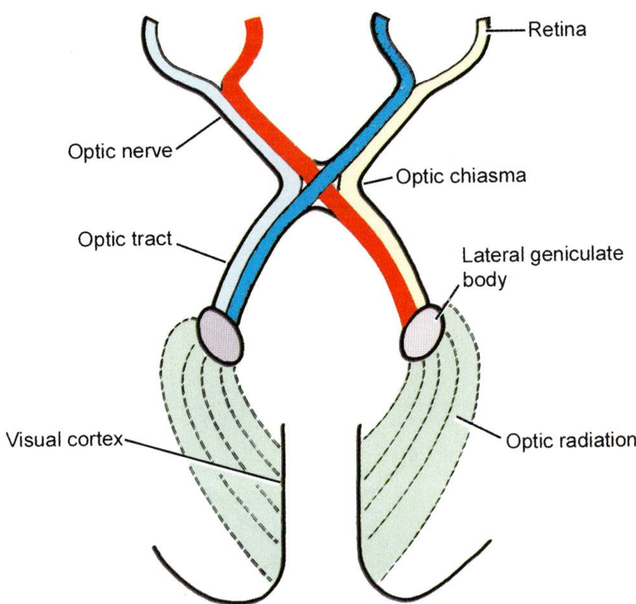


**54.1:** The visual pathway. Note that the fibres from the medial (or nasal) half of each retina cross to the optic tract of the opposite side

4. The difference though slight, is of considerable importance as it forms the basis for the perception of depth (***stereoscopic vision***).
5. For convenience of description, the visual field is divided into right and left halves.
6. It may also be divided into upper and lower halves so that the visual field can be said to consist of four quadrants (54.2).
7. In a similar manner, each retina can also be divided into quadrants.
8. Images of objects in the field of vision are formed on the retina by the lens of the eyeball.
   a. As with any convex lens the image is inverted.
   b. If an object is placed in the ***right*** half of the field of vision, its image is formed on the ***left*** half of the retina and ***vice versa.*** Instead of using the words right and left, the two halves of the retina are usually referred to as ***nasal*** (= medial) and ***temporal*** (= lateral) halves. The image of an object placed in the right half of the field of vision falls on the temporal half of the left retina, and on the nasal half of the right retina.

## Optic Nerve, Optic Chiasma and Optic Tract

1. The optic nerve is made up of axons of the ganglion cells of the retina.
2. These axons are at first unmyelinated. After passing through the sclera (in the region of the lamina cribrosa) each fibre acquires a myelin sheath.
3. The fibres of the nerve arising from the four quadrants of the retina maintain the same relative position within the nerve.
4. The fibres arising from the macula are numerous and form the ***papillomacular bundle***. Close to the eyeball, the macular fibres occupy the lateral part of the nerve, but by the time they reach the chiasma they lie in the central part of the nerve.
5. a. The fibres of the optic nerve arising in the nasal half of each retina enter the optic tract of the opposite side after crossing in the chiasma.
   b. Fibres from the temporal half of each retina enter the optic tract of the same side (54.1).

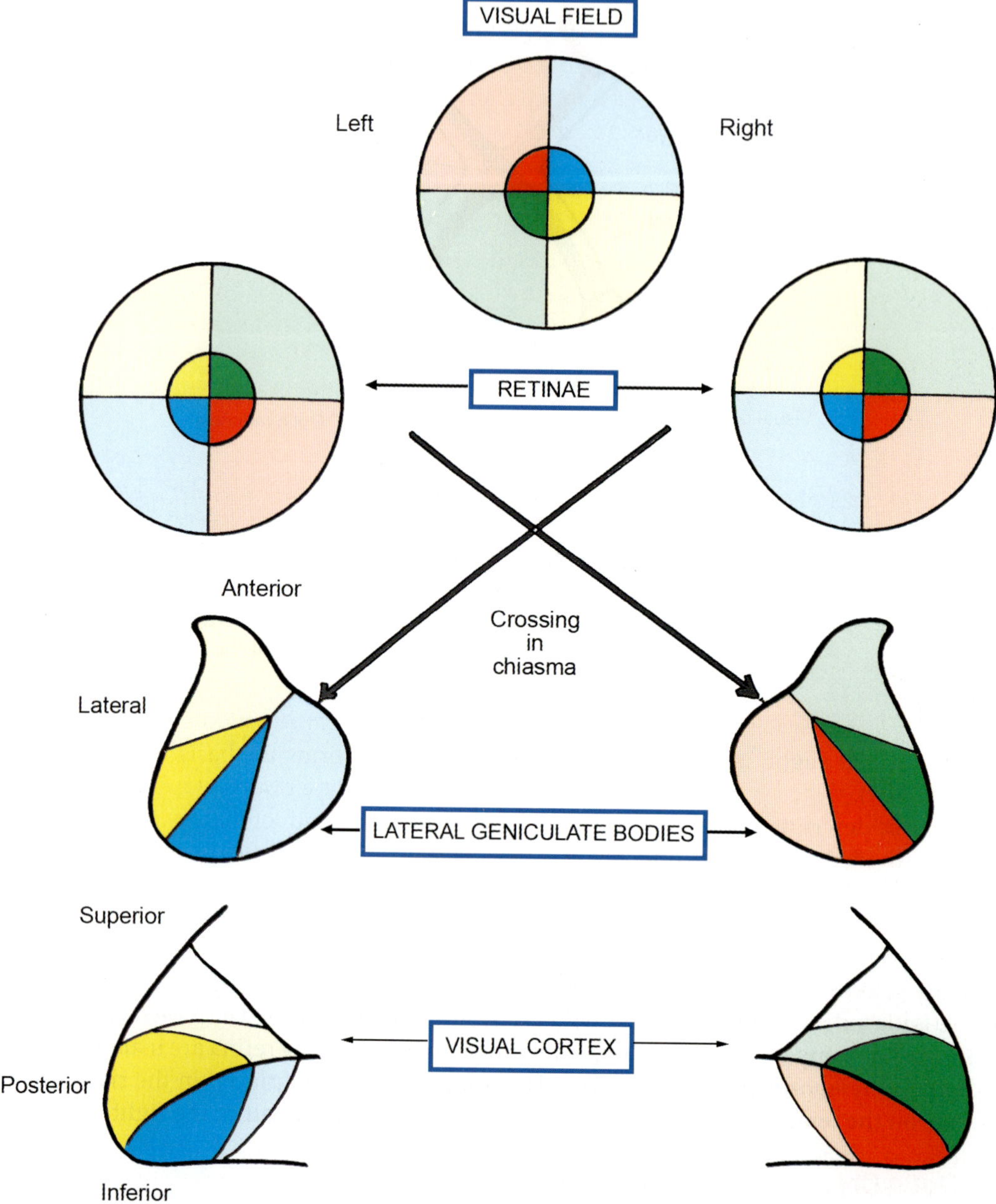


**54.2:** Scheme to show the representation of the visual field in the retinae, the lateral geniculate bodies, and the visual cortex of the two sides. The retinal quadrants for the peripheral parts of the field of vision are shown in light colour, while the corresponding macular areas are shown in dark colour

6. Thus, the right optic tract comes to contain fibres from the right halves of both retinae, and the left tract from the left halves.
7. In other words, all optic nerve fibres carrying impulses relating to the left half of the field of vision are brought together in the right optic tract and ***vice versa.***
8. We have already noted that each optic tract carries these fibres to the lateral geniculate body of the corresponding side.

## The Lateral Geniculate Body

1. Some aspects of the structure of the lateral geniculate body have been considered in chapter 53.
2. Sections through the lateral geniculate body show that its grey matter is split into six laminae.
   a. These layers are numbered one to six from ventral to dorsal side.
   b. Fibres from the eye of the same side end in laminae 2, 3, and 5.
   c. While those from the opposite eye end in laminae 1, 4, and 6.
3. The macular fibres end in the central and posterior part of the lateral geniculate body, and this area is relatively large (54.2).
4. Fibres from the peripheral parts of the retina end in the anterior part of the lateral geniculate body.
   a. The upper half of the retina is represented laterally, and the lower half of the retina is represented medially.
   b. Specific points on the retina project to specific points in the lateral geniculate body.
   c. In turn, specific points of the lateral geniculate body project to specific points in the visual cortex.
   d. In this way a point-to-point relationship is maintained between the retinae and the visual cortex.

## Geniculocalcarine Tract and Visual Cortex

1. Fibres arising from cells of the lateral geniculate body constitute the ***geniculocalcarine tract*** or ***optic radiation.***
2. These fibres pass through the retrolentiform part of the internal capsule.
3. The optic radiation ends in the visual areas of the cerebral cortex (areas 17, 18, 19).
4. The cortex of each hemisphere receives impulses from the retinal halves of the same side (i.e., from the opposite half of the field of vision).
   a. The upper quadrants of the retina are represented above the calcarine sulcus, and the lower quadrants below it (54.2).
   b. The cortical area for the macula is larger than that for peripheral areas. It occupies the posterior part of the visual area.
   c. The cortical area for the peripheral part of the retina is situated anterior to the area for the macula.

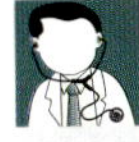

### CLINICAL CORRELATION

*Testing the Optic Nerve*

1. To test the optic nerve first ask the patient if his vision is normal.
2. Acuity (sharpness) of vision can be tested by making the patient read letters of various sizes printed on a chart from a fixed distance. It must be remembered that loss of acuity of vision can be caused by errors of refraction, or by the presence of opacities in the cornea or the lens (cataract).
3. As part of a normal clinical examination, the field of vision can be tested as follows:
   a. Ask the patient to sit opposite you (about half a meter away) and look straight forwards at you.
   b. As one eye to be tested at a time ask the patient to place a hand on one eye so that he can see only with the other eye.
   c. Stretch out one of your arms laterally so that your hand is about equal distance from your face and that of the patient.
   d. Keep moving your index finger and gradually bring the hand towards yourself until you can just see the movements of the finger. This gives you an idea of the extent of your own visual field in that direction.
   e. By asking the patient to tell you as soon as he can see the moving finger (making sure that he does not turn his head) you can get an idea of the patient's field of vision in the direction of your hand.
   f. By repeating the test placing your hand in different directions a good idea of the field of vision of the patient can be obtained.
   g. If an abnormality is suspected detailed testing can be done using a procedure called ***perimetry***.

4. If there is any doubt about the integrity of optic nerve, the retina is examined using an ophthalmoscope. With this instrument we can see the interior of the eye through the pupil of the eye. The optic disc and blood vessels radiating from it can be seen.

*Effects of Injury to Visual Pathway*

1. Injuries to different parts of the visual pathway can produce various kinds of defects.
2. Loss of vision in one half (right or left) of the visual field is called ***hemianopia***.
3. If the same half of the visual field is lost in both eyes the defect is said to be ***homonymous*** and if different halves are lost the defect is said to be ***heteronymous***.
4. Note that the hemianopia is named in relation to the visual field and not to the retina.
5. Injury to the optic nerve produces total blindness in the eye concerned.
6. Damage to the central part of the optic chiasma (e.g., by pressure from an enlarged hypophysis) interrupts the crossing fibres derived from the nasal halves of the two retinae resulting in ***bitemporal heteronymous hemianopia***.
7. It has been claimed that macular fibres are more susceptible to damage by pressure than peripheral fibres and are affected first.
8. When the lateral part of the chiasma is affected, a ***nasal hemianopia*** results. This may be unilateral or bilateral.
9. Complete destruction of the optic tract, the lateral geniculate body, the optic radiation or the visual cortex of one side, results in loss of the opposite half of the field of vision.
10. A lesion on the right side leads to ***left homonymous hemianopia***. Lesions anterior to the lateral geniculate body also interrupt fibres responsible for the pupillary light reflex.

## PATHWAY FOR HEARING

1. The peripheral organ for hearing is the ear that is described in chapter 44.
2. We have seen that sound waves travelling through air enter the external acoustic meatus and produce vibrations in the tympanic membrane.
3. These vibrations are transmitted through the chain of ossicles present in the middle ear to reach the internal ear.
4. Pressure waves set up in the perilymph reach the spiral organ (of Corti) present in intimate relationship to the cochlea.
5. Hair cells present in the spiral organ convert these vibrations into nervous impulses.
6. The first neurons of the pathway of hearing lie in the spiral ganglion located in a bony tunnel running along the cochlea.
   a. These neurons are bipolar.
   b. Peripheral processes of neurons lying in this ganglion innervate the hair cells of the spiral organ (of Corti).
   c. The central processes of the neurons form the cochlear nerve.
7. The fibres of the cochlear nerve terminate in the dorsal and ventral cochlear nuclei (54.3). The neurons in these nuclei are, therefore, second order neurons.
   a. Their axons pass medially in the dorsal part of the pons.
   b. Most of them cross to the opposite side, but some remain uncrossed (54.3).
   c. The crossing fibres of the two sides form a conspicuous mass of fibres called the ***trapezoid body***.
8. The large majority of fibres from the cochlear nuclei terminate in the superior olivary complex (made up of a number of nuclei).
9. Third order neurons arising in this complex form an important ascending bundle called the ***lateral lemniscus***.
10. Some cochlear fibres that do not relay in the superior olivary nucleus join the lemniscus after relaying in scattered cells lying within the trapezoid body: these cells constitute the ***trapezoid nucleus (nucleus of the trapezoid body)***.
11. Still other cochlear fibres relay in cells that lie within the lemniscus itself: these neurons form the ***nucleus of the lateral lemniscus***.

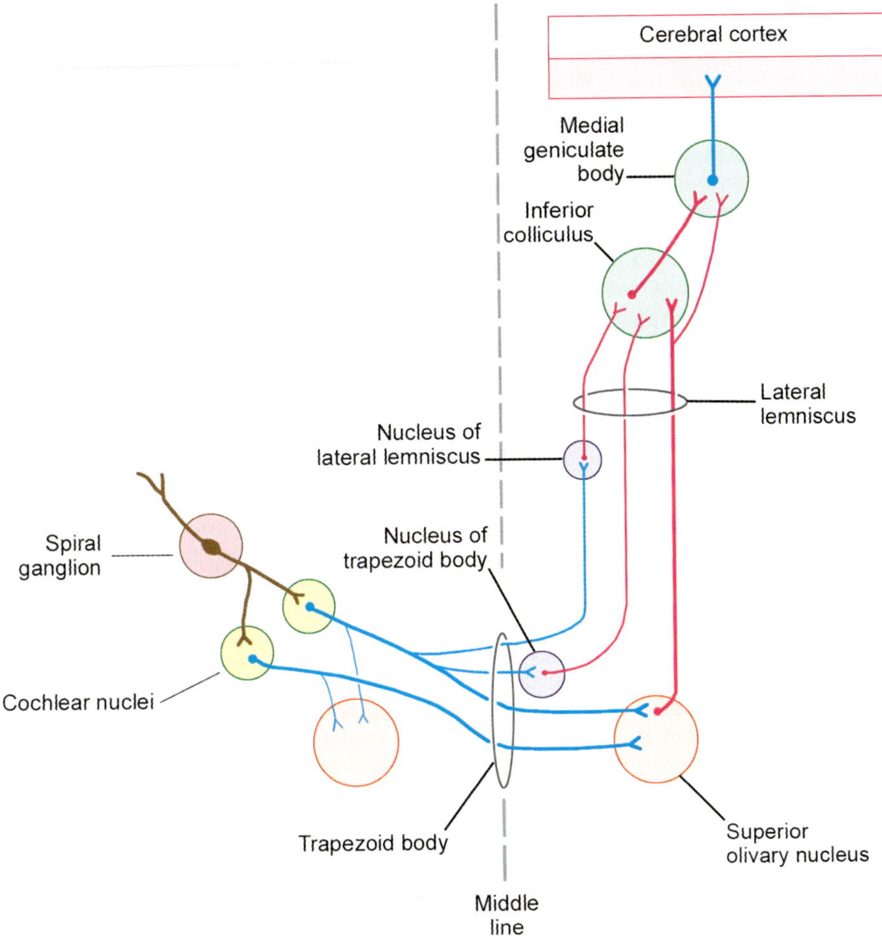


**54.3:** Scheme to show the pathway for hearing

12. The fibres of the lateral lemniscus ascend to the midbrain and terminate in the inferior colliculus (54.3).
13. Fibres arising in the colliculus enter the inferior brachium to reach the medial geniculate body. Some fibres in the lemniscus reach this body without relay in the inferior colliculus.
14. Fibres arising in the medial geniculate body form the ***acoustic radiation*** that ends in the acoustic area of the cerebral cortex.
15. It may be stressed that each lateral lemniscus carries impulses arising in both the right and left cochleae. The medial and lateral geniculate bodies are described in chapter 53.

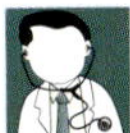

## CLINICAL CORRELATION

*Testing the Vestibulocochlear Nerve*

This nerve is responsible for hearing (cochlear part) and for equilibrium (vestibular part). Normally, we test only the cochlear part.

1. The hearing of the patient can be tested by using a watch.
   a. First place the watch near one ear so that the patient knows what he is expected to hear.
   b. Next ask him to close his eyes and say so when he hears the ticking of the watch.

c. The watch should be held away from the ear and then gradually brought towards it.
d. The distance at which the sounds are first heard should be compared with the other ear.

2. In doing this test it must be remembered that loss of hearing can occur from various causes such as the presence of wax in the ear, or middle ear disease.
3. Nerve deafness can be distinguished from deafness due to a conduction defect (as in middle ear disease) by noting the following:
   a. Sounds can be transmitted to the internal ear through air (normal way), and can also be transmitted through bone. Normally conduction through air is better than that through bone, but in defects of conduction the sound is better heard through bone.
   b. Air conduction and bone conduction of sound can be compared by using a tuning fork.
   c. Strike the tuning fork against an object so that it begins to vibrate producing sound.
   d. Place the tuning fork near the patient's ear and then immediately put the base of the tuning fork on the mastoid process. Ask the patient where he hears the sound better. (This is called ***Rinne's test***).
   e. In another test, the base of a vibrating tuning fork is placed on the forehead. The sound is heard in both ears but is clearer in the ear with a conduction defect. (This is ***Weber's test***).
4. Defects in the vestibular apparatus or in the vestibular nerve are difficult to test and such cases need to be examined by a specialist.

## PATHWAYS FOR TASTE

1. The end organs for taste are taste buds located mainly on the tongue.
   a. They are most numerous in relation to vallate papillae.
   b. Some taste buds are present in the mucosa of the soft palate, and of the epiglottis.
2. Sensations of taste arising in the taste buds travel through a number of different pathways as follows:
   a. Sensations of taste from the anterior two-thirds of the tongue (the part of the tongue lying anterior to the sulcus terminalis, but excluding the vallate papillae) travel through the lingual nerve, the chorda tympani and the facial nerve.
   b. Sensations of taste from the posterior one-third of the tongue (part of the tongue posterior to the sulcus terminalis, and including the vallate papillae) are carried by the glossopharyngeal nerve.
   c. Taste fibres from the posterior most part of the tongue (just in front of the epiglottis), and from taste buds on the epiglottis, are carried by the superior laryngeal branch of the vagus nerve.
   d. The course of taste fibres from the soft palate is shown in 43.56.
   e. On entering the brainstem all fibres of taste (travelling through the facial, glossopharyngeal and vagus nerves) end in the upper part of the nucleus of the tractus solitarius.
   f. New fibres arising in this nucleus travel to the thalamus through the solitariothalamic tract (54.4). The fibres reach the ventral posteromedial nucleus of the thalamus.
   g. From here they are relayed to the cerebral cortex (areas 3, 2, 1). The fibres form part of the superior thalamic radiation passing through the posterior limb of the internal capsule.

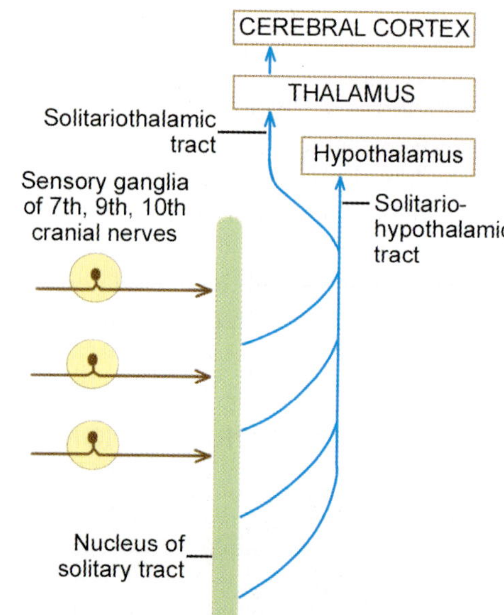


**54.4:** Connections of the nucleus of the solitary tract

## PATHWAY FOR SMELL

The peripheral organ for smell is the olfactory mucosa, and the cranial nerve concerned is the olfactory nerve.

A complete description of olfactory pathways is given in chapter 52.

55

CHAPTER

# Ventricles of the Brain and Cerebrospinal Fluid

1. The interior of the brain contains a series of cavities (55.1).
   a. The cerebrum contains a median cavity: the ***third ventricle;*** and two ***lateral ventricles***: one in each hemisphere.
   b. Each lateral ventricle opens into the third ventricle through an ***interventricular foramen.***
   c. The third ventricle is continuous, caudally, with the ***cerebral aqueduct*** that traverses the midbrain and opens into the fourth ventricle.
   d. The ***fourth ventricle*** is situated dorsal to the pons and medulla, and ventral to the cerebellum.
   e. It communicates, inferiorly, with the ***central canal*** that traverses the lower part of the medulla, and the spinal cord.
2. The entire ventricular system is lined by an epithelium layer called the ***ependyma.***

## THE LATERAL VENTRICLES

1. The lateral ventricles are two cavities, one situated within each cerebral hemisphere.
2. Each ventricle consists of a central part that gives off three extensions called the anterior, posterior and inferior horns (55.1).

### The Central Part

1. The central part of the lateral ventricle is elongated anteroposteriorly.
2. Anteriorly, it becomes continuous with the anterior horn, at the level of the interventricular foramen.
3. Posteriorly, the central part reaches the splenium of the corpus callosum.
4. The central part is triangular in cross section (55.2). It has a roof, a floor, and a medial wall. The roof and floor meet on the lateral side.
5. The ***roof*** of the central part is formed by the trunk of the corpus callosum.
6. The ***medial wall*** is formed by the septum pellucidum and by the body of the fornix. It is common to the two lateral ventricles.
7. The ***floor*** is formed mainly by:
   a. The superior surface of the thalamus (medially)
   b. The caudate nucleus (laterally).
8. Between these two structures, there are:
   a. The stria terminalis (laterally).
   b. The thalamostriate vein (medially).
9. From 55.2, it will be seen that there is a space between the fornix and the upper surface of the thalamus.
   a. This is the choroid fissure.
   b. A fold of pia mater, the tela choroidea, invaginates into the ventricle through the fissure and covers part of the thalamus.
10. The tela choroidea is common to the two lateral ventricles, and to the third ventricle. Within each lateral edge of the tela choroidea, there are plexuses of blood vessels that constitute the ***choroid plexus*** (55.2).
11. The tela choroidea and other structures forming the walls of the ventricle are lined by ependyma.

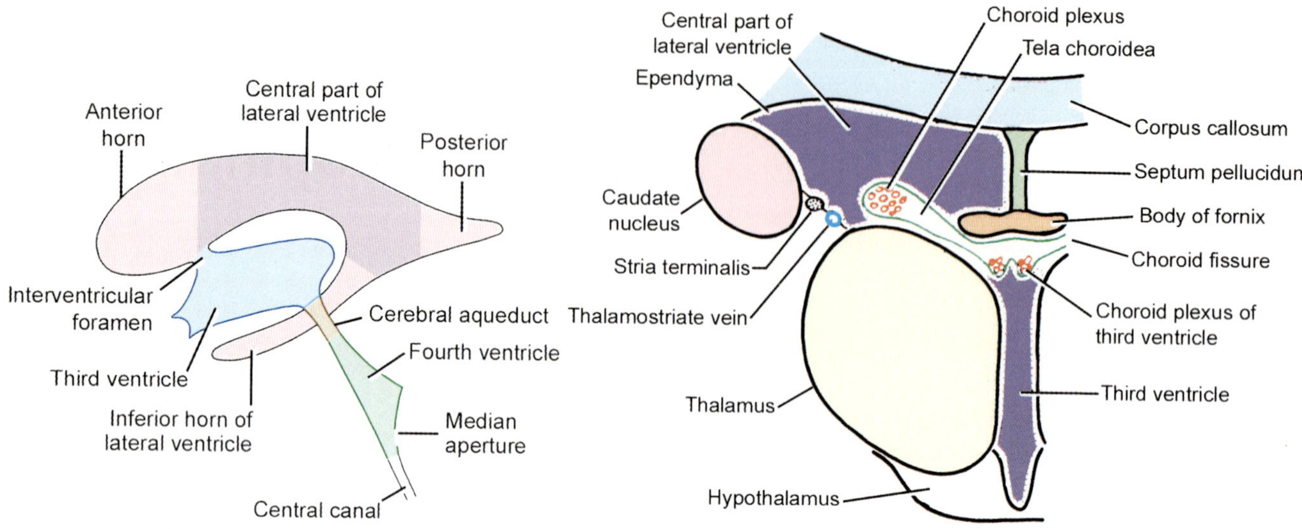


**55.1:** The ventricular system of the brain. Lateral view

**55.2:** Boundaries of the central part of the lateral ventricle and of the third ventricle. Note the relationship of the tela choroidea and choroid plexuses to these ventricles

## The Anterior Horn

1. The anterior horn of the lateral ventricle, lies anterior to its central part, the two being separated by an imaginary vertical line drawn at the level of the interventricular foramen (55.1).
2. This horn is triangular in section. It has a roof, a floor and a medial wall.
3. It is closed, anteriorly, by the genu and rostrum of the corpus callosum.
4. The ***roof*** is formed by the most anterior part of the trunk of the corpus callosum.
5. The floor is formed, mainly, by the head of the caudate nucleus. A small part of the floor, near the middle line, is formed by the upper surface of the rostrum of the corpus callosum.
6. The ***medial wall*** (common to the two sides) is formed by the septum pellucidum.
7. It may be noted that the tela choroidea and the choroid plexus ***do not*** extend into the anterior horn.

## The Posterior Horn

1. The posterior horn of the lateral ventricle extends backwards into the occipital lobe.
2. It has a roof, a lateral wall, and a medial wall.
3. The ***roof*** and ***lateral wall*** are formed by the tapetum.
4. The ***medial wall*** shows two elevations.
   a. The upper of these is the ***bulb of the posterior horn***, which is produced by fibres of the forceps major as they run backwards from the splenium of the corpus callosum.
   b. The lower elevation is called the ***calcar avis***. It represents white matter 'pushed in' by formation of the calcarine sulcus.

## The Inferior Horn

1. The inferior horn of the lateral ventricle begins at the posterior end of the central part.
2. It runs downwards and forwards into the temporal lobe, its anterior end reaching close to the uncus.
3. In considering the structures to be seen in the walls of the inferior horn it is useful to note that:
   a. The anterior horn, the central part, and the inferior horn form one continuous C-shaped cavity (55.1).

   b. The floor of the central part of the ventricle is continuous with the roof of the inferior horn.
   c. The body of the fornix divides, posteriorly, into two crura which become continuous with the fimbria and hippocampus.
4. In the central part of the ventricle, the choroid fissure lies below the fornix.
   a. When traced into the inferior horn, the fissure lies ***above*** the fimbria and hippocampus.
   b. The choroid plexus extends into the inferior horn through the choroid fissure.
5. In cross section, the inferior horn is seen to have a narrow cavity (55.3).
   a. The cavity is bounded above, and laterally, by the ***roof.***
   b. Below, and medially, by the ***floor.***
6. Because of this orientation, the lateral part of the roof is sometimes called the ***lateral wall,*** and the medial part of the floor is called the ***medial wall.***
7. The lateral part of the roof (or lateral wall) is formed by fibres of the tapetum. The medial part of the roof is formed by the tail of the caudate nucleus (laterally) and the stria terminalis (medially).
8. These structures are continued into the roof of the inferior horn from the floor of the central part.
9. Anteriorly, the tail of the caudate nucleus and the stria terminalis end in relation to the amygdaloid complex, which lies in the most anterior part of the roof.
10. The floor of the inferior horn is formed mainly by the hippocampus, along with the alveus and fimbria.
11. In the lateral part of the floor there is an elevation, the ***collateral eminence,*** produced by inward bulging of the white matter that lies deep to the collateral sulcus.

## THE THIRD VENTRICLE

1. The third ventricle is the cavity of the diencephalon. It is a median cavity situated between the right and left thalami (55.2).
2. It communicates, on either side, with the lateral ventricle through the interventricular foramen (55.1 and 55.4).
3. Posteriorly, it continues into the cerebral aqueduct that connects it to the fourth ventricle.
4. The ventricle has two lateral walls, an anterior wall, a posterior wall, a floor and a roof.
5. Each ***lateral wall*** is marked by the ***hypothalamic sulcus*** (55.4) that follows a curved course from the interventricular foramen to the aqueduct.
   a. Above the sulcus, the wall is formed by the medial surface of the thalamus. The two thalami are usually connected by a band of grey matter called the ***interthalamic connexus,*** which passes through the ventricle.
   b. The lateral wall, below the hypothalamic sulcus, is formed by the medial surface of the hypothalamus.

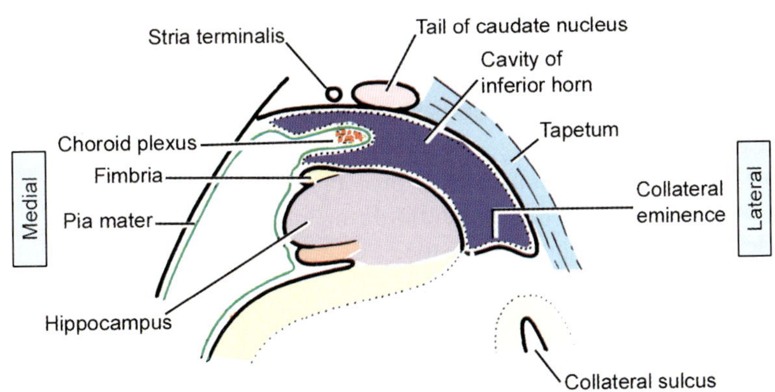


**55.3:** Boundaries of the inferior horn of the lateral ventricle

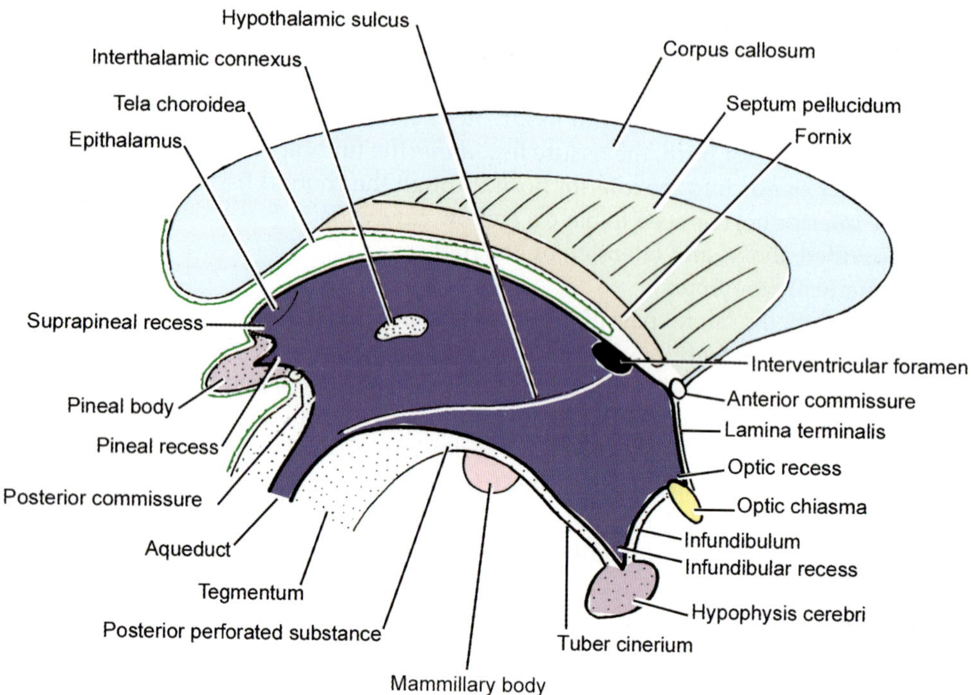


**55.4:** Boundaries and recesses of the third ventricle. Note the mode of formation of the tela choroidea that lies in the roof of the ventricle

  c. A small part of the lateral wall, above and behind the thalamus, is formed by the epithalamus.
  d. The interventricular foramen is seen on the lateral wall, just behind the column of the fornix.
6. The ***anterior wall*** of the third ventricle is formed mainly by the lamina terminalis. Its upper part is formed by the anterior commissure, and by the columns of the fornix as they diverge from each other.
7. The ***posterior wall*** is formed by the pineal body and the posterior commissure.
8. The ***floor*** is formed by:
   a. The optic chiasma
   b. The tuber cinereum and the infundibulum
   c. The mammillary bodies
   d. The posterior perforated substance
   e. The tegmentum of the midbrain.
9. The ***roof*** of the ventricle is formed by the ependyma that stretches across the two thalami (55.2).
   a. Above the ependyma, there is the tela choroidea.
   b. Within the tela choroidea, there are two plexuses of blood vessels (one on either side of the middle line) which bulge downwards into the cavity of the third ventricle. These are the choroid plexuses of the third ventricle (See below).
10. The cavity of the third ventricle shows a number of prolongations or recesses (55.4).
   a. The ***infundibular recess*** extends into the infundibulum.
   b. The ***optic recess*** lies just above the optic chiasma.
   c. The ***pineal recess*** lies between the superior and inferior lamina of the stalk of the pineal body.
   d. The ***suprapineal recess*** lies above the pineal body in relation to the epithalamus.

## Tela Choroidea of the Third and Lateral Ventricles

1. The tela choroidea is a double-layered fold of pia mater that occupies the interval between the splenium of the corpus callosum and fornix, above, and the two thalami below.

**WANT TO KNOW MORE?**

2. It is triangular in shape. Its posterior end is broad and lies in the gap between the splenium (above) and the posterior part of the roof of the third ventricle (below) (55.4). This gap is called the ***transverse fissure***.
3. The anterior end (representing the apex of the triangle) lies near the right and left interventricular foramina.
   a. The median part of the tela choroidea lies over the roof of the third ventricle.
   b. Its right and left lateral edges project into the central parts of the corresponding lateral ventricles (55.2).
4. When traced posteriorly, the two layers of pia mater forming the tela choroidea separate.
   a. The upper layer curves upwards over the posterior aspect of the splenium.
   b. The lower layer turns downwards over the pineal body and tectum (55.4).

### Choroid Plexuses

1. The choroid plexuses are highly vascular structures that are responsible for the formation of cerebrospinal fluid.

**WANT TO KNOW MORE?**

2. The surface of each plexus is lined by a membrane formed by fusion of the ventricular ependyma with the pia mater of the tela choroidea.
3. Deep to this membrane, there is a plexus of blood vessels.
4. Microscopic examination shows that the surface of the choroid plexus has numerous villous processes.
   a. Each process contains a plexus of capillaries that are connected to afferent and efferent vessels.
   b. Because of the presence of these processes, the surface area of the choroid plexuses is considerable.
   c. It is further increased by the presence of microvilli (seen with the EM) present on the ependymal cells.
5. Four choroid plexuses are to be seen in relation to the tela choroidea of the third and lateral ventricles.
   a. Two of these (one right and one left) lie along the corresponding lateral margins, and project into the central part of the corresponding lateral ventricle.
   b. Two other plexuses run parallel to each other, one on either side of the middle line. These are the choroid plexuses of the third ventricle.
6. At each posterolateral angle of the tela choroidea, the choroid plexus of the lateral ventricle continues into the inferior horn.
7. The tela choroidea and choroid plexuses of the fourth ventricle are considered later in this chapter.

## THE FOURTH VENTRICLE

### Preliminary Remarks

1. For a proper understanding of the anatomy of the fourth ventricle, it is necessary that some features of the gross anatomy of the cerebellum and of related structures be clearly understood.
2. Reference to 55.5 will show that the cerebellum is intimately related to the ventricle.
3. The upper part of the ventricle is related to the ***superior medullary velum.*** When traced inferiorly (and posteriorly) the velum merges into the white matter of the cerebellum.
4. The lower part of the ventricle is related to the nodule (55.5). It will be recalled that the nodule forms the most anterior part of the inferior vermis.
5. Immediately lateral to the nodule, there is the tonsil of the cerebellum. If the tonsil is lifted away, we see that the nodule is continuous laterally with a membrane called the ***inferior medullary velum***.

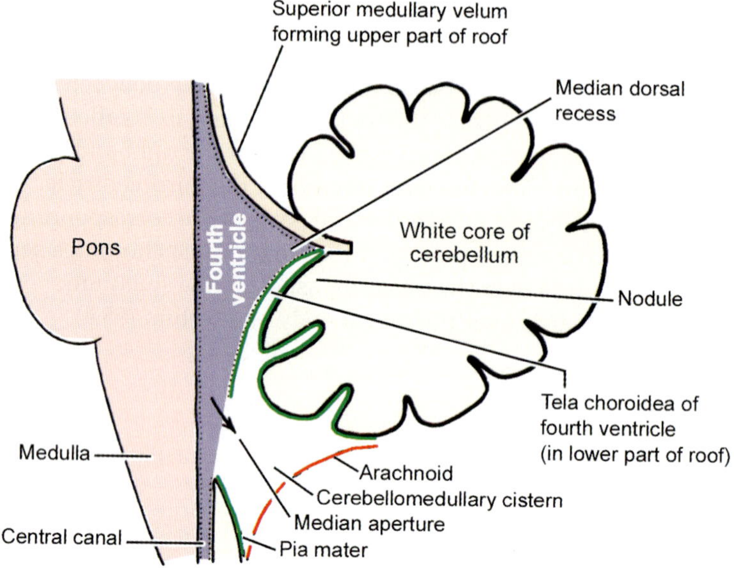


**55.5:** Midsagittal section through the fourth ventricle and related structures. Note how the tela choroidea is formed. The pia mater is shown in green

6. Posteriorly, the inferior velum merges into the white matter of the cerebellum.
7. The inferior medullary velum has a thickened free edge that connects the nodule to the flocculus. This edge is the peduncle of the flocculus.

## Boundaries of Fourth Ventricle

1. The fourth ventricle is a space situated dorsal to the pons and to the upper part of the medulla; and ventral to the cerebellum.
2. For descriptive purposes, the ventricle may be considered as having a cavity, a floor, a roof and lateral walls.

### *The Cavity*

1. The cavity of the ventricle is continuous, inferiorly, with the central canal; and, superiorly, with the cerebral aqueduct.
2. It communicates with the subarachnoid space through three apertures, one median, and two lateral (55.5).
3. A number of extensions from the main cavity are described.
   a. The largest of these are two ***lateral recesses,*** one on either side.
   b. Each lateral recess passes laterally in the interval between the inferior cerebellar peduncle (ventrally), and the peduncle of the flocculus (dorsally).
   c. The lateral extremity of the recess reaches the flocculus. At this extremity, the recess opens into the subarachnoid space at the ***lateral aperture.***
4. Another recess present in the middle line, is called the ***median dorsal recess.*** It extends into the white core of the cerebellum and lies just cranial to the nodule (55.5).
5. Immediately lateral to the nodule, another recess projects dorsally, on either side, above the inferior medullary velum. This is the ***lateral dorsal recess.***

### *The Floor*

1. Because of its shape, the floor of the fourth ventricle is often called the ***rhomboid fossa*** (55.6).

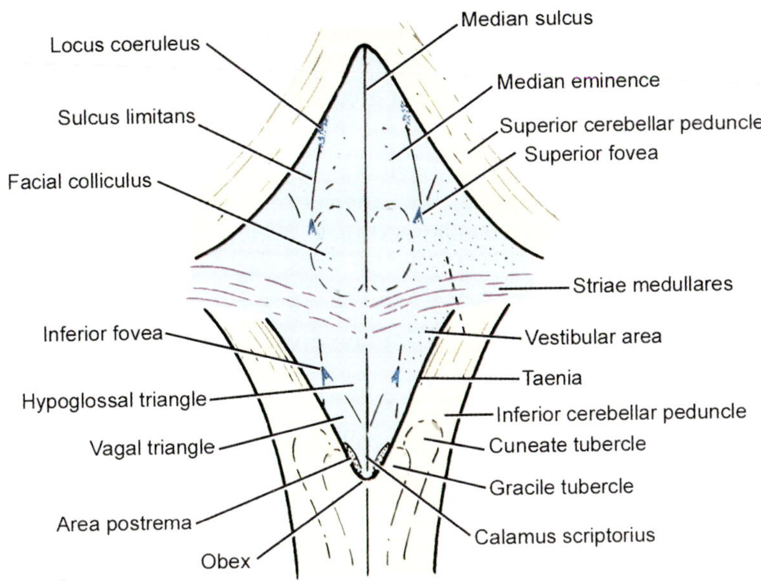


**55.6:** Structures in the floor of the fourth ventricle

2. It is divisible into an upper triangular part formed by the posterior surface of the pons; a lower triangular part formed by the upper part of the posterior surface of the medulla; and an intermediate part at the junction of the medulla and pons.
3. The intermediate part is prolonged laterally over the inferior cerebellar peduncle as the floor of the lateral recess.
4. Its surface is marked by the presence of delicate bundles of transversely running fibres. These bundles are the ***striae medullares.***
5. The entire floor is divided into right and left halves by a ***median sulcus.***
6. Next to the middle line, there is a longitudinal elevation called the ***median eminence***.
7. The eminence is bounded laterally by the ***sulcus limitans.***
8. The region lateral to the sulcus limitans is the ***vestibular area*** that overlies the vestibular nuclei. The vestibular area lies partly in the pons and partly in the medulla.
9. The pontine part of the floor shows some features of interest in close relation to the sulcus limitans and the median eminence.
10. The uppermost part of the sulcus limitans overlies an area that is bluish in colour and is called the ***locus coeruleus*** (Deep to the locus coeruleus, there is the nucleus coeruleus that extends upwards into the tegmentum of the midbrain. It is regarded as part of the reticular formation).
11. Somewhat lower down, the sulcus limitans is marked by a depression, the ***superior fovea.***
12. At this level, the median eminence shows a swelling, the ***facial colliculus***.
13. The medullary part of the floor also shows some features of interest in relation to the median eminence and the sulcus limitans.
14. The sulcus limitans is marked by a depression, the ***inferior fovea.***
15. Descending from the fovea, there is a sulcus that runs obliquely towards the middle line. This sulcus divides the median eminence into two triangles.
16. These are the ***hypoglossal triangle***, medially; and the ***vagal triangle***, laterally.
17. Between the vagal triangle (above) and the gracile tubercle (below), there is a small area called the ***area postrema.***
18. Finally mention must be made of two terms often used in relation to the medulla.
    a. The lowest part of the floor of the fourth ventricle is called the ***calamus scriptorius,*** because of its resemblance to a nib.

   b. Each inferolateral margin of the ventricle is marked by a narrow white ridge or ***taenia.***
   c. The right and left taeniae meet at the inferior angle of the floor to form a small fold called the ***obex.***
   d. The term obex is often used to denote the inferior angle itself.

### *The Lateral Walls*

1. The upper part of each lateral wall is formed by the superior cerebellar peduncle.
2. The lower part is formed by the inferior cerebellar peduncle, and by the gracile and cuneate tubercles.

### *The Roof*

1. The roof of the fourth ventricle is tent-shaped and can be divided into upper and lower parts that meet at an apex (55.5).
2. The apex extends into the white core of the cerebellum.
3. The upper part of the roof is formed by the superior cerebellar peduncles and the superior medullary velum.
4. The inferior part of the roof is devoid of nervous tissue in most of its extent.
   a. It is formed by a membrane consisting of ependyma and a double fold of pia mater that constitutes the ***tela choroidea of the fourth ventricle.***
   b. Laterally, on each side, this membrane reaches and fuses with the inferior cerebellar peduncles.
   c. The lower part of the membrane has a large aperture in it. This is the ***median aperture*** of the fourth ventricle through which the ventricle communicates with the subarachnoid space in the region of the cerebello-medullary cistern.
   d. In the region of the lateral recess, the membrane is prolonged laterally and helps to form the wall of the recess.
   e. The inferior medullary velum forms a small part of the roof in the region of the lateral dorsal recess.

**WANT TO KNOW MORE?**

5. The ***choroid plexuses of the fourth ventricle*** are similar in structure to those of the lateral and third ventricles.
   a. They lie within the folds of pia mater that form the tela choroidea, and project into the cavity of the ventricle from the lower part of the roof.
   b. Each plexus (right or left) consists of a vertical limb lying next to the midline, and a horizontal limb extending into the lateral recess.
   c. The vertical limbs of the two plexuses lie side by side so that the whole structure is T-shaped.
   d. The lower ends of the vertical limbs reach the median aperture and project into the subarachnoid space through it.
   e. The lateral ends of the horizontal limbs reach the lateral apertures, and can be seen on the surface of the brain, near the flocculus.

## THE CEREBROSPINAL FLUID

1. The cerebrospinal fluid (CSF) fills the subarachnoid space. It also extends into the ventricles of the brain, and into the central canal of the spinal cord.
2. The CSF provides a fluid cushion that protects the brain from injury. It also helps to carry nutrition to the brain, and to remove waste products.
3. CSF is formed by the choroid plexuses of the ventricles.
   a. The fluid formed in each lateral ventricle flows into the third ventricle through the interventricular foramen.
   b. From the third ventricle, it passes through the aqueduct into the fourth ventricle.
   c. Here it passes through the median and lateral apertures in the roof of this ventricle to enter the part of the subarachnoid space that forms the cerebello-medullary cistern.
   d. From here the fluid enters other parts of the subarachnoid space.

4. In passing from the posterior cranial fossa into the upper (supratentorial) part of the cranial cavity, the CSF traverses the narrow interval between the free margin of the tentorium cerebelli and the brainstem.
5. It leaves the subarachnoid space by entering the venous sinuses through arachnoid villi.

## WANT TO KNOW MORE?

6. The total volume of CSF is about 140 ml of which about 25 ml is in the ventricles. The CSF is constantly replaced.
7. The CSF consists of water, sodium chloride, potassium, glucose and proteins. The proportions of these substances differ considerably in blood and CSF and hence, it is believed that CSF is formed by an active secretory process, and not by passive filtration.
8. The epithelium and other tissues of the choroid plexuses form an effective barrier between the blood and the CSF. This blood CSF barrier allows selective passage of substances from blood to CSF, but not in the reverse direction.
9. The arachnoid villi provide a valvular mechanism for flow of CSF into blood without permitting back flow of blood into the CSF.

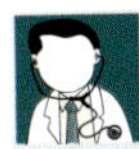

## CLINICAL CORRELATION

1. An abnormal increase in the quantity of CSF can lead to enlargement of the head in children. This condition is called ***hydrocephalus.***
2. Abnormal pressure of CSF leads to degeneration of brain tissue.
3. Hydrocephalus may be caused by:
   a. Excessive production of CSF
   b. By obstruction to its flow
   c. By impaired absorption through the arachnoid villi.
4. It is classified as ***obstructive*** when there is obstruction to flow of CSF from the ventricular system to the subarachnoid space, or as ***communicating*** when such obstruction is not present.
5. Obstruction is most likely to occur where CSF has to pass through narrow passages e.g.,
   a. The interventricular foramina
   b. The aqueduct
   c. The apertures of the fourth ventricle.
6. In each of the above instances, dilatation is confined to cavities proximal to the obstruction.
7. Occasionally, meningitis may lead to obstruction of the narrow interval between the tentorium cerebelli and the brainstem.
8. Meningitis may also lead to hydrocephalus by affecting the arachnoid villi, thus hampering the reabsorption of CSF.
9. Samples of CSF are often required for help in clinical diagnosis. They are obtained most easily by ***lumbar puncture.*** In this procedure, a needle is introduced into the subarachnoid space through the interval between the third and fourth lumbar vertebrae.
10. Under exceptional circumstances, CSF may be obtained by ***cisternal puncture*** in which a needle is passed into the cerebello-medullary cistern.

***Blood-Brain Barrier***

1. It has been observed that while some substances can pass from the blood into the brain with ease, others are prevented from doing so. This has given rise to the concept of a selective barrier between blood and the brain.

2. Anatomically, the structures that could constitute the barrier are as follows:
   a. Capillary endothelium
   b. Basement membrane of the endothelium
   c. Closely applied to the vessels, there are numerous processes of astrocytes. It has been estimated that these processes cover about eighty five percent of the capillary surface.
3. Some areas of the brain (and related structures) appear to be devoid of a blood-brain barrier. These include:
   a. The pineal body
   b. The hypophysis cerebri
   c. The choroid plexus and certain other regions.

## Ventriculography

The ventricles of the brain can be studied in living subjects by taking radiographs after injecting a radio-opaque dye into the ventricular system. The procedure is called ventriculography. Parts of the ventricles can also be seen using CT scans and magnetic resonance imaging (See chapter 56).

56

CHAPTER

# Blood Supply of the Brain and Some Investigative Procedures for Neurological Diagnosis

1. The nervous system is richly supplied with blood. Interruption of blood supply even for a short period can result in damage to nervous tissue. It is interesting to note that lymphatic vessels are not present in nervous tissue.
2. The blood supply of the spinal cord has been described in chapter 40. Here we will consider the blood supply of the brain.

## ARTERIES THAT SUPPLY THE BRAIN

The arteries that supply the brain are derived from the internal carotid and vertebral arteries.

### Internal Carotid Artery (Cerebral Part)

1. The internal carotid artery has been described in chapter 42.
   a. We have seen that the artery ascends up through the neck.
   b. After reaching the skull the artery follows a complicated course through the carotid canal, the foramen lacerum, and the cavernous sinus.
   c. Finally, it pierces the duramater forming the roof of the cavernous sinus, medial to the anterior clinoid process, and comes into relationship with the brain.
2. The artery turns backwards to reach the anterior perforated substance of the brain, and terminates here by dividing into the ***anterior cerebral*** and ***middle cerebral*** arteries.
3. Other branches given off by the internal carotid artery in the intracranial part of its course are shown in 42.8. Two of these branches may be noted.
   a. These are the anterior choroidal artery
   b. The posterior communicating artery which takes part in supply of the brain. These branches are described briefly below. Further details will be mentioned when we take up the blood supply of different parts of the brain.

#### *Anterior Cerebral Artery*

1. We have seen that the anterior cerebral artery arises from the internal carotid artery below the anterior perforated substance, lateral to the optic chiasma (56.1A and 56.2).
2. From here it runs forwards and medially crossing above the optic chiasma to reach the median longitudinal fissure.
3. Here the arteries of the two sides lie close together and are united to each other by the ***anterior communicating artery***.
4. The anterior cerebral artery now turns sharply to reach the medial surface of the cerebral hemisphere.
   a. Here, it runs upwards to reach the genu of the corpus callosum (56.1B).
   b. It winds round the front of the genu and then runs backwards just above the body of the corpus callosum, ending near its posterior part.

5. The distribution of the artery is considered below, along with that of the middle cerebral and posterior cerebral arteries.
6. The anterior cerebral artery gives off a ***recurrent branch*** (also called the ***artery of Heubner***). This branch runs backwards and laterally to enter the anterior perforated substance (56.2).

### Middle Cerebral Artery

1. After its origin from the internal carotid artery (just below the anterior perforated substance), the middle cerebral artery runs laterally on the inferior aspect of the cerebral hemisphere lying deep within the stem of the lateral sulcus (56.1A).
2. Reaching the superolateral surface of the hemisphere it runs backwards deep within the posterior ramus of the lateral sulcus (56.1C).
3. Along its course the artery gives off several branches to the brain. Their distribution is considered below along with that of the anterior and posterior cerebral arteries.

### Posterior communicating artery

1. This artery arises from the internal carotid artery just before the termination of the latter (56.2).
2. The artery runs backwards crossing inferior to the optic tract, and ends by joining the posterior cerebral artery, thus helping to form an arterial circle in relation to the base of the brain (see below).
3. It gives off some central branches that enter the cerebral hemisphere and supply part of the thalamus.

### Anterior choroidal artery

1. This artery arises from the internal carotid artery near the termination of the latter.
2. It runs backwards in relation to the uncus and the optic tract (56.2).
3. It ends in the choroid plexus in the inferior horn of the lateral ventricle.
4. This artery also gives off branches to several parts of the brain including the internal capsule.

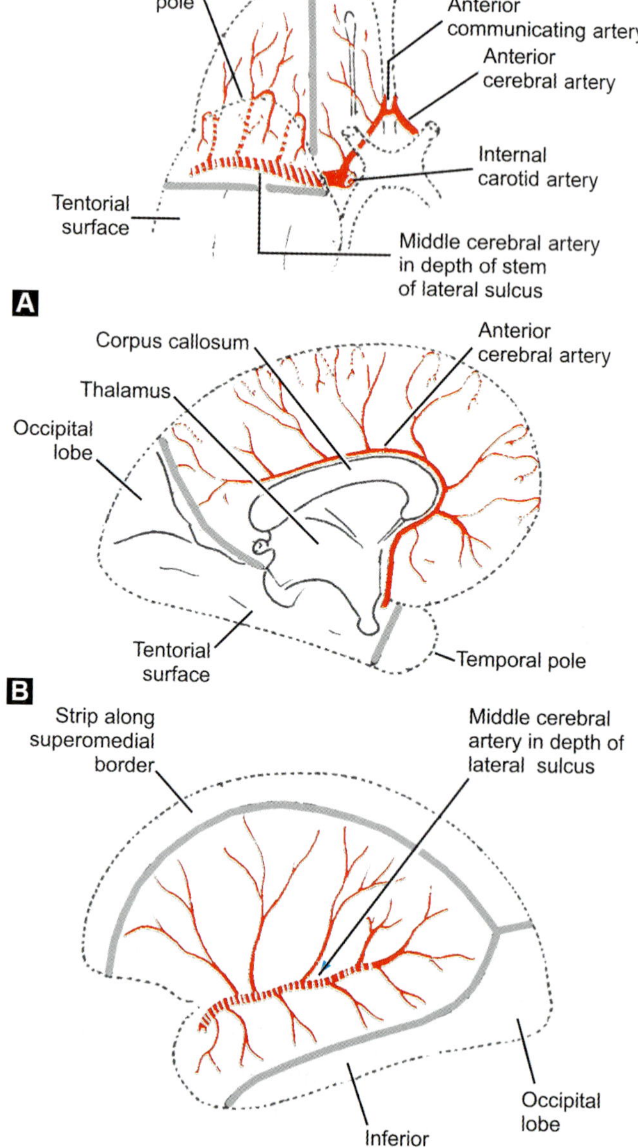


**56.1A to C:** (A) Initial parts of the anterior and middle cerebral arteries (seen from below); (B) Course of anterior cerebral artery (medial view); (C) Course of middle cerebral artery (lateral view). The thick grey lines demarcate areas supplied

### Vertebral Arteries

1. The vertebral artery has been described on page 850 (chapter 42).
2. We have seen that it is a branch of the subclavian artery.
3. It ascends up the neck passing through foramina transversaria of the upper six cervical vertebrae, runs through the suboccipital region and enters the upper part of the vertebral canal.
4. It then passes upwards to enter the cranial cavity through the foramen magnum, and comes to lie lateral to the lower part of the medulla oblongata.

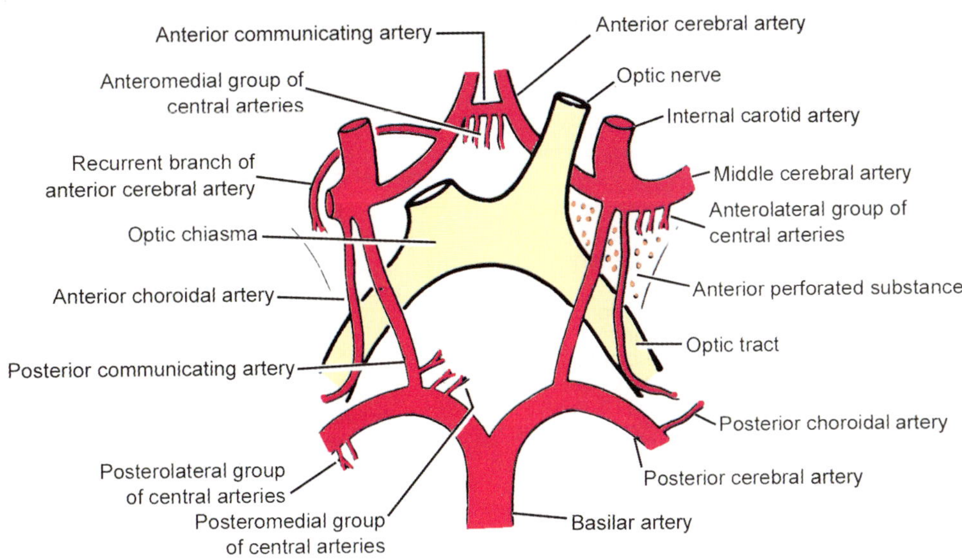


**56.2:** The circulus arteriosus and related structures

5. Continuing its ascent it gradually passes forwards and medially over the medulla and ends at the lower border of the pons by anastomosing with the opposite vertebral artery to form the ***basilar artery*** (56.3).
6. The vertebral artery gives off several branches along its course. The branches that take part in supplying the brain are as follows.

### *Anterior and posterior spinal arteries*

These are described on page 852 (42.30). They are meant for supply of the spinal cord, but they also give some branches to the medulla. See 56.10.

### *Posterior inferior cerebellar artery*

1. This is the largest branch of the vertebral artery.
2. It first runs backwards in relation to the lateral aspect of the medulla, and then ramifies into branches over the posterior part of the inferior surface of the cerebellum (56.3).

## The Basilar Artery

1. The basilar artery is formed by the union of the right and left vertebral arteries at the lower border of the pons.
2. It ascends in the middle line, ventral to the pons, and ends at its upper border by dividing into the right and left posterior cerebral arteries.
3. The branches of the basilar artery are as follows (56.4).

### *Posterior Cerebral Artery*

1. The posterior cerebral artery is a terminal branch of the basilar artery.
2. It passes backwards winding round the midbrain to reach the tentorial surface of the cerebral hemisphere (56.5).
3. Near its origin it is joined by the posterior communicating branch of the internal carotid artery.
4. The posterior cerebral artery gives off cortical and central branches to the cerebral hemisphere. They are considered below along with those of the anterior and middle cerebral arteries.

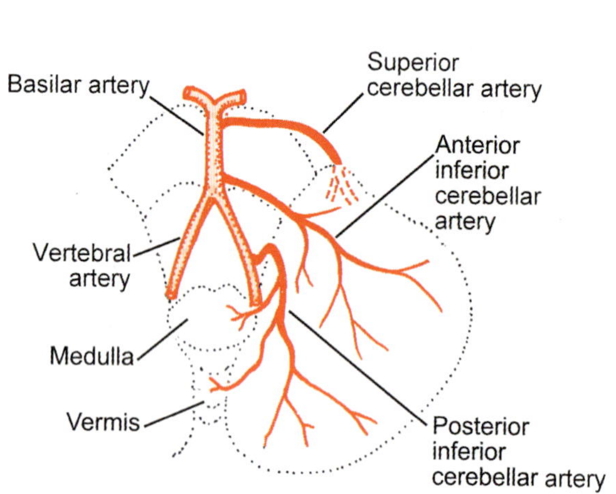


**56.3:** Arteries supplying the cerebellum

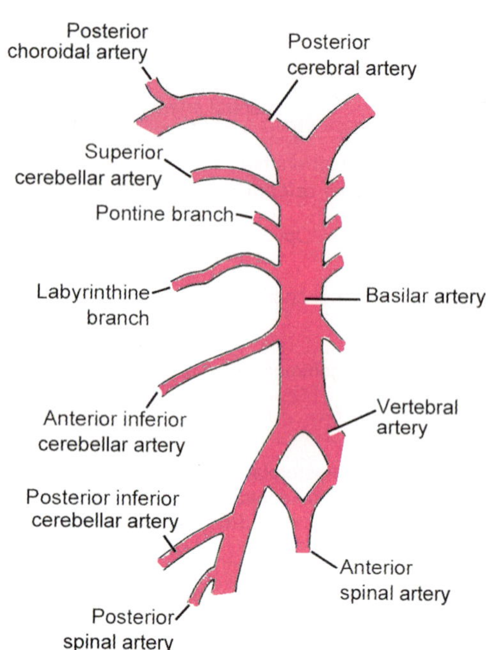


**56.4:** Branches of the basilar artery. Some branches of the vertebral artery are also shown

5. The ***posterior choroidal artery*** is a branch of the posterior cerebral artery (56.2).
   a. It supplies the choroid plexuses of the lateral and third ventricles.
   b. It also supplies the lateral geniculate body.

### *Superior Cerebellar Artery*

This artery arises from the basilar artery just proximal to the termination of the latter. It winds round the midbrain to reach the superior surface of the cerebellum that it supplies (56.3).

### *Anterior Inferior Cerebellar Artery*

This artery arises from the basilar artery near its lower end. It runs backwards and laterally to reach the anterior part of the inferior surface of the cerebellum which it supplies (56.3).

### *Other Branches of Basilar Artery*

1. The basilar artery gives off some small ***pontine branches*** to the pons (56.4).
2. It also gives off the ***labyrinthine artery*** that accompanies the facial nerve into the internal acoustic meatus to reach the internal ear.

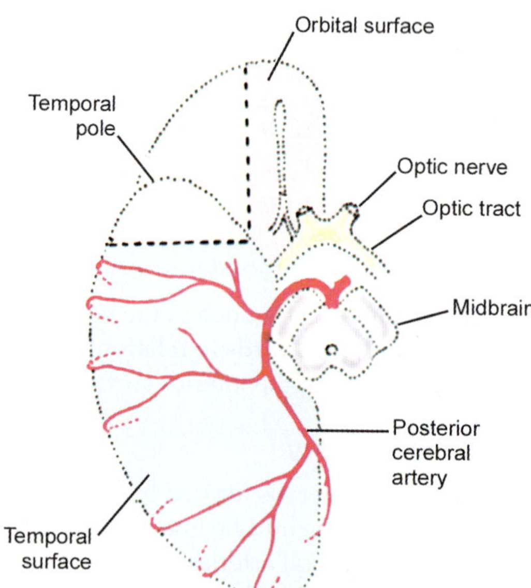


**56.5:** Course and distribution of the posterior cerebral artery

### *Circulus Arteriosus*

1. From 56.2 we see that some of the arteries supplying the brain form an arterial circle that is present in relation to the base of the brain (in the region of the interpeduncular fossa).

2. Anteriorly, the circle is formed by the right and left anterior cerebral arteries, and the anterior communicating artery that unites them.
3. On either side, the arterial ring is formed by the internal carotid artery and its posterior communicating branch.
4. Posteriorly, the ring is completed by the bifurcation of the basilar artery into the right and left posterior cerebral arteries.
5. The posterior communicating artery joins the posterior cerebral artery to complete the ring.
6. Because of anastomoses between the major arteries supplying the brain, blood supply of the area supplied by one artery can be taken over by another artery in the event of it becoming blocked. This remark applies, however, only to the main arteries, and ***not*** to their smaller branches (see below).

## ARTERIAL SUPPLY OF THE CEREBRAL CORTEX

1. The anterior, middle and posterior cerebral arteries give rise to two sets of branches, ***cortical*** and ***central***. The distribution of cortical branches is given below. The central branches are also described below.
2. The cortical branches ramify on the surface of the cerebral hemispheres and supply the cortex. Details of supply on each surface of the cerebral hemispheres are as follows.

### Superolateral Surface

1. The greater part of the superolateral surface of the cerebral hemisphere is supplied by the ***middle cerebral artery*** (56.6). The areas ***not*** supplied by this artery are as follows:
   a. A strip half to one inch wide along the superomedial border extending from the frontal pole to the parieto-occipital sulcus is supplied by the anterior cerebral artery.
   b. The area belonging to the occipital lobe is supplied by the posterior cerebral artery.
   c. The inferior temporal gyrus (excluding the part adjoining the temporal pole) is also supplied by the posterior cerebral artery.

Anterior cerebral artery
Middle cerebral artery
Posterior cerebral artery

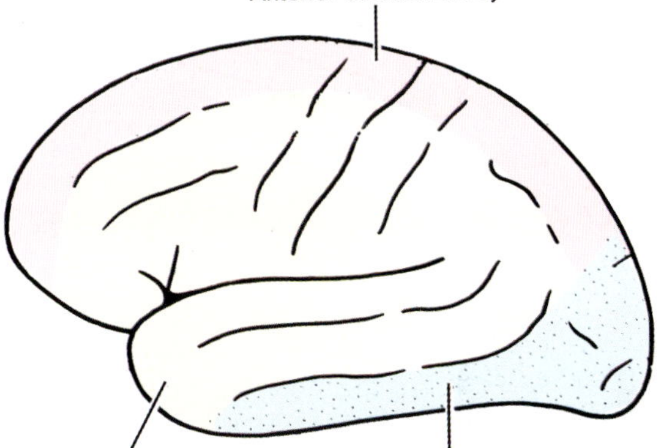

**56.6:** Distribution of the anterior, posterior and middle cerebral arteries on the superolateral surface of the cerebral hemisphere

### Medial Surface

1. The main artery supplying the medial surface is the ***anterior cerebral*** (56.7).
2. The part of the medial surface belonging to the occipital lobe is supplied by the posterior cerebral artery.

### Inferior Surface

1. The ***orbital surface*** is supplied, in its lateral part, by the middle cerebral artery, and in its medial part by the anterior cerebral artery (56.8).
2. The ***tentorial surface*** is supplied by the posterior cerebral artery.
3. The temporal pole is, however, supplied by the middle cerebral artery (56.8).

### Additional Points of Interest

1. From the description given above it will be clear that the main somatic motor and sensory areas are supplied by the middle cerebral artery except in their uppermost parts (leg areas) which are supplied by the anterior cerebral.
2. The acoustic area is supplied by the middle cerebral artery, and the visual area by the posterior cerebral.

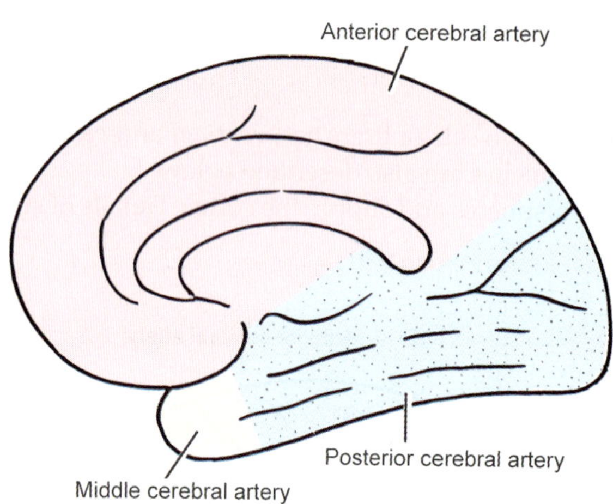


**56.7:** Arteries supplying the medial surface of the cerebral hemisphere

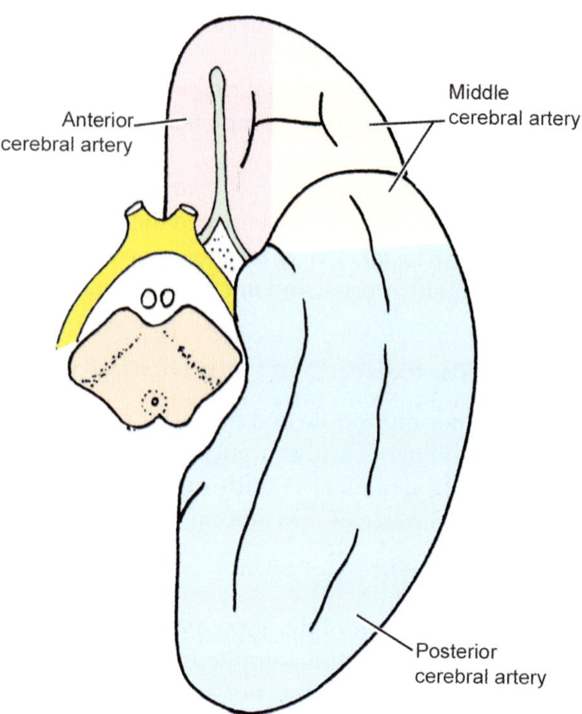


**56.8:** Arteries supplying the orbital and tentorial surfaces of the cerebral hemisphere

**WANT TO KNOW MORE?**

3. The part of the visual area responsible for macular vision lies in the region where the territories of supply of the middle and posterior cerebral arteries meet.
   a. It may receive a supply from the middle cerebral artery, either directly, or through anastomoses with branches of the posterior cerebral artery.
   b. This is one explanation for the observation that macular vision is often spared in cases of thrombosis of the posterior cerebral artery.
   c. The phenomenon can also be explained by the observation that dye injected into the carotid system (for angiographic studies) often passes into the posterior cerebral artery through the posterior communicating artery.

4. The cortical arteries give off branches that run perpendicularly into the substance of the cerebral hemisphere.
   a. Some of these are short and end within the grey matter of the cortex.
   b. Others are longer and penetrate into the subjacent white matter.
5. While cortical branches may anastomose with each other on the surface of the brain, the perpendicular branches (both long and short) behave as terminal or end arteries.
   a. Each branch supplies a limited area of brain tissue, and does not anastomose with neighbouring arteries.
   b. As a result, blockage of such a branch leads to death (necrosis) of brain tissue in the region of supply.

## ARTERIES SUPPLYING THE INTERIOR OF THE CEREBRAL HEMISPHERE

### Central or Perforating Arteries

1. Structures in the interior of the cerebral hemisphere are supplied by central (or perforating) branches that arise from arteries lying in relation to the base of the brain.
2. They consist of six main groups:
   a. Anteromedial
   b. Posteromedial (which are median and unpaired)
   c. Right and left anterolateral
   d. Right and left posterolateral (56.2).
3. The arteries of the ***anteromedial group*** arise from the anterior cerebral and anterior communicating arteries. They enter the most medial part of the anterior perforated substance.
4. The arteries of the ***anterolateral group*** are the so-called ***striate arteries***.
   a. They arise mainly from the middle cerebral artery.
   b. Some of them arise from the anterior cerebral artery.
   c. The anterolateral group of perforating arteries pierce the anterior perforated substance and divide into two sets, medial and lateral.
   d. The ***medial striate arteries*** ascend through the lentiform nucleus. They supply this nucleus and also the caudate nucleus and the internal capsule.
   e. The ***lateral striate arteries*** ascend lateral to the lower part of the lentiform nucleus; they then turn medially and pass through the substance of the lentiform nucleus to reach the internal capsule and the caudate nucleus.
   f. One of these lateral striate arteries is usually larger than the others. It is called ***Charcot's artery***, or ***artery of cerebral haemorrhage***.
5. The ***posteromedial group*** of central arteries take origin from the posterior cerebral and posterior communicating arteries. They enter the interpeduncular region.
6. The central branches of the ***posterolateral group*** arise from the posterior cerebral artery, as it winds around the cerebral peduncle.

### WANT TO KNOW MORE?

**Arterial Supply of Individual Structures**

***Internal capsule***

1. The main arteries supplying the internal capsule are:
   a. The medial and lateral striate branches of the middle cerebral artery
   b. The recurrent branch of the anterior cerebral
   c. The anterior choroidal artery.
2. The internal capsule may also receive direct branches from the internal carotid artery, and branches from the posterior communicating artery (56.9).
3. The ***upper parts*** of the anterior limb, the genu, and the posterior limb of the internal capsule are supplied by striate branches of the middle cerebral artery.
4. The ***lower parts*** of these regions are supplied as follows:
   a. The lower part of the anterior limb of the internal capsule is supplied by the recurrent branch of the anterior cerebral artery.
   b. The lower part of the genu of the internal capsule is supplied by direct branches from the internal carotid, and from the posterior communicating artery.
   c. The lower part of the posterior limb of the internal capsule is supplied by the anterior choroidal artery.

5. The entire ***retrolentiform part*** of the capsule is supplied by the anterior choroidal artery. The ***sublentiform part*** is probably supplied by the anterior choroidal artery.

*Thalamus*

1. The thalamus is supplied mainly by perforating branches of the posterior cerebral artery.
   a. The posteromedial group of branches (also called ***thalamoperforating*** arteries) supply the medial and anterior part.
   b. The posterolateral group (also called ***thalamogeniculate*** branches) supply the posterior and lateral parts of the thalamus.
   c. The thalamus also receives some branches from the posterior communicating, anterior choroidal, posterior choroidal, and middle cerebral arteries.

*Hypothalamus*

1. The anterior part of the hypothalamus is supplied by central branches of the anteromedial group (arising from the anterior cerebral artery).
2. The posterior part is supplied by central branches of the posteromedial group (arising from the posterior cerebral and posterior communicating arteries).

*Corpus striatum*

1. The main arterial supply of the ***caudate nucleus*** and ***putamen*** is derived from the medial and lateral striate branches of the middle cerebral artery.
2. a. In addition, their most anterior parts (including the head of the caudate nucleus) receive their blood supply through the recurrent branch of the anterior cerebral artery.
   b. Their posterior parts (including the tail of the caudate nucleus) through the anterior choroidal artery.
3. The main supply of the ***globus pallidus*** is from the anterior choroidal artery.
   a. Its lateral segment also receives blood through the striate arteries.
   b. The most medial part of the globus pallidus receives branches from the posterior communicating artery.

## Arterial Supply of the Brainstem

### *Medulla*

1. The medulla is supplied by various branches of the vertebral arteries. These are:
   a. The anterior and posterior spinal arteries
   b. The posterior inferior cerebellar artery
   c. Small direct branches.

**WANT TO KNOW MORE?**

2. The anterior spinal artery supplies a triangular area next to the middle line (56.10). This area includes:
   a. The pyramid
   b. The medial lemniscus
   c. The hypoglossal nucleus.
3. The posterior spinal artery supplies a small area including the gracile and cuneate nuclei.
4. The posterior inferior cerebellar artery supplies the retro-olivary region. This region contains several important structures including:
   a. The spinothalamic tracts
   b. The rubrospinal tract
   c. The nucleus ambiguus

   d. The dorsal vagal nucleus
   e. Descending autonomic fibres.

   The posterior inferior cerebellar artery also supplies part of the inferior cerebellar peduncle.

5. The rest of the medulla is supplied by direct bulbar branches of the vertebral arteries.
6. Thrombosis in an artery supplying the medulla produces symptoms depending upon the structures involved.
7. Two characteristic syndromes are:
   a. The ***medial medullary syndrome*** produced by thrombosis in the anterior spinal artery.
   b. The ***lateral medullary syndrome*** produced by thrombosis in the posterior inferior cerebellar artery.

### Pons

1. The pons is supplied by branches from the basilar artery.

### WANT TO KNOW MORE?

2. The medial portion of the ventral part of the pons is supplied by ***paramedian branches.***
3. The lateral portion of the ventral part is supplied by ***short circumferential branches.***
4. The dorsal part of the pons is supplied by ***long circumferential branches.***
5. The dorsal part also receives branches from the anterior inferior cerebellar and superior cerebellar arteries.
6. The paramedian branches of the basilar artery may extend into this region from the ventral part of the pons.

### Midbrain

1. The midbrain is supplied mainly by branches of the basilar artery. These are:
   a. The posterior cerebral and superior cerebellar arteries.
   b. Direct branches from the basilar artery.
2. Branches are also received from the posterior communicating and anterior choroidal arteries.

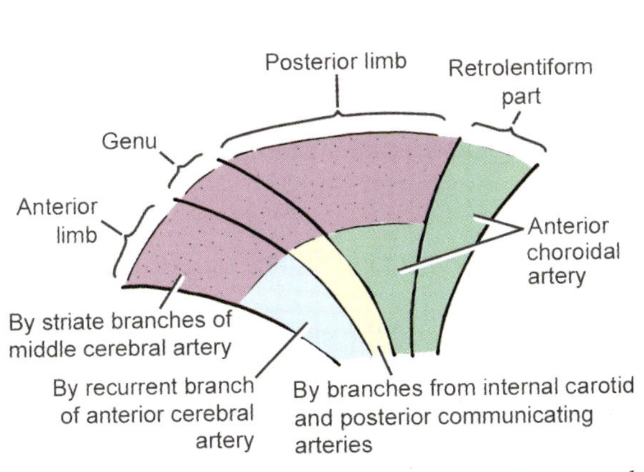


**56.9:** Scheme to show the arterial supply of the internal capsule

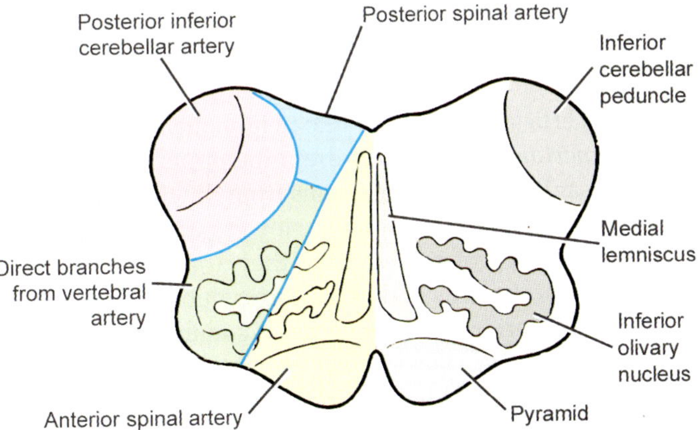


**56.10:** Cross-section through the medulla to show regions supplied by different arteries

**WANT TO KNOW MORE?**

3. Branches arising from these vessels may either be:
   a. ***Paramedian,*** which supply parts near the midline
   b. ***Circumferential*** which wind round the midbrain to supply lateral and dorsal parts.
4. One of the latter arteries is called the ***quadrigeminal artery.*** It is the main source of blood to the colliculi.

### Arteries Supplying the Cerebellum

1. The superior surface of the cerebellum is supplied by the ***superior cerebellar*** branches of the basilar artery (56.3).
2. The anterior part of the inferior surface is supplied by the ***anterior inferior cerebellar*** branches of the same artery.
3. The posterior part of the inferior surface is supplied by the ***posterior inferior cerebellar*** branch of the vertebral artery.

## VENOUS DRAINAGE OF THE BRAIN

1. The veins draining the brain open into the dural venous sinuses (56.11A to C). These are:
   a. Superior sagittal
   b. Inferior sagittal
   c. Straight
   d. Transverse
   e. Sigmoid
   f. Cavernous
   g. Sphenoparietal
   h. Petrosal
   i. Occipital sinuses.
2. They have been described in detail in chapter 42. Ultimately, the blood from all these sinuses reaches the sigmoid sinus that becomes continuous with the internal jugular vein.
3. The drainage of individual parts of the brain is as follows.

### Veins of the Cerebral Hemisphere

The veins of the cerebral hemisphere consist of two sets: Superficial and deep.

#### *Superficial Veins*

1. The superficial veins drain into neighbouring venous sinuses.
2. The ***superior cerebral veins*** drain the upper parts of the superolateral and medial surfaces, and end in the superior sagittal sinus. Some veins from the medial surface join the inferior sagittal sinus.
3. ***Inferior cerebral veins*** drain the lower part of the hemisphere.
   a. On the superolateral surface, they drain into the ***superficial middle cerebral vein*** that lies superficially along the lateral sulcus and its posterior ramus.
   b. The posterior end of this vein is connected to the superior sagittal sinus by the ***superior anastomotic vein***; and to the transverse sinus by the ***inferior anastomotic vein*** (56.11A).
4. The superficial middle cerebral vein terminates in the cavernous sinus.
5. Veins from the inferior surface of the cerebral hemisphere drain into the transverse, superior petrosal, cavernous and sphenoparietal sinuses. Some may ascend to join the inferior sagittal sinus.

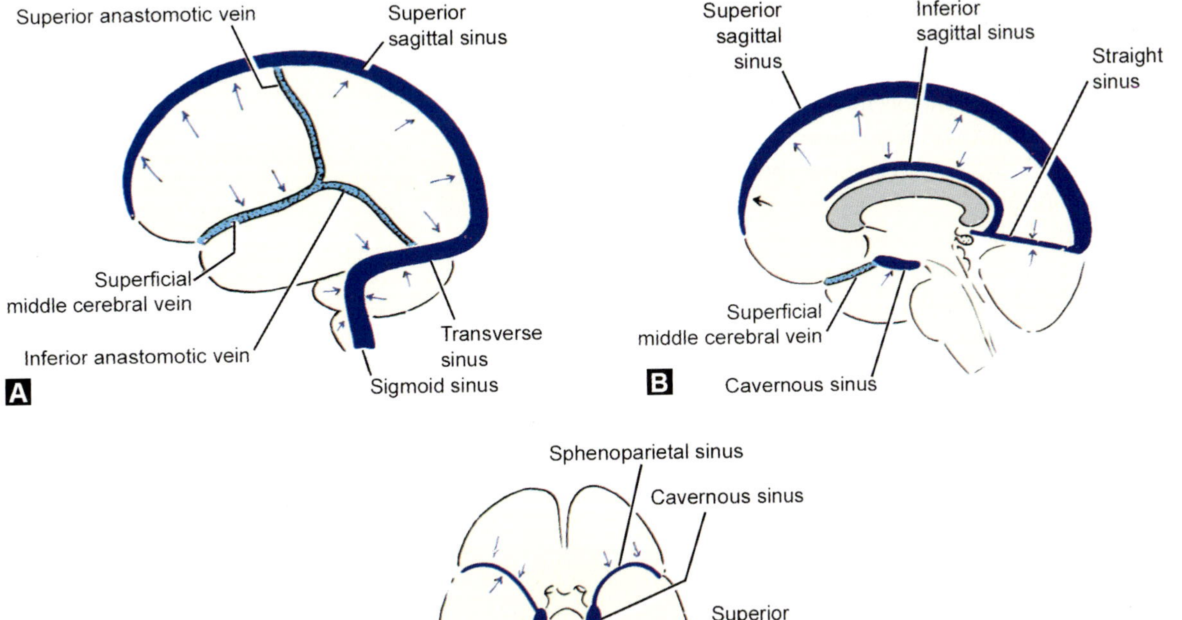


**56.11A to C:** Diagrams to show the position of the intracranial venous sinuses in relation. (A) Lateral; (B) Medial; (C) Inferior aspects of the brain

### *Deep Veins*

1. The deep veins of the cerebral hemisphere are:
   a. The two ***internal cerebral veins***, that join to form the ***great cerebral vein***.
   b. The two ***basal veins,*** that wind round the midbrain to end in the great cerebral vein.
2. Each internal cerebral vein begins at the interventricular foramen, and runs backwards in the tela choroidea, in the roof of the third ventricle. It has numerous tributaries. One of these is the ***thalamostriate vein*** that lies in the floor of the lateral ventricle (between the thalamus, medially, and the caudate nucleus, laterally).

#### WANT TO KNOW MORE?

3. Each basal vein begins near the anterior perforated substance. It is formed by union of the following:
   a. The anterior cerebral vein, which accompanies the anterior cerebral artery.
   b. The deep middle cerebral vein, which lies deep in the stem and posterior ramus of the lateral sulcus.
   c. Some ***inferior striate veins*** that emerge from the anterior perforated substance.

4. The great cerebral vein, formed by union of the two internal cerebral veins, passes posteriorly beneath the splenium of the corpus callosum, to end in the straight sinus. It receives:
   a. The basal veins
   b. Some veins from the occipital lobes
   c. Some from the corpus callosum.
5. The deep cerebral veins described above are responsible for draining:
   a. The thalamus
   b. The hypothalamus
   c. The corpus striatum
   d. The internal capsule
   e. The corpus callosum
   f. The septum pellucidum
   g. The choroid plexuses.

**WANT TO KNOW MORE?**

6. Many tributaries of the internal cerebral veins extend beyond the corpus striatum into the white matter of the hemispheres.
   a. Here they establish communications with superficial veins.
   b. They can thus serve as alternative channels for draining parts of the cerebral cortex.
7. a. The upper part of the ***thalamus*** is drained by the tributaries of the internal cerebral vein (including the thalamostriate vein).
   b. The lower part of the thalamus, and the hypothalamus, are drained by veins that run downwards to end in a plexus of veins present in the interpeduncular fossa.
   c. This plexus drains into the cavernous and sphenoparietal sinuses, and into the basal veins.
8. The ***corpus striatum*** and ***internal capsule*** are drained by two sets of striate veins.
   a. The ***superior striate veins*** run dorsally and drain into tributaries of the internal cerebral vein.
   b. The ***inferior striate veins*** run vertically downwards and emerge on the base of the brain through the anterior perforated substance. Here they end in the basal vein.

## Veins of the Cerebellum and Brainstem

1. The veins from the upper surface of the ***cerebellum*** drain into:
   a. The straight
   b. Transverse
   c. Superior petrosal venous sinuses.
2. Veins from the inferior surface drain into:
   a. The right and left sigmoid, and inferior petrosal sinuses.
   b. The occipital sinus and the straight sinus.
3. The veins of the ***midbrain*** drain into the great cerebral vein or into the basal vein.
4. The ***pons*** and ***medulla*** drain into:
   a. The superior and inferior petrosal sinuses.
   b. The transverse sinus and the occipital sinus.
5. Inferiorly, the veins of the medulla are continuous with the veins of the spinal cord.

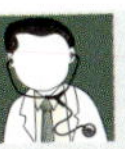

## CLINICAL CORRELATION

### Some Investigative Procedures used for Neurological Diagnosis

Considerable help in localisation of neurological lesions and in diagnosis of their nature, may be obtained by the use of certain investigative procedures that are briefly mentioned below.

*Lumbar Puncture*

1. A needle can be introduced into the subarachnoid space through the interval between the third and fourth lumbar vertebrae. This procedure, called lumbar puncture, is useful for several purposes.
   a. The pressure of CSF can be estimated, roughly, by counting the rate at which drops flow out of the needle; or more accurately, by connecting the needle to a manometer.
   b. Samples of CSF can be collected for examination. The important points to note about CSF are its colour, its cellular content, and its chemical composition (specially the protein and sugar content).
   c. Lumbar puncture may be used for introducing air or radio-opaque dyes into the subarachnoid space for certain investigative procedures (see below). Drugs may also be injected for treatment.
   d. Mention may be made here of a use of lumbar puncture, not related to neurological diagnosis. Anaesthetic drugs injected into the subarachnoid space act on the lower spinal nerve roots and render the lower part of the body insensitive to pain. This procedure, called ***spinal anaesthesia***, is frequently used for operations on the lower abdomen or on the lower extremities.

*Radiological Procedures*

1. Plain radiographs of the skull may give evidence of disease when the skull bones are affected, or when there are areas of calcification.
2. Air injected into the subarachnoid space through lumbar puncture ascends in the spinal subarachnoid space to the cranial cavity. The air can be seen in radiographs. This procedure is called ***pneumoencephalography.*** The air injected may enter the ventricles. Their outlines can then be seen. (This procedure is no longer used and is of historical interest only).
3. The ventricles can be visualised by injecting radio-opaque dyes directly into the lateral ventricle (***ventriculography)*** (56.12). Abnormal dilatations of the ventricular system (hydrocephalus) can be detected.
4. The vascular system of the brain can be visualised by injecting radio-opaque material into the common carotid or vertebral arteries (***Cerebral angiography).*** Radiographs taken immediately after the injection reveal the arterial pattern (56.13). The capillary and venous patterns can be seen after brief intervals.
5. The spinal subarachnoid space can be visualised by injecting radio-opaque material (***myelography***). Abnormal appearances seen with the procedures mentioned above help in determining the nature and location of tumours or other masses present in relation to the brain or spinal cord.

*Electrophysiological Methods*

1. Information about the functioning of the brain can be obtained by a study of the patterns of electrical activity within it. Electrodes are applied over the scalp at various points. These are connected to a machine that records the electrical potentials. The procedure is called ***electroencephalography*** or EEG).
2. Electrical activity precedes or accompanies muscle contraction. This can be recorded by suitable machines. The procedure is called ***electromyography*** or EMG. It is employed for the study of various disorders of skeletal muscle. It is also a valuable tool for investigating the normal actions of muscles.
3. The rate of conduction in nerve fibres can also be measured by electrical methods.
4. One of the standard methods of neurophysiological investigation has been to stimulate a particular part of the nervous system and to record ***evoked potentials*** from other regions.
   a. Most such experiments have been done on animals after exposing the regions concerned.
   b. Sophisticated instruments are now available that enable similar studies to be done in human subjects through surface electrodes.
   c. Using such methods it is possible to determine the integrity (or otherwise) of various pathways.

*Ultrasound Methods*

1. Ultrasound waves applied to any part of the body are reflected back by various structures.
2. The reflected waves (or echo) can be picked up and visualised on a screen.
3. Images of internal organs can be obtained in this way.
4. In the field of neurology, ultrasound waves can be used to detect a shift of midline structures e.g., the falx cerebri. The technique is called ***echoencephalography.***

*Computed Tomography*

1. The term ***tomography*** has been applied to radiological methods in which tissues lying in a particular plane are visualised.
2. In recent years a technique has been developed in which a series of levels studied in this way are analysed using computers.
   a. Such analysis provides images giving a remarkable degree of detail.
   b. The procedure is called ***computerised tomography*** or CT scan.
   c. The technique has revolutionised neurological diagnosis, and has rendered many older techniques obsolete.
   d. Tumours, areas of haemorrhage, and various other lesions can be identified with confidence.

*Magnetic Resonance Imaging*

1. This is a technique that produces images of outstanding clarity, of structures inside the body (56.14).
2. The technique uses very powerful magnetic fields, radiofrequency waves and sophisticated computer analysis to form the images.
3. Disadvantages are very high cost, long time taken, and the need for the patient to keep very still for many minutes.

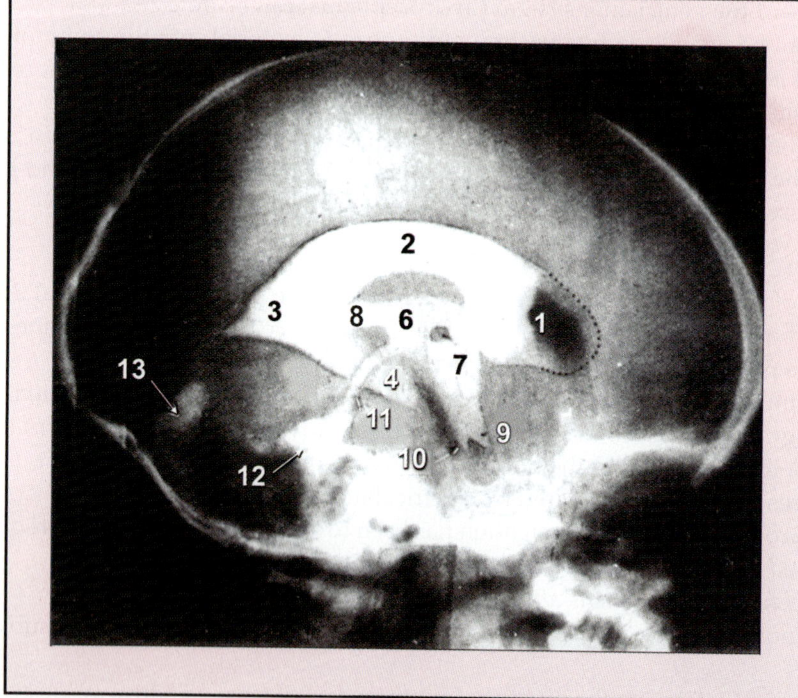


**56.12:** Ventriculogram. Lateral view. A radiograph of the head was taken after injecting a radio-opaque dye into the ventricular system. The parts of the lateral ventricle seen are: (1) Anterior horn (part of which appears dark as air has entered it during injection); (2) Central part; (3) Posterior horn; (4) Inferior horn. In relation to (6) The third ventricle, we can identify: (8) The suprapineal recess; (9) The optic recess and (10) The infundibular recess: The interthalamicconnexus is seen as, (7) A dark area. Other structures seen are: (11) The aqueduct and (12) The fourth ventricle. Some dye that has reached the cisterna magna (through the apertures of the fourth ventricle is also seen (13).
*Courtesy*: Prof SC Srivastava

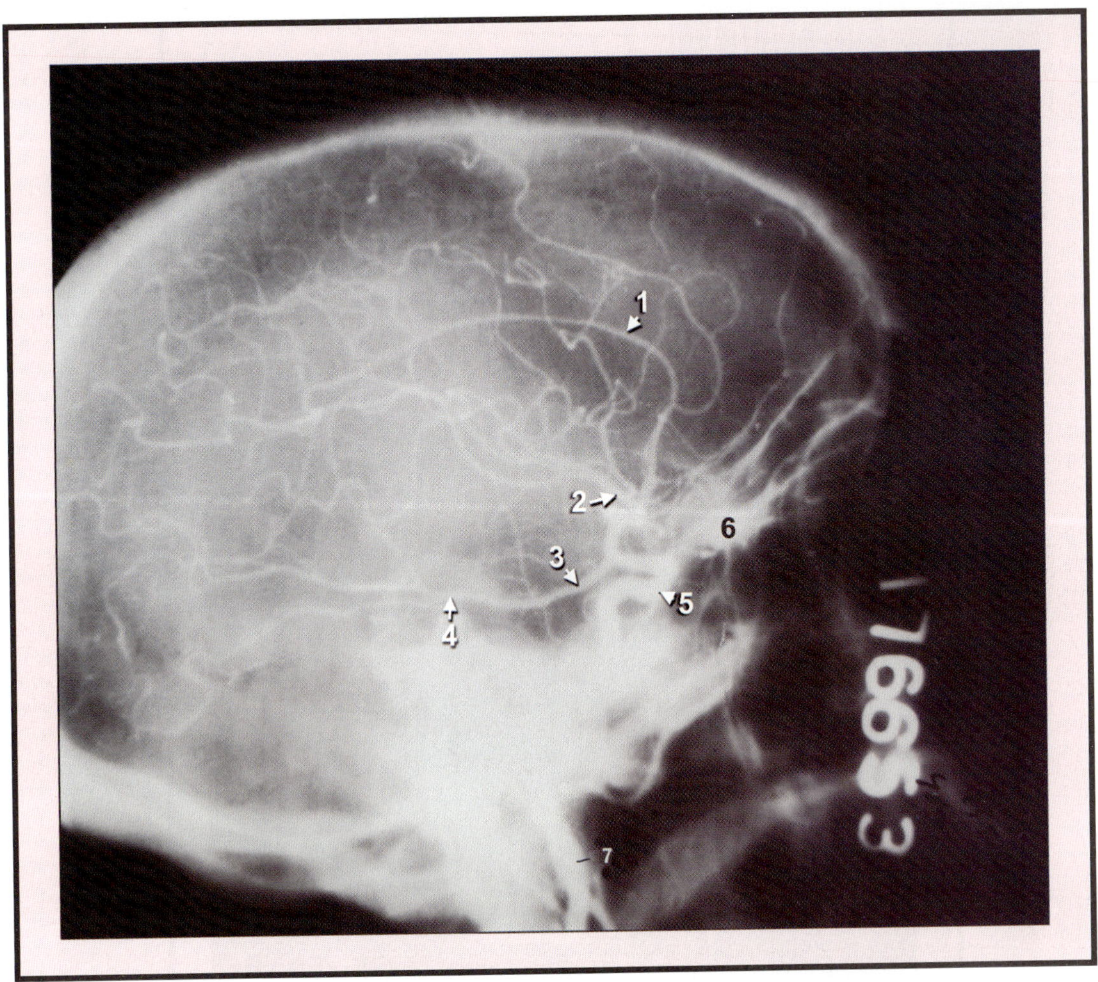


**56.13:** Arteries of the brain visualised in a living person by the technique of carotid angiography. Lateral view:(1) Anterior cerebral artery; (2) Middle cerebral artery; (3) Posterior communicating artery. In this patient this artery appears to continue into the posterior cerebral artery; (4) This is unusual; (5) Internal carotid artery in the cavernous sinus; (6) Branches of ophthalmic artery; (7) Internal carotid artery in the neck. *Courtesy*: Dr RK Yadav

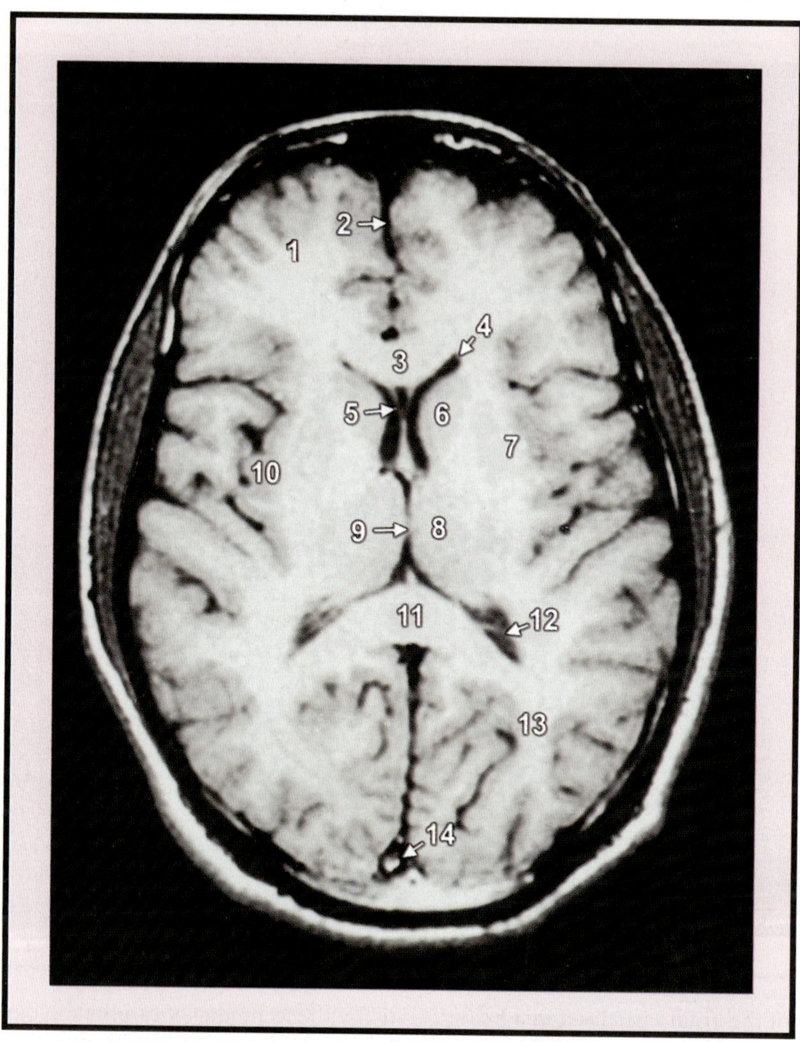


**56.14:** Sectional view of cerebral hemisphere obtained in a living person by the technique of magnetic resonance imaging (MRI). 1. Frontal lobe; 2. Median longitudinal fissure; 3. Genu of corpus callosum; 4. Anterior horn of lateral ventricle; 5. Septum pellucidum (double layered); 6. Caudate nucleus; 7. Lentiform nucleus; 8. Thalamus; 9. Third ventricle; 10. Insula; 11. Splenium of corpus callosum; 12. Posterior horn of lateral ventricle; 13. Occipital lobe; 14. Superior sagittal sinus

# Index

Page numbers followed by *f* refer to figures, and those followed by *t* refer to tables

## A

## B

## C

## D

## E

## M

## P

## Q



## R

## S

## U

## V



## W



## X



## Z